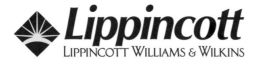

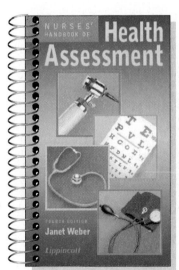
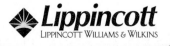

Health Assessment in Nursing

Health Assessment in Nursing

Second Edition

Janet Weber   RN, EdD

Professor
Department of Nursing
Southeast Missouri State University
Cape Girardeau, Missouri

Jane Kelley   RN, PhD

Professor
School of Nursing
University of Mississippi Medical Center
Jackson, Mississippi

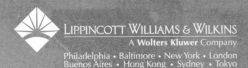

LIPPINCOTT WILLIAMS & WILKINS
A **Wolters Kluwer** Company

Philadelphia · Baltimore · New York · London
Buenos Aires · Hong Kong · Sydney · Tokyo

Acquisitions Editor: Elizabeth Nieginski
Development Editor: Deedie McMahon
Senior Project Editor: Tom Gibbons
Senior Production Manager: Helen Ewan
Design Coordinator: Doug Smock
Manufacturing Manager: William Alberti
Indexer: Ellen Brennan
Compositor: Circle Graphics
Printer: R. R. Donnelley

2nd Edition

9 8 7 6 5 4 3 2 1

Library of Congress Cataloging-in Publication Data

Weber, Janet.
  Health assessment in nursing / Janet Weber, Jane Kelley.—2nd ed.
    p. ; cm.
  Includes bibliographical references and index.
  ISBN 0-7817-3207-7 (cloth : alk. paper)
   1. Nursing assessment. I. Kelley, Jane, 1944-II. Title.
   [DNLM: 1. Nursing Assessment. WY 100.4 W374h 2002]
  RT48 .W43 2003
  610.73—dc21

2001050698

Care has been taken to confirm the accuracy of the information presented and to describe generally accepted practices. However, the authors, editors, and publisher are not responsible for errors or omissions or for any consequences from application of the information in this book and make no warranty, express or implied, with respect to the content of the publication.

The authors, editors, and publisher have exerted every effort to ensure that drug selection and dosage set forth in this text are in accordance with the current recommendations and practice at the time of publication. However, in view of ongoing research, changes in government regulations, and the constant flow of information relating to drug therapy and drug reactions, the reader is urged to check the package insert for each drug for any change in indications and dosage and for added warnings and precautions. This is particularly important when the recommended agent is a new or infrequently employed drug.

Some drugs and medical devices presented in this publication have Food and Drug Administration (FDA) clearance for limited use in restricted research settings. It is the responsibility of the health care provider to ascertain the FDA status of each drug or device planned for use in his or her clinical practice.

DEDICATION

My husband, children, mother, father, and grandmothers who shared their wisdom in special ways

Janet

My husband, mother, father, and grandmother, each of whom has helped me to see the world through new eyes

Jane

But there's no vocabulary
For love within a family, love that's lived in
But not looked at, love within the light of which
All else is seen, the love within which
All other love finds speech.
This love is silent.

From ***The Elder Statesman***, T. S. Eliot (1888–1964)

Contributors

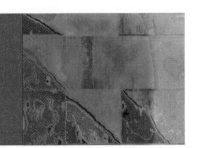

Linda Bugle, RN, PhD
Assistant Professor
Southeast Missouri State University
Department of Nursing
Cape Girardeau, Missouri
Chapter 28, Community Assessment

Jill C. Cash, RN, CS, MSN, FNP
Southern Illinois OB-GYN Associates
Carbondale, Illinois
Chapter 24, Assessment of Infants, Children,
    and Adolescents
Chapter 25, Assessment of the Childbearing Woman

Kathy Casteel, RN, MSN, CS, FNP
Family Nurse Practitioner
Prompt Care
Jackson, Missouri
Chapter 22, Musculoskeletal Assessment

Nancy Collins, RN, MSN
Lipid Nurse Clinician
Midwest Heart Specialists
Naperville, Illinois
Chapter 18, Abdominal Assessment

Linda Garner, RN, MSN
Director of Nursing
Southern Seven Health Department
Ulliri, Illinois
Chapter 23, Neurologic Assessment

Brenda P. Johnson, RN, PhD
Assistant Professor
Southeast Missouri State University
Department of Nursing
Cape Girardeau, Missouri
Chapter 26, Assessment of the Frail Elderly Client

Cheryl Kieffer, RN, MSN
Assistant Professor
Southeast Missouri State University
Department of Nursing
Cape Girardeau, Missouri
Section of Chapter 1, Nurse's Role in Health
    Assessment: Collecting and Analyzing Data

Bobbi Morris, RN, MSN, CS, FNP
Assistant Professor and Family Nurse Practitioner
Southeast Missouri State University
Department of Nursing
Cape Girardeau, Missouri
Chapter 16, Heart and Neck Vessel Assessment

Ann Sprengel, RN, EdD
Associate Professor
Southeast Missouri State University
Department of Nursing
Cape Girardeau, Missouri
Chapter 17, Peripheral Vascular Assessment

Sharon C. Wahl, MS, EdD
Professor
San Jose State University School of Nursing
San Jose, California
Chapter 8, General Survey and Nutritional Assessment
Chapter 22, Musculoskeletal Assessment
Case Studies

Terri Woods, RN, EdD
Assistant Professor
Southeast Missouri State University
Department of Nursing
Cape Girardeau, Missouri
Chapter 10, Head and Neck Assessment
Chapter 11, Eye Assessment
Chapter 12, Ear Assessment

Cathy Young, RN, MSN, CS, FNP
Assistant Professor
Southeast Missouri State University
Cape Girardeau, Missouri
Chapter 19, Male Genitalia Assessment
Chapter 20, Female Genitalia Assessment
Chapter 21, Anus, Rectum, and Prostate Assessment

Reviewers for the Second Edition

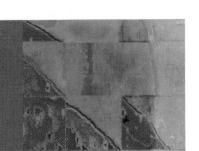

Stasia Arcarese, RN, MS
Clinton Community College
Plattsburgh, New York

Connie Booth, RN, MSN
Des Moines Area Community College
Boone, Iowa

Patricia Brien, RN, MSN, MEd
Berkshire Community College
Pittsfield, Massachusetts

Michelle M. Byrne, RN, MS, PhD, CNOR
Independent Nurse Consultant
Acworth, Georgia

Teresa L. Cervantez-Thompson, RN, PhD, CRRN-A
Assistant Professor
Oakland University
Rochester, Michigan

Patricia Collins, RN, MSN, EdD candidate
West Shore Community College
Scottville, Michigan

Sally P. Cummings, RN, EdD, CS, FNP
University of North Carolina—Wilmington
Wilmington, North Carolina

Rosie Dawker, RN, CDE
St. Francis Medical Center
Cape Girardeau, Missouri

Margaret Downey, RN, MSN, CCRN
Boise State University
Boise, Idaho

Nancy Fishwick, RN, PhD, CS
University of Maine School of Nursing
Orono, Maine

Jean Jackson, RN, MEd, BSCN
Durham College
Oshawa, Ontario, Canada

Laurie Kaudewitz, RNC, MSN
East Tennessee State University
Johnson City, Tennessee

Shauntell Kline, RN, BSN
Baptist Hospital
Jackson, Mississippi

Diana S. Knox, RN, MS
Southwestern Oklahoma State University
Weatherford, Oklahoma

Marcy Lashley, RN, PhD, CRNP
Towson State University
Towson, Maryland

Nancy Logue, RN, MN
University of New Brunswick,
Saint John, New Brunswick, Canada

Lenore Mangles, RN, MSN
Nicole Area Technical College
Rhinelander, Wisconsin

Donna Mitchell, RN, PhD, CNS
Chair, School of Nursing
University of Rio Grande
Rio Grande, Ohio

Ellen M. Moore, RN, MEd, MScN, MHSN, CS, FNP
Purdue University—Calumet
Hammond, Indiana

Phyllis Murray, BNC-C
University of New Brunswick
Fredericton, New Brunswick, Canada

Sandy Nettina, RN, MSN, CS, ANP
Nurse Practitioner
Glenelg, Maryland
Adjunct Faculty, George Washington University
Washington, DC

Louiselle L. Ouellet, RN, MSN
University of New Brunswick
Fredericton, New Brunswick, Canada

Thena E. Parrott, RNCS, PhD
Blinn College
Bryan, Texas

Charles Ramirez, RN, MN
Saint Luke's College
Kansas City, Missouri

Kathy Reavy, RN, MSN, PhDc
Boise State University
Boise, Idaho

Sally S. Roach, RN, MSN
Associate Professor
University of Texas at Brownsville
   and Texas Southmost College
Brownsville, Texas

Carol Roe, RN, MSN
Kalamazoo Valley Community College
Kalamazoo, Michigan

Kristen Rogers, RN, MSN
Washington Hospital School of Nursing
Washington, Pennsylvania

Mary C. Shoemaker, RN, PhD
Saint Francis Medical Center College of Nursing
Peoria, Illinois

Lori Stewart, RN, MSN
Southwestern Oklahoma State University
Weatherford, Oklahoma

Margaret M. Tolbert, MSN, ARNP-CS
University of Miami
Miami, Florida

Linda Van Days, RN, MSN, ACNP
Midlands Technical College
Columbia, South Carolina

Kim Webb, RN, MN
Northern Oklahoma College
Tonkawa, Oklahoma

Michael Williams, RN, MSN, CCRN
Eastern Michigan University
Ypsilanti, Michigan

Paulette Worchester, RN, DNF, FNP-C
Miami University
Miami, Ohio

Preface

Our second edition of *Health Assessment in Nursing* continues the tradition of helping students acquire the skills they need to perform assessments in today's health care environment. As nurses provide more and more care in more and more settings—acute care agencies, clinics, family homes, rehabilitation centers, and long-term care facilities—they need to be better prepared than ever before to perform accurate and timely health assessments. And no matter where a nurse practices, the two components of an accurate collection of client data are essential: a comprehensive knowledge base and expert physical assessment skills.

Besides physical assessment skills, today's nurses also need expert critical thinking skills to analyze the data they collect and to detect client problems—whether they are nursing problems that can be treated independently by nurses, collaborative problems that can be treated in conjunction with other health care practitioners, or medical problems that require referral to other appropriate professionals. The second edition of *Health Assessment in Nursing* has been updated and expanded to highlight applicable critical thinking skills.

In-depth, accurate information, illustrations, and learning tools fill these pages to help the student develop expert subjective and objective assessment skills built upon a comprehensive knowledge base. Initial chapters of *Health Assessment in Nursing* discuss the nurse's role of critical thinking and data analysis as it relates to health assessment.

Following the early chapters, the text is devoted primarily to assessment of the adult from head to toe, system by system. The final chapters are devoted to health assessment of the pediatric client, the childbearing woman, the frail elderly adult, the family, and the community.

Text Walks Students Through Physical Assessment

Unique features of the text include baseline nursing process applications (detailed in the first seven chapters and highlighted in each chapter thereafter), clear explanations of anatomic structures and physiologic function, sample health history questions and rationale, and special

COLDSPA

CHARACTER: Describe the sign or symptom. How does it feel, look, sound, smell, and so forth?
ONSET: When did it begin?
LOCATION: Where is it? Does it radiate?
DURATION: How long does it last? Does it recur?
SEVERITY: How bad is it?
PATTERN: What makes it better? What makes it worse?
ASSOCIATED FACTORS: What other symptoms occur with it?

mnemonics to guide the thorough investigation of client complaints.

Risk factors and risk reduction teaching tips for many major health conditions are among the key elements of each chapter, as are "Tips From the Experts" and relevant

RISK FACTORS
Lung Cancer

Lung cancer is the leading cause of cancer death in the United States, and rates for lung cancer continue to increase. However, the rates for men and women have changed: cancer in 2000 than died in 1999, with fewer men the drop in the numbers of young men who smoke.

RISK FACTORS

- Cigarette smoking
- Genetic predisposition, possibly associated with an interaction of genetics and smoking (Humphrey et al., 1995)
- Asbestos exposure
- Radon exposure

RISK REDUCTION TEACHING TIPS

- Do not start smoking, and stop smoking if you do smoke.
- Join a smoking cessation program.
- Eat a healthy, low-cholesterol diet with adequate

PALPATE THE POSTERIOR TIBIAL PULSES

Palpate behind and just below the medial malleolus (in the groove between the ankle and the Achilles tendon). Palpating both posterior tibial pulses at the same time aids in making comparisons. Assess amplitude bilaterally.

The posterior tibial pulses should be strong bilaterally. However, in about 15% of healthy clients, the posterior tibial pulses are absent.

A weak or absent pulse indicates partial or complete arterial occlusion.

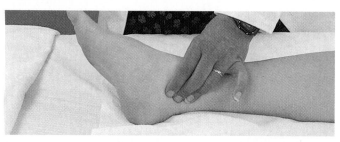

Palpating the posterior tibial pulse. (© B. Proud.)

cultural and gerontologic considerations, which are integrated throughout the text.

Part One of the chapter text presents the physiologic concepts that the student needs to review and explains how the information relates to a particular physical assessment. The physical examination procedures are then presented and photographically illustrated in step-by-step fashion across three columns. The first column shows how to perform specific aspects of the examination, the second column reveals normal findings, and the third column identifies abnormal findings.

The student reads on to find out what to do with the information collected and how to analyze it. A case study and working examples of data are provided along with various displays, tables, and guidelines of normal and abnormal findings, which further illustrate and complement the learning experience.

Units Structured for Comprehensive Coverage

Health Assessment in Nursing has three units:

- Overview of the Health Assessment Process
- Nursing Assessment of the Adult
- Nursing Assessment of Special Groups

The seven chapters in **Unit One** present the steps of health assessment as it is based in the nursing process. The unit starts by discussing the nurse's role in Health Assessment and Collecting and Analyzing Data. The chapter is followed by chapters covering Assessment Frameworks, The Client in the Context of Culture, Family and Community, Collecting Subjective Data, Collecting Objective Data, Validating and Documenting Data, and, most importantly, Using Diagnostic Reasoning Skills to Analyze Data. These concepts are then carried through Units 2 and 3 as examples that students can use to model their own data collections, analyses, and formulation of nursing diagnoses, collaborative problems, or referrals.

The 16 chapters of **Unit Two** immerse the student in actual assessment techniques, starting with a General Survey and Nutritional Assessment and progressing to Head and Neck Assessment, Thoracic and Lung Assessment, Peripheral Vascular Assessment, Abdominal Assessment, Neurologic Assessment, and many others. **Unit Three,** Nursing Assessment of Special Groups, focuses on infants, children, frail elderly adults, families, and communities.

Positive Concepts Emphasize Health and Wellness

Health promotion and client wellness are important baseline concepts in *Health Assessment in Nursing*. Asking the

---

Q Do you wheeze when you cough or when you are active?

R Wheezing indicates narrowing of the airways due to spasm or obstruction. Wheezing is associated with congestive heart failure (CHF), asthma (reactive airway disease), or excessive secretions.

PAST HISTORY

Q Have you had prior respiratory problems?

R A history of respiratory disease increases the risk for a recurrence, and some respiratory diseases may imitate other disorders. For example, asthma symptoms may mimic symptoms associated with emphysema or heart failure.

Q Have you ever had any thoracic surgery, biopsy, or trauma?

R Previous surgeries may alter the appearance of the thorax and cause changes in respiratory sounds. Trauma to the thorax can result in lung tissue changes.

Diagnostic Reasoning: Case Study

The case study presents assessment data for a specific client. It is followed by an analysis of the data, working through the steps involved in diagnostic reasoning to arrive at specific conclusions.

Josephine Carmino is a 57-year-old woman who lives alone in a small urban apartment. She lives on a fixed income from her deceased husband's Social Security pension. She has come to the clinic for her routine checkup. During the initial interview, you notice that she does not always answer your questions appropriately and she talks very softly when she offers information spontaneously. When you check her hearing with the whisper test, she asks you to repeat the word several times, and finally tells you, with annoyance in her voice, "You just have to speak up if you expect people to hear you!" When you do the Rinne test, the results show BC>AC. When you question her about problems, she denies having any hearing loss. She says she has never had audiometric studies and she can't afford them now. She also tells you that she doesn't talk to friends on the telephone anymore, because they don't talk loudly enough.

1 Identify abnormal data and strengths (in both subjective and objective data).

SUBJECTIVE DATA

- Denies any hearing loss
- Never has had audiometry and can't afford it
- Doesn't talk to friends on telephone anymore
- Friends do not talk loud enough on the telephone

OBJECTIVE DATA

- Does not answer questions appropriately
- Speaks very softly
- Fails whisper test
- Rinne test: BC>AC

2 Cue Clusters	**3** Inferences	**4** Possible Nursing Diagnoses	**5** Defining Characteristics	**6** Confirm or Rule Out
A • Does not answer questions appropriately • Fails whisper test • Speaks very softly • Friends do not talk loud enough on the telephone • Rinne test: BC>AC	Data suggest a conduction hearing loss. Soft speaking voice indicates that she hears her own voice loudly, which also points to conductive loss in the middle ear	Impaired Verbal Communication related to lack of understanding of hearing deficit	*Major:* Inappropriate response does not answer nurse's questions appropriately *Minor:* Does not talk to friends on telephone because she cannot hear them (not understanding)	Confirm because it meets the major and minor defining characteristic

types of questions exemplified in the "Nursing History" sections of the chapters provides the nurse with an opportunity to promote health and healthful practices to clients—particularly in regard to nutrition, activity and exercise, sleep and rest, medication use and abuse, self-care responsibilities, social activities, family relationships, education and careers, stress levels and coping strategies, and adaptation to the environment and community.

Risk Factors

In addition, the Risk Factor displays are excellent resources for creative health education activities, some of which are integrated into the text—for example, how to perform self-examinations. Directions for a skin self-examination are in Chapter 9, and breast and testicular self-examinations appear in Appendix C. These pages can be copied and distributed to clients and others.

Culture

In today's health care environment, both health care providers and health care recipients bring vast cultural variation to the marketplace, which in turn presents new ideas, practices, and challenges for nursing assessment. Consideration of culture is a high priority in *Health Assessment in Nursing*. It is not an aside to assessment—it is an integral part of it, which is why normal and abnormal findings related to culture are integrated throughout the text and among the risk factors displays exactly where the student would expect to find the information during an actual assessment. These displays are highlighted by a special icon.

Clients from some cultures (eg, Islam) may accept subjective or physical assessment only by a same-gender nurse, especially when genital and/or sexual issues are being addressed.

Lifespan

People today are living longer and healthier lives, making it more important than ever to meet the health needs of an aging population. The text explains how to adapt the assessment process to elderly clients, particularly frail elderly adults. Moreover, the text describes how some physical changes are actually normal adaptations to aging rather than abnormal health findings.

> Body weight may decrease with aging because of a loss of muscle or lean body tissue.

However, special individual chapters provide comprehensive discussions of the differences inherent in assessing very young and very old clients, as well as childbearing women. The uniqueness of these differences in regard to body structures and functions, interview techniques, growth and development, and physical examination techniques is explained and illustrated.

Family and Community

Chapters devoted to assessment of families and communities complete the text. Among topics covered are theories of family function, family communication styles, nursing interview techniques, internal and external family structuring, and family development stages and tasks.

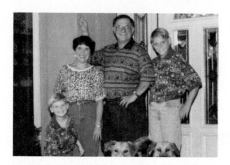

Community assessment addresses the theme of the kinds of communities families and individuals live in and how the community enhances health or presents a barrier to effective healthful functioning. How the physical environment of a community interacts with community health and social services is also explained and illustrated.

New and Special Features of the Second Edition

New features of the second edition of *Health Assessment in Nursing* include two new chapters: The Client in Context: Culture, Family, and Community; and Assessment

of the Frail Elderly Adult. In addition, the chapter on Eye and Ear Assessment in the first edition has been separated into two new chapters. The new chapters further complement the first edition's comprehensive text and colorful step-by-step images of the physical assessment process. Assessment theory and technique is fully disclosed—from health history interviewing to hands-on examination to sequential analysis of assessment findings

- **Full color** line art and photographs and type faces complement the sturdy hardbound text to highlight proper techniques for eliciting obtaining normal and abnormal findings.
- **Chapter Outlines** begin each chapter and present the major points of the chapter.
- **Cultural Considerations** as they relate to physical assessment are interspersed throughout the text.
- **Gerontologic Considerations,** like Cultural Considerations, are interspersed throughout the text to highlight age-related adaptations and abnormalities. They are highlighted with an icon of reading glasses.
- **Risk Factors** displays define risk factors for major diseases and disorders as well as risk-reduction measures and related cultural considerations.
- **Tips From the Experts** are also interspersed throughout the text. They alert the reader to shortcuts or variations of techniques and special tips that can help the student refine his or her assessments skills.

> **Tip From the Experts** If you place the client's arm across the chest while palpating pulse, you can also count respirations. Do this by keeping your fingers on the client's pulse even after you have finished taking it.

- **Diagnostic Reasoning and Case Study materials,** based on real-life situations, are contained in each physical assessment chapter. They present a scenario of client findings obtained during a nursing interview and physical assessment. The scenario is followed by a detailed, lively analysis that requires critical thinking used to analyze data in actual practice. The reader progresses from the client's situation to the analysis by grouping assessment findings into subjective and objective data clusters and then formulating and confirming nursing diagnoses, collaborative problems, or referrals that are specific to the data collected.
- **Appendices and Glossary** round out the text. **Appendix A** is an example of all the components of a complete adult assessment—nursing health history and physical assessment. **Appendix B** lists potential Collaborative Problems that may be identified during assessment and that require treatment not only with nursing interventions but with the services of other health care providers as well. **Appendix C,** an illustrated step-by-step self-examination guide for detecting breast and/or testicular abnormalities, can be reproduced to give to clients as a reference re-

source. **Appendix D** is a mini-nutritional assessment and is followed by a glossary of commonly used assessment terms and abbreviations.

Additional Materials

STUDENT LAB MANUAL

A significant resource to enhance learning and prepare the student for practice is the combined study guide and lab manual that is available for purchase at the student bookstore. Known as the *Student Lab Manual to Accompany Health Assessment in Nursing*, this soft-cover book offers self-test activities and interactive student group exercises that help students apply and retain the knowledge gained from the textbook.

INSTRUCTOR'S MANUAL AND TESTBANK

The *Instructor's Resource CD-ROM to Accompany Health Assessment in Nursing* contains what every instructor needs to bring health assessment to life for the student. It is available on CD-ROM upon adoption of the text.

Janet Weber
Jane Kelley

Acknowledgments

With love, appreciation and many thanks, we would like to acknowledge the following people for their help in making the second edition of *Health Assessment in Nursing* a reality.

JW:

- To Jane, my coauthor, for all your support and for sharing your research and cultural expertise throughout the text
- To Bill, my husband, for your encouragement on a long-term project and belief that it could be done
- To Joey and Wesley, my sons, for your humor and distractions to refresh my mind with what is really important in life.
- To my mom, for your support and persistence with copying and child-sitting.

JK:

- To Janet, precious friend, loyal colleague, and primary author, for encouraging my participation and for making the challenge a delightful experience
- To Arthur, my husband, for your sense of humor, creative outlook, and encouragement over the years
- To my mother, for inspiring me with an eagerness to learn

JW and JK:

- To Ilze Rader and Elizabeth Nieginski, acquisitions editors, for all your encouragement
- To Deedie McMahon, for your patience, perseverance, and special insights
- To all of our colleagues and contributors who have shared their expertise to make this book a reality
- To our students who give us insight as to how one learns best
- To our friends who give us endless hope and encouragement
- To Tom Mondeau, Mark Hill, Dr. Stanley Sides, Dr. Richard Martin, Dr. Michael Bennett, and Dr. Terri Woods for all your wonderful photography
- To Barbara Proud for your excellent professional photography that is present throughout the text
- To Larry Ward for your outstanding illustrations throughout the text
- To Jill Cash and clients for your time, assessment, expertise, and participation in photo shoots. The beautiful photographs in Assessment of the Childbearing Woman and Assessment of Infants, Children, and Adolescents would not have been possible without you
- To ElderNet of Lower Merion—Narberth, Bryn Mawr, Pennsylvania, for your professionalism and kind assistance in eldercare

Contents

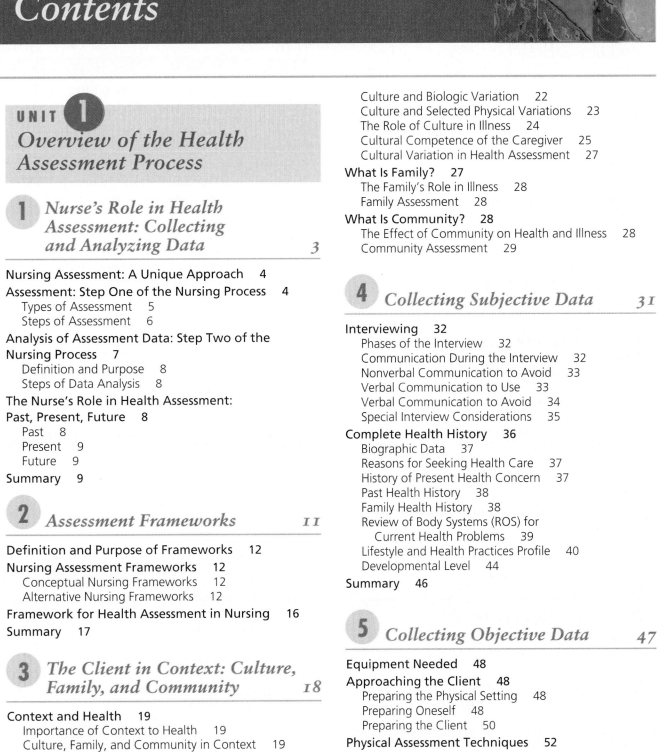

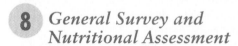
UNIT 2
Nursing Assessment of the Adult

UNIT 3
Nursing Assessment of Special Groups

Health Assessment in Nursing

Overview of the Health Assessment Process

Nurse's Role in Health Assessment: Collecting and Analyzing Data

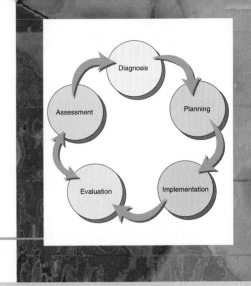

1

Picture yourself in the following situations:

- You walk into Mrs. Smith's room for the first time and see her sitting on the edge of the bed crying. She is still in her street clothes and has not changed into a hospital gown. You introduce yourself and say, "You seem very upset." Mrs. Smith tells you that she is concerned about her husband being left at home alone while she is in the hospital for colon surgery.
- You are making a follow-up visit to a new mother and her 3-day-old infant. You arrive at the address that was provided to you and find the mother and infant living in a worn-down trailer. The mother appears very tired. When asked about this, she says that she has been unable to rest because of several visitors. "I don't mind the attention, but I'm sorta worried that my baby is gonna get sick because a lot of the people that have been coming over are sick with colds." She also tells you that she has had trouble breast-feeding. You see the infant in a crib and notice that his breathing is labored.
- While shopping in a grocery store, you notice a mother with three young children. The youngest, a boy, is in the grocery cart attempting to climb from the cart to the checkout counter. The child does not have on a safety belt, and there is none available on the cart. The mother is gathering her coupons together and has her back to the boy to chide her two girls who are fighting with each other.

As a professional nurse, you constantly observe situations and collect information to make nursing judgments. This occurs no matter what the setting: hospital, clinic, home, community, or long-term care. Each of the previous situations requires you to collect additional data before making a nursing judgment. For example, is Mr. Smith capable of caring for himself? What is the physical health status of the infant in the trailer home? Does the community grocery store have any carts with child safety seat belts on them? Additional information may be gathered from further direct observations of the client and surroundings. In addition, you may also collect data by talking with the client, mother, or store manager.

You probably conduct many informal assessments every day. For example, when you get up in the morning, you may check the weather and determine what would be the most appropriate clothing to wear. You assess whether you are hungry. Do you need a light or heavy breakfast? When will you be able to eat next? You may even assess the physical condition of your skin. Do you need moisturizing lotion? The assessments you make each day determine many of your actions and influence your comfort and success for the remainder of the day. Likewise, the professional nursing assessments you make on a client, family, or community determine nursing interventions that directly or indirectly influence the health status of your client.

Nursing Assessment: A Unique Approach

Virtually every health care professional performs assessments to make professional judgments related to his or her clients. However, the purpose of a nursing history and physical examination differs greatly from that of a medical or other type of health care examination (eg, dietary assessment or examination for physical therapy).

The purpose of a nursing assessment is to collect subjective and objective data to determine a client's overall level of functioning in order to make a professional clinical judgment. The nurse collects physiologic, psychological, sociocultural, developmental, and spiritual data *about* the client. Thus, a holistic data collection is performed. The mind, body, and spirit are considered to be interdependent factors that affect a person's level of health.

The nurse, in particular, focuses on how the client's health status affects his or her activities of daily living and how the client's activities of daily living affect his or her health.

The physician performing a medical examination focuses primarily on the client's physiologic development status. Little attention is given to his or her psychological, sociocultural, or spiritual well-being. Similarly, a physical therapist would focus more on the client's musculoskeletal system and ability to perform activities of daily living.

Another disciplinary distinction is the framework used to collect nursing assessment data. This framework differs from that used by other professionals. Using a nursing framework helps to organize information and promotes the collection of holistic data. This, in turn, provides clues that help to determine human responses. Several different types of nursing frameworks and the framework used for this text are discussed in Chapter 2.

The end result of a nursing assessment is the formulation of nursing diagnoses (wellness, risk, or actual) that require nursing care, the identification of collaborative problems that require interdisciplinary care, and the identification of problems that require immediate referral. Physicians typically use a body systems framework that focuses on the client's chief complaint, medical symptoms, past medical history, and so forth to determine his or her physiologic status. How these physiologic symptoms affect the client's function, spirit, or relationships is often ignored. The end result of the medical assessment is to make a medical diagnosis and prescribe treatment.

Assessment: Step One of the Nursing Process

Assessment is the first and most critical phase of the nursing process. If data collection is inadequate or inaccurate, incorrect nursing judgments may be made that adversely affect the remaining phases of the process: diagnosis, planning, implementation, and evaluation (Table 1-1). Although the assessment phase of the nursing process precedes the other phases in the formal nursing process, nurses are always aware that assessment is ongoing and continuous throughout all the phases of the nursing process. The nursing process should be thought of as circular, not linear (Fig. 1-1).

TYPES OF ASSESSMENT

The four basic types of assessment are:

- Initial comprehensive assessment
- Ongoing or partial assessment
- Focused or problem-oriented assessment
- Emergency assessment

Each varies with the amount and type of data collected.

Initial Comprehensive Assessment

An initial comprehensive assessment requires the nurse to collect subjective data about the client's perception of his or her health of all body parts or systems, past history, family history, and lifestyle and health practices (which includes information related to the client's overall function) as well as objective data gathered during a step-by-step physical examination.

The nurse typically collects the subjective data, especially those related to the client's overall function. However, depending on the setting (hospital, community, clinic, or home), other members of the health care team may participate in various parts of the objective data collection. For example, in a hospital setting, the physician usually performs a total physical examination when the client is admitted (if this was not previously done in the physician's office). A physical therapist may perform a musculoskeletal examination, as in the case of a stroke patient, and a dietitian may take anthropometric measurements in addition to a subjective nutritional assessment. In a community

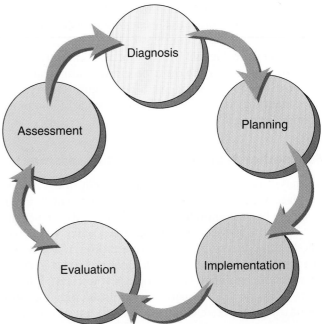

FIGURE 1-1. Each step of the nursing process depends on the accuracy of the preceding step. The steps are also overlapping because you may have to move more quickly for some problems than others. While *Evaluation* involves examining all the previous steps, it especially focuses on achieving desired outcomes. The arrow between *Assessment* and *Evaluation* goes in both directions because assessment and evaluation are ongoing processes as well as separate phases. When the outcomes are not as anticipated, the nurse needs to revisit (reassess) all the steps, collect new data, and formulate adjustments to the plan of care. (Based on Alfaro, R. [1997]. *Applying nursing process: A step-by-step guide* [4th ed.]. Philadelphia: Lippincott Williams & Wilkins.)

clinic, a nurse practitioner may perform the entire physical examination. The nurse is usually responsible for performing most of the physical examination in the home setting.

Regardless of who collects the data, a total health assessment (subjective and objective data regarding functional health and body systems) is needed when the client first enters a health care system and periodically thereafter to establish baseline data against which future health status changes can be measured and compared. Frequency of comprehensive assessments depends on the client's age, risk factors, health status, health promotion practices, and lifestyle.

Ongoing or Partial Assessment

An ongoing or partial assessment of the client consists of data collection that occurs after the comprehensive database is established. This consists of a mini-overview of the client's body systems and holistic health patterns as a follow-up on his or her health status. Any problems that were initially detected in the client's body system or holistic health patterns are reassessed in less depth to determine any major

TABLE 1-1. Phases of the Nursing Process

Phase	Title	Description
I	**A**ssessment	Collecting subjective and objective data
II	**D**iagnosis	Analyzing subjective and objective data to make a professional nursing judgment (nursing diagnosis, collaborative problem, or referral)
III	**P**lanning	Determining outcome criteria and developing a plan
IV	**I**mplementation	Carrying out the plan
V	**E**valuation	Assessing whether outcome criteria have been met and revising the plan as necessary

changes (deterioration or improvement) from the baseline data. In addition, a brief reassessment of the client's normal body system or holistic health patterns is performed to detect any new problems. This type of assessment is usually performed whenever the nurse or another health care professional has an encounter with the client. This type of assessment may be performed in the hospital, community, or home setting.

Focused or Problem-Oriented Assessment

A focused or problem-oriented assessment does not take the place of the comprehensive health assessment. It is performed when a comprehensive database exists for a client, but he or she arrives at the health care agency with a specific health concern. It consists of a thorough assessment of a particular client problem and does not cover areas not related to the problem. For example, if your client, John P., tells you that he has ear pain, you would ask him questions about the pain, possible hearing loss, dizziness, ringing in his ears, and personal ear care. Asking questions about his sexual functioning or his normal bowel habits would be unnecessary and inappropriate. The physical examination should focus on his ears, nose, mouth, and throat. It would not be appropriate to repeat all system examinations, such as the heart and neck vessel or abdominal assessment, at this time.

Emergency Assessment

An emergency assessment is a very rapid assessment performed in life-threatening situations. In such situations (choking, cardiac arrest, drowning), an immediate diagnosis is needed to provide prompt treatment. An example of an emergency assessment is the evaluation of the client's airway, breathing, and circulation (known as the ABCs) when cardiac arrest is suspected. The major and only concern during this type of assessment is to determine the status of the client's life-sustaining physical functions.

STEPS OF ASSESSMENT

The assessment phase of the nursing process has four major steps:

1. Subjective data collection
2. Objective data collection
3. Validation of data
4. Documentation of data

Although there are four steps, they tend to overlap, and you may perform two or three steps concurrently. For example, you may ask your client, Jane Q., if she has dry skin while you are inspecting the condition of the skin. If she answers no, but you notice that the skin on her hands is very dry, validation with the client may be performed at this point.

Each part of assessment is discussed briefly in the following sections. However, Chapters 4, 5, and 6 of this text provide an in-depth explanation of the four assessment steps. In addition, the four steps of the assessment process format are carried thematically throughout this text. All nursing assessment chapters contain the following sections: Collecting Subjective Data, Collecting Objective Data, and a combined Validation and Documentation section.

Preparation Before Assessment

Before you actually meet the client and begin your nursing assessment, there are several things you should do to prepare. It is helpful to review the client's record, if available. Knowing the client's basic biographical data (age, sex, religion, occupation) is useful. Also useful is documented information regarding the client's medical diagnoses and progress notes. These give you an opportunity to verify what you read with what the client tells you and to ask further questions as needed. Reviewing the client's status with other health care team members who have taken care of or interacted with him or her is also helpful.

However, after reviewing the record or discussing the client's status with others, remember to keep an open mind and to avoid premature judgments that may alter your ability to collect accurate data. For example, do not assume a 30-year-old female nurse knows everything regarding hospital routine and medical care, or that a 60-year-old male client with diabetes mellitus needs client teaching regarding diet. Keep an open mind. Validate information with the client, and be prepared to collect additional data.

Also use this time to educate yourself about the client's diagnoses or tests performed. The client may have a medical diagnosis that you have never heard of or that you have not dealt with in the past. Perhaps you review the record and find that the client had a special blood test and the results were abnormal, and you are not familiar with this test. At that time, you could consult the necessary resources (laboratory manual, textbook, or blood laboratory) to learn about the test and the implications of its findings.

Once you have gathered some basic data about the client, take a minute to reflect on your own feelings regarding your initial encounter with the client. For example, the client may be a 22-year-old with a drug addiction. If you are 22 years old and are a very health-conscious person who does not drink, smoke, take illegal drugs, or drink caffeine, you need to take time to examine your own feelings so you avoid biases, judgmentalism, and the tendency to project your own feelings onto the client. You must be as objective and open as possible. Other client situations that may require more reflection time include those involving sexually transmitted diseases, terminal illnesses, amputation, paralysis, early teenage pregnancies, human immunodeficiency virus (HIV) infection or acquired immunodeficiency syndrome (AIDS), and abortion.

Finally, remember to obtain and organize materials that you will need for the assessment. The materials may be assessment tools, such as a guide to interview questions or forms on which to record data collected during the nursing history interview and physical examination, and any equipment (eg, stethoscope, thermometer, otoscope) necessary to perform a nursing health assessment.

Collecting Subjective Data

Subjective data are sensations or symptoms (eg, pain, hunger), feelings (eg, happiness, sadness), perceptions, desires, preferences, beliefs, ideas, values, and personal information that can be elicited and verified only by the client. To elicit accurate subjective data, the nurse must learn to use effective interviewing skills with a variety of clients in different settings. The major areas of subjective data include biographical information (name, age, religion, occupation), physical symptoms related to each body part or system (eg, eyes and ears, abdomen), past and family history, and holistic information regarding the client's health (eg, health practices that put the client at risk, nutrition, activity, relationships). The skills of interviewing and the complete health history are discussed in Chapter 4.

Collecting Objective Data

Objective data are directly observed or indirectly observed through measurements. These data can be physical characteristics (skin color, posture), body functions (heart rate, respiratory rate), appearance (dress and hygiene), behavior (mood, affect), measurements (blood pressure, temperature, height, weight), or the results of laboratory testing (platelet count, x-ray findings).

This type of data is obtained by general observation and by using the four physical examination techniques: inspection, palpation, percussion, and auscultation. Another source of objective data is the client's medical/health record, which is the document that contains information about what other health care professionals (ie, nurses, physicians, physical therapists, dietitians, social workers, clergy) observed about him or her. Objective data may also be observations noted by the family or significant others about the client. See Table 1-2 for a comparison of objective and subjective data.

Validation of Assessment Data

Validation of assessment data is a crucial part of assessment that often occurs along with collection of subjective and objective data. It serves to ensure that the assessment process is not ended before all relevant data have been collected, and it helps prevent documentation of inaccurate data. What types of assessment data should be validated, the different ways to validate data, and identifying areas where data are missing are all parts of the process. Validation of data is discussed in detail in Chapter 6.

TABLE 1-2. Comparing Subjective and Objective Data

	Subjective	Objective
Description	Data elicited and verified by the client	Data directly or indirectly observed through measurement
Sources	Client Family and significant others Client record Other health care professionals	Observations and physical assessment findings of the nurse or other health care professionals Documentation of assessments made in client record Observations made by the client's family or significant others
Methods used to obtain data	Client interview	Observation and physical examination
Skills needed to obtain data	Interview and therapeutic communication skills Caring ability and empathy Listening skills	Inspection Palpation Percussion Auscultation
Examples	"I have a headache." "It frightens me." "I am not hungry."	Respirations 16 per minute BP 180/100, apical pulse 80 and irregular X-ray film reveals fractured pelvis

Documentation of Data

Documentation of assessment data is an important step of assessment because it forms the database for the entire nursing process and provides data for all other members of the health care team. Thorough and accurate documentation is vital to ensure valid conclusions are made when the data are analyzed in the second step of the nursing process. The types of documentation, purpose of documentation, what to document, guidelines for documentation, and different types of documentation forms are discussed in Chapter 6.

Analysis of Assessment Data: Step Two of the Nursing Process

Analysis of the collected data goes hand in hand with the rationale for performing a nursing assessment. The purpose of assessment is to arrive at conclusions about the client's health. To arrive at conclusions, the nurse must analyze the assessment data. Indeed, the nurse often begins to analyze the data in his or her mind while performing assessment. To achieve the goal or anticipated outcome of the assessment, the nurse makes sure that the data collected are as accurate and thorough as possible.

DEFINITION AND PURPOSE

Analysis of data (often called nursing diagnosis) is the second phase of the nursing process. During this phase, you analyze and synthesize data to determine whether the data reveal a nursing concern (nursing diagnosis), a collaborative concern (collaborative problem), or a concern that needs to be referred to another discipline (referral).

A nursing diagnosis is defined by the North American Nursing Diagnosis Association (NANDA) as "a clinical judgment about individuals, family or community responses to actual and potential health problems and life processes" (NANDA, 2001–2002). A nursing diagnosis provides the basis for selection of nursing interventions to achieve outcomes for which the nurse is accountable. Collaborative problems are defined as certain "physiological complications that nurses monitor to detect their onset or changes in status" (Carpenito, 2000). Nurses manage collaborative problems by implementing both physician- and nurse-prescribed interventions to reduce further complications. Referrals occur because nurses assess the "whole" (physical, psychological, social, cultural, and spiritual) client and therefore often identify problems that require the assistance of other health care professionals. Nursing diagnoses, collaborative problems, and referrals are discussed in Chapter 7.

STEPS OF DATA ANALYSIS

To arrive at nursing diagnoses, collaborative problems, or referral, you must go through the steps of data analysis. This process requires diagnostic reasoning skills, often called critical thinking. The process can be divided into seven major steps.

1. Identify abnormal data and strengths.
2. Cluster the data.
3. Draw inferences and identify problems.
4. Propose possible nursing diagnoses.
5. Check defining characteristics.
6. Confirm or rule out.
7. Document conclusions.

Each of these steps is explained in detail in Chapter 7. In addition, each assessment chapter in this text contains a section called "Part Three: Analysis of Data," which uses these steps to analyze the assessment data presented in a specific client case study related to chapter content.

The Nurse's Role in Health Assessment: Past, Present, Future

The nurse's role in health assessment has changed significantly over the years. In the 21st century, the nurse's role in assessment continues to expand, becoming more crucial than ever before.

PAST

Her long skirt swished with her stride and the flame of the oil lamp flickered as she approached the last bed in the dark and crowded infirmary. The tall, thin and frail man lay still on his back with his sunken eyes barely open. She spoke softly as she moved the light near him and gazed at his pale face. She placed the top of her hand over his fevered brow and felt the weak pulsation at his wrist. She wiped the beads of sweat from his temples, watched his heavy chest movements, and counted his loud breathing. She pressed a moist cloth to his dry lips, straightened his pillow, then moved to the window to write her notes.—N. Collins

As the previous passage indicates, physical assessment has been an integral part of nursing since the days of Florence Nightingale. Nurses relied on their natural senses; the patient's face and body would be observed for "changes in color, temperature, muscle strength, use of limbs, body output, and degrees of nutrition, and hydration" (Nightingale, 1992). Palpation was used to measure pulse rate and quality and to locate the fundus of the puerperal woman (Fitzsimmons & Gallagher, 1978).

Examples of independent nursing practice using inspection, palpation, and auscultation have been recorded in nursing journals since 1901. Some examples reported in the *American Journal of Nursing* (1901–1938) include gastrointestinal palpation, testing eighth cranial nerve function, and examination of children in school systems. In addition, the *American Journal of Public Health* documents routine patient and home inspection by public health nurses in the 1930s. This role of case finding, prevention of communicable diseases, and routine use of assessment skills in poor inner-city areas was performed through the Frontier Nursing Service and the Red Cross (Fitzsimmons & Gallagher, 1978). Nurses were also hired to conduct preemployment health stories and physical examinations for major companies, such as New York Telephone, from 1953 through 1960 (Bewes & Baillie, 1969; Cipolla & Collings, 1971).

Despite historical documentation of the use of assessment skills by nurses, it is generally recognized that the depth and scope of nursing assessment have expanded significantly over the past several decades because of rapid advances in biomedical knowledge and technology and through the promotion of primary health care. The early 1970s prompted nurses to develop an active role in the provision of primary health services and expanded the professional nurse role in conducting health histories and physical and psychological assessments (Holzemer, Barkauskas, & Ohlson, 1980; Lysaught, 1970).

Joint statements of the American Nurses Association and the American Academy of Pediatrics agreed that in-depth patient assessments and on-the-spot diagnostic judgments would enhance the productivity of nurses and the health care of patients (Bullough, 1976; Fagin & Goodwin, 1972).

Acute care nurses in the 1980s employed the "primary care" method of delivery of care. Each nurse was autonomous in making comprehensive initial assessments from which individualized plans of care were established. In the 1990s, critical pathways or care maps guided the client's progression, with each stage based on specific protocols that the nurse was responsible for assessing and validating.

Over the last 20 years, the movement of health care from the acute care setting to the community and the proliferation of baccalaureate and graduate education solidified the nurses' role in holistic assessment. Advanced practice nurses have been increasingly used in the hospital as clinical nurse specialists and in the community as nurse practitioners. While state legislators and the American Medical Association struggled with issues of reimbursement and prescriptive services by nurses, government and societal recognition of the need for greater cost accountability in the health care industry brought the advent of diagnosis-related groups (DRGs) and promotion of health care coverage plans such as health maintenance organizations (HMOs) and preferred provider organizations (PPOs). Downsizing, budget cuts, and restructuring were the priorities of the 1990s. In turn, there was a demand for documentation of client assessments by all health care providers to justify health care services.

PRESENT

The current focus on managed care and internal case management has had a dramatic impact on the assessment role of the nurse. The acute care nurse increasingly performs a focused assessment and then incorporates assessment findings from a multidisciplinary team to develop a comprehensive plan of care. Ambulatory care nurses assess and screen clients to determine the need for physician referrals. Home health nurses make independent diagnostic judgments. Public health nurses assess the needs of communities, school nurses monitor the growth and health of our children, and hospice nurses assess the needs of the dying and their families. In all settings, the nurse increasingly documents and retrieves assessment data through sophisticated computerized information systems. Nursing health assessment courses with informatics content are becoming the norm in baccalaureate programs. As the scope and environment for nursing assessment diversify, nurses must be prepared to assess populations of clients not only across the continuum of health but also by way of telecommunication systems with online data retrieval and documentation capabilities.

FUTURE

Picture the nurse assessing a client who has "poor circulation." While in the client's home, the nurse can refresh his or her knowledge of the differences between arterial and venous occlusions, using a "point of need" learning file accessed over the Internet. Also immediately available are the agency's policies, procedures, and care maps. Digital pictures of the client's legs can be forwarded to the off-site nurse practitioner or physician for analysis. These networks have already been prototyped and will allow nurses to transmit and receive information by video cameras attached to portable computers or television sets in the client's home. The nurse can then discuss and demonstrate assessments with other health care professionals as clearly and quickly as if they were in the same room. Assessment data and findings can be documented over the Internet or in computerized medical records—some small enough to fit into a laboratory coat pocket and many activated by the nurse's voice.

The future will see increased specialization and diversity of assessment skills for nurses. While patient acuity increases and technology advances, bedside nurses are challenged to make in-depth physiologic and psychosocial assessments while correlating clinical data from multiple technical monitoring devices. Bedside computers increasingly access individual patient data as well as informational libraries and clinical resources (Graves, 2000). The communication of health assessment and clinical data will span a myriad of electronic interactivities and research possibilities. Health care networks already comprise a large hospital or medical center with referrals from smaller community hospitals; subacute, rehabilitation, and extended care units; HMOs; and home health services. These structures provide diverse settings and levels of care in which nurses will assess clients and facilitate their progress. New delivery systems such as "integrated clinical practice" for surgical care may require the nurse to assess and follow a client from the preoperative visit to a multidisciplinary outpatient clinic and even into the home by way of remote technology.

Nursing leaders envision tremendous growth of the nursing role in the managed care environment. The most marketable nurses will continue to be those with strong assessment and patient teaching abilities and also those who are technologically savvy. The following factors will continue to promote opportunities for nurses with advanced assessment skills:

- Rising educational costs and focus on primary care, affecting the numbers and availability of medical students
- Increasing complexity of acute care
- Growing aging population with complex comorbidities
- Expanding health care needs of single parents
- Increasing impact of children and the homeless on communities
- Intensifying mental health issues
- Expanding health service networks
- Increasing reimbursement for health promotion and preventive care services

Summary

Nursing assessment differs in purpose, framework, and end result from all other types of professional health care assessment. Assessment is the first and most critical step of the nursing process. Accuracy of assessment data affects all other phases of the nursing process. There are four types of nursing assessment: initial comprehensive, ongoing or partial, focused or problem-oriented, and emergency. Nursing assessment can be divided into four steps: collecting subjective data, collecting objective data, validation of data, and documentation of data.

It is difficult to discuss nursing assessment without taking the process one step further. Data analysis is the second step of the nursing process and the end result of nursing assessment. The purpose of data analysis is to reach conclusions concerning the client's health. These conclusions are in the form of nursing diagnoses, collaborative problems, or a need for referral. To arrive at conclusions, the nurse must go through seven steps of diagnostic reasoning or critical thinking.

The role of the nurse in health assessment has expanded drastically from the days of Florence Nightingale, when the nurse used the senses of sight, touch, and hearing to assess clients. Today, communication and physical assessment techniques are used independently by nurses to arrive at professional clinical judgments concerning the client's health. In addition, advances in technology have expanded the role of assessment, and the development of managed care has increased the necessity of assessment skills. Expert clinical assessment and informatics skills are absolute necessities for the future as nurses continue to expand their role in all health care settings.

REFERENCES AND SELECTED READINGS

Alfaro-LeFevre, R. (2000). *Applying the nursing process: A step-by-step guide* (4th ed.). Philadelphia: Lippincott Williams & Wilkins.

Anderson, L. (1998). Exploring the diagnostic reasoning process to improve advanced physical assessments. *Perspectives, 22*(1), 17–22.

Archibald, G. (2000). A post-modern nursing model. *Nursing Standard, 14*(34), 40–42.

Attree, M., & Murphy, G. (1999). Commentary: Nursing process: Paradigm, paradox, or Pandora's box? *Nurse Education Today, 19*(7), 592–597.

Bachman, J. (2000). Information technology: A world wide web–based health resource: Survey of Missouri school nurses to determine priority health information resources for SchoolhealthLink. *Journal of School Nursing, 16*(1), 28–33.

Beck, L. H. (1999). Clinical experience. Periodic health examination and screening tests in adults. *Hospital Practice, 34*(12), 117–118.

Bewes, D., & Baillie, J. (1969). Pre-placement health screening by nurses. *The Journal of Public Health, 12*(59), 2178–2184.

Britton, B. (2000). Measuring costs and quality of telehomecare. *Home Health Care Management and Practice, 12*(4), 27–32.

Brocht, D., Abbott, P., Smith, C., Valus, K., & Berry, S. (1999). A clinic on wheels: A paradigm shift in the provision of care and the challenges of the information infrastructure. *Computers in Nursing, 17*(3), 109–113.

Bullough, B. (1976). Influences on role expansion. *American Journal of Nursing, 9*(76), 1476–1481.

Carpenito, L. J. (2000). *Nursing diagnosis: Application to clinical practice* (8th ed.). Philadelphia: Lippincott Williams & Wilkins.

Cipolla, J., & Collings, G. (1971). Nurse clinicians in industry. *American Journal of Nursing, 8*(71), 1530–1534.

Darbyshire, P. (2000). User-friendliness of computerized information systems. *Computers in Nursing, 18*(2), 93–99.

Fagin, C., & Goodwin, B. (1972). Baccalaureate preparation for primary care. *Nursing Outlook, 4*(20), 240–244.

Fitzsimmons, V., & Gallagher, L. (1978). Physical assessment skills: A historical perspective. *Nursing Forum, 4*(17), 345–355.

Frauman, A. C., & Skelly, A. H. (1999). Evolution of the nursing process. *Clinical Excellence for Nurse Practitioners, 3*(4), 238–244.

Geyer, N., & Naude, S. (1998). Getting the full picture of physical assessment. *Nursing News (South Africa), 22*(2), 40–42.

Goodfellow, L. M. (1997). Physical assessment: A vital nursing tool in both developing and developed countries. *Critical Care Nursing Quarterly, 20*(2), 6–8.

Graves, R. (2000). What are the literature indexes? *Sigma Theta Tau International.* Available: www.stti.iupui.edu/library/nki_what.html.

Harris, R., Wilson-Barnett, J., Griffiths, P., & Evans, A. (1998). Patient assessment: Validation of a nursing instrument. *International Journal of Nursing Studies, 35*(6), 303–313.

Hesselgrave, B. (2000). Healthcare informatics international: A global perspective on health informatics today and tomorrow. *Healthcare Informatics, 17*(4), 54, 56, 58.

Holzemer, W., Barkauskas, V., & Ohlson, V. (1980). A program evaluation of four workshops designed to prepare nurse faculty in health assessment. *Journal of Nursing Education, 4*(19), 7–18.

Langer, S. (2000). Architecture of an image capable, web-based, electronic medical record. *Journal of Digital Imaging, 13*(2), 82–89.

Lillibridge, J., & Wilson, M. (1999). Registered nurses' descriptions of their health assessment practices. *International Journal of Nursing Practice, 5*(1), 29–37.

Lysaught, J. (1970). *An abstract for action.* New York: McGraw-Hill.

McManus, B. (2000). A move to electronic patient records in the community: A qualitative case study of a clinical data collection system. *Topics in Health Information Management, 20*(4), 23–37.

Nightingale, F. (1992). Role expansion or role extension. *Nursing Forum, 4*(9), 380–390.

Nightingale Tracker Field Test Nurse Team. (1999). Designing an information technology application for use in community-focused nursing education . . . the Nightingale Tracker. *Computers in Nursing, 17*(2), 73–81.

North American Nursing Diagnosis Association. (2001–2002). *Nursing diagnoses: Definitions and classification, 2001–2002* (4th ed.). Philadelphia: Author.

Peterson, H. (1997). What's new in health care screening. *Patient Care, 21*(11), 109–110, 115, 118–119.

Rapsilber, L., & Anderson, E. (2000). Understanding the reimbursement process. *Nurse Practitioner: American Journal of Primary Health Care, 25*(5), 36, 43, 46.

Rushforth, H., Bliss, A., Burge, D., & Glasper, E. A. (2000). Nurse-led preoperative assessment: A study of appropriateness. *Paediatric Nursing, 12*(5), 15–20.

Simpson, R. (2000). Nursing informatics: Toward a new millennium. *Nursing Administration Quarterly, 24*(1), 93–97.

Snyder-Halpern, R. (2000). Informatics nurse specialist: A role for the new century in health care. *Aspen's Advisor for Nurse Executives, 15*(4), 3–5.

Stricklin, M., Jones, S., & Niles, S. (2000). Home talk/healthy talk: Improving patients' health status with telephone technology. *Home Healthcare Nurse, 18*(1), 53–62.

Werfel, P. A. (2000). 20 tips to perfect your assessment skills. *Journal of Emergency Medical Services, 25*(1), 68–70, 72–73.

For additional information on this book, be sure to visit http://connection.lww.com.

Assessment
Frameworks

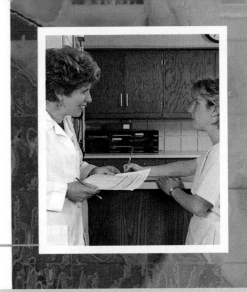

2

The purpose of assessment is to identify patterns of functioning that conform to or deviate from baseline or accepted norms. The assessment process begins with data collection, and a systematic approach to data collection is essential to ensure comprehensiveness and efficiency (Mattison, McConnell & Linton, 1997).

Definition and Purpose of Frameworks

Assessment frameworks offer a systematic approach to identifying patterns of functioning. They are organizational tools developed to enable the systematic collection of data. Physicians use a medical model as their assessment framework. The medical goal is to gather data related to symptoms, body systems findings, medical history, and family history; to then diagnose a medical problem; and to intervene with medical treatment of the problem.

Nurses also collect information regarding symptoms, body systems findings, medical history, and family history. However, the focus is on the client's health behaviors and response to disease. In collecting data, nurses consider holistic aspects of the client, including developmental, psychosocial, spiritual, and other functional areas. The nurse's goal in collecting data differs from the physician's in that nurses collect data to determine areas in which they can independently assist the client with nursing interventions. The nurse's approach to assessment may vary depending on the objectives of the practice setting and the needs of the population served.

Nursing Assessment Frameworks

As a result of this difference in objectives and approaches, many nursing-based assessment frameworks have been developed. The two basic groups of assessment frameworks are those based on conceptual nursing theories and those developed to stand alone or to be used with a nursing theory.

A nurse chooses a particular framework for a variety of reasons. The choice may be based on philosophical orientation, facilitation of research, nursing needs of a particular client population, what was learned in nursing school, or what is used in a particular health care institution. All frameworks effectively capture the essence of nursing's unique contribution to health care. However, nurses who embrace different frameworks perceive nursing differently.

CONCEPTUAL NURSING FRAMEWORKS

Conceptual nursing theories or models were developed to provide a basis to help the nurse make decisions regarding which types of information and observations are essential to ensure accurate evaluative judgments. A conceptual theory or model is a set of abstract, interrelated statements describing the nurse, the client, the nature of nurse–client interaction, definitions of health, the goals of nursing, and nursing interventions. It specifies the focus of nursing. Theorists initially believed that if nurses could agree on one conceptual model, nursing's unique body of knowledge could be defined and communication could be facilitated. Consensus on a particular model was never achieved, but nurses today are comfortable with a pluralist approach to conceptualizing nursing. Table 2-1 provides a summary of several common nursing theories.

Assessment frameworks based on conceptual theories have been developed for use as tools for organizing the assessment data. One example of an assessment framework based on a nursing assessment theory is the nine human response patterns of the unitary person. Kim, McFarland, and McLane (1984) based this framework on Martha Rogers' Science of Unitary Human Beings nursing theory. This model gives the nurse a way to assess the client holistically and is useful for the nurse who is trying to group data to make a nursing diagnosis. The nine human response patterns of this framework are explained in Display 2-1.

ALTERNATIVE NURSING FRAMEWORKS

Although conceptual theories are abstract, nursing frameworks based on assessment guidelines are specific and focus on the structure of nursing assessment or, in other words, what data are to be gathered. The domain of nursing responsibility and accountability is clearly specified, and foci for nursing research can be readily identified. The ways in which assessment data are subsequently interpreted and used would differ according to the nurse's preferred conceptual theory.

Functional Health Patterns

Marjorie Gordon (1987) proposes that, although nurses are unable to agree on one conceptual model, they can agree on which "common areas of information about the client are needed to implement any model of nursing." Despite the diversity in theoretical perspectives, nurses could achieve uniformity in practice by agreeing that certain health-related behavior patterns should be assessed by all. Gordon emphasizes that "at a basic level, all frameworks require similar assessment data." Based on this belief, Gordon developed an assessment framework based on 11 functional health patterns.

Gordon proposes that the central focus of nursing is human functioning. She delineates 11 functional health pattern areas that provide a standardized assessment format for a basic database and encompass a "holistic approach to human functional assessment in any setting and with any age group at any point in the health-illness continuum."

TABLE 2-1. Comparison of Nursing Conceptual Models

Model	Client	Nurse	Nursing	Health	Goal of Nursing
Betty Neuman's (1995) Health Care Systems Model	An open system in which repeated cycles of input, process, output, and feedback constitute a dynamic, organizational pattern. Client may be an individual, group, family, community, or other aggregate.	Provides the linkage between client system, environment, health, and nursing.	Implementation of a three-step nursing process: 1. Nursing diagnosis • Determines existing state of wellness and actual or potential reaction to stressors 2. Nursing goals • Negotiated with the recipient of care • Identified with interventions based on primary, secondary, and tertiary levels of prevention 3. Nursing outcomes • Validates that anticipated or prescribed changes have occurred	Optimum system stability. A dynamic continuum from wellness to illness. Wellness is determined by assessing actual or potential effects of invading stressors on the system's energy levels. Client system moves toward illness when more energy is needed than is available; system moves toward wellness when more energy is available than is needed.	To help the client system to attain, maintain, or retain system stability.
Sister Callista Roy's (Roy & Andrews, 1991) Adaptation Model	Holistic, adaptive system in constant interaction with the environment. The adaptive system has inputs of stimuli and adaptation levels. Outputs are internal and external responses of the person that can be either adaptive or ineffective. Client may be a person, family, group, community, or society.	Manipulates focal, conceptual, and residual stimuli to promote adaptive responses.	Activities/interventions that promote adaptive responses in situations of health and illness: • Behavioral assessment of four adaptive modes • Assessment of stimuli • Nursing diagnosis using Roy's typology • Plan for implementation • Evaluation	State and process of being and becoming an integrated, whole person.	Promotion of adaptive responses in relation to four adaptive modes: • Physiologic • Self-concept • Role function • Interdependence. Nurse seeks to reduce ineffective responses and promote adaptive ones.
Imogene King's (1990) Theory of Goal Attainment	The client is viewed as a personal system. The concepts relevant to the personal system are perception, self, growth and development, body image, space, learning, and time. The client may also be an interpersonal system (dyad, triad, small or large group) or a social system (health care delivery system).	Professional who is concerned with human beings interacting with their environment in ways that lead to self-fulfillment and to maintenance of health.	A major system within health care systems. A process of action, reaction, and interaction whereby nurse and client share information about their perceptions in the nursing situation. Through communication, nurse and client set and agree on means to achieve goals.	A dynamic state that may be viewed as the ability to function in one's usual roles. It is not a continuum but rather a holistic state with genetic, subjective, relative, dynamic, environmental, functional, cultural, and perceptual characteristics.	Mutual interaction with the client to identify problems and establish and meet goals to achieve the client's maximum potential for daily living.
Martha Roger's (1970) Science of Unitary Human Beings	A unified whole possessing integrity and characteristics more and different from the sum of the parts; an energy field continuously exchanging mat-	Promotes symphonic interaction of human beings and their environments to strengthen the coherence and integrity of the human field and	Study of irreducible human beings and their environments; humanistic and humanitarian science directed toward describing and explaining	A value judgment that is individually defined.	To participate in the process of change so people may benefit.

(continued)

TABLE 2-1. Comparison of Nursing Conceptual Models (Continued)

Model	Client	Nurse	Nursing	Health	Goal of Nursing
	ter and energy with the environment and evolving unidirectionally along a space–time continuum.	to direct and redirect patterning of the human and environmental fields for the realization of maximum health.	the human being in synergistic wholeness and in developing the hypothetical generalizations and predictive principles basic to knowledgeable service.		
Jean Watson's (1988) Science of Human Caring	A valued person to be cared for; a fully functioning integrated self greater than or different from the sum of his parts.	Combines care factors derived from a humanistic perspective with a scientific knowledge base to promote health, prevent illness, care for the sick, and restore health.	A human science of persons and human health–illness experiences that are mediated by professional, scientific, esthetic, and ethical human care transactions.	Accepts WHO's definition of health but adds three more elements: • High level of overall physical, mental, and social functioning • General adaptive maintenance level of daily functioning • Absence of illness or presence of efforts that lead to absence	Through the caring process, help people gain a high degree of harmony within the self to promote self-knowledge and self-healing or to gain insight into the meaning of the happenings in life.
Myra Estrin Levine's (1971) Model of Adaptation—Conservation—Integrity (see Levine, 1991)	A human being continuously adapting in his or her interactions with the environment. The process of adaptation results in conservation.	Supports adaptation to achieve conservation and integrity.	Client care guided by concepts of adaptation, conservation, and integrity. Assessment data are in relation to conservation of energy, structural integrity, personal integrity, and social integrity.	Health is the goal of conservation, successful patterns of adaptive change. Defined by each individual for himself or herself.	Development of nursing care judgments or diagnoses that focus on areas in which adaptation needs to be supported to achieve conservation and integrity.
Dorothea Orem's (1991) General Theory of Nursing • Theory of Self-Care • Theory of Nursing Systems	A self-care agent who performs or practices activities to maintain life, health, and well-being, is affected by age, gender, developmental state, health state, sociocultural factors, health system factors, environment, and resource adequacy and availability.	Performs and regulates self-care tasks of client, coordinates self-care task performance to system of care coordinated with other components of care. Guides, directs, and supports clients in their exercise of self-care agency. Nurses use five methods of helping: • Acting for/doing for • Guiding and directing • Providing physical or psychological support • Providing and maintaining an environment that supports personal development • Teaching. Designs are wholly compensatory, partly compensatory, and supportive/educative nursing systems.	Human service distinguished from other human services by its focus on persons to maintain the continuous provision of health care. Nursing is needed when adults are unable to maintain the amount and quality of self-care needed to sustain life and health, recover from disease or injury, or cope with their effects. Children require nursing when their parents or guardians are unable to maintain their requisite care.	WHO definition: A state of physical, mental, and social well-being.	Helping others meet their therapeutic self-care demands by exercising or developing their own self-care agency.

Adapted from George, J. D. (1995). *Nursing theories: The base for professional nursing practice* (4th ed.). Norwall: CT: Appleton & Lange.

DISPLAY 2-1. Nine Patterns of the Unitary Person

EXCHANGING

Mutual exchanging; giving and receiving (eg, oxygenation, intake and output, body temperature)

COMMUNICATING

Sending messages; speech

RELATING

Developing bonds; social interactions, roles, sexual functions, parenting, finances

VALUING

Assignment of relative worth; religious preference and practices, cultural beliefs and practices, belief in a higher being

CHOOSING

Choosing from alternatives; decision making, acceptance of help from others, denial of problems

MOVING

Activity; self-care abilities, diversional and recreational activities, sleep habits, breastfeeding, safety, and environment

PERCEIVING

Reception of information; seeing, smelling, hearing, feeling, perception of self-control of situation

KNOWING

Meaning of information; knowledge of condition and health, cognitive abilities, level of orientation, memory ability

FEELING

Subjective consciousness or perception of information; anxiety and other emotions, pain, or other subjective symptoms, grief

Patterns are described as sequences of behavior over time that serve as the basis for clinical judgment. All people share certain functional health patterns that contribute to health, quality of life, and achievement of human potential. During data collection, an overview of the client's patterns is constructed from the client's descriptions and the nurse's observations. Dysfunctional patterns yield nursing diagnoses (Gordon, 1987). If unaltered, dysfunctional patterns lead to disease processes. Together, they provide a set—or typology—of assessment categories and systematize the assessment process. Clients are not bombarded with disorganized sets of questions; the rationale for collecting different types of data is clear.

Gordon emphasizes that the 11 functional health patterns artificially divide integrated human functioning. In reality, the patterns are interrelated, interactive, and interdependent. The 11 categories provide a structure for analyzing problems within one pattern and for searching other patterns for causes and contributory factors. For example, a dysfunctional role—relationship pattern could result from conflicts in values and beliefs.

These functional health patterns can be used across all specialties. Basic historical and current information is collected about each health pattern. The resulting database serves as a baseline against which future changes are measured. In healthy clients, changes may give evidence of developmental transitions or health alterations that should be closely monitored. In chronically ill clients, changes alert the nurse to effectiveness of symptom management or to disease progression. The client provides the nurse with a description of his or her patterns as well as with perceptions about them. By listening to the client's explanations, the nurse can identify knowledge deficits, risk factors for disease, and problems with health management. Gordon's 11 functional health patterns are described in Display 2-2.

When Gordon's functional health pattern format for assessment is adapted for use with individuals of any age, patterns must be assessed according to developmental norms. Similarly, when the health pattern approach is used for community assessment, that community's norms must be considered. Once initial assessment is complete, dysfunctional patterns that become nursing diagnoses can be identified. Subsequent steps of the nursing process are guided by the nurse's preferred conceptual theory.

Mnemonic Devices

Mnemonic devices are frequently used by nurses to organize rapid, initial client assessment. FANCAPES is one example of an assessment mnemonic. Each letter of the mnemonic represents an area of client assessment: Fluid intake, Aeration, Nutrition, Communication, Activity, Pain, Elimination, Socialization. In this textbook, the nurse can use the COLDSPA mnemonic—Character, Onset, Location, Duration, Severity, Pattern, and Associated symptoms—to investigate any sign or symptom reported by a client (see Chapter 4 for more information).

Five Dimensions of Wellness

Another means of organizing client assessment is the five dimensions of wellness identified by Travis and Ryan (1988). These five dimensions include:

DISPLAY 2-2. Eleven Functional Health Patterns

HEALTH PERCEPTION/HEALTH MANAGEMENT

How the client perceives and manages his or her health; compliance with health care practices

NUTRITIONAL/METABOLIC

Client's dietary habits and metabolic needs

ELIMINATION

Client's bowel and bladder function

ACTIVITY/EXERCISE

Activities of daily living, including work, recreation, exercise, and leisure

SEXUALITY/REPRODUCTIVE

Sexual functioning, needs, and perceived level of satisfaction

SLEEP/REST

Quality of sleep, rest, and relaxation periods

COGNITIVE/PERCEPTUAL

Knowledge, thought, perception, and language; sensory perception (hearing, sight, smell, touch, and taste)

ROLE/RELATIONSHIP

Roles and relationships within family, at work, and in society

SELF-PERCEPTION/SELF-CONCEPT

Client's perception of identity, abilities, body image, and self-worth

COPING/STRESS

Stressors in client's life, tolerance levels, and methods of coping

VALUE/BELIEF

Client's life values, goals, philosophical beliefs, religious beliefs, and spiritual beliefs

- Physical fitness
- Nutritional awareness
- Stress management
- Environmental sensitivity
- Self-responsibility for health

Physical fitness refers to flexibility, strength, endurance, and aerobic capacity. Nutritional awareness relates to the client's knowledge of and compliance with the recommended dietary allowances for her or his age. Stress management addresses coping styles and behaviors. The concept of environmental sensitivity addresses the extent to which the environment places demands on the individual. *Environment* is defined broadly as the physical environments in which the person resides, works, and recreates, as well as the interpersonal environment composed of family, friends, and associates. Self-responsibility for health concerns the degree to which the client feels a sense of accountability and mastery concerning his or her health status.

Framework for Health Assessment in Nursing

Because there are so many nursing assessment frameworks available for organizing data, it was thought that picking one assessment framework would limit the use of this text and ignore many other valid nursing assessment framework methods. Therefore, the objective of this textbook is to provide the reader with the essential raw material necessary to perform a thorough nursing assessment without locking into one particular nursing assessment framework. The reader can take the information in this book and adapt it to the nursing assessment framework of her or his choice.

The book is organized around a head-to-toe assessment of body parts and systems. In each chapter, the nursing history is organized according to a "generic" nursing history framework, which is an abbreviated version of the complete nursing history detailed in Chapter 4. The questions asked in each chapter concentrate on that particular body part or system and are broken down into four sections:

- Current symptoms
- Past history
- Family history
- Lifestyle and health practices

The rationale for the first three sections may be medical, nursing related, or both. The lifestyle and health practices section concentrates on information particularly important to nursing. The questions in this section fall into one of the following four categories:

- What lifestyle or health practices does the client follow that may put him or her at risk for alterations in health?
- What effect does the client's health have on the ability to function in his or her activities of daily living?
- How does the client's health affect his or her psychological or social well-being, or how does the client's social or psychological state affect his or her health?
- Does the client self-treat health concerns, adhere to prescribed treatment, or have adequate knowledge about his or her state of health?

After the nursing history, the physical assessment section provides the procedure, normal findings, and abnormal findings for each step of examination of a particular body part or system. The collected data based on the client's answers to the types of questions asked in the nursing history, along with the objective data gathered during the hands-on physical assessment, enable the nurse to make judgments concerning nursing diagnoses, collaborative problems, referral, and need for client teaching.

Summary

The nurse may choose from a variety of approaches to organize client assessment data. Many nurses are committed to a particular conceptual theory. Some of these theorists propose specific assessment tools for use with their model, for example, Rogers' nine human response patterns of unitary beings. Some nurses may elect to use such tools, if available, to organize their assessment. Others may prefer to use Gordon's 11 functional health patterns by themselves or in conjunction with a conceptual framework. Simpler approaches include the use of mnemonic acronyms or analyzing the components of a single concept, such as wellness, which is integrally linked to nursing diagnosis and nursing care.

This second edition of *Health Assessment in Nursing* presents a head-to-toe approach for assessing body parts or systems. In each chapter, the nursing history and physical assessment are organized in a "generic" nursing framework in a straightforward, logical manner that teaches the reader how to perform a complete nursing health assessment. After learning what should be included in a complete nursing health assessment from the data presented in this text, the reader can adapt the information to the nursing assessment framework of her or his choice.

REFERENCES AND SELECTED READINGS

Fitzpatrick, J., & Whall, A. (1989). *Conceptual models of nursing: Analysis and application* (2nd ed.). Norwalk, CT: Appleton & Lange.

George, J. B. (1995). *Nursing theories: The base for professional nursing* (4th ed.) Norwalk, CT: Appleton & Lange.

Gordon, M. (1987). *Nursing diagnosis: Process and application* (2nd ed.). New York: McGraw-Hill.

Kim, M. J., McFarland, G. K., & McLane, A. M. (1984). *Classification of nursing diagnoses: Proceedings of the fifth national conference*. St. Louis, MO: C. V. Mosby.

King, I. (1990). *A theory for nursing: Systems, concepts, process*. Albany, NY: Delmar.

Levine, M. E. (1991). The conservation principles: A model for health. In K. M. Schaefer & J. B. Pond (Eds.). *Levine's conservation model: A framework for nursing practice* (pp. 101–117). Philadelphia, PA: F. A. Davis.

———. (1973). *Introduction to clinical nursing* (2nd ed.). Philadelphia, PA: F. A. Davis.

Malinski, V. M. (Ed.). (1986). *Explorations on Martha Rogers' science of unitary human beings*. Norwalk, CT: Appleton & Lange.

Mattison, M. A., McConnell, E. S., & Linton, A. D. (1997). *Gerontological nursing: Concepts and practice* (2nd ed.). Philadelphia, PA: W. B. Saunders.

Neuman, B. (1995). *The Neuman systems model* (3rd ed.). Norwalk, CT: Appleton & Lange.

Orem, D. E. (1991). *Nursing: Concepts of practice* (4th ed.). St. Louis, MO: C. V. Mosby.

———. (1980). *Nursing: Concepts of practice* (2nd ed.). New York, NY: McGraw-Hill.

Rogers, M. E. (1970). *The theoretical basis of nursing*. Philadelphia, PA: F. A. Davis.

Roy, C., & Andrews, H. A. (Eds.). (1991). *The Roy adaptation model: The definitive statement*. Norwalk, CT: Appleton & Lange.

Travis, J., & Ryan, R. (1988). *Wellness workbook* (2nd ed.). Berkeley, CA: Ten Speed Press.

Watson, J. (1988). *Human science and human care: A theory of nursing*. New York, NY: National League for Nursing.

For additional information on this book, be sure to visit http://connection.lww.com.

The Client in Context: Culture, Family, and Community

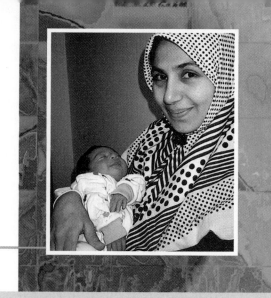

3

Why does a text on health assessment include sections that deal with culture, family assessment, and community assessment? Well, let us look at a nurse and client encounter and see if the reason becomes clear.

Context and Health

Mrs. Gutierrez, age 52, arrives at the clinic for diabetic teaching. She appears distracted and sad, uninterested in the teaching. The nurse suspects that Mrs. G. is upset by her diagnosis of diabetes. As the assessment progresses, the nurse learns that Mrs. G. has no appetite and no energy, wants to stay in bed all day, misses her sisters in Mexico, and cannot do her normal housekeeping or cooking. The nurse thinks that Mrs. G. is probably suffering from depression. But when the nurse asks Mrs. G. what she believes is causing her lack of appetite and low energy, Mrs. G. says that she was given a shock when her husband was arrested for drunk driving. She says she is suffering from *susto* and that a few days in bed will help her recover her soul and her health. The nurse decides to reschedule the diabetic teaching for a later time and just provide essential information for Mrs. G. at this visit.

IMPORTANCE OF CONTEXT TO HEALTH

What can we conclude from this scenario? Many systems are operating to create the context in which the client exists and functions. The nurse sees an individual client, but accurate interpretation of what the nurse sees depends on perceiving the client in context. Culture, family, and community operate as systems interacting to form the context.

CULTURE, FAMILY, AND COMMUNITY IN CONTEXT

A health assessment textbook for nurses focuses on providing a solid baseline for determining normal versus abnormal data gathered in a health history and physical assessment. This text must be supported by knowledge or concurrent instruction in medical–surgical and psychosocial nursing and, of course, a strong command of anatomy and physiology. The text can provide only a review of key concepts of these subjects.

As with anatomy and physiology, medical–surgical nursing, and psychosocial nursing content, a health assessment textbook can only provide key concepts related to culture, family, and community. Texts on transcultural nursing, family nursing, family therapy, social work, and community nursing should provide the knowledge base, concurrent instruction, or resources needed for exhaustive information. This assessment text emphasizes the need to consider the client in context for best practice in health assessment.

When completing a health assessment, the nurse must be aware of the key elements of assessment that are presented in this text. If the nurse notes a finding that is perplexing, she or he should explore with the client or seek further resources to determine whether culture, family, or community factors affect the finding. This text presents basic principles and some examples of how to perceive and explore findings that may result from the influence of the three systems: culture, family, and community.

SYSTEMS AND THEIR RELATIONSHIP TO THE INDIVIDUAL

The authors of this text believe that individual clients cannot be assessed thoroughly unless they are perceived in context—in the context of the various systems of which they are a part. The scenario involving the interaction between the nurse and Mrs. G. illustrates how looking at one client as an isolated individual sitting in an examination room can be quite misleading if the contexts of the many systems of which the client is a part are not considered.

A system is an interacting whole formed from many parts, but when the parts constantly interact, the system is more complex and has more dimensions than the individual parts. The individual, subgroups, and other parts of the system constantly interact to greater or lesser degree at any point in time, but the influences are operating at all times. To make the picture even more complex, various systems are interacting with one another constantly, too.

When a nurse meets a client, the client brings to the encounter the influence of several systems. For the purposes of this text, the systems to be considered are the client's culture, family, and community of residence and work. These systems have enormous influence on health and illness, and their influence is essential to understanding a client's health status and risk factors for illness. Indeed, some of the assessment findings cannot be interpreted at all—or they may be interpreted inaccurately—if the nurse lacks knowledge of cultural variation, family patterns, and community factors.

CULTURE, FAMILY, AND COMMUNITY AS SYSTEMS

Culture, family, and community are systems. But it is very difficult to separate the three systems to examine each because the systems constantly interact and change based on the interaction. A cultural group that is entirely isolated would not be known by outsiders. So, the introduction of outsiders into the group begins to influence the isolated culture, and the outsiders begin to effect small to large changes of the culture. Within the "isolated" culture, there are norms for the family pattern (who belongs to the family, what the purpose of the family is, how family members relate to nonfamily members of the cultural group, and so forth). Once outside influence is introduced, the amount of the influence may determine what level of change will occur in the cultural group's beliefs and practices regarding family and nonfamily interaction. The size of the community in which the cultural group lives, how many subgroups of different cultures reside within the community, whether the cultural group is more or less affiliated with the dominant cultural group of the community, and the resources available for the cultural group to remain somewhat isolated while living within the community will certainly affect the likelihood of change.

Consider an example of a cultural group that has been able to remain somewhat isolated while residing within a larger community. There are many Orthodox Jewish communities in the United States that maintain a strict cultural group with cultural norms for individuals' daily life practices, family patterns and practices, and limited interaction of designated individuals with the community at large. Many of these groups reside in large metropolitan areas, yet maintain their own cultural patterns and family structure. Does the larger community affect these cultural groups? Of course it does. The environment, government and social resources, and many points of interaction with the larger community affect the cultural group. The group's acceptance within the larger community affects many aspects of the group's well-being. Think of Orthodox Jews living in St. Louis as opposed to those living in Moscow or Tel Aviv.

So, the community can influence cultural change, and we are all aware of how community values can affect norms for family and how the influence of strong cultural groups within a community can affect the community at large. None of the three systems functions in isolation, even within the small isolated cultural group. The more isolated group culture affects or dictates family structure and function, and culture and family affect the community development, which, in turn, affects the culture and family.

Before further discussion, it is necessary to look at the three systems separately to understand more about culture, family, and community.

CULTURE AND VARIATIONS

Within a culture there are many variations of beliefs and practices, and these variations are defined as normal (Display 3-1). The same is true for biologic variations. For example,

heights and weights may vary significantly, yet the variations are normal. Only the extremes of height and weight are considered abnormal (Display 3-2).

What Is Culture?

Culture, an anthropologic term that is widely used in many fields of study, is difficult to define. Exact definitions are hard to determine and are still debated. Purnell and Paulanka (1998, p. 2) provide a useful definition capturing the sense of many others' by defining culture as "the totality of socially transmitted behavioral patterns, arts, beliefs, values, customs, lifeways, and all other products of human work and thought characteristic of a population or people that guide their worldview and decision making." Based on this definition, culture is composed of all verbal and behavioral systems that transmit meaning.

BASIC CHARACTERISTICS

Culture is learned. It is transmitted from one generation to the next through socialization. It is learned through life experiences within one's own cultural group and as one experiences contact with other cultural groups.

Culture is shared. Norms for behaviors, values, and beliefs are shared by the cultural group to a great extent, and it is the sharing of these through interaction and socialization that forms the cultural group.

Culture is associated with adaptation to the environment. As environmental circumstances change, the group changes to improve its ability to survive or to make maximal use of the environment in which it lives. Culture is, therefore, ever changing.

Culture is universal. Cultures may vary, but humans cannot exist without culture. The only humans without socially transmitted culture would be those known as feral children who are separated from all human contact (some raised by animals in the wild; rarely, children left in the

---

DISPLAY 3-1.   Cultural Beliefs and Practices: Normal or Abnormal?

Quiz: Of the following beliefs and practices, which are normal variations and which are abnormal findings?

- The request for anointing by a priest before surgery
- The request for a shaman (witch doctor) to treat the client along with the medical doctor
- Placement in a room with a bed pointing toward Mecca in Saudi Arabia
- Having family members present at a family member's death
- An obstetric patient refusing care by a male physician
- Refusing iced drinks while ill
- Claiming that a child's illness is due to evil eye

Conclusion: All of the above beliefs and practices are based on cultural practices of different cultural groups. Therefore, all may be considered normal variations.

DISPLAY 3-2. Normal Variations and Abnormal Findings

Sometimes, distinguishing normal from abnormal findings becomes particularly difficult, especially when the finding is peculiar to a particular cultural or ethnic group. Compare, for example, mongolian spots, which are normal in dark-skinned infants, with bruises, which are not normal findings.

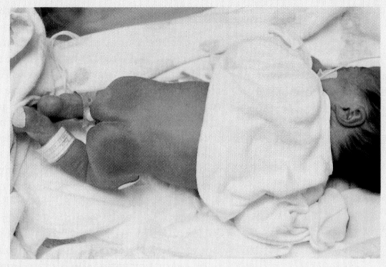

Mongolian spots.

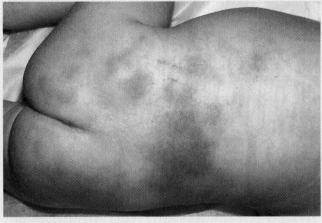

Bruised buttocks.

Other reasonably common findings that may be difficult to define as normal or abnormal because of cultural factors include lip pits (genetic variations) and cheilosis (a lip condition characterized by chapping and fissures) and Beau's lines (lines in the nails from acute and severe illness) and nail streaks (lines in the nails that are normal in darker-skinned people).

wilderness who survive), for example, Romulus and Remus or, more recently, Nell.

In summary, Agar (1994) suggests that culture serves as an ever-changing frame for interpreting information and understanding how the world works. The culture defines values (learned beliefs about what is held to be good or bad) and norms (learned behaviors that are perceived to be appropriate or inappropriate). The world view that each of us forms based on our own culture becomes, for us, reality.

If we have limited interaction with other cultural groups, our cultural world view is the limit of our experience. The perception that our world view is the only acceptable truth and that our beliefs, values, and sanctioned behaviors are superior to all others is called ethnocentrism.

Many people are aware of other cultures and the different beliefs, values, and accepted behaviors but do not recognize the great variation that can exist within any cultural group. When a person fails to recognize this variation, he or she tends to stereotype all members of the particular culture, expecting group members to hold the same beliefs and behave in the same way.

A term commonly associated with culture is ethnicity. Lipson (1996, p. 8) defines ethnicity as identification with a "socially, culturally, and politically constructed group of individuals that holds a common set of characteristics not shared by others with whom its members come in contact."

CULTURE AND BIOLOGIC VARIATION

Physical anthropologists have studied human variation for many decades. The study of the effects on health and illness of these variations has been a more recent endeavor, especially of biomedical anthropologists and some transcultural nurses. Three questions arise about the significance of biologic variation.

- What are the mechanisms that cause humans to vary?
- What effects do the variations have on individual and group health?
- Which of the variations are important to health assessment for nurses?

Mechanisms of Variation: Genetics and Environment

The mechanisms that cause humans to vary biologically are genetics and environment and the interaction of the two. Gene variations cause obvious differences, such as eye color, and genetic diseases, such as trisomy 21. Increasingly, however, genes are identified as playing a role in most diseases, even if only to increase or decrease a person's susceptibility to infectious or chronic diseases.

Of course, environment has been proved to cause disease. But modern thought on disease causation leans toward a mingling of genetics and environment. If, for example, a person has lungs that are genetically "hardy," then exposure to smoking may not cause lung cancer or chronic lung disease.

So, students of anatomy and physiology, disease etiology, and such need a strong grounding in genetics and the sciences of environment. But what do nurses need to know to assess humans effectively to differentiate the normal from the abnormal? They need to be able to distinguish characteristics that have risen in some groups but not in others, characteristics that are physical, genetic, and behavioral, so that they can separate the differences that are of no consequence from differences that signify abnormality.

Race and Ethnicity

First, examine how genetic changes occur. Mutations occur in genes, and interbreeding groups whose members mate mostly within the group develop distinct biologic characteristics. The concept of race is based on genetics. Overfield (1995) provides a discussion of race and why anthropolo-

gists argue against the concept. Race indicates a breeding population that mates largely within its group, so that small genetic differences exist between the group and other groups, and the group members share some distinct biologic characteristics. However, genetic variations do not necessarily occur together, and, when looking worldwide, most characteristics vary from high frequency to low frequency across a continuum. For instance, blond hair has a high frequency in northern Europe, and hair tends to become increasingly darker as you move south and east. But what of the blond, wavy hair of some Australian aboriginal children? Their hair color and texture are not from intermarriage with Caucasians, but may predate the earliest Caucasians. But the pale skin color of northern Europeans with blond hair is not found in the aborigines, whose skin color is very dark.

The genetic background of the client affects the genetic-based characteristics seen. The amount of genetic admixture will affect which genes are expressed. For example, African Americans in the United States generally have a genetic background of West African origin mixed with Western European admixture. The isolation from the African continent and mating within the African American and European American gene pools have resulted in a fairly large amount of variation within the African American population. There is still likelihood of finding variations associated with West African genes, however, such as more frequent malaria-associated genetic diseases (eg, sickle cell); dark brown skin, hair and eyes; tightly curled, fragile hair; and dry scalp. Body shapes vary greatly as they do in West African populations.

All characteristics so readily associated with racial differences have the same complex patterns and cannot be identified with any one "race." But what other word can be used? Overfield (1995) notes that "ethnic group" is often substituted but is usually inappropriate because it is concerned with learned behavior, independent of genetics and nationality.

Perhaps the concept of human variation is best for discussing group differences. The nurse assessing a client is challenged to look beyond the individual person and include the contexts of culture, family, and community. This section on human variation is included under culture, because we so often associate the two.

Other Factors Affecting Variation

Discussion of human variations associated with behaviors is included in Chapter 4 and throughout this book. The physical variations (resulting from genetics or cultural behaviors) are included directly in the normal and abnormal findings discovered during the assessment process. The authors believe that integrating the information helps the nurse attend to the possible variations during all assessments, rather than having to seek the information elsewhere if the client appears to be from a different culture.

One limitation of this approach has to be acknowledged. Because characteristics vary along a continuum with many possible points of reference, it would be cumbersome to include every possible variation as the point from which a characteristic varies. Acknowledging that this is an imperfect approach, the authors have used the U.S. population majority group as the point from which variation is assessed. As U.S. population demographics change, the baseline point will have to change in future texts.

CULTURE AND SELECTED PHYSICAL VARIATIONS

In his model of cultural competence, Purnell (Purnell & Paulanka, 1998) includes a category called biocultural ecology. This category refers to the client's physical, biologic, and physiologic variations, such as variations in drug metabolism, disease, and health conditions. The term biocultural ecology presents an interesting perspective. However, this text uses the term biologic variation to include human variation of a biologic and physiologic nature. Overfield (1995) divides the discussion of biologic variation into sections as follows:

I. Surface variations and anatomic differences
   A. Surface variation
      1. Color
      2. Secretions
      3. Surface anatomy
   B. Anatomic variation
      1. Body proportions
      2. Bones
      3. Pelvic measurements and newborn size
      4. Pulmonary function
      5. Teeth
      6. Soft tissue
II. Developmental variation in childhood
   A. Body size and proportion differences
   B. Developmental maturity differences
   C. Environmental effects
   D. Surface features
   E. Common clinical measurements
   F. Disease differential
   G. Other variations
III. Developmental variation in adulthood
   A. Body size, shape, and composition
   B. Surface manifestations
   C. Developmental changes
   D. Disease susceptibility
IV. Biochemical variation and differential disease susceptibility
V. Environmentally related variation
   A. Climate
   B. Altitude
   C. Diet
VI. Sexual variation

Additionally, there are culturally based syndromes of diseases that are perceived to exist in some cultures but not perceived to exist in other cultures (nor by the health care providers of other cultures).

Obviously, an assessment text cannot discuss all of the topics in biologic variation. Only a sampling is included in this text. The variations selected for inclusion are among the most often seen or most likely to be interpreted incorrectly as normal or abnormal. A sampling of variation associated with selected diseases is included in the risk factors display for selected diseases included in most physical assessment chapters.

Surface Variation: Secretions

Secretions as an example of a surface variation (from Overfield, above) refers to the variation in apocrine and eccrine sweat secretions and the apocrine secretion of ear wax. Sebaceous gland activity and secretion composition do not show significant variation.

Eccrine glands, distributed over the entire body, show no variation in number or distribution but do vary in activity based on environmental and individual adaptations (not by race). Persons born in the tropics have more functioning glands than those born in other areas, and than those who move to the tropics later in life. Studies of Japanese and Solomon Islanders have noted this pattern (Overfield, 1995, p. 16). Eskimos have been noted to sweat less on their trunks and extremities but more on their faces than do Caucasians, which is believed to be an adaptation to allow thermoregulation without dampening clothes (Overfield, 1995, p. 16).

The amount of chloride excreted by sweat glands differs by ethnic or racial group and by environment. The sweat of people of black African origin has a low salt concentration, but the sweat of Caucasians acclimatized to the tropics also has a lower salt–chloride concentration than does the sweat of nonacclimatized Caucasians (Overfield, 1995, p. 16).

Apocrine glands, opening into the hair follicles in the axilla, groin, and pubic regions, around the anus, umbilicus, and breast areola, and in the external auditory canal, vary much in the number of functioning glands. Asians and Native Americans have fewer functioning apocrine glands than do most Caucasians and blacks (Overfield, 1995, p. 16). The amount of sweating and body odor are directly related to the function of apocrine glands, although the odor is probably related to the decomposition of lipids in the secretions. Prepubescent children, Asians, and Native Americans have no or limited underarm sweat and body odor.

Ear wax, produced by the apocrine glands in the external ear, varies between dry and wet wax based on a genetic trait. About 85% of Asians and Native Americans have dry ear wax, and about 97% of Caucasians and 99% of blacks have wet ear wax (Overfield, 1995, p. 17). Reasons for the genetic variation are thought to include climate and disease susceptibility. For instance, women with dry ear wax have a lower incidence of breast cancer.

Anatomic Variation

Lower extremity venous valves vary between Caucasians and black Africans. Black Africans have been noted to have fewer valves in the external iliac veins but many more valves lower in the leg than do Caucasians. The additional valves may account for the lower prevalence of varicose veins in blacks (Overfield, 1995, p. 28).

Developmental Variation

Maturity differences appear to be related to both genetics and environment. African American infants and children tend to be ahead of other American groups in motor development. However, studies of the effect of socioeconomic status show that lower-status children show earlier motor development than do higher-status children, irrespective of racial group (Overfield, 1995, p. 45). Overfield cautions those using the Denver Developmental Screening Test (DDST) because its development was based primarily on white American children. She suggests that any African American child who lags below the 50th percentile on motor development items should have further diagnostic procedures.

Biochemical Variation and Differential Disease Susceptibility

Drug metabolism differences, lactose intolerance, and malaria-related conditions, such as sickle cell disease, thalassemia, glucose-6-phosphate dehydrogenase (G6PD) deficiency, and Duffy blood group, are considered biochemical variations. Both Overfield (1995) and Campinha-Bacote (1998b) provide extensive reviews of ethnic–racial group differences in drug metabolism. As far as lactose intolerance is concerned, most of the world's population is lactose intolerant. The ability to digest lactose after childhood relates to a mutation that occurs mainly in those of North and Central European ancestry and in some Middle Eastern populations (Overfield, p. 104). The malaria-related conditions would obviously occur in populations living in or originating from mosquito-infested locales such as the Mediterranean and Africa.

These brief examples show that health status and health assessment are greatly influenced by biologic variations. Many of the chapters in this text include physical characteristics to be assessed that have normal variations or that vary in the way abnormalities are expressed. These variations are inserted into the physical assessment discussions. Also, many of the chapters include risk factor discussions addressing common illnesses associated with the content of the chapter. The epidemiology of the condition and the cultural or biologic variations associated with the illness are included.

THE ROLE OF CULTURE IN ILLNESS

Group behaviors have developed around beliefs about health and illness and about norms for human interaction. Health care is interactive. Most human behavioral variations that are useful to nurses performing assessments concern communication; these are considered in Chapter 4. A few behaviors associated with treating illness are included in the physical assessment tables.

A special facet of illness and culture involves cultural and behavioral variations considered to be culture-based syndromes. These are perceived to be separate illnesses within certain cultures. They typically have both behavioral and physical characteristics, and they pose a special challenge to the nurse performing a health assessment.

Culture-bound syndromes are illnesses that are defined as such by a specific cultural group, but they are interpreted differently or not perceived as illnesses by other groups. Many of these illnesses have an emotional component or a spiritual cause.

Selected Culture-Bound Syndromes in Hispanic Groups

Four culture-bound syndromes recognized in some Hispanic populations are *susto, mal ojo, empacho,* and *caida de la mollera*. Campinha-Bacote (1998b, p. 21) and Purnell (1998, p. 414) provide brief highlights of these syndromes.

- *Susto* (soul loss or magical fright) is believed to be caused by a shock or fright causing the spirit to leave the body. Symptoms, real or fabricated, may include anorexia, listlessness, apathy, and withdrawal, or the symptoms may be nonspecific. The sufferer is released from work or life responsibilities and is allowed to assume the sick role.
- *Mal ojo* (evil eye) has many manifestations in many cultures around the world. In Hispanic cultures, *mal ojo* has a basis in the belief that social relationships contain dangers for an individual, especially for women and children. *Mal ojo* is caused by a strong person exerting a negative power over a weaker person, causing that person to become ill. Symptoms may appear abruptly, and they include fever, rashes, nervousness, and irritability.
- *Empacho* (blocked intestines) may be caused by a hot–cold food imbalance, causing a lump of food to stick to the intestinal wall. Massaging the stomach and back to dislodge the food lump is often the treatment for *empacho* in children.
- *Caida de la mollera* (fallen fontanelle) is thought to result from mishandling an infant. For instance, removing an infant too harshly from the nipple may cause this syndrome. Symptoms range from irritability to failure to thrive. Treatment is holding the infant upside down by the legs.

Selected Culture-Bound Syndromes in African American–Caribbean Groups

Two culture-bound syndromes identified with some African American and Caribbean cultural groups are "falling out" and voodoo illness (Campinha-Bacote, 1998a, p. 65; 1998b, p. 21).

- *Falling out* involves sudden collapse and paralysis, inability to see or speak, but, at the same time, the person's hearing and understanding remain intact. This condition is a cultural response to hearing of the death of a family member and is not a medical condition requiring emergency treatment.
- *Voodoo illness* (often called rootwork, hex, fix, witchcraft, spell, black magic, or a trick) is based on the belief that illness or death may be caused by an individual by means of a supernatural force. Symptoms include both gastrointestinal and behavioral disorders, such as nausea, vomiting, diarrhea, complaints that food doesn't taste right, convulsions, muscle weakness, paralysis, or complaints that animals are living in the person's body.

Because culture-bound syndromes often are similar to psychological illnesses, the health care provider needs to be especially careful to avoid a misdiagnosis. Clarifying the client's belief about symptoms and causes can help to identify some culture-bound illnesses.

CULTURAL COMPETENCE OF THE CAREGIVER

The primary reason for including culture and biologic variation in a text about health assessment is to recognize the importance of the cultural competence needed by the caregiver who is assessing a client. As noted above, culture is part of the context in which assessment findings must be evaluated. The level of competence of the caregiver affects the level of accuracy of the assessment findings. But how does a caregiver determine cultural competence? Perhaps an answer to that question is provided by Campinha-Bacote (1998b), who presents a brief historical review of cultural assessment tools and an overview of her culturally competent model of care. She describes the process of cultural competence in the delivery of health care services (Fig. 3-1) as dynamic and reflective of the complexity of the cyclic process of becoming culturally competent. There are five constructs in the process: cultural awareness, cultural knowledge, cultural skill, cultural encounter, and cultural desire (1998b, p. 9).

Cultural Awareness

Cultural awareness is the "deliberate, cognitive process in which the healthcare provider becomes appreciative and sensitive to the values, beliefs, life ways, practices and problem-solving strategies of a client's culture" (Campinha-Bacote, 1998b, p. 10). Health care providers are challenged to examine their own prejudices and biases toward other cultures

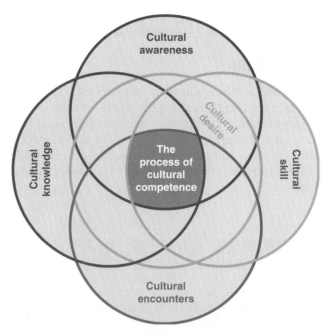

FIGURE 3-1. The process of cultural competence in the delivery of health care services. (With permission from Campinha-Bacote, J. [1998b]. *The process of cultural competence in the delivery of health care services: A culturally competent model of care* [3rd ed.]. Cincinnati, OH: Transcultural C.A.R.E Associates.)

and explore their own cultural background. The stages of cultural awareness are:

- *Unconscious incompetence* (not aware that one lacks cultural knowledge; not aware that cultural differences exist)
- *Conscious incompetence* (aware that one lacks knowledge about another culture; aware that cultural differences exist, but not knowing what they are or how to communicate effectively with clients from different cultures)
- *Conscious competence* (consciously learning about the client's culture and providing culturally relevant interventions; aware of differences; able to have effective transcultural interactions)
- *Unconscious competence* (able to automatically provide culturally congruent care to clients from a different culture; having much experience with a variety of cultural groups and having an intuitive grasp of how to communicate effectively in transcultural encounters)

Cultural Knowledge

Cultural knowledge is "the process of seeking and obtaining a sound educational foundation concerning the various world views of different cultures" (Campinha-Bacote, 1998b, p. 17). The client's world view is the basis for his or her behaviors and interpretations of the world. For instance, the client's world view will help clarify his or her belief about what causes illness, what symptoms are defined as illness, and what are considered appropriate interactions within cultural groups. These characteristics based on world view, along with biologic (physical and pharmacologic) variations, make up the content of cultural knowledge useful for the nurse assessing a client from a different culture.

Cultural Skill

Cultural skill is "the ability to collect relevant cultural data regarding the client's health history and presenting problem as well as accurately performing a physical assessment" (Campinha-Bacote, 1998b, p. 26). Cultural skill involves learning how to complete cultural assessments and culturally based physical assessments and to interpret the data accurately.

Cultural Encounter

A cultural encounter is "the process that allows the health-care provider to engage directly in cross-cultural interactions . . ." (Campinha-Bacote, 1998b, p. 39). This process requires going beyond the study of a culture and limited interaction with three or four members of the culture. Repeated face-to-face encounters help to refine or modify the nurse's knowledge of the culture. The nurse must seek out many such encounters with the desire to understand more and more about the culture. For more information, see Display 3-3.

DISPLAY 3-3. Do's and Don'ts for Cultural Encounters

DO'S

- Develop a cultural habit—the desire to effectively build relationships with people from different cultural backgrounds.
- Recognize that intra-ethnic variation exists among all cultural and ethnic groups. Specifically recognize that there are more differences within ethnic groups than across ethnic groups. This will help prevent stereotyping and labeling.
- Remember that cultural competence is a journey, not a destination; a process, not an event; and a state of becoming, not of being.
- Become sensitive to nonverbal cues and communication. Be aware that some nonverbal communication may be insulting to specific cultures.
- Remember that ethnicity is only one aspect of cultural diversity. Many factors other than ethnicity constitute a cultural group. Geographic location, gender, age, socioeconomic status, religious affiliation, and occupation are a few of the variables that constitute a distinct cultural group.
- Keep in mind that, when conflict exists between two people, each should examine whether the source of conflict is self-generated.
- Engage in many direct cultural encounters; seek out evaluative feedback on cross-cultural interactions. Be receptive to constructive criticism, and avoid becoming defensive.
- Appreciate differences, but build on similarities. When people recognize and value differences, they will realize that they are more alike than different.
- Remember that communication is inevitable. One cannot not communicate. Culturally sensitive communication, however, requires not only many cultural encounters but also cultural knowledge, cultural skill, and an awareness of the role one's own cultural values play in communicating.

DON'TS

- Do not assume that because someone looks and behaves much the same as you do that there are no cultural differences or barriers to communication.
- Avoid relying solely on textbooks and other written materials for information on cultural groups. Direct cross-cultural interactions will help a person gain accurate information about a cultural group.
- Never assume that you understand any nonverbal communication unless you are familiar with a particular culture.
- Do not personalize all negative communication. Some cultures may respond to you based on "what you represent" and not necessarily on who you truly are. Make a genuine good first impression of who you truly are.
- Avoid judging others based on your personal cultural values and rules. People live by different rules and priorities that are valid according to their cultural beliefs.
- Do not be content with just respecting and understanding another culture's view of the world. Challenge yourself to enter into cultural synergy, which involves a serious commitment to internalize and incorporate selected values, practices, beliefs, lifestyles, and problem-solving skills of another culture into one's own world view. Remember, "the whole is greater than the sum of its parts."

(Adapted from Campinha-Bacote, J. [1998b]. *The process of cultural competence in the delivery of health care services: A culturally competent model of care* [3rd ed.] Cincinnati, OH: Transcultural C.A.R.E. Associates.)

Cultural Desire

The motivation to want to engage in intercultural encounters and to acquire cultural competence is known as cultural desire. In summary, to be a culturally competent health care provider, the nurse must sincerely desire to acquire the cultural knowledge and skill necessary for effectively assessing the client. The nurse must also seek repeated encounters with people of the culture so knowledge and skill continually increase.

CULTURAL VARIATION IN HEALTH ASSESSMENT

To be successful in completing a health assessment, the nurse must develop skill in the many areas of cultural competence. The variations in communication style and content, the different beliefs and behaviors that result from different world views, the effects of environment and genetics all affect behavioral, physical, and pharmacologic variation. Recognizing the possible influence of culture on assessment skill and findings is essential for the nurse as-

sessing any client, not just the client who comes from a culture obviously different from the nurse's own. Culture is one of the contexts to be considered when interacting with a client.

What Is Family?

Look at Figure 3-2. Which image represents a family? Once you have selected an image that meets your criteria for family, think about what criteria you use for determining family. For family health assessment purposes, the most effective way to work with clients is to accept the client's definition of family rather than the nurse's. So, the family is whatever the client says it is. Nurses may hold different beliefs about what makes a family, but the therapeutic approach holds that the nurse focus on assessing rather than valuing. Rather than valuing whether the grouping makes up a "good kind" of family, the nurse focuses on determining whether the family functions

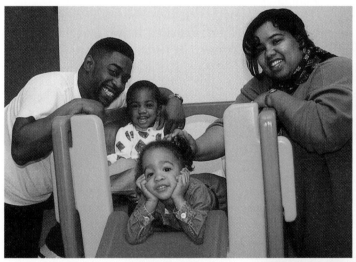
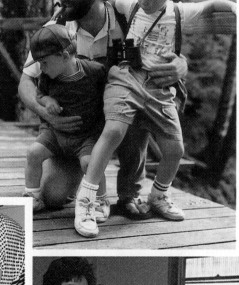
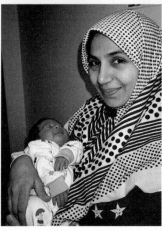
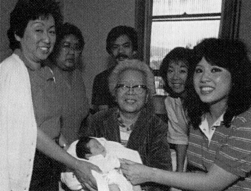

FIGURE 3-2. Families.

supportively to promote the client's and other members' well-being.

Look again at the pictures. Which of these are supportive families?

Can you tell just by looking at the family members? Of course not. Perhaps the traditional family of mother, father, and two children has a child abuser or spouse abuser, an alcoholic member, or other aberration. Many other possibilities can be imagined, but the only way to get a real idea of how a family functions is to assess.

An individual client cannot be completely separated from the family, nor can the family be considered with any member omitted. The family works as a system of interactions. The client's beliefs about human interaction, about roles, and about illness and its effect on lives are all interrelated with family beliefs. The culture in which the family operates and the specific culture developed within the family unit interact to form a context for the client. Moreover, for the nurse to meaningfully interpret the collected data, elements of the culture and the family's beliefs are so much a part of the client that he or she cannot be considered apart from them.

THE FAMILY'S ROLE IN ILLNESS

Think about the family's role in illness in the following examples:

- Mr. Thomas drinks excessively. He also smokes and eats whatever he wants (high-fat, calorie-rich diet). His risks for cardiovascular disease are very high. Why does he not maintain a preventive lifestyle? His family believes that men are strong and that it is a sign of weakness to practice preventive care.
- Mr. and Mrs. Phillips are exhausted after several years of caring for their disabled son, John. When the suggestion is made that they take a vacation, they refuse even to consider it. Such a break would be considered selfish and uncaring and not responsible behavior for good parents.
- Susie Hanes is making no progress getting over a bout of hepatitis. She has had several illnesses in her young life but does not seem to be regaining her strength after this one. Her parents tell you that is to be expected because youngest daughters are always sickly in their family.
- There is apparently much anger and unsupportive behavior in the Evans family. The children are spiteful to their brother, Jim, and talk back to their parents. After family assessment, it becomes clear that the parents believe that, if they do not focus family energy on Jim, who has diabetes, his condition might get worse or he may die. The other children can take care of themselves. Jim is very dependent in his diabetic regimen. The siblings are rebellious. The parents are anxious and perplexed.

FAMILY ASSESSMENT

Because of the need to understand client as integrated with family, a chapter dedicated to assessment of the family (Chapter 27) is included in this textbook. The chapter considers family as context and family as client, although intervening with a family system as the client is a higher-level psychiatric–mental health nursing function. However, maintaining the perspective of family as client and understanding the dynamics that must be considered can help the nurse to perceive the family as a system and as context. Concepts of family structure, development, and function are presented. Assessment strategies and tools are described.

What Is Community?

Which of the images in Figure 3-3 show normal communities and which show abnormal patterns within a community? Which images did you determine to be communities? Which did you determine to indicate normal patterns for a community? Which suggest abnormal patterns?

Community can be defined in several ways. For purposes of this text, *community* is defined in two ways: geopolitical communities determined by natural boundaries, and communities organized based on the relationship among a group of people. So, all of the examples represent communities. But those that do not provide a healthful environment are noted to have an abnormal pattern.

THE EFFECT OF COMMUNITY ON HEALTH AND ILLNESS

The community is a system, and the cultures and family patterns represented in the community form a larger system, no part of which can be separated from the whole. The community affects the families, and the families affect the community, just as family cultures and larger cultural groups affect each other and the community as a whole. To assess a client, be it a single person, family, or community, the nurse must maintain a perspective of the system. The nurse will need to assess how the community is affecting the client, the health and illness of the client, and the community itself.

Consider the following examples:

- The primary economic base of the community is an industry that puts residue into the local waterways. If the economic base is lost, the community will lose income and, therefore, the means for citizens to support themselves without moving to another community. If the pollution is to be stopped, the industry might have to go out of business. The residents are under great emotional stress, from the new regulations, and under physical stress, from the water pollution. Illness rates are increasing in the community.

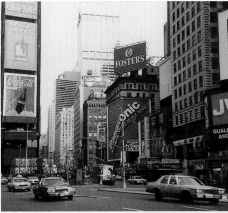
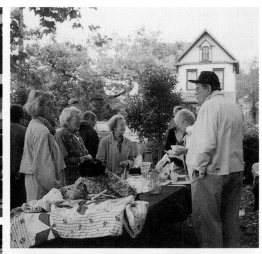
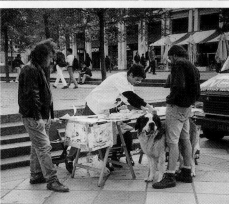
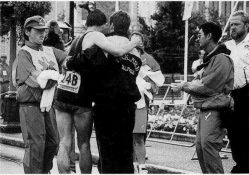
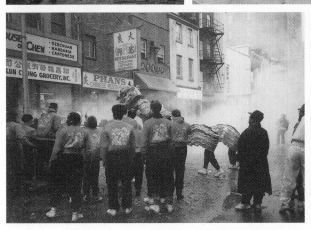
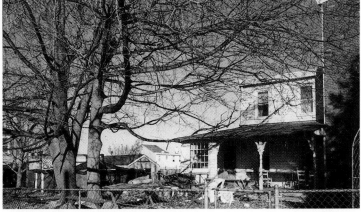

FIGURE 3-3. Communities. (Middle right by Paul Johnson, courtesy of Sandy Gelmour.)

- A group of like-minded citizens have banded together to form a small community to combat drug use in a medium-sized town. The group has a great sense of mission and is beginning to see a decline in drug use among teens. The group has also noted an improvement in the group members' health during their cooperative efforts.
- Men from a village have to leave home and live in another state for long periods of time to make a living to support their families. Many of these men set up households in the new location, ultimately leaving their families and no longer providing support.

COMMUNITY ASSESSMENT

The examples provide evidence that the emotional and physical health of individuals and families are affected by the communities in which they live. It is important for the nurse to assess the effect of community on the client to complete an effective assessment. This textbook includes a chapter on assessment of the community (Chapter 28) to assist the nurse to maintain this systems perspective. As noted before, this assessment text cannot provide the entire content of a community nursing course; it only provides the highlights.

REFERENCES AND SELECTED READINGS

Agar, M. (1994). The intercultural frame. *International Journal of Intercultural Relations, 18* (2), 221–237.

Campinha-Bacote, J. (1998a). African-Americans. In L. Purnell & B. J. Paulanka (Eds.), *Transcultural health care: A culturally competent approach* (pp. 53–73). Philadelphia: F. A. Davis.

———. (1998b). *The process of cultural competence in the delivery of healthcare services [monograph].* Cincinnati: Transcultural C.A.R.E. Associates.

Lipson, J. (1996). Diversity issues. In J. Lipson, S. Dibble & P. Minarik (Eds.), *Culture and nursing care: A pocket guide* (pp. 7–10). San Francisco: UCSF Nursing Press.

Overfield, T. (1995). *Biological variation in health and illness: Race, age, and sex differences* (2nd ed.). Boca Raton, FL: CRC Press.

Purnell, L. D. (1998). Mexican-Americans. In L. Purnell & B. J. Paulanka (Eds.), *Transcultural health care: A culturally competent approach* (pp. 397–421). Philadelphia: F. A. Davis.

Purnell, L. D., & Paulanka, B. J. (Eds.). (1998). *Transcultural health care: A culturally competent approach.* Philadelphia: F.A. Davis.

For additional information on this book, be sure to visit http://connection.lww.com.

Collecting Subjective Data

4

COLDSPA

Character
Onset
Location
Duration
Severity
Pattern
Associated Factors

Collecting subjective data is an integral part of nursing health assessment. Subjective data consist of sensations or symptoms, feelings, perceptions, desires, preferences, beliefs, ideas, values, and personal information. These types of data can be elicited and verified only by the client. Subjective data provide clues to possible physiologic, psychological, and sociologic problems. They also provide the nurse with information that may reveal a client's risk for a problem, as well as areas of strengths for the client.

When a client is having a complete, head-to-toe physical assessment, collection of subjective data usually requires that the nurse take a complete health history. The complete health history is modified or shortened when necessary. For example, if the physical assessment will focus on the heart and neck vessels, the subjective data collection would be limited to the data relevant to the heart and neck vessels. Regardless of whether a complete or modified nursing history is performed, the information is obtained through interviewing. Therefore, effective interviewing skills are vital to accurate and thorough collection of subjective data.

Interviewing

Key to obtaining a valid nursing health history are professional, interpersonal, and interviewing skills. The nursing interview is a communication process that has two focuses: (1) establishing rapport and a trusting relationship with the client to elicit accurate and meaningful information, and (2) gathering information on the client's developmental, psychological, physiologic, sociocultural, and spiritual status to identify deviations that can be treated with nursing and collaborative interventions, or strengths that can be enhanced through nurse–client collaboration.

PHASES OF THE INTERVIEW

The nursing interview has three basic phases: introductory, working, and summary and closure phases. These phases are briefly explained by describing the roles of the nurse and the client during each one.

Introductory Phase

After introducing himself or herself to the client, the nurse explains the purpose of the interview, discusses the types of questions that will be asked, explains the reason for taking notes, and assures the client that confidential information will remain confidential. The nurse also makes sure that the client is comfortable (physically and emotionally) and has privacy. It is also essential for the nurse to develop trust and rapport at this point in the interview. Developing rapport depends heavily on verbal and nonverbal communication on the part of the nurse. These types of communication are discussed later in the chapter.

Working Phase

The nurse elicits the client's comments about major biographic data, reasons for seeking care, history of present health concern, past health history, family health history, review of body systems for current health problems, lifestyle and health practices, and developmental level. The nurse then listens and observes cues in addition to using critical thinking skills to interpret and validate information received from the client. The nurse and client collaborate to identify the client's problems and goals. The facilitating approach may be free-flowing or more structured with specific questions, depending on the time available and the type of data needed.

Summary and Closure Phase

The nurse summarizes information obtained during the working phase and validates problems and goals with the client (see Chapter 6). Possible plans to resolve the problem (nursing diagnoses and collaborative problems) are identified and discussed with the client (see Chapter 7). Finally, the nurse makes sure to ask whether anything else concerns the client and whether there are any further questions.

COMMUNICATION DURING THE INTERVIEW

Two types of communication are used during the client interview—nonverbal and verbal. Several special techniques and certain general considerations will improve both types of communication and promote an effective and productive interview.

Nonverbal Communication to Use

Nonverbal communication is as important as verbal communication. Your appearance, demeanor, posture, facial expressions, and attitude strongly influence how the client perceives the questions you ask. Never overlook this type of communication or take it for granted.

APPEARANCE

First, take care to ensure that your appearance is professional. The client is expecting to see a health professional; therefore, you should look the part. Wear comfortable, neat clothes and a laboratory coat or a uniform. Be sure your name tag, including credentials, is clearly visible. Your hair should be neat and not in any extreme style; some nurses like to wear long hair pulled back. Fingernails should be short and neat; jewelry should be minimal.

DEMEANOR

Your demeanor should also be professional. When you enter a room to interview a client, aim for composure. Focus on the client and the upcoming interview and assessment. Do not enter the room laughing loudly, yelling to a coworker, or muttering under your breath. This appears unprofessional to the client and will have an effect on the entire interview process. Greet the client calmly and focus your full attention on him or her. Do not be overwhelmingly friendly or "touchy"; many clients are uncomfortable with this type of behavior. It is best to maintain a professional distance.

FACIAL EXPRESSION

Facial expressions are often an overlooked aspect of communication. Because your facial expression often shows what you are truly thinking, regardless of what you are saying, keep a close check on your facial expression. No matter what you think about a client or what kind of day you are having, keep your expression neutral and friendly. If your face shows anger or anxiety, the client will sense it and may think it is directed toward him or her. If you cannot effectively hide your emotions, you may want to explain that you are angry or upset about a personal situation. Admitting this to the client may also help in developing a trusting relationship and genuine rapport.

Portraying a neutral expression does not mean that your face lacks expression. It means using the right expression at the right time. If the client looks upset, you should appear, and be, understanding and concerned. Conversely, smiling when the client is on the verge of tears will cause the client to believe that you do not care about his or her problem.

ATTITUDE

One of the most important nonverbal skills to develop as a health care professional is a nonjudgmental attitude. All clients should be accepted, regardless of beliefs, ethnicity, lifestyle, and health care practices. Do not act superior to the client or appear shocked, disgusted, or surprised at what you are told. These attitudes will cause the client to feel uncomfortable opening up to you, and important data concerning his or her health status could be withheld.

Being nonjudgmental involves not "preaching" to the client or imposing your own sense of ethics or morality on him or her. Focus on health care and how you can best help the client achieve the highest possible level of health. For example, if you are interviewing a client who smokes, avoid lecturing condescendingly about the dangers of smoking. Also avoid telling the client he or she is foolish or portraying an attitude of disgust. This will only harm the nurse–client relationship and do nothing to improve the client's health. The client is, no doubt, already aware of the dangers of smoking. Forcing guilt on him or her is unhelpful. Accept the client, be understanding of the habit, and work together to improve the client's health. This does not mean you should not encourage the client to quit; it means that how you approach the situation makes a difference. Let the client know you understand that it is hard to quit smoking, support efforts to quit, and offer suggestions on the latest methods available to help kick the smoking habit.

SILENCE

Another nonverbal technique to use during the interview process is silence. Periods of silence allow you and the client to reflect and organize thoughts, which facilitates more accurate reporting and data collection.

Nonverbal Communication to Avoid

Several nonverbal affects or attitudes may hinder effective communication. They may promote discomfort or distrust.

EXCESSIVE OR INSUFFICIENT EYE CONTACT

Avoid extremes in eye contact. Some clients feel very uncomfortable with too much eye contact; others believe that you are hiding something from them if you do not look them in the eye. Therefore, it is best to use a moderate amount of eye contact. For example, establish eye contact when the client is speaking to you, but look down at your notes from time to time. A client's cultural background often determines how he or she feels about eye contact (see Cultural Variations in Communication for more information).

DISTRACTION AND DISTANCE

Another nonverbal communication style to avoid is being occupied with something else while you are asking questions during the interview. This behavior makes the client believe that the interview may be unimportant to you. Avoid appearing mentally distant as well. The client will sense your distance and will be less likely to answer your questions thoroughly. Also try to avoid physical distance exceeding 2 to 3 feet during the interview. Rapport and trust are established when the client senses your focus and concern are solely on the client and the client's health. Physical distance may portray a noncaring attitude or a desire to avoid close contact with the client.

STANDING

Finally, avoid standing while the client is seated during the interview. Standing puts you and the client at different levels. You may be perceived as the superior, making the client feel inferior. Care of the client's health should be an equal partnership between the health care provider and the client. If the client is made to feel inferior, he or she will not feel empowered to be an equal partner, and the potential for optimal health may be lost. In addition, vital information may not be revealed if the client believes that the interviewer is untrustworthy, judgmental, or disinterested.

Verbal Communication to Use

Effective verbal communication is essential to a client interview. The goal of the interview process is to elicit as much data about the client's health status as possible. Several types of questions and techniques to use during the interview are discussed in the following sections.

OPEN-ENDED QUESTIONS

Open-ended questions are used to elicit the client's feelings and perceptions. They typically begin with the words "how" or "what." An example of this type of question is "How have you been feeling lately?" These types of questions are important because they require more than a one-word response from the client and, therefore, encourage description. Asking open-ended questions may help to reveal significant data about the client's health status.

The following example shows how open-ended questions work. Imagine yourself interviewing an elderly male client who is at the physician's office because of diabetic complications. He mentions casually to you, "Today is the 2-month anniversary of my wife's death from cancer." Failure to follow up with an open-ended question such as "How does this make you feel?" may result in the loss of important data that could provide clues to the client's current state of health.

CLOSED-ENDED QUESTIONS

Use closed-ended questions to obtain facts and to zero in on specific information. The client can respond with one or two words. The questions typically begin with the words "when" or "did." An example of this type of question is "When did your headache start?" Closed-ended questions are useful in keeping the interview on course. They can also be used to clarify or obtain more accurate information about issues disclosed in response to open-ended questions. For example, in response to the open-ended question "How have you been feeling lately?" the client says, "Well, I've been feeling really sick at my stomach, and I don't feel like eating because of it." You may be able to follow up and learn more about the client's symptom with a closed-ended question, such as "When did the nausea start?"

LAUNDRY LIST

Another way to ask questions is to provide the client with a choice of words to choose from in describing symptoms, conditions, or feelings. This laundry list approach helps you obtain specific answers and reduces the likelihood of the client's perceiving or providing an expected answer. For example, "Is the pain severe, dull, sharp, mild, cutting, or piercing?" "Does the pain occur once every year, day, month, or hour?" Repeat choices as necessary.

REPHRASING

Rephrasing information the client has provided is an effective way to use statements during the interview. This technique helps you to clarify information the client has stated; it also enables you and the client to reflect on what was said. For example, your client, Mr. G., tells you that he has been really tired and nauseated for 2 months and that he is scared because he fears that he has some horrible disease. You might rephrase the information by saying, "You are thinking that you have a serious illness?"

WELL-PLACED PHRASES

Client verbalization can be encouraged by well-placed phrases from the nurse. If the client is in the middle of explaining a symptom or feeling and believes that you are not paying attention, you may fail to get all the necessary information. Listen closely to the client during his or her description and use phrases such as "um-hum," "yes," or "I agree" to encourage the client to continue.

INFERRING

Inferring information from what the client tells you and what you observe in the client's behavior may elicit more data or verify existing data. Be careful not to lead the client to answers that are not true (see Verbal Communication to Avoid for more information). An example of inferring information follows: Your client, Mrs. J., tells you that she has bad pain. You ask where the pain is, and she says, "My stomach." You notice the client has a hand on the right side of her lower abdomen and seems to favor her entire right side. You say, "It seems you have more difficulty with the right side of your stomach" (use the word "stomach" because that is the term the client used to describe the abdomen). This technique, if used properly, helps to elicit the most accurate data possible from the client.

PROVIDING INFORMATION

Another important thing to consider throughout the interview is to provide the client with information as questions and concerns arise. Make sure you answer every question as well as you can. If you do not know the answer, explain that you will find out for the client. The more clients know about their own health, the more likely they are to become equal participants in caring for their health.

Verbal Communication to Avoid

BIASED OR LEADING QUESTIONS

Avoid using biased or leading questions. These cause the client to provide answers that may or may not be true. The way you phrase a question may actually lead the client to think you want him or her to answer in a certain way. For example, if you ask "You don't feel bad, do you?" the client may conclude that you do not think he or she should feel bad and will answer "no" even if this is not true.

RUSHING THROUGH THE INTERVIEW

Rushing the client is something else you should avoid. If you ask the client questions on top of questions, several things may occur. First, the client may answer "no" to a series of closed-ended questions when he or she would have answered "yes" to one of the questions if it was asked individually. This may occur because the client did not hear the individual question clearly or because the answers to most were "no" and the client forgot about the "yes" answer in the midst of the others. With this type of interview technique, the client may believe that his or her individual situation is of little concern to the nurse. Taking time with clients shows that you are concerned about their health and helps them to open up. Finally, rushing someone through the interview process undoubtedly causes important information to be left out of the health history. A client will usually sense that you are rushed and may try to help hurry the interview by providing abbreviated or incomplete answers to questions.

READING THE QUESTIONS

Avoid reading questions from the history form. This deflects attention from the client and results in an impersonal interview process. As a result, the client may feel ill at ease opening up to formatted questions.

SPECIAL INTERVIEW CONSIDERATIONS

Three variations in communication must be considered as you interview clients: gerontologic, cultural, and emotional. These variations affect the nonverbal and verbal techniques you use during the interview. Imagine, for example, that you are interviewing an 82-year-old woman and you ask her to describe how she has been feeling. She does not answer you, and she looks confused. This older client may have some hearing loss. In such a case, you may need to modify the verbal technique of asking open-ended questions by following the guidelines provided under Gerontologic Variations in Communication (see Domarad & Buschmann, 1995).

Gerontologic Variations in Communication

Age affects and commonly slows all body systems to varying degrees. However, normal aspects of aging do not necessarily equate with a health problem, so it is important not to approach an interview with an elderly client assuming that there is a health problem. Older clients have the potential to be as healthy as younger clients.

The first thing to do when interviewing an elderly client is to assess hearing acuity. Hearing loss occurs normally with age, and undetected hearing loss is often misinterpreted as mental slowness or confusion. If you detect hearing loss, speak slowly, face the client at all times during the interview, and speak on the side on which hearing is more accurate. Do not yell at the client.

Older clients may have more health concerns than younger clients and may seek health care more often. Many times, older clients with health problems feel vulnerable and scared. They need to believe that they can trust you before they will open up to you about what is bothering them. That is why establishing and maintaining trust, privacy, and partnership with the older client is particularly important (Fig. 4-1). It is not unusual for elderly clients to be taken for granted and their health complaints ignored, causing them to become fearful of complaining. Equally discon-

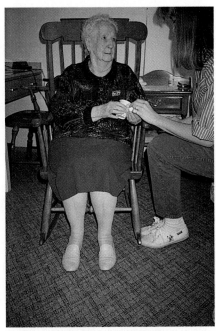

FIGURE 4-1. Establishing and maintaining trust, privacy, and partnership with older adults sets the tone for effectively collecting data and sharing concerns.

certing is that their health problems may be discussed openly among many people, including health care providers and family members. Assure your elderly clients that you are concerned, that you see them as equal partners in health care, and that what is discussed will be between you, their primary care provider, and themselves.

Speak clearly and use straightforward language during the interview with the elderly client. Ask questions in simple terms. Avoid medical jargon and modern slang. However, do not talk down to the client. Being older physically does not mean the client is slower mentally. Showing respect is very important. However, if the older client is mentally confused or forgetful, it is important to have a significant other (eg, spouse, child, close friend) present during the interview to provide or clarify the data.

Cultural Variations in Communication

Ethnic variations in communication and self-disclosure styles may significantly affect the information obtained (Andrews & Boyle, 1999; Giger & Davidhizar, 1995; Luckmann, 2000). Be aware of possible variations in the communication styles of yourself and the client. If misunderstanding or difficulty in communicating is evident, seek help from an expert, what some professionals call a "culture broker." This is someone who is thoroughly familiar not only with the client's language, culture, and related health care practices but also with the health care setting and system of the dominant culture. Frequently noted variations in communication styles include:

- Reluctance to reveal personal information to strangers for various culturally based reasons
- Variation in willingness to openly express emotional distress or pain
- Variation in ability to receive information (listen)
- Variation in meaning conveyed by language. For example, a client who does not speak the predominant language may not know what a certain medical term or phrase means and, therefore, will not know how to answer your question. Use of slang with non-native speakers is discouraged as well. Keep in mind that it is hard enough to learn proper language, let alone the idiom vernacular. The non-native speaker will likely have no idea what you are trying to convey.
- Variation in use and meaning of nonverbal communication: eye contact, stance, gestures, demeanor. For example, direct eye contact may be perceived as rude, aggressive, or immodest by some cultures, but lack of eye contact may be perceived as evasive, insecure, or inattentive by other cultures. A slightly bowed stance may indicate respect in some groups; size of personal space affects one's comfortable interpersonal distance; touch may be perceived as comforting or threatening.
- Variation in disease/illness perception: Culture-specific syndromes or disorders are accepted by some groups (eg, in Latin America, *susto* is an illness caused by a sudden shock or fright).
- Variation in past, present, or future time orientation (eg, the dominant U.S. culture is future oriented; other cultures vary)
- Variation in family decision-making process: A person other than the client or the client's parent may be the major decision maker about appointments, treatments, or follow-up care for the client.

You may have to interview a client who does not speak your language. To perform the best interview possible, it is necessary to use an interpreter. Possibly the best interpreter would be a culture expert (or culture broker). Consider the relationship of the interpreter to the client. If the interpreter is the client's child or a person of a different sex, age, or social status, interpretation may be impaired. Also, keep in mind that communication through use of pictures may be helpful when dealing with some clients.

Emotional Variations in Communication

Not every client you encounter will be calm, friendly, and eager to participate in the interview process. Clients' emotions vary for a number of reasons. They may be scared or anxious about their health or about disclosing personal information, angry that they are sick or about having to have an examination, depressed about their health or other life events, or they may have an ulterior motive for having an assessment performed. Clients may also have some sensitive issues with which they are grappling and may turn to you for help. Some helpful ways to deal with various clients with various emotions follow:

- *Anxious client:* Approach this client with simple, organized information. Explain your role and purpose.
- *Angry client:* Approach this client in a calm, reassuring, in-control manner. Allow him or her to ventilate feelings. Avoid arguing and facilitate personal space.
- *Depressed client:* Express interest and understanding in a neutral manner.
- *Manipulative client:* Provide structure and set limits.
- *Client and sensitive issues* (eg, sexuality, dying, spirituality): First, be aware of your own thoughts and feelings regarding dying, spirituality, and sexuality; then, recognize that these factors may affect the client's health and may need to be discussed with someone. If you do not feel comfortable or competent discussing personal, sensitive topics, you may make referrals as appropriate, for example, to a pastoral counselor for spiritual concerns or other specialists as needed.

Complete Health History

The health history is an excellent way to begin the assessment process because it lays the groundwork for identifying nursing problems and provides a focus for the physical examination. The importance of the health history lies in its ability to provide information that will assist the examiner in identifying areas of strength and limitation in the individual's lifestyle and current health status. Data from the health history also provide the examiner with specific cues to health problems that are most apparent to the client. Then, these areas may be more intensely examined during the physical assessment.

Taking a health history should begin with an explanation to the client of why the information is being requested, for example, "so that I will be able to plan individualized nursing care with you." This section of the chapter explains the rationale for collecting the data, discusses each portion of the health history, and provides sample questions. The health history has eight sections:

- Biographic data
- Reasons for seeking health care
- History of present health concern
- Past health history
- Family health history
- Review of body systems (ROS) for current health problems
- Lifestyle and health practices profile
- Developmental level

As discussed in Chapter 2, which focuses on nursing frameworks, the organization for collecting data in this text is a generic nursing framework that the nurse can use as is or adapt to use with any nursing assessment framework. A sample tool for subjective data collection based on this generic format is provided in Appendix A.

BIOGRAPHIC DATA

Biographic data usually include information that identifies the client, such as his or her name, address, phone number, gender, and who provided the information—the client or significant others. The client's birth date, Social Security number, medical record number, or similar identifying data may be included in the biographic data section.

When students are collecting the information and sharing it with instructors, addresses and phone numbers should be deleted and initials used to protect the client's privacy. The name of the person providing the information needs to be included, however, to assist in determining its accuracy. The client is considered the primary source, and all others (including the client's medical record) are secondary sources. In some cases, the client's immediate family or caregiver may be a more accurate source of information than the client. An example would be an elderly client's wife who has kept the client's medical records for years, or the legal guardian of a mentally compromised client. In any event, validation of the information by a secondary source may be helpful.

The client's culture, ethnicity, and subculture may begin to be determined by collecting data about date and place of birth, nationality or ethnicity, marital status, religious or spiritual practices, and primary and secondary languages spoken, written, and read. This information helps the nurse examine special needs and beliefs that may affect the client or family's health care. A person's primary language is usually the one spoken in the family during early childhood and the one in which the person thinks. However, if the client was educated in another language from kindergarten on, it may be the primary language, and the birth language would be secondary.

Gathering information about the client's educational level, occupation, and working status at this point in the health history assists the examiner to tailor questions to the client's level of understanding. In addition, this information can help to identify possible client strengths and limitations affecting health status. For example, if the client was recently downsized from a high-power, high-salary position, the effects of overwhelming stress may play a large part in his or her health status.

Finally, asking who lives with the client and identifying significant others points out the availability of potential caregivers and support people for the client. Absence of support people would alert the examiner to the (possible) need for finding external sources of support.

REASONS FOR SEEKING HEALTH CARE

Two questions are included in this category: "What is your major health problem or concerns at this time?" and "How do you feel about having to seek health care?" The first question assists the client to focus on his or her most significant health concern and answers the nurse's question, "Why are you here?" or "How can I help you?" Physicians call this the client's chief complaint (CC), but a more holistic approach for phrasing the question may draw out concerns that reach beyond just a physical complaint and may address stress or lifestyle changes.

The second question, "How do you feel about having to seek health care?", can encourage the client to discuss fears or other feelings about having to see a health care provider. For example, a woman visiting a nurse practitioner states her major health concern: "I found a lump in my breast." This woman may be able to respond to the second question by voicing fears that she has been reluctant to share with her significant others. This question may also draw out descriptions of previous experiences—both positive and negative—with other health care providers.

HISTORY OF PRESENT HEALTH CONCERN

This section of the health history takes into account several aspects of the health problem and asks questions whose answers can provide a detailed description of the concern. The nurse first encourages the client to explain the health problem or symptom in as much detail as possible by focusing on the onset, progression, and duration of the problem; signs and symptoms and related problems; and what the client perceives as causing the problem. The nurse may also ask the client to evaluate what makes the problem worse, what makes it better, which treatments have been tried, what effect the problem has had on daily life or lifestyle, what expectations are held about recovery, and what is the client's ability to provide self-care.

The following questions are examples of what the nurse would ask a client with back pain. (*Note:* Although the questions presented here are clustered together for presentation purposes, keep in mind that you should ask only one question at a time.)

- "When did you first notice the pain in your back? How long have you experienced it? Has it become worse, better, or stayed the same since it first occurred?"
- "What does the pain feel like? Where does it hurt the most? Does it radiate or go to any other part of your body? How intense is the pain? Rate the pain on a scale of 1 to 10, with 1 being barely noticeable and 10 being the worst pain you have ever experienced. Do you have any other problems that seem related to this back pain?"
- "What do you think caused this problem to start?"
- "What makes your back hurt more? What makes it feel better? Have you tried any treatments to relieve the pain, such as aspirin or acetaminophen (Tylenol) or anything else?"
- "How does the pain affect your life and daily activities?"

- "What do you think will happen with this problem? Do you expect to get well? What about your job? Do you think you will be able to continue working?"

The client's answers to the questions provide the nurse with a great deal of information about the client's problem and especially how it affects lifestyle and activities of daily living. This helps the nurse to evaluate the client's insight into the problem and the client's plans for managing it. The nurse can also begin to postulate nursing diagnoses from this initial information.

Exploring the Signs and Symptoms of the Present Health Concern

Problems or symptoms particular to body parts or systems are covered in the Nursing History section under Current Symptoms in the physical assessment chapters. Each identified symptom must be described for clear understanding of probable cause and significance.

COLDSPA

Because there are many characteristics to be explored for each symptom, a memory helper—known as a mnemonic—can help the nurse complete the assessment of the sign, symptom, or health concern. Many mnemonics have been developed for this purpose (eg, PQRST, COLDSPAR, COLDSTER, LOCSTAAM). The mnemonic used in this text is COLDSPA.

COLDSPA

CHARACTER: Describe the sign or symptom. How does it feel (sharp, dull, aching, throbbing), look (shiny, bumpy, red, swollen, bruised), sound (loud, soft, rasping), smell (foul, sweet, pungent), and so forth?
ONSET: When did it begin?
LOCATION: Where is it? Does it radiate?
DURATION: How long does it last? Does it recur?
SEVERITY: How bad is it?
PATTERN: What makes it better: What makes it worse?
ASSOCIATED FACTORS: What other symptoms occur with it?

PAST HEALTH HISTORY

At this point in the health history, the nurse asks questions related to the client's past, from the earliest beginnings to the present. These questions elicit data related to the client's strengths and weaknesses in his or her health history. The data may also point to trends of unhealthy behaviors, such as being accident prone. Information covered in this section includes questions about birth, growth, development, childhood diseases, immunizations, allergies, previous health

problems, hospitalizations, surgeries, pregnancies, births, previous accidents, injuries, pain experiences, and emotional or psychiatric problems.

- "Can you tell me how your mother described your birth? Were there any problems? As far as you know, did you progress normally as you grew to adulthood? Were there any problems that your family told you about or that you experienced?"
- "What diseases did you have as a child, such as measles or mumps? What immunizations did you get, and are you up to date now?"
- "What illnesses or allergies have you had?"
- "Have you ever been pregnant and delivered a baby?"
- "Have you ever been hospitalized or had surgery?"
- "What about accidents or injuries?"
- "Have you experienced pain in any part of your body?"
- "Have you ever been treated for emotional or mental problems?"

The information gained from these questions assists the nurse to identify risk factors to the client and to his or her significant others. The risk factors are those stemming from previous health problems.

How clients frame their previous health concerns suggests how they feel about themselves and is an indication of their sense of responsibility for their own health. Some clients are very forthcoming about their past health status; others are not. It is helpful to have a series of alternative questions for less responsive clients and for those who may not understand what is being asked.

FAMILY HEALTH HISTORY

As researchers discover more and more health problems that seem to run in families and are genetically based, the family health history assumes greater importance. In addition to genetic predisposition, it is also helpful to see other health problems that may have affected the client by virtue of having grown up in the family and being exposed to these problems. For example, a gene for smoking has not yet been discovered, but a family with smoking members can affect other members in at least two ways. First, the second-hand smoke can compromise the physical health of nonsmoking members; second, the smoker can be a negative role model for children, inducing them to take up the habit as well. Another example involves obesity; recognizing it in the family history can alert the nurse to a potential risk factor.

The family history should include as many genetic relatives as the client can recall. Include maternal and paternal grandparents, aunts and uncles on both sides, parents, siblings, and the client's children. Such thoroughness usually identifies those diseases that may skip a generation, such as autosomal recessive disorders. Include the client's spouse, but indicate that there is no genetic link (unless there is). Identifying the spouse's health problems could explain disorders in the client's children not indicated in the client's family history.

A genogram should be drawn to represent the client's family history. Use a standard format so others can easily understand the information. Also provide a key to the symbols used. Usually, female relatives are indicated by a circle and male relatives by a square. A deceased relative is noted by marking an X in the circle or square and listing the age at death and the cause of death. Identify all relatives, living or dead, by age and provide a brief list of diseases or conditions. If the relative has no problems, the letters "A/W" (alive and well) should be placed next to the age. Straight vertical and horizontal lines are used to show relationships. A horizontal dotted line can be used to indicate the client's spouse; a vertical dotted line can be used to indicate adoption. A sample genogram is illustrated in Figure 4-2.

After the diagrammatic family history, prepare a brief summary of the kinds of health problems present in the family. For example, the client in the genogram represented by Figure 4-2 has longevity, obesity, heart disease, hypertension (HTN), arthritis, thyroid disorders, non–insulin-dependent diabetes mellitus (NIDDM, also known

as type 2 diabetes), alcoholism, smoking, myopia, learning disability, hyperactivity disorder, and cancer (one relative) on his maternal side. On the client's paternal side are obesity, heart disease, hypercholesterolemia, back problems, arthritis, myopia, and cancer. The paternal history is not as extensive as the maternal history because the client's father was adopted. In addition, the client's sister is obese and has Graves' disease and hypercholesterolemia. His wife has arthritis; his children are both A/W.

REVIEW OF BODY SYSTEMS (ROS) FOR CURRENT HEALTH PROBLEMS

In this part of the health history, each body system is addressed and the client is asked specific questions to draw out current health problems or problems from the recent past that may still affect the client or that are recurring. Care must be taken in this section to include only the client's subjective information, and not the examiner's observations. There is a tendency, especially with more expe-

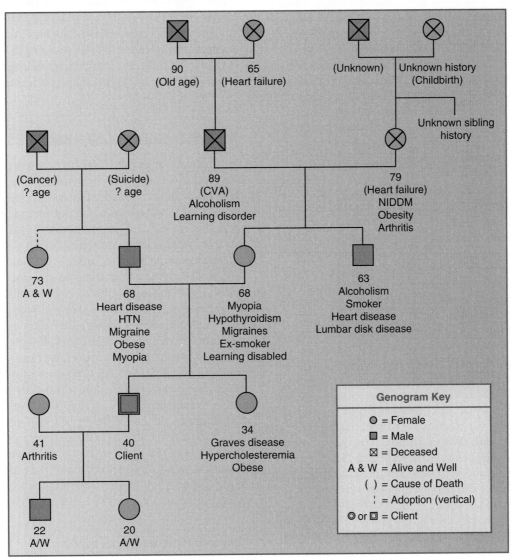

FIGURE 4-2. Genogram of a 40-year-old male client.

rienced nurses, to fill up the spaces with observations, such as "lungs clear" or "skin warm and dry."

What should be documented in the review of body systems are the client's descriptions of his or her health status for each body system and a notation of the client's denial of signs, symptoms, diseases, or problems that the nurse asks about but are not experienced by the client. For example, under the area "Head and Neck," the client may respond that there are no problems, but, on questioning from the nurse about headaches, stiffness, pain, or cracking in the neck with motion, swelling in the neck, difficulty swallowing, sore throat, enlarged lymph nodes, and so on, the client may suddenly remember that he did have a sore throat a week ago that he self-treated with zinc lozenges. This information might not have emerged without specific questions. Also, if the lone entry "no problems" is entered on the health history form, other health care professionals reviewing the history cannot even ascertain what specific questions had been asked, if any.

The questions about problems and signs or symptoms of disorders should be asked in terms that the client understands, but findings may be recorded in standard medical terminology. If the client appears to have a limited vocabulary, the nurse may need to ask questions in several different ways and use very basic lay terminology. If the client is well educated and seems familiar with medical terminology, the nurse should not insult him or her by talking at a much lower level. The most obvious information to collect for each body part or system is listed below. See the physical assessment chapters for in-depth questions and rationales for each particular body part or system.

- *Skin, hair, and nails:* Skin color, temperature, condition, excessive sweating, rashes, lesions, balding, dandruff, condition of nails
- *Head and neck:* Headache, swelling, stiffness of neck, difficulty swallowing, sore throat, enlarged lymph nodes
- *Eyes:* Vision, eye infections, redness, excessive tearing, halos around lights, blurring, loss of side vision, moving black spots/specks in visual fields, flashing lights, double vision, and eye pain
- *Ears:* Hearing, ringing or buzzing, earaches, drainage from ears, dizziness, exposure to loud noises
- *Mouth, throat, nose, and sinuses:* Condition of teeth and gums; sore throats; mouth lesions; hoarseness; rhinorrhea; nasal obstruction; frequent colds; sneezing or itching of eyes, ears, nose, or throat; nose bleeds; snoring
- *Thorax and lungs:* Difficulty breathing, wheezing, pain, shortness of breath during routine activity, orthopnea, cough or sputum, hemoptysis, respiratory infections
- *Breasts and regional lymphatics:* Lumps or discharge from nipples, dimpling or changes in breast size, swollen or tender lymph nodes in axilla
- *Heart and neck vessels:* Last blood pressure, ECG tracing or findings, chest pain or pressure, palpitations, edema
- *Peripheral vascular:* Swelling, or edema, of legs and feet; pain; cramping; sores on legs; color or texture changes on the legs or feet

- *Abdomen:* Indigestion, difficulty swallowing, nausea, vomiting, abdominal pain, gas, jaundice, hernias
- *Male genitalia:* Excessive or painful urination, frequency or difficulty starting and maintaining urinary stream, leaking of urine, blood noted in urine, sexual problems, perineal lesions, penile drainage, pain or swelling in scrotum, difficulty achieving an erection and/or difficulty ejaculating, exposure to sexually transmitted infections
- *Female genitalia:* Sexual problems; sexually transmitted diseases; voiding problems (eg, dribbling, incontinence); reproductive data, such as age at menarche, menstruation (length and regularity of cycle), pregnancies, and type of or problems with delivery, abortions, pelvic pain, birth control, menopause (date or year of last menstrual period), and use of hormone replacement therapy
- *Anus, rectum, and prostate:* Bowel habits, pain with defecation, hemorrhoids, blood in stool, constipation, diarrhea
- *Musculoskeletal:* Swelling, redness, pain, stiffness of joints, ability to perform activities of daily living, muscle strength
- *Neurologic:* General mood, behavior, depression, anger, concussions, headaches, loss of strength or sensation, coordination, difficulty speaking, memory problems, strange thoughts and/or actions, difficulty learning

LIFESTYLE AND HEALTH PRACTICES PROFILE

This is a very important section of the health history because it deals with the client's human responses, which include nutritional habits, activity and exercise patterns, sleep and rest patterns, use of medications and substances, self-concept and self-care activities, social and community activities, relationships, values and beliefs system, education and work, stress level and coping style, and environment.

Here, clients give the nurse an account of how they are managing their lives, their awareness of healthy versus toxic living patterns, and the strengths and supports they have or use. When assessing this area, use open-ended questions to promote a dialogue with the client. Follow up with specific questions to guide the discussion and clarify the information as necessary. Be sure to pay special attention to the cues the client may provide that point to possibly more significant content. Take brief notes so that pertinent data are not lost and so there can be follow-up if some information needs clarification or expansion. If clients give permission and it does not seem to cause anxiety or inhibition, using an audiocassette recorder frees the nurse from the need to write while clients talk. In this section, each area is discussed briefly and then followed by a few sample questions.

Description of Typical Day

This information is necessary to elicit an overview of how the client sees his or her usual pattern of daily activity. The questions you ask should be vague enough to allow the client to provide the orientation from which the day is viewed, for example, "Please tell me what an average or typical day is for you. Start with awakening in the morning and continue until bedtime." Encourage the client to discuss a usual day, which, for most people, includes work or school. If the client gives minimal information, additional specific questions may be asked to draw out more details.

Nutrition and Weight Management

Ask the client to recall what consists of an average 24-hour intake for him or her with emphasis on what foods are eaten and in what amounts. Also ask about snacks, fluid intake, and other substances consumed. Depending on the client, you may want to ask who buys and prepares the food and when and where meals are eaten. Food habits that are health promoting, as well as those that are less desirable, are uncovered in this area. The client's answers about food intake should be compared with the guidelines illustrated in the "food pyramid" (Fig. 4-3). The food pyramid, developed by the U.S. Department of Agriculture, is designed to teach people what types and amounts of food to eat to ensure a balanced diet, to promote health, and to prevent disease. Consider reviewing the food pyramid with the client and explaining what a serving size is. The client's fluid intake should be compared with the general recommendation of six to eight glasses of water or noncaffeinated fluids daily. It is also important to ask about the client's bowel and bladder habits at this time (included in review of symptoms). Examples follow:

"What do you usually eat during a typical day? Please tell me the kinds of foods you prefer, how often you eat throughout the day, and how much you eat."

"Do you eat out at restaurants frequently?"

"Do you eat only when hungry? Do you eat because of boredom, habit, anxiety, depression?"

"Who buys and prepares the food you eat?"

"Where do you eat your meals?"

"How much and what types of fluids do you drink?"

Activity Level and Exercise

Next, the nurse needs to assess how active the client is during an average week, either at work or at home. Inquire about regular exercise. Some clients believe that if they do heavy physical work at their job, they do not need additional exercise. Make it a point to distinguish between activity done when working, which may be stressful and fatiguing, and exercise, which is designed to reduce stress and strengthen the individual. Compare the client's answers with the recommended exercise regimen of regular aerobic exercise for 20 to 30 minutes at least three times a week. Explain to the client that regular exercise reduces the

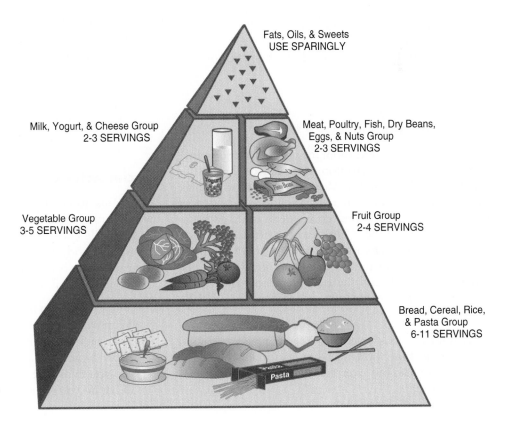

FIGURE 4-3. The Food Guide Pyramid. (U.S. Department of Agriculture.)

risk of heart disease, strengthens heart and lungs, reduces stress, and manages weight.

"What is your daily pattern of activity?"

"Do you follow a regular exercise plan? What types of exercise do you do?"

"Are there any reasons why you cannot follow a moderately strenuous exercise program?"

"What do you do for leisure and recreation?"

"Do your leisure and recreational activities include exercise?"

Sleep and Rest

The nurse should inquire whether the client feels he or she is getting enough sleep and rest. Questions should focus on specific sleep patterns, such as how many hours a night the person sleeps, interruptions, whether the client feels rested, problems sleeping (eg, insomnia), rituals the client uses to promote sleep, and concerns the client may have regarding sleep habits. Some of this information may have already been presented by the client, but it is useful to gather data in a more systematic and thorough manner at this time. Inquiries about sleep can bring out problems, such as anxiety, which manifests as sleeplessness, or inadequate sleep time, which can predispose the client to accidents. Compare the client's answers with the normal sleep requirement for adults, which is usually between 5 and 8 hours a night. However, sleep requirements vary depending on age, health, and stress levels.

"Tell me about your sleeping patterns."

"Do you have trouble falling asleep or staying asleep?"

"How much sleep do you get each night?"

"Do you feel rested when you awaken?"

"Do you nap during the day? How often and for how long?"

"What do you do to help you fall asleep?"

Medication and Substance Use

The information gathered about medication and substance use provides the nurse with information concerning lifestyle and a client's self-care ability. Medication and substance use can affect the client's health and cause loss of function or impaired senses. In addition, certain medications and substances can increase the client's risk for disease. Because many people use vitamins or a variety of herbal supplements, it is important to ask which and how often. Prescription medications and these supplements may interact (eg, garlic decreases coagulation and interacts with warfarin [Coumadin]).

"What medications have you used in the recent past and currently, both those that your doctor prescribed and those you can buy over the counter at a drug or grocery store?"

"How much beer, wine, or other alcohol do you drink on the average?"

"Do you drink coffee or other beverages containing caffeine (eg, cola)?"

"Do you now or have you ever smoked cigarettes or used any other form of nicotine, or used drugs not prescribed by your physician?"

"Have you ever used, or do you now use, recreational drugs?"

"Do you take vitamins or herbal supplements?"

Self-Concept and Self-Care Responsibilities

This should include assessment of how the client views himself or herself and investigation of all behaviors that a person does to promote his or her health. Examples of subjects to be addressed include sexual responsibility; basic hygiene practices; regularity of health care checkups (ie, dental, visual, medical); breast/testicular self-examination; and accident prevention and hazard protection (eg, seat belts, smoke alarms, and sunscreen).

You can correlate answers to questions in this area with health-promotion activities discussed previously and with risk factors from the family history. This will help to point out client strengths and needs for health maintenance. Questions to the client can be open-ended, but the client may need prompting to cover all areas.

"What do you see as your talents or special abilities?"

"How do you feel about yourself? About your appearance?"

"Can you tell me what activities you do to keep yourself safe, healthy, or to prevent disease?"

"Do you practice safe sex?"

"How do you keep your home safe?"

"Do you drive safely?"

"How often do you have medical checkups or screenings?"

"How often do you see the dentist or have your eyes (vision) examined?"

Social Activities

Questions about social activities help the nurse discover which outlets the client has for support and relaxation, and whether the client is involved in the community beyond family and work. Information in this area also helps determine the client's current level of social development and his or her progression to it.

"What do you do for fun and relaxation?"

"With whom do you socialize most frequently?"

"Are you involved in any community activities?"

"How do you feel about your community?"

"Do you think that you have enough time to socialize?"

"What do you see as your contribution to society?"

Relationships

Ask clients to describe the composition of the family into which they were born and about past and current relationships with these family members. In this way, you can assess problems and potential support from the client's family of origin. In addition, similar information should be sought about the client's current family (Fig. 4-4). If the client does not have any family by blood or marriage, then information should be gathered about any significant others (including pets) that may constitute the client's "family."

> "Who is (are) the most important person(s) in your life?"
> "What was it like growing up in your family?"
> "What is your relationship like with your spouse?"
> "What is your relationship like with your children?"
> "Describe any relationships you have with significant others."
> "Do you get along with your in-laws?"
> "Are you close to your extended family?"
> "Do you have any pets?"
> "What is your role in your family? Is it an important role?"
> "Are you satisfied with your current sexual relationships? Have there been any recent changes?"

Values and Belief System

Client values should be assessed. In addition, the clients' philosophical, religious, and spiritual beliefs should be discussed. Some clients may not be comfortable discussing values or beliefs. Their feelings should be respected. However, data can help to identify important problems or strengths.

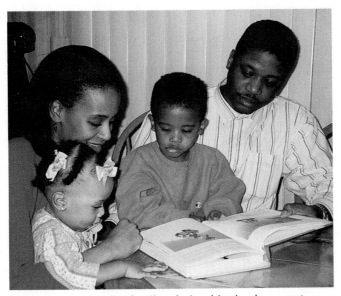

FIGURE 4-4. Discussing family relationships is a key way to assess support systems.

> "What is most important to you in life?"
> "What do you hope to accomplish in your life?"
> "Do you have a religious affiliation? Is this important to you?"
> "Is a relationship with God (or another higher power) an important part of your life?"
> "What gives you strength and hope?"

Education and Work

Questions about education and work help to identify areas of stress and satisfaction in the client's life. If the client does not perceive that he has enough education or his work is not what he enjoys, he may need assistance or support to make changes. Sometimes, providing information in this area will help the client feel good about what he has accomplished and promote his sense of life satisfaction. Questions should bring out data about the kind and amount of education the client has, whether the client enjoyed school, whether it is perceived as satisfactory or whether there were problems, and what plans the client may have for further education, either formal or informal. Similar questions should be asked about work history.

> "Tell me about your experiences in school or what it is like getting an education."
> "Are you satisfied with the level of education you have? Do you have future educational plans?"
> "What can you tell me about your work? What are your responsibilities at work?"
> "Do you enjoy your work?"
> "How do you feel about your coworkers?"
> "What kind of stress do you have that is work related? Any major problems?"
> "Who is the main financial supporter in your family?"
> "Does your current income meet your needs?"

Stress Levels and Coping Styles

To investigate what clients see as the amount of stress they are under and how they cope with it, ask questions that address what events cause stress for the client and how they usually respond. In addition, find out what the client does to relieve stress and whether these behaviors or activities can be construed as adaptive or maladaptive. To avoid denial responses, nondirective questions or observations regarding previous information provided by the client may be an easy way to get the client to discuss this subject.

> "What types of things make you angry?"
> "How would you describe your stress level?"
> "How do you manage anger or stress?"
> "What do you see as the greatest stressors in your life?"
> "Where do you usually turn for help in a time of crisis?"

Environment

Questions regarding the client's environment are asked to assess health hazards unique to the client's living situation and lifestyle. Look for physical, chemical, or psychological situations that may put the client at risk. These may be found in the client's neighborhood, home, work, or recreational environment. They may be controllable or uncontrollable.

> "What risks are you aware of in your environment, such as in your home, neighborhood, on the job, or any other activities in which you participate?"
>
> "What types of precautions do you take, if any, when playing contact sports, using harsh chemicals or paint, or operating machinery?"
>
> "Do you believe you are ever in danger of becoming a victim of violence? Explain."

DEVELOPMENTAL LEVEL

Determining the client's developmental level is essential to complete the client's portrait. You do not need to ask the client additional questions unless major gaps in the data collection were found or clarification is needed. Instead, group and analyze the data obtained during the health history and compare them with normal developmental parameters (eg, height, weight, Erikson's psychosocial developmental stages; see Schuster & Asburn, 1992). This requires integrating all that has been learned about the client by the health history and using critical thinking to position the client on a developmental continuum. This will help you as a nurse to determine any developmental impairments. Standard growth charts can be used to determine physical development. However, when assessing adults, the area most likely to yield delays or unresolved problems occurs in the psychosocial domain of development. The theorist Erik Erikson developed a psychosocial theory that identifies a number of dichotomous concepts to describe growth from birth to death (Table 4-1). Although there are implied age ranges attached to these stages and it is hoped that a person might move through them in an or-

derly fashion, this does not always occur. Thus, it is important to look at the client's behavior rather than age to identify the stage of development currently in progress.

Strong indicators that the client is functioning much below the usual behavior for his or her age range point to areas for possible nursing diagnoses (developmental delay) and nursing intervention. Sometimes, a person skips one or more developmental levels and, at a later stage of maturity, goes back and successfully works through the missed levels. A thorough knowledge of the behaviors and approximate age levels provides the nurse with a powerful tool for assessing and helping a client grow to his or her full potential. Although accomplishment of all of the tasks in the stage before moving on is ideal, it is believed that partial resolution is adequate for health, growth, and development.

The psychosocial developmental stages of the young adult, middle-aged adult, and older adult are discussed in detail in the following sections. Each section is followed by important questions to ask yourself about the client to determine if he or she has accomplished all of the required tasks in a particular psychosocial developmental stage. If the adult client does not seem even to have advanced psychologically to the intimacy versus isolation stage, refer to the earlier stages discussed in Chapter 24.

Young Adult: Intimacy Versus Isolation

The young adult should have achieved self-efficacy during adolescence and is now ready to open up and become intimate with others. Although this stage focuses on the desire for a special and permanent love relationship, it also includes the ability to have close, caring relationships with friends of both sexes and a variety of ages. Spiritual love also develops during this stage. Having established an identity apart from the childhood family, the young adult is now able to form adult friendships with his or her parents and siblings. However, the young adult will always be a son or daughter.

If the young adult cannot express emotion and trust enough to open up to others, social and emotional isolation may occur. Loneliness may cause the young adult to

TABLE 4-1. Erik H. Erikson's Psychosocial Developmental Levels

Developmental Level	Basic Task	Negative Counterpart	Basic Virtues
1. Infant	Basic trust	Basic mistrust	Drive and hope
2. Toddler	Autonomy	Shame and doubt	Self-control and will power
3. Preschooler	Initiative	Guilt	Direction and purpose
4. Schoolager	Industry	Inferiority	Method and competence
5. Adolescent	Identity	Role confusion	Devotion and fidelity
6. Young adult	Intimacy	Isolation	Affiliation and love
7. Middlescent	Generativity	Stagnation	Production and care
8. Older adult	Ego-integrity	Despair	Renunciation and wisdom

(Erikson, E. H. [1963]. *Childhood and society* [2nd ed]. New York: Norton.)

turn to addictive behaviors such as alcoholism, drug abuse, or sexual promiscuity. Some people try to cope with this developmental stage by becoming very spiritual or social, playing an acceptable role, but never fully sharing who they are or becoming emotionally involved with others. When adults successfully navigate this stage and they have stable and satisfying relationships with important others, they are freed to express themselves through others as they move into the next stage.

Accept self: physically, cognitively, and emotionally?

Have independence from the parental home?

Express love responsibly, emotionally, and sexually?

Have close or intimate relationships with a partner?

Have a social friendship group?

Have a philosophy of living and life?

Have a profession or a life's work that provides a means of contribution?

Solve problems of life that accompany independence from the parental home?

Middlescent: Generativity Versus Stagnation

The middle-aged adult is now able to share self with others and establish nurturing relationships. During this stage, the adult will be able to extend self and possessions to others. Although traditionalists tend to think of generativity in terms of raising one's children and guiding their lives, generativity can be realized in several ways, even without having children. Generativity implies mentoring and giving to future generations. This can be accomplished by producing ideas, products, inventions, paintings, writings, books, films, or any other creative endeavors that are then given to the world for the unrestricted use of its people.

Generativity also includes teaching others, children or adults, mentoring young workers, or providing experience and wisdom to assist a new business to survive and grow. Also implied in this stage is the ability to guide and then let go of one's creations. Without this important step, the gift is not given and the stage does not come to successful completion. Stagnation occurs when the middle-aged person has not accomplished one or more of the previous developmental tasks and is unable to give to future generations. Sometimes, severe losses may result in withdrawal and stagnation. In these cases, the person may have total dependency on work, a favorite child, or even a pet, and be incapable of giving to others. A project may never be finished or schooling completed because the person cannot let go and move on. Without a creative outlet, a paralyzing stagnation sets in. Successful movement through this stage results in a fuller and more satisfying life and prepares the mature adult for the next stage.

Ask yourself . . . Does the client

Have healthful life patterns?

Derive satisfaction from contributing to growth and development of others?

Have an abiding intimacy and long-term relationship with a partner?

Maintain a stable home?

Find pleasure in an established work or profession?

Take pride in self and family accomplishments and contributions?

Contribute to the community to support its growth and development?

Older Adult: Ego Integrity Versus Despair

When the middle-aged adult has accomplished at least partial resolution of the previous developmental tasks, he or she moves into the ego integrity versus despair stage. According to Erikson, a person in this stage looks back and either finds that life was good or despairs that goals were not accomplished. This stage can extend over a long time and include excursions into previous stages to complete unfinished business. Successful movement through this stage does not mean that one day a person wakes up and says, "My life has been good"; rather, it encompasses a series of reminiscences in which the person may be able to see past events in a new and more positive light.

This can be a very rich and rewarding time in a person's life, especially if there are others with whom to share memories and who can assist with reframing life experiences (Fig. 4-5). For some people, resolution and acceptance do not come until the final weeks of life, but this still allows for a peaceful death. If the older person cannot feel grateful for his or her life, cannot accept those less desirable aspects as merely part of living, or cannot integrate all of the experiences of life, then the person will spend his or her last days in bitterness and regret and will ultimately die in despair.

Obviously, mental or physical developmental delays can affect the smooth movement through Erikson's tasks.

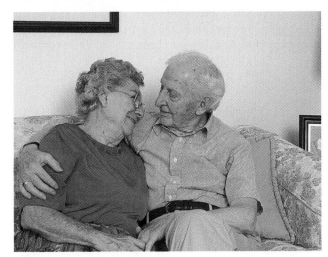

FIGURE 4-5. Older adulthood can be a rich and rewarding time to review life events. (© B. Proud.)

In fact, some may be entirely unachievable. However, it is important not to assume data not in evidence and assign a person to a lower level just because of other problems in development. Many such people are quite capable of advancing through all psychological stages. Rely on data collected, not on age or physical/mental accomplishments.

Ask yourself . . . Does the client

Adjust to the changing physical self?

Recognize changes present as a result of aging, in relationships and activities?

Maintain relationships with children, grandchildren, and other relatives?

Continue interests outside of self and home?

Complete transition from retirement at work to satisfying alternative activities?

Establish relationships with others his or her own age?

Adjust to deaths of relatives, spouse, and friends?

Maintain a maximum level of physical functioning through diet, exercise, and personal care?

Find meaning in past life and face inevitable mortality of self and significant others?

Integrate philosophical or religious values into self-understanding to promote comfort?

Review accomplishments and recognize meaningful contributions he or she has made to community and relatives?

Summary

Collecting subjective data is a key step of nursing health assessment. Subjective data consist of information elicited and verified only by the client. Interviewing is the means by which subjective data are gathered. Two types of communication are useful for interviewing: nonverbal and verbal. Variations in communication, such as gerontologic, cultural, and emotional variations, may be encountered during the client interview.

The complete health history is performed to collect as much subjective data about a client as possible. It consists of eight sections: biographic data, reasons for seeking health care, history of present health concern, past health history, family health history, review of body systems (ROS) for current health problems, lifestyle and health practices, and developmental level.

REFERENCES AND SELECTED READINGS

Adams, C. E., Johnson, J. E., & Moore, J. F. (1996). Patients' health problems: Differences in perceptions between home health patients and nurses. *Home Healthcare Nurse, 14* (12), 932–938.

Andrews, M., & Boyle, J. (1999). *Transcultural concepts in nursing care* (3rd ed.). Philadelphia: Lippincott Williams & Wilkins.

Brush, B. L. (2000). Assessing spirituality in primary care practice: Is there time? *Clinical Excellence for Nurse Practitioners, 4* (2), 67–71.

DiMartino, G. (2000). Legal issues: The patient history. *Dynamic Chiropractic, 18* (14), 26.

Domarad, B. R., & Buschmann, M. T. (1995). Interviewing older adults: Increasing the credibility of interview data. *Journal of Gerontological Nursing, 21* (9), 14–20.

Fareed, A. (1996). The experience of reassurance: Patients' perspectives. *Journal of Advanced Nursing, 23* (2), 272–279.

Giger, J., & Davidhizar, R. (1995). *Transcultural nursing: Assessment and intervention* (2nd ed.). St. Louis: Mosby–Year Book.

Goldfinger, S. (1998). Off to the races—a graphic patient history. *New England Journal of Medicine, 339* (10), 707.

Heery, K. (2000). Straight talk about the patient interview. *Nursing 2000, 20* (6), 66–67.

Hill, M. J. (1998). Another piece of the patient history puzzle. *Dermatology Nursing, 10* (5), 320.

Holm, K., Cohen, F., Dudas, S., Medema, P. G., & Allen, B. L. (1999). Effect of personal pain experience on pain assessment. *Image, 21* (2), 72–75.

Luckmann, J. (2000). *Transcultural communication in health care.* Albany, NY: Delmar.

Owens, M., McConvey, G. G., Weeks, D., & Zeisberg, L. (2000). Pain and symptom management. A pilot program to evaluate pain assessment skills of hospice nurses. *American Journal of Hospice and Palliative Care, 17* (1), 44–48.

Performing that initial assessment: Know your patient's drugs, lifestyle. (2000). *Home Care Quality Management, 6* (7), 83–84.

Schuster, C. S., & Asburn, S. S. (1992). *The process of human development: A holistic life-span approach* (3rd ed.). Philadelphia: J. B. Lippincott.

For additional information on this book, be sure to visit http://connection.lww.com.

Collecting Objective Data

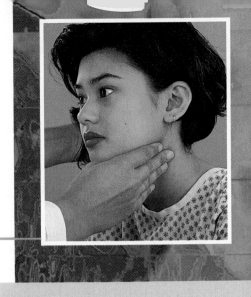

5

A complete nursing assessment includes both the collection of subjective data (discussed in Chapter 4) and the collection of objective data. Objective data include information about the client that the nurse directly observes during interaction with him or her or information that is elicited through physical assessment (examination) techniques. To become proficient with physical assessment skills, the nurse must have basic knowledge in three areas:

- The pieces of equipment needed for the particular examination (eg, penlight, sphygmomanometer, otoscope, tuning fork, stethoscope) and how to use each piece
- Preparation of the setting, oneself, and the client for the physical assessment
- Performance of the four assessment techniques: inspection, palpation, percussion, and auscultation

Equipment Needed

Each part of the physical examination requires specific pieces of equipment. Table 5-1 lists what is necessary for each part of the examination and describes the general purpose of each piece of equipment. More detailed descriptions of each piece of equipment and the procedures for using them are provided in the chapters on the body systems where each piece is used. However, because the stethoscope is used during the assessment of many body systems, this chapter includes a description of it and guidelines on how to use it.

The necessary equipment should be collected and available in the area where the examination will be performed. This promotes organization and prevents the nurse from leaving the client to search for a piece of equipment.

Approaching the Client

Preparing and approaching the client for physical assessment are crucial aspects of objective data collection. How well you prepare the physical setting, yourself, and the client can affect the quality of the data you elicit. As an examiner, you must make sure that you have prepared for all three aspects before beginning an examination. Practicing with a friend, relative, or classmate will help you achieve proficiency in all three aspects of preparation.

PREPARING THE PHYSICAL SETTING

The physical examination may be performed in a variety of physical settings, such as a hospital room, outpatient clinic, physician's office, school health office, employee health office, or a client's home. It is important that the nurse strive to ensure that the following conditions characterize the examination setting:

- Comfortable, warm room temperature—Provide a warm blanket if the room temperature cannot be adjusted.
- Private area free of interruptions from others—Close the door or pull the curtains if possible.
- Quiet area free of distractions—Turn off the radio, television, or other noisy equipment.
- Adequate lighting—It is best to use sunlight (when available). However, good overhead lighting is sufficient. A portable lamp is helpful for illuminating the skin and for viewing shadows or contours.
- Firm examination table or bed at a height that prevents stooping—A roll-up stool may be useful when it is necessary for the examiner to sit for parts of the assessment.
- A bedside table tray to hold the equipment needed for the examination.

PREPARING ONESELF

As a beginning examiner, it is helpful to assess your own feelings and anxieties before examining the client. Anxiety is easily conveyed to the client, who may already feel uneasy and self-conscious about the examination. Self-confidence in performing a physical assessment can be achieved by practicing the techniques on a classmate, friend, or relative. Your "pretend client" should be encouraged to simulate the client role as closely as possible. It is also important to perform some of your practice assessments with an experienced instructor or practitioner who can give you helpful hints and feedback on your technique.

Another important aspect of preparing yourself for the physical assessment examination involves preventing the transmission of infectious agents. In 1997, the Centers for Disease Control and Prevention (CDC) and the Hospital Infection Control Practices Advisory Committee (HICPAC) updated Standard Precautions to be followed for all clients (CDC & HICPAC, 1997). These Standard Precautions appear in Display 5-1; they are a modified combination of the original Universal Precautions and Body Substance Isolation Guidelines. General principles to keep in mind while performing a physical assessment include the following:

- Wash your hands before beginning the examination, immediately after accidental direct contact with blood or other body fluids (you should wear gloves if there is a chance that you will come in direct contact with blood or other body fluids), and after completing the physical examination. If possible, wash your hands in the examining room in front of the client. This assures your client that you are concerned about his or her safety.
- Wear gloves if you have an open cut or skin abrasion, if the client has an open or weeping cut, if you are collecting body fluids (eg, blood, sputum, wound drainage, urine, or stools) for a specimen, if you are handling contaminated surfaces (eg, linen, tongue blades, vaginal speculum), and when you are performing an examination of the mouth, an open wound, genitalia, vagina, or rectum.

TABLE 5-1. Equipment Needed for Physical Examinations

Equipment Needed	Purpose
For All Examinations	
Gloves	Protection for any part of the examination when the examiner may have contact with blood, body fluids, secretions, excretions, and contaminated items or when disease-causing agents could be transmitted to or from the client
For Vital Signs	
Sphygmomanometer	To measure diastolic and systolic blood pressure
Stethoscope	To auscultate blood sounds when measuring blood pressure
Thermometer (oral, rectal, tympanic)	To measure body temperature
Watch with second hand	To time heart rate, pulse rate
For Anthropometric Measurements	
Skinfold calipers	To measure skinfold thickness of subcutaneous tissue
Flexible tape measure	To measure mid-arm circumference
Platform scale with height attachment	To measure height and weight
For Skin, Hair, and Nail Examination	
Ruler with centimeter markings	To measure size of skin lesions
Magnifying glass	To enlarge visibility of lesion
Wood's light	To test for fungus
For Head and Neck Examination	
Small cup of water	To help client swallow during examination of the thyroid gland
For Eye Examination	
Penlight	To test pupillary constriction
Snellen chart	To test distant vision
Ophthalmoscope	To view the red reflex and to examine the retina of the eye
Cover card	To test for strabismus
Newspaper or Rosenbaum Pocket Screener	To test near vision
For Ear Examination	
Otoscope	To view the ear canal and tympanic membrane
Tuning fork	To test for bone and air conduction of sound
For Mouth, Throat, Nose, and Sinus Examination	
Penlight	To provide light to view the mouth and throat and to transilluminate the sinuses
Tongue depressor	To depress tongue to view throat, check looseness of teeth, view cheeks, and check strength of tongue
Piece of small gauze	To grasp tongue to examine mouth
Otoscope with wide-tip attachment	To view the internal nose
For Thoracic and Lung Examination	
Stethoscope (diaphragm)	To auscultate breath sounds
Marking pencil and centimeter ruler	To measure diaphragmatic excursion
For Heart and Neck Vessel Examination	
Stethoscope (bell and diaphragm)	To auscultate heart sounds
Two centimeter rulers	To measure jugular venous pressure
For Abdominal Examination	
Stethoscope	To detect bowel sounds
Marking pencil and tape measure with centimeter markings	To mark area of percussion of organs to measure size
Two small pillows	To place under knees and head to promote relaxation of abdomen
For Genitalia Examination	
Vaginal speculum and lubricant	To inspect cervix through dilatation of the vaginal canal
Slides or specimen container, bifid spatula, and cotton-tipped applicator	To obtain endocervical swab and cervical scrape and vaginal pool sample

TABLE 5-1. Equipment Needed for Physical Examinations (Continued)

Equipment Needed	Purpose
For Anus, Rectum, Prostate Examination	
Lubricating jelly	To promote comfort for client
Specimen container	To test for occult blood
For Peripheral Vascular Examination	
Stethoscope and sphygmomanometer	To auscultate vascular sounds and measure blood pressure
Flexible tape measure	To measure size of extremities for edema
Cotton ball and paper clip	To detect light, blunt, and sharp touch
Tuning fork	To detect vibratory sensation
Doppler ultrasound probe blood	To detect pressure and weak pulses not easily heard with a stethoscope
For Musculoskeletal Examination	
Tape measure	To measure size of extremities
Goniometer	To measure degree of flexion and extension of joints
For Neurologic Examination	
Tuning fork	To test for vibratory sensation
Cotton wisp, paper clip	To test for light, sharp, and dull touch and two-point discrimination
Soap, coffee	To test for smelling perception
Salt, sugar, lemon, pickle juice	To test for taste perception
Tongue depressor	To test for rise of uvula and gag reflex
Reflex hammer	To test deep tendon reflexes
Coin or key	To test for stereognosis (ability to recognize objects by touch)

- If a pin or other sharp object is used to assess sensory perception, discard the pin and use a new one for your next client.
- Wear a mask and protective eye goggles if you are performing an examination in which you are likely to be splashed with blood or other body fluid droplets (eg, if you are performing an oral examination on a client who has a chronic productive cough).

PREPARING THE CLIENT

An initial nurse–client relationship should be established during the client interview, before the physical examination takes place. This is important because it helps to alleviate any tension or anxiety that the client is experiencing. At the end of the interview, explain to the client that the physical assessment will follow, and describe what the examination will involve. For example, you might say to a client, "Mr. Smith, based on the information you have given me, I believe that a complete physical examination should be performed so I can better assess your health status. This will require you to remove your clothing and to put on this patient gown. You may leave on your underwear until it is time to perform the genital examination."

The client's desires and requests related to the physical examination must be respected. Some client requests may be simple, such as asking to have a family member or friend present during the examination. Another request may involve not wanting certain parts of the examination (eg, breast, genitalia) to be performed. In this situation, you should explain to the client the importance of the examination and the risk of missing important information if any part of the examination is omitted. Ultimately, however, whether to have the examination is the client's decision. Some health care providers ask the client to sign a consent form before a physical examination, especially in situations where a vaginal or rectal examination will be performed.

If a urine specimen is necessary, explain to the client the purpose of a urine sample and the procedure for giving a sample, and provide him or her with a container to use. If a urine sample is not necessary, ask the client to urinate before the examination to promote an easier and more comfortable examination of the abdomen and genital areas. Ask the client to undress and put on an examination gown. Allow him or her to keep on underwear until just before the genital examination to promote comfort and privacy. Leave the room while the client changes into the gown and knock before reentering the room to ensure the client's privacy.

Begin the examination with the less intrusive procedures, such as measuring the client's temperature, pulse, blood pressure, height, and weight. These nonthreatening procedures allow the client to feel more comfortable with you and help to ease client anxiety about the examination. Continue to explain what procedure you are performing and why you are performing it throughout the examination. This also helps to ease your client's anxiety. It is usually helpful to integrate health teaching and health promotion during the examination (eg, breast self-examination technique).

DISPLAY 5-1. Standard Precautions

Use Standard Precautions, or the equivalent, for the care of all patients—Category 1B.*

GUIDELINES

A. HANDWASHING

1. Wash hands after touching blood, body fluids, secretions, excretions, and contaminated items, whether or not gloves are worn. Wash hands immediately after gloves are removed, between patient contacts, and when otherwise indicated to avoid transfer of microorganisms to other patients or environments. It may be necessary to wash hands between tasks and procedures on the same patient to prevent cross-contamination of different body sites—Category 1B.
2. Use a plain (nonantimicrobial) soap for routine handwashing—Category 1B.
3. Use an antimicrobial agent or a waterless antiseptic agent for specific circumstances (eg, control of outbreaks or hyperendemic infections), as defined by the infection control program—Category 1B.

B. GLOVES

Wear gloves (clean, nonsterile gloves are adequate) when touching blood, body fluids, secretions, excretions, and contaminated items. Put on clean gloves just before touching mucous membranes and nonintact skin. Change gloves between tasks and procedures on the same patient after contact with material that may contain a high concentration of microorganisms. Remove gloves promptly after use, before touching noncontaminated items and environmental surfaces, and before going to another patient. Wash hands immediately to avoid transfer of microrganisms to other patients or environments—Category 1B.

C. MASK, EYE PROTECTION, FACE SHIELD

Wear a mask and eye protection or a face shield to protect mucous membranes of the eyes, nose, and mouth during procedures and patient care activities that are likely to generate splashes or sprays of blood, body fluids, secretions, and excretions—Category 1B.

D. GOWN

Wear a gown (a clean, nonsterile gown is adequate) to protect skin and to prevent soiling of clothing during procedures and patient care activities that are likely to generate splashes or sprays of blood, body fluids, secretions, or excretions. Select a gown that is appropriate for the activity and amount of fluid likely to be encountered. Remove a soiled gown as promptly as possible, and wash hands to avoid transfer of microorganisms to other patients or environments—Category 1B.

E. PATIENT CARE EQUIPMENT

Handle used patient care equipment soiled with blood, body fluids, secretions, and excretions in a manner that prevents skin and mucous membrane exposures, contamination of clothing, and transfer of microorganisms to other patients and environments. Ensure that reusable equipment is not used for the care of another patient until it has been cleaned and reprocessed appropriately. Ensure that single-use items are discarded properly—Category 1B.

F. ENVIRONMENTAL CONTROL

Ensure that the hospital has adequate procedures for the routine care, cleaning, and disinfection of environmental surfaces, beds, bedrails, bedside equipment, and other frequently touched surfaces, and ensure that these procedures are being followed—Category 1B.

G. LINEN

Handle, transport, and process used linen soiled with blood, body fluids, secretions, and excretions in a manner that prevents skin and mucous membrane exposures and contamination of clothing, and that avoids transfer of microorganisms to other patients and environments—Category 1B.

H. OCCUPATIONAL HEALTH AND BLOODBORNE PATHOGENS

1. Take care to prevent injuries when using needles, scalpels, and other sharp instruments or devices; when handling sharp instruments after procedures; when cleaning used instruments;

(continued)

DISPLAY 5-1. **Standard Precautions** (Continued)

and when disposing of used needles. Never recap used needles, or otherwise manipulate them using both hands, or use any other technique that involves directing the point of a needle toward any part of the body; rather, use either a one-handed "scoop" technique or a mechanical device designed for holding the needle sheath. Do not remove used needles from disposable syringes by hand, and do not bend, break, or otherwise manipulate used needles by hand. Place used disposable syringes and needles, scalpel blades, and other sharp items in appropriate puncture-resistant containers, which are located as close as practical to the area in which the items were used. Place reusable syringes and needles in a puncture-resistant container for transport to the reprocessing area—Category 1B.

2. Use mouthpieces, resuscitation bags, or other ventilation devices as an alternative to mouth-to-mouth resuscitation methods in areas where the need for resuscitation is predictable—Category 1B.

I. PATIENT PLACEMENT

Place a patient who contaminates the environment or who does not (or cannot be expected to) assist in maintaining appropriate hygiene or environmental control in a private room. If a private room is not available, consult with infection control professionals regarding patient placement or other alternatives—Category 1B.

*Category 1B: Strongly recommended for all hospitals and reviewed as effective by experts in the field and a consensus of the Hospital Injection Control Practices Advisory Committee (HICPAC) based on strong rationale and suggestive evidence, even though definitive scientific studies have not been done.

(From CDC & HICPAC, [1997]. *Guidelines for isolation precautions in hospitals: Category IP.* Atlanta: Author.)

The client should be approached from the right-hand side of the examination table or bed because most examination techniques are performed with the examiner's right hand (even if the examiner is left-handed). You may ask the client to change positions frequently, depending on the part of the examination being performed. Prepare the client for these changes at the beginning of the examination by explaining that these position changes are necessary to ensure a thorough examination of each body part and system. Many clients need assistance getting into the required position. Display 5-2 illustrates various positions and provides guidelines for using them during the examination.

Older Adult Considerations

Some positions may be very difficult or impossible for the older client to assume or maintain because of decreased joint mobility and flexibility (see Display 5-2). Therefore, try to perform the examination in a manner that minimizes position changes. Also, it is a good idea to allow rest periods for the older adult, if needed. Some older clients may process information at a slower rate. Therefore, explain the procedure and integrate teaching in a clear and slow manner.

Physical Assessment Techniques

Four basic techniques must be mastered before you can perform a thorough and complete assessment of the client. These techniques are *inspection, palpation, percussion,* and *auscultation.* Each technique is described, and guidelines

on how to perform the basic technique are given. How to use each technique for assessing specific body systems is described in the appropriate chapter. After performing each of the four assessment techniques, the examiner needs to think of certain questions that will facilitate analysis of the data and determine areas in which more data may be needed. These questions include:

- Did I inspect, palpate, percuss, or auscultate any deviations from the normal findings? (Normal findings are listed in the second column of the Physical Assessment sections in the body systems chapters.)
- If there is a deviation, is it a normal physical, gerontologic, or cultural finding; an abnormal adult finding; or an abnormal physical, gerontologic, or cultural finding? (Normal gerontologic and cultural findings are in the second column of the Physical Assessment sections in the body systems chapters. Abnormal adult, gerontologic, and cultural findings can be found in the third column of the Physical Assessment sections.)
- Based on my findings, do I need to ask the client more questions to validate or obtain more information about my inspection, palpation, percussion, or auscultation findings?
- Do I need to zero in and focus my physical assessment on other related body systems based on my observations and data?
- Should I validate my inspection, palpation, percussion, or auscultation findings with my instructor or another practitioner?
- Should I refer the client and data findings to a primary care provider?

(*text continues on page 56*)

DISPLAY 5-2. Positioning the Client

GUIDELINES

SITTING POSITION

The client should sit upright on the side of the examination table. In the home or office setting, the client can sit on the edge of a chair or bed. This position is good for evaluating the head, neck, lungs, chest, back, breasts, axillae, heart, vital signs, and upper extremities. This position is also useful because it permits full expansion of the lungs and it allows the examiner to assess symmetry of upper body parts. Some clients may be too weak to sit up for the entire examination. They may need to lie down (supine position) and rest throughout the examination. Other clients may be unable to tolerate the position for any length of time. An alternative position is for the client to lie down with his or her head elevated.

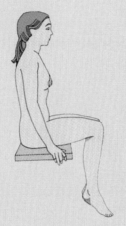

Sitting position.

SUPINE POSITION

Ask the client to lie down with the legs together on the examination table (or bed if in a home setting). A small pillow may be placed under the head to promote comfort. If the client has trouble breathing, the head of the bed may need to be raised. This position allows the abdominal muscles to relax and provides easy access to peripheral pulse sites. Areas assessed with the client in this position may include head, neck, chest, breasts, axillae, abdomen, heart, lungs, and all extremities.

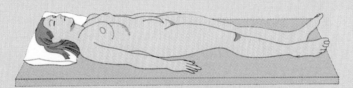

Supine position.

(continued)

DORSAL RECUMBENT POSITION

The client lies down on the examination table or bed with the knees bent, the legs separated, and the feet flat on the table or bed. This position may be more comfortable than the supine position for clients with pain in the back or abdomen. Areas that may be assessed with the client in this position include head, neck, chest, axillae, lungs, heart, extremities, breasts, and peripheral pulses. The abdomen should not be assessed because the abdominal muscles are contracted in this position.

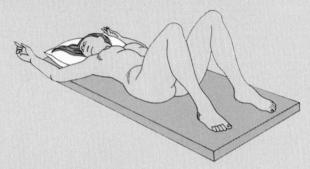

Dorsal recumbent position.

SIMS' POSITION

The client lies on his or her right or left side with the lower arm placed behind the body and the upper arm flexed at the shoulder and elbow. The lower leg is slightly flexed at the knee while the upper leg is flexed at a sharper angle and pulled forward. This position is useful for assessing the rectal and vaginal areas. The client may need some assistance getting into this position. Clients with joint problems and elderly clients may have some difficulty assuming and maintaining this position.

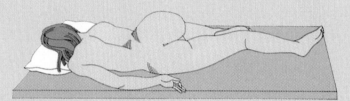

Sims' position.

STANDING POSITION

The client stands still in a normal, comfortable, resting posture. This position allows the examiner to assess posture, balance, and gait. This position is also used for examining the male genitalia.

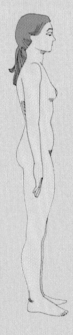

Standing position.

(continued)

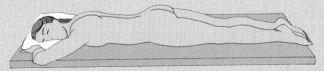

PRONE POSITION

The client lies down on his or her abdomen with the head to the side. The prone position is used primarily to assess the hip joint. The back can also be assessed with the client in this position. Clients with cardiac and respiratory problems cannot tolerate this position.

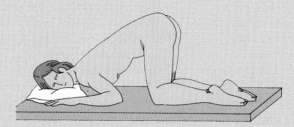

Prone position.

KNEE–CHEST POSITION

The client kneels on the examination table with the weight of the body supported by the chest and knees. A 90-degree angle should exist between the body and the hips. The arms are placed above the head, with the head turned to one side. A small pillow may be used to provide comfort. The knee–chest position is useful for examining the rectum. This position may be embarrassing and uncomfortable for the client, and, therefore, the client should be kept in the position for as limited a time as possible. Elderly clients and clients with respiratory and cardiac problems may be unable to tolerate this position.

Knee–chest position.

LITHOTOMY POSITION

The client lies on his or her back with the hips at the edge of the examination table and the feet supported by stirrups. The lithotomy position is used to examine the female genitalia, reproductive tracts, and the rectum. The client may require assistance getting into this position. It is an exposed position, and clients may feel embarrassed. In addition, elderly clients may not be able to assume this position for very long or at all. Therefore, it is best to keep the client well draped during the examination and to perform the examination as quickly as possible.

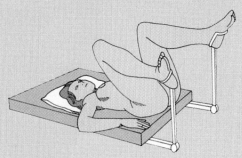

Lithotomy position.

INSPECTION

Inspection involves using the senses of vision, smell, and hearing to observe and detect any normal or abnormal findings in the client. This technique is used from the moment that you meet the client and continues throughout the examination. Inspection precedes palpation, percussion, and auscultation because the latter techniques can potentially alter the appearance of what is being inspected. Although most of the inspection involves the use of the senses only, a few body systems require the use of special equipment (eg, ophthalmoscope for the eye inspection, otoscope for the ear inspection).

Use the following guidelines as you practice the technique of inspection:

- Make sure the room is a comfortable temperature. A too-cold or too-hot room can alter the normal behavior of the client and the appearance of the client's skin.
- Use good lighting, preferably sunlight. Fluorescent lights can alter the true color of the skin. In addition, abnormalities may be overlooked with dim lighting.
- Look and observe before touching. Touch can alter appearance and distract you from a complete, focused observation.
- Completely expose the body part you are inspecting while draping the rest of the client as appropriate.
- Note the following characteristics while inspecting the client: color, patterns, size, location, consistency, symmetry, movement, behavior, odors, or sounds.
- Compare the appearance of symmetric body parts (eg, eyes, ears, arms, hands) or both sides of any individual body part.

PALPATION

Palpation consists of using parts of the hand to touch and feel for the following characteristics: *texture* (rough/smooth), *temperature* (warm/cold), *moisture* (dry/wet), *mobility* (fixed/movable/still/vibrating), *consistency* (soft/hard/fluid filled), *strength of pulses* (strong/weak/thready/bounding), *size* (small/medium/large), *shape* (well defined/irregular), and *degree of tenderness.*

Three different parts of the hand—the fingerpads, ulnar/palmar surface, and dorsal surface—are used during palpation. Each part of the hand is particularly sensitive to certain characteristics. Determine which characteristic you are trying to palpate and refer to Table 5-2 to find which part of the hand is best to use. Several types of palpation can be used to perform an assessment; they include light, moderate, deep, or bimanual palpation. The depth of the structure being palpated and the thickness of the tissue overlying that structure determine whether you should use light, moderate, or deep palpation. Bimanual palpation is the use of both hands to hold and feel a body structure.

TABLE 5-2. **Parts of Hand to Use When Palpating**	
Hand Part	*Sensitive To*
Fingerpads	Fine discriminations: pulses, texture, size, consistency, shape, crepitus
Ulnar or palmar surface	Vibrations, thrills, fremitus
Dorsal (back) surface	Temperature

In general, the examiner's fingernails should be short and the hands should be a comfortable temperature. Standard precautions should be followed if applicable. Proceed from light palpation, which is safest and the most comfortable for the client, to moderate palpation, and finally to deep palpation. Specific instructions on how to perform the four types of palpation follow:

- *Light palpation:* To perform light palpation (Fig. 5-1), place your dominant hand lightly on the surface of the structure. There should be very little or no depression (less than 1 cm). Feel the surface structure using a circular motion. Use this technique to feel for pulses, tenderness, surface skin texture, temperature, and moisture.
- *Moderate palpation:* Depress the skin surface 1 to 2 cm (0.5 to 0.75 inch) with your dominant hand, and use a circular motion to feel for easily palpable body organs and masses. Note the size, consistency, and mobility of structures you palpate.
- *Deep palpation:* Place your dominant hand on the skin surface and your nondominant hand on top of your dominant hand to apply pressure (Fig. 5-2). This should result in a surface depression between 2.5 and 5 cm (1 and 2 inches). This allows you to feel very deep organs or structures that are covered by thick muscle.

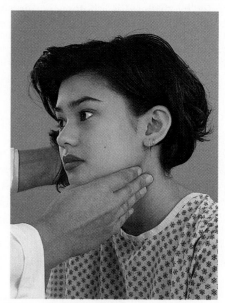

FIGURE 5-1. Light palpation.

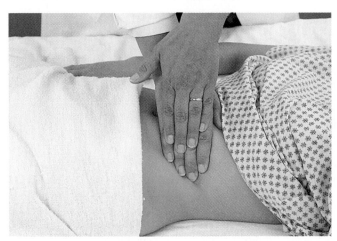

FIGURE 5-2. Deep palpation.

- *Bimanual palpation:* Use two hands, placing one on each side of the body part (eg, uterus, breasts, spleen) being palpated (Fig. 5-3). Use one hand to apply pressure and the other hand to feel the structure. Note the size, shape, consistency, and mobility of the structures you palpate.

PERCUSSION

Percussion involves tapping body parts to produce sound waves. These sound waves or vibrations enable the examiner to assess underlying structures. Percussion has several different assessment uses, including:

- *Eliciting pain:* Percussion helps to detect inflamed underlying structures. If an inflamed area is percussed, the client's response may indicate or the client will report that the area feels tender, sore, or painful.
- *Determining location, size, and shape:* Percussion note changes between borders of an organ and its neighbor can elicit information about location, size, and shape.
- *Determining density:* Whether an underlying structure is filled with air or fluid or is a solid structure can be determined through percussion.

- *Detecting abnormal masses:* Superficial abnormal structures or masses can be detected using percussion. Percussion vibrations penetrate approximately 5 cm deep. Deep masses do not produce any change in the normal percussion vibrations.
- *Eliciting reflexes:* Deep tendon reflexes are elicited using the percussion hammer.

The three types of percussion are *direct, blunt,* and *indirect.* Direct percussion (Fig. 5-4) is the direct tapping of a body part with one or two fingertips to elicit possible tenderness (eg, tenderness over the sinuses). Blunt percussion (Fig. 5-5) is used to detect tenderness over organs (eg, kidneys) by placing one hand flat on the body surface and using the fist of the other hand to strike the back of the hand flat on the body surface. Indirect or mediate percussion (Fig. 5-6) is the most commonly used method of percussion. The tapping done with this type of percussion produces a sound or tone that varies with the density of underlying structures. As density increases, the sound of the tone becomes quieter. Solid tissue produces a soft tone, fluid produces a louder tone, and air produces an even louder tone. These tones are referred to as percussion notes and are classified according to origin, quality, intensity, and pitch (Table 5-3).

The following techniques help develop proficiency in the technique of indirect percussion:

- Place the middle finger of your nondominant hand on the body part you are going to percuss.
- Keep your other fingers off the body part being percussed because they will damp the tone you elicit.
- Use the pad of your middle finger of the other hand (ensure that this fingernail is short) to strike the middle finger of your nondominant hand that is placed on the body part.

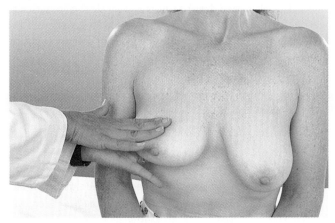

FIGURE 5-3. Bimanual palpation of the breast.

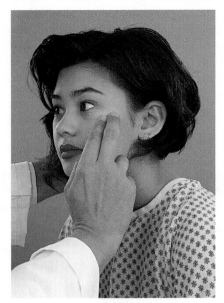

FIGURE 5-4. Direct percussion of sinuses.

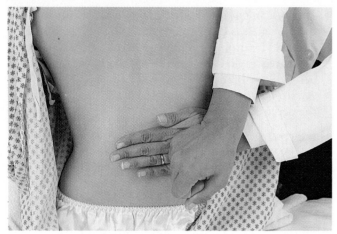

FIGURE 5-5. Blunt percussion of kidneys.

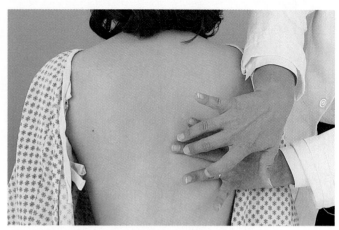

FIGURE 5-6. Indirect or mediate percussion of lungs. (Photos © 1996 by B. Proud.)

- Withdraw your finger immediately to avoid damping the tone.
- Deliver two quick taps, and listen carefully to the tone.
- Use quick, sharp taps by quickly flexing your wrist, not your forearm.

Practice percussing by tapping your thigh to elicit a flat tone and your puffed-out cheek to elicit a tympanic tone. A good way to detect changes in tone is to fill a carton halfway with fluid and practice percussing on it. The tone will change from resonance over air to a duller tone over the fluid.

AUSCULTATION

Auscultation is a type of assessment technique that requires the use of a stethoscope to listen for heart sounds, movement of blood through the cardiovascular system, movement of the bowel, and movement of air through the respiratory tract. A stethoscope is used because these body sounds are not audible to the human ear. The sounds that are detected using auscultation are classified according to the intensity (loud or soft), pitch (high or low), duration (length), and quality (musical, crackling, raspy) of the sound (Display 5-3).

The following guidelines should be followed as you practice the technique of auscultation:

- Eliminate distracting or competing noises from the environment (eg, radio, television, machinery).

- Expose the body part you are going to auscultate. Do not auscultate through the client's clothing or gown. Rubbing against the clothing obscures the body sounds.
- Use the diaphragm of the stethoscope to listen for high-pitched sounds, such as normal heart sounds, breath sounds, and bowel sounds, and press the diaphragm firmly on the body part being auscultated.
- Use the bell of the stethoscope to listen for low-pitched sounds, such as abnormal heart sounds and bruits (abnormal loud, blowing, or murmuring sounds heard during auscultation). Hold the bell lightly on the body part being auscultated.

Summary

Collecting objective data is essential for a complete nursing assessment. The nurse must have knowledge of and skill in three basic areas to become proficient in collecting objective data—necessary equipment and how to use it; preparing the setting, oneself, and the client for the examination; and how to perform the four basic assessment techniques. Collecting objective data requires a great deal of practice to become proficient. Proficiency is needed because how the data are collected can affect the accuracy of the information elicited.

TABLE 5-3. Sounds (Tones) Elicited by Percussion

Sound	Intensity	Pitch	Length	Quality	Example of Origin
Resonance (heard over part air and part solid)	Loud	Low	Long	Hollow	Normal lung
Hyper-resonance (heard over mostly air)	Very loud	Low	Long	Booming	Lung with emphysema
Tympany (heard over air)	Loud	High	Moderate	Drumlike	Puffed-out cheek, gastric bubble
Dullness (heard over more solid tissue)	Medium	Medium	Moderate	Thudlike	Diaphragm, pleural effusion, liver
Flatness (heard over very dense tissue)	Soft	High	Short	Flat	Muscle, bone, sternum, thigh

DISPLAY 5-3. How to Use the Stethoscope

The stethoscope is used to listen for (auscultate) body sounds that cannot ordinarily be heard without amplification (eg, lung sounds, bruits, bowel sounds, and so forth). To use a stethoscope, follow these guidelines:

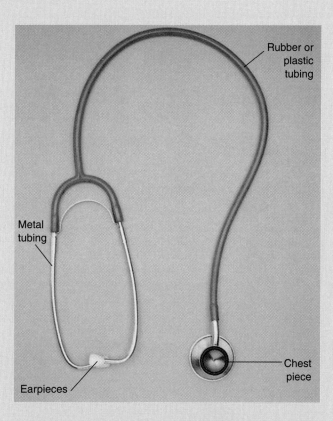

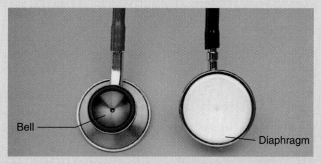

1. Place the earpieces into the outer ear canal. They should fit snugly but comfortably to promote effective sound transmission. The earpieces are connected to binaurals (metal tubing), which connect to rubber or plastic tubing. The rubber or plastic tubing should be flexible and no more than 12 inches long to prevent the sound from diminishing.

2. Angle the binaurals down toward your nose. This will ensure that sounds are transmitted to your eardrums.

3. Use the diaphragm of the stethoscope to detect high-pitched sounds. The diaphragm should be at least 1.5 inches wide for adults and smaller for children. Hold the diaphragm firmly against the body part being auscultated.

4. Use the bell of the stethoscope to detect low-pitched sounds. The bell should be at least 1 inch wide. Hold the bell lightly against the body part being auscultated.

(continued)

DISPLAY 5-3. How to Use the Stethoscope (Continued)

SOME DO'S AND DON'TS

● Warm the diaphragm or bell of the stethoscope before placing it on the client's skin.

● Explain what you are listening for and answer any questions the client has. This will help to alleviate anxiety.

● Do not apply too much pressure when using the bell—too much pressure will cause the bell to work like the diaphragm.

● Avoid listening through clothing, which may obscure or alter sounds.

REFERENCES AND SELECTED READINGS

Basfield-Holland, E. S. (1997). Home health. Assessing pulmonary status: It's more than listening to breath sounds. *Nursing 97, 27*(8), 32–39.

Byers, V. B. (1973). *Nursing observation* (2nd ed.). St. Louis: C. V. Mosby.

Centers for Disease Control and Prevention (CDC) and the Hospital Infection Control Practices Advisory Committee (HICPAC). (1997, February). *Guidelines for isolation precautions in hospitals: Category 1B.* Atlanta: Author.

Fitzgerald, M. A. (1991). The physical exam. *RN, 54*(11), 34–39.

Fleury, J., & Keller, C. (2000). Assessment. Cardiovascular risk assessment in elderly individuals. *Journal of Gerontological Nursing 26*(5), 30–37.

Gaskin, P. R. A., Ownes, S. E., Tainer, N. S., Sanders, S. P., & Li, J. S. (2000). Clinical auscultation skills in pediatric residents. *Pediatrics, 105* (6), 1184–1186.

King, R. C. (1983). Refining your assessment techniques. *RN, 46,* 43–47.

Littman, D. (1972). Stethoscopes and auscultation. *American Journal of Nursing, 72*(7), 1238–1241.

O'Hanlon-Nichols, T. (1998a). Basic assessment series: A review of the adult musculoskeletal system. *American Journal of Nursing, 98*(6), 48–52.

———. (1998b). Basic assessment series: A review of the adult pulmonary system. *American Journal of Nursing, 98*(2), 39–45.

———. (1998c). Basic assessment series: Gastrointestinal system. *American Journal of Nursing, 98*(4), 48–53.

Schiff, L. Stethoscopes. (2000). *RN, 63*(7), 63–64.

Shub, C. (1999). Cardiac physical examination: Clinical "pearls" and application. *ACC Current Journal Review, 8*(6), 9–13.

Smith, G. R. (2000). Devices for measuring blood pressure. *Professional Nurse, 15*(5), 337–340.

Torrance, C., & Elley, K. (1997). Practical procedures for nurses. 4.1 Respiration technique and observation. *Nursing Times, 93*(43), S1–S2.

For additional information on this book, be sure to visit http://connection.lww.com.

Validating and
Documenting Data

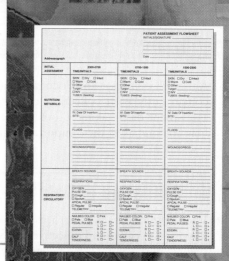

6

Although validation and documentation of data often occur concurrently with collection of subjective and objective assessment data, taking a look at each step separately can help to emphasize their importance in the realm of nursing assessment.

Validation of Data

Validation of data is the process of confirming or verifying that the subjective and objective data you have collected are reliable and accurate. The steps of validation include deciding whether the data require validation, determining ways to validate the data, and identifying areas where data are missing. Failure to validate data may result in premature closure of the assessment or collection of inaccurate data. Errors during assessment cause judgments to be made on unreliable data, which result in diagnostic errors during the second part of the nursing process—analysis of data. Thus, validation of the data collected during assessment of the client is crucial to the first step of the nursing process.

DATA REQUIRING VALIDATION

Not every piece of data you collect must be verified. For example, you would not need to verify or repeat the client's pulse, temperature, or blood pressure unless certain conditions exist. Conditions that require data to be rechecked and validated include:

- Discrepancies or gaps between the subjective and objective data. For example, a male client tells you that he is very happy despite learning that he has terminal cancer.
- Discrepancies or gaps between what the client says at one time and then at another time. For example, your female patient says she has never had surgery, but later in the interview she mentions that her appendix was removed at a military hospital when she was in the Navy.
- Findings that are very abnormal and inconsistent with other findings. For example, the client has a temperature of 104°F. The client is resting comfortably. The client's skin is warm to the touch and not flushed.

METHODS OF VALIDATION

There are several ways to validate your data:

- Recheck your own data through a repeat assessment. For example, take the client's temperature again with a different thermometer.
- Clarify data with the client by asking additional questions. For example, if a client is holding his abdomen the nurse may assume he is having abdominal pain, when actually the client is very upset about his diagnosis and is feeling nauseated.
- Verify the data with another health care professional. For example, ask a more experienced nurse to listen to the abnormal heart sounds you think you have just heard.
- Compare your objective findings with your subjective findings to uncover discrepancies. For example, if the

client states that she "never gets any time in the sun," yet has dark, wrinkled, suntanned skin, you need to validate the client's perception of never getting any time in the sun.

IDENTIFICATION OF AREAS WHERE DATA ARE MISSING

Once you establish an initial database, you can identify areas where more data are needed. You may have overlooked certain questions, or you were not able to complete the entire database on the form provided (eg, foods consumed in a typical day). In addition, as data are examined in a grouped format, you may realize that additional information is needed. For example, if an adult client weighs only 98 lb, you would explore further to see whether the client recently lost weight or whether this has been the usual weight for an extended time. If a client tells you he or she lives alone, you may need to identify the existence of a support system, his or her degree of social involvement with others, and his or her ability to function independently.

Documentation of Data

In addition to validation, documentation of assessment data is another crucial part of the first step in the nursing process. The significance of this aspect of assessment is addressed specifically by various state nurse practice acts, accreditation and/or reimbursement agencies (eg, The Joint Commission on Accreditation of Healthcare Organizations [JCAHO], Medicare, Medicaid), professional organizations (local, state, and national), and institutional agencies (acute, transitional, long-term, and home care). JCAHO, for example, has specific standards that address documentation for assessments. The preamble states:

> [The] care provided to each patient is based on a determination of the patient's needs. This determination is based on an assessment of the patient's relevant physical, psychological, and social status needs. The assessment includes the collection and analysis of data about the patient to determine the need for any additional data, the patient's care needs, and the care to be provided (Marrellin, 1996).

Health care institutions have developed assessment and documentation policies and procedures that provide not only the criteria for documenting but also assistance in completing the forms. The categories of information on the forms are designed to ensure that the nurse gathers pertinent information needed to meet the standards and guidelines of the specific institutions mentioned previously and to develop a plan of care for the client.

PURPOSE OF DOCUMENTATION

The primary reason for documenting the initial assessment is to provide the health care team with a database that becomes the foundation for the entire nursing process. It helps in the identification of health problems and aids in the formulation of nursing diagnostic statements to plan immediate and ongoing interventions. If the nursing diagnosis is made without supporting assessment data, incorrect conclusions may result.

The initial and ongoing assessment documentation database also establishes a way to communicate with the multidisciplinary team members. With the advent of computer-based documentation systems, this database can link to other documents and health care departments, eliminating repetition of similar data collection by other health team members. The many other purposes that assessment documentation serves are described in Display 6-1.

In the past nurses tended to overdocument, believing that the more data they documented, the safer they were legally. Today, nurses use comprehensive and systematic nursing databases that streamline data collection and organization yet maintain a concise record that satisfies legal standards.

INFORMATION NECESSARY FOR DOCUMENTATION

Every institution is unique when it comes to documenting assessments. However, two key elements are always included in every documentation—nursing history and physical examination, also known as subjective and objective data. Most data collection starts with subjective data and ends with objective data.

Subjective data consist of the information that the client or significant others tell the nurse, and objective data are what the nurse observes through inspection, palpation, percussion, or auscultation. It is important to remember to document only what the client tells you and what you observe—not what you interpret or infer from the data.

Interpretation or inference is performed during the analysis phase of the nursing process.

Subjective Data

Subjective data typically consist of biographic data, current symptoms (or the client's chief complaint or concerns), past history, family history, and lifestyle and health practices information.

Biographic data typically consist of the client's name, age, occupation, ethnicity, and support systems or resources. A review of information is recorded in statements that reflect the client's current symptoms. Statements should begin, "Client (or significant other) states. . . ." Describe items as accurately and descriptively as possible. For example, if a client complains of difficult breathing, report how the client describes the problem, when the problem started, what started it, how long it occurred, and what makes the breathing better or worse. Keep a memory help, such as COLDSPA, in mind for every symptom or sign reported by the client.

COLDSPA

CHARACTER: Describe the sign or symptom. How does it feel, look, sound, smell, and so forth?

ONSET: When did it begin?

LOCATION: Where is it? Does it radiate?

DURATION: How long does it last? Does it recur?

SEVERITY: How bad is it?

PATTERN: What makes it better: What makes it worse?

ASSOCIATED FACTORS: What other symptoms occur with it?

DISPLAY 6-1. Purposes of Assessment Documentation

- Provides a chronologic source of client assessment data and a progressive record of assessment findings that outline the client's course of care.
- Ensures that information about the client and family is easily accessible to members of the health care team; provides a vehicle for communication; and prevents fragmentation, repetition, and delays in carrying out the plan of care.
- Establishes a basis for screening or validating proposed diagnoses.
- Acts as a source of information to help diagnose new problems.
- Offers a basis for determining the educational needs of the client, family, and significant others.
- Provides a basis for determining eligibility for care and reimbursement. Careful recording of data can support financial reimbursement or gain additional reimbursement for transitional or skilled care needed by the client.
- Constitutes a permanent legal record of the care that was or was not given to the client.
- Forms a component of client acuity system or client classification systems (Eggland & Heinemann, 1994). Numeric values may be assigned to various levels of care to help determine the staffing mix for the unit.
- Provides access to significant epidemiologic data for future investigations and research and educational endeavors.
- Promotes compliance with legal, accreditation, reimbursement, and professional standard requirements.

This information provides the health care team members with details that help in diagnosis and clinical problem solving. Sometimes, you may need to record the absence of specific signs and symptoms (eg, no vomiting, diarrhea, or constipation).

Past history data tell the nurse about events that happened before the client's admission to the health care facility or the current encounter with the client. The data may be about previous hospitalizations, surgeries, treatment programs, acute illness, chronic illnesses, and injuries.

Family history data include information about the client's biologic family (eg, family history of diseases or behaviors that may be genetic or familial).

The lifestyle and health practices information typically details risk behaviors such as past or present smoking; alcohol use; medication (prescribed, over-the-counter, or illicit) use; environmental factors that may affect health; social and psychological factors that may affect the client's health; client and family health education needs; family and other relationships; and treatment and disease data.

Objective Data

After you complete the nursing history, the physical examination begins. This examination includes inspection, palpation, percussion, and auscultation. These data help further define the client's problems, establish baseline data for ongoing assessments, and validate the subjective data obtained during the nursing history interview. A variety of systematic approaches may be used, namely, head-to-toe, major body systems, functional health patterns, or human response patterns.

No matter which approach is used, general rules apply. Make notes as you perform the assessments, and document as concisely as possible. Avoid general nondescriptive terms such as normal, abnormal, good, fair, satisfactory, or poor. Instead, use specific descriptive terms about what you inspected, palpated, percussed, and auscultated.

GUIDELINES FOR DOCUMENTATION

The way that the nursing assessments are recorded varies among practice settings. However, several general guidelines apply to all settings. They include:

- *Document legibly or print neatly in unerasable ink.* Errors in documentation are usually corrected by drawing one line through the entry, writing "error," and initialing the entry. Never obliterate the error with white paint or tape, an eraser, or a marking pen. Keep in mind that the health record is a legal document.
- *Use correct grammar and spelling.* Use only abbreviations that are acceptable and approved by the institution. Avoid slang, jargon, or labels unless they are direct quotes.
- *Avoid wordiness that creates redundancy.* For example, do not record: "Auscultated gurgly bowel sounds in right upper, right lower, left upper, and left lower abdominal quadrants. Heard 36 gurgles per minute."

Instead record: "Bowel sounds present in all quadrants at 36/minute."
- *Use phrases instead of sentences to record data.* For example, avoid recording: "The client's lung sounds were clear both in the right and left lungs." Instead record: "Bilateral lung sounds clear."
- *Record data findings, not how they were obtained.* For example, do not record: "Client was interviewed for past history of high blood pressure, and blood pressure was taken." Instead record: "Has 3-year history of hypertension treated with medication. BP sitting right arm 140/86, left arm 136/86."
- *Write entries objectively without making premature judgments or diagnoses.* Use quotation marks to identify clearly the client's responses. For example, record: "Client crying in room, refuses to talk, husband has gone home" instead of "Client depressed due to fear of breast biopsy report and not getting along well with husband." Avoid making inferences and diagnostic statements until you have collected and validated all data with client and family.
- *Record the client's understanding and perception of problems.* For example, record: "Client expresses concern regarding being discharged soon after gallbladder surgery because of inability to rest at home with six children."
- *Avoid recording the word "normal" for normal findings.* For example, do not record: "Liver palpation normal." Instead record: "Liver span 10 cm in right MCL and 4 cm in MSL. No tenderness on palpation." In some health care settings, however, only abnormal findings are documented if the policy is to chart by exception only. In that case, no normal findings would be documented in any format.
- *Record complete information and details for all client symptoms or experiences.* For example, do not record: "Client has pain in lower back." Instead record: "Client has had aching-burning pain in lower back for 2 weeks. Pain worsens after standing for several hours. Rest and ibuprofen used to take edge off pain. No radiation of pain. Rates pain as 7 on scale of 1 to 10."
- *Include additional assessment content when applicable* (eg, include information about the caregiver or last physician contact).
- *Support objective data with specific observations obtained during the physical examination.* For example, when describing the emotional status of the client as depressed, follow it with a description of the ways depression is demonstrated, such as "dressed in dirty clothing, avoids eye contact, unkempt appearance, and slumped shoulders."

ASSESSMENT FORMS USED FOR DOCUMENTATION

Standardized assessment forms have been developed to ensure that content in documentation and assessment data meets regulatory requirements and provides a thorough database. The type of assessment form used for documentation varies according to the health care institution. In fact, a variety of assessment forms may even be used within an institution. Typically, however, three types of assessment forms are used to document data: an initial assessment form, frequent or ongoing assessment forms, and focused or specialized assessment forms.

Initial Assessment Form

An initial assessment form is called a nursing admission or admission database. Four types of frequently used initial assessment documentation forms are known as open-ended, cued or checklist, integrated cued checklist, and nursing minimum data set (NMDS) forms. Display 6-2 describes each type of initial assessment form. In addition, Figure 6-1

is an example of the cued or checklist admission documentation form used in an acute care setting.

Frequent or Ongoing Assessment Form

Various institutions have created flow charts that help staff record and retrieve data for frequent reassessments. Examples of two types of flow charts are the frequent vital signs sheet, which allows for vital signs to be recorded in a graphic format that promotes easy visualization of abnormalities, and the assessment flow chart, which allows for rapid comparison of recorded assessment data from one time period to the next (Fig. 6-2).

Progress notes may be used to document unusual events, responses, significant observations, or interactions because
(*text continues on page 70*)

DISPLAY 6-2. Types of Initial Assessment Documentation Forms

OPEN-ENDED FORMS: FEATURES
- Traditional form
- Calls for narrative description of problem and listing of topics
- Provides lines for comments
- Individualizes information
- Provides "total picture," including specific complaints and symptoms in the client's own words
- Increases risk of failing to ask a pertinent question because questions are not standardized
- Requires a lot of time to complete the database

CUED OR CHECKLIST FORMS: FEATURES
- Standardizes data collection
- Lists (categorizes) information that alerts the nurse to specific problems or symptoms that are assessed for each client (see Fig. 6-1)
- Usually includes a comment section after each category to allow for individualization
- Prevents missed questions
- Promotes easy, rapid documentation
- Makes documentation somewhat like data entry because it requires nurse to place checkmarks in boxes instead of writing narrative
- Poses chance that a significant piece of data may be missed because the checklist does not include the area of concern

INTEGRATED CUED CHECKLIST
- Combines assessment data with identified nursing diagnoses
- Helps cluster data, focuses on nursing diagnoses, assists in validating nursing diagnosis labels, and combines assessment with problem listing in one form
- Promotes use by different levels of caregivers, resulting in enhanced communication among the disciplines

NURSING MINIMUM DATA SET
- Comprises format commonly used in long-term care facilities
- Has a cued format that prompts nurse for specific criteria; usually computerized
- Includes specialized information, such as cognitive patterns, communication (hearing and vision) patterns, physical function and structural patterns, activity patterns, restorative care, and the like
- Meets the needs of multiple data users in the health care system
- Establishes comparability of nursing data across clinical populations, settings, geographic areas, and time

SOUTHEAST MISSOURI HOSPITAL	ADULT NURSING HEALTH HISTORY	Name: Sex: Phys:	Account #: Med Rec #: DOB: Age:

(May be completed by patient, family, or significant other)

Unable to take history ☐ Patient confused/unresponsive
☐ Patient not accompanied by family/significant other(s)   ☐ History taken from previous medical record

YES NO

HEALTH MANAGEMENT   COMMENTS
Barriers to learning:
☐ ☐ Vision problems: _____
☐ ☐ Hearing problems: _____
        Where do you live: ☐ home ☐ other _____
☐ ☐ Live alone _____
        Primary support person: _____
☐ ☐ Have you ever smoked? _____
        Packs per day _____ # Years _____ Date quit _____
☐ ☐ Drink alcohol? Drinks per day _____

NUTRITIONAL/METABOLIC
☐ ☐ Diet restrictions followed at home _____
☐ ☐ Undesired weight loss _____
☐ ☐ Undesired weight gain _____
☐ ☐ Recent loss of appetite _____
☐ ☐ Difficulty eating/swallowing _____
        ☐ Onset during the last 7 days _____
☐ ☐ Recent vomiting (more than 3 days) _____
☐ ☐ Have you ever had cancer _____
☐ ☐ Diabetes - For how long: _____
☐ ☐ Metal or foreign objects in body
        (i.e. shrapnel, metal slivers) _____
☐ ☐ Mechanical devices on or implanted
        in the body _____
☐ ☐ Medication pump   Company: _____
☐ ☐ Feeding tube   Company: _____

RESPIRATORY/CIRCULATORY
☐ ☐ Asthma or emphysema _____
☐ ☐ COPD _____
☐ ☐ Shortness of breath _____
☐ ☐ Taking breathing treatments _____
☐ ☐ Uses oxygen Company: _____
☐ ☐ Uses CPAP or other device Company: _____
☐ ☐ CHF (Congestive heart failure) _____
☐ ☐ Mitral valve prolapse _____
☐ ☐ Chest pain or heart attack _____
☐ ☐ Pacemaker _____
☐ ☐ Bleeding or bruising tendency _____

ELIMINATION
☐ ☐ Kidney or urinary problems _____
☐ ☐ Stomach or intestinal problems _____
☐ ☐ Uses a catheter _____
☐ ☐ Ostomy
Previous surgeries: (Type, date, and facility) _____
_____
_____

YES NO

SEXUALITY/REPRODUCTIVE
Female:
        Number of pregnancies _____
        Number of live births _____
        Date of last menstrual period _____
☐ ☐ Is there a chance you are pregnant _____

ACTIVITY/EXERCISE
☐ ☐ Arm/leg weakness/paralysis _____
        ☐ Onset during last 7 days
☐ ☐ Needs help with self care _____
        ☐ Onset during last 7 days
☐ ☐ Problems with walking _____
        ☐ Onset during last 7 days
☐ ☐ Recent fracture or surgical procedure involving the
        arms, legs or spine: _____
        Use of special equipment
☐ ☐ Walker   Company obtained from: _____
☐ ☐ Wheelchair Company obtained from: _____
☐ ☐ Cane   Company obtained from: _____
☐ ☐ Crutches   Company obtained from: _____

COGNITIVE/PERCEPTUAL
☐ ☐ Stroke _____
☐ ☐ Memory loss or confusion _____
☐ ☐ Difficulty speaking or communicating _____
        ☐ Onset during last 7 days
☐ ☐ Fainting spells or dizziness _____
☐ ☐ Convulsions, seizures or epilepsy _____
☐ ☐ Nervous or mental disorders _____
☐ ☐ Claustrophobia - If yes, how bad: _____

VALUE/BELIEF
☐ ☐ Is there anything in your religious or cultural belief that
        affects the care we provide or how we teach you?
        Explain: _____
☐ ☐ Would you like hospital chaplain to visit? _____
        Is there anything you would like to learn about your
        condition? Explain: _____
What are your goals for this hospitalization? _____
_____

INFECTIOUS DISEASE
☐ ☐ Confirmed HIV positive
☐ ☐ Ever had Hepatitis? Type: A B C Year: _____
☐ ☐ Ever had ☐ MRSA ☐ VRE   Year: _____
☐ ☐ Ever had Tuberculosis (TB)   Year: _____

ALLERGEN: DRUGS, LATEX, FOOD, TAPE

ALLERGEN	SYMPTOMS	ALLERGEN	SYMPTOMS

Signature of person completing this form: _____   Date: _____

FIGURE 6-1. Admission record. (Used with permission of Southeast Missouri Hospital, Cape Girardeau, MO.)

| SOUTHEAST MISSOURI HOSPITAL | ADULT NURSING HEALTH HISTORY | Name: | Account #:
Med Rec #: |

TO BE COMPLETED BY HOSPITAL STAFF

Family Physician: _____   Town: _____

Most Recent Hospitalization: (When and where) _____

☐ YES ☐ NO Nutritional status appears adequate?   ☐ YES ☐ NO Multiple bruising
☐ YES ☐ NO Patient is clean on admission?   ☐ YES ☐ NO Frequent, untreated injuries
☐ YES ☐ NO Is abuse or neglect suspected?   ☐ YES ☐ NO Pt/family makes appropriate eye contact

Receives		Needs		
yes	no	yes	no	
☐	☐	☐	☐	Nutrition Services _____
☐	☐	☐	☐	Discharge Planning _____ (Home Health, Hospice, Meals on Wheels, Home IV care, Homemaker Services, Home Oxygen, Equipment)
☐	☐	☐	☐	Social Services _____ (Nursing home placement, Financial Assistance, Transportation, Transfers, Rehab, Chemical Dependency
☐	☐	☐	☐	Rehab Services _____ (Occupational Therapy, Physical Therapy, Speech Therapy)
				PATIENT EDUCATION
☐	☐	☐	☐	Patient Education ☐ unstable diabetes ☐ diabetic needs ☐ pressure ulcers ☐ Other: _____
☐	☐	☐	☐	Cardiac Rehab ☐ Congestive Heart Failure... _____
☐	☐	☐	☐	Diet Instruction _____
☐	☐	☐	☐	Respiratory Therapy ☐ Asthma... _____
☐	☐	☐	☐	Pulmonary Rehab/Instruction _____

CURRENT MEDICATIONS, Include: Alternative Medications, Herbs, and Over-the-Counter Medications

NAME	DOSE/ROUTE/FREQUENCY	LAST DOSE	NAME	DOSE/ROUTE/FREQUENCY	LAST DOSE

MEDICATION
☐ Sent to pharmacy ☐ Sent home ☐ Not here

MEDICATION INFORMATION FROM
☐ Bottles
☐ Transfer Record
☐ Verbally
☐ Written List
☐ Other _____

PATIENT'S PHARMACY _____

_____   _____   Entered into Computer: _____
Staff Signature   Date   Date/Time

FIGURE 6-1. (CONTINUED)

PATIENT ASSESSMENT FLOWSHEET

INITIALS/SIGNATURE _____

_____

_____

_____

_____

Date _____

Addressograph

INITIAL ASSESSMENT	2300-0700 TIME/INITIALS _____	0700-1500 TIME/INITIALS _____	1500-2300 TIME/INITIALS _____
NUTRITION/ METABOLIC	SKIN: ☐ Dry ☐ Intact ☐ Warm ☐ Cold ☐ Other _____ Turgor: _____ ☐ N/V _____ TUBES: (feeding) _____ IV: Date Of Insertion: _____ SITE: _____ FLUIDS: _____ WOUNDS/DRSGS: _____	SKIN: ☐ Dry ☐ Intact ☐ Warm ☐ Cold ☐ Other _____ Turgor: _____ ☐ N/V _____ TUBES: (feeding) _____ IV: Date Of Insertion: _____ SITE: _____ FLUIDS: _____ WOUNDS/DRSGS: _____	SKIN: ☐ Dry ☐ Intact ☐ Warm ☐ Cold ☐ Other _____ Turgor: _____ ☐ N/V _____ TUBES: (feeding) _____ IV: Date Of Insertion: _____ SITE: _____ FLUIDS: _____ WOUNDS/DRSGS: _____
RESPIRATORY/ CIRCULATORY	BREATH SOUNDS: _____ RESPIRATIONS: _____ OXYGEN: _____ PULSE OX: _____ ☐ Cough _____ ☐ Sputum _____ APICAL PULSE: _____ ☐ Regular ☐ Irregular TELEMETRY: _____ NAILBED COLOR: ☐ Pink ☐ Pale ☐ Blue PEDAL PULSES: R ☐— ☐+ L ☐— ☐+ EDEMA: R ☐— ☐+ L ☐— ☐+ CALF TENDERNESS: R ☐— ☐+ L ☐— ☐+	BREATH SOUNDS: _____ RESPIRATIONS: _____ OXYGEN: _____ PULSE OX: _____ ☐ Cough _____ ☐ Sputum _____ APICAL PULSE: _____ ☐ Regular ☐ Irregular TELEMETRY: _____ NAILBED COLOR: ☐ Pink ☐ Pale ☐ Blue PEDAL PULSES: R ☐— ☐+ L ☐— ☐+ EDEMA: R ☐— ☐+ L ☐— ☐+ CALF TENDERNESS: R ☐— ☐+ L ☐— ☐+	BREATH SOUNDS: _____ RESPIRATIONS: _____ OXYGEN: _____ PULSE OX: _____ ☐ Cough _____ ☐ Sputum _____ APICAL PULSE: _____ ☐ Regular ☐ Irregular TELEMETRY: _____ NAILBED COLOR: ☐ Pink ☐ Pale ☐ Blue PEDAL PULSES: R ☐— ☐+ L ☐— ☐+ EDEMA: R ☐— ☐+ L ☐— ☐+ CALF TENDERNESS: R ☐— ☐+ L ☐— ☐+

FIGURE 6-2. Assessment flow sheet. (Used with permission of Southeast Missouri Hospital, Cape Girardeau, MO.)

PATIENT ASSESSMENT FLOWSHEET, Page 2

Addressograph

Date _____

INITIAL ASSESSMENT	2300-0700 TIME/INITIALS _____	0700-1500 TIME/INITIALS _____	1500-2300 TIME/INITIALS _____
ELIMINATION	ABDOMEN: ☐ Soft ☐ Firm ☐ Nondistended ☐ Distended BOWEL SOUNDS: ☐ Normoactive ☐ Hyperactive ☐ Hypoactive ☐ Absent LBM: _____ TUBES: _____ _____ _____ _____	ABDOMEN: ☐ Soft ☐ Firm ☐ Nondistended ☐ Distended BOWEL SOUNDS: ☐ Normoactive ☐ Hyperactive ☐ Hypoactive ☐ Absent LBM: _____ TUBES: _____ _____ _____ _____	ABDOMEN: ☐ Soft ☐ Firm ☐ Nondistended ☐ Distended BOWEL SOUNDS: ☐ Normoactive ☐ Hyperactive ☐ Hypoactive ☐ Absent LBM: _____ TUBES: _____ _____ _____ _____
ACTIVITY/ EXERCISE	MAE: ☐ Full ☐ Impaired _____ Fall Prevention _____	MAE: ☐ Full ☐ Impaired _____ Fall Prevention _____	MAE: ☐ Full ☐ Impaired _____ Fall Prevention _____
COGNITIVE/ PERCEPTUAL	LOC: ☐ Alert ☐ Lethargic ☐ Unresponsive ORIENTATION: ☐ Person ☐ Place ☐ Time ☐ Pain _____ _____ _____ _____	LOC: ☐ Alert ☐ Lethargic ☐ Unresponsive ORIENTATION: ☐ Person ☐ Place ☐ Time ☐ Pain _____ _____ _____ _____	LOC: ☐ Alert ☐ Lethargic ☐ Unresponsive ORIENTATION: ☐ Person ☐ Place ☐ Time ☐ Pain _____ _____ _____ _____
PLAN OF CARE	Discussed Plan of Care with: ☐ Patient ☐ Family/Significant Other(s) _____ _____	Discussed Plan of Care with: ☐ Patient ☐ Family/Significant Other(s) _____ _____	Discussed Plan of Care with: ☐ Patient ☐ Family/Significant Other(s) _____ _____
CARE PER STANDARD			
ONGOING PATIENT TEACHING (Time and Initial each entry)	☐ Video ☐ Handout/Booklet _____ ☐ Verbal - See Nurses Notes _____ _____ ☐ Pt/Family Response: _____ _____	☐ Video ☐ Handout/Booklet _____ ☐ Verbal - See Nurses Notes _____ _____ ☐ Pt/Family Response: _____ _____	☐ Video ☐ Handout/Booklet _____ ☐ Verbal - See Nurses Notes _____ _____ ☐ Pt/Family Response: _____ _____
EDUCATIONAL (To be completed on Admission and PRN)	Motivation: ☐ Appears Interested ☐ Seems Uninterested ☐ Denies Need for Education Factors Affecting Teaching: _____ _____	Motivation: ☐ Appears Interested ☐ Seems Uninterested ☐ Denies Need for Education Factors Affecting Teaching: _____ _____	Motivation: ☐ Appears Interested ☐ Seems Uninterested ☐ Denies Need for Education Factors Affecting Teaching: _____ _____

FIGURE 6-2. (CONTINUED)

the data are inappropriate for flow records (Fig. 6-3). Flow sheets streamline the documentation process and prevent needless repetition of data. Emphasis is placed on quality, not quantity, of documentation.

Focused or Specialty Area Assessment Form

Assessment forms that are focused on one major area of the body may be used in some institutions for clients who have a particular problem. Examples include cardiovascular or neurologic assessment documentation forms. In addition, forms may be customized. For example, a form may be used as a screening tool to assess specific concerns or risks, such as falling or skin problems. These forms are usually abbreviated versions of admission data sheets, with specific assessment data related to the purpose of the assessment (Fig. 6-4).

> 12/15/97 Client short of breath with labored respirations of 32/minute. Chest barrel shaped. Skin reddish. Decreased tactile fremitus percussed bilaterally. Bilateral hyperresonance. Respiratory and diaphragmatic excursion decreased. Has nonproductive cough, decreased breath sounds with wheezing and prolonged expirations. Client states, "I'm so short of breath."

FIGURE 6-3. Documentation of assessment findings on a narrative progress note.

Summary

Validation and documentation are two crucial aspects of nursing health assessment. Nurses need to concentrate on learning how to perform these two steps of assessment thoroughly and accurately.

Validation of data is verification of the assessment data that you have gathered from the client. It consists of deter-

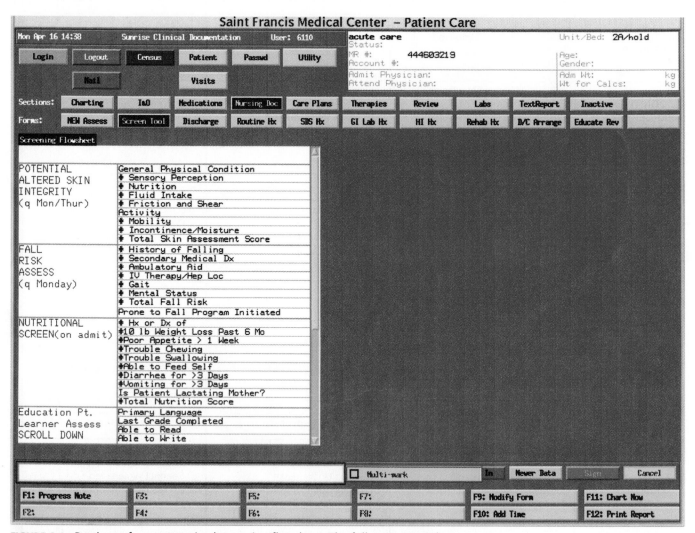

FIGURE 6-4. Portions of a computerized screening flowsheet. The full assessment document includes cells for systemic findings as well as functional data, such as nutrition, activities of daily living, and client education needs. (Used with permission of Saint Francis Medical Center, Cape Girardeau, MO.)

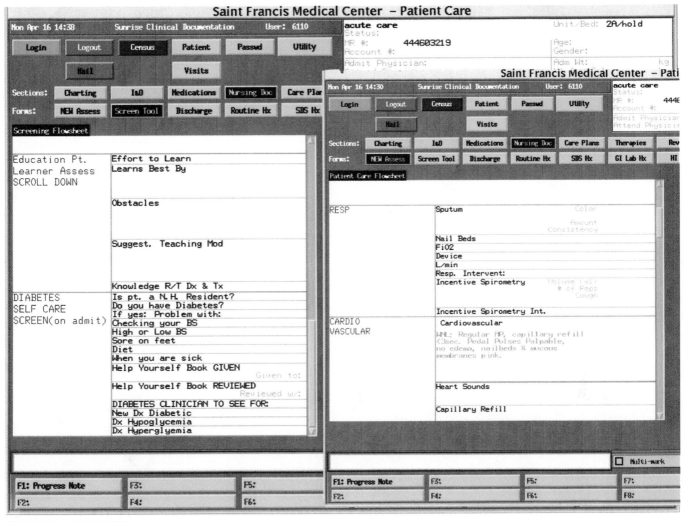

FIGURE 6-4. (CONTINUED)

mining which data require validation, implementing techniques to validate, and identifying areas that require further assessment data.

Documentation of data is the act of recording the client assessment findings. Nurses first need to understand the purpose of documentation, next learn which information to document, and then be aware of and follow the individual documentation guidelines of their particular health care facility. In addition, it is important for nurses to be familiar with the different documentation forms that are used in other health care institutions.

REFERENCES AND SELECTED READINGS

Allen, J., & Englebright, J. (2000). Patient-centered documentation: An effective and efficient use of clinical information systems. *Journal of Nursing Administration, 30* (2), 90–95.

Behrend, S. W. (1994). Documentation in the ambulatory setting. *Seminars in Oncology Nursing, 10* (4), 264–280.

Burke, L. J., & Murphy, J. (1995). *Charting by exception applications: Making it work in clinical settings.* Albany, NY: Delmar Publications.

Butler, M., & Bender, A. (1999). Intensive care unit bedside documentation systems: Realizing cost savings and quality improvements. *Computers in Nursing, 17* (1), 32–41.

Cameron, S., Regalado, M., Quitoles, M., & Ordonez, L. (1999). Harnessing technology: The creation of an electronic care management record in a social health maintenance organization. *Managed Care Quarterly, 7* (10), 11–15.

Carpenito, L. J. (1999). *Nursing care plans and documentation: Nursing diagnoses and collaborative problems* (3rd ed.). Philadelphia: Lippincott Williams & Wilkins.

Eggland, E. T., & Heinemann, D. S. (1994). *Nursing documentation: Charting, recording, and reporting.* Philadelphia: J. B. Lippincott.

Joint Commission for the Accreditation of Healthcare Organizations. (1999). *Mastering documentation* (2nd ed.). Spring House, PA: Springhouse Corp.

————. (1994). *UPDATE. Accreditation manual for hospitals.* Chicago: Author.

Marrellin, T. M. (1996). *Nursing documentation handbook.* St. Louis: C. V. Mosby.

McManus, B. (2000). A move to electronic patient records in the community: A qualitative case study of a clinical data collection system. *Topics in Health Information Management, 20* (4), 23–37.

Stephens, S., & Mason, S. (1999). Putting it together: A documentation system that works. *Nursing Management, 30* (3), 43–47.

For additional information on this book, be sure to visit http://connection.lww.com.

Using Diagnostic Reasoning Skills to Analyze Data

IDENTIFY

Cluster

Infer

Propose diagnoses

Check

Confirm / Rule out

Document

7

Data analysis is often referred to as the diagnostic phase because the end result or purpose of this phase is the identification of a nursing diagnosis (wellness, actual, or risk), collaborative problem, or need for referral to another health care professional.

Analysis of Data and Critical Thinking—Step Two of the Nursing Process

As the second step or phase of the nursing process, data analysis is a very difficult step because the nurse is required to use diagnostic reasoning skills to interpret data accurately. Diagnostic reasoning is a form of critical thinking. Because of the complex nature of nursing as both a science and an art, the nurse must think critically—in a rational, self-directed, intelligent, and purposeful manner.

Critical thinking is the way in which the nurse processes information using knowledge, past experiences, intuition, and cognitive abilities to formulate conclusions or diagnoses. Several characteristics must be developed to think critically. An open mind and exploration of alternatives are essential when making judgments and plans. Judgments and ideas are supported by sound rationale; hurried decisions are to be avoided. The critical thinker reflects on thoughts and gathers more information when necessary. Then, too, the critical thinker uses each clinical experience to learn new information and to add to the knowledge base. Another important aspect of critical thinking involves awareness of human interactions and the environment, which provide cues and directly influence decisions and judgments (Display 7-1). Ask yourself the following questions to determine whether you are a critical thinker:

1. Do you reserve your final opinion or judgment until you have collected more or all of the information?
2. Do you support your opinion or comments with supporting data, sound rationale, and literature?
3. Do you explore and consider other alternatives before making a decision?

DISPLAY 7-1. Essential Elements of Critical Thinking

- Keep an open mind.
- Use rationale to support opinions or decisions.
- Reflect on thoughts before reaching a conclusion.
- Use past clinical experiences to build knowledge.
- Acquire an adequate knowledge base that continues to build.
- Be aware of the interactions of others.
- Be aware of the environment.

---

4. Can you distinguish between a fact, opinion, cue, or inference?
5. Do you ask your client for more information or clarification when you do not understand?
6. Do you validate your information and judgments with experts in the field?
7. Do you use your past knowledge and experiences to analyze data?
8. Do you try to avoid biases or preconceived ways of thinking?
9. Do you try to learn from past mistakes in your judgments?
10. Are you open to the fact that you may not always be right?

If you answered "yes" to most of these questions, you have already started to develop a critical thinking mindset. Many books (some with practice exercises) are available on how to think critically as a nurse. Such books can help the nurse learn, and continue to develop, critical thinking skills.

The Diagnostic Reasoning Process

Before you begin analyzing data, make sure you have accurately performed the steps of the assessment phase of the nursing process (collection and organization of assessment data, validation of data, and documentation of data). This information will have a profound effect on the conclusions you reach in the analysis step of the nursing process.

If you are confident of your work during the assessment phase, you are ready to analyze your data—the diagnostic phase of the nursing process. This phase consists of the following essential components: grouping and organizing data, validating data and comparing the data with norms, clustering data to make inferences, generating possible hypotheses regarding the client's problems, formulating a professional clinical judgment, and validating the judgment with the client. These basic components have been organized in various ways to break the process of diagnostic reasoning into easily understood steps. Regardless of how the information is organized, or the title of the steps, diagnostic reasoning always consists of these basic components.

Seven distinct steps have been developed for this text to provide a clear, concise explanation of how to perform data analysis. Each of these steps is described in detail. In addition, these seven steps are used throughout the text in the Part Three: Analysis of Data sections of the assessment chapters (see Analysis of Data Throughout Health Assessment in Nursing later in this chapter).

STEP ONE—IDENTIFY ABNORMAL DATA AND STRENGTHS

Identifying abnormal findings and strengths requires the nurse to have and use a knowledge base of anatomy and physiology, psychology, and sociology. In addition, collected assessment data should be compared with findings in reliable charts and reference resources that provide standards and values for physical and psychological norms (ie, height, nutritional requirements, growth and development). Additionally, the nurse should have a basic knowledge of risk factors for the client. Risk factors are based on client data such as gender, age, cultural background, and occupation. Therefore, the nurse needs to have access to both the data supplied by the client and the known risk factors for specific diseases or disorders.

The nurse's knowledge of anatomy and physiology, psychology, and sociology; use of reference materials; and attention to risk factors help to identify strengths, risks, and abnormal findings. Identified strengths are used in formulating wellness diagnoses. Identified potential weaknesses are used in formulating risk diagnoses, and abnormal findings are used in formulating actual nursing diagnoses.

STEP TWO—CLUSTER DATA

During step two, the nurse looks at the identified abnormal findings and strengths for cues that are related. Both abnormal cues and strength cues should be clustered, and a particular nursing framework should be used as a guide when possible. The following is an example of how to cluster data after assessing a client who reports the subjective information defined below and whose physical examination discloses the objective findings listed below:

Identified Abnormal Data and Strengths: Subjective

- "Hair falling out in chunks"
- Red rash on face and chest, "looks like a bad case of acne"
- "So ugly"
- Concerned that she may lose her job because of how she looks
- Surfer—out in the sun all day on weekends—minimal use of sunscreen
- Sought out occupational health nurse

Identified Abnormal Data and Strengths: Objective

- Anxious appearing
- Diagnosed with discoid lupus erythematosus
- Red, raised plaques on face, neck, shoulders, back, and chest
- Patchy alopecia

A cue cluster based on these data would be:

- Rash on face, neck, chest, and back
- Patchy alopecia
- "So ugly"

While you are clustering the data during this step, you may find that certain cues are pointing toward a problem but that more data are needed to support the problem. For example, a client may have a nonproductive cough with labored respirations at a rate of 24/min. However, you have gathered no data on the status of breath sounds. In such a situation, you would need to assess the client's breath sounds to formulate an appropriate nursing diagnosis or collaborative problem.

STEP THREE—DRAW INFERENCES

Step three requires the nurse to write down hunches about each cue cluster. For example, based on the cue cluster presented in step two—rash on face, neck, chest, and back; patchy alopecia; "so ugly"—you would write down what you think these data are saying and determine whether it is something that the nurse can treat independently. Your hunch about this data cluster might be "Changes in physical appearance are affecting self-perception." This is something for which the nurse would intervene and treat independently. Therefore, the nurse would move to step four—analysis of data to formulate a nursing diagnosis.

However, if the inference you draw from a cue cluster suggests the need for both medical and nursing interventions to resolve the problem, you would attempt to generate collaborative problems. Collaborative problems are defined as "certain physiological complications that nurses monitor to detect their onset or changes in status; nurses manage collaborative problems using physician-prescribed and nursing-prescribed interventions to minimize the complications of events" (Carpenito, 2000).

Collaborative problems are equivalent in importance to nursing diagnoses but represent the interdependent or collaborative role of nursing. A list of collaborative problems is given in Appendix C.

Another purpose of step three is the referral of identified problems for which the nurse cannot prescribe definitive treatment. Referring can be defined as connecting clients with other professionals and resources. For example, if the collaborative problem for which the nurse is monitoring occurs, an immediate referral to the client's physician or nurse practitioner is necessary for implementing medical treatment. Another example may be a diabetic client who is having trouble understanding the exchange diet. Although the nurse has knowledge in this area, referral to a dietitian can provide the client with updated materials and allow the nurse more time to deal with client problems within the nursing domain. Another important reason for referral is the identification or suspicion of a medical problem based on the subjective and objective data collected. In such cases, referral to the client's physician, nurse practitioner, or another specialist is necessary.

The referral process differs from health care setting to health care setting. Sometimes, the nurse makes a direct referral; other times, it may be the policy to notify the nurse practitioner or physician who, if they cannot intervene, will make the referral. To save time and to provide high-quality care for the client, make sure you are familiar with the referral process used in your health care setting.

STEP FOUR—PROPOSE POSSIBLE NURSING DIAGNOSES

If resolution of the situation requires primarily nursing interventions, you would hypothesize and generate possible nursing diagnoses. The nursing diagnoses may be wellness diagnoses, risk diagnoses, or actual diagnoses (Kelley, Frisch & Avant, 1995). A wellness diagnosis indicates that the client has the opportunity for enhancement of a health state. There are occasions when clients are ready to improve an already healthy level of function. When such an opportunity exists, the nurse can support the client's movement toward greater health and wellness by identifying "opportunities for enhancement."

A risk diagnosis indicates the client does not currently have the problem but is at high risk for developing it (ie, Risk for Impaired Skin Integrity related to immobility, poor nutrition, and incontinence).

An actual nursing diagnosis indicates the client is currently experiencing the stated problem or has a dysfunctional pattern (ie, Impaired Skin Integrity: reddened area on right buttocks). An example of how to generate possible nursing diagnoses from a cue cluster: The cue cluster from step two was determined to be something for which the nurse could intervene. Changes in physical appearance are affecting self-perception. Possible nursing diagnoses based on this inference include (1) Body Image Disturbance related to changes in physical appearance and (2) Risk for Ineffective Individual Coping related to changes in physical appearance and newly diagnosed disease. Table 7-1 provides a comparison of wellness, risk, and actual nursing

diagnoses. Appendix C provides a list of common nursing diagnoses.

STEP FIVE—CHECK FOR DEFINING CHARACTERISTICS

At this point in analyzing the data, the nurse must check for defining characteristics for the data clusters and hypothesized diagnoses in order to choose the most accurate diagnoses and delete those diagnoses that are not valid or accurate for the client. This step is often difficult because diagnostic labels overlap, making it hard to identify the most appropriate diagnosis. For example, the diagnostic categories of Impaired Gas Exchange, Ineffective Airway Clearance, and Ineffective Breathing Patterns all reflect respiratory problems, but each is used to describe a very different human response pattern and set of defining characteristics.

Reference texts such as North American Nursing Diagnosis Association (NANDA) *Nursing Diagnoses: Definitions and Classifications 2001–2002* can assist the nurse to determine when and when not to use each nursing diagnostic category (NANDA, 2001). It assists with ruling out invalid diagnoses and selecting valid diagnoses. Thus, both the definition and defining characteristics should be compared with the client's set of data (cues) to make sure that the correct diagnoses are chosen for the client. For an example of how to check for defining characteristics, consider the two nursing diagnoses hypothesized in step four. For the first nursing diagnosis, a major defining characteristic is "verbal negative response to actual change in structure." A minor defining characteristic is negative feelings. There are no major or minor defining characteristics for the second nursing diagnosis.

STEP SIX—CONFIRM OR RULE OUT

If the cue cluster data do not meet the defining characteristics, you can rule out that particular diagnosis. If the cue

---

TABLE 7-1. Comparison of Wellness, Risk, and Actual Nursing Diagnoses

	Wellness Diagnoses	Risk Diagnoses	Actual Diagnoses
Client status	State of harmony and balance	State of risk for identified problem	State of health problems
Format for stating	Opportunity to enhance . . . or for enhanced	"Risk for . . . ."	Nursing diagnoses and "related to" clause
Examples	Opportunity to enhance body image	Risk for Altered Body Image	Altered Body Image related to hand wound that is not healing
	Opportunity to enhance family processes	Risk for Altered Family Processes	Altered Family Processes related to hospitalization of patient
	Opportunity to enhance effective breast-feeding	Risk for Ineffective Breast-feeding	Ineffective Breast-feeding related to poor mother–infant attachment
	Opportunity to enhance skin integrity	Risk for Impaired Skin Integrity	Impaired Skin Integrity related to immobility

cluster data do meet the defining characteristics, the diagnosis should be verified with the client and other health care professionals who are caring for the client. Tell the client what you perceive his or her diagnosis to be. Often, nursing diagnosis terminology is difficult for the client to understand. For example, you would not tell the client that you believe that he has Impaired Nutrition: Less Than Body Requirements. Instead, you might say that you believe that current nutritional intake is not adequate to promote healing of body tissues. Then you would ask the client if this seemed to be an accurate statement of the problem. It is essential that the client understand the problem so treatment can be properly implemented. If the client is not in a coherent state of mind to help validate the problem, you can consult with family members or significant others or even other health care professionals.

Validation is also important with the client who has a collaborative problem or who requires a referral. If the client has a collaborative problem, you need to inform him or her about which signs you are monitoring. For example, you might tell the client you will be monitoring blood pressure and level of consciousness every 30 minutes for the next several hours. It is also important to collaborate with the client regarding referrals to determine what is needed to resolve the problem and to discuss possible resources to help the client. List possible resources (including availability and cost) for the client when possible. Help the client make the contact by phone or letter. Then follow up to determine whether the referral was made and whether the client was connected to the appropriate resources.

STEP SEVEN—DOCUMENT CONCLUSIONS

Be sure to document all of your professional judgments and the data that support those judgments. Documentation of data collection before analysis is described in Chapter 6. Guidelines for correctly documenting nursing diagnoses, collaborative problems, and referrals are described in the sections that follow.

Nursing Diagnoses and Collaborative Problems

Nursing diagnoses are often documented and worded in different formats. The most useful formats for wellness, risk, and actual nursing diagnoses are described below.

WELLNESS NURSING DIAGNOSES

Wellness diagnoses represent those situations in which the client does not have a problem, but is at a point where he or she can attain a higher level of health. Only eight wellness nursing diagnoses labels are on the NANDA list (see Appendix B). When documenting these diagnoses, it is best to use the following format:

Opportunity to enhance + diagnostic label + related to (r/t) + etiology + as manifested by (AMB) + symptoms (defining characteristics)

Example: Opportunity to Enhance Effective Breast-feeding r/t confident mother, full-term healthy infant, and normal breast structure AMB infant contentment after feeding and mother's request to continue to breast-feed

Wellness diagnoses other than those for which NANDA has labels may be formulated by using the following format:

Opportunity to enhance + NANDA problem-oriented diagnostic label minus the modifiers + r/t + etiology + AMB + symptoms (defining characteristics)

Example: Opportunity to Enhance Parenting r/t effective bonding with children and effective basic parenting skills AMB parent's verbalized concern to continue effective parenting skills during child's illness

RISK NURSING DIAGNOSES

A risk diagnosis describes a situation in which an actual diagnosis will most likely occur if the nurse does not intervene. In this case, the client does not have any symptoms or defining characteristics that are manifested, and thus a shorter statement is sufficient:

Risk for + diagnostic label + related to (r/t) + etiology

Example: Risk for Infection r/t presence of dirty knife wound, leukopenia, and lack of client knowledge of how adequately to care for the wound

ACTUAL NURSING DIAGNOSES

The most useful format for an actual nursing diagnosis is:

NANDA label (for problem) + r/t + etiology + AMB + defining characteristics

Example: Fatigue r/t an increase in job demands and personal stress AMB client's statements of feeling exhausted all of the time and inability to perform usual work and home responsibilities (eg, cooking, cleaning).

Shorter formats are often used to describe client problems. However, this format provides all of the necessary information and provides the reader with the clearest and most accurate description of the client's problem.

COLLABORATIVE PROBLEMS AND REFERRALS

Collaborative problems should be documented as Potential Complication (PC): _____ (what the problem is). Nursing goals for the collaborative problem should be documented, as well as which parameters the nurse must monitor and how often they should be monitored. The nurse also needs to indicate when the physician or nurse practitioner should be notified and to identify nursing interventions to help prevent the complication from occurring and nursing interventions to be initiated if a change occurs. If a referral is indicated, document the problem (or suspected problem), the need for immediate referral, and to whom the client is being referred. The major conclusions of a nursing assessment are compared in Table 7-2.

Developing Diagnostic Reasoning Expertise and Avoiding Pitfalls

A diagnosis or judgment is considered to be highly accurate if the diagnosis is consistent with all of the cues, supported by highly relevant cues, and as precise as possible (Lunney, 1990). Developing expertise with making professional judgments comes with accumulation of both knowledge and experience. One does not become an expert diagnostician overnight. It is a process that develops with time and practice. A beginning nurse attempts to make accurate diagnoses but, because of a lack of knowledge and experience, often finds that he or she has made diagnostic errors. Experts have an advantage because they know when exceptions can be applied to the rules that the novice is so accustomed to using and applying. Beginning nurses tend

to see things as right or wrong, whereas experts realize there are shades of gray or areas between right and wrong. Novices also tend to focus on details and may miss the big picture, whereas experts have a broader perspective in examining situations.

Although beginning nurses lack the depth of knowledge and expertise that expert nurses have, they can still learn to increase their diagnostic accuracy by becoming aware of, and avoiding, the several pitfalls of diagnosing. These pitfalls decrease the reliability of cues and decrease diagnostic accuracy. There are two sets of pitfalls—those that occur during the assessment phase and those that occur during the analysis of data phase.

The first set of pitfalls is discussed in detail in Chapter 6. They include too many or too few data, unreliable or invalid data, and an insufficient number of cues available to support the diagnoses.

The second set of pitfalls occurs during the analysis phase. Cues may be clustered yet unrelated to each other. For example, the client may be very quiet and appear depressed. A nurse may assume the client is grieving because her husband died a year ago, but the client may just be fatigued because of all the diagnostic tests she has just undergone.

Another common error is quickly diagnosing a client without hypothesizing several diagnoses. For example, a

TABLE 7-2. Major Conclusions of Assessment

	Wellness Nursing Diagnosis	Actual Problem Nursing Diagnosis	Potential Problem Nursing Diagnosis	Collaborative Problem	Problem for Referral
Who identifies the concern?	Nurse	Nurse	Nurse	Nurse or other provider	Nurse or other provider
Who deals with the concern?	Nurse (independent practice)	Nurse (independent practice)	Nurse (independent practice)	Nurse (interdependent practice)	Other provider
What content knowledge is needed?	Nursing science Sciences Basic studies	Nursing science Sciences Basic studies	Nursing science Sciences Basic studies	Nursing science Sciences Basic studies Domain of other providers	Nursing science Sciences Basic studies Domain of other providers
What minimum work experience is needed?	Average	Average	Better than average	Average	Average
What does first part of conclusion statement look like?	Opportunity to enhance . . .	Taxonomy label or other descriptive label	Usually taxonomy label of "Risk for . . ."	Potential Complication	N/A
Are related factors included?	Yes (but not mandatory)	Yes, unless unknown	Yes (mandatory)	Sometimes	N/A
What might complete statement look like?	Opportunity to Enhance Effective Breast-feeding r/t confident mother, full-term healthy infant, and normal breast structure	Self-Esteem Disturbance r/t knowledge deficit, ineffective coping as new mother, and loss of job	Risk for Impaired Skin Integrity r/t immobility, incontinence and fragile skin	PC: Rejection of kidney transplant	Unsafe housing (referral is necessary)

nurse may assume that a readmitted diabetic client with hyperglycemia has a knowledge deficit concerning the exchange diet. However, further exploration of data reveals that the client has low self-esteem and feelings of powerlessness and hopelessness in controlling a labile, fluctuating blood glucose level. The nurse's goal is to avoid making diagnoses too quickly without taking sufficient time to process the data.

Another pitfall to avoid is incorrectly wording the diagnostic statement. This leads to an inaccurate picture of the client for others caring for him or her. Finally, do not overlook consideration of the client's cultural background when analyzing data. Clients from other cultures may be misdiagnosed because the defining characteristics and labels for specific diagnoses do not accurately describe the human responses in their culture. Therefore, it is essential to look closely at cultural norms and responses for various clients.

Analysis of Data Throughout Health Assessment in Nursing

The whole purpose of assessing a client's health status is to analyze the subjective and objective data that are collected. Therefore, because analysis of data is such a natural next step, the importance of illustrating the link between assessment and analysis for each body part or system assessment chapter is apparent. In the clinical assessment chapters of this textbook, Part Three: Analysis of Data was developed to help the reader visualize, understand, and practice analyzing data (diagnostic reasoning).

Part Three: Analysis of Data consists of four sections. The first section, called Diagnostic Reasoning: Key Steps, contains a succinct definition of each of the seven key steps of analysis that were described earlier in this chapter. Repeating the definitions throughout the text enables the reader to become familiar with each step of diagnostic reasoning and serves as a handy reference tool while formulating nursing diagnoses.

The second section is called Diagnostic Reasoning: Possible Conclusions. This section contains possible nursing diagnoses, collaborative problems, and referrals for the material covered in the particular chapter. This list is presented so that the reader becomes familiar with common possible conclusions seen with the particular body part or system. It also provides a convenient list for the reader to refer to while working through the case study in section three or completing the critical thinking exercise in the study guide/laboratory manual that is a companion piece for the textbook.

The third section is entitled Diagnostic Reasoning: Case Study. This section consists of a case study followed by the seven key steps of analysis and the accompanying data for each step based on the case study. This section illustrates exactly how to analyze data and which information to include in each of the seven key steps of diagnostic reasoning. It helps the reader grasp the concepts of critical thinking and data analysis.

A critical thinking exercise, based on an actual case, is presented in the study guide/laboratory manual. Blank spaces are provided under each key step. This exercise encourages the reader to build critical thinking and data analysis skills. The reader can do this by working through the seven key steps of diagnostic reasoning based on the information in the case study and by documenting data and conclusions in the space provided.

Summary

Analysis of data is the second step of the nursing process. It is the purpose and end result of assessment. It is often called the diagnostic phase because the purpose of this phase is identification of nursing diagnoses, collaborative problems, or need for referral to another health care professional. The thought process required for data analysis is called diagnostic reasoning—a form of critical thinking. Therefore, it is important to develop the characteristics of critical thinking in order to analyze the data as accurately as possible.

Seven key steps have been developed for this text that clearly explain how to analyze assessment data. These steps include:

1. Identify abnormal data and strengths
2. Cluster data
3. Draw inferences
4. Propose possible nursing diagnoses
5. Check for presence of defining characteristics
6. Confirm or rule out
7. Document conclusions

Keep in mind that developing expertise in formulating nursing diagnoses requires much knowledge and experience as a nurse. However, the novice nurse can learn to increase diagnostic accuracy by becoming aware of, and avoiding, the pitfalls of diagnosing.

Because analysis of data is so closely linked to assessment, a special part on analysis of data is included in each body part or system assessment chapter.

REFERENCES AND SELECTED READINGS

American Nurses Association. (1991). *Standards of clinical nursing practice*. Kansas City, MO: Author.

Anderson, L. (1998). Exploring the diagnostic reasoning process to improve advanced physical assessments. *Perspectives, 22*(1), 17–22.

Aquilino, M. L., & Keenan, G. (2000). Having our say: Nursing's standardized nomenclatures. *American Journal of Nursing, 100*(7), 33–38.

Bond, E. O., & Urick, J. (1999). Nursing diagnosis at work. From metaphors to nursing diagnoses. *Nursing Diagnosis: The Journal of Nursing Language and Classification, 10*(2), 81–83.

Carpenito, L. J. (2000). *Nursing diagnosis: Application to clinical practice* (8th ed.). Philadelphia: Lippincott Williams & Wilkins.

Collier, I. C., McCash, K. E., & Bartram, J. M. (1996). *Writing nursing diagnoses: A critical thinking approach.* St. Louis: C. V. Mosby.

Duchscher, J. E. B. (1999). Catching the wave: Understanding the concept of critical thinking. *Journal of Advanced Nursing, 29*(3), 577–583.

Glaser, V. (2000). Five diagnostic controversies. *Patient Care, 34*(3), 179–182, 185–186, 191–194.

Green, C. (2000). *Critical thinking in nursing.* Upper Saddle River, NJ: Prentice Hall.

Johnson, M., Bulechek, G., McCloskey, J., Maas, M., & Moorhead, S. (2001). *Nursing diagnoses, outcomes and interventions: NANDA, NOC, and NIC linkages.* St. Louis: C. V. Mosby.

Kelley, J., Frisch, N., & Avant, K. (1995). A trifocal model of nursing diagnoses: Wellness reinforced. *Nursing Diagnosis, 6*(3), 123–128.

Lunney, M. (1990). Accuracy of nursing diagnoses: Concept development. *Nursing Diagnosis, 1*(1), 12–17.

McCloskey, J. C., & Bulechek, G. M. (2000). *Nursing interventions classification (NIC)* (2nd ed.). St. Louis: C. V. Mosby.

North American Nursing Diagnosis Association. (2001). *Nursing diagnoses: Definitions and classification, 2001–2002* (4th ed.). Philadelphia: NANDA.

Rubenfeld, M. G., & Scheffer, B. K. (1999). *Critical thinking in nursing: An interactive approach* (2nd ed.). Philadelphia: Lippincott Williams & Wilkins.

Wilkinson, J. M. (1996). *Nursing process: A critical thinking approach* (2nd ed.). St. Louis: C. V. Mosby.

For additional information on this book, be sure to visit http://connection.lww.com.

Nursing Assessment
of the Adult

General Survey and Nutritional Assessment

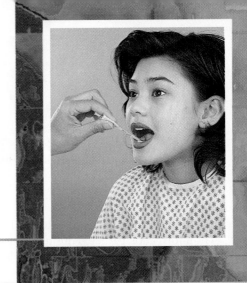

8

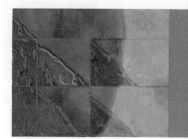

Preassessment Overview

The general survey is the first step in the assessment process. The information gathered during the general survey provides clues about the overall health of the client. The general survey includes:

Impression of the client: This requires your skills of objective observation concerning the client's appearance, mobility, body build, and behavior.

Vital signs: Pulse, respiration, blood pressure and temperature are the body's indicators of health. Usually when a vital sign (or signs) is abnormal, something is wrong in at least one of the body systems.

Anthropometric measurements including nutritional status: This part of the general survey includes measuring the client's height and wrist circumference to determine body frame; weighing the client to determine body mass index and ideal body weight; and measuring the waist-to-hip ratio, mid-arm circumference (MAC), triceps skinfold (TSF) thickness, and mid-arm muscle circumference (MAMC). The information from these measurements presents a good picture of overall physical and nutritional health and helps the examiner determine where to focus during the body systems assessment. Keep in mind how culture and ethnic variations may affect your impressions.

Impression of the Client

The first time you meet a client, you tend to remember certain obvious characteristics. These characteristics form your impression of the client. This part of the examination consists of a systematic examination and recording of these general impressions of the client. If possible, try to observe the client and environment quickly before interacting with the client. This gives you the opportunity to "see" the client before he or she assumes a social face or behavior and allows you to glimpse any distress, sadness, or pain before the client covers it up.

When you meet the client for the first time, observe any significant abnormalities in the client's skin color, dress, hygiene, posture, gait, and body build. If you observe abnormalities, you may need to perform an in-depth assessment of the body area that appears to be affected (eg, an unusual gait may prompt you to perform a detailed mus-

culoskeletal assessment). You should also generally assess the client's level of consciousness, level of comfort, behavior, body movements, affect, facial expression, speech and mental acuity. If you detect any abnormalities during your general impression examination, you will need to do an in-depth mental status examination. This examination is described in Chapter 23. Additional preparation involves creating a comfortable, nonthreatening atmosphere to relieve anxiety in the client. You do not need any special equipment.

Vital Signs

The nurse usually begins the "hands-on" physical examination by taking vital signs. This is a common, nonthreatening physical assessment procedure that most clients are accustomed to. Vital signs provide data that reflect the status of several body systems, including but not limited to the cardiovascular, neurologic, peripheral vascular, and respiratory systems. Measure the client's temperature first, followed by pulse, respirations, and blood pressure. Measuring the temperature puts the client at ease and causes him or her to remain still for several minutes. This is important because pulse, respirations, and blood pressure are influenced by anxiety and activity. By easing the client's anxiety and keeping him or her still, you help to increase the accuracy of the data.

TEMPERATURE

For the body to function on a cellular level, a core body temperature between 36.5°C and 37.7°C (96.0°F and 99.9°F, orally) must be maintained. An approximate reading of core body temperature can be taken at various anatomic sites. None of these is completely accurate; they are simply a good reflection of the core body temperature.

Several factors may cause normal variations in the core body temperature. Strenuous exercise, stress, and ovulation can raise temperature. Body temperature is lowest early in the morning (4 to 6 AM) and highest late in the evening (8 PM to midnight). Hypothermia (lower than 36.5°C or 96.0°F) may be seen in prolonged exposure to the cold, hypoglycemia, hypothyroidism, or starvation. Hyperthermia (higher than 38.0°C or 100°F) may be seen in viral or bacterial infections, malignancies, trauma, and various blood, endocrine, and immune disorders.

In the older adult, temperature may range from 95.0°F to 97.5°F. Therefore, the older client may not have an obviously elevated temperature with an infection or be considered hypothermic below 96°F.

PULSE

A shock wave is produced when the heart contracts and forcefully pumps blood out of the ventricles into the aorta. The shock wave travels along the fibers of the arteries and is commonly called the *arterial* or *peripheral pulse*. The body has many arterial pulse sites. One of them—the radial pulse—gives a good overall picture of the client's health status. Several characteristics should be assessed when measuring the radial pulse—rate, rhythm, amplitude and contour, and elasticity.

Of the various characteristics, amplitude can be quantified as follows:

1+ Thready or weak (easy to obliterate)
2+ Normal (obliterate with moderate pressure);
3+ Bounding (unable to obliterate or requires very firm pressure)

If abnormalities are noted during assessment of the radial pulse, further assessment should be performed. For more information on assessing pulses and abnormal pulse findings, refer to Chapters 16 and 17.

RESPIRATIONS

The respiratory rate and character are additional clues to the client's overall health status. Respirations can be easily observed without alerting the client by watching chest movement before removing the stethoscope after you have completed counting the apical beat. Notable characteristics of respiration are rate, rhythm, and depth.

BLOOD PRESSURE

Blood pressure reflects the pressure that is exerted on the walls of the arteries. This pressure varies with the cardiac cycle, reaching a high point with systole and a low point with diastole (Fig. 8-1). Therefore, blood pressure is a measurement of the pressure of the blood in the arteries when the ventricles are contracted (systolic blood pressure) and when the ventricles are relaxed (diastolic blood pressure). Blood pressure is expressed as the ratio of the systolic pressure over the diastolic pressure. A client's blood pressure is determined by several factors:

- *Cardiac output*—Blood pressure increases with increased cardiac output and decreases with decreased cardiac output.

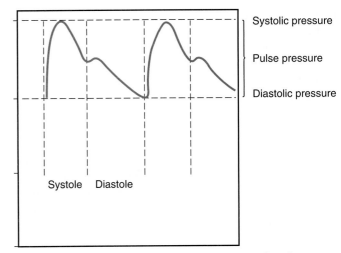

FIGURE 8-1. Blood pressure measurement identifies the amount of pressure in the arteries when the ventricles of the heart contract (systole) and when they relax (diastole).

- *Distensibility of the arteries*—Blood pressure increases when more effort is required to push blood through stiffened arteries.
- *Blood volume*—Blood pressure increases with increased volume and decreases with decreased volume.
- *Blood velocity*—Blood pressure increases when blood flow is slowed due to resistance and decreases when blood flow meets no resistance.
- *Blood viscosity (thickness)*—Blood pressure increases when the blood is thickened and decreases with thinning of the blood.

A client's blood pressure will normally vary throughout the day due to external influences. These include the time of day, caffeine or nicotine intake, exercise, emotions, pain, and temperature. The difference between systolic and diastolic pressure is termed the *pulse pressure*. The pulse pressure should be determined after the blood pressure is measured because it reflects the stroke volume—the volume of blood ejected with each heart beat.

Blood pressure may also vary depending on the position of the body and of the arm. Blood pressure in a normal person who is standing is usually slightly higher to compensate for the effects of gravity. Blood pressure in a normal reclining person is slightly lower because of decreased resistance.

Nutritional Assessment and Anthropometric Measurements

Anthropometric measurements are used to evaluate the client's physical growth, development, and nutritional status. First, the client's height and wrist circumferences are measured to determine frame size to use to compare to standard tables and norms. The client is then weighed, and formulas are used to determine his or her ideal body weight and body mass index. Then the waist-to-hip ratio may be calculated to estimate the client's risk for development of obesity-related diseases.

The client's mid-arm circumference is measured to assess skeletal muscle mass. Next, the triceps skinfold is measured to evaluate subcutaneous fat stores. Finally, the mid-arm circumference and triceps skinfold are used in a formula to calculate the mid-arm muscle circumference to evaluate muscle reserve stores. These measurements are also used to evaluate the client's nutritional status. Additional nutritional data are collected during the complete health history and during assessment of the skin, mouth, thyroid, abdomen, lungs, heart, and neurologic systems.

GENERAL STATUS

The nutrition assessment should begin with questions regarding the client's dietary habits. Questions should solicit information about average daily intake of food and fluids, types and quantities consumed, where and when food is eaten, and any conditions or diseases that affect intake or absorption. Collection of these data can add to the evaluation of the client's risk factors as well as point to health education needs. A variety of tools for assessing food habits and nutrition are available. Among them are checklists to use for nutritional screening (Display 8-1), the U.S. Department of Agriculture Food Guide Pyramid (see also Chapter 4), and other food pyramids, such as those for a traditional Asian diet and a traditional Latin American diet (Fig. 8-2).

MALNUTRITION AND BIOCHEMICAL INDICATORS

Certain diseases, disorders, or lifestyle behaviors can place clients at risk for malnutrition, and malnutrition can exacerbate or facilitate disease processes. The following is a selected list of risk factors:

- Lowest socioeconomic status whereby nutritious foods are unaffordable
- Lifestyle of long work hours and obtaining one or more meals from a fast-food chain or vending machine
- Poor food choices by both adults and teens, including lots of fatty or fried meats, sugary foods, but few fruits and vegetables
- Chronic dieting, particularly with fad diets, to meet perceived societal norms for weight and appearance
- Chronic diseases (eg, Crohn's disease, cirrhosis, cancer, or diabetes) that may interfere with absorption or use of nutrients
- Dental and other factors, such as difficulty chewing, loss of taste sensation, depression

---

DISPLAY 8-1. Speedy Checklist for Nutritional Health

Some warning signs of poor nutritional health are noted in this checklist. Use it to find out if your client is at nutritional risk. Read the statements below. Circle the number in the yes column for those that apply to the client. For each yes answer, score the number in the box. Total the nutrition score.

	YES
Illness or condition that made client change the kind and/or amount of food eaten	2
Eats fewer than two meals per day	3
Eats few fruits or vegetables, or milk products	2
Has three or more drinks of beer, liquor or wine almost every day	2
Tooth or mouth problems that make it hard to eat	2
Does not always have enough money to buy the food needed	4
Eats alone most of the time	1
Takes three or more different prescribed or over-the-counter drugs a day	1
Without wanting to, has lost or gained 10 lb in the last 6 months	2
Not physically able to shop, cook, and/or feed self	2
TOTAL	

Total the nutritional score.

0–2	Good. Recheck the score in 6 months.
3–5	Moderate nutritional risk. See what can be done to improve eating habits and lifestyle. Recheck score in 3 months.
6 or more	High nutritional risk. Consult with physician, dietitian, or other qualified health or social service professional.

Note: Remember that warning signs suggest risk but do not represent diagnosis of any condition.

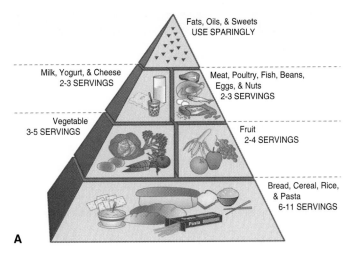

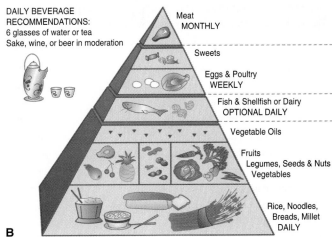

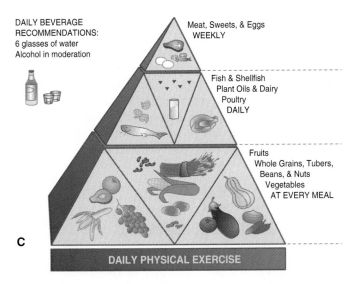

FIGURE 8-2. Most Americans are familiar with the USDA's official food pyramid for a healthy American diet (**A**), but compare it with other pyramid guides for healthful nutrition, for example (**B**) the traditional healthy Asian diet pyramid and (**C**) the traditional healthy Latin American diet pyramid.

- Limited access to sufficient food regardless of socioeconomic status
- Diseases whereby food is refused (eg, anorexia nervosa, bulimia, depression or other psychiatric disorders)
- Illness or trauma that increases client's nutritional needs dramatically but that interferes with his or her ability to ingest adequate nourishment

The clinical signs and symptoms of malnutrition are often confused with those of other diseases or conditions. In addition, the signs and symptoms may not manifest until the malnutrition is profound. The nurse needs to collect as much data as possible, especially in clients who are at risk for malnutrition or show some early clinical signs. Then, all of the information should be evaluated in context to avoid making judgments based on one or two isolated signs or symptoms. Table 8-1 compares indicators of good nutritional status with indicators of poor nutritional status.

An assessment of certain laboratory studies can yield valuable information about the client's nutritional status.

These can identify malnutrition, especially subtle changes before they are clinically evident. If a person is obese and malnourished because of poor food choices, these studies may also provide useful information. High cholesterol and triglyceride values can indicate risk factors in undernourished, normal, and obese people because these factors can be related to inherited tendencies, stress, lack of exercise, and unhealthful dietary habits.

When people are suffering from malnutrition, the body's protein stores are affected. The proteins usually sacrificed early are those that the body considers to be less essential to survival: albumen and globulins, transport proteins, skeletal muscle proteins, blood proteins, and immunoglobulins. These can be evaluated easily by blood tests. Additional tests to evaluate general immunity consist of small-dose intradermal injections of antigens, such as those used to test for tuberculosis, measles, and *Candida* (yeast). Because everyone has been exposed to at least one of these, an absence of reaction can indicate immunosuppression resulting from malnutrition. Table 8-2 summarizes laboratory values and

TABLE 8-1. General Indicators of Nutritional Status

Good Nutritional Status	Poor Nutritional Status
Alert, energetic, good endurance, good posture	Withdrawn, apathetic easily fatigued, stooped posture
Good attention span, psychological stability	Inattentive, irritable
Weight within range for height, age, body size	Overweight or underweight
Firm, well-developed muscles, healthy reflexes	Flaccid muscles, wasted appearance, paresthesias, diminished reflexes
Skin glowing, elastic, good turgor, smooth	Skin dull, pasty, scaly, dry, bruised
Eyes bright, clear without fatigue circles	Eyes dull, conjunctiva pale, discoloration under eyes
Hair shiny, lustrous, minimal loss	Hair brittle, dull, falls out easily
Mucous membranes:	Mucous membranes:
pink-red, gums pink and firm, tongue pink and moderately smooth, no swelling	pale, gums are red, boggy and bleed easily, tongue bright dark red and swollen
Abdomen flat, firm	Abdomen flaccid or distended (ascites)
No skeletal changes	Skeletal malformations

other tests that alert health care professionals to possible malnutrition.

OVERNUTRITION

Too much food, and especially food high in fat and sugar, can contribute to being "over fat" or to obesity. The health risks of obesity—heart disease, cancers, musculoskeletal disorders—are well known to most adults. Generally, a person who is 10% over his or her ideal body weight (IBW) is considered to be overfat, whereas one who is 20% over IBW is considered obese (see Table 8-3 for a determination of obesity based on body mass index). However, weight alone is not a completely reliable criterion because muscle is heavier than fat. A heavily muscled person may be inaccurately evaluated as obese in such a case.

Bioelectrical impedance testing or water-weight evaluation, with various anthropometric assessments, can discriminate the amount of body fat from muscle. Bioelectrical impedance testing involves passing a minute electrical current through the extremities and obtaining values that are then used to evaluate the relative amounts of fat and muscle. Water-weight evaluation involves submerging a person in a tub of water, having him or her completely exhale while under the water, and weighing the person. Because equal volumes of fat weigh less than muscle, the difference between the weight measured underwater and the weight measured in a dry setting distinguishes fat weight from muscle weight. In practical terms, this means that a thin client may have a high percentage of fat, putting him or her at risk, whereas a husky client may be heavy-boned and muscled with a healthy percentage of fat stores. Therefore, although evaluating nutritional status by a client's weight can inform the nurse about obvious alterations in either end of the weight–nutrition scale, the client with subtle deviations from a healthy-appearing body may benefit from more extensive and varied examination.

Researchers in the field of nutrition still use height–weight charts (Table 8-4) as a beginning reference point but insist that decisions about malnutrition and obesity are better determined by anthropometric evaluations that describe percentages of fat versus muscle (Office of Disease Prevention and Health Promotion, 2000). In addition, malnutrition can be evaluated more accurately by specific laboratory tests.

Hydration Assessment

Hydration is another important indicator of the general health status of the client but may be overlooked or confused with the signs and symptoms of nutritional changes. The signs of hydration changes may also be confused with certain disease states if only one or two indicators are evaluated. For this reason, the nurse needs to look for clusters of signs and symptoms that may indicate changes in hydration status. Adequate hydration can be affected by various situations in all age groups. Some examples in adults include:

- Exposure to excessively high environmental temperatures
- Inability to access adequate fluids, especially water (eg, clients who are unconscious or physically or mentally disabled)
- Excessive intake of alcohol or other diuretic fluids (coffee, sugar-rich and/or caffeine-rich soft drinks)
- People with impaired thirst mechanisms
- People taking diuretic medications
- Diabetic clients with severe hyperglycemia
- People with high fevers

Dehydration can have a seriously damaging effect on body cells and the execution of body functions. Because the

TABLE 8-2. Laboratory Values That Reflect Malnutrition

Laboratory Value	Normal Range	Abnormal Range
Hemoglobin and Hematocrit		
Hemoglobin (identifies iron-carrying capacity of the blood; test helps identify anemia and malnutrition)	Males: 13–18 g/dL Females: 12–16 g/dL	Males: <12 g/dL Females: <11 g/dL
Hematocrit (identifies volume of red blood cells/liter of blood)	Males: 40%–52% Females: 36%–48% (Normal is usually about three times the hemoglobin level [ie., the Hct–Hgb ratio is 1:3])	Males: <36% Females: <33%
Visceral Proteins		
Serum albumin level	3.5–5.5 g/dL	Mild depletion: 2.8–3.5 Moderate depletion: 2.1–2.7 Severe depletion <2.1
Total protein level (includes globulins)	6–8 g/dL	<5.0 g/dL
Prealbumin: Transport protein for thyroxin (T4); short half-life makes it more sensitive to changes in protein stores	15–25 mg/dL	Mild depletion: 10–15 Moderate depletion: 5–10 Severe depletion: <5
Serum transferrin: Transport protein for iron; may be more sensitive indicator of visceral protein stores than albumin	170–250	Mild depletion: 150–170 Moderate depletion: 100–150 Severe depletion: <100
Creatinine Height Index (CHI)		
CHI: Measures skeletal muscle mass	80%–100%	Moderate depletion: 60%–80% Severe depletion: <60%
Immune Function Tests		
Total lymphocyte count (TLC): % of lymphocytes in the white blood cell count with differential multiplied by 100	> 2000 mm³	Mild immuno-incompetence: 1200–2000 Moderate immuno-incompetence: 800–1199 Severe immuno-incompetence: <800
Delayed cutaneous hypersensitivity (to common antigens injected intradermally and observed after 24 to 48 hours)	>5–10 mm	<5 mm induration indicates immuno-incompetence

thirst mechanism is poorly developed in humans, dehydration can develop unnoticed in normal persons under adverse conditions. Often, a person may experience a sense of thirst only after dangerous excess or deficit of various serum electrolyte levels has occurred. A chronically and seriously ill client who is not receiving adequate fluids either orally or parenterally is at high risk for dehydration unless monitored carefully.

Overhydration in a healthy person is usually not a problem because the body is effective in maintaining a correct fluid balance. It does this by shifting fluids in and out of physiologic third spaces, such as extracellular tissues, the pleural and pericardial spaces, the tongue and the eyeball, and by excreting fluid in the urine, stool, and through respiration and perspiration. Clients at risk for overhydration or fluid retention are those with kidney, liver, and cardiac disease in which the fluid dynamic mechanisms are impaired.

In addition, seriously ill clients who are on humidified ventilation or who are receiving large volumes of parenteral fluids without close monitoring of their hydration status are also at risk. The health history interview is an ideal time to teach home care clients and their caregivers how to monitor hydration by keeping records of fluid intake and output.

TABLE 8-3. Determining Degree of Obesity by Body Mass Index

BMI	Weight Classification
25.0–29.9	Overweight (pre-obese)
30.0–34.9	Class 1 obesity
35.0–39.9	Class 2 obesity
≥ 40	Class 3 obesity

TABLE 8-4. Height and Weight Table: Weights for Persons 25 to 59 years According to Build*

Men					Women				
Height		Small Frame	Medium Frame	Large Frame	Height†		Small Frame	Medium Frame	Large Frame
Feet	Inches				Feet	Inches			
5	2	128–134	131–141	138–150	4	10	102–111	109–121	118–131
5	3	130–136	133–143	140–153	4	11	103–113	111–123	120–134
5	4	132–138	135–145	142–156	5	0	104–115	113–125	122–137
5	5	134–140	137–148	144–160	5	1	106–118	115–129	125–140
5	6	136–142	139–151	146–164	5	2	108–121	118–132	128–143
5	7	138–145	142–154	149–168	5	3	111–124	121–135	131–147
5	8	140–148	145–157	152–172	5	4	114–127	124–138	134–151
5	9	142–151	148–160	155–176	5	5	117–130	127–141	137–155
5	10	144–154	151–163	158–180	5	6	120–133	130–144	140–159
5	11	146–157	154–166	161–184	5	7	123–136	133–147	143–163
6	0	149–160	157–170	164–188	5	8	126–139	136–150	146–167
6	1	152–164	160–174	168–192	5	9	129–142	139–153	149–170
6	2	155–168	164–178	172–197	5	10	132–145	142–156	152–173
6	3	158–172	167–182	176–202	5	11	135–148	145–159	155–176
6	4	162–176	171–187	181–207	6	0	138–151	148–162	158–179

Courtesy Metropolitan Life Insurance Company, Statistical Bulletin, 2000.
* Indoor clothing weighing 5 lb for men and 3 lb for women.
† Shoes with 1-inch heels.

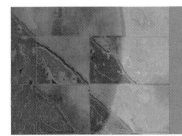

Nursing Assessment

Collecting Subjective Data: Nursing History

During the general survey or the nutritional assessment, the COLDSPA mnemonic may be particularly helpful in exploring unusual signs and symptoms or problems reported as you and the client ask and answer various questions during the health history interview.

COLDSPA

CHARACTER: Describe the sign or symptom. How does it feel, look, sound, smell, and so forth?
ONSET: When did it begin?
LOCATION: Where is it? Does it radiate?
DURATION: How long does it last? Does it recur?
SEVERITY: How bad is it?
PATTERN: What makes it better: What makes it worse?
ASSOCIATED FACTORS: What other symptoms occur with it?

Question What is your name, address, and telephone number?

Rationale Answers to these questions provide verifiable and accurate identification data about the client. They also provide baseline information about level of consciousness, memory, speech patterns, articulation, or speech defects.

Q How old are you?

R Establishes baseline for comparing appearance and development to chronologic age.

Q Do you know what your usual blood pressure is?

R Knowing blood pressure indicates client is involved in own health care.

Q When and where did you last have your blood pressure checked?

R Answer indicates whether client consults professionals for health care, whether client relies on possibly erroneous equipment in public places (eg, drug stores), or whether client has approved equipment at home that he or she is trained to use.

Q Have you had any high fevers that occur often or persistently?

R A pattern of elevated temperatures may indicate a chronic infection or blood disorder, such as leukemia.

Q What is your height and usual weight?

R Answer provides a baseline for comparing client's perception with actual and current measurements. Answer also indicates client's knowledge of own health status.

Q Have you lost or gained a considerable amount of weight recently?

R Weight changes may point to changes in nutrition or hydration status or to an illness causing weight changes.

Q Are you now or have you been on a diet recently? How did you decide on the diet you are following?

R Whether or not the client is following his or her own diet or a medically prescribed diet, the answer to the question helps identify chronic dieters and clients with eating disorders.

Q How much fluid do you drink each day? How much of it is water? How many sugary, caffeinated, or alcoholic beverages do you have each day?

R Answers to these questions identify clients in terms of adequate, moderate, or excessive consumption of various kinds of fluids; they also identify those at risk for dehydration.

Q Can you recall what you ate in the last 24 hours? In the last 72 hours?

R The client's typical daily diet indicates his or her level of nourishment, likes and dislikes, and dietary habits. As such, it provides a basis for planning healthful menu choices.

Collecting Objective Data

CLIENT PREPARATION

After the interview, ask the client to put on an examination gown. The client should be in a comfortable sitting position on the examination table (or on a bed in the home setting). The usual general survey begins with a measurement of vital signs, which may be taken with the client in the supine position, if necessary.

Unless the client is bed bound in the hospital, nursing home, or home care setting, explain that he or she will need to both stand and sit during the assessment—particularly during anthropometric assessments. Keep in mind that some clients may be embarrassed to be measured like this, especially if they are overweight or underweight. To reassure the client, explain that the examination is necessary for evaluating overall health status. It will be helpful to proceed with the examination in a straightforward, nonjudgmental manner.

EQUIPMENT AND SUPPLIES

- One of the following thermometers: mercury-in-glass oral, axillary, or rectal thermometer; electronic thermometer; tympanic thermometer

- Protective, disposable covers for each type of thermometer
- An aneroid or mercury sphygmomanometer or electronic blood pressure–measuring equipment (Displays 8-2 and 8-3)
- Stethoscope (see How to Use the Stethoscope in Chapter 5)
- Watch with a second hand
- Balance beam scale with height attachment
- Metric measuring tape
- Marking pencil
- Skinfold calipers

KEY ASSESSMENT POINTS

- Perform the parts of the general survey in order.
- Observe and evaluate the client's general status effectively.
- Identify the equipment needed to measure vital signs and its proper use.
- Identify the equipment needed to take anthropometric measurements and its proper use.
- Explain the importance of anthropometric measurements to general health status.
- Educate the client regarding nutritional concerns and health-related risks.

(*text continues on page 107*)

DISPLAY 8-2. Measuring Blood Pressure

GUIDELINES

1. Assemble your equipment so that the sphygmomanometer, stethoscope, and your pen and recording sheet are within easy reach.
2. Assist the client into a comfortable, quiet, restful position for 5 to 10 minutes. Client may lie down or sit.
3. Remove client's clothing from the arm and palpate the pulsations of the brachial artery. (If the client's sleeve can be pushed up to make room for the cuff, make sure that the clothing is not so constrictive that it would alter a correct pressure reading.)
4. Place the blood pressure cuff so the midline of the bladder is over the arterial pulsation, and wrap the appropriate-sized cuff smoothly and snugly around the upper arm, 1 inch above the antecubital area so there is enough room to place the bell of the stethoscope. The bladder inside the cuff should encircle 80% of the arm circumference in adults and 100% of the arm circumference in children younger than age 13.

 Tip From the Experts A cuff that is too small may give a false or abnormally high blood pressure reading.

---

5. Hold the client's arm slightly flexed at heart level with the palm up.
6. Put the ear pieces of the stethoscope in your ears; then, palpate the brachial pulse again and place the stethoscope lightly over this area. Position the mercury gauge on the manometer at eye level.
7. Adjust the screw above the bulb to tighten the valve on the air pump, and make sure that the tubing is not kinked or obstructed.

(continued)

DISPLAY 8-2. Measuring Blood Pressure (Continued)

8. Inflate the cuff by pumping the bulb to about 30 mmHg above the point at which the brachial pulse disappears. This will help you avoid missing an auscultatory gap (see Display 8-3).

9. Deflate the cuff slowly—about 2 mm per second—by turning the valve in the opposite direction while listening for the first of Korotkoff's sounds.

10. Read the point, closest to an even number, on the mercury gauge at which you hear the first faint but clear sound. Record this number as the systolic blood pressure. This is phase I of Korotkoff's sounds.

11. Next, note the point, closest to an even number, on the mercury gauge at which the sound becomes muffled (phase IV of the Korotkoff's sounds). Finally, note the point where the sound subsides completely (phase V of the Korotkoff's sounds). When both a change in sounds and a cessation of the sounds are heard, record the numbers at which you hear phase I, IV, and V sounds. Otherwise, record the first and last sounds.

12. Finally, deflate the cuff at least another 10 mmHg to make sure you hear no more sounds. Then, deflate completely and remove.

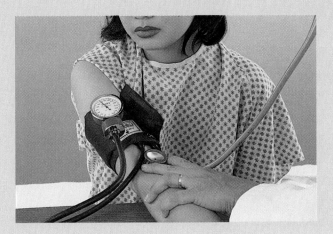

(American Heart Association. [1994]. *Human blood pressure determination by sphygmo-manometry* [6th ed.]. Publication No. 70-1061 [SA]. Dallas: Author.)

DISPLAY 8-3. Identifying Korotkoff's Sounds

PHASE I

Characterized by the first appearance of clear, repetitive, tapping sounds. This coincides approximately with the resumption of a palpable pulse. The number on the pressure gauge at which you hear the first tapping sound is the systolic pressure.

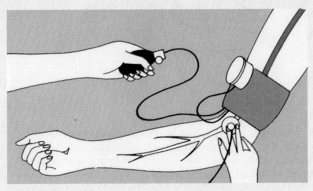

Initial silence.

(continued)

DISPLAY 8-3. **Identifying Korotkoff's Sounds** (Continued)

PHASE II

Characterized as muffled or swishing, these sounds are softer and longer than phase I sounds. They also have the quality of an intermittent murmur. They may temporarily subside, especially in hypertensive people. The loss of the sound during the latter part of phase I and during phase II is called the auscultatory gap. The gap may cover a range of as much as 40 mmHg; failing to recognize this gap may cause serious errors of underestimating systolic pressure or overestimating diastolic pressure.

PHASE III

Characterized by distinct, crisp, and louder sounds as the blood flows relatively freely through an increasingly open artery.

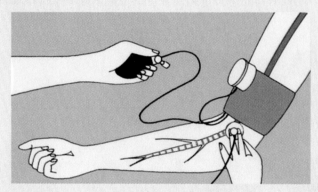

Turbulence.

PHASE IV

Characterized by sounds that are muffled, less distinct, and softer (with a blowing quality).

PHASE V

Characterized by sounds subsiding completely. The last sound heard before this period of continuous silence is the onset of phase V and is the pressure commonly considered to define the diastolic measurement. (Some clinicians still consider the last sounds of phase IV the first diastolic value.)

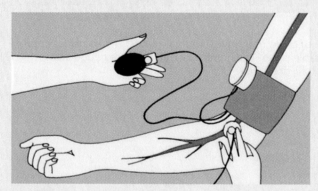

Final silence.

Note: The American Heart Association recommends that values in phase IV and phase V be recorded when both a change in the sounds and a cessation in the sounds occur.

These recommendations apply particularly to children under age 13, pregnant women, and clients with high cardiac output or peripheral vasodilation. For example, such a blood pressure would be recorded as 120/80/64.

(Adapted from American Heart Association. [1994] *Human blood pressure determination by sphygmomanometry* [6th ed.]. Publication No. 70-1061 [SA]. Dallas, TX: Author.)

PHYSICAL ASSESSMENT

ASSESSMENT PROCEDURE	NORMAL FINDINGS	ABNORMAL FINDINGS
Observe physical and sexual development.	Client appears to be his or her stated chronologic age.	Client appears older than actual chronologic age (ie, hard life, manual labor, chronic illness, alcoholism, smoking).
Compare client's stated age with his or her apparent age and developmental stage.	Sexual development is appropriate for gender and age.	Delayed puberty, male client with female characteristics, female client with male characteristics.
Observe skin and color. **Tip From the Experts** Keep in mind that underlying red tones from good circulation give a liveliness or healthy glow to all shades of skin color.	Color is even without obvious lesions: light to dark beige-pink in light-skinned client. Light tan to dark brown or olive in dark-skinned clients.	Extreme pallor, flushed, or yellow in light-skinned client. Loss of red tones, ashen gray in cryanosis in dark-skinned client. See abnormal skin colors and their significance in Chapter 9.
Observe dress. **Tip From the Experts** Be careful not to make premature judgments regarding the client's dress. Styles and clothing fads (e.g, torn jeans, oversized clothing, baggy pants), developmental level, socioeconomic level, and culture all influence a person's dress (eg, Indian women wear saris; Hasidic Jewish men wear black suits and black skull caps).	Dress is appropriate for occasion and weather. Dress varies considerably from person to person, depending on individual preference. There may be several normal dress variations depending on the client's developmental level, age, socioeconomic level, and culture or subculture. Some older adults may wear excess clothing because of slowed metabolism and loss of subcutaneous fat, resulting in cold intolerance.	Uncoordinated clothing, extremely light clothing, or extremely warm clothing for the weather conditions may be seen on mentally ill, grieving, depressed, or poor clients. This may also be noted in clients with heat or cold intolerances. Extremely loose clothing held up by pins or a belt may suggest recent weight loss. Clients wearing long sleeves in warm weather may be protecting themselves from the sun or covering up needle marks secondary to drug abuse. Soiled clothing may indicate homelessness, elderly vision deficits, or mental illness.
Observe hygiene. Asians and Native Americans have fewer sweat glands and, therefore, less obvious body odor than most Caucasians and black Africans who have more sweat glands. Additionally, some cultures do not use deodorant products (see Chapter 9 for more information).	Clean and groomed appropriately for occasion. The nurse must determine what the normal level of hygiene is for the client's developmental and socioeconomic level and cultural background. Stains on hands and dirty nails may reflect certain occupations, such as mechanic or gardener.	A dirty, unshaven, unkempt appearance with a foul body odor may reflect depression, drug abuse, or low socioeconomic level (ie, homeless client). Poor hygiene may be seen in dementia or other conditions that indicate a self-care deficit. If the client is cared for by others, poor hygiene may reflect neglect by caregiver or caregiver role strain. Breath odors from smoking or from drinking alcoholic beverages may be noted as may diet-related odors, such as garlic or soy products.

(continued)

ASSESSMENT PROCEDURE	NORMAL FINDINGS	ABNORMAL FINDINGS
Observe posture and gait.	Posture is erect and comfortable for age. Gait is rhythmic and coordinated with arms swinging at side.	Curvatures of the spine (lordosis, scoliosis, or kyphosis) may indicate a musculoskeletal disorder. Stiff, rigid movements are common in arthritis or Parkinson's disease (see Chapter 20). Slumped shoulders may signify depression. Clients with chronic pulmonary obstructive disease tend to lean forward, brace themselves with arms. Tense or anxious clients may elevate shoulders toward their ears and hold the entire body stiffly. 👓 In older adults, osteoporotic thinning and collapse of the vertebrae secondary to bone loss may result in kyphosis. In older men, gait may be wider based with arms held outward. Older women tend to have a narrow base and may waddle to compensate for a decreased sense of balance. Steps shorten, with decreased speed and arm swing. Mobility may be decreased, and gait may be rigid.
Observe body build as well as muscle mass and fat distribution	A wide variety of body types fall within a normal range—from small amounts of both fat and muscle to large amounts of muscle and/or fat. In general, the normal body is proportional. Bilateral muscles are firm and well developed. There is equal distribution of fat with some subcutaneous fat. Body parts are intact and appear equal without obvious deformities.	A lack of subcutaneous fat with prominent bones is seen in the undernourished. Abdominal ascites is seen in starvation and liver disease. Abundant fatty tissue is noted in obesity. 👓 Muscle tone and mass decrease with aging. There is a loss of subcutaneous fat, making bones and muscles more prominent. Fat is also redistributed with aging. Fat is lost from the face and neck and redistributed to the arms, abdomen, and hips.

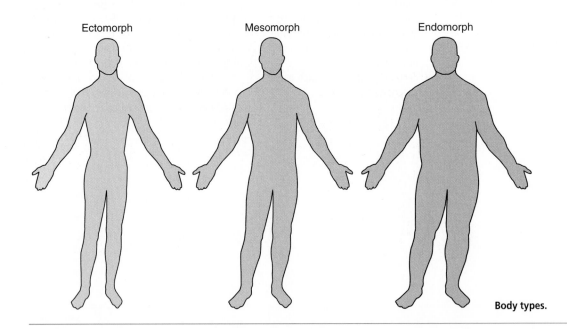

Ectomorph   Mesomorph   Endomorph

Body types.

(continued)

ASSESSMENT PROCEDURE	NORMAL FINDINGS	ABNORMAL FINDINGS
Observe the client's level of consciousness. This can be determined by asking the client his or her name, address, and phone number. 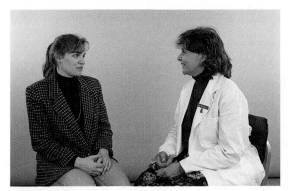 **Assessing level of consciousness. (© B. Proud.)**	Client is alert and oriented to what is happening at the time of the interview and physical assessment. Client responds to your questions and interacts appropriately. Although the older client's response and ability to process information may be slower, he or she is normally alert and oriented.	If the client does not respond appropriately, refer to Chapter 23 to further assess level of consciousness. Lethargy, obtundation, stupor, and coma are seen in various conditions, such as neurologic disorders and cerebrovascular disease.
Observe comfort level.	Client assumes a relatively relaxed posture without excessive position shifting. Facial expression is alert and pleasant.	Facial expression indicates discomfort (grimacing, frowning). Client may brace or holds body part that is painful. Breathing pattern indicates distress (shortness of breath, shallow, rapid breathing).
Observe behavior, body movements, and affect.	Client is cooperative and purposeful in his or her interactions with others. Mild to moderate anxiety may be normal in a client who is having a health assessment performed. Affect is appropriate for the client's situation.	Uncooperative, bizarre behavior may be seen in the angry, mentally ill, or violent client. Anxious clients are often fidgety and restless. Some degree of anxiety is often seen in ill clients. Apathy or crying may be seen with depression. Incongruent behavior may be seen in clients who are in denial of problems or illness. In the older adult, purposeless movements, wandering, aggressiveness, or withdrawal may indicate neurologic deficits.
Observe facial expression.	Facial features are symmetric with movement. Client establishes good eye contact when conversing with others. Smiles and frowns appropriately.	Poor eye contact is seen in depressed clients. An expressionless, masklike face is common in Parkinson's disease. Staring, watchfulness appears in metabolic disorders and anxiety. Inappropriate facial expressions (eg, smiling when expressing sad thoughts) may indicate mental illness. Drooping or gross asymmetry occurs with neurologic disorder or injury (eg, Bell's palsy or stroke).
Listen to speech. Note style and pattern.	Speech is clear, moderately paced, and culturally appropriate. Normally, in older adults, responses may be slowed, but speech should be clear and moderately paced.	Disorganized speech, consistent (nonstop) speech, or long periods of silence may indicate mental illness or a neurologic disorder (eg, dysarthria, dysphasia, speech defect, garbled speech).

ASSESSMENT PROCEDURE	NORMAL FINDINGS	ABNORMAL FINDINGS

TAKE VITAL SIGNS

Oral Temperature

Use a mercury-in-glass or electronic thermometer with a disposable protective cover. Use your wrist to shake the mercury in a glass thermometer down to below the 35.5°C (96°F) level. Then, place the thermometer under the client's tongue, to the right or left of the frenulum. Ask the client to keep lips tightly closed around the glass thermometer for 5 minutes. To record the temperature, hold the thermometer at eye level and read the number that coincides with the mercury level.

Electronic thermometers give a digital reading in about 2 minutes.

Oral temperature 36.5°C to 37.0°C (96.0°F to 99.9°F)

Oral temperature below 36.5°C and over 37.0°C

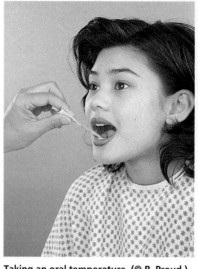 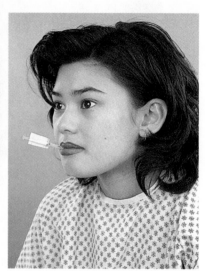

Taking an oral temperature. (© B. Proud.)

Axillary Temperature

Hold the glass or electronic thermometer under the axilla firmly by having the client hold the arm down and across the chest for 10 minutes.

The axillary temperature is 0.5°C (1°F) lower than the oral temperature.

Rectal Temperature

Use this route only if other routes are not practical (ie, client cannot cooperate, is comatose, cannot close mouth, or tympanic thermometer is unavailable). Cover the glass thermometer with a disposable, sterile sheath, and lubricate the thermometer. Wear gloves, and insert thermometer 1 inch into rectum. Hold a glass thermometer in place for 3 minutes; hold an electronic thermometer in place until the temperature appears in the display window.

The rectal temperature is between 0.4°C and 0.5°C (0.7°F and 1°F) higher than the normal oral temperature.

Tip From the Experts Never force the thermometer into the rectum or use a rectal thermometer for clients with severe coagulation disorders.

(continued)

ASSESSMENT PROCEDURE	NORMAL FINDINGS	ABNORMAL FINDINGS

Tympanic Temperature

An electronic tympanic thermometer measures the temperature of the tympanic membrane quickly and safely. It is also a good device for measuring core body temperature because the tympanic membrane is supplied by a tributary of the artery (internal carotid) that supplies the hypothalamus (the body's thermoregulatory center). Place the probe very gently at the opening of the ear canal for 2 to 3 seconds until the temperature appears in the digital display.

The tympanic membrane temperature is about 0.8°C (1.4°F) higher than the normal oral temperature.

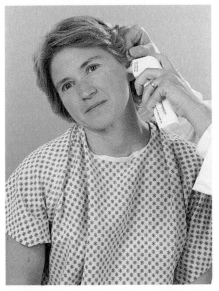

Taking a tympanic temperature. (© B. Proud.)

Take Pulse

To measure the radial pulse rate, use the pads of your two middle fingers and lightly palpate the radial artery on the lateral aspect of the client's wrist. Count the number of beats you feel for 30 seconds if the pulse rhythm is regular. Multiply by two to get the rate. Count for a full minute if the rhythm is irregular. Then, verify by taking an apical pulse as well.

A pulse rate ranging from 60 to 100 beats/min is normal for adults. Tachycardia may be normal in clients who have just finished strenuous exercise. Bradycardia may be normal in well-conditioned athletes.

Tachycardia: Greater than 100 beats/min. May occur with fever, certain medications, stress, and other abnormal states, such as cardiac dysrhythmias.

Bradycardia: Less than 60 beats/min. Sitting or standing for long periods may cause the blood to pool and decrease the pulse rate. Heart block or dropped beats can also manifest as bradycardia. Abnormal findings should be followed up with cardiac auscultation of the apical pulse (see Chapter 16 for more detail).

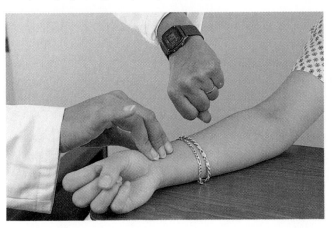

Timing the radial pulse rate. (© B. Proud.)

(continued)

ASSESSMENT PROCEDURE	NORMAL FINDINGS	ABNORMAL FINDINGS
Evaluate pulse rhythm.	Regular intervals between beats	Irregular intervals between beats, which should be followed up with auscultation of the apical pulse (see Chapter 16). When describing irregular beats, indicate whether they are regular irregular or irregular irregular.
Assess amplitude and contour.	Normally, pulsation is equally strong in both wrists. Upstroke is smooth and rapid with a more gradual downstroke.	A bounding or weak and thready pulse is not normal. Delayed upstroke is also abnormal. Follow up on abnormal amplitude and contour findings by palpating the carotid arteries, which provides the best assessment of amplitude and contour (see Chapter 16).
Palpate arterial elasticity.	Artery feels straight, resilient, and springy. The older client's artery may feel more rigid, hard, and bent.	Rigid

Monitor Respirations

Monitor the respiratory rate by observing the client's chest rise and fall with each breath. Count respirations for 30 seconds and multiply by 2 (refer to Chapter 14, Thoracic and Lung Assessment).	Between 12 and 20 breaths/min is normal. In the older adult, the respiratory rate may range from 15 to 22. The rate may increase with a shallower inspiratory phase because vital capacity and inspiratory reserve volume decrease with aging.	Fewer than 12 breaths/min; more than 20 breaths/min.

Tip From the Experts If you place the client's arm across the chest while palpating pulse, you can also count respirations. Do this by keeping your fingers on the client's pulse even after you have finished taking it.

Observe respiratory rhythm.	Regular (if irregular, count for one full minute).	Irregular (see Chapter 12 for more detail).
Observe respiratory depth.	Equal bilateral chest expansion of 1 to 2 inches.	Unequal, shallow, or extremely deep chest expansion (see Chapter 14 for more detail) and labored or gasping breaths are abnormal.

Measure Blood Pressure

Follow guidelines for measuring blood pressure (See Display 8-2), and take blood pressure in both arms when recording it for the first time.	Systolic: 100 to 130 mmHg Diastolic: 60 to 80 mmHg; varies with individuals. A pressure difference of 10 mmHg between arms is normal.	Higher or lower than normal systolic and diastolic readings. (See Tables 8-5 and 8-6 for blood pressure classifications and recommended follow-up criteria.) More than a 10-mmHg pressure difference between arms may indicate coarctation of the aorta or cardiac disease. More rigid, arteriosclerotic arteries account for higher systolic blood pressure in older adults. Systolic pressure over 140 but diastolic pressure under 90 is called isolated systolic hypertension.

(continued)

ASSESSMENT PROCEDURE	NORMAL FINDINGS	ABNORMAL FINDINGS
If the client takes antihypertensives or has a history of fainting or dizziness, assess for possible orthostatic hypotension. Measure blood pressure with the client in a standing or sitting position after taking the pressure with the client in a supine position.	A drop of less than 20 mmHg from recorded sitting position.	A drop of 20 mmHg or more from the recorded sitting blood pressure may indicate orthostatic (postural) hypotension. Orthostatic hypotension may be related to a decreased baroreceptor sensitivity, fluid volume deficit (eg, dehydration), or certain medications (ie, diuretics, antihypertensives). Symptoms of orthostatic hypotension include dizziness, lightheadedness, and falling. Further evaluation and referral to the client's primary care provider are necessary.

🌸 **Tip From the Experts** An ill client may not be able to stand, and sitting is usually adequate to detect whether the client truly has orthostatic hypotension.

Finally, assess the pulse pressure—the difference between the systolic and diastolic blood pressure levels. Record in mmHg. For example, if the blood pressure was 120/80, then the pulse pressure would be 120–80 or 40 mmHg.	Pulse pressure is 30 to 50 mmHg. 👓 Widening of the pulse pressure is seen with aging due to less elastic peripheral arteries.	A pulse pressure lower than 30 mmHg or higher than 50 mmHg may indicate cardiovascular disease.

NUTRITION AND ANTHROPOMETRIC MEASUREMENTS

Measure Height

Measure the client's height by using the L-shaped measuring attachment on the balance scale. Instruct the client to stand on the balance scale platform with heels together and back straight, and to look straight ahead. Raise the attachment above the client's head. Then lower it to the top of the client's head. Record the client's height.

Height is within range for age, ethnic and genetic heritage. Children are usually within the range of parents' height.

👓 Height begins to wane in the fifth decade of life because the intervertebral discs become thinner and spinal kyphosis increases.

Extreme shortness is seen in achondroplastic dwarfism and Turner's syndrome. Extreme tallness is seen in gigantism (excessive secretion of growth hormone) and in Marfan's syndrome.

🌸 **Tip From the Experts** Without a scale, have the client stand shoeless with the back and heels against the wall. Balance a straight, level object (ruler) atop the client's head—parallel to the floor—and mark the object's position on the wall. Measure the distance between the mark and the floor. If the client cannot stand, measure the arm span to estimate height. Have the client stretch arms straight out sideways. Measure from the tip of one middle finger to the tip of the opposite middle finger. Record the arm span height. (See Display 8-4.)

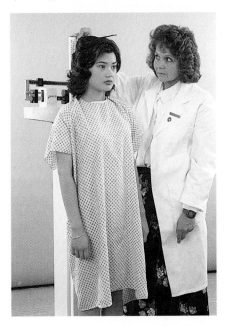

Measuring height. (© B. Proud.)

(continued)

ASSESSMENT PROCEDURE	NORMAL FINDINGS	ABNORMAL FINDINGS

Measure Weight

Level the balance beam scale at zero before weighing the client. Do this by moving the weights on the scale to zero and adjusting the knob by turning it until the balance beam is level. Ask the client to remove shoes and heavy outer clothing and to stand on the scale. Adjust the weights to the right and left until the balance beam is level again. Record weight (1 lb = 2.2 kg). If you are weighing a client at home, you may have to use a scale with an automatically adjusting true zero.

Desirable weights for men and women are listed in Table 8-4.

Body weight may decrease with aging because of a loss of muscle or lean body tissue.

Weight does not fall within range of desirable weights for women and men.

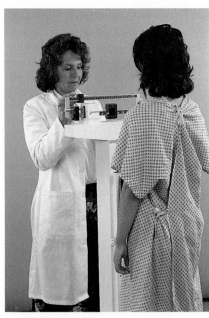

Measuring weight. (© B. Proud.)

Determine Ideal Body Weight (IBW) and Percentage of IBW

Use this formula to calculate the client's IBW:

Female: 100 lb for 5 ft + 5 lb for each inch over 5 ft ±10% for small or large frame

Male: 106 lb for 5 ft + 6 lb for each inch over 5 ft ± 10% for small or large frame.

Calculate the client's percentage of IBW by the following formula:

$$actual\ weight \times 100 = \%\ IBW.$$

Body weight is within 10% of ideal range.

A current weight that is 80% to 90% of IBW indicates a lean client and possibly mild malnutrition. Weight that is 70% to 80% indicates moderate malnutrition; less than 70% may indicate severe malnutrition possibly from systemic disease, eating disorders, cancer therapies, and other problems. Weight exceeding 10% of the IBW range is called overweight; weight exceeding 20% of IBW is called obesity.

Measure Body Mass Index (BMI)

Determine BMI using one of these formulas:

$$\frac{Weight\ in\ kilograms}{Height\ in\ meters^2} = BMI$$

or

$$\frac{Weight\ in\ pounds}{Height\ in\ inches^2} \times 705 = BMI$$

BMI between 20 and 25

BMI <20 is associated with health problems in some people. BMI between 25 and 27 may lead to health problems in some people. BMI > 27 indicates increased risk of developing health problems.

(continued)

ASSESSMENT PROCEDURE	NORMAL FINDINGS	ABNORMAL FINDINGS

Determine Waist-to-Hip Ratio

Have the client stand. Measure the waist. Then measure the hips midway between the iliac crest and the greater trochanter.

Use this formula to calculate the waist-to-hip ratio:

$$\text{Waist-to-hip ratio} = \frac{\text{waist circumference}}{\text{hip circumference}}$$

Females: Waist 20% smaller than hips or waist-to-hip ratio less than or equal to 0.80

Males: Waist-to-hip ratio less than or equal to 1.0

Females with a waist-to-hip ratio greater than 0.80 and males with a waist-to-hip ratio greater than 1.0 have a three to five times greater risk for having a heart attack or stroke.

Measure Mid-Arm Circumference (MAC)

The MAC measurement evaluates skeletal muscle mass and fat stores.

Have the client dangle the nondominant arm freely next to the body. Locate the arm's midpoint (halfway between the top of the acromion process and the olecranon process). Mark the midpoint and measure the MAC, holding the tape measure firmly around, but not pinching, the arm.

Compare the client's current MAC to prior measurements and compare to the standard mid-arm circumference measurements for the client's age and sex listed in Table 8-7.

Measurements that are significantly higher or lower than the 50th percentile on the standard reference charts indicate that further assessment of the client's nutritional status is needed. The MAC may increase with obesity to the upper percentiles and decrease to the lower percentiles in malnutrition.

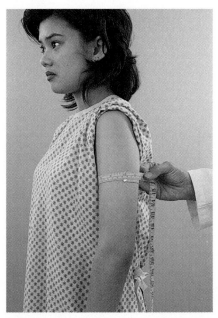

Measuring mid-arm circumference.
(© B. Proud.)

(continued)

ASSESSMENT PROCEDURE	NORMAL FINDINGS	ABNORMAL FINDINGS

Measure Triceps Skinfold Thickness (TSF)

Take the TSF measurement to evaluate the degree of fat stores. Instruct the client to stand and hang the non-dominant arm freely. Grasp the skinfold and subcutaneous fat between the thumb and forefinger 1 cm above the midpoint mark. Pull the skin away from the muscle (ask client to flex arm—if you feel a contraction with this maneuver, you still have the muscle) and apply the calipers. Repeat three times and average the three measurements.

Compare the client's current measurement to past measurements and to the standard TSF measurements for the client's age and sex, listed in Tables 8-8 and 8-9.

Fat stores decrease in malnutrition and increase in obesity.

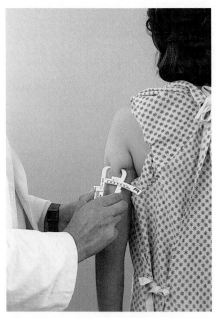

Measuring triceps skinfold thickness.
(© B. Proud.)

🎗 **Tip From the Experts** A more accurate measurement can be obtained from the suprailiac region of the abdomen or the subscapular area.

Calculate Mid-Arm Muscle Circumference (MAMC)

The MAMC calculation determines skeletal muscle reserves from MAC and TSF measurements by this formula:

$$\text{MAMC (cm)} = \text{MAC (cm)} - (0.314 \times \text{TSF}).$$

Compare the client's current MAMC to past measurements and to the data for MAMCs for the client's age and sex, listed in Table 8-7.

The MAMC decreases to the lower percentiles with malnutrition and in obesity if TSF is high. If the MAMC is in a lower percentile and the TSF is in a higher percentile, the client may benefit from muscle-building exercises that increase muscle mass and decrease fat.

(continued)

ASSESSMENT PROCEDURE	NORMAL FINDINGS	ABNORMAL FINDINGS

Calculate Mid-Arm Muscle Area (MAMA)

To determine skeletal muscle reserves and evaluate malnourishment in clients, calculate the midarm muscle area (MAMA). MAMA is more sensitive than MAMC for malnutrition, particularly for growing children and clients with long-term malnutrition. MAMA is derived from MAC and MAMC by the following formula:

$$\frac{\left(MAC - MAMC\right)^2}{4\pi\left(12.56\right)} = MAMA$$

See Table 8-7 for normal values.

Malnutrition
Mild — MAMA of 90%
Moderate — MAMA 60% to 90%
Severe — MAMA <60%

Tip From the Experts When evaluating anthropometric data, base conclusions on a data cluster, not on individual findings. Factor in any special considerations and general health status. Although general standards are useful for making estimates, the client's overall health and well-being may be equal or more useful indicators of nutritional status.

HYDRATION

Measure Intake and Output (I & O) in Inpatient Settings

Measure all fluids taken in by oral and parenteral routes, through irrigation tubes, as medications in solution, and through tube feedings.
   Also measure all fluid output (urine, stool, drainage from tubes, perspiration). Calculate insensible loss at 800 to 1000 mL daily, and add to total output.

Intake and output are closely balanced over 72 hours when insensible loss is included.

Tip From the Experts
   Fluid is normally retained during acute stress, illness, trauma, and surgery. Expect diuresis to occur in most clients in 48 to 72 hours.

Imbalances in either direction suggest impaired organ function and fluid overload or inability to compensate for losses resulting in dehydration.

Monitor Fluid-Related Changes in Any Setting

Weight: Weigh clients at risk for hydration changes daily.

Weight is stable or changes less than 2 to 3 lb over 1 to 5 days.

Weight gains or losses of 6 to 10 lb in 1 week or less indicate a major fluid shift. A change of 2.2 lb (1 kg) is equal to a loss or gain of 1 L of fluid.

Skin: Check skin turgor by pinching a small fold of skin, observing elasticity, and watching how quickly the skin returns to its original position.

No tenting, and skin returns to original position.

Tenting can indicate fluid loss but is also present in malnutrition and loss of collagen in aged individuals. This finding must be correlated with other hydration findings.

Check for pitting edema.

No edema

Pitting edema is a sign of fluid retention especially in cardiac and renal disease.

Observe skin for moisture.

Skin is not excessively dry.

Abnormally dry and flaky skin. Corroborate such a finding with other findings because heredity and cholesterol and hormone levels determine skin moistness.

(continued)

ASSESSMENT PROCEDURE	NORMAL FINDINGS	ABNORMAL FINDINGS
Venous filling: Lower the client's arm or leg and observe how long it takes to fill. Then raise the arm or leg and watch how long it takes to empty.	Veins fill in 3 to 5 seconds. Veins empty in 3 to 5 seconds.	Filling or emptying that takes more than 6 to 10 seconds suggests fluid volume deficit.
Observe neck veins with client in the supine position and then with the head elevated above 45 degrees.	Neck veins are softly visible in supine position. With head elevated above 45 degrees, the neck veins flatten or are slightly visible but soft.	Flat veins in supine client may indicate dehydration. Visible firm neck veins indicate distention possibly resulting from fluid retention and heart disease.
Tongue: Inspect the tongue's condition and furrows.	Tongue is moist, plump with central sulcus and no additional furrows.	Tongue is dry with visible papillae and several longitudinal furrows, suggesting loss of normal third-space fluid and dehydration.
Eyeballs: Gently palpate eyeball.	Moderately firm to touch but not hard.	Eyeball is boggy and lacks normal tension, suggesting loss of normal third-space fluid and dehydration.

> **Tip From the Experts** A hard eyeball is more indicative of eye disease than of hydration abnormalities.

ASSESSMENT PROCEDURE	NORMAL FINDINGS	ABNORMAL FINDINGS
Observe eye position and surrounding coloration.	Eyes are not sunken, and no dark circles appear under them.	Sunken eyes, especially with deep dark circles point to dehydration.
Lungs: Auscultate lung sounds.	No crackles, friction rubs, or harsh lung sounds	Loud or harsh breath sounds indicate decreased pleural fluid. Friction rubs may also be heard. Crackling indicates increased fluid, as in interstitial fluid sequestration, (ie, pulmonary edema).
Blood pressure and pulse: Take blood pressure with client in standing, sitting, and lying positions. Also palpate radial pulse.	No orthostatic changes; blood pressure and pulse rate remain within normal range for client's activity level and status.	Blood pressure registers lower than usual and/or drops more than 20 mmHg from lying to standing position, thereby indicating fluid volume deficit, especially if the pulse rate is also elevated. Radial pulse rate +1 and thready denotes dehydration. Elevated pulse rate and blood pressure indicate overhydration.

TABLE 8-5. Classification of Blood Pressure for Adults Age 18 and Older*

Category	Systolic (mmHg)		Diastolic (mmHg)
Optimal	<120	and	<80
Normal†	<130	and	<85
High-normal	130–139	or	85–89
Hypertension‡			
Stage 1	140–159	or	90–99
Stage 2	160–179	or	100–109
Stage 3	≥180	or	≥110

* Not taking antihypertensive drugs and not acutely ill. When systolic and diastolic blood pressures fall into different categories, the higher category should be selected to classify the individual's blood pressure status. For example, 160/92 mm Hg should be classified as stage 2 hypertension, and 174/120 mm Hg should be classified as stage 3 hypertension. Isolated systolic hypertension is defined as SBP of 140 mm Hg or greater and DBP below 90 mm Hg and staged appropriately (eg. 170/82 mm Hg is defined as stage 2 isolated systolic hypertension). In addition to classifying stages of hypertension on the basis of average blood pressure levels, clinicians should specify presence or absence of target organ disease and additional risk factors. This specificity is important for risk classification and treatment.

† Optimal blood pressure with respect to cardiovascular risk is below 120/80 mm Hg. However, unusually low readings should be evaluated for clinical significance.

‡ Based on the average of two or more readings taken at each of two or more visits after an initial screening.

(From the Report of the Sixth Joint National Committee on Prevention, Detection, Evaluation, and Treatment of High Blood Pressure, (1997). *Archives of Internal Medicine, 157,* 2413–2446.)

TABLE 8-6. Recommendations for Follow-up Based on Initial Blood Pressure Measurements for Adults

Initial Blood Pressure (mm Hg)*		
Systolic	Diastolic	Follow-up Recommended†
<130	<85	Recheck in 2 years
130–139	85–89	Recheck in 1 year‡
140–159	90–99	Confirm within 2 months
160–179	100–109	Evaluate or refer to source of care within 1 month
≥180	≥110	Evaluate or refer to source of care immediately or within 1 week depending on clinical situation

* If systolic and diastolic categories are different, follow recommendations for shorter time follow-up (eg. 160/86 mm Hg should be evaluated or referred to source of care within 1 month).

† Modify the scheduling of follow-up according to reliable information about past blood pressure measurements, other cardiovascular risk factors, or target organ disease.

‡ Provide advice about lifestyle modifications.

(From the Report of the Sixth Joint National Committee on Prevention, Detection, Evaluation, and Treatment of High Blood Pressure. [1997]. *Archives of Internal Medicine, 157,* 2413–2446.)

Validation and Documentation of Normal Findings

EXAMPLE OF SUBJECTIVE DATA

Ann Sanchez appears to be a 30- to 35-year-old Hispanic female. She is neatly and appropriately dressed for the time of year. Posture is erect and gait smooth. Well-developed body build for age with even distribution of fat and firm muscle. Client is alert, friendly, cooperative, and answers questions with good eye contact. Speech is fluent, clear, and moderately paced.

EXAMPLE OF OBJECTIVE DATA

Oral temperature: 98.6°F; radial pulse: 84/min regular, bilateral, equally strong, and resilient; respirations: 16/min regular, equal bilateral chest expansion; blood pressure: sitting position—120/78 right arm, 124/80 left arm; standing position—124/80, RA; 126/82, LA.

Height: 5 feet, 5 inches (165 cm); body frame: medium; weight: 128 lb (58 kg); BMI: 24; ideal body weight: 125; waist-to-hip ratio: .6; MAC: 28 cm; TSF: 16.8 mm; MAMC: 22.7 cm.

DISPLAY 8-4. Estimating Frame Size

To better use the height–weight charts, estimate the client's frame either by a wrist–height comparison (less precise but easy) or an evaluation of elbow breadth.

Wrist–Height Comparison

Use a tape measure to measure the wrist distal to the styloid process in inches. Then identify the client's height in inches. Compare results with the table below to get the approximate frame size.

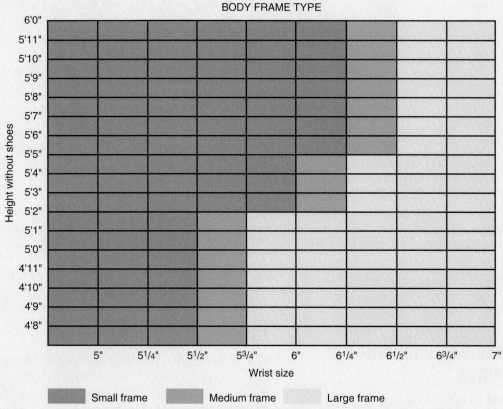

BODY FRAME TYPE

Height without shoes (vertical axis): 6'0", 5'11", 5'10", 5'9", 5'8", 5'7", 5'6", 5'5", 5'4", 5'3", 5'2", 5'1", 5'0", 4'11", 4'10", 4'9", 4'8"

Wrist size (horizontal axis): 5", 5¼", 5½", 5¾", 6", 6¼", 6½", 6¾", 7"

Small frame   Medium frame   Large frame

The wrist is measured distal to styloid process of radius and ulna at smallest circumference. Use height without shoes and inches for wrist size to determine frame type from this chart.

You can also calculate the frame using the following formula:

$$\frac{\text{height in centimeters or inches}}{\text{wrist in centimeters or inches}} = r$$

Results of the above formula may be interpreted as follows:

Males	Females
Small: r > 10.4	Small: r > 11.0
Medium: r = 9.6 – 10.4	Medium: r = 10.1 – 11.0
Large: r < 9.6	Large: r > 10.1

Elbow Breadth

For greatest accuracy, use flat-blade sliding calipers or a broad-blade anthropometer. For estimating purposes, however, you can use calipers used to measure fat stores. Ask the client to hold the right arm in front of the body and bend the elbow at a 90-degree angle. Place the calipers or the anthropometer on the outside of the condoyles of the humerus, and measure the distance between the condoyles. Identify the frame size by comparing findings with the table below in relationship to age.

(continued)

DISPLAY 8-4. Estimating Frame Size (Continued)

Frame Size by Elbow Breadth of Male and Female Adults in the United States

| Age (yr) | Frame Size (cm) | | |
	Small	Medium	Large
Males			
18–24	≤6.6	>6.6 and <7.7	≥7.7
25–34	≤6.7	>6.7 and <7.9	≥7.9
35–44	≤6.7	>6.7 and <8.0	≥8.0
45–54	≤6.7	>6.7 and <8.1	≥8.1
55–64	≤6.7	>6.7 and <8.1	≥8.1
65–74	≤6.7	>6.7 and <8.1	≥8.1
Females			
18–24	≤5.6	>5.6 and <6.5	≥6.5
25–34	≤5.7	>5.7 and <6.8	≥6.8
35–44	≤5.7	>5.7 and <7.1	≥7.1
45–54	≤5.7	>5.7 and <7.2	≥7.2
55–64	≤5.8	>5.8 and <7.2	≥7.2
65–74	≤5.8	>5.8 and <7.2	≥7.2

(From Frisancho, A. R. [1984]. New standards of weight and body composition by frame size and height for assessment of nutritional status of adults and the elderly. (*American Journal of Clinical Nutrition*, 808–819. © American Society for Clinical Nutrition.)

TABLE 8-7. Percentiles of Upper Arm Circumference (mm) and Estimated Upper Arm Muscle Circumference (mm)

| Age (yr) | Arm Circumference (mm) | | | | | | | Arm Muscle Circumference (mm) | | | | | | |
	5	10	25	50	75	90	95	5	10	25	50	75	90	95
Male														
1–1.9	142	146	150	159	170	176	183	110	113	119	127	135	144	147
2–2.9	141	145	153	162	170	178	185	111	114	122	130	140	146	150
3–3.9	150	153	160	167	175	184	190	117	123	131	137	143	148	153
4–4.9	149	154	162	171	180	186	192	123	126	133	141	148	156	159
5–5.9	153	160	167	175	185	195	204	128	133	140	147	154	162	169
6–6.9	155	159	167	179	188	209	228	131	135	142	151	161	170	177
7–7.9	162	167	177	187	201	223	230	137	139	151	160	168	177	190
8–8.9	162	170	177	190	202	220	245	140	145	154	162	170	182	187
9–9.9	175	178	187	200	217	249	257	151	154	161	170	183	196	202
10–10.9	181	184	196	210	231	262	274	156	160	166	180	191	209	221
11–11.9	186	190	202	223	244	261	280	159	165	173	183	195	205	230
12–12.9	193	200	216	232	254	282	303	167	171	182	195	210	223	241
13–13.9	194	211	228	247	263	286	301	172	179	196	211	226	238	245
14–14.9	220	226	237	253	283	303	322	189	199	212	223	240	260	264
15–15.9	222	229	244	264	284	311	320	199	204	218	237	254	266	272
16–16.9	244	248	262	278	303	324	343	213	225	234	249	269	287	296
17–17.9	246	253	267	285	308	336	347	224	231	245	258	273	294	312

(continued)

TABLE 8-7. Percentiles of Upper Arm Circumference (mm) and Estimated Upper Arm Muscle Circumference (mm) (Continued)

Age (yr)	Arm Circumference (mm)							Arm Muscle Circumference (mm)						
	5	10	25	50	75	90	95	5	10	25	50	75	90	95
Male (continued)														
18–18.9	245	260	276	297	321	353	379	226	237	252	264	283	298	324
19–24.9	262	272	288	308	331	355	372	238	245	258	273	289	309	321
25–34.9	271	282	300	319	342	362	375	243	250	264	279	298	314	326
35–44.9	278	287	305	326	345	363	374	247	255	269	286	302	318	327
45–54.9	267	281	301	322	342	362	376	239	249	265	281	300	315	326
55–64.9	258	273	296	317	336	355	269	236	245	260	278	295	310	320
65–74.9	248	263	285	307	325	344	355	223	235	251	268	284	298	306
Female														
1–1.9	138	142	148	156	164	172	177	105	111	117	124	132	139	143
2–2.9	142	145	152	160	167	176	184	111	114	119	126	133	142	147
3–3.9	143	150	158	167	175	183	189	113	119	124	132	140	146	152
4–4.9	149	154	160	169	177	184	191	115	121	128	136	144	152	157
5–5.9	153	157	165	175	185	203	211	125	128	134	142	151	159	165
6–6.9	156	162	170	176	187	204	211	130	133	138	145	154	166	171
7–7.9	164	167	174	183	199	216	231	129	135	142	151	160	171	176
8–8.9	168	172	183	195	214	247	261	138	140	151	160	171	183	194
9–9.9	178	182	194	211	224	251	260	147	150	158	167	180	194	198
10–10.9	174	182	193	210	228	251	265	148	150	159	170	180	190	197
11–11.9	185	194	208	224	248	276	303	150	158	171	181	196	217	223
12–12.9	194	203	216	237	256	282	294	162	166	180	191	201	214	220
13–13.9	202	211	223	243	271	301	338	169	175	183	198	211	226	240
14–14.9	214	223	237	252	272	304	322	174	179	190	201	216	232	247
15–15.9	208	221	239	254	279	300	322	175	178	189	202	215	228	244
16–16.9	218	224	241	258	283	318	334	170	180	190	202	216	234	249
17–17.9	220	227	241	264	295	324	350	175	183	194	205	221	239	257
18–18.9	222	227	241	258	281	312	325	174	179	191	202	215	237	245
19–24.9	221	230	247	265	290	319	345	179	185	195	207	221	236	249
25–34.9	233	240	256	277	304	342	368	183	188	199	212	228	246	264
35–44.9	241	251	267	290	317	356	378	186	192	205	218	236	257	272
45–54.9	242	256	274	299	328	362	384	187	193	206	220	238	260	274
55–64.9	243	257	280	303	335	367	385	187	196	209	225	244	266	280
65–74.9	240	252	274	299	326	356	373	185	195	208	225	244	264	279

(From Frisancho, A. R. [1981]. New norms of upper limb fat and muscle areas for assessment of nutritional status. *American Journal of Clinical Nutrition, 30*, 2540–2548. © American Society for Clinical Nutrition.)

TABLE 8-7. Selected Percentiles of Triceps Skinfold Thickness and Bone-Free Upper Arm Area by Height in U.S. Women, Age 25 to 54 yr, with Small, Medium, and Large Frames

Height		Triceps (mm)							Bone-Free MAMA (cm²)						
		5	10	15	50	85	90	95	5	10	15	50	85	90	95
Small Frame															
in	cm														
58	147		12	13	24	30	33			22	24	29	36	44	
59	150	8	11	14	21	29	36	37	17	20	22	28	38	39	43
60	152	8	11	12	21	28	29	33	19	21	22	28	36	40	44
61	155	11	12	14	21	28	31	34	20	21	23	28	28	39	42
62	157	10	12	14	20	28	31	34	20	21	21	27	33	35	37
63	160	10	11	13	20	27	30	36	20	21	22	27	33	35	38
64	163	10	13	13	20	28	30	34	22	23	23	28	34	38	42
65	165	12	13	14	22	29	31	34	21	22	23	28	37	39	47
66	168			12	19	30						23	27	35	
67	170				18							26			
68	173				20							25			
69	175														
70	178														
Medium Frame															
in	cm														
58	147			20	25	40					24	35	42		
59	150	15	19	21	30	37	40	40	23	24	26	33	43	45	49
60	152	14	15	17	26	35	37	41	22	25	25	32	42	45	49
61	155	11	14	15	25	34	36	42	21	24	25	31	42	45	51
62	157	12	14	16	24	34	36	40	21	23	25	31	40	43	48
63	160	12	13	15	24	33	35	38	22	23	25	32	41	43	50
64	163	11	14	15	23	33	36	40	21	23	24	31	40	43	48
65	165	12	14	15	22	31	34	38	21	23	24	31	40	43	49
66	168	11	13	14	22	31	33	37	21	23	24	30	39	41	44
67	170	12	13	15	21	29	30	35	22	24	25	30	40	43	48
68	173	10	14	15	22	31	32	36	22	24	25	30	37	38	39
69	175		11	12	19	29	31				23	24	30	36	39
70	178				19							32			
Large Frame															
in	cm														
58	147														
59	150				36							45			
60	152				38							44			
61	155		25	26	36	48	50			29	33	41	62	74	
62	157	16	19	22	34	48	48	50	26	28	31	44	56	63	72
63	160	18	20	22	34	48	48	50	27	30	32	43	60	65	77
64	163	16	20	21	32	43	45	49	26	28	29	39	50	55	63
65	165	17	20	21	31	43	46	48	27	28	29	39	56	59	67
66	168	13	17	18	27	40	43	45	23	24	27	35	49	53	69
67	170	13	16	17	30	41	43	49	25	28	30	37	50	53	55
68	173		16	20	29	37	40			28	30	38	51	54	
69	175			21	30	42					27	35	49		
70	178				20							37			

MAMA = mid-arm muscle area. (Adapted from Frisancho, A.R. [1984]. New standards of weight and body composition by frame size and height for assessment of nutritional status of adults and the elderly. *American Journal of Clinical Nutrition, 40*, 808–809. © American Society for Clinical Nutrition.)

TABLE 8-8. Selected Percentiles of Triceps Skinfold Thickness and Bone-Free Upper Arm Area by Height in US Men, Age 25 to 54 yr, with Small, Medium, and Large Frames

Height		Triceps (mm)							Bone-Free MAMA (cm²)						
		5	10	15	50	85	90	95	5	10	15	50	85	90	95
Small Frame															
in	cm														
62	157				11							52			
63	160			6	10	17				32		48	54		
64	163		5	5	10	16	18			37	38	49	58	63	
65	165	4	5	6	11	17	19	21	31	35	37	47	60	63	71
66	168	5	6	6	11	18	18	20	31	36	38	49	60	62	71
67	170	5	6	6	11	18	20	22	35	39	41	49	58	60	62
68	173	5	6	6	10	15	16	20	33	37	40	49	59	62	69
69	175		6	6	11	17	20			36	40	58	61	63	
70	178			7	10	17					35	48	57		
71	180			7	10	16					39	47	52		
72	183				10							45			
73	185														
74	188														
Medium Frame															
in	cm														
62	157				15							58			
63	160				11							55			
64	163		6	6	12	18	20			43	47	56	67	71	
65	165	5	7	8	12	20	22	25	40	43	45	56	67	69	70
66	168	5	6	7	11	16	18	22	38	42	44	55	69	72	78
67	170	5	7	7	13	21	23	28	39	42	44	53	66	69	73
68	173	4	5	7	11	18	20	24	41	44	45	55	67	71	76
69	175	5	6	7	12	18	20	24	38	41	44	54	66	69	73
70	178	5	6	7	12	18	20	23	39	42	43	55	65	68	72
71	180	4	5	7	12	19	21	25	37	41	44	54	67	68	73
72	183	5	7	7	12	20	22	26	40	42	44	56	65	67	74
73	185	6	7	8	12	20	24	27	39	42	43	55	67	69	73
74	188		6	9	13	21	23			43	43	55	62	63	
Large Frame															
in	cm														
62	157														
63	160														
64	163														
65	165				14							62			
66	168			9	14	30					48	58	76		
67	170		7	7	11	23	27			50	52	61	73	78	
68	173		9	10	14	22	23			51	53	65	78	86	
69	175	6	7	8	15	25	29	31	46	48	49	61	73	78	83
70	178	7	7	7	14	23	25	30	43	47	50	61	75	77	86
71	180	6	8	10	15	25	27	31	47	48	50	62	75	81	83
72	183	5	6	7	12	20	22	25	45	48	50	61	77	80	86
73	185	5	6	7	13	19	22	31	47	49	51	66	79	83	86
74	188			8	12	19					53	66	78		

MAMA = mid-arm muscle area. (Adapted from Frisancho, A. R. [1984]. New standards of weight and body composition by frame size and height for assessment of nutritional status of adults and the elderly. *American Journal of Clinical Nutrition, 40,* 808–819, © American Society for Clinical Nutrition.)

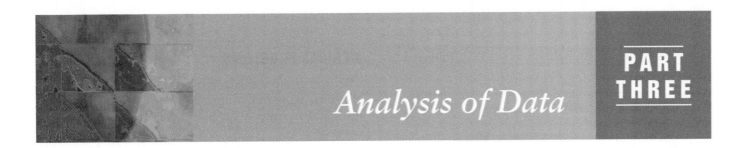

After you have collected your assessment data, you will need to analyze the data, using diagnostic reasoning skills discussed in Chapters 6 and 7. Diagnostic Reasoning: Case Study shows you how to analyze data from a general survey for a specific client. Finally, you have an opportunity to analyze data in the critical thinking exercise in the study guide/laboratory manual that accompanies this text.

Diagnostic Reasoning: Possible Conclusions

Below are some possible conclusions related to your general survey.

SELECTED NURSING DIAGNOSES

After collecting subjective and objective data pertaining to the general survey, you will need to identify abnormals and cluster the data to reveal any significant patterns or abnormalities. These data will then be used to make clinical judgments (nursing diagnoses: wellness, risk, or actual) about the status of the client's general survey. Following is a list of selected nursing diagnoses that you may identify when analyzing data for this part of the assessment.

Nursing Diagnoses (Wellness)

- Opportunity to Enhance Health-Seeking Behaviors related to desire and request to learn more about health promotion

Nursing Diagnoses (Risk)

- Risk for Hyperthermia related to impending dehydration secondary to nausea and vomiting
- Risk for Hyperthermia related to lack of adequate home cooling system and high environmental temperatures forecasted
- Risk for Hypothermia related to decreased tactile sensations, decreased cardiac output, and decreased subcutaneous tissue secondary to the aging process

Nursing Diagnoses (Actual)

- Impaired Verbal Communication related to foreign language barrier (inability to speak English or accepted dominant language)
- Impaired Verbal Communication related to hearing loss
- Impaired Verbal Communication related to inability to clearly express self or understand others (aphasia)
- Dressing/Grooming Self-Care Deficit related to impaired upper-extremity mobility and lack of resources
- Bathing/Hygiene Self-Care Deficit related to inability to wash body parts or inability to obtain water
- Hyperthermia related to vigorous exercise and exposure to high temperatures
- Hyperthermia related to dehydration or increased metabolic rate
- Hyperthermia related to decreased ability to sweat
- Hypothermia related to malnutrition, consumption of alcohol, low body weight, and unprotected exposure to cold, sleet, and snow
- Imbalanced Nutrition: More Than Body Requirements related to excessive caloric intake and sedentary lifestyle
- Imbalanced Nutrition: Less Than Body Requirements related to inadequate caloric/nutrient intake secondary to lack of access and ability to prepare or obtain nutritious foods to meet caloric and nutritive requirements
- Ineffective Thermoregulation related to decreased ability to adapt to cold or heat secondary to aging process (eg, decreased circulation, decreased metabolism, decreased subcutaneous tissue)

SELECTED COLLABORATIVE PROBLEMS

After you group the data, it may become apparent that certain collaborative problems emerge. Remember, collaborative problems differ from nursing diagnoses in that they cannot be prevented by nursing interventions. However, these physiologic complications of medical conditions can be detected and monitored by the nurse. In addition, the nurse can use physician- and nurse-prescribed interventions to minimize the complications of these problems. The nurse may also have to refer the client in such situations for further treatment of the problem. Following is a list of collaborative problems that may be identified when obtaining a general impression. These problems are worded as Potential Complications (or PC), followed by the problem.

- PC: Hypertension
- PC: Hypotension
- PC: Dysrhythmias

MEDICAL PROBLEMS

After you group the data, it may become apparent that the client has signs and symptoms that require medical diagnosis and treatment. Refer to a primary care provider as necessary.

Diagnostic Reasoning: Case Study

The case study presents assessment data for a specific client. It is followed by an analysis of the data, working out the seven key steps to arrive at specific conclusions.

Mrs. Helen Jones, 78 years old, has a history of insulin-dependent diabetes mellitus (IDDM), also known as type 1 diabetes. When you weigh her during your weekly home visit, you find that she weighs 98 lb, which is 12 lb less than she weighed at your last visit. You try to weigh her at the same time of day each week—9:30 AM. She usually has breakfast at 6:30 AM and takes her morning NPH insulin, 40 units, at 7:30 AM. Today, she tells you that she has been urinating "a lot," and that she feels like she has had the flu for about 3 days, with nausea and "just a little vomiting." She says she has not been eating well but adds, "I'm keeping my blood sugar up by drinking orange juice."

On assessment, you find that she has soft, sunken eyeballs and her tongue is dry and furrowed. Her blood pressure is 104/86 (usual is 150/88); her pulse is 92, and respirations are 22. Her temperature is 99.4°F. Her blood glucose level, tested by fingerstick, is 468 mg/dL (usual is 250–300 mg/dL). Mrs. Jones refuses to check her blood glucose level herself. When asked why she did not call the nurse or doctor when she be-

came ill, she stated, "I didn't think it was that serious—I didn't have a high temperature."

1 Identify abnormal data and strengths (in both subjective and objective data).

SUBJECTIVE DATA

- "Urinating a lot"
- Feels like she had the flu for 3 days
- Nausea and vomiting
- Not eating well
- "Keeping blood sugar up by drinking orange juice"
- Did not think illness serious because she didn't have a high temperature

OBJECTIVE DATA

- Diagnosed with IDDM
- Weight loss of 12 lb in 1 week
- Soft, sunken eyeballs and dry, furrowed tongue
- BP 104/86
- Temperature 99.4°F
- Blood glucose level (by fingerstick test) is 468 mg/dL
- Takes 40 U NPH insulin every morning
- Did not notify physician or nurse of illness

2 Cue Clusters	3 Inferences	4 Possible Nursing Diagnoses	5 Defining Characteristics	6 Confirm or Rule Out
A • Weight loss—12 lb in 1 week • Soft, sunken eyeballs • Dry, furrowed tongue • Systolic BP down 46 points • Blood glucose level 468 mg/dL • Nausea and vomiting	Dehydration due to the osmotic diuretic effect of the high blood sugar. Short-term weight loss indicative of fluid loss.	Fluid Volume Deficit related to oral intake inadequate to balance excessive urinary output secondary to nausea, vomiting and high blood glucose.	*Major:* Weight loss and dry mucous membranes *Minor:* Excessive urine output	Accept diagnosis if validated by client since it meets defining characteristic.

	2 Data Clusters	3 Inferences	4 Possible Nursing Diagnoses	5 Presence of Defining Characteristics	6 Confirm or Rule Out
B	• Weight loss—12 lb in 1 week • Not eating well • Nausea and vomiting	Not eating because of nausea and vomiting could contribute to weight loss as well.	Imbalanced Nutrition: Less Than Body Requirements related to decreased desire to eat secondary to flu symptoms and nausea and vomiting	*Major:* Reported inadequate food intake; weight loss *Minor:* None	Confirm, because it meets defining characteristic. However, because of her diabetic status, collect more data when flu symptoms subside. This may be a temporary situation that can be corrected when glucose level returns to a more normal range.
C	• Does not self-test blood glucose level • Drank orange juice when not eating • Did not report illness • Did not think illness serious because temperature not high (99.4°F)	Is at risk for increased complications of diabetes due to not knowing when to notify nurse or physician and not checking own blood glucose level. Also, does not seem to know that older clients may not have a high fever with illness.	Ineffective Management of Therapeutic Regimen related to inadequate knowledge of how to manage diabetes when ill and to belief that seriousness of illness is directly proportional to degree of fever.	*Major:* Verbalizes difficulty with integration of one of the prescribed regimens for treatment of illness (refusing to monitor blood glucose level and not calling nurse/physician when ill) *Minor:* Acceleration of illness symptoms (blood glucose level 468 mg/dL)	Accept diagnosis since it meets both major and minor defining characteristics and is validated by client. Collect more information about knowledge and ability to manage diabetes with weekly nursing visits. There may be other areas in which client needs information and help.
D	• Diagnosis of IDDM • Flu for 3 days • Takes 40 U NPH daily • Blood glucose level 468 mg/dL • Temperature 99.4°F	Diabetes is out of control due to hyperglycemia—current insulin dosage may be inadequate. Client's status needs to be reevaluated by physician.			

7 Document conclusions.

All three of the alternative diagnoses are appropriate for Mrs. Jones at this time:

- Fluid Volume Deficit related to oral intake inadequate to balance excessive urinary output secondary to nausea and vomiting and high blood glucose
- Imbalanced Altered Nutrition: Less Than Body Requirements related to decreased desire to eat secondary to flu symptoms and nausea and vomiting

- Ineffective Management of Therapeutic Regimen related to inadequate knowledge of how to manage diabetes when ill and that seriousness of illness is directly proportional to degree of fever

In addition, collaborative problems to be alert for include ketoacidosis, hyperglycemic hyperosmolar nonketotic (HHNK) syndrome, infection, vascular disease, diabetic retinopathy, diabetic neuropathy, and nephropathy. Mrs. Jones needs an immediate referral to her physician to manage the acute episode of hyperglycemia, to treat her "flu," and to evaluate her diabetic treatment regimen.

REFERENCES AND SELECTED READINGS

Academy of Sciences—National Research Council, Food & Nutrition Board. (1989). *Recommended dietary allowances, selected standard heights in adults.* Washington, DC: Author.

Amara, A. M., & Cerrato, P. L. (1996). Eating disorders—still a threat. *RN, 59* (6), 30–35.

American Heart Association. (1987). *Recommendations for measuring human blood pressure determination by sphygmomanometer.* Publication No. 7001005. Dallas, TX: Author.

Armstrong, L., Maresh, C., Castellani, J., Bergeron, M. M., Kenefick, R., Lagrasse, K., & Reibe, D. (1994). Urinary indices of hydration status. *International Journal of Sport Nutrition, 4* (3), 265–279.

Bishop, C. W., Bowen, P. E., & Ritchey, S. J. (1981). Reference data (percentiles) for midarm circumference, triceps skinfold, and mid-arm muscle circumference. *American Journal of Clinical Nutrition, 34,* 25–30.

Cole, F. L. (1993). Temporal variation in the effects of iced water on oral temperature. *Research in Nursing Health, 16* (2), 107–111.

Cooper, K. M. (1992). Measuring blood pressure the right way. *Nursing 92, 22* (4), 75.

Corbett, J. V. (2000). *Laboratory tests and diagnostic procedures* (5th ed.). Upper Saddle River, NJ: Prentice Hall.

Erickson, R. (1976). Thermometer placement for oral temperature measurement in febrile adults. *International Journal of Nursing Studies, 38,* 671–675.

Frisancho, A. R. (1984). New standards of weight and body composition by frame size and height for assessment of nutritional status of adults and the elderly. *American Journal of Clinical Nutrition, 40,* 808–819.

Garcia, C., & Gibner, J. (1990). A comparative study of temperatures in the elderly. *Nursing Homes, 39* (5/6), 21–23.

Geyer, N. (1995). Continuing education: Clinical vital signs: Assessment of body temperature. Part 3. *Nursing News* (South Africa), *19* (6), 18–20.

Hill, M. N. (1991). How to take a precise blood pressure. *American Journal of Nursing, 91* (2), 38–42.

Hollerbach, A., & Sneed, N. (1990). Accuracy of radial pulse assessment by length of counting interval. *Heart and Lung, 19* (3), 258–264.

Kittler, P. G., & Sucher, K. (2001). *Food and culture.* Belmont, CA: West-Wadsworth.

Konopad, E., Kerr, J. R., Noseworthy, T., & Grace, H. (1994). A comparison of oral, axillary, rectal, and tympanic membrane temperatures of intensive care patients with and without an oral endotracheal tube. *Journal of Advanced Nursing, 20* (1), 77–84.

Ludwig, D. S., Majzoub, J. A., Al-Zahrani, A., Dallal, G. E., Blanco, I., & Roberts, S. (1999, March). High glycemic-index foods, overeating, and obesity. *Pediatrics, 103.*

Lyke, E. M. (1992). *Assessing for nursing diagnosis: A human needs approach.* Philadelphia: J. B. Lippincott.

Mentes, J. C. (2000). Hydration management protocol. *Journal of Gerontological Nursing, 26* (10), 6–15.

Metropolitan Life Insurance Company. (1988). Data from Build Study 1979, Society of Actuaries and Association of Life Insurance Medical Directors of America. New York: Author.

Murphy, L., & Linn, L. (1996). Managing vital sign monitoring problems. *Nursing, 26* (1), 32.

Nowazels, V., & Neeley, M. A. (1996). Health assessment of the older patient. *Critical Care Nursing Quarterly, 19* (2), 1–6.

Office of Disease Prevention and Health Promotion, US Department of Health and Human Services. (2000). *Healthy people 2010: Understanding and improving health* (2nd ed.). Washington, DC: Author.

Report of the Sixth Joint National Committee on Prevention, Detection, Evaluation and Treatment of High Blood Pressure. (1997). *Archives of Internal Medicine, 157,* 2413–2446.

Roper, M. (1996). Back to basics: Assessing orthostatic vital signs. *American Journal of Nursing, 96* (8), 43–46.

Ross Laboratories. (1988). *Nutritional assessment of the elderly through anthropometry.* Columbus, OH: Author.

For additional information on this book, be sure to visit http://connection.lww.com.

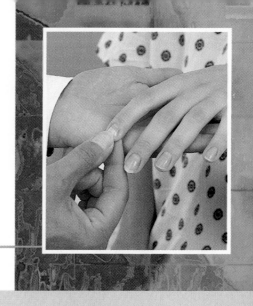

Skin, Hair, and Nail Assessment

9

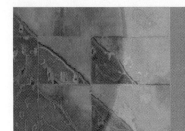

Structure and Function

PART ONE

The skin, hair, and nails are external structures that serve a variety of specialized functions. The sebaceous and sweat glands originating within the skin also have many vital functions. Each of these structures and their function is described separately.

Skin

The skin is composed of three layers, the epidermis, dermis, and subcutaneous tissue (Fig. 9-1). The skin is thicker on the palms of the hands and soles of the feet and is continuous with the mucous membranes at the orifices of the body. Subcutaneous tissue, which contains varying amounts of fat, connects the skin to underlying structures.

The skin is a physical barrier that protects the underlying tissues and structures from microorganisms, physical trauma, ultraviolet radiation, and dehydration. It plays a vital role in temperature maintenance, fluid and electrolyte balance, absorption, excretion, sensation, immunity, and vitamin D synthesis. The skin also provides an individual identity to a person's appearance.

EPIDERMIS

The epidermis, the outer layer of skin, is composed of four distinct layers (see Fig. 9-1): the stratum corneum, stratum lucidum, stratum granulosum, and stratum germinativum. The outermost layer consists of dead, keratinized cells that render the skin waterproof. (Keratin is a scleroprotein that is insoluble in water. The epidermis, hair, nails, dental enamel, and horny tissues are composed of keratin.) The epidermal layer is almost completely replaced every 3 to 4 weeks. The innermost layer of the epidermis (stratum germinativum) is the only layer that undergoes cell division and contains melanin (brown pigment) and keratin-forming cells. Skin color depends on the amount of melanin and carotene (yellow pigment) contained in the skin and the volume of blood containing hemoglobin, the oxygen-binding pigment that circulates in the dermis.

DERMIS

The inner layer of skin is the dermis (see Fig. 9-1). It is connected to the epidermis by means of papillae. These papillae form the base for the visible swirls or friction ridges that provide the unique pattern of fingerprints with which we

are familiar. Ridges also appear on the palms of the hands, the toes, and the soles of the feet. The dermis is a well-vascularized connective tissue layer containing collagen and elastic fibers, nerve endings, and lymph vessels. It is also the origin of hair follicles, sebaceous glands, and sweat glands.

Sebaceous Glands

The sebaceous glands (see Fig. 9-1) develop from hair follicles and, therefore, are present over most of the body, excluding the soles and palms. They secrete an oily substance called sebum that lubricates hair and skin and reduces water loss through the skin. Sebum also has some fungicidal and bactericidal effects.

Sweat Glands

Sweat glands (see Fig. 9-1) are of two types, eccrine and apocrine. The eccrine glands are located over the entire skin surface and secrete an odorless, colorless fluid, the evaporation of which is vital to the regulation of body temperature. The apocrine glands are concentrated in the axillae, perineum, and areolae of the breast and usually open through a hair follicle. They secrete a milky sweat. The interaction of sweat with skin bacteria produces a characteristic body odor. Apocrine glands are dormant until puberty, at which time they become active. In women, apocrine secretions are linked with the menstrual cycle.

SUBCUTANEOUS TISSUE

Merging with the dermis is the subcutaneous tissue, which is a loose connective tissue containing fat cells, blood vessels, nerves, and the remaining portions of sweat glands and hair follicles (see Fig. 9-1). The subcutaneous tissue assists with heat regulation and contains the vascular pathways for the supply of nutrients and removal of waste products from the skin.

Hair

Hair consists of layers of keratinized cells found over much of the body except for the lips, nipples, soles of the feet, palms of the hands, labia minora, and penis. Hair develops within a sheath of epidermal cells called the hair follicle. Hair growth occurs at the base of the follicle, where cells in the hair bulb are nourished by dermal blood vessels. The hair shaft is visible above the skin; the hair root is surrounded by the hair follicle (see Fig. 9-1). Attached to the follicle are the erector pili muscles, which contract in response to cold or fright, decreasing skin surface area and causing the hair to stand erect.

There are two general types of hair: vellus and terminal. Vellus hair is short, pale, and fine and is present over much of the body. The terminal hair (particularly scalp and eyebrows) is longer, generally darker, and coarser than the vellus hair. Puberty initiates the growth of additional terminal hair in both sexes on the axillae, perineum, and legs. Hair color varies and is determined by the type and amount of pigment production. The absence of pigment or the inclusion of air spaces within the layers of the hair shaft results in gray or white hair.

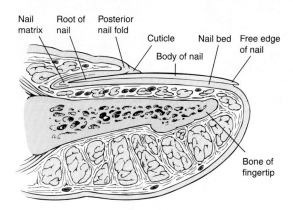

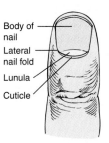

FIGURE 9-2. The nail and related structures.

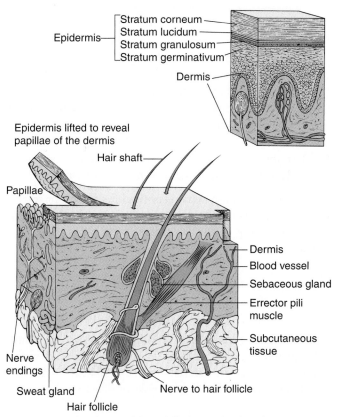

FIGURE 9-1. The skin and hair follicles and related structures.

Hair serves useful functions. Scalp hair is a protective covering. Nasal hair and ear hair, as well as eyelashes and eyebrows, filter dust and other airborne debris.

Nails

The nails, located on the distal phalanges of fingers and toes, are hard, transparent plates of keratinized epidermal cells that grow from a root underneath the skin fold called the cuticle (Fig. 9-2). The nail body extends over the entire nailbed and has a pink tinge as a result of the rich blood supply underneath. At the base of the nail is the lunula, a paler, crescent-shaped area. The nails protect the distal ends of the fingers and toes.

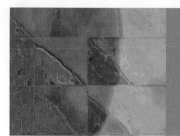

Nursing Assessment

PART TWO

Collecting Subjective Data

Diseases and disorders of the skin, hair, and nails can be local, or they may be caused by an underlying systemic problem. To perform a complete and accurate assessment, the nurse needs to collect data about current symptoms, the client's past and family history, and lifestyle and health practices. The information obtained provides clues to the client's overall level of functioning in relation to the skin, hair, and nails. (See Risk Factors—Skin Cancer for more information.)

INTERVIEW APPROACH

When interviewing a client for information regarding skin, hair, and nails, ask questions in a straightforward manner. Keep in mind that a nonjudgmental and sensitive approach is needed if the client has abnormalities that may be associated with poor hygiene or unhealthful behaviors. Also, some skin disorders might be highly visible and potentially damaging to the person's body image and self-concept.

Remember, if the client reports any symptom, you need to explore it further with a symptom analysis. Use the COLDSPA mnemonic as a guide:

COLDSPA

CHARACTER: Describe the sign or symptom. How does it feel, look, sound, smell, and so forth?

ONSET: When did it begin?

LOCATION: Where is it? Does it radiate?

DURATION: How long does it last? Does it recur?

SEVERITY: How bad is it?

PATTERN: What makes it better: What makes it worse?

ASSOCIATED FACTORS: What other symptoms occur with it?

Nursing History
HISTORY OF CURRENT SYMPTOMS

Question Are you experiencing any current skin problems, such as rashes, lesions, dryness, oiliness, drainage, bruising, swelling, or increased pigmentation? What aggravates the problem? What relieves it?

Tip From the Experts Because of differences in education, language, or cultural background, some clients may provide vague or confusing answers. Be sure to state questions clearly and use words that the client can understand; avoid medical jargon.

Rationale Any of these symptoms may be related to a pathologic skin condition and may affect the client's response. Bruises, welts, or burns may indicate accidents or trauma or abuse. If these injuries cannot be explained or the client's explanation seems unbelievable or vague, physical abuse should be suspected.

Q Describe any birthmarks, tattoos, or moles you now have. Have any of them changed color, size, or shape?

R You need to know what is normal for the client so that future variations can be detected. A change in the appearance or bleeding of any skin mark, especially a mole, may indicate cancer.

Q Have you noticed any change in your ability to feel pain, pressure, light touch, or temperature changes? Are you experiencing any pain, itching, tingling, or numbness?

R Changes in sensation may indicate vascular or neurologic problems, such as peripheral neuropathy related to diabetes mellitus or arterial occlusive disease. Sensation problems may put the client at risk for developing pressure ulcers.

Q Have you had any hair loss or change in the condition of your hair? Describe.

R Patchy hair loss may accompany infections, stress, hairstyles that put stress on hair roots, and some types of chemotherapy. Generalized hair loss may be seen in various systemic illnesses such as hypothyroidism and in clients receiving certain types of chemotherapy or radiation therapy.

 A receding hair line or male pattern baldness may occur with aging.

RISK FACTORS
Skin Cancer

OVERVIEW

Skin cancer is the most common of cancers. It occurs in three types: melanoma, basal cell carcinoma (BCC), and squamous cell carcinoma (SCC). BCC and SCC are nonmelanomas. It was estimated that 92,000 new melanoma cases and 2.75 million nonmelanocyte cases occur worldwide each year (Armstrong & Dricker, 1995). The American Cancer Society predicted that there would be 1,900 deaths from nonmelanoma skin cancers and 7,700 deaths from melanoma during the year 2000.

The incidence of melanoma (new cases per 100,000 population) increased from 5.7 to 13.8 between 1973 and 2000. Melanoma accounts for 4% of skin cancers but 79% of skin cancer deaths. Nonmelanocyte skin cancers are the most common and are also increasing in populations that are heavily exposed to sunlight, especially in areas of ozone depletion. Davidowitz, Belafsky, and Amedee (1999) state that melanoma will develop in 1 in 70 white Americans.

Intermittent exposure to the sun or ultraviolet radiation is associated with greatest risk for melanoma and for BCC, but overall amount of exposure is thought to be associated with SCC. SCC is most common on body sites with very heavy sun exposure, whereas BCC is most common on sites with moderate exposure (ie, upper trunk or women's lower legs).

Precursor lesions occur for some melanomas (benign or dysplastic nevi) and for invasive SCC (actinic keratoses or SCC in situ), but there are no precursor lesions for BCC (Gloster & Brodland, 1995).

RISK FACTORS

- Sun exposure, especially intermittent pattern with sunburn; risk increases if excessive sun exposure began in childhood
- Nonsolar sources of ultraviolet radiation (tanning booth, sunlamps)
- Medical therapies, such as PUVA and ionizing radiation
- Family history and genetic susceptibility (especially for malignant melanoma)
- Moles, especially atypical lesions
- Pigmentation irregularities (albinism, burn scars)
- Fair skin that burns and freckles easily; light hair
- Immunosuppression
- Age; risk increases with increasing age
- Male gender (for nonmelanoma cancers)
- Chemical exposure (arsenic, tar, coal, paraffin, some oils for nonmelanoma cancers)
- Human papillomavirus (nonmelanoma cancers)
- Xeroderma pigmentosum (rare, inherited condition)
- Long-term skin inflammation or injury (nonmelanoma)

RISK REDUCTION TEACHING TIPS

- Reduce sun exposure.
- Always use sunscreen (SPF 15 or higher) when sun exposure is anticipated.
- Wear long-sleeved shirts and wide-brimmed hats.
- Avoid sunburns.
- Avoid intermittent tanning.
- Understand the link between sun exposure and skin cancer and the accumulating effects of sun exposure on developing cancers.
- Examine the skin for suspect lesions. If there is anything unusual, seek professional advice as soon as possible.

 ### CULTURAL CONSIDERATIONS

The darkness of skin pigmentation affects the incidence of all skin cancers, with the lowest rates occurring in Asians and the highest rates in white Australians. The most susceptible are people with pale white, freckled skin and red hair. Australians have mounted an intense campaign that emphasizes wearing sunscreen, long sleeves, and hats any time they are in the sun. Although less susceptible to skin cancer, African Americans have two additional risk factors beside the ones listed previously. These are higher incidences of chronic inflammatory skin diseases and chronic discoid lupus erythematosus (Halder & Bridgeman-Shah, 1995). Teaching about skin cancer prevention and diagnosis should be provided to African Americans and Asians, even though they have a lower incidence than whites (Hall & Rogers, 1999).

Q Have you had any change in the condition or appearance of your nails? Describe.

R Nail changes may be seen in systemic disorders such as malnutrition or with local irritation (eg, nail biting).

Q Do you have trouble controlling body odor? How much do you perspire?

R Uncontrolled body odor or excessive or insufficient perspiration may indicate an abnormality with the sweat glands or an endocrine problem such as hypothyroidism or hyperthyroidism. Poor hygiene practices may account for body odor, and health education may be indicated.

 Perspiration decreases with aging because sweat gland activity decreases.

Because of decreased sweat production, most Asians and Native Americans have mild to no body odor, whereas Caucasians and African Americans tend to have a strong body odor (Andrews & Boyle, 1999), unless they use antiperspirant or deodorant products. Any strong body odor may indicate an abnormality.

PAST HISTORY

Q Describe any previous problems with skin, hair, or nails, including any treatment or surgery and its effectiveness.

R Current problems may be a recurrence of previous ones. Visible scars may be explained by previous problems.

Q Have you ever had any allergic skin reactions to food, medications, plants, or other environmental substances?

R Various types of allergens can precipitate a variety of skin eruptions.

Q Have you had a fever, nausea, vomiting, gastrointestinal (GI), or respiratory problems?

R Some skin rashes or lesions may be related to viruses or bacteria.

FAMILY HISTORY

Q Has anyone in your family had a recent illness, rash, or other skin problem or allergy? Describe.

R Acne and atopic dermatitis tend to be familial. Viruses (eg, chickenpox, measles) can be highly contagious. Some allergies may be identified from family history.

Q Has anyone in your family had skin cancer?

R A genetic component is associated with skin cancer, especially malignant melanoma.

LIFESTYLE AND HEALTH PRACTICES

Q Do you sunbathe? How much sun or tanning-booth exposure do you get? What type of protection do you use?

R Sun exposure can cause premature aging of skin and increase the risk of cancer. Hair can also be damaged by too much sun.

Q In your daily activities, are you regularly exposed to chemicals that may harm the skin (eg, paint, bleach, cleaning products, weed killers, insect repellents, petroleum)?

R Any of these substances have the potential to irritate or damage the skin, hair, or nails.

Q Do you spend long periods of time sitting or lying in one position?

R Older, disabled, or immobile clients who spend long periods of time in one position are at risk for pressure ulcers.

Q Have you had any exposure to extreme temperatures?

R Temperature extremes affect the blood supply to the skin and can damage the skin layers. Examples include frostbite and burns.

Q What is your daily routine for skin, hair, and nail care? What products do you use (eg, soaps, lotions, oils, cosmetics, self-tanning products, razor type, hair spray, shampoo, coloring, nail enamel)? How do you cut your nails?

R Regular habits provide information on hygiene and lifestyle. The products used may also be a cause of an abnormality. Improper nail-cutting technique can lead to ingrown nails or infection.

Decreased flexibility and mobility may impair the ability of some elderly clients to maintain proper hygiene practices, such as nail cutting, bathing, and hair care.

Q What kinds of foods do you consume in a typical day? How much fluid do you drink each day?

R A balanced diet is necessary for healthy skin, hair, and nails. Adequate fluid intake is required to maintain skin elasticity.

Q *For female clients:* Are you pregnant? Are your menstrual periods regular?

R Some skin and hair conditions can result from hormonal imbalance.

Q Do skin problems limit any of your normal activities?

R Certain activities such as hiking, camping, and gardening may expose the client to allergens such as poison ivy. Moreover, exposure to the sun can aggravate conditions such as scleroderma. In addition, general home maintenance (eg, cleaning, car washing) may expose the client to certain cleaning products to which he or she is sensitive or allergic.

Q Describe any skin disorder that prevents you from enjoying your relationships.

R Skin, hair, or nail problems, especially if visible, may impair the client's ability to interact comfortably with others because of embarrassment or rejection by others.

Q How much stress do you have in your life? Describe.

R Stress can cause or exacerbate skin abnormalities.

Q Do you perform a skin self-examination once a month?

R If clients do not know how to inspect the skin, teach them how to recognize suspicious lesions early (Display 9-1).

DISPLAY 9-1. How to Examine Your Own Skin

GUIDELINES

You can systematically and regularly assess your skin for abnormalities by using the following recommended procedure for skin assessment from the American Cancer Society.

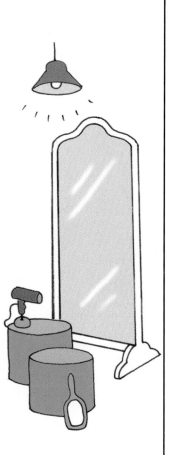

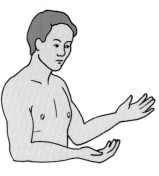

Step 2

Hold your hands with the palms face up, as shown in the drawing. Look at your palms, fingers, spaces between the fingers, and forearms. Then turn your hands over and examine the backs of your hands, fingers, spaces between the fingers, fingernails, and forearms.

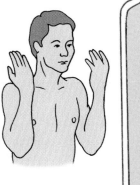

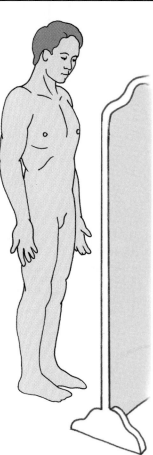

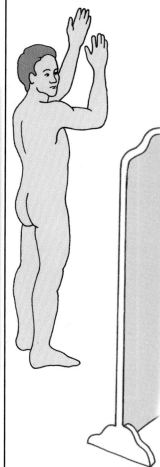

Step 1

Make sure the room is well-lighted, and that you have nearby a full-length mirror, a hand-held mirror, a hand-held blow dryer, and two chairs or stools. Undress completely.

Step 3

Now position yourself in front of the full-length mirror. Hold up your arms, bent at the elbows, with your palms facing you. In the mirror, look at the backs of your forearms and elbows.

Step 4

Again, using the full-length mirror, observe the entire front of your body. In turn, look at your face, neck, and arms. Turn your palms to face the mirror and look at your upper arms. Then look at your chest and abdomen; pubic area; thighs and lower legs.

Step 5

Still standing in front of the mirror, lift your arms over your head with the palms facing each other. Turn so that your right side is facing the mirror and look at the entire side of your body: your hands and arms, underarms, sides of your trunk, thighs, and lower legs. Then turn, and repeat the process with your left side.

DISPLAY 9-1. How to Examine Your Own Skin (Continued)

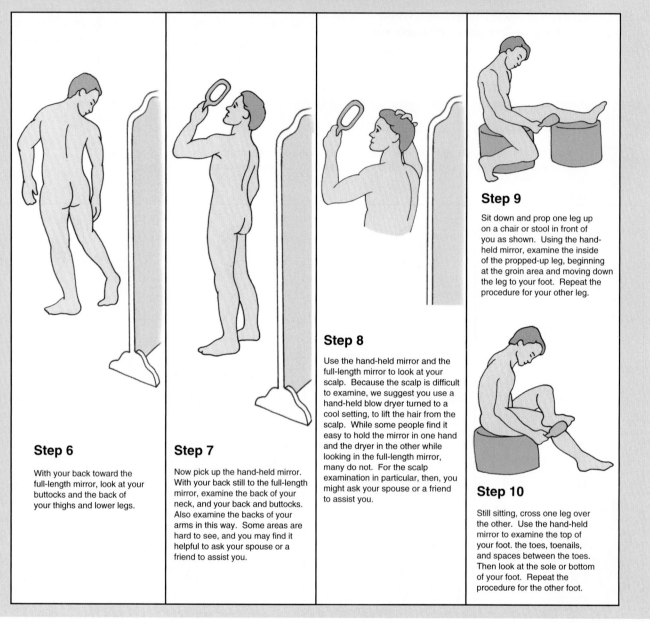

Step 6

With your back toward the full-length mirror, look at your buttocks and the back of your thighs and lower legs.

Step 7

Now pick up the hand-held mirror. With your back still to the full-length mirror, examine the back of your neck, and your back and buttocks. Also examine the backs of your arms in this way. Some areas are hard to see, and you may find it helpful to ask your spouse or a friend to assist you.

Step 8

Use the hand-held mirror and the full-length mirror to look at your scalp. Because the scalp is difficult to examine, we suggest you use a hand-held blow dryer turned to a cool setting, to lift the hair from the scalp. While some people find it easy to hold the mirror in one hand and the dryer in the other while looking in the full-length mirror, many do not. For the scalp examination in particular, then, you might ask your spouse or a friend to assist you.

Step 9

Sit down and prop one leg up on a chair or stool in front of you as shown. Using the hand-held mirror, examine the inside of the propped-up leg, beginning at the groin area and moving down the leg to your foot. Repeat the procedure for your other leg.

Step 10

Still sitting, cross one leg over the other. Use the hand-held mirror to examine the top of your foot. the toes, toenails, and spaces between the toes. Then look at the sole or bottom of your foot. Repeat the procedure for the other foot.

Courtesy of the American Cancer Society.

Collecting Objective Data

Physical assessment of the skin, hair, and nails provides the nurse with data that may reveal local or systemic problems or alterations in a client's self-care activities. Local irritation, trauma, or disease can alter the condition of the skin, hair, or nails. Systemic problems related to impaired circulation, endocrine imbalances, allergic reactions, or respiratory disorders may also be revealed with alterations in the skin, hair, or nails. The appearance of the skin, hair, and nails also provides the nurse with data related to health maintenance and self-care activities such as hygiene, exercise, and nutrition.

A separate, comprehensive skin, hair, and nail examination, preferably at the beginning of a comprehensive physical examination, ensures that you do not inadvertently omit part of the examination. As you inspect and palpate the skin, hair, and nails, pay special attention to lesions and growths.

CLIENT PREPARATION

To prepare for the skin, hair, and nail examination, ask the client to remove all clothing and jewelry and put on an examination gown. In addition, ask the client to remove nail enamel, artificial nails, wigs, toupees, or hairpieces as appropriate.

Have the client sit comfortably on the examination table or bed for the beginning of the examination. The client may remain in a sitting position for most of the examination. However, to assess the skin on the buttocks and dorsal surfaces of the legs properly, the client may lie on his or her side or abdomen.

During the skin examination, ensure privacy by exposing only the body part being examined. Make sure that the room is a comfortable temperature. If available, sunlight is best for inspecting the skin. However, a bright light that can be focused on the client works just as well. Keep the room door closed or the bed curtain drawn to provide privacy as necessary. Explain what you are going to do, and answer any questions the client may have. Wear gloves when palpating any lesions because you may be exposed to drainage.

Clients from conservative religious groups (eg, Orthodox Jews or Muslims), may require that the nurse be the same sex as the client. Also, to respect the client's modesty or desire for privacy, provide a long examination gown or robe.

EQUIPMENT AND SUPPLIES

- Examination light
- Penlight
- Mirror for client's self-examination of skin
- Magnifying glass
- Centimeter ruler
- Gloves
- Wood's light
- Examination gown or drape

KEY ASSESSMENT POINTS

- Inspect skin color, temperature, moisture, texture
- Check skin integrity
- Be alert for skin lesions
- Evaluate hair condition; loss or unusual growth
- Note nailbed condition and capillary refill

(*text continues on page 132*)

PHYSICAL ASSESSMENT

ASSESSMENT PROCEDURE	NORMAL FINDINGS	ABNORMAL FINDINGS

SKIN INSPECTION

Inspect general skin coloration. Keep in mind that the amount of pigment in the skin accounts for the intensity of color as well as hue. Small amounts of melanin are common in whiter skins, while large amounts of melanin are common in olive and darker skins. Carotene accounts for a yellow cast. A blue hue may be from cyanosis, a sign of illness. 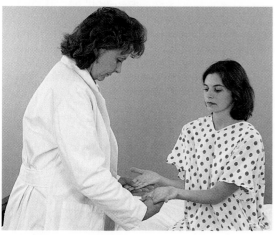 **Inspecting the palms is an opportunity to assess overall coloration. (© B. Proud.)**	Evenly colored skin tones without unusual or prominent discolorations. The older client's skin becomes pale due to decreased melanin production and decreased dermal vascularity.	**Pallor** (loss of color) is seen in arterial insufficiency, decreased blood supply, and anemia. Pallid tones vary from pale to ashen without underlying pink. **Cyanosis** makes white skin appear blue-tinged, especially in the perioral, nailbed, and conjunctival areas. Dark skin appears blue, dull and lifeless in the same areas. Central cyanosis results from a cardiopulmonary problem whereas peripheral cyanosis may be a local problem resulting from vasoconstriction. To differentiate between central and peripheral cyanosis, look for central cyanosis in the oral mucosa. **Jaundice** in light- and dark-skinned people is characterized by yellow skin tones, from pale to pumpkin, particularly in the sclera, oral mucosa, palms, and soles. **Acanthosis nigricans,** roughening and darkening of skin in localized areas, especially the posterior neck (Stuart, et al., 1999).
While inspecting skin coloration, note any odors emanating from the skin.	Slight or no odor of perspiration, depending on activity.	A strong odor of perspiration or foul odor may indicate disorder of sweat glands. Poor hygiene practices may indicate a need for client teaching or assistance with activities of daily living.

(continued)

ASSESSMENT PROCEDURE	NORMAL FINDINGS	ABNORMAL FINDINGS

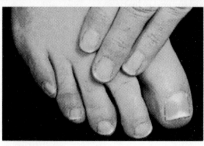
A

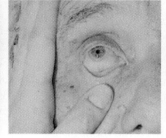
B

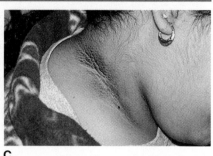
C

(A) Bluish cyanotic skin associated with oxygen deficiency. (B) Jaundice associated with hepatic dysfunction. (C) Acanthosis nigricans (AN), a linear streaklike pattern in dark-skinned people, suggests diabetes mellitus. (With permission from Goodheart, H. P. [1999]. *A photo guide of common skin disorders: Diagnosis and management.* Baltimore: Williams & Wilkins.)

Inspect for Color Variations

Inspect localized parts of the body, noting any color variation. Keep in mind that some clients have sun-tanned areas, freckles, or white patches known as vitiligo (Display 9-2). The variations are due to different amounts of melanin in certain areas. A generalized loss of pigmentation is seen in albinism. Dark-skinned clients have lighter-colored palms, soles, nailbeds, and lips. Frecklelike or dark streaks of pigmentation are also common in the sclera and nailbeds of dark-skinned clients.

White-skinned clients have darker pigment around nipples, lips, and genitalia.

Mongolian spots on the lower back, buttocks, or even on the upper back, arms, thighs, or abdomen occur in most blacks, Asians, Native Americans, and some whites. These bluish, bruiselike markings usually fade by 2 years of age (Overfield, 1995).

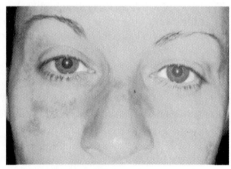
Characteristic butterfly rash of lupus erythematosus.

Rashes, such as the reddish (in light-skinned people) or darkened (in dark-skinned people) butterfly rash across the bridge of the nose and cheeks, characteristic of discoid lupus erythematosus (DLE).

Albinism is a generalized loss of pigmentation.

Erythema (skin redness and warmth) is seen in inflammation, allergic reactions, or trauma.

Erythema in the dark-skinned client may be difficult to see. However, the affected skin feels swollen and warmer than the surrounding skin.

(continued)

ASSESSMENT PROCEDURE	NORMAL FINDINGS	ABNORMAL FINDINGS
Inspect for Skin Integrity Check skin integrity, especially carefully in pressure point areas (eg, sacrum, hips, elbows). If any skin breakdown is noted, use a scale to document the degree of skin breakdown.	Skin is intact, and there are no reddened areas.	Skin breakdown is initially noted as a reddened area on the skin that may progress to serious and painful pressure ulcers (Display 9-3). Depending on the color of the client's skin, reddened areas may not be prominent, although the skin may feel warmer in the area of breakdown than elsewhere.
Inspect for Lesions Observe the skin surface to detect abnormalities. 🎗 **Tip From the Experts** When examining female or obese clients, lift the breasts (or ask the client to lift them) and skin folds to inspect all areas for lesions. Note color, shape, and size of lesion. For very small lesions, use a magnifying glass to note these characteristics.	Smooth, without lesions. Stretch marks (striae), healed scars, freckles, moles, or birthmarks are common findings (see Display 9-2). 👓 Older clients may have skin lesions because of aging. Some examples are seborrheic or senile keratoses, senile lentigines, cherry angiomas, purpura, and cutaneous tags and horns.	Lesions may indicate local or systemic problems. Primary lesions (Display 9-4) arise from normal skin due to irritation or disease. Secondary lesions (Display 9-5) arise from changes in primary lesions. Vascular lesions (Display 9-6), reddish-bluish lesions, are seen with bleeding, venous pressure, aging, liver disease, or pregnancy. Skin cancer lesions can be either primary or secondary lesions and are classified as squamous cell carcinoma, basal cell carcinoma, or malignant melanoma (Display 9-7).
If you suspect a fungus, shine a Wood's light (an ultraviolet light filtered through a special glass) on the lesion.	Lesion does not fluoresce.	Blue-green fluorescence indicates fungal infection.
If you observe a lesion, note its location, distribution, and configuration.	Normal lesions may be moles, freckles, birthmarks, and the like. They may be scattered over the skin in no particular pattern.	In abnormal findings, distribution may be diffuse (scattered all over), localized to one area, or in sun-exposed areas. Configuration may be discrete (separate and distinct), grouped (clustered), confluent (merged), linear (in a line), annular and arciform (circular or arcing), or zosteriform (linear along a nerve route; Display 9-8).
Palpate Skin to Assess Texture Use the palmar surface of your three middle fingers to palpate skin texture.	Skin is smooth and even.	Rough, flaky, dry skin is seen in hypothyroidism.
Palpate to Assess Thickness If lesions are noted when assessing skin thickness, put gloves on and palpate the lesion between the thumb and finger. Observe for drainage or other characteristics. Measure the lesion with a centimeter ruler.	Skin is normally thin, but calluses (rough, thick sections of epidermis) are common on areas of the body that are exposed to constant pressure.	Very thin skin may be seen in clients with arterial insufficiency or in those on steroid therapy.

(continued)

ASSESSMENT PROCEDURE	NORMAL FINDINGS	ABNORMAL FINDINGS

Palpate to Assess Moisture

Some nurses believe that using the dorsal surfaces of the hands to assess moisture leads to a more accurate result. Check under skin folds and in unexposed areas.

👓 The older client's skin may feel dryer than a younger client's skin because sebum production decreases with age.

Skin surfaces vary from moist to dry depending on the area assessed. Recent activity or a warm environment may cause increased moisture.

Increased moisture or diaphoresis (profuse sweating) may occur in conditions such as fever or hyperthyroidism. Decreased moisture occurs with dehydration or hypothyroidism. Clammy skin is typical in shock or hypotension.

Palpate to Assess Temperature

Use the dorsal surfaces of your hands to palpate the skin. You may also want to palpate with the palmar surfaces of your hands because current research indicates that these surfaces of the hands and fingers may be more sensitive to temperature (Cantwell-Gaw, 1996).

Skin is normally a warm temperature.

Cold skin may accompany shock or hypotension. Cool skin may accompany arterial disease. Very warm skin may indicate a febrile state or hyperthyroidism.

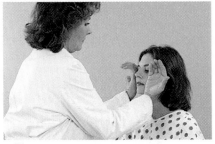

Assessing temperature and moisture. (© B. Proud.)

Palpate to Assess Mobility and Turgor

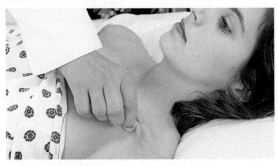

Palpating to assess skin turgor and mobility. (© B. Proud.)

Skin pinches easily and immediately returns to its original position.

👓 The older client's skin loses its turgor because of a decrease in elasticity and collagen fibers. Sagging or wrinkled skin appears in the facial, breast, and scrotal areas.

Decreased mobility is seen with edema. Decreased turgor (a slow return of the skin to its normal state taking longer than 30 seconds) is seen in dehydration.

Ask the client to lie down. Using two fingers, gently pinch the skin on the sternum or under the clavicle. *Mobility* refers to how easily the skin can be pinched. *Turgor* refers to the skin's elasticity and how quickly the skin returns to its original shape after being pinched.

Palpate to Detect Edema

Use your thumbs to press down on the skin of the feet or ankles to check for edema (swelling related to accumulation of fluid in the tissue).

Skin rebounds and does not remain indented when pressure is released.

Indentations on the skin may vary from slight to great and may be in one area or all over the body. See Chapter 17, Peripheral Vascular Assessment, for a full discussion of edema.

(continued)

ASSESSMENT PROCEDURE	NORMAL FINDINGS	ABNORMAL FINDINGS

SCALP AND HAIR: CONDITION AND TEXTURE

Have the client remove any hair clips, hair pins, or wigs. Wear gloves if lesions are suspected or if hygiene is poor. Then inspect the scalp and hair.

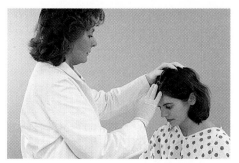

Inspecting the scalp and hair. (© B. Proud.)

Inspect amount and distribution of scalp, body, axillae, and pubic hair. Look for unusual growth elsewhere on the body.

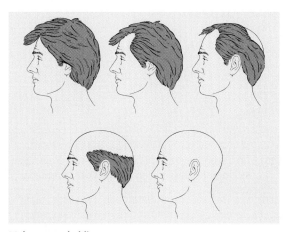

Male pattern balding.

At 1-inch intervals, separate the hair from the scalp and inspect and palpate the hair and scalp for cleanliness, dryness or oiliness, parasites, and lesions.

Natural hair color, as opposed to chemically colored hair, varies among clients from pale blond to black to gray or white. The color is determined by the amount of melanin present.

Varying amounts of terminal hair cover the scalp, axillary, body, and pubic areas according to normal gender distribution. Fine vellus hair covers the entire body except for the soles, palms, lips, and nipples. Normal male pattern balding is symmetric.

Older clients have thinner hair because of a decrease in hair follicles. Pubic, axillary, and body hair also decrease with aging. Alopecia is seen, especially in men. Hair loss occurs from the periphery of the scalp and moves to the center.
Elderly women may have terminal hair growth on the chin owing to hormonal changes.

Scalp is clean and dry. Sparse dandruff may be visible. Hair is smooth and firm, somewhat elastic. However, as people age, hair feels coarser and drier.

Individuals of black African descent often have very dry scalps and dry, fragile hair, which the client may condition with oil or a petroleum jelly like product. (This kind of hair is of genetic origin and not related to thyroid disorders or nutrition. Such hair needs to be handled very gently.)

Excessive generalized hair loss may occur with infection, nutritional deficiencies, hormonal disorders, thyroid or liver disease, drug toxicity, hepatic or renal failure (Sabbagh,1999). It may also result from chemotherapy or radiation therapy.

Nutritional deficiencies may cause patchy gray hair in some clients. Severe malnutrition in African-American children may cause a copper-red hair color (Andrews & Boyle, 1999).

Hirsutism (facial hair on females) is a characteristic of Cushing's disease and results from an imbalance of adrenal hormones, or it may be a side effect of steroids.

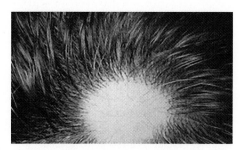

Patchy hair loss may result from infections of the scalp, discoid or systemic lupus erythematosus, and some types of chemotherapy. (Courtesy Neutrogena Skin Care Institute.)

Excessive scaliness may indicate dermatitis. Raised lesions may indicate infections or tumor growth. Dull, dry hair may be seen with hypothyroidism and malnutrition. Poor hygiene may indicate a need for client teaching or assistance with activities of daily living.

(continued)

ASSESSMENT PROCEDURE	NORMAL FINDINGS	ABNORMAL FINDINGS

NAILS

ASSESSMENT PROCEDURE	NORMAL FINDINGS	ABNORMAL FINDINGS
Inspect nail grooming and cleanliness.	Clean and manicured.	Dirty, broken, or jagged fingernails may be seen with poor hygiene. They may also result from the client's hobby or occupation.
Inspect nail color and markings.	Pink tones should be seen. Some longitudinal ridging is normal. Dark-skinned clients may have freckles or pigmented streaks in their nails.	Pale or cyanotic nails may indicate hypoxia or anemia. Splinter hemorrhages may be caused by trauma. Beau's lines occur after acute illness and eventually grow out. Yellow discoloration may be seen in fungal infections or psoriasis. Nail pitting is common in psoriasis (Display 9-9).
Inspect shape of nails.	There is normally a 160-degree angle between the nail base and the skin (see Display 9-9).	Early clubbing (180-degree angle with spongy sensation) and late clubbing (greater than 180-degree angle) can occur from hypoxia. Spoon nails (concave) may be present with iron deficiency anemia (see Display 9-9).
Palpate nail to assess texture.	Nails are hard and basically immobile. Dark-skinned clients may have thicker nails. Older clients' nails may appear thickened, yellow, and brittle because of decreased circulation in the extremities.	Thickened nails (especially toenails) may be caused by decreased circulation.
Palpate to assess texture and consistency, noting whether nailplate is attached to nailbed.	Smooth and firm; nailplate should be firmly attached to nailbed.	Paronychia (inflammation) indicates local infection. Detachment of nailplate from nailbed (onycholysis) is seen in infections or trauma.
Test capillary refill in nailbeds by pressing the nail tip briefly and watching for color change.	Pink tone returns immediately to blanched nailbeds when pressure is released.	There is slow (greater than 2 seconds) capillary nailbed refill (return of pink tone) with respiratory or cardiovascular diseases that cause hypoxia.

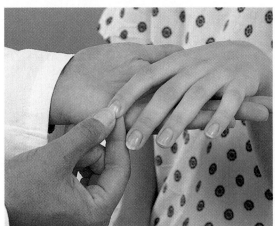

Testing capillary refill. (© B. Proud.)

DISPLAY 9-2. Common Skin Variations

COMMON
VARIATIONS

Many skin assessment findings are considered normal variations in that they are not health- or life-threatening. For example, freckles are common variations in fair-skinned clients, whereas unspotted skin is considered the ideal. Scars and vitiligo, on the other hand, are not exactly normal findings because scars suggest a healed injury or surgical intervention and vitiligo may be related to a dysfunction of the immune system. However, they are common and usually insignificant. Other common findings appear below.

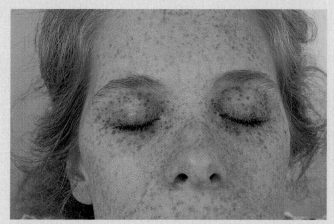

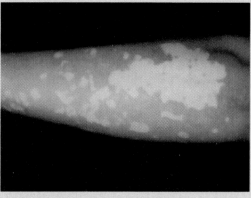

Vitiligo of forearm in an African American client. (Courtesy Neutrogena Care Institute.)

Freckles—flat, small macules of pigment that appear following sun exposure. (© B. Proud.)

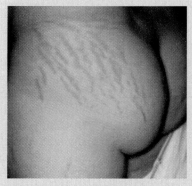

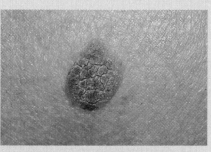

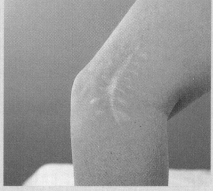

Scar.

Striae (sometimes called stretch marks). (Courtesy E. R. Squibb.)

Seborrheic keratosis, a warty or crusty pigmented lesion. (With permission from Goodheart, H. P. [1999]. *A photo guide of common skin disorders: Diagnosis and management.* Baltimore: Williams & Wilkins.)

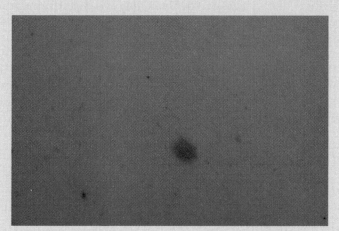

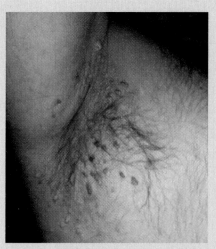

Mole (also called nevus), a flat or raised tan/brownish marking up to 6 mm wide.

Cutaneous tags, raised yellow papules with a depressed center. (Courtesy of Steifel Laboratories, Inc.)

(continued)

DISPLAY 9-2. **Common Skin Variations** (Continued)

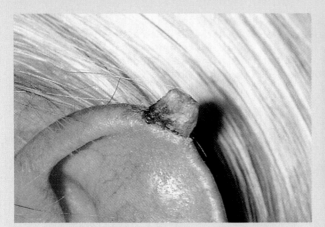

Cutaneous horn.

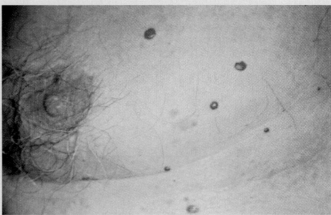

Cherry angiomas, small raised spots (1–5 mm wide) typically seen with aging.

Validation and Documentation of Findings

Validate your normal and abnormal findings with the client, other health care workers, or your instructors. Next, document the skin, hair, and nail assessment data that you have collected on the appropriate form your school or agency uses. The following is a summary of areas of coverage and findings that are considered normal in a skin, hair, and nail assessment. Of course, abnormal findings would be carefully documented too. Normal findings can act as a baseline for findings that may change later.

EXAMPLE OF SUBJECTIVE DATA

Thirty-five-year-old woman with no history of skin lesions, excessive hair loss, or nail disorders. Reports one episode of fine, raised, reddened rash on trunk after taking ampicillin for ear infection. Rash cleared within 3 days after discontinuation of ampicillin and administration of antihistamine. Showers in AM and bathes in PM with deodorant soap. Shampoos with baby shampoo each AM. Applies moisturizer to skin after each cleansing; conditions hair after shampoo. Uses antiperspirant twice daily. Shaves legs and axillae with electric razor twice weekly. Weekly, trims toenails and fingernails and applies

nail enamel to fingernails. Denies exposure to chemicals, abrasives, or excessive sunlight.

EXAMPLE OF OBJECTIVE DATA

Skin pink, warm, dry, and elastic. No lesions or excoriations noted. Old appendectomy scar right lower abdomen, 4 inches long, thin, and white. Sprinkling of freckles noted across nose and cheeks. Hair brown, shoulder-length, clean, shiny. Normal distribution of hair on scalp and perineum. Hair has been removed from legs, axillae. Nails form 160-degree angle at base; are hard, smooth, and immobile. Nailbeds pink without clubbing. Cuticles smooth; no detachment of nail plate. Fingernails well manicured with clear enamel. Toenails clean and well trimmed.

After you have collected your assessment data, analyze the data, using diagnostic reasoning skills. You can review the key steps in diagnostic reasoning in Chapter 7. Then, read on to "Diagnostic Reasoning: Possible Conclusions." This discussion features an overview of common conclusions that you may reach from raw data after a skin, hair, and nail assessment. Then, "Diagnostic Reasoning: Case Study" shows you how to analyze skin, hair, and nail assessment data for a specific client. Finally, you will have an opportunity to analyze data in your laboratory manual/study guide in the "Critical Thinking Exercise."

DISPLAY 9-3. Stages of Pressure Ulcers

During any skin assessment, the nurse remains watchful for signs of skin breakdown, especially in cases of limited mobility or fragile skin (eg, in elderly or bedridden clients). Pressure ulcers, which lead to complications such as infection, are easier to prevent than to treat. Some risk factors for skin breakdown leading to pressure ulcers include poor circulation, poor hygiene, infrequent position changes, dermatitis, infection, or traumatic wounds. The stages of pressure ulcers appear below.

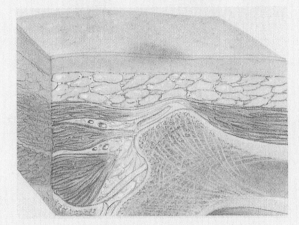

Stage I. Skin is unbroken but appears red; no blanching when pressed.

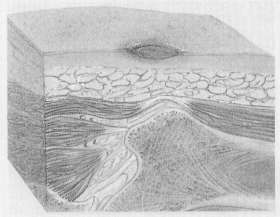

Stage II. Skin *is* broken, and there is superficial skin loss involving the epidermis alone or also the dermis. The lesion resembles a vesicle, erosion, or blister.

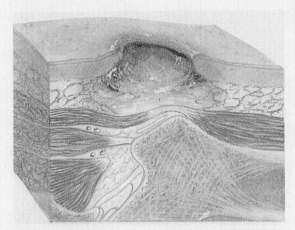

Stage III. Pressure area involves epidermis, dermis, and subcutaneous tissue. The ulcer resembles a crater. Hidden areas of damage may extend through the subcutaneous tissue beyond the borders of the external lesion but not through underlying fascia.

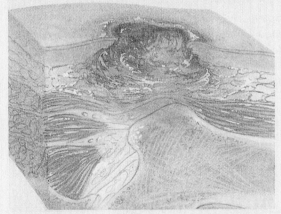

Stage IV. Pressure area involves epidermis, dermis, subcutaneous tissue, bone, and other support tissue. The ulcer resembles a massive crater with hidden areas of damage in adjacent tissue.

(Illustrations with permission from Maklebust, J., & Sieggreen, M. Y. [2001]. *Pressure ulcers: Guidelines for prevention and management.* Springhouse, PA: Springhouse Corporation.)

DISPLAY 9-4. Primary Skin Lesions

ABNORMAL
FINDINGS

Primary skin lesions are original lesions arising from previously normal skin. Secondary lesions can originate from primary lesions.

MACULE, PATCH

- *Macule:* <1 cm, circumscribed border
- *Patch:* >1 cm, may have irregular border
- Flat, nonpalpable skin color change (color may be brown, white, tan, purple, red)

Examples:

Freckles, flat moles, petechiae, rubella, vitiligo, port wine stains, ecchymosis

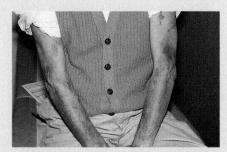

Ecchymoses (from prolonged topical cortico-steroid use).

Macule.

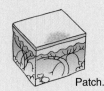

Patch.

PAPULE, PLAQUE

- *Papule:* <0.5 cm
- *Plaque:* >0.5 cm
- Elevated, palpable, solid mass
- Circumscribed border
- Plaque may be coalesced papules with flat top

Examples:

Papules: Elevated nevi, warts, lichen planus
Plaques: Psoriasis, actinic keratosis

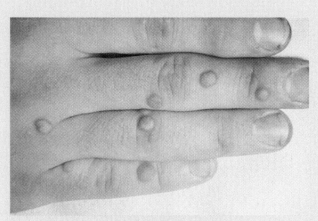

Warts, circumscribed elevations caused by a virus. (Courtesy of Reed and Carnick Pharmaceuticals.)

Papule.

Plaque.

(continued)

NODULE, TUMOR

- *Nodule:* 0.5–2 cm
- *Tumor:* >1–2 cm
- Elevated, palpable, solid mass
- Extends deeper into the dermis than a papule
- Nodules circumscribed
- Tumors do not always have sharp borders

Examples:

Nodules: Lipoma, squamous cell carcinoma, poorly absorbed injection, dermatofibroma

Tumors: Larger lipoma, carcinoma

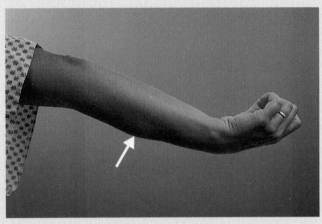

Lipoma.

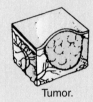

Tumor.

VESICLE, BULLA

- *Vesicle:* <0.5 cm
- *Bulla:* >0.5 cm
- Circumscribed, elevated, palpable mass containing serous fluid

Examples:

Vesicles: Herpes simplex/zoster, chickenpox, poison ivy, second-degree burn (blister)

Bulla: Pemphigus, contact dermatitis, large burn blisters, poison ivy, bullous impetigo

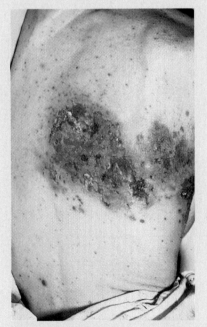

Herpes zoster (shingles), an acute, inflammatory, infectious skin disease caused by a herpes virus.

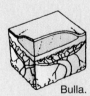

Bulla.

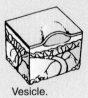

Vesicle.

(continued)

DISPLAY 9-4. **Primary Skin Lesions** (Continued)

WHEAL

- Elevated mass with transient borders
- Often irregular
- Size, color varies
- Caused by movement of serous fluid into the dermis
- Does not contain free fluid in a cavity (eg, a vesicle)

Examples:

Urticaria (hives), insect bites

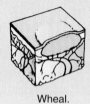

Wheal.

Insect bites.

PUSTULE

- Pus-filled vesicle or bulla

Examples:

Acne, impetigo, furuncles, carbuncles

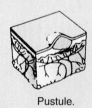

Pustule.

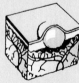

Acne. (Hoechst-Roussel Pharmaceuticals, Inc.)

CYST

- Encapsulated fluid-filled or semisolid mass
- In the subcutaneous tissue or dermis

Examples:

Sebaceous cyst, epidermoid cyst

Cyst.

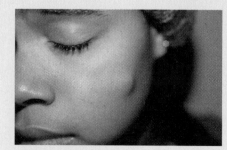

Epidermoid cysts are nodular.

DISPLAY 9-5. Secondary Skin Lesions

ABNORMAL
FINDINGS

Secondary skin lesions result from changes in primary lesions.

EROSION

- Loss of superficial epidermis
- Does not extend to dermis
- Depressed, moist area

Examples:
Ruptured vesicles, scratch marks, aphthous ulcer

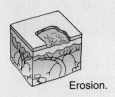

Erosion.

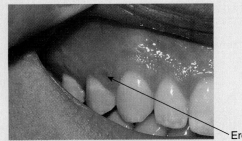

Erosion

Aphthous ulcer. (With permission from Goodheart, H. P. [1999]. *A photo guide of common skin disorders: Diagnosis and management.* Baltimore: Williams & Wilkins.)

ULCER

- Skin loss extending past epidermis
- Necrotic tissue loss
- Bleeding and scarring possible

Examples:
Stasis ulcer of venous insufficiency, pressure ulcer

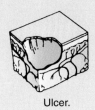

Ulcer.

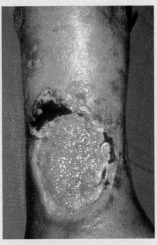

Ulcer from venous stasis.

SCAR [CICATRIX]

- Skin mark left after healing of a wound or lesion
- Represents replacement by connective tissue of the injured tissue
- Young scars: red or purple
- Mature scars: white or glistening

Examples:
Healed wound or surgical incision

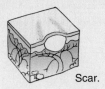

Scar.

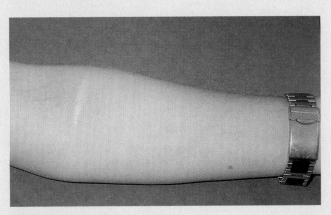

Mature healed wound.

(continued)

FISSURE

- Linear crack in the skin
- May extend to dermis

Examples:

Chapped lips or hands, athlete's foot

Fissure.

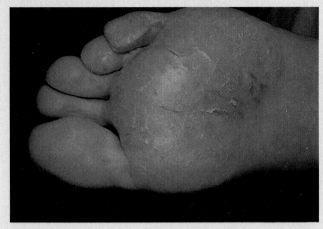

Athlete's foot.

SCALES

- Flakes secondary to desquamated, dead epithelium
- Flakes may adhere to skin surface
- Color varies (silvery, white)
- Texture varies (thick, fine)

Examples:

Dandruff, psoriasis, dry skin, pityriasis rosea

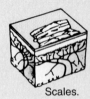

Scales.

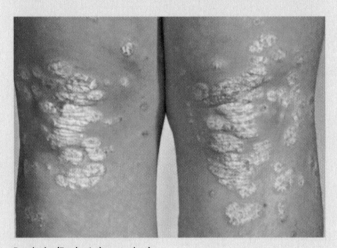

Psoriasis. (Roche Laboratories.)

CRUST

- Dried residue of serum, blood, or pus on skin surface
- Large adherent crust is a scab

Examples:

Residue left after vesicle rupture: impetigo, herpes, eczema

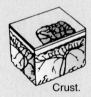

Crust.

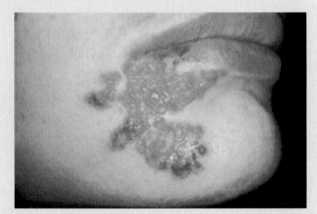

Ruptured vesicles of herpes simplex. (Dermik Laboratories, Inc.)

(continued)

DISPLAY 9-5. Secondary Skin Lesions (Continued)

KELOID

- Hypertrophied scar tissue
- Secondary to excessive collagen formation during healing
- Elevated, irregular, red
- Greater incidence in African Americans

Example:

Keloid of ear piercing or surgical incision

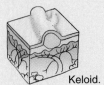
Keloid.

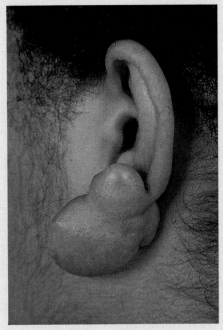
Ear keloid. (© 1992 J. Barabe.)

ATROPHY

- Thin, dry, transparent appearance of epidermis
- Loss of surface markings
- Secondary to loss of collagen and elastin
- Underlying vessels may be visible

Examples:

Aged skin, arterial insufficiency

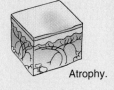
Atrophy.

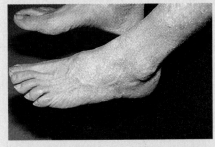
Dry, translucent, aged skin. (With permission from Goodheart, H. P. [1999]. *A photo guide of common skin disorders: Diagnosis and management.* Baltimore: Williams & Wilkins.)

LICHENIFICATION

- Thickening and roughening of the skin
- Accentuated skin markings
- May be secondary to repeated rubbing, irritation, scratching

Examples:

Contact dermatitis, often resulting from exposure to aero allergens, chemicals, foods, and emotional stress

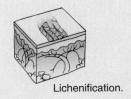
Lichenification.

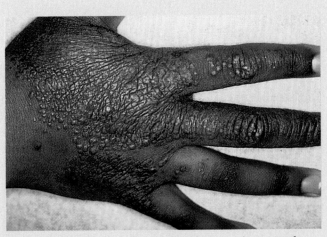
Contact dermatitis, chronic inflammation of the skin. (Courtesy of Geigy Pharmaceuticals.)

DISPLAY 9-6. Vascular Skin Lesions

Vascular skin lesions are associated with bleeding, aging, circulatory conditions, diabetes, pregnancy and hepatic disease, among other problems.

PETECHIA (*PL.* PETECHIAE)

- Round red or purple macule
- Small: 1–2 mm
- Secondary to blood extravasation
- Associated with bleeding tendencies or emboli to skin

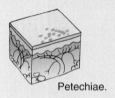

Petechiae.

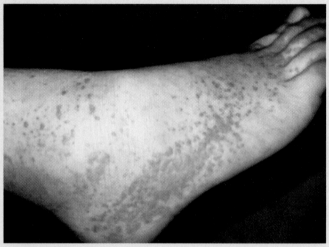

Petechiae. (Dermik Laboratories.)

ECCHYMOSIS (*PL.* ECCHYMOSES)

- Round or irregular macular lesion
- Larger than petechia
- Color varies and changes: black, yellow, and green hues
- Secondary to blood extravasation
- Associated with trauma, bleeding tendencies

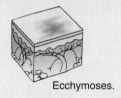

Ecchymoses.

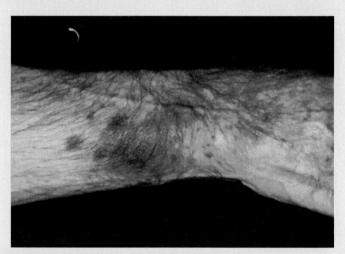

Purpura (hemorrhagic disease that produces ecchymoses and petechiae). (Syntex Laboratories, Inc.)

HEMATOMA

- A localized collection of blood creating an elevated ecchymosis
- Associated with trauma

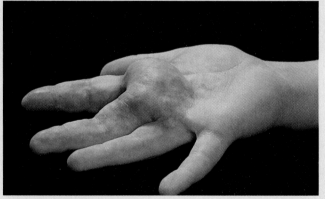

Hematoma. (© 1991 Patricia Barbara, RBP.)

(continued)

DISPLAY 9-6. **Vascular Skin Lesions** (Continued)

CHERRY ANGIOMA

- Papular and round
- Red or purple
- Noted on trunk, extremities
- May blanch with pressure
- Normal age-related skin alteration
- Usually not clinically significant

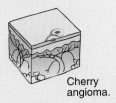

Cherry angioma.

SPIDER ANGIOMA

- Red, arteriole lesion
- Central body with radiating branches
- Noted on face, neck, arms, trunk
- Rare below the waist
- May blanch with pressure
- Associated with liver disease, pregnancy, vitamin B deficiency

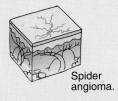

Spider angioma.

Spider angioma. (Dr. H. C. Robinson/Science Photo Library.)

TELANGIECTASIS (VENOUS STAR)

- Shape varies: spiderlike or linear
- Color bluish or red
- Does not blanch when pressure is applied
- Noted on legs, anterior chest
- Secondary to superficial dilation of venous vessels and capillaries
- Associated with increased venous pressure states (varicosities)

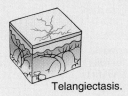

Telangiectasis.

DISPLAY 9-7. Cancerous Skin Lesions

With the exception of malignant melanoma, most skin cancers are easily seen and easily cured, or at least controlled. Malignant melanoma can be deadly if not discovered and treated early, which is one reason why professional health assessment and skin self-assessment can be life-saving procedures. The most commonly detected skin cancers are illustrated below.

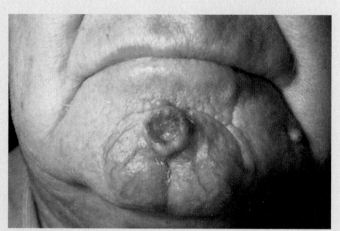

Squamous cell carcinoma.

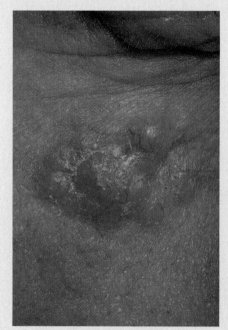

Basal cell carcinoma on patient's face. (CMSP Paul Parker/Science Photo Library.)

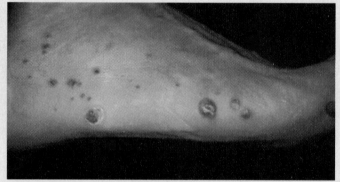

Kaposi's sarcoma of foot. (Owen/Calderma.)

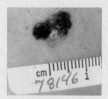

Asymmetrical

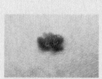

Borders irregular

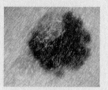

Color varied
Diameter more than
6 mm
Elevated

Malignant melanoma is usually evaluated according to the mnemonic ABCDE: A for asymmetrical; B for borders that are irregular; C for color variations; D for diameter exceeding 6 mm; and E for elevated, not flat. Danger signs of malignant melanoma include asymmetry of pigmented lesions, irregular borders (margins), varying colors (black, blue, red brown, tan, white) and diameter greater than 6 mm. However, smaller areas may indicate early stage melanomas. Other warning signs include itching, burning, and a change in size or bleeding of a mole. New pigmentations are also warning signs. (American Cancer Society; American Academy of Dermatology.)

DISPLAY 9-8. Configurations of Skin Lesions

Describing lesions by shape, distribution, or configuration is one way to communicate specific characteristics that can help to identify causes and treatments. Some common configurations include the following:

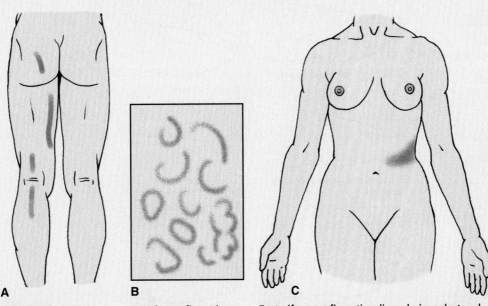

A

Linear configuration: straight line as in a scratch or streak.

B

Annular configuration: circular lesions.

C

Zosteriform configuration: linear lesions clustered along a nerve route.

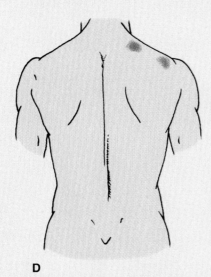

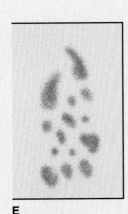

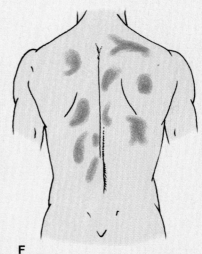

D

Discrete configuration: individual and distinct lesions.

E

Polycyclic configuration: circular lesions that tend to run together.

F

Confluent configuration: lesions run together.

DISPLAY 9-9. Common Nail Disorders

Many clients have nails with lines, ridges, spots, and uncommon shapes that suggest an underlying disorder. Some examples follow:

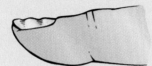

A Beau's lines (acute illness)

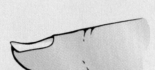

B Spoon nails (iron deficiency anemia)

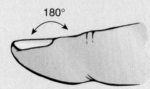

C Early clubbing (oxygen deficiency)

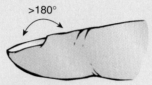

D Late clubbing (oxygen deficiency)

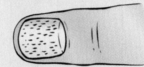

E Pitting (psoriasis)

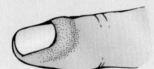

F Paronychia (local infection)

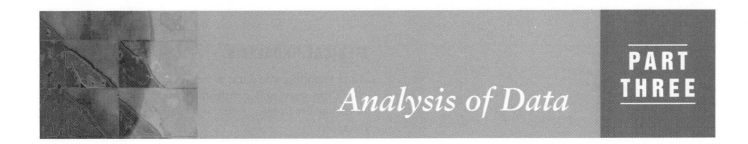

Diagnostic Reasoning: Possible Conclusions

Listed below are some possible conclusions that the nurse may make after assessing a client's skin, hair, and nails.

SELECTED NURSING DIAGNOSES

After compiling subjective and objective data related to the client's skin, hair, and nails, you will need to identify abnormalities and cluster the data to reveal any significant patterns or abnormalities. These data may then be used to make clinical judgments (nursing diagnoses: wellness, risk, or actual) about the status of the client's skin, hair, and nails. The following is a list of selected nursing diagnoses that may be identified when analyzing data from a skin, hair, and nail assessment.

Nursing Diagnoses (Wellness)

- Opportunity to enhance skin, hair, and nail integrity related to healthy hygiene and skin care practices, avoidance of overexposure to sun
- Health-Seeking Behavior: Requests information on skin reactions and effects of using a sun-tanning booth

Nursing Diagnoses (Risk)

- Risk for Impaired Skin Integrity related to excessive exposure to cleaning solutions and chemicals
- Risk for Impaired Skin Integrity related to prolonged sun exposure
- Risk for Impaired Skin Integrity related to immobility, decreased production of natural oils, and thinning skin
- Risk for Impaired Skin Integrity of toes related to thickened, dried toenails
- Risk for Altered Body Temperature related to severe diaphoresis
- Risk for Infection related to scratching of rash
- Risk for Impaired Nail Integrity related to prolonged use of nail polish

- Risk for Altered Nutrition: Less Than Body Requirements related to increased vitamin and protein requirements necessary for healing of a wound

Nursing Diagnoses (Actual)

- Altered Health Maintenance related to lack of hygienic care of the skin, hair, and nails
- Impaired Skin Integrity related to immobility and decreased circulation
- Impaired Skin Integrity related to poor nutritional intake and bowel/bladder incontinence
- Body Image Disturbance related to scarring, rash, or other skin condition that alters skin appearance
- Sleep Pattern Disturbance related to persistent itching of the skin
- Fluid Volume Deficit related to excessive diaphoresis secondary to excessive exercise and high environmental temperatures

SELECTED COLLABORATIVE PROBLEMS

After grouping the data, certain collaborative problems may become apparent. Remember that collaborative problems differ from nursing diagnoses in that they cannot be prevented or managed with independent nursing interventions. However, these physiologic complications of medical conditions can be detected and monitored by the nurse. In addition, the nurse can use physician- and nurse-prescribed interventions to minimize the complications of these problems. The nurse may also have to refer the client in such situations for further treatment of the problem. The following is a list of collaborative problems that may be identified when assessing the skin, hair, and nails. These problems are worded as Potential Complications (or PC), followed by the problem.

- PC: Allergic reaction
- PC: Skin rash
- PC: Insect/animal bite
- PC: Septicemia
- PC: Hypovolemic shock
- PC: Skin infection

- PC: Skin lesion
- PC: Ischemic skin ulcers
- PC: Graft rejection
- PC: Hemorrhage
- PC: Burns

MEDICAL PROBLEMS

After grouping the data, it may become apparent that the client has signs and symptoms that require medical diagnosis and treatment. Referral to a primary care provider is necessary.

Diagnostic Reasoning: Case Study

The case study presents assessment data for a specific client. It is followed by an analysis of the data, by following the seven key steps found in Chapter 7, to arrive at specific conclusions.

Mary Michaelson, a 29-year-old divorced woman, works as an office manager for a large, prestigious law firm. She reports she recently went to see a doctor because "my hair was falling out in chunks, and I have a red rash on my face and chest. It looks like a bad case of acne." After doing some blood work, her physician diagnosed her condition as discoid lupus erythematosus (DLE). She says she has come to see you, the occupational health nurse, because she feels "so ugly," and she is concerned that she may lose her job because of how she looks.

During the interview, she tells you that she is a surfer and is out in the sun all day nearly every weekend. She shares that she uses sunscreen but forgets to put it on at regular intervals during the day.

Your physical examination reveals an attractive, tanned, thin, anxious-appearing young woman. You note confluent and nonconfluent maculopapular lesions on her neck, chest above the nipple line, and over the shoulders and upper back to about the level of the T5 vertebra. Many of the lesions appear as red, scaling plaques with depressed, pale centers. A few of the lesions on her forehead and cheeks appear blistered. Patchy alopecia is also present. Her vital signs are within normal limits, and no other abnormalities are apparent at this time.

1 Identify abnormal data and strengths (in both subjective and objective data).

SUBJECTIVE DATA

- "Hair falling out in chunks"
- Red rash on face and chest—"looks like a bad case of acne"
- "So ugly"
- Concerned that she may lose her job because of how she looks
- Surfer—out in the sun all day on weekends—minimal use of sunscreen
- Sought out occupational health nurse

OBJECTIVE DATA

- Anxious appearing
- Diagnosed with discoid lupus erythematosus
- Red, raised plaques on face, neck, shoulders, back, and chest
- Patchy alopecia

2 Cue Clusters	**3** Inferences	**4** Possible Nursing Diagnoses	**5** Defining Characteristics	**6** Confirm or Rule Out
A • Diagnosed with DLE • Discoid lesions apparent on face, neck, chest, back—raised red patches with some blistering	Textbook picture for DLE as diagnosed by physician Monitor for collaborative problems	Body Image Disturbance related to changes in physical appearance	*Major:* Verbal negative response to actual change in structure *Minor:* Negative feelings about body	Accept diagnosis because it meets defining characteristics and is validated by client.
B • Rash on face, neck, chest, and back • Patchy alopecia • "So ugly"	Changes in physical appearance are affecting self-perception	Ineffective Individual Coping related to changes in physical appearance and newly diagnosed disease	*Major:* None *Minor:* None	Rule out diagnosis because it has none of the defining characteristics; however, more data should be collected regarding her support systems and coping behaviors.

Cue Clusters	Inferences	Possible Nursing Diagnoses	Defining Characteristics	Confirm or Rule Out
2	**3**	**4**	**5**	**6**
• Surfer, out in sunlight weekly • Inadequate applications of sunscreen	Excessive sun exposure can worsen lesions causing blistering, weeping, and scarring Does not seem to know about these effects	Risk for Altered Health Maintenance related to knowledge deficit of effects of sunlight on skin lesions	*Major:* Reports unhealthy practice (not using sunscreen effectively) *Minor:* None	Confirm diagnosis because it meets major defining characteristics and is validated by client.
C • Sought out occupational health nurse	Possibly seeking information about managing her illness	Health-Seeking Behavior	*Major:* Sought out occupational health nurse *Minor:* None	This is ambiguous. The client sought out the occupational health nurse for more information, but after she was already diagnosed, rather than for health promotion before the fact. Collect more data before accepting this diagnosis.
D • Anxious appearing • Concerned that she may lose her job because of how she looks • Office manager in large, prestigious law firm	Perceives current position depends on attractive appearance	Anxiety related to possible loss of work position secondary to perceived unattractiveness	*Major:* Physical appearance (unspecified anxiety) and self-deprecation (about physical appearance) *Minor:* None	Accept diagnosis because it meets defining characteristics, but collect more data to confirm this diagnosis. Fear may be more appropriate, but data needed for that as well.

7 **Document conclusions.**

The following nursing diagnoses are appropriate for Ms. Michaelson at this time:

- Body Image Disturbance related to changes in physical appearance
- Risk for Altered Health Maintenance related to knowledge deficit of effects of sunlight on skin lesions
- Anxiety related to possible loss of work position secondary to perceived unattractiveness

Collaborative problems related to the medical diagnosis could include:

- PC: Skin Infection/Scarring
- PC: Ischemic Ulcers
- PC: Systemic Lupus Erythematosus (SLE) and all related complications (1 in 20 people diagnosed with discoid lupus erythematosus [DLE] progress to systemic lupus erythematosus [SLE])

REFERENCES AND SELECTED READINGS

Andrews, M., & Boyle, J. (1999). *Transcultural concepts in nursing care* (3rd ed.). Philadelphia: Lippincott Williams & Wilkins.

Conditions of the skin. (1999). *American Family Physician, 60*(4), 1258–1261.

Correale, C. E., & Walker, C. (1999). Atopic dermatitis: A review of diagnosis and treatment. *American Family Physician, 60*(4), 1191–1198.

Guttman, C. (2000). Nail exam should be routine in elderly patients. *Dermatology Times, 21*(4), 40.

———. (1999). Practical approach provides key clues to hair disorder diagnosis. *Dermatology Times, 19*(10), 14.

Kuznar, W. (1997). Skin holds clues to many systemic disorders. *Dermatology Times, 18*(4), 11.

McMichael, A. J. (1999). A review of cutaneous disease in African-American patients. *Dermatology Nursing, 11*(1), 35–36, 41–47.

Muirhead, G. (1999). Common dermatologic problems in people of color. *Patient Care, 33*(20), 97.

National Institutes of Health. (1992). The NIH Consensus Development Panel on Melanoma: Diagnosis and treatment of early melanoma. *Journal of the American Medical Association, 268*, 1314–1319.

Noronha, P., & Zubkov, B. (1997). Nails and nail disorders in children and adults. *American Family Physician, 55*(6), 21–29.

Overfield, T. (1995). *Biologic variation in health and illness: Race, age, and sex differences* (2nd ed.). Boca Raton, FL: CRC Press.

Parhizgar, B. (2000). Skin signs of systemic disease. *Cortlandt Forum, 13*(1), 169.

Passchier, J. (1998). Quality of life issues in male pattern hair loss. *Dermatology, 197*(3), 217–218.

Rudikoff, D., & Lebwohl, M. (1998). Atopic dermatitis. *Lancet, 351* (9117), 1715.

Sabbagh, L. (1999). Hair loss in women should be taken seriously. *Dermatology Times, 20*(12), 24–25.

Sinclair, R. (1998). Male pattern androgenetic alopecia. *British Medical Journal, 317*(7162), 865.

Smoker, A. (1999). Skin care in old age. *Nursing Standard, 13*(48), 47–54.

Stuart, C., Driscoll, M., Lundquist, K., Gilkison, C., Shaheb, S., & Smith, M. (1999). Acanthosis nigricans. *Journal of Basic Clinical Physiology and Pharmacology, 9*(2–4), 407–418.

Wysocki, A. B. (1999). Skin anatomy, physiology, and pathophysiology. *Nursing Clinics of North America, 34*(4), 777–797.

Risk Factors–Skin Cancer

American Cancer Society (ACS). (2000). *Cancer Resource Center.* Available: www.cancer.org.

Armstrong, B., & Dricker, A. (1995). Skin cancer. *Dermatology Clinics, 13,* 583–594.

Davidowitz, S., Belafsky, P., & Amedee, R. (1999). The epidemiology of malignant melanoma in Louisiana and beyond. *Journal of the Louisiana State Medical Society, 15*(10), 493–499.

Gloster, H., & Brodland, D. (1995). The epidemiology of skin cancer. *Dermatology Surgery, 22,* 217–226.

Goodheart, H. P. (1999). *A photoguide of common skin disorders: Diagnosis and management.* Baltimore, MD: Williams & Wilkins.

Halder, R., & Bridgeman-Shah, S. (1995). Skin cancer in African Americans. *Cancer, 75*(Suppl. 2), 667–673.

Hall, H., & Rogers, J. (1999). Sun protection behaviors among African Americans. *Ethnic Diseases, 9*(1), 126–131.

Nicol, N., & Penske, N. (1993). Photodamage: Cause, clinical manifestations, and prevention. *Dermatology Nursing, 5,* 263–277, 326.

For additional information on this book, be sure to visit http://connection.lww.com.

Head and Neck Assessment

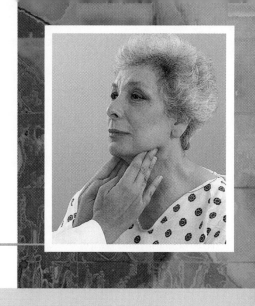

10

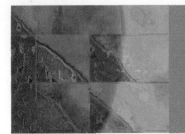

PART ONE

Structure and Function

A head and neck assessment focuses on the cranium, face, thyroid gland, and lymph node structures contained within the head and neck.

The Head

The framework of the head is the skull, which can be divided into two subsections, the cranium and the face (Fig. 10-1).

CRANIUM

The cranium consists of eight bones:

- Frontal (1)
- Parietal (2)
- Temporal (2)
- Occipital (1)
- Ethmoid (1)
- Sphenoid (1)

In the adult client the cranial bones are joined together by immovable sutures: the sagittal, coronal, squamosal, and lambdoid sutures. The cranium houses and protects the brain and major sensory organs.

FACE

The face consists of 14 bones:

- Maxilla (2)
- Zygomatic (cheek) (2)
- Inferior conchae (2)
- Nasal (2)
- Lacrimal (2)
- Palatine (2)
- Vomer (1)
- Mandible (jaw) (1)

All of the facial bones are immovable except for the mandible, which is allowed free movement at the temporomandibular joint. These bones give shape to the face. The face also consists of many muscles that produce facial movement and expressions. A major artery, the temporal artery, is located between the eye and the top of the ear. Two other important structures located in the facial region are the parotid and submandibular salivary glands. The parotid glands are located on each side of the face, anterior and inferior to the ears and behind the mandible. The submandibular glands are located inferior to the mandible, underneath the base of the tongue (see Fig. 10-1).

The Neck

The structure of the neck is composed of muscles, ligaments, and the cervical vertebrae. Contained within the neck are the hyoid bone, several major blood vessels, the larynx, trachea, and the thyroid gland, which is in the anterior triangle of the neck (Fig. 10-2).

MUSCLES AND CERVICAL VERTEBRAE

The sternomastoid (sternocleidomastoid) and trapezius muscles are two of the paired muscles that allow movement and provide support to the head and neck (Fig. 10-3). The sternomastoid muscle rotates and flexes the head, whereas the trapezius muscle extends the head and moves the shoulders. The eleventh cranial nerve is responsible for muscle movement that permits shrugging of the shoulders by the trapezius muscles and turning the head against resistance by the sternomastoid muscles. These two major muscles also form two triangles that provide important landmarks for assessment. The anterior triangle is located under the mandible, anterior to the sternomastoid muscle. The posterior triangle is located between the trapezius and sternomastoid muscles (see Fig. 10-3). The cervical vertebrae (C1 through C7) are located in the posterior neck and support the cranium (Fig. 10-4). The vertebra prominens is C7, which can easily be palpated when the neck is flexed. Using C7 as a landmark will help you locate other vertebrae.

BLOOD VESSELS

The internal jugular veins and carotid arteries are located bilaterally, parallel and anterior to the sternomastoid muscles. The external jugular vein lies diagonally over the surface of these muscles. The purpose and assessment of these major blood vessels are discussed in Chapter 17. However, you need to know the location of the carotid arteries when assessing the neck to avoid bilateral compression of the vessels, which can reduce the blood supply to the brain.

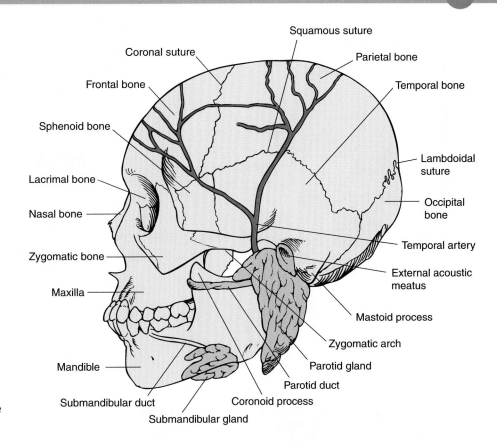

FIGURE 10-1. Bones and sutures of the skull (face and cranium).

THYROID GLAND

The thyroid gland is the largest endocrine gland in the body. It produces thyroid hormones that increase the metabolic rate of most body cells. The thyroid gland is surrounded by several structures that are important to palpate for accurate location of the thyroid gland. The trachea, through which air enters the lungs, is composed of C-shaped hyaline cartilage rings. The first upper tracheal ring, called the cricoid cartilage, has a small notch in it. The thyroid cartilage (Adam's apple) is larger and located just above the cricoid cartilage. The hyoid bone, which is at-tached to the tongue, lies above the thyroid cartilage and under the mandible (see Fig. 10-2).

The thyroid gland consists of two lateral lobes that curve posteriorly on both sides of the trachea and esophagus and are mostly covered by the sternomastoid muscles. These

FIGURE 10-2. Structures of the neck.

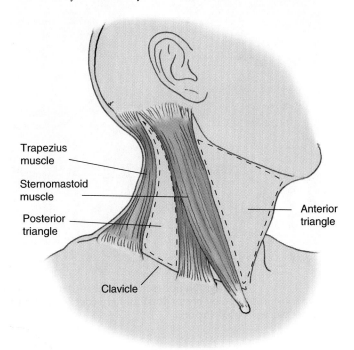

FIGURE 10-3. Neck muscles and landmarks.

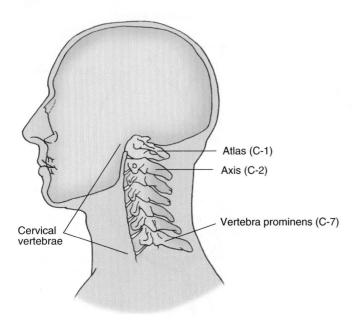

FIGURE 10-4. Cervical vertebrae.

two thyroid lobes are connected by an isthmus that overlies the second and third tracheal rings below the cricoid cartilage. In about one third of the population, there is a third lobe that extends upward from the isthmus or from one of the two lobes.

Lymph Nodes of the Head and Neck

Several lymph nodes are located in the head and neck (Fig. 10-5). Lymph nodes filter lymph, a clear substance composed mostly of excess tissue fluid, after the lymphatic vessels collect it but before it returns to the vascular system. This filtering action removes bacteria and tumor cells from lymph. In addition, lymphocytes and antibodies are produced in the lymph nodes as a defense against invasion by foreign substances. The size and shape of lymph nodes vary, but most are less than 1 cm long and are buried deep in the connective tissue, which makes them nonpalpable in normal situations. They usually appear in clusters that vary in size from 2 to 100 individual nodes.

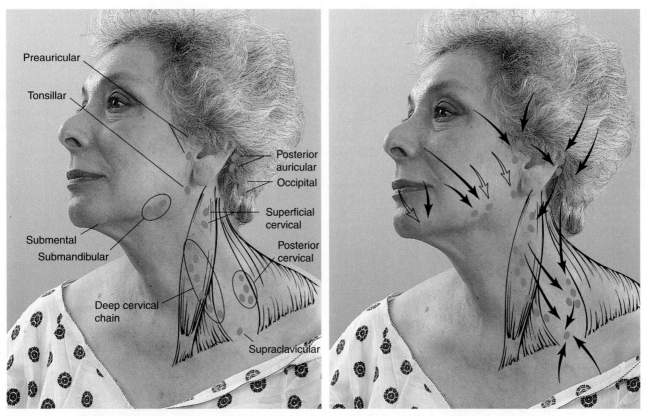

FIGURE 10-5. (Left) Lymph nodes in the neck. (Right) Direction of lymph flow. *Note:* Lymph nodes (represented by *green dots*) that are covered by hair may be palpated in the scalp under the hair. (© B. Proud.)

If the nodes become overwhelmed by microorganisms, as happens with an infection such as mononucleosis, they swell and become painful, but, if cancer metastasizes to the lymph nodes, they may enlarge but not be painful. Normally, lymph nodes are either not palpable or they may feel like a very small bead. Sources vary in their reference to the names of lymph nodes. The most common head and neck lymph nodes are referred to as follows:

- Preauricular
- Postauricular
- Tonsillar
- Occipital
- Submandibular
- Submental
- Superficial cervical
- Posterior cervical
- Deep cervical
- Supraclavicular

Drainage from various parts of the head and neck flows into a lymph node in the neck (see Fig. 10-5). When an enlarged lymph node is detected during assessment, the nurse needs to know from which part of the head or neck the lymph node receives drainage to assess whether an abnormality (eg, infection, disease) is in that area.

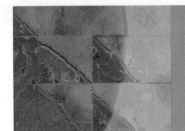

Collecting Subjective Data

The nursing history is important in assessing the head and neck because abnormalities that cannot be directly observed in the physical appearance of the head and neck are often detected in the client's history. For example, a client may have no visible signs of any problems but may complain of frequent headaches. A detailed description of the type of headache pain and its location, intensity, and duration provides the nurse with valuable clues as to what the underlying problem might be.

COLDSPA

CHARACTER: Describe the sign or symptom. How does it feel, look, sound, smell, and so forth?

ONSET: When did it begin?

LOCATION: Where is it? Does it radiate?

DURATION: How long does it last? Does it recur?

SEVERITY: How bad is it?

PATTERN: What makes it better: What makes it worse?

ASSOCIATED FACTORS: What other symptoms occur with it?

In addition, because of the overlap of several body systems in this area, a thorough nursing history is needed to detect the cause of possible underlying systemic problems. For example, the client experiencing dizziness, spinning, lightheadedness, or loss of consciousness may perceive the problems as related to his or her head. However, these symptoms may indicate problems with the heart and neck vessels, peripheral vascular system, or neurologic system (inner ear).

The nursing history assessment also provides an opportunity for the nurse to evaluate activities of daily living that may affect the condition of the client's head and neck. Stress, tension, poor posture while performing work, and lack of proper exercise may lead to head and neck discomfort. To prevent head and neck injuries, the nurse may inform the client of protective measures, such as wearing helmets, seat belts, and hard hats, during the history portion of the assessment.

Finally, when discussing the client's head, neck, and facial structures, recognize that the appearance of these structures often has a great influence on the client's self-image.

Nursing History

The following is a selection of questions you may ask and areas you may cover with an average client.

CURRENT SYMPTOMS

Question Have you noticed any lumps or lesions on your head or neck that do not heal or disappear? Explain.

Rationale Lumps and lesions that do not heal or disappear may indicate cancer.

Q Do you have any difficulty moving your head or neck?

R Diseases and disorders involving head and neck muscles may limit mobility and affect daily functioning.

Q Do you experience neck pain?

R Neck pain may accompany muscular problems or cervical spinal cord problems. Stress and tension may increase neck pain. Sudden head and neck pain seen with elevated temperature and neck stiffness may be a sign of meningeal irritation or inflammation.

Older clients who have arthritis or osteoporosis may experience neck pain and a decreased range of motion.

Q Do you experience headaches? Describe.

R A precise description of the symptoms can help determine possible causes of the discomfort. Temporomandibular joint syndrome is a major cause of chronic headaches. See Table 10-1 for a discussion of typical findings for migraine, tension, cluster, and tumor-related headaches.

Q Do you have any facial pain? Describe.

R Trigeminal neuralgia (tic douloureux) is manifested by sharp, shooting, piercing facial pains that last from seconds to minutes. Pain occurs over the divisions of the fifth trigeminal cranial nerve (the ophthalmic, maxillary, and mandibular areas).

TABLE 10-1. Kinds and Characteristics of Headaches

Migraine	Cluster	Tension	Tumor Related
Character			
Accompanied by nausea, vomiting, and sensitivity to noise or light	May be accompanied by tearing, eyelid drooping, reddened eye, or runny nose	Symptoms of anxiety, tension, and depression may be present	Neurologic and mental symptoms and nausea and vomiting may develop
Onset and Precipitating Factors			
• May have prodromal stage (visual disturbances, vertigo, tinnitus, numbness or tingling of fingers or toes) • Precipitated by emotional disturbances, anxiety, or ingestion of alcohol, cheese, chocolate, or other foods and substances to which client is sensitive	• Sudden onset • May be precipitated by ingesting alcohol	• No prodromal stage • May occur with stress, anxiety, or depression	• No prodromal stage • May be aggravated by coughing, sneezing, or sudden movements of the head
Location			
Located around eyes, temples, cheeks, or forehead	Localized in the eye and orbit and radiating to the facial and temporal regions	Usually located in the frontal, temporal, or occipital region	Varies with location of tumor
Duration			
Lasts up to 3 days	Typically occurs in the late evening or night	Lasts days, months, or years	Commonly occurs in the morning and lasts for several hours
Severity			
Throbbing, severe, recurring	Intense and stabbing	Dull, aching, tight, diffuse	Aching, steady, variable in intensity
Pattern			
Rest may bring relief	Movement or walking back and forth may relieve the discomfort	Symptomatic relief may be obtained by local heat, massage, analgesics, antidepressants, and muscle relaxants	Headache usually subsides later in the day.
Associated Factors			
Migraines occur more often in women	Cluster headaches occur more in young males	Tension headaches affect women more often than men	

Q Have you experienced any dizziness, lightheadedness, spinning sensation, or loss of consciousness? Explain.

R Problems with the heart and neck vessels or neurologic system, such as carotid artery occlusion or inner ear disease, may cause these symptoms. Symptoms imply risk for injury.

Q Have you noticed a change in the texture of your skin, hair, or nails?

Have you noticed changes in your energy level, sleep habits, or emotional stability?

Have you experienced any palpitations, blurred vision or changes in bowel habits?

R Alterations in thyroid function are manifested in several ways. An increase in thyroid hormone production (hyperthyroidism) can result in insomnia, thinning hair, palpitations, and weight loss. A decrease in thyroid hormone production (hypothyroidism) can result in insomnia and will have the opposite effects of thickening skin and nails, decreased energy levels, and constipation.

PAST HISTORY

Q Describe any previous head or neck problems (trauma, injury) you have had. How were they treated (surgery, medication, physical therapy)? What were the results?

R Previous head and neck trauma may cause chronic pain and limitation of movement. This may affect functioning.

Q Have you ever undergone radiation therapy for a problem in your neck region?

R Radiation therapy has been linked to the development of thyroid cancer.

FAMILY HISTORY

Q Is there a history of head and neck cancer in your family?

R Genetic predisposition is a risk factor for head and neck cancers.

Q Is there a history of migraine headaches in your family?

R Migraine headaches commonly have a familial association.

LIFESTYLE AND HEALTH PRACTICES

Q Do you smoke or chew tobacco? If yes, how much?

R Tobacco use increases the risk of head and neck cancer. See "Risk Factors—Cancer of the Oral Cavity" in Chapter 13.

Q Do you wear a helmet when riding a horse, bicycle, motorcycle, or other open sports vehicle (eg, four-wheeler, go-cart)? Do you wear a hard hat for hazardous occupations? (See Risk Factors—Traumatic Brain Injury for more information.)

R Failure to use safety precautions increases the risk for head and neck injury.

Q What is your typical posture when relaxing, during sleep, and when working?

R Poor posture or body alignment can lead to or exacerbate head and neck discomfort.

Q In what kinds of recreational activity do you participate? Describe the activity.

R Contact or aggressive sports may increase the risk for a head or neck injury.

Q Have any problems with your head or neck interfered with your relationships with others or the role you occupy at home or at work?

R Head and neck pain may interfere with relationships or prevent clients from completing their usual activities of daily living.

Collecting Objective Data

Examining the head allows the nurse to evaluate the overlying protective structures (cranium and facial bones) before evaluating the underlying special senses (vision, hearing, smell, and taste) and the functioning of the neurologic system. This examination can detect head and facial shape abnormalities, asymmetry, structural changes, or tenderness.

Assessment of both the head and neck assists the nurse to detect enlarged or tender lymph nodes. By palpating the thyroid gland, thyroid enlargement, nodules, masses, or tenderness may be detected. Abnormalities of the neck and facial muscles may also be detected by palpation.

Take care to consider cultural norms for touch when assessing the head. Some cultures (eg, Southeast Asian) prohibit touching the head or touching the feet before touching the head (Lipson, Dibble & Minarik, 1996).

Be aware that some clients may be anxious as you palpate the neck for lymph nodes, especially if they have a history of cancer that caused lymph node enlargement. Tell the client what you are doing and share your assessment findings. Another important thing to keep in mind as you examine the head and neck is that normal facial structures and features tend to vary widely among individuals and cultures.

CLIENT PREPARATION

Prepare the client for the head and neck examination by instructing him or her to remove any wig, hat, hair ornaments, pins, rubber bands, jewelry, and head or neck scarves. Ask the client to sit in an upright position, with the back and shoulders held back and straight. Explain to him or her the importance of remaining still during most of the inspection and palpation of the head and neck. However, explain that he or she will be requested to move and bend the neck for examination of muscles and for palpation of the thyroid gland.

EQUIPMENT AND SUPPLIES

- Gloves
- Small cup of water
- Stethoscope

KEY ASSESSMENT POINTS

- Inform client of risk factors and risk reduction measures related to traumatic brain injury (TBI).
- Observe size, shape, configuration, and mobility of head, face, and neck.
- Evaluate size shape and function of neck, trachea, and thyroid gland.
- Palpate lymph nodes of head and neck.

(*text continues on page 167*)

RISK FACTORS
Traumatic Brain Injury

OVERVIEW

In 2000, the Centers for Disease Control and Prevention (CDC) estimated that the yearly impact of traumatic brain injury (TBI) in the United States is 1 million people treated and released from emergency rooms, 230,000 people hospitalized and surviving, and 50,000 dead (CDC, 2000). The average TBI incidence rate for hospitalization and mortality is 95 per 100,000 population. Highest risks are among adolescents, young adults, and those over age 75 years. Males have twice as much risk as females. The leading causes of TBI are motor vehicle accidents, violence, and falls. Firearm-related incidents are high in the violence category, and nearly two thirds of firearm-related TBIs are classified as suicidal in intent. The leading causes vary by age; falls are the leading cause for people age 65 years and older. Motor vehicle, bicycle, and other modes of transport are the leading causes for people from age 5 to 64 years.

Outcomes of these injuries vary depending on cause: 91% of firearm-related TBIs result in death; 11% of fall-related TBIs are fatal. Each year, however, more than 80,000 Americans survive TBI to be discharged from the hospital with disabilities. Approximately 5.3 million Americans are alive today with TBI-related disabilities, which include impaired cognition (concentration, memory, judgment, and mood), movement (strength, coordination, and balance), and sensation (tactile sensation and special senses such as vision), seizure activity, or persistent unconsciousness (1% of TBI survivors; CDC, 2000).

RISK FACTORS

- Transportation accidents
- Violence (often firearm related)
- Falls (especially in people above age 65)
- Male gender
- Failure to use protective equipment (helmets, seat belts)
- Participation in contact and other sports, such as soccer

RISK REDUCTION TEACHING TIPS

- Use safe driving techniques.
- Wear protective gear such as helmets and seat belts, especially when riding a bicycle or motorcycle.
- Avoid violent or potentially violent environments when possible.
- Work with community agencies to modify violent environments; develop anger management programs, drug-free programs, and firearm safety programs.
- Modify one's residence to prevent falls.
- Acquire and learn safe use of adaptive equipment for safe mobility inside and outside the home.
- Avoid dangerous contact sports likely to cause brain injury; wear protective equipment when engaging in such activity.

CULTURAL CONSIDERATIONS

The few cultural considerations that come into play are related to dependence on poorly maintained automobiles or bicycles, lack of use of protective gear, inadequate and unsafe housing, unsafe celebratory practices (such as shooting guns to welcome the new year) and such norms within societies, especially less developed societies.

PHYSICAL ASSESSMENT

ASSESSMENT PROCEDURE	NORMAL FINDINGS	ABNORMAL FINDINGS

THE HEAD AND FACE

Inspect the Head

Inspect for size, shape, and configuration.

Head size and shape vary, especially in accord with ethnicity. Usually the head is symmetric, round, erect, and in midline. No lesions are visible.

The skull and facial bones are larger and thicker in acromegaly, which occurs when there is an increased production of growth hormone (Display 10-1).

Acorn-shaped, enlarged skull bones are seen in Paget's disease of the bone.

Inspect for involuntary movement.

Head should be held still and upright.

Tremors associated with neurologic disorders may cause a horizontal jerking movement. An involuntary nodding movement may be seen in patients with aortic insufficiency. Head tilted to one side may indicate unilateral vision or hearing deficiency or shortening of the sternomastoid muscle.

Palpate the Head

Palpate the head to assess consistency.

The head is normally hard and smooth without lesions.

Lesions or lumps on the head may indicate recent trauma or cancer.

 Tip From the Experts Wear gloves to protect yourself from possible drainage.

Inspect the Face

Inspect for symmetry, features, movement, expression, and skin condition.

The face is symmetric with a round, oval, elongated, or square appearance. No abnormal movements noted.

In older clients, facial wrinkles are prominent because subcutaneous fat decreases with age. In addition, the lower face may shrink and the mouth may be drawn inward as a result of resorption of mandibular bone, also an age-related process.

Asymmetry in front of the earlobes occurs with parotid gland enlargement from an abscess or tumor. Unusual or asymmetric orofacial movements may be from an organic disease or neurologic problem, which should be referred for medical follow-up.

Drooping of one side of the face may result from a stroke—or cerebrovascular accident (CVA)—or a neurologic condition known as Bell's palsy.

A "masklike" face marks Parkinson's disease; a "sunken" face with depressed eyes and hollow cheeks is typical of cachexia (emaciation or wasting); and a pale, swollen face may result from nephrotic syndrome.

Tip From the Experts The nasolabial folds and palpebral fissures are ideal places to check facial features for symmetry.

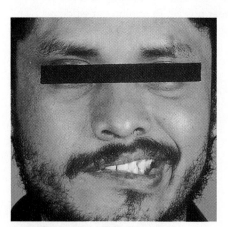

One-sided facial paralysis characterizes Bell's palsy. (© Chet Childs/CMSP.)

(continued)

ASSESSMENT PROCEDURE	NORMAL FINDINGS	ABNORMAL FINDINGS

Palpate the Temporal Artery

Palpate the temporal artery, which is located between the top of the ear and the eye.

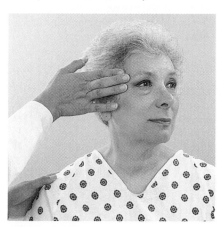

Palpating the temporal artery. (© B. Proud.)

The temporal artery is elastic and not tender.

> The strength of the pulsation of the temporal artery may be decreased in the older client.

The temporal artery is hard, thick, and tender with inflammation, as seen with temporal arteritis (inflammation of the temporal arteries that may lead to blindness).

Palpate the Temporomandibular Joint

To assess the temporomandibular joint (TMJ), place your index finger over the front of each ear as you ask the client to open his or her mouth.

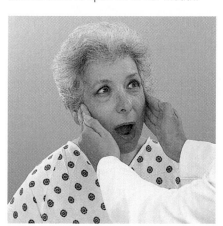

Palpating the TMJ. (© B. Proud.)

Normally, there is no swelling, tenderness, or crepitation with movement. Mouth opens and closes fully (3 to 6 cm between upper and lower teeth). Lower jaw moves laterally 1 to 2 cm in each direction.

Limited range of motion, swelling, tenderness, or crepitation may indicate TMJ syndrome.

> **Tip From the Experts** When assessing TMJ syndrome, be sure to explore the client's history of headaches, if any.

(continued)

ASSESSMENT PROCEDURE	NORMAL FINDINGS	ABNORMAL FINDINGS

THE NECK

Inspect the Neck

Observe the client's slightly extended neck for position, symmetry, and lumps or masses. Shine a light from the side of the neck across to highlight any swelling.

Neck is symmetric with head centered and without bulging masses.

Swelling, enlarged masses, or nodules may indicate an enlarged thyroid gland, inflammation of lymph nodes, or a tumor.

Inspect Movement of the Neck Structures

Ask the client to swallow a small sip of water. Observe the movement of the thyroid cartilage, thyroid gland.

The thyroid cartilage, cricoid cartilage, and thyroid gland move upward symmetrically as the client swallows.

Asymmetric movement or generalized enlargement of the thyroid gland is considered abnormal.

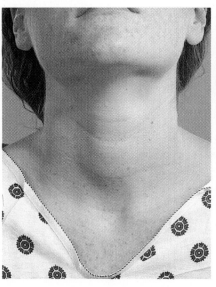 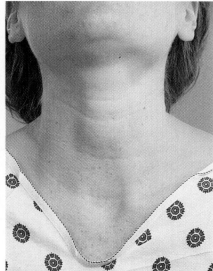

(Left) Slightly extended neck discloses internal structure. **(Right)** Neck structures move (rise and fall). (© B. Proud.)

Inspect the Cervical Vertebrae

Ask the client to flex the neck (chin to chest, ear to shoulder, twist left to right and right to left, and backward and forward).

C7 (vertebrae prominens) is usually visible and palpable.

In older clients, cervical curvature may increase because of kyphosis of the spine. Moreover, fat may accumulate around the cervical vertebrae (especially in women). This is sometimes called a "dowager's hump."

Prominence or swellings other than the C7 vertebrae may be abnormal.

(continued)

ASSESSMENT PROCEDURE	NORMAL FINDINGS	ABNORMAL FINDINGS

Inspect Neck Range of Motion

Ask the client to turn the head to the right and to the left (chin to shoulder), touch each ear to the shoulder, touch chin to chest, and lift the chin to the ceiling.

Normally, neck movement should be smooth and controlled with 45-degree flexion, 55-degree extension, 40-degree lateral abduction, and 70-degree rotation.

> Older clients usually have somewhat decreased flexion, extension, lateral bending, and rotation of the neck. This is usually due to arthritis.

Muscle spasms, inflammation, or cervical arthritis may cause stiffness, rigidity, and limited mobility of the neck, which may affect daily functioning.

Palpate the Trachea

Place your finger in the sternal notch. Feel each side of the notch and palpate the tracheal rings. The first upper ring above the smooth tracheal rings is the cricoid cartilage.

Trachea is midline.

The trachea may be pulled to one side in cases of a tumor, thyroid gland enlargement, aortic aneurysm, pneumothorax, atelectasis, or fibrosis.

Palpating the trachea. (© B. Proud.)

Palpate the Thyroid Gland

Locate key landmarks with your index finger and thumb:

Hyoid bone (arch-shaped bone that does not articulate directly with any other bone; located high in anterior neck).

Thyroid cartilage (under the hyoid bone; the area that widens at the top of the trachea), also known as the "Adam's apple."

Cricoid cartilage (smaller upper tracheal ring under the thyroid cartilage; see Fig. 10-2).

Landmarks are positioned midline.

Landmarks deviate from midline or are obscured because of masses or abnormal growths.

(continued)

ASSESSMENT PROCEDURE	NORMAL FINDINGS	ABNORMAL FINDINGS
To palpate the thyroid, use a posterior approach. Stand behind the client and ask her or him to lower the chin to the chest and turn the neck slightly to the right. This will relax the client's neck muscles. Then place your thumbs on the nape of the client's neck with your other fingers on either side of the trachea below the cricoid cartilage. Use your left fingers to push the trachea to the right. Then use your right fingers to feel deeply in front of the sternomastoid muscle.	Unless the client is extremely thin with a long neck, the thyroid gland is usually not palpable. However, the isthmus may be palpated in midline. If the thyroid can be palpated, the lobes are smooth, firm, and nontender. The right lobe is often 25% larger than the left lobe.	In cases of diffuse enlargement; such as hyperthyroidism, Graves' disease, or an endemic goiter, the thyroid gland may be palpated. An enlarged, tender gland may result from thyroiditis. Multiple nodules of the thyroid may be seen in metabolic processes. However, rapid enlargement of a single nodule suggests a malignancy and must be evaluated further.

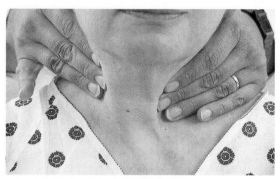

Palpating the thyroid. (© B. Proud.)

If palpable, the older client's thyroid may feel more nodular or irregular because of fibrotic changes that occur with aging; the thyroid may also be felt lower in the neck because of age-related structural changes.

Ask the client to swallow as you palpate the right side of the gland. Reverse the technique to palpate the left lobe of the thyroid.	Glandular thyroid tissue may be felt rising underneath your fingers. Lobes should feel smooth, rubbery, and free of nodules.	Coarse tissue or irregular consistency may indicate an inflammatory process. Nodules should be described in terms of location, size, and consistency (Display 10-2).

Auscultate an Enlarged Thyroid Gland

You will auscultate the thyroid only if you find an enlarged thyroid gland during inspection or palpation. Do so with the bell of the stethoscope placed over the lateral lobes of the thyroid gland. Ask the client to hold his or her breath (to obscure any tracheal breath sounds while you auscultate).	No bruits are auscultated.	A soft, blowing, swishing sound auscultated over the thyroid lobes is often heard in hyperthyroidism because of an increase in blood flow through the thyroid arteries.

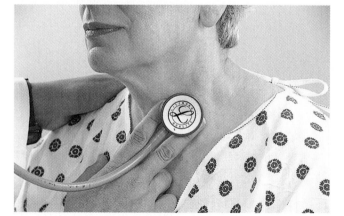

Auscultating for bruits over the thyroid gland. (© B. Proud.)

(continued)

ASSESSMENT PROCEDURE	NORMAL FINDINGS	ABNORMAL FINDINGS

LYMPH NODES OF THE HEAD AND NECK

Have the client remain seated upright. Then palpate the lymph nodes with your fingerpads in a slow walking, gentle, circular motion. Ask the client to bend the head slightly toward the side being palpated to relax the muscles in that area. Compare lymph nodes that occur bilaterally. As you palpate each group of nodes, assess their size and shape, delimitation (whether they are discrete or confluent), mobility, consistency, and tenderness (see Display 10-2). Choose a particular palpation sequence. Here, the sequence chosen proceeds in a superior to inferior order (from 1 to 10).

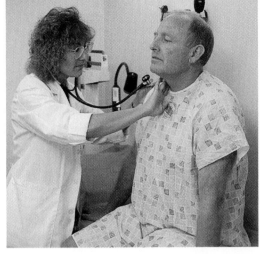

© Susan Van Etten, Stock Boston.

Tip From the Experts Which sequence you choose is not important. What is important is that you establish a specific sequence that does not vary from assessment to assessment. This helps guard against skipping over a group of nodes.

Palpate the
1. **Preauricular nodes** in front of the ear
2. **Postauricular nodes** behind the ears
3. **Occipital nodes** at the posterior base of the skull

No swelling or enlargement and no tenderness

Enlarged nodes

Palpate the
4. **Tonsillar nodes** at the angle of the mandible on the anterior edge of the sternomastoid muscle

Palpate the
5. **Submandibular nodes** located on the medial border of the mandible

No swelling, no tenderness, no hardness

Swelling, tenderness, hardness, immobility

Tip From the Experts Do not confuse the submandibular nodes with the lobulated submandibular gland.

Palpate the
6. **Submental nodes,** which are a few centimeters behind the tip of the mandible

Tip From the Experts It is easier to palpate these nodes using one hand.

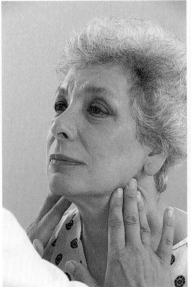
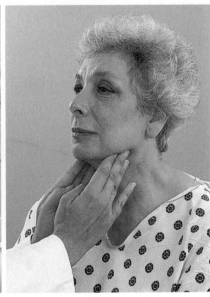

Palpating the tonsillar nodes. (© B. Proud.)

Palpating the submandibular nodes. (© B. Proud.)

(continued)

ASSESSMENT PROCEDURE	NORMAL FINDINGS	ABNORMAL FINDINGS

Palpate the

7. **Superficial cervical nodes** in the area superficial to the sternomastoid muscle

Palpate the

8. **Posterior cervical nodes** in the area posterior to the sternomastoid and anterior to the trapezius in the posterior triangle

Palpate the

9. **Deep cervical chain nodes** deeply within and around the sternomastoid muscle

Palpate the

10. **Supraclavicular nodes** by hooking your fingers over the clavicles and feeling deeply between the clavicles and the sternomastoid muscles

No enlargement or tenderness

An enlarged, hard, nontender node, particularly on the left side, may indicate a metastasis from a malignancy in the abdomen or thorax.

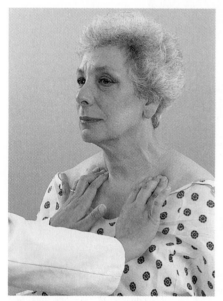

Palpating the supraclavicular nodes.
(© B. Proud.)

Display 10-1. Head and Neck Abnormalities

During any physical examination of the head, the nurse may encounter many variations from normal as well as many abnormalities. Some of the most common abnormalities are pictured here.

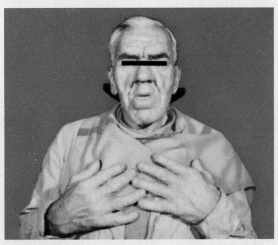

Acromegaly is characterized by enlargement of the facial features (nose, ears) and the hands and feet.

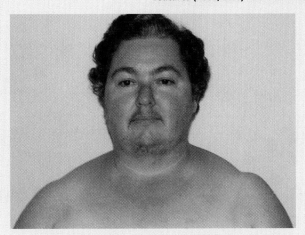

A moon-shaped face with reddened cheeks and increased facial hair may indicate Cushing's syndrome.

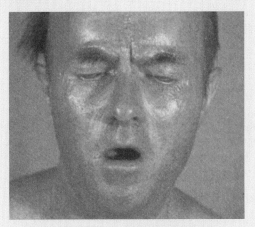

A tightened-hard face with thinning facial skin is seen in scleroderma. (With permission from Clements, P. J., & Furst, D. E. [1996]. *Systemic sclerosis.* Baltimore: Williams & Wilkins.)

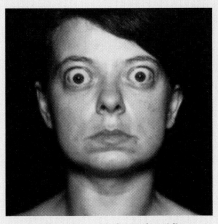

Exophthalmos is seen in hyperthyroidism.

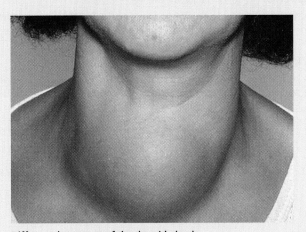

Diffuse enlargement of the thyroid gland.

Display 10-2. Characteristics of Lymph Nodes

While palpating the lymph nodes, note the following:

- Size and shape
- Delimitation
- Mobility
- Consistency
- Tenderness and location

NORMAL SIZE AND SHAPE

Normally, lymph nodes, which are round and smaller than 1 cm, are not palpable. In older clients, especially, the lymph nodes become fibrotic, fatty, and smaller because of a loss of lymphoid elements related to aging. (This may decrease the older person's resistance to infection.)

ABNORMAL SIZE AND SHAPE

When lymph node enlargement exceeds 1 cm, the client is said to have lymphadenopathy, which may be caused by acute or chronic infection, an auto-immune disorder, or metastatic disease. If one or two lymphatic groups enlarge, the client is said to have *regional lymphadenopathy*. Enlargement of three or more groups is *generalized lymphadenopathy*. Generalized lymphadenopathy that persists for more than 3 months may be a sign of human immunodeficiency virus (HIV) infection.

DELIMITATION

Normally, lymph node delimitation (the lymph node's position or boundary) is discrete. In chronic infection, however, the lymph nodes become confluent (they merge). In acute infection, they remain discrete.

MOBILITY

Typical lymph nodes are mobile both from side to side and up and down. In metastatic disease, the lymph nodes enlarge and become fixed in place.

CONSISTENCY

Somewhat more fibrotic and fatty in older clients, the normal lymph node is soft, whereas the abnormal node is hard and firm. Hard, firm, unilateral nodes are seen with metastatic cancers.

TENDERNESS AND LOCATION

Tender, enlarged nodes suggest acute infections; normally, lymph nodes are not sore or tender. Of course, you need to document the location of the lymph node being assessed.

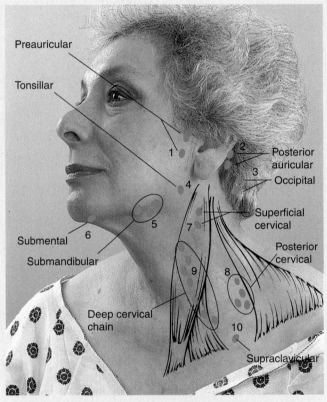

Location of the lymph nodes of the head and neck. (© B. Proud.)

(continued)

Validation and Documentation of Findings

Validate the head and neck assessment data that you have collected. This is necessary to verify that the data are reliable and accurate. Document the assessment data following the health care facility or agency policy.

EXAMPLE OF SUBJECTIVE DATA

No history of head or neck problems, trauma, or surgery. No head or facial pain. Has not experienced episodes of lightheadedness or dizziness. Does not chew or smoke tobacco. Works as secretary. Has good work setting and equipment to promote correct posture. Rides bikes 10 miles four times a week to relieve stress. Wears a bike helmet. Has no complaints about current condition of head and neck.

EXAMPLE OF OBJECTIVE DATA

Head symmetrically round, hard, and smooth without lesions or bumps. Face oval, smooth, and symmetric. Temporal artery elastic and nontender. Temporomandibular joint palpated with full range of motion without tenderness. Neck symmetric with centered head position and no bulging masses. C7 is visible and palpable with neck flexed. Has smooth, controlled, full range of motion of neck. Thyroid gland nonvisible but palpable when swallowing. Trachea in midline. Lymph nodes nonpalpable except for a few deep cervical less than 1 cm bilaterally.

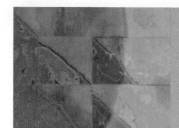
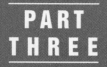
After collecting the assessment data, you will need to analyze the data, using the diagnostic reasoning skills discussed in Chapter 7.

Diagnostic Reasoning: Possible Conclusions

Listed below are some possible conclusions and nursing diagnoses resulting from assessment of the client's head and neck.

SELECTED NURSING DIAGNOSES

After collecting subjective and objective data pertaining to the head and neck assessment, you will need to identify abnormal findings and cluster the data to reveal any significant patterns or abnormalities. These data will then be used to make clinical judgments (nursing diagnoses: wellness, risk, or actual) about the status of the client's head and neck. The following lists of selected nursing diagnoses may be some that you identify when analyzing data for this part of the assessment.

Nursing Diagnoses (Wellness)

- Opportunity to enhance the posture and mobility of the head and neck
- Health-Seeking Behavior: Requests assistance information on how to quit smoking

Nursing Diagnoses (Risk)

- Risk for Injury to head and neck related to poor posture
- Risk for Injury to head and neck related to not wearing protective devices (eg, head gear during contact sports, seat belts, eye goggles)

Nursing Diagnoses (Actual)

- Ineffective Health Maintenance related to lack of knowledge of the importance of wearing protective gear during contact sports and wearing seat belt while driving or riding as a passenger
- Ineffective Health Maintenance related to lack of knowledge of the effects and dangers associated with smoking and using smokeless tobacco

- Ineffective Tissue Perfusion: Cerebral related to impaired circulation to brain
- Imbalanced Nutrition: More Than Body Requirements related to increased metabolism secondary to hyperthyroidism
- Imbalanced Nutrition: Less Than Body Requirements related to decreased metabolism secondary to hypothyroidism
- Imbalanced Nutrition: Less Than Body Requirements related to irritated oral cavity that prevents consumption of food
- Activity Intolerance related to fatigue and weakness secondary to slowed metabolic rate secondary to hypothyroidism or surgery of head, neck, or face
- Risk for Constipation or Diarrhea related to hyperthyroidism or hypothyroidism
- Disturbed Body Image related to injury
- Impaired Physical Mobility of head and neck related to cervical injury
- Impaired Swallowing related to mechanical obstruction of the head and neck secondary to tissue swelling, tracheostomy, or abnormal growth
- Impaired Swallowing related to lack of gag reflex, paralysis of facial muscles, or decreased cognition

SELECTED COLLABORATIVE PROBLEMS

After grouping the data, certain collaborative problems may become apparent. Remember, collaborative problems differ from nursing diagnoses in that they cannot be prevented by nursing interventions. However, these physiologic complications of medical conditions can be detected and monitored by the nurse. In addition, the nurse can use physician- and nurse-prescribed interventions to minimize the complications of these problems. The nurse may also have to refer the client in such situations for further treatment of the problem. Following is a list of collaborative problems that may be identified when assessing the head and neck of a patient. These problems are worded as Potential Complications (or PC) followed by the problem.

- PC: Lymphedema
- PC: Hypocalcemia
- PC: Hypercalcemia
- PC: Corneal abrasion (related to inability to close eyelids secondary to exophthalmos)
- PC: Thyroid crisis

- PC: Thyroid dysfunction
- PC: Cerebral vascular accident
- PC: Seizures
- PC: Cranial nerve impairment (fifth trigeminal, seventh facial, eleventh spinal accessory)
- PC: Increased intracranial pressure

MEDICAL PROBLEMS

After the data are grouped, it may become apparent that the client has signs and symptoms that may require medical diagnosis and treatment. Referral to a primary care provider is necessary.

Diagnostic Reasoning: Case Study

The case study presents assessment data for a specific client. It is followed by an analysis of the data, working out the seven key steps to arrive at specific conclusions.

You are volunteering to do health screening assessments at a neighborhood clinic. As you observe Margy Kase, who is 19 years old, you notice a diffuse swelling of her anterior neck. Margy is thin and fidgety; she has beads of perspiration on her forehead and upper lip, even though the room is cool. She denies any throat pain or difficulty swallowing, but she says that she is hungry all of the time lately and thinks she has lost some weight. She says she has come to the clinic today for a physical examination because she wants to stay healthy, even though she doesn't have health insurance and cannot afford a doctor. She tells you that somehow she manages to obtain a yearly checkup.

Margy's height is 5 ft 9 in, and her weight is 110 lb. She states that "This is about 7 pounds lower than my normal weight." As you consult the standard weight charts, you discover that she is in about the fifth percentile for her age, with a medium frame. Her vital signs: BP 132/78, pulse 96, respirations 18. She does not know what her usual blood pressure is. Her thyroid gland appears slightly enlarged when pal-pated, and a bruit is detected upon auscultation. The rest of the physical examination findings appear to be within normal limits.

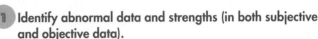 **Identify abnormal data and strengths (in both subjective and objective data).**

SUBJECTIVE DATA

- 7-lb weight loss
- Does not know her usual blood pressure
- Hungry all the time
- Came to clinic for physical examination because she wants to stay healthy
- No health insurance and cannot afford a doctor
- Usually obtains a yearly checkup

OBJECTIVE DATA

- Thin, 19-year-old woman
- Weight at 110 lb is in fifth percentile for height
- Excessive perspiration and fidgeting
- Diffuse swelling of anterior neck
- Slightly enlarged thyroid on palpation
- BP 132/82, P 96, R 18

2 Cue Clusters	3 Inferences	4 Possible Nursing Diagnoses	5 Defining Characteristics	6 Confirm or Rule Out
A • Weight decreased by 7 lb, thin • Diffuse swelling, anterior neck • Increased perspiration, fidgeting • Slightly enlarged thyroid on palpation • Bruit auscultated over thyroid • BP 132/82, P 96, R 18 • Hungry all the time	May have medical problem related to hyperthyroidism May not be eating enough for her energy output	Imbalanced Nutrition: Less Than Body Requirements related to possible inability to consume enough food to meet metabolic demands	*Major:* None *Minor:* None	Does not meet the defining characteristics with the data available. Collect more information about actual intake and type of food ingested.

2 Cue Clusters	**3** Inferences	**4** Possible Nursing Diagnoses	**5** Defining Characteristics	**6** Confirm or Rule Out
B • No health insurance • Can't afford physician visit	May be placing her health in jeopardy because of finances	Ineffective Health Maintenance related to inadequate resources to meet health needs	*Major:* None *Minor:* None	Rule out this diagnosis because it does not have any of the defining characteristics. In fact, even though the client does not have health insurance, she has come to the clinic seeking health care.
C • Wants to stay healthy • Doesn't know usual BP	Finding ways to check up on health status even when she cannot afford a private physician	Health-Seeking Behaviors related to verbalization of coming to clinic to stay healthy	*Major:* Expressed desire to seek information for health promotion *Minor:* None observed lack of knowledge of usual BP and presenting signs and symptoms.	Confirm because client meets defining characteristics and client validated data.

 Document conclusions.

Only one nursing diagnosis is selected at this time:

- Health-Seeking Behaviors

Because there is no medical diagnosis, there are no collaborative problems at this time.

This client does need a referral to a primary care provider because the findings from the physical examination suggest that she may have a thyroid problem. She needs a referral for a thorough evaluation for diagnosis and treatment, if applicable.

REFERENCES AND SELECTED READINGS

Argueta, R. (2000). When a thyroid abnormality is palpable. Symposium. First of four articles on thyroid diseases. *Postgraduate Medicine, 107*(1), 100–104, 109–110, 155–156.

Brach, J. (1999). Not all facial paralysis is Bell's palsy: A case report. *Archives of Physical Medicine and Rehabilitation, 80*(7), 857–859.

Carr, K. K., & Clark, N. (1995). Physical assessment (7-part series). *American Journal of Nursing* [Video].

Diamond, S. (1999). Headache of the month: Evaluating chronic headaches. *Consultant, 39*(9), 2482, 2485–2486.

Duchro, P. N., Chibnall, J. T., & Greenberg, M. S. (1995). Myofacial involvement in chronic post-traumatic headache. *Headache Quarterly, Current Treatment and Research, 6*(1), 34–38.

Geyer, N., & Naude, S. (1996). Continuing education: Clinical, diagnostic skills: Assessment of the head and neck. *Nursing News (South Africa), 20*(3), 50–51.

Gilkison, C. R. (1993). Differential diagnosis: A case of a swollen thyroid. *American Journal of Nursing, 93*(12), 16F–16J.

Heitman, B., & Irizarry, A. (1995). Hypothyroidism: Common complaints, perplexing diagnosis. *Nurse Practitioner, 20*(3), 54–60.

Kunkel, R. (2000). Managing primary headache symptoms. *Patient Care, 34*(2), 100–117.

Lipson, J., Dibble, S., & Minarik, P. (Eds.). (1996). *Culture and nursing care: A pocket guide.* San Francisco: UCSF Nursing Press.

Moloney, M. (2000). Caring for the women with migraine headaches. *Nurse Practitioner: American Journal of Primary Health Care, 25*(2), 17–18, 21–22, 24.

Paulson, G. W., & Gill, W. W. (1993). Oral and facial movements in the aged. *Journal of Neuro-science Nursing, 25,* 246–248.

Pinkowish, M. (1998). The clinical challenge of chronic daily headaches. *Patient Care Nurse Practitioner, 1*(5), 41–45.

Siminoski, K. (1995). The rational clinical examination: Does this patient have a goiter? *Journal of the American Medical Association, 273*(10), 813–817.

Weiss, J. (1999). Assessing and managing the patient with headaches. *Nurse Practitioner: American Journal of Primary Health Care 24*(7) 18–29.

Young, J. (1999). Actionstat. Thyroid storm. *Nursing 99, 29*(8), 33.

Risk Factors—Traumatic Brain Injury

Centers for Disease Control and Prevention (CDC). National Center for Injury Prevention and Control. (2000). *Epidemiology of traumatic brain injury in the United States.* Available: www.cdc.gov/ncipc.

For additional information on this book, be sure to visit http://connection.lww.com.

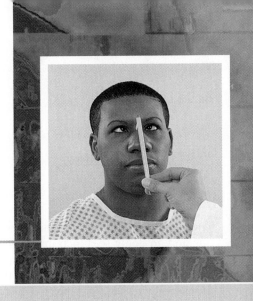

Eye Assessment

11

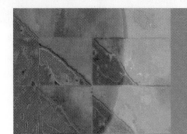

Structure and Function

The eye transmits visual stimuli to the brain for interpretation and, in doing so, functions as the organ of vision. The eyeball is located in the eye orbit, a round, bony hollow formed by several different bones of the skull. In the orbit, the eye is surrounded by a cushion of fat. The bony orbit and fat cushion protect the eyeball.

Parts of the Eye

To perform a thorough assessment of the eye, the nurse should have a good understanding of the external structures of the eye, the internal structures of the eye, the visual fields and pathways, and the visual reflexes.

EXTERNAL STRUCTURES

The *eyelids* (upper and lower) are two movable structures composed of skin and two types of muscle—striated and smooth. Their purpose is to protect the eye from foreign bodies and limit the amount of light entering the eye. In addition, they serve to distribute tears that lubricate the surface of the eye (Fig. 11-1). The upper eyelid is larger, more mobile, and contains *tarsal plates* made up of connective tissue. These plates contain the *meibomian glands,* which secrete an oily substance that lubricates the eyelid.

The eyelids join at two points—the *lateral (outer) canthus* and *medial (inner) canthus*. The medial canthus contains the puncta, two small openings that allow drainage of tears into the lacrimal system, and the *caruncle,* a small, fleshy mass that contains sebaceous glands. The white space between open eyelids is called the *palpebral fissure*. When closed, the eyelids should touch. When open, the upper lid position should be between the upper margin of the iris and the upper margin of the pupil. The lower lid should rest on the lower border of the iris. No sclera should be seen above or below the limbus (the point where the sclera meets the cornea).

Eyelashes are projections of stiff hair curving outward along the margins of the eyelids that filter dust and dirt from air entering the eye.

The *conjunctiva* is a thin, transparent, continuous membrane that is divided into two portions—a *palpebral* and a *bulbar* portion. The palpebral conjunctiva lines the inside of the eyelids, and the bulbar conjunctiva covers most of the anterior eye, merging with the cornea at the limbus.

The point at which the palpebral and bulbar conjunctivae meet creates a folded recess that allows movement of the eyeball. This transparent membrane allows for inspection of underlying tissue and serves to protect the eye from foreign bodies.

The *lacrimal apparatus* consists of glands and ducts that serve to lubricate the eye (Fig. 11-2). The *lacrimal gland,* located in the upper outer corner of the orbital cavity just above the eye, is responsible for tear production. Tears are washed across the eye as the lid blinks and then drain into the *puncta,* which is visible on the upper and lower lids at the inner canthus. Tears are then channeled into the *nasolacrimal sac,* through the *nasolacrimal duct.* They drain into the nasal meatus.

The *extraocular muscles* are the six muscles attached to the outer surface of each eyeball. These muscles control six different directions of eye movement. Four rectus muscles are responsible for straight movement, and two oblique muscles are responsible for diagonal movement. Each muscle coordinates with a muscle in the opposite eye. This allows for parallel movement of the eyes and thus the binocular vision characteristic of humans (Fig. 11-3). Innervation for these muscles is supplied by three cranial nerves, the oculomotor (III) trochlear (IV), and abducens (VI).

INTERNAL STRUCTURES

The eyeball is composed of three separate coats or layers (Fig. 11-4). The outermost layer consists of the *sclera* and *cornea*. The sclera is a dense, protective, white covering that physically supports the internal structures of the eye. It is continuous anteriorly with the transparent cornea (the "window of the eye"). The cornea permits the entrance of light, which passes through the lens to the retina. It is well supplied with nerve endings, making it responsive to pain and touch. Because of this sensory property, contact with a wisp of cotton stimulates a blink in both eyes known as the *corneal reflex.* This reflex is supported by the trigeminal nerve, which carries the afferent sensation into the brain, and the facial nerve, which carries the efferent message that stimulates the blink.

The middle layer is known as the *choroid layer.* This layer contains the vascularity necessary to provide nourishment to the inner aspect of the eye and prevents light from reflecting internally. Anteriorly, this layer is continuous with the ciliary body and the iris. The *ciliary body* consists

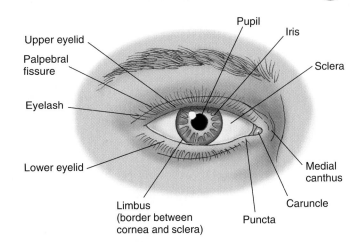

FIGURE 11-1. Eyelids are structured to protect the eyes from foreign matter, distribute tears, and shield the eye from excessive light.

of muscle tissue that controls the thickness of the lens, which must be adapted to focus on objects near and far away.

The *iris* is a circular disc of muscle that contains pigments that determine eye color. The central aperture of the iris is called the pupil. Its size is adjusted by the muscles in the iris, which, therefore, controls the amount of light entering the eye. The muscle fibers of the iris also decrease the size of the pupil to accommodate for near vision and dilate the pupil when far vision is needed.

The *lens* is a biconvex, transparent, avascular, encapsulated structure located immediately posterior to the iris. Suspensory ligaments attached to the ciliary body support the position of the lens. The lens functions to refract (bend) light rays onto the retina. Adjustments must be made in re-

fraction depending on the distance of the object being viewed. Refractive ability of the lens can be changed by a change in shape of the lens (which is controlled by the ciliary body). The lens bulges to focus on close objects and flattens to focus on far objects.

The innermost layer, the *retina*, extends only to the ciliary body anteriorly and consists of numerous layers of nerve cells, including the cells commonly called rods and cones. These specialized nerve cells are often referred to as "photoreceptors" because they are responsive to light. The rods are highly sensitive to light, regulate black and white vision, and function in dim light. The cones function in bright light and are sensitive to color.

The *optic disc* is a cream-colored, circular area located on the retina toward the medial or nasal side of the eye (Fig. 11-5). At this location, the optic nerve enters the eyeball. The optic disc can be seen with the use of an ophthalmoscope and is normally round or oval in shape, with distinct

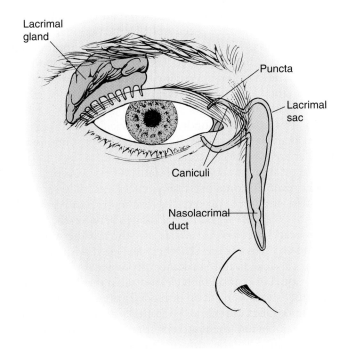

FIGURE 11-2. The lacrimal apparatus consists of tear (lacrimal) glands and ducts.

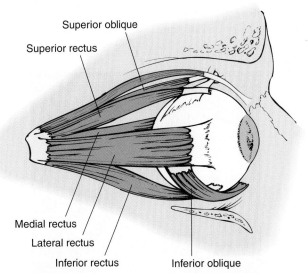

FIGURE 11-3. Extraocular muscles control the direction of eye movement.

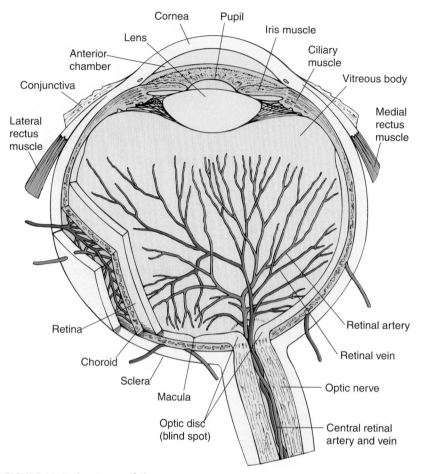

FIGURE 11-4. Anatomy of the eye.

margins. A smaller circular area that appears slightly depressed is referred to as the *physiologic cup*. This area is approximately one third the size of the entire optic disc and appears somewhat whiter than the disc borders.

The *retinal vessels* can be readily viewed with the aid of an ophthalmoscope. Four sets of *arterioles* and *venules* travel through the optic disc, bifurcate, and extend to the periph-ery of the fundus. Vessels are dark red and grow progressively narrower as they extend out to the peripheral areas. Arterioles carry oxygenated blood and appear brighter red and narrower than the veins. The general background, or fundus, varies in color, depending on skin color. A retinal depression known as the fovea centralis is located adjacent to the optic disc in the temporal section of the fundus (see Fig. 11-5). This area is surrounded by the macula, which appears darker than the rest of the fundus. The fovea centralis and macular area are highly concentrated with cones and form the area of highest visual resolution and color vision.

The eyeball contains several chambers that serve to maintain structure, protect against injury, and transmit light rays. The *anterior chamber* is located between the cornea and iris, and the *posterior chamber* is the area between the iris and the lens. These chambers are filled with aqueous humor, a clear liquid substance produced by the ciliary body. Aqueous humor helps cleanse and nourish the cornea and lens, as well as maintain intraocular pressure. The aqueous humor filters out of the eye from the posterior to the anterior chamber and then into the *canal of Schlemm* through a filtering site called the *trabecular meshwork*. Another chamber, the *vitreous chamber,* is located in the area behind the lens to the retina. It is the largest of the chambers and is filled with vitreous humor, a clear, gelatinous substance.

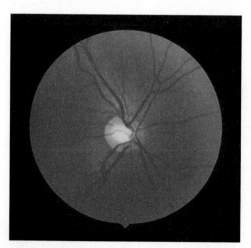

FIGURE 11-5. Normal ocular fundus. (© 1994, CMSP.)

Visual Fields and Visual Pathways

A visual field refers to what a person sees with one eye. The visual field of each eye can be divided into four quadrants—upper temporal, lower temporal, upper nasal, and lower nasal (Fig. 11-6). The temporal quadrants of each visual field extend farther than the nasal quadrants. Thus, each eye sees a slightly different view, but their visual fields overlap quite a bit. As a result of this, humans have binocular vision ("two-eyed" vision) in which the visual cortex fuses the two slightly different images and provides depth perception or three-dimensional vision.

Visual perception occurs as light rays strike the retina, where they are transformed into nerve impulses, conducted to the brain through the optic nerve, and interpreted. In the eye, light must pass through transparent media (cornea, aqueous humor, lens, and vitreous body) before reaching the retina. The cornea and lens are the main eye components that refract (bend) light rays on the retina. The image that is projected on the retina is upside down and reversed right to left from the actual image. For example, an image from the lower temporal visual field strikes the upper temporal quadrant of the retina. At the point where the optic nerves from each eyeball cross—the *optic chiasma*—the nerve fibers from the nasal quadrant of each retina (from both temporal visual fields) cross over to the opposite side. At this point, the right optic tract contains only nerve fibers from the right side of the retina and the left optic tract contains only nerve fibers from the left side of the retina. Therefore, the left side of the brain views the right side of the world.

Visual Reflexes

The *pupillary light reflex* causes pupils immediately to constrict when exposed to bright light. This can be seen as a *direct reflex*, in which constriction occurs in the eye exposed to the light, or as an *indirect or consensual reflex*,

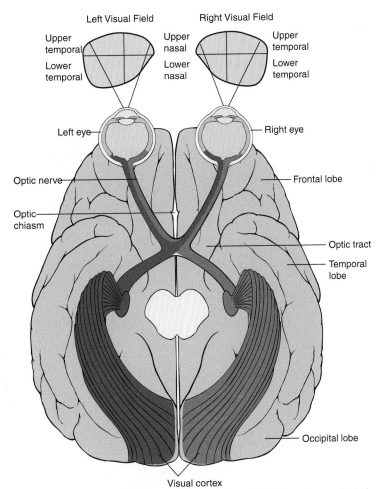

FIGURE 11-6. Visual fields and visual pathways. Each eye has a slightly different view of the same field. However, the views overlap significantly, which accounts for binocular vision.

in which exposure to light in one eye results in constriction of the pupil in the opposite eye (Fig. 11-7). These protective reflexes, mediated by the oculomotor nerve, prevent damage to the delicate photoreceptors by excessive light.

Accommodation is a functional reflex allowing the eyes to focus on near objects. This is accomplished through movement of the ciliary muscles causing an increase in the curvature of the lens. This change in shape of the lens is not visible. However, convergence of the eyes and constriction of the pupils occur simultaneously, and can be seen.

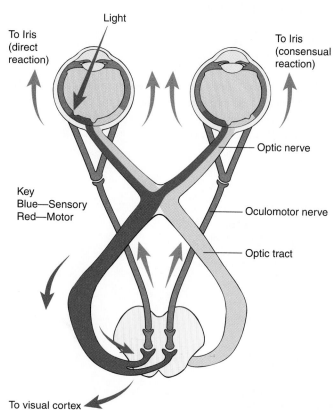

FIGURE 11-7. The pupils admit light that travels over the visual pathways. If a light focuses on only one eye, the pupil responds to ensure that the light needed for vision can enter but not so much that eye damage would result. The other pupil responds in the same manner. This phenomenon of direct pupillary response and consensual pupillary response is a reflex governed by the oculomotor nerve.

Collecting Subjective Data

Beginning when the nurse first meets the client, assessment of vision provides important information about the client's ability to interact with the environment. Changes in vision are often gradual and go unrecognized by clients until a severe problem develops. Therefore, asking the client specific questions about his or her vision may help with early detection of disorders. With recent advances in medicine and surgery, early detection and intervention are increasingly important.

First, gather data from the client about his or her current level of eye health. Also discuss any past and family history problems that are related to the eye. Collecting data concerning environmental influences on vision as well as how any problems are influencing or affecting the client's usual activities of daily living is also important. Answers to these types of questions help to evaluate a client's risk for vision loss and, in turn, present ways that the client may modify or reduce the risk of eye problems.

Nursing History

When interviewing a client about eye health and vision, remember to investigate and analyze any reported symptoms or signs further. Use the COLDSPA mnemonic as a guide.

COLDSPA

CHARACTER: Describe the sign or symptom. How does it feel, look, sound, smell, and so forth?
ONSET: When did it begin?
LOCATION: Where is it? Does it radiate?
DURATION: How long does it last? Does it recur?
SEVERITY: How bad is it?
PATTERN: What makes it better: What makes it worse?
ASSOCIATED FACTORS: What other symptoms occur with it?

CURRENT SYMPTOMS

Question Describe any recent changes in your vision.

Rationale Sudden changes in vision are associated with acute problems, such as head trauma or increased intracranial pressure. Gradual changes in vision may be related to aging, diabetes, hypertension, or neurologic disorders.

Q Do you see spots or floaters in front of your eyes?

R Spots or floaters are common among clients with myopia or in clients over age 40. In most cases, they are due to normal physiologic changes in the eye associated with aging and require no intervention.

Q Do you experience blind spots?

R A scotoma is a blind spot that is surrounded by either normal or slightly diminished peripheral vision. It may be from glaucoma. Intermittent blind spots may be associated with vascular spasms (ophthalmic migraines) or pressure on the optic nerve by a tumor or intracranial pressure. Consistent blind spots may indicate retinal detachment. Any report of a blind spot requires immediate attention and referral to a physician.

Q Do you see halos or rings around lights?

R Seeing halos around lights is associated with narrow-angle glaucoma.

Q Do you have trouble seeing at night?

R Night blindness is associated with optic atrophy, glaucoma, and vitamin A deficiency.

Q Do you experience double vision?

R Double vision (diplopia) may indicate increased intracranial pressure due to injury or a tumor.

Q Do you have any eye pain? Describe.

R Burning or itching pain is usually associated with allergies or superficial irritation. Throbbing, stabbing, or deep, aching pain suggests a foreign body in the eye or changes within the eye. Most common eye disorders are not associated with actual pain; therefore, any reported eye pain should be referred immediately.

Q Do you have any redness or swelling in your eyes?

R Redness or swelling of the eye is usually related to an inflammatory response caused by allergy, foreign body, or bacterial or viral infection.

Q Do you experience excessive watering or tearing of the eye? One eye or both eyes?

R Excessive tearing (epiphora) is caused by exposure to irritants or obstruction of the lacrimal apparatus. Unilateral epiphora is often associated with foreign body or obstruction. Bilateral epiphora is often associated with exposure to irritants, such as makeup or facial cleansers, or it may be a systemic response.

Q Have you had any eye discharge? Describe.

R Discharge other than tears from one or both eyes suggests a bacterial or viral infection.

PAST HISTORY

Q Have you ever had problems with your eyes or vision?

R A history of eye problems or changes in vision provides clues to the current health of the eye.

Q Have you ever had eye surgery?

R Surgery may alter the appearance of the eye and the results of future examinations.

Q Describe any past treatments you have received for eye problems (medication, surgery, laser treatments, corrective lenses). Were these successful? Were you satisfied?

R Client may not be satisfied with past treatments for vision problems.

FAMILY HISTORY

Q Is there a history of eye problems or vision loss in your family?

R Many eye disorders have familial tendencies. Examples include glaucoma, refraction errors, and allergies.

LIFESTYLE AND HEALTH PRACTICES

Q Are you exposed to conditions or substances in the workplace or home that may harm your eyes or vision (eg, chemicals, fumes, smoke, dust, or flying sparks)? Do you wear safety glasses during exposure to harmful substances?

R Injuries or diseases may be related to exposure in the workplace or home. These problems can be minimized or avoided altogether with hazard identification and implementation of safety measures.

Q Do you wear sunglasses during exposure to the sun?

R Exposure to ultraviolet radiation puts the client at risk for the development of cataracts (opacities of the lenses of the eyes; see Risk Factors—Cataracts). Consistent use of sunglasses during exposure minimizes the client's risk.

Q What types of medications do you take?

R Some medications have ocular side effects, such as corticosteroids, lovastatin, pyridostigmine, quinidine, risperidone, and rifampin.

Q Has your vision loss affected your ability to care for yourself? To work?

R Vision problems may interfere with the client's ability to perform usual activities of daily living. The client may be unable to read medication labels or fill insulin syringes. If the vision problem is severe, the client's ability to perform hygiene practices or prepare food may be affected. Vision problems may affect a client's ability to work if the job is one that depends on sight, such as pilot or bus driver.

Q When was your last eye examination?

R A thorough eye examination is recommended for healthy clients every 2 years. Clients with eye disorders or vision problems should be examined more frequently according to their physician's recommendations.

Q Do you have a prescription for corrective lenses (glasses or contacts)? Do you wear them regularly? If you wear contacts, how long do you wear them? How do you clean them?

R The amount of time the client wears the corrective lenses provides information on the severity of the visual problem. Clients who do not wear the prescribed corrective lenses are susceptible to eye strain. Improper cleaning or prolonged wearing of contact lenses can lead to infection and corneal damage.

Collecting Objective Data

The purpose of the eye and vision examination is to identify any changes in vision or signs of eye disorders in an effort to initiate early treatment or corrective procedures. Collected objective data should include assessment of eye function through specific vision tests, inspection of the external eye, and inspection of the internal eye using an ophthalmoscope.

For the most part, inspection and palpation of the external eye are straightforward and simple to perform. The vision tests and use of the ophthalmoscope require a great deal of skill, and thus practice, for the examiner to be capable and confident during the examination. It is a good idea for the beginning examiner to practice on friends, family, or classmates to gain experience and to become comfortable performing the examinations.

CLIENT PREPARATION

The client should be seated comfortably during the eye examination. Client participation during the examination is very important. Therefore, the test should be thoroughly explained to guarantee accurate results. During examination of the internal eye with the ophthalmoscope, the examiner must move very close to the client's face to view the retina and internal structures. Explain to the client that this may be slightly uncomfortable. To ease any client anxiety, explain in detail what you will be doing and answer any questions the client may have.

RISK FACTORS
Cataracts

OVERVIEW

Cataract is the name given to opacity or clouding of the eye's lens. The opacity can develop in various parts of the lens. Cataracts are the leading cause of blindness worldwide with 20 million people blind from cataracts (World Health Organization, 2000).

RISK FACTORS

- Increasing age, especially over age 50
- Exposure to ultraviolet B (UV-B) light, especially at latitudes closer to the equator
- Diabetes mellitus
- Cigarette smoking
- Alcohol use
- Diet low in antioxidant vitamins (Heseker, 1995)
- High blood pressure

POSSIBLE RISK FACTORS

- Being female
- Persistent diarrhea
- Gout for 10 to 20 years' duration or use of allopurinol
- Use of phenothiazines
- Abdominal obesity
- Use of beta blockers
- Arthritis
- Myopia
- Family history in parent or sibling

(Christen et al., 2000; Heseker, 1995; Leske et al., 1999; McCarty et al., 2000; Rowe et al., 2000; West & Valmadrid, 1995; WHO, 1997, 2000).

RISK REDUCTION TEACHING TIPS

- Wear sunglasses and hats in the sun. This is important because even on bright cloudy days, ultraviolet light can penetrate clouds. Squinting does not eliminate ultraviolet light entering the eye.
- Quit smoking
- Limit alcohol intake
- Eat a diet high in antioxidant vitamins

CULTURAL CONSIDERATIONS

Cataract is the major cause of visual impairment and blindness reported in studies of various populations around the world. Most of the 20 million people blind from cataracts live in Third World countries (WHO, 1997, 2000). An interesting pattern of 3% increase in cataracts for each 1-degree decrease in (more southerly) latitude has been correlated with ultraviolet content of sunlight (Javitt & Taylor, 1994–1995). The major worldwide difference in blindness caused by cataracts is access to equipment and trained professionals to perform cataract surgeries. WHO Vision 2020 is targeting the financial and cultural barriers to accessing these services in poorer countries of the developing world (WHO, 2000).

EQUIPMENT AND SUPPLIES

- Snellen or E chart (Display 11-1)
- Hand-held Snellen card or near vision screener
- Penlight
- Opaque cards
- Ophthalmoscope (Display 11-2)
- Disposable gloves (wear as needed to prevent spreading infection or coming in contact with exudate)

KEY ASSESSMENT POINTS

Review and recognize structures and functions of the eyes.

- Explain risks related to excessive sun exposure.
- Administer vision tests competently, and record the results.
- Use the ophthalmoscope correctly and confidently.
- Recognize and distinguish normal variations from abnormal finding.

(*text continues on page 192*)

DISPLAY 11-1. Understanding and Using Vision Charts

SNELLEN CHART

Used to test distant visual acuity, the Snellen chart consists of lines of different letters stacked one on top of the other. The letters are large at the top and decrease in size from top to bottom. The chart is placed on a wall or door at eye level in a well-lighted area. The client stands 20 feet from the chart and covers one eye with an opaque card (which prevents the client from peeking through the fingers). Then, the client reads each line of letters until he or she can no longer distinguish them.

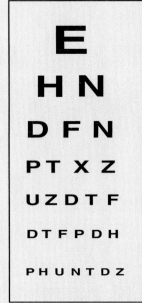 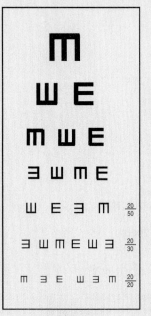

E CHART

If the client cannot read or has a handicap that prevents verbal communication, the E chart is used. The E chart is configured just like the Snellen chart, but the characters on it are only Es, which face in all directions. The client is asked to indicate by pointing which way the open side of the E faces. If the client wears glasses, they should be left on, unless they are reading glasses (reading glasses blur distance vision).

TEST RESULTS

Acuity results are recorded somewhat like blood pressure readings—in a manner that resembles a fraction (but in no way is interpreted as a fraction). A common example of an acuity test score is 20/20. The top, or first, number is always 20, indicating the distance from the client to the chart. The bottom, or second, number refers to the last full line the client could read. Usually, the last line on the chart is the 20/20 line. The examiner needs to document whether the client wore glasses during the test. If any letters on a line are missed, encourage the client to continue reading until he or she cannot distinguish any letters, but record the number of letters missed by using a minus sign. If the client missed two letters on the 20/30 line, the recorded score would be 20/30 −2.

DISPLAY 11-2. How to Use the Ophthalmoscope

The ophthalmoscope is a hand-held instrument that allows the examiner to view the fundus of the eye by the projection of light through a prism that bends the light 90 degrees. There are several lenses arranged on a wheel that affect the focus on objects in the eye. The examiner can rotate the lenses with his or her index finger. Each lens is labeled with a negative or positive number, a unit of strength called a diopter. Red numbers indicate a negative diopter and are used for myopic (nearsighted) clients. Black numbers indicate a positive diopter and are used for hyperopic (farsighted) clients. The zero lens is used if neither the examiner nor the client has refractive errors.

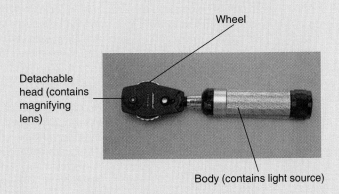

Wheel

Detachable head (contains magnifying lens)

Body (contains light source)

BASICS OF OPERATION

1. Turn the ophthalmoscope "on" and select the aperture with the large round beam of white light. The small round beam of white light may be used if the client has smaller pupils. There are other apertures, but they are not typically used for basic ophthalmologic screening.
2. Ask the client to remove eyeglasses but keep contact lenses in place. You should also remove your glasses. Any refractive errors can be accommodated for by rotating the lenses (if errors are severe, glasses should be left on). Removing glasses enables you to get closer to the client's eye, allowing for a more accurate inspection. Keep your contact lenses in place.
3. Ask the client to fix his or her gaze on an object that is straight ahead and slightly upward.
4. Darken the room to allow pupils to dilate (for a more thorough examination, eyedrops are used to dilate pupils).
5. Hold the ophthalmoscope in your right hand with your index finger on the lens wheel and place it to your right eye (braced between the eyebrow and the nose) if you are examining the client's right eye. Use your left hand and left eye if you are examining the client's left eye. This allows you to get as close to the client's eye as possible without bumping noses with the client.

SOME DO'S AND DON'TS

Do

- Begin about 10 to 15 inches from the client at a 15-degree angle to the client's side.
- Pretend that the ophthalmoscope is an extension of your eye. Keep focused on the red reflex as you move in closer, then rotate the diopter setting to see the optic disk.

Don't

- Do not use your right eye to examine the client's left eye or your left eye to examine the client's right eye (your noses will bump).
- Do not move the ophthalmoscope around; ask the client to look into light to view the fovea and macula.
- Do not get frustrated—the ophthalmologic examination requires practice.

PHYSICAL ASSESSMENT

ASSESSMENT PROCEDURE	NORMAL FINDINGS	ABNORMAL FINDINGS

VISION TESTS

Distant Visual Acuity Test

Position the client 20 feet from the Snellen or E chart (see Display 11-1) and ask her to read each line until she cannot decipher the letters or their direction. Document the results. If the client wears glasses, they should be left on unless they are reading glasses (reading glasses blur distance vision).

Tip From the Experts During this vision test, note any client behaviors (ie, leaning forward, head tilting or squinting) that could be unconscious attempts to see better.

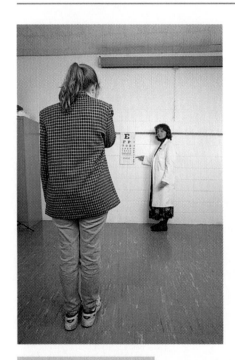

Testing distant visual acuity from 20 feet. (© B. Proud.)

Normal distant visual acuity is 20/20 with or without corrective lenses. This means the client can distinguish what the person with normal vision can distinguish from 20 feet away.

Myopia (impaired far vision) is present when the second number in the test result is larger than the first (20/40). The higher the second number, the poorer the vision. A client is considered legally blind when vision in the better eye with corrective lenses is 20/200 or less. Any client with vision worse than 20/30 should be referred for further evaluation.

Visual acuity varies by race in US populations. Japanese and Chinese Americans have the poorest corrected visual acuity (especially myopia), followed by African Americans and Hispanics. Native Americans and Caucasians have the best corrected acuity. Eskimos are undergoing an epidemic of myopia (Overfield, 1995).

Near Visual Acuity Test

Use this test for middle-aged clients and others who complain of difficulty reading.

Give the client a hand-held vision chart (eg, Jaeger reading card, Snellen card, or comparable chart) to hold 14 inches from the eyes. Have the client cover one eye with an opaque card before reading from top (largest print) to bottom (smallest print). Repeat test for other eye.

Tip From the Experts The client who wears glasses should keep them on for this test.

Normal near visual acuity is 14/14 (with or without corrective lenses). This means the client can read what the normal eye can read from a distance of 14 inches.

Presbyopia (impaired near vision) is indicated when the client moves the chart away from the eyes to focus on the print. It is caused by decreased accommodation.

Presbyopia is a common condition in clients over age 45.

(continued)

ASSESSMENT PROCEDURE	NORMAL FINDINGS	ABNORMAL FINDINGS

Visual Fields Test for Gross Peripheral Vision

To perform the confrontation test, position yourself approximately 2 feet away from the client at eye level. Have the client cover his left eye while you cover your right eye. Look directly at each other with your uncovered eyes. Next, fully extend your left arm at midline and slowly move one finger (or a pencil) upward from below until the client sees your finger (or pencil). Test the remaining three visual fields of the client's right eye (ie, superior, temporal, and nasal). Repeat the test for the opposite eye.

With normal peripheral vision, the client should see the examiner's finger at the same time the examiner sees it. Normal visual field degrees are approximately as follows:
Inferior: 70 degrees
Superior: 50 degrees
Temporal: 90 degrees
Nasal: 60 degrees

A delayed or absent perception of the examiner's finger indicates reduced peripheral vision (Display 11-3). The client should be referred for further evaluation.

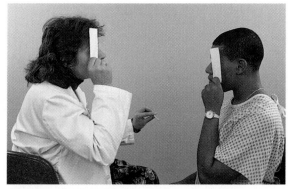

Performing confrontation test to assess visual fields. (© B. Proud.)

EXTRAOCULAR MUSCLE FUNCTION

Corneal Light Reflex Test

This test assesses parallel alignment of the eyes. Hold a penlight approximately 12 inches from the client's face. Shine the light toward the bridge of the nose while the client stares straight ahead. Note the light reflected on the corneas.

The reflection of light on the corneas should be in the exact same spot on each eye, which indicates parallel alignment.

Asymmetric position of the light reflex indicates deviated alignment of the eyes. This may be due to muscle weakness or paralysis (Display 11-4).

Cover Test

The cover test detects deviation in alignment or strength and slight deviations in eye movement by interrupting the fusion reflex that normally keeps the eyes parallel.

Ask the client to stare straight ahead and focus on a distant object. Cover one of the client's eyes with an opaque card. As you cover the eye, observe the uncovered eye for movement. Now, remove the opaque card and observe the previously covered eye for any movement. Repeat test on the opposite eye.

The uncovered eye should remain fixed straight ahead. The covered eye should remain fixed straight ahead after being uncovered.

The uncovered eye will move to establish focus when the opposite eye is covered. When the covered eye is uncovered, movement to reestablish focus occurs. Either of these findings indicates a deviation in alignment of the eyes and muscle weakness.
Phoria is a term used to describe misalignment that occurs only when fusion reflex is blocked.
Strabismus is constant malalignment of the eyes.
Tropia is a specific type of misalignment: *esotropia* is an inward turn of the eye, and *exotropia* is an outward turn of the eye (see Display 11-4).

(continued)

ASSESSMENT PROCEDURE	NORMAL FINDINGS	ABNORMAL FINDINGS

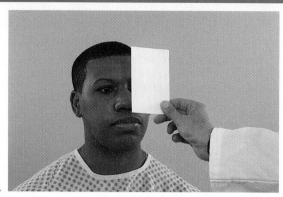 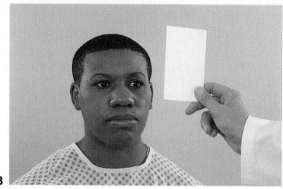

A **B**

Performing cover test with (*A*) eye covered and (*B*) eye uncovered. (© B. Proud.)

Positions Test

The positions test assesses eye muscle strength and cranial nerve function.

Instruct the client to focus on an object that you are holding (approximately 12 inches from the client's face). Move the object through the six cardinal positions of gaze in a clockwise direction, and observe the client's eye movements.

Eye movement should be smooth and symmetric throughout all six directions.

Failure of eyes to follow movement symmetrically in any or all directions indicates a weakness in one or more extraocular muscles or dysfunction of the cranial nerve that innervates the particular muscle (see Display 11-4).

Nystagmus, an oscillating (shaking) movement of the eye may be associated with an inner ear disorder, multiple sclerosis, brain lesions, or narcotics use.

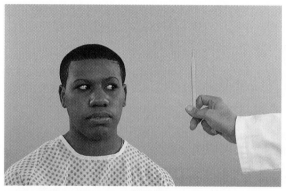

Performing positions test. (© B. Proud.)

EXTERNAL EYE STRUCTURES

Inspect Eyelids and Eyelashes

Inspect the eyelids and eyelashes, noting
- Width and position of palpebral fissures
- Discharge

The upper lid margin should be between the upper margin of the iris and the upper margin of the pupil. The lower lid margin rests on the lower border of the iris. No white sclera is seen above or below the iris. Palpebral fissures may be horizontal.

Drooping of the upper lid, called *ptosis,* may be attributed to oculomotor nerve damage, myasthenia gravis, weakened muscle or tissue, or a congenital disorder. Retracted lid margins, which allow for viewing of the sclera when the eyes are open, suggest hyperthyroidism.

Check ability of eyelids to close.

The upper and lower lids close easily and meet completely when closed.

Failure of lids to close completely puts client at risk for corneal damage.

(continued)

ASSESSMENT PROCEDURE	NORMAL FINDINGS	ABNORMAL FINDINGS
Note the position of the eyelids in comparison with the eyeballs. Also note any unusual • Turnings • Color • Swelling • Lesions • Discharge	The lower eyelid is upright with no inward or outward turning. Eyelashes are evenly distributed and curve outward along the lid margins. Xanthelasma, raised yellow plaques located most often near the inner canthus, are a normal variation associated with increasing age and high lipid levels.	An inverted lower lid is a condition called an *entropion,* which may cause pain and injure the cornea as the eyelash brushes against the conjunctiva and cornea. *Ectropion,* an everted lower eyelid, results in exposure and drying of the conjunctiva. Both conditions interfere with normal tear drainage. Though usually abnormal, entropion and ectropion are common in older clients.
Observe for redness, swelling, discharge, or lesions.	Skin on both eyelids is without redness, swelling, or lesions.	Redness and crusting along the lid margins suggest seborrhea or blepharitis, an infection caused by *Staphylococcus aureus.* Hordeolum (stye), a hair follicle infection, causes local redness, swelling, and pain. A chalazion, an infection of the meibomian gland (located in the eyelid), may produce extreme swelling of the lid, moderate redness, but minimal pain (Display 11-5).

Inspect Eyeball Position

Observe the position and alignment of the eyeball in the eye socket.	Eyeballs are symmetrically aligned in sockets without protruding or sinking. The eyes of blacks protrude more than those of whites, and blacks of both sexes may have eyes protruding beyond 21 mm (Overfield, 1995).	Protrusion of the eyeballs accompanied by retracted eyelid margins is termed *exophthalmos* and is characteristic of Graves' disease (a type of hyperthyroidism). A sunken appearance of the eyes may be seen with severe dehydration or chronic wasting illnesses (see Display 11-5).

Inspect the Bulbar Conjunctiva and Sclera

To inspect the clear bulbar conjunctiva and the underlying sclera, have the client keep his or her head straight while looking from side to side and then up toward the ceiling. Observe clarity, color, and texture. 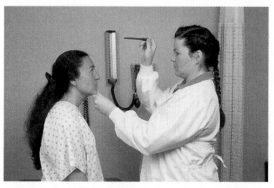 **To inspect the bulbar conjunctiva, have the client look upward.**	Bulbar conjunctiva is clear, moist, and smooth. Underlying structures are clearly visible. Sclera is white. Yellowish nodules on the bulbar conjunctiva are called *pinguecula.* These harmless nodules are common in older clients and appear first on the medial side of the iris and then on the lateral side. Darker-skinned clients may have sclera with yellow or pigmented freckles.	Generalized redness of the conjunctiva suggests *conjunctivitis* (pink eye). Areas of dryness are associated with allergies or trauma. *Episcleritis* is a local, noninfectious inflammation of the sclera. The condition is usually characterized by either a nodular appearance or by redness with dilated vessels (see Display 11-5).

(continued)

ASSESSMENT PROCEDURE	NORMAL FINDINGS	ABNORMAL FINDINGS

Inspect the Palpebral Conjunctiva

First, inspect the palpebral conjunctiva of the lower eyelid by placing your thumbs bilaterally at the level of the lower bony orbital rim and gently pulling down to expose the palpebral conjunctiva. Avoid pressuring the eye. Ask the client to look up as you observe the exposed areas. (See Display 11-6 for more information.)

🌹 **Tip From the Experts** This procedure is stressful and uncomfortable for the client, It is usually only done if the client complains of pain or "something in the eye."

The lower and upper palpebral conjunctivae are clear and free of swelling or lesions.

Cyanosis of the lower lid suggests a heart or lung disorder.

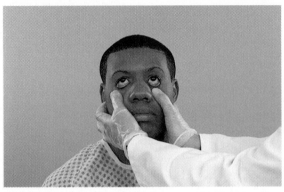

Inspecting palpebral conjunctiva: lower eyelid. (© B. Proud.)

Inspect the Lacrimal Apparatus

Inspect the areas over the lacrimal glands (lateral aspect of upper eyelid) and the puncta (medial aspect of lower eyelid).

No swelling or redness should appear over areas of the lacrimal gland. The puncta is visible without swelling or redness and is turned slightly toward the eye.

Swelling of the lacrimal gland may be visible in the lateral aspect of the upper eyelid. This may be caused by blockage, infection, or an inflammatory condition. Redness or swelling around the puncta may indicate an infectious or inflammatory condition. Excessive tearing may indicate a nasolacrimal sac obstruction.

Palpate the Lacrimal Apparatus

Put on disposable gloves to palpate the nasolacrimal duct to assess for blockage. Use one finger and palpate just inside the lower orbital rim.

No drainage should be noted from the puncta when palpating the nasolacrimal duct.

Expressed drainage from the puncta on palpation occurs with duct blockage.

Palpating the lacrimal apparatus. (© B. Proud.)

(continued)

ASSESSMENT PROCEDURE	NORMAL FINDINGS	ABNORMAL FINDINGS

Inspect the Cornea and Lens

Shine a light from the side of the eye for an oblique view. Look through the pupil to inspect the lens.

The cornea is transparent with no opacities. The oblique view shows a smooth and overall moist surface; the lens is free of opacities.

Arcus senilis, a normal condition in older clients, appears as a white arc around the limbus. The condition has no effect on vision.

Areas of roughness or dryness on the cornea are often associated with injury or allergic responses. Opacities of the lens cataracts (Display 11-7).

Inspect the Iris and Pupil

Inspect shape and color of iris and size and shape of pupil. Measure pupils against a chart if they appear larger or smaller than normal or if they appear to be two different sizes.

Pupil Gauge (mm)

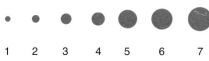

1 2 3 4 5 6 7

Pupillary gauge measures pupils (dilation or constriction) in millimeters (mm). (© B. Proud.)

The iris is typically round, flat, and evenly colored. The pupil, round with a regular border, is centered in the iris. Pupils are normally equal in size (3–5 mm). An inequality in pupil size of less than 0.5 mm occurs in 20% of clients. This condition, called *anisocoria,* is normal.

Typical abnormal findings include irregularly shaped irises, miosis, mydriasis, and anisocoria. (For a description of these abnormalities and their implications, see Display 11-8).

If the difference in pupil size changes throughout pupillary response tests, the inequality of size is abnormal.

Test Pupillary Reaction to Light

Test pupillary reaction for direct response by darkening the room and asking the client to focus on a distant object. To test direct pupil reaction, shine a light obliquely into one eye and observe the pupillary reaction. Shining the light obliquely into the pupil and asking the client to focus on an object in the distance ensures that pupillary constriction is a reaction to light and not a near reaction.

The normal direct and consensual pupillary response is constriction.

Monocular blindness can be detected when light directed to the blind eye results in no response in either pupil. When light is directed into the unaffected eye, both pupils constrict.

Tip From the Experts Use a pupillary gauge to measure the constricted pupil. Then, document the finding in a format similar to (but not) a fraction. The top (or first) number indicates the pupil's eye at rest, and the bottom (or second) number indicates the constricted size; for example, O.S. (left eye, *oculus sinister*) 3/2; O.D. (right eye, *oculus dexter*) 3/1.

(continued)

ASSESSMENT PROCEDURE	NORMAL FINDINGS	ABNORMAL FINDINGS
Assess consensual response at the same time as direct response by shining a light obliquely into one eye and observing the pupillary reaction in the opposite eye.	The normal and consensual pupillary response is constriction.	Pupils do not react at all to direct and consensual pupillary testing.

> **Tip From the Experts** When testing for consensual response, place your hand or another barrier to light (eg, index card) between the client's eyes to avoid an inaccurate finding.

Test Accommodation of Pupils

Accommodation occurs when the client moves his or her focus of vision from a distant point to a near object, causing the pupils to constrict. Hold your finger or a pencil about 12 to 15 inches from the client. Ask the client to focus on your finger or pencil and to remain focused on it as you move it closer in toward the eyes.	The normal pupillary response is constriction of the pupils and convergence of the eyes when focusing on a near object (accommodation and convergence).	Pupils do not constrict; eyes do not converge.

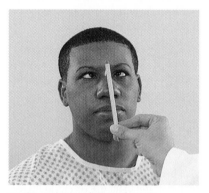

Testing accommodation of pupils.
(© B. Proud.)

Internal Eye Structures and Red Reflex

Using an ophthalmoscope (see Display 11-2), inspect the internal eye. To observe the red reflex, set the diopter at zero and stand 10 to 15 inches from the client's right side at a 15-degree angle. Place your free hand on the client's head, which helps limit head movement. Shine the light beam toward the client's pupil.	The red reflex should be easily visible through the ophthalmoscope. The red area should appear round with regular borders.	Abnormalities of the red reflex most often result from cataracts. These usually appear as black spots against the background of the red light reflex. Two types of age-related cataracts are nuclear cataracts and peripheral cataracts (see Display 11-7).

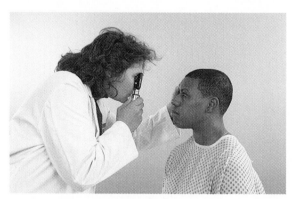

Inspecting the red reflex. (© B. Proud.)

(continued)

ASSESSMENT PROCEDURE	NORMAL FINDINGS	ABNORMAL FINDINGS

Inspect the Optic Disc

To inspect the optic disc, keep the light beam focused on the pupil and move closer to the client from a 15-degree angle. You should be very close to the client's eye (about 3–5 cm), almost touching the eyelashes. Rotate the diopter setting to bring the retinal structures into sharp focus. The diopter should be zero if neither the examiner nor the client has refractive errors. Note shape, color, size, and physiologic cup.

Tip From the Experts The diameter of the optic disc (DD) is used as the standard of measure for the location and size of other structures and any abnormalities or lesions within the ocular fundus. When documenting a structure within the ocular fundus, also note the position of the structure as it relates to numbers on the clock. For example, lesion is at 2:00, 1 DD in size, 2 DD from disc.

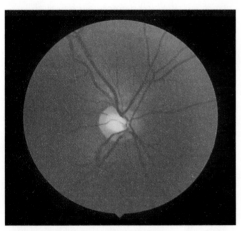

Normal ocular fundus (also called the optic disc).

The optic disc should be round to oval with sharp, well-defined borders.

The nasal edge of the optic disc may be blurred. The disc is normally creamy, yellow-orange to pink, and approximately 1.5 mm wide.

The physiologic cup, the point at which the optic nerve enters the eyeball, appears on the optic disc as slightly depressed and a lighter color than the disc. The cup occupies less than half of the disc's diameter. The disc's border may be surrounded by rings and crescents, consisting of white sclera or black retinal pigment. These normal variations are not considered in the optic disc's diameter.

Optic nerve discs are larger in blacks, Asians, and Native Americans than in Hispanics and non-Hispanic whites (Overfield, 1995).

Papilledema, or swelling of the optic disc, appears as a swollen disc with blurred margins, a hyperemic (blood-filled) appearance, more visible and more numerous disc vessels, and lack of visible physiologic cup. The condition may result from hypertension or increased intracranial pressure.

The intraocular pressure associated with *glaucoma* interferes with the blood supply to optic structures and results in the following characteristics: an enlarged physiologic cup that occupies more than half of the disc's diameter, pale base of enlarged physiologic cup, and obscured or displaced retinal vessels.

Optic atrophy is evidenced by the disc being white in color and a lack of disc vessels. This condition is caused by the death of optic nerve fibers (Display 11-9).

Inspect the Retinal Vessels

Remain in the same position as described previously. Inspect the sets of retinal vessels by following them out to the periphery of each section of the eye. Note the number of sets of arterioles and venules.

Also note color and diameter of the arterioles.

Four sets of arterioles and venules should pass through the optic disc.

Arterioles are bright red and progressively narrow as they move away from the optic disc. Arterioles have a light reflex that appears as a thin, white line in the center of the arteriole. Venules are darker red and larger than arterioles. They also progressively narrow as they move away from the optic disc.

Changes in the blood supply to the retina may be observed in constricted arterioles, dilated veins, or absence of major vessels.

Initially, hypertension may cause a widening of the arterioles' light reflex, and the arterioles take on a copper color. With long-standing hypertension, arteriole walls thicken and appear opaque or silver.

(continued)

ASSESSMENT PROCEDURE	NORMAL FINDINGS	ABNORMAL FINDINGS
Observe the arteriovenous (AV) ratio.	The ratio of arteriole diameter to vein diameter (AV ratio) is 2:3 or 4:5.	
Look at AV crossings.	In a normal AV crossing, the vein passing underneath the arteriole is seen right up to the column of blood on either side of the arteriole (the arteriole wall itself is normally transparent).	Arterial nicking, tapering, and banking are abnormal AV crossings caused by hypertension or arteriosclerosis (Display 11-10).

Inspect Retinal Background

Remain in the same position described previously and search the retinal background from the disc to the macula, noting the color and the presence of any lesions.	General background appears consistent in texture. The red-orange color of the background is lighter near the optic disc.	Cotton-wool patches (soft exudates) and hard exudates from diabetes and hypertension appear as light-colored spots on the retinal background. Hemorrhages and micro-aneurysms appear as red spots and streaks on the retinal background (see Display 11-10).

Inspect Fovea (Sharpest Area of Vision) and Macula

Remain in the same position described previously. Shine the light beam toward the side of the eye or ask the client to look directly into the light. Observe the fovea and the macula that surrounds it.	The macula is the darker area, one disc diameter in size, located to the temporal side of the optic disc. Within this area is a starlike light reflex called the fovea.	Excessive clumped pigment appears with detached retinas or retinal injuries. Macular degeneration may be due to hemorrhages, exudates, or cysts.

Inspect Anterior Chamber

Remain in the same position and rotate the lens wheel slowly to +10, +12, or higher to inspect the anterior chamber of the eye.	The anterior chamber is transparent.	*Hyphemia* occurs when injury causes red blood cells to collect in the lower half of the anterior chamber. *Hypopyon* usually results from an inflammatory response in which white blood cells accumulate in the anterior chamber produce cloudiness in front of the iris.

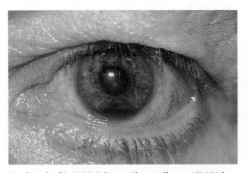

Hyphemia. (© 1995 Science Photo Library/CMSP.)

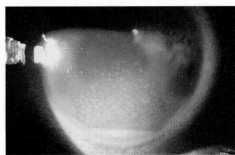

Hypopyon.

DISPLAY 11-3. Visual Field Defects

ABNORMAL FINDINGS

When a client reports losing full or partial vision in one or both eyes, the nurse can usually anticipate a lesion as the cause. Some abnormal findings associated with visual field defects are illustrated here. The darker areas signify vision loss.

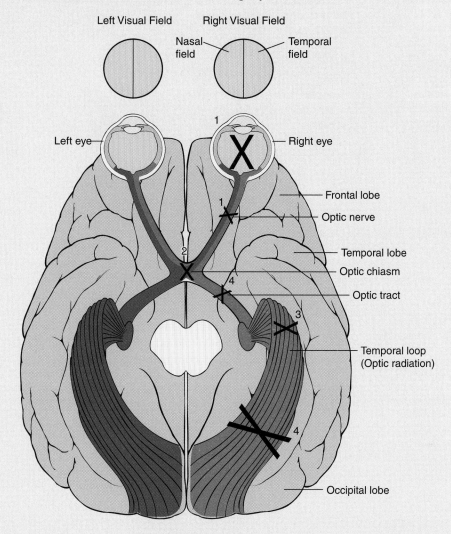

FINDING	POSSIBLE SOURCE	EXAMPLE Left Eye	Right Eye
Unilateral blindness (eg, blind right eye)	Lesion in (right) eye or (right) optic nerve		
Bitemporal hemianopia (loss of vision in both temporal fields)	Lesion of optic chiasm		

(continued)

DISPLAY 11-3. **Visual Field Defects** (Continued)

FINDING	POSSIBLE SOURCE	EXAMPLE
		Left Eye Right Eye
Left superior quadrant anopia or similar loss of vision (homonymous) in quadrant of each field	Partial lesion of temporal loop (optic radiation)	
Right visual field loss—right homonymous hemianopia or similar loss of vision in half of each field	Lesion in right optic tract or lesion in temporal loop (optic radiation)	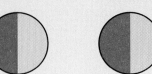

Validation and Documentation of Findings

Validate the eye assessment data that you have collected. This is necessary to verify that the data are reliable and accurate. Document the assessment data following the health care facility or agency policy.

EXAMPLE OF SUBJECTIVE DATA

Client denies recent changes in vision. No excessive tearing, redness, swelling, or pain of eyes. Denies spots, floaters, or blind spots. States no problem with seeing at night. No previous eye surgeries. No family history of eye problems. Denies exposure to conditions or substances that harm the eyes. Wears sunglasses regularly. Does not wear corrective lenses. Last eye examination was 1 year ago.

EXAMPLE OF OBJECTIVE DATA

Acuity tested by Snellen chart: O.D. (right eye) 20/20, O.S. (left eye) 20/20. Visual fields full by confrontation. Corneal light reflex shows equal position of reflection. Eyes remain fixed throughout cover test. Extraocular movements smooth and symmetric with no nystagmus. Eyelids

in normal position with no abnormal widening or ptosis. No redness, discharge, or crusting noted on lid margins. Conjunctiva and sclera appear moist and smooth. Sclera white with no lesions or redness. No swelling or redness over lacrimal gland; puncta is visible without swelling or redness; no drainage noted when nasolacrimal duct is palpated. Cornea is transparent, smooth, and moist with no opacities; lens is free of opacities. Irises are round, flat, and evenly colored. Pupils are equal in size and reactive to light and accommodation. Pupils converge evenly. Red reflex present bilaterally. Both optic discs visualized easily, creamy white in color, with distinct margins and vessels noted with no crossing defects. Retinal background free of lesions and orange-red in color. Macula visualized within normal limits. Anterior chamber is transparent.

After you have collected your assessment data, you will need to analyze the data, using the diagnostic reasoning skills delineated in Chapter 6. After that, in Diagnostic Reasoning: Possible Conclusions, you will see an overview of common conclusions that you may reach after eye assessment. Next, Diagnostic Reasoning: Case Study shows you how to analyze eye assessment data for a specific client. In the laboratory manual/study guide that accompanies the text, you have opportunity to analyze data in the critical thinking exercise.

(*text continues on page 205*)

DISPLAY 11-4. **Extraocular Muscle Dysfunction**

ABNORMAL FINDINGS

Abnormalities found during an assessment of extraocular muscle function are described below:

CORNEAL LIGHT REFLEX TEST ABNORMALITIES

Pseudostrabismus

Normal in young children, the pupils will appear at the inner canthus (due to the epicanthic fold).

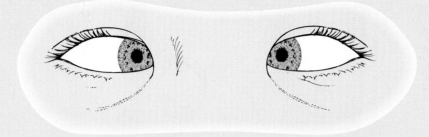

Strabismus (or Tropia)

A constant malalignment of the eye axis, strabismus is defined according to the direction toward which the eye drifts and may cause amblyopia.

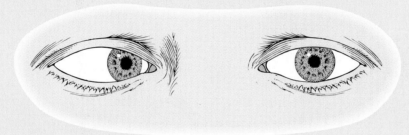

Esotropia (eye turns inward).

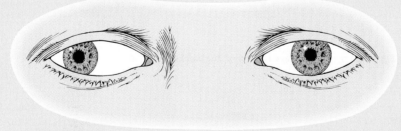

Exotropia (eye turns outward).

(continued)

DISPLAY 11-4. Extraocular Muscle Dysfunction (Continued)

COVER TEST ABNORMALITIES

Phoria (Mild Weakness)

Noticeable only with the cover test, phoria is less likely to cause amblyopia than strabismus. Esophoria is an inward drift and exophoria an outward drift of the eye.

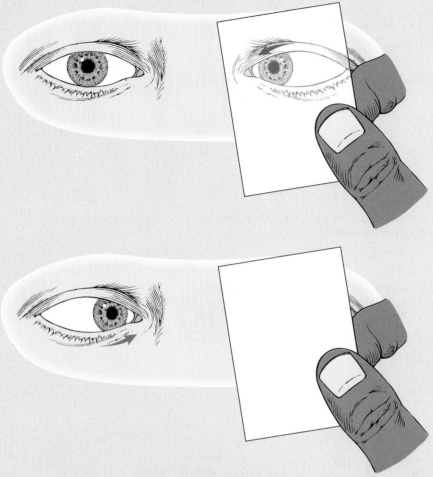

The uncovered eye is weaker; when the stronger eye is covered; the weaker eye moves to refocus.

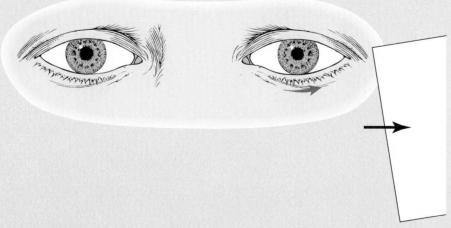

When the weaker eye is covered, it will drift to a relaxed position. Once the eye is uncovered, it will quickly move back to reestablish fixation.

(continued)

DISPLAY 11-4. Extraocular Muscle Dysfunction (Continued)

POSITIONS TEST ABNORMALITIES

Paralytic Strabismus

Noticeable with the positions test, paralytic strabismus is usually the result of weakness or paralysis of one or more extraocular muscles. The nerve affected will be on the same side as the eye affected (for instance, a right eye paralysis is related to a right-side cranial nerve). The position in which the maximum deviation appears indicates the nerve involved.

6th nerve paralysis: The eye cannot look to the outer side.

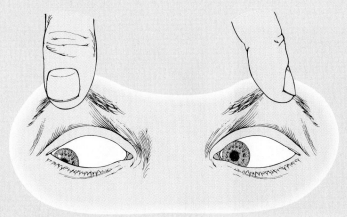

In left 6th nerve paralysis, the patient tries to look to the left. The right eye moves left, but the left eye cannot move left.

4th nerve paralysis: The eye cannot look down when turned inward.

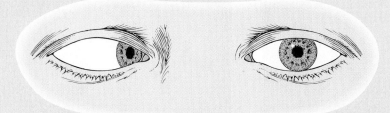

A client with left 4th nerve paralysis looks down and to the right.

3rd nerve paralysis: Upward, downward, and inward movements are lost. Ptosis and pupillary dilation may also occur.

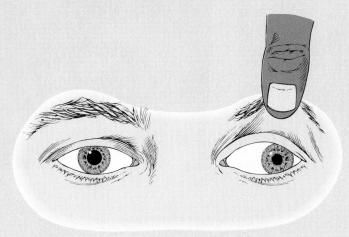

A client with left 3rd nerve paralysis looks straight ahead.

ABNORMAL FINDINGS

DISPLAY 11-5. **Abnormalities of the External Eye**

Some easily recognized abnormalities that affect the external eye are ptosis (drooping eyelid), entropion (inwardly turned lower eyelid that irritates the conjunctiva), ectropion (outwardly turned lower eyelid that exposes the conjunctiva, allowing it to dry), blepharitis (a staphylococcal infection of the eyelid), hordeolum (stye, an infection of the hair follicles), chalazion (an infected meibomian gland), exophthalmos (protruding eyeballs and retracted eyelids), conjunctivitis (generalized inflammation of the conjunctiva, also called pink eye), and episcleritis (local inflammation of the sclera).

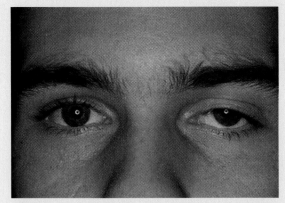

Ptosis.

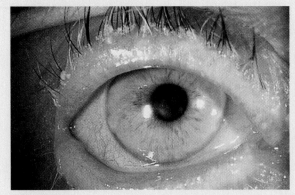

Blepharitis.

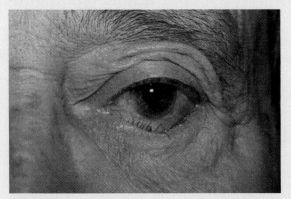

Entropion.

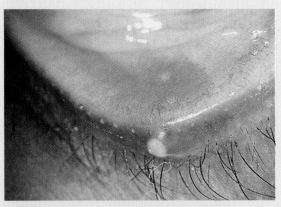

Hordeolum [stye].

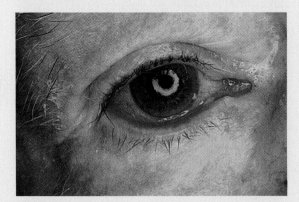

Ectropion.

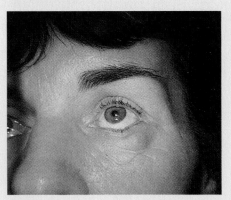

Chalazion.

(continued)

DISPLAY 11-5. **Abnormalities of the External Eye** (Continued)

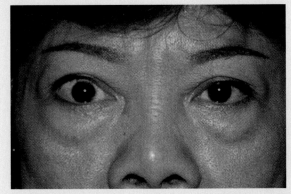

Exophthalmos.

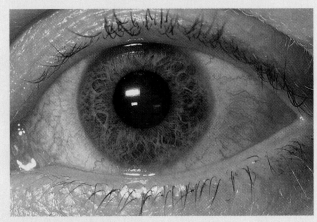

Conjunctivitis. (© 1995 Dr. P. Marazzi/Science Photo Library/CMSP.)

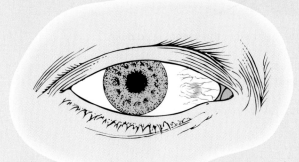

Episcleritis.

DISPLAY 11-6. **Everting the Upper Eyelid**

GUIDELINES

1. Ask the client to look down with his or her eyes slightly open.
2. Gently grasp the client's upper eyelashes and pull the lid downward.

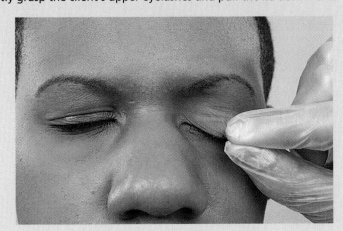

(continued)

DISPLAY 11-6. Everting the Upper Eyelid (Continued)

GUIDELINES

3. Place a cotton-tipped applicator approximately 1 cm above the eyelid margin and push down with the applicator while still holding the eyelashes.

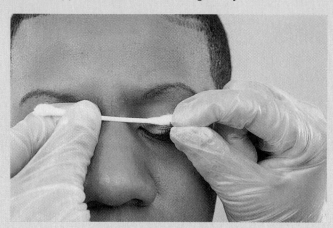

4. Hold the eyelashes against the upper ridge of the bony orbit, just below the eyebrow, to maintain the everted position of the eyelid.

5. Examine the palpebral conjunctiva for swelling, foreign bodies, or trauma.

6. Return the eyelid to normal by moving the lashes forward and asking the client to look up and blink. The eyelid should return to normal.

7. Hold the eyelashes against the upper ridge of the bony orbit, just below the eyebrow, to maintain the everted position of the eyelid.

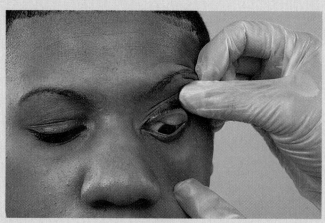

(Photos © B. Proud.)

8. Examine the palpebral conjunctiva for swelling, foreign bodies, or trauma.

9. Return the eyelid to normal by moving the eyelashes forward and asking the client to look up and blink. The eyelid should return to normal.

DISPLAY 11-7. Abnormalities of the Cornea and Lens

Representative abnormalities of the cornea are illustrated below as a corneal scar and a pterygium. Lens abnormalities are represented by a nuclear cataract and a peripheral cataract. Usually, cataracts are most easily seen by the naked eye.

CORNEAL ABNORMALITIES

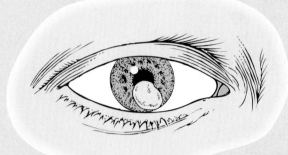

A corneal scar, which appears grayish white, usually is due to an old injury or inflammation.

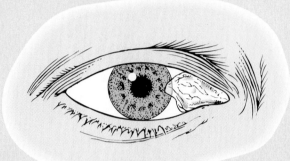

A pterygium is a thickening of the bulbar conjunctiva that extends across the cornea from the nasal side.

LENS ABNORMALITIES

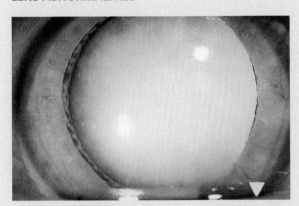

Nuclear cataracts appear gray when seen with a flashlight; they appear as a black spot against the red reflex when seen through an ophthalmoscope.

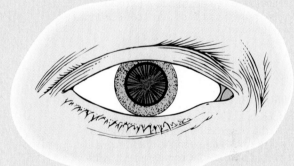

Peripheral cataracts look like gray spokes that point inward when seen with a flashlight; they look like black spokes that point inward against the red reflex when seen through an ophthalmoscope.

DISPLAY 11-8. Abnormalities of the Iris and Pupils

IRREGULARLY SHAPED IRIS

An irregularly shaped iris causes a shallow anterior chamber, which may increase the risk for narrow-angle (closed-angle) glaucoma.

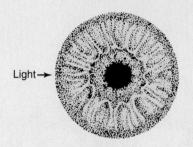 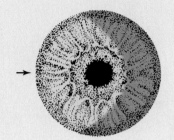

Light→

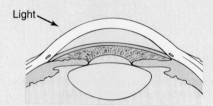 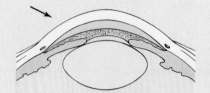

Light→

MIOSIS

Also known as pinpoint pupils, miosis is characterized by constricted and fixed pupils—possibly a result of narcotic drugs or brain damage.

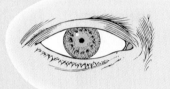 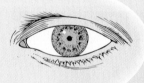

ANISOCORIA

Anisocoria is pupils of unequal size. In some cases, the condition is normal; in other cases, it is abnormal. For example, if anisocoria is greater in bright light compared with dim light, the cause may be trauma, tonic pupil (caused by impaired parasympathetic nerve supply to iris), and oculomotor nerve paralysis. If anisocoria is greater in dim light compared with bright light, the cause may be Horner's syndrome (caused by paralysis of the cervical sympathetic nerves and characterized by ptosis, sunken eyeball, flushing of the affected side of the face, and narrowing of the palpebral fissure).

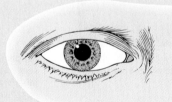 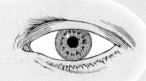

MYDRIASIS

Dilated and fixed pupils, typically resulting from central nervous system injury, circulatory collapse, or deep anesthesia.

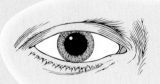 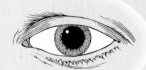

DISPLAY 11-9. Abnormalities of the Optic Disc

ABNORMAL
FINDINGS

Characteristic abnormal findings during an ophthalmoscopic examination include signs and symptoms of papilledema, glaucoma, and optic atrophy as described below.

PAPILLEDEMA

- Swollen optic disc
- Blurred margins
- Hyperemic appearance from accumulation of excess blood
- Visible and numerous disc vessels
- Lack of visible physiologic cup

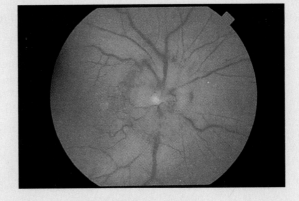

GLAUCOMA

- Enlarged physiologic cup occupying more than half of the disc's diameter
- Pale base of enlarged physiologic cup
- Obscured and/or displaced retinal vessels

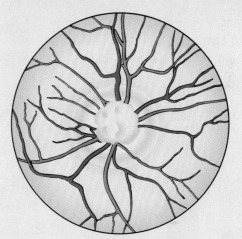

OPTIC ATROPHY

- White optic disc
- Lack of disc vessels

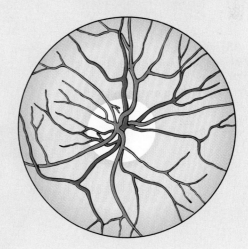

DISPLAY 11-10. Abnormalities of the Retinal Vessels and Background

Characteristic abnormal findings during an ophthalmoscopic examination of the retinal vessels include constricted arterioles, copper wire arterioles, silver wire arteriole arteriovenous (AV) nicking, AV tapering, and AV banking. Signs and symptoms are described below.

CONSTRICTED ARTERIOLE

Narrowing of the arteriole, which occurs with hypertension.

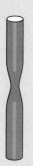

COPPER WIRE ARTERIOLE

- Widening of the light reflex and a coppery color.
- Occurs with hypertension.

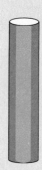

SILVER WIRE ARTERIOLE

- Opaque or silver appearance caused by thickening of arteriole wall.
- Occurs with long-standing hypertension.

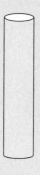

ARTERIOVENOUS NICKING

- Arteriovenous crossing abnormality characterized by vein appearing to stop short on either side of arteriole.
- Caused by loss of arteriole wall transparency from hypertension.

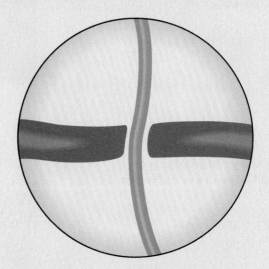

ARTERIOVENOUS TAPERING

- Arteriovenous crossing abnormality characterized by vein appearing to taper to a point on either side of the arteriole.
- Caused by loss of arteriole wall transparency from hypertension.

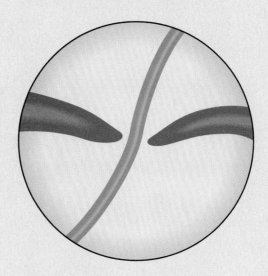

DISPLAY 11-10. **Abnormalities of the Retinal Vessels and Background** (Continued)

ARTERIOVENOUS BANKING

- Arteriovenous crossing abnormality characterized by twisting of the vein on the arteriole's distal side and formation of a dark, knuckle-like structure.
- Caused by loss of arteriole wall transparency from hypertension.

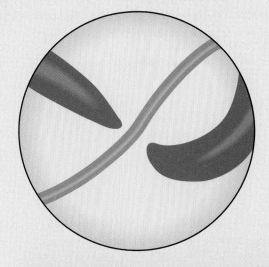

COTTON WOOL PATCHES

- Also known as *soft exudates*, cotton wool patches have a fluffy cotton ball appearance with irregular edges.
- Appear as white or gray moderately sized spots on retinal background.
- Caused by arteriole microinfarction.
- Associated with diabetes mellitus and hypertension.

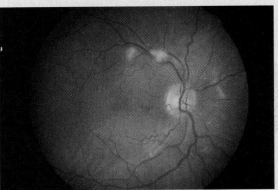

HARD EXUDATE

- Solid, smooth surface and well-defined edges.
- Creamy yellow-white, small, round spots typically clustered in circular, linear, or star pattern.
- Associated with diabetes mellitus and hypertension.

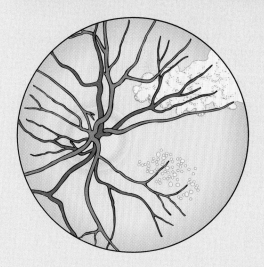

(continued)

SUPERFICIAL (FLAME-SHAPED) RETINAL HEMORRHAGES

- Appear as small, flame-shaped, linear red streaks on retinal background.
- Hypertension and papilledema are common causes.

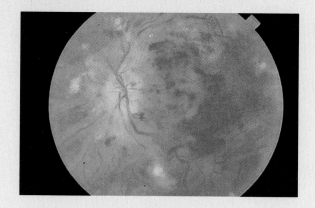

DEEP (DOT-SHAPED) RETINAL HEMORRHAGES

- Appear as small, irregular red spots with blurred edges on retinal background.
- Lie deeper in retina than superficial retinal hemorrhages.
- Associated with diabetes mellitus.

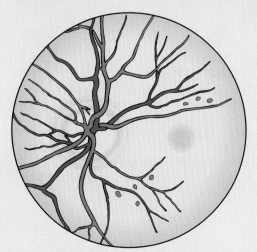

MICROANEURYSMS

- Round, tiny red dots with smooth edges on retinal background.
- Localized dilations of small vessels in retina, but vessels are too small to see.
- Associated with diabetic retinopathy.

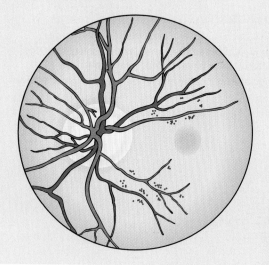

Diagnostic Reasoning: Possible Conclusions

Listed below are some possible conclusions reached after assessment of the client's eyes.

SELECTED NURSING DIAGNOSES

After collecting subjective and objective data pertaining to the eyes, you will need to identify abnormal findings and cluster the data to reveal any significant patterns or abnormalities. These data will then be used to make clinical judgments (nursing diagnoses: wellness, risk, or actual) about the status of the client's eyes. Following is a listing of selected nursing diagnoses that you may identify when analyzing data for this part of the assessment.

Nursing Diagnoses (Wellness)

- Opportunity to enhance visual integrity

Nursing Diagnoses (Risk)

- Risk for Eye Injury related to hazardous work area or participation in high-level contact sports
- Risk for Injury related to impaired vision secondary to the aging process
- Risk for Eye Injury related to decreased tear production secondary to the aging process
- Risk for Self-Care Deficit (specify) related to vision loss

Nursing Diagnoses (Actual)

- Ineffective Health Maintenance related to lack of knowledge of necessity for eye examinations
- Self-Care Deficit (specify) related to poor vision
- Acute Pain related to injury from eye trauma, abrasion, or exposure to chemical irritant
- Social Isolation related to inability to interact effectively with others secondary to vision loss

SELECTED COLLABORATIVE PROBLEMS

After grouping the data, it may become apparent that certain collaborative problems emerge. Remember, collaborative problems differ from nursing diagnoses in that they cannot be prevented by nursing interventions. However, these physiologic complications of medical conditions can be detected and monitored by the nurse. In addition, the nurse can use physician- and nurse-prescribed interventions to minimize the complications of these problems. The nurse may also have to refer the client in such situations for further treatment of the problem. Following is a list of collaborative problems that may be identified when assessing the eye. These problems are worded as Potential Complications (PC), followed by the problem.

- PC: Increased intraocular pressure
- PC: Corneal ulceration or abrasion

MEDICAL PROBLEMS

After grouping the data, it may become apparent that the client has signs and symptoms that may require medical diagnosis and treatment. Referral to a primary care provider is necessary.

Diagnostic Reasoning: Case Study

You are preparing to discharge Mr. Luther Johnson (LJ), a 68-year-old African American man, after a 2-day hospital stay for management of an acute asthma attack. His history indicates that he has been taking oral and inhaled corticosteroids intermittently for the last 17 years for asthma. You ask him if he has any other concerns he wants to discuss before he leaves. "Yes," he says, "I have noticed some strange things that are happening with my vision. I'm concerned, although my doctor says it's nothing to worry about—but I am worried." When you ask for an example of what is unusual about his vision, he tells you that he doesn't always see stairs in front of him ("I trip a lot lately.") and when he is reading, words on the page seem to be missing sometimes. "At first I thought I was just distracted, but then I almost hit another car when I made a left turn—I didn't see it at all. I got more concerned after that. My wife says that she has noticed more problems with my driving but didn't want to upset me by saying something." He indicates he does a lot of driving for his work as a computer hardware trouble-shooter. "I have to work to pay the rent and support my wife."

When you examine his eyes, you note the following: conjugate gaze without ptosis; slight protrusion of eyeballs and firm to touch; pupils are small, equal, round and constrict with both direct and consensual illumination 2/1 OU (each eye). Corneas appear smooth with normal corneal light reflex and spontaneous blink reflex; sclera slightly yellow (appropriate for ethnicity), iris dark brown without defect; EOMs—parallel tracking through six cardinal positions of gaze; with confrontation, defects noted in left, right, and inferior peripheral visual fields; central and superior visual fields appear intact; visual acuity 20/30 OU (using a vision screener). Negative for pain, redness, discharge, swelling.

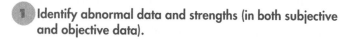

1 **Identify abnormal data and strengths (in both subjective and objective data).**

SUBJECTIVE DATA

- "Strange things are happening with my vision"
- Can't always see stairs in front of him
- "I trip a lot lately"
- Words missing on page when reading
- Almost hit a car making a left turn—didn't see car
- Wife noticed problems with his driving
- Worried about vision; has mentioned to doctor
- Work involves much driving—trouble-shooting computer hardware
- Financial support for wife and home

OBJECTIVE DATA

- African American man, 68 years old
- Recent hospitalization with acute asthma attack
- On oral and inhaled corticosteroids for almost 20 years
- Visual acuity 20/30 OU with gross screening
- PERRL 2/1 OU
- Conjugate gaze, parallel tracking
- Intact corneal light and blink reflexes
- Sclera slightly yellow, iris dark brown
- Visual field defects in right, left, and inferior peripheral fields
- Intact central and superior visual fields
- Slight protrusion of eyeballs, firm to touch

2 Cue Clusters	**3** Inferences	**4** Possible Nursing Diagnoses	**5** Defining Characteristics	**6** Confirm or Rule Out
A • African American 63 y/o • Nearly 20-year corticosteroid use • Peripheral vision loss • Can't see stairs; "Trip a lot" • Missing words when reading • Problems with driving • Eyeballs firm to touch	Has risk factors for and late symptoms of primary open-angle glaucoma. Should be referred to ophthalmologist before discharge.	Collaborative problem		
B • Worried about vision • Near accident—didn't see other car • Wife notes driving problems • Some problems with reading, seeing stairs	Subtle visual changes put client at risk for accidents. Implied concern about safety.	Fear related to unknown progression of visual impairment Risk for Injury related to lack of awareness of potential dangers due to changes in vision	*Major:* Feelings of apprehension *Minor:* Verbal report of worry Not needed with risk diagnosis	Confirm: Meets major and minor defining characteristics. Confirm, but need to evaluate the degree of understanding of danger to self and others.
C • Drives a lot for work • Computer hardware trouble-shooter • Financial support for wife and home	Ability to drive and to have good visual acuity essential for current occupation. Client's role as wage earner for family is at risk.	Ineffective Individual Coping related to perceived loss of ability to work Self-Concept Disturbance related to potential altered role performance secondary to visual loss	*Major:* None noted *Minor:* Worry Not defined for this diagnosis	Rule out, but collect more data. Confirm diagnosis but collect more data regarding actual impact on client and family if glaucoma diagnosis is confirmed.

7 **Document conclusions.**

The following nursing diagnoses are appropriate for Mr. Johnson at this time:

- Fear related to unknown progression of visual impairment
- Risk for Injury related to lack of awareness of potential dangers due to changes in vision
- Self-Concept Disturbance related to potential altered role performance secondary to visual loss

Collaborative problems related to the ophthalmic disorders may include:

- PC: Blindness
- PC: Increased intraocular pressure

Medical diagnosis is yet to be made. Client should be referred to an ophthalmologist for further examination.

REFERENCES AND SELECTED READINGS

Beckerman, B. (1999). Prehospital management of ocular trauma. *Emergency Medical Services, 28*(3), 63–66, 78.

Cleary, M. (1995). Helping the person who is visually impaired: Concerns, questions, remedies, and resources. *Journal of Ophthalmic Nursing and Technology, 14*(5), 205–211.

Curl, A. (1999). Seeing red. A review of subconjunctival hemorrhage. *Advance for Nurse Practitioners, 7*(3), 77–78.

Cutarelli, P. (1999). The painful eye: External and anterior segment causes. *Clinics in Geriatric Medicine, 15*(1), 103–112.

El Mallah, M. (2000). Amblyopia: Is visual loss permanent? *British Journal of Ophthalmology, 84*(9), 952–956.

Glenn, G. (2000). Risk factors, screening and treatment of diabetic eye disease. *Journal of Diabetes Nursing, 4*(1), 28–31.

Goldschmidt, L. (2000). Multimedia patient education in the office: Going where few patients have gone before. *Ophthalmology Clinics of North America, 13*(2), 239–247.

Harris, E. (2000). Bacterial subretinal abscess: A case report and review of the literature. *American Journal of Ophthalmology, 129*(6), 778–785.

Kushner, F. (2000). The usefulness of the cervical range of motion device in the ocular motility examination. *Archives of Ophthalmology, 118*(7), 946–950.

Laio, J. (1999). Eye injuries in sports. *Athletic Therapy Today, 4*(5), 36–41.

Lewis, L. (1999). Early clues to vision loss. *Patient Care, 33*(7), 220–237.

McCarty, C., & Taylor, H. (2000). Age-specific causes of bilateral visual impairment. *Archives of Ophthalmology, 118*(2), 264–269.

Moss, S. (2000). Prevalence of and risk factors for dry eye syndrome. *Archives of Ophthalmology, 118*(9), 1264–1268.

Parver, D. (1999). Recognizing diseases and disorders of the eye. *Athletic Therapy Today, 4*(5), 22–33, 63.

Quillen, D. (1999). Common causes of vision loss in elderly patients. *American Family Physician, 60*(1), 99–108.

Rapaport, M. (2000). Eyelid dermatitis. *Dermatology Nursing, 12*(5), 352–354.

Schaumberg, D. (2000). Demographic predictors of eye care utilization among women. *Medical Care, 38*(6), 638–646.

Weih, L., Van Newkirk, M., & Stickler, G. (2000). Are yearly physical examinations in adolescents necessary? *Journal of the American Board of Family Practice, 13*(3), 172–177.

Wingate, S. (1999). Treating corneal abrasions. *Nurse Practitioner: American Journal of Primary Health Care, 24*(6), 53–54, 57, 60.

Yawn, B. (1996). Is school vision screening effective? *Journal of School Health, 66*(5), 171.

Zabel, K. (1996). Accurate tests play critical role. *Ophthalmology Times, 21*(13), 12.

Risk Factors—Cataracts

Christen, W., Glynn, R., Ajani, U., Schaumberg, D., Buring, J., et al. (2000). Smoking cessation and risk of age-related cataract in men. *Journal of the American Medical Association, 284*(6), 713–716.

Heseker, H. (1995). Antioxidative vitamins and cataracts in the elderly. *Zeitschrift fur Ernahrungswissenschaft, 34*(3), 167–176.

Javitt, J., & Taylor, H. (1994–1995). Cataract and latitude. *Documenta Ophthalmologica, 88*(3–4), 307–325.

Leske, M., Wu, S., Hennis, A., Connell, A., Hyman, L., & Schachat, A. (1999). Diabetes, hypertension, and central obesity as cataract risk factors in a black population: The Barbados Study. *Ophthalmology, 106*(1), 35–46.

McCarty, C. A., Nanjan, M., & Taylor, H. (2000). Attributable risk estimates for cataract to prioritize medical and public health action. *Investigative Ophthalmology and Visual Science, 41*(12), 3720–3725.

Rowe, N., Mitchell, P., Cumming, R., & Wans, J. (2000). Diabetes, fasting blood glucose and age-related cataract: The Blue Mountains Eye Study. *Ophthalmic Epidemiology, 7*(2), 103–114.

West, S., & Valmadrid, C. (1995). Epidemiology of risk factors for age-related cataract. *Survey of Ophthalmology, 39*(4), 323–334.

World Health Organization (WHO). (2000). Control of major blinding diseases and disorders (2): Vision 2020 [On-line]. Available: http://www.who.int/inf-fs/en/fact 214.html.

———. (1997). Blindness and visual disability: Part II of VII: Major causes worldwide [On-line]. Available: http://www.who.int/inf-fs/en/fact 143.html.

For additional information on this book, be sure to visit http://connection.lww.com.

Ear Assessment

12

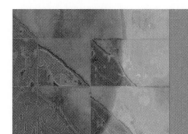

The ear is the sense organ of hearing and equilibrium. It consists of three distinct parts—the external ear, the middle ear, and the inner ear. The tympanic membrane separates the external ear from the middle ear. Both the external ear and the tympanic membrane can be assessed by direct inspection and by using an otoscope. However, the middle and inner ear cannot be directly inspected. Instead, these parts of the ear are assessed by testing hearing acuity and the conduction of sound.

External Ear Structures

The external ear is composed of the auricle or pinna and the external auditory canal (Fig. 12-1). The external auditory canal is S-shaped in the adult. The outer part of the canal curves up and back and the inner part of the canal curves down and forward. Modified sweat glands in the external ear canal secrete cerumen, a waxlike substance that keeps the tympanic membrane soft. The stickiness of cerumen serves as a defense against foreign bodies. A translucent, pearly gray, concave membrane, the tympanic membrane, or eardrum, serves as a partition stretched across the inner end of the auditory canal, separating it from the middle ear. The distinct landmarks (Fig. 12-2) of the tympanic membrane include:

- Handle and short process of the malleus
- Umbo
- Cone of light
- Pars flaccida
- Pars tensa

Middle Ear Structures

The middle ear, or tympanic cavity, is a small, air-filled chamber in the temporal bone. It is separated from the external ear by the eardrum and from the inner ear by a bony partition containing two openings, the round and oval windows. The middle ear contains three auditory ossicles: The malleus, the incus, and the stapes. These tiny bones are responsible for transmitting sound waves from the eardrum to the inner ear through the oval window. Air pressure is equalized on both sides of the tympanic mem-

brane by means of the eustachian tube, which connects the middle ear to the nasopharynx (see Fig. 12-1).

Inner Ear Structures

The inner ear, or labyrinth, is fluid filled and is made up of the bony labyrinth and an inner membranous labyrinth. The bony labyrinth has three parts: the cochlea, the vestibule, and the semicircular canals. The inner cochlear duct contains the spiral organ of Corti, which is the sensory organ for hearing. Sensory receptors, located in the vestibule and in the membranous semicircular canals, sense position and head movements to help maintain both static and dynamic equilibrium. Nerve fibers from these areas form the vestibular nerve, which connects with the cochlear nerve to form the eighth cranial nerve (acoustic or vestibulocochlear nerve).

Hearing Pathways

Sound vibrations traveling through air are collected by and funneled through the external ear and cause the eardrum to vibrate. Sound waves are then transmitted through bone as the vibration of the eardrum causes the malleus, incus, and then the stapes to vibrate. As the stapes vibrates at the oval window, the sound waves are passed to the fluid in the inner ear. The movement of this fluid stimulates the hair cells of the spiral organ of Corti and initiates the nerve impulses that travel to the brain by way of the acoustic nerve.

The transmission of sound waves through the external and middle ear is referred to as "conductive hearing," and the transmission of sound waves in the inner ear is referred to as "perceptive" or "sensorineural hearing." Therefore, a conductive hearing loss would be related to a dysfunction of the external or middle ear (eg, impacted ear wax, otitis media, foreign object, perforated eardrum, drainage in the middle ear, or otosclerosis). A "sensorineural loss" would be related to dysfunction of the inner ear (ie, organ of Corti, cranial nerve VIII, or temporal lobe of brain).

In addition to the usual pathway for sound vibrations detailed previously, the bones of the skull also conduct sound waves. This bone conduction serves to augment the usual pathway of sound waves through air, bone, and finally fluid (Fig. 12-3).

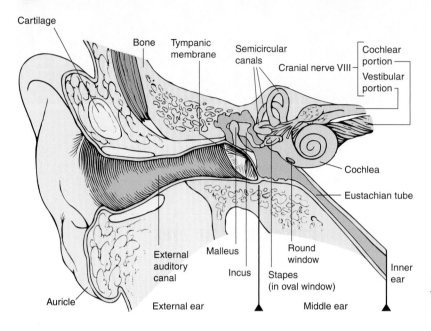

FIGURE 12-1. Lines anchored by triangles set the boundaries for the external, middle, and inner ear.

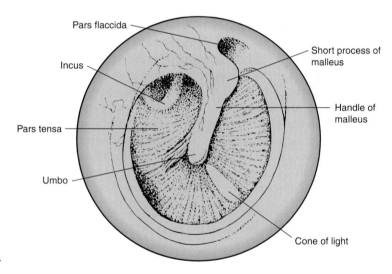

FIGURE 12-2. Right tympanic membrane.

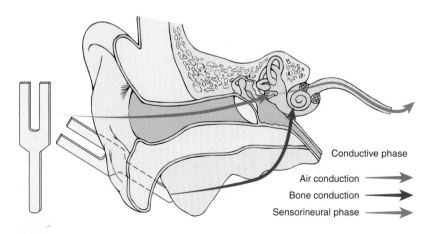

Conductive phase

Air conduction →

Bone conduction →

Sensorineural phase →

FIGURE 12-3. Pathways of hearing.

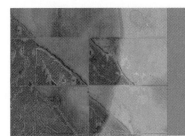
Beginning when the nurse first meets the client, assessment of hearing provides important information about the client's ability to interact with the environment. Changes in hearing are often gradual and go unrecognized by clients until a severe problem develops. Therefore, asking the client specific questions about hearing may help in detecting disorders at an early stage.

Collecting Subjective Data

First, it is important to gather data from the client about the current level of hearing and ear health as well as past and family health history problems that are related to the ear. Collecting data concerning environmental influences on hearing and how these problems affect the client's usual activities of daily living is also important. Answers to these types of questions help you evaluate a client's risk for hearing loss and, in turn, present ways that the client may modify or lower the risk of ear and hearing problems. If the client complains of or reports a history of ear infections or suspects hearing loss, collect as much related data as possible. Use the COLDSPA mnemonic as your guide.

COLDSPA

CHARACTER: Describe the sign or symptom. How does it feel, look, sound, smell, and so forth?

ONSET: When did it begin?

LOCATION: Where is it? Does it radiate?

DURATION: How long does it last? Does it recur?

SEVERITY: How bad is it?

PATTERN: What makes it better: What makes it worse?

ASSOCIATED FACTORS: What other symptoms occur with it?

Nursing History

CURRENT SYMPTOMS

Question Describe any recent changes in your hearing.

Rationale A sudden decrease in ability to hear in one ear may be associated with otitis media. A client reporting any sudden hearing loss should be referred to a physician for evaluation.

 Presbycusis, a gradual hearing loss, is common after the age of 50 years.

Q Are all sounds affected with this change, or just some sounds?

R Presbycusis often begins with a loss of the ability to hear high-frequency sounds.

Q Do you have any ear drainage? Describe the amount and any odor.

R Drainage (otorrhea) usually indicates infection. Purulent, bloody drainage suggests an infection of the external ear (external otitis). Purulent drainage associated with pain and a popping sensation is characteristic of otitis media with perforation of the tympanic membrane.

Q Do you have any ear pain? If so, do you have an accompanying sore throat, sinus infection, or problem with your teeth or gums?

R Earache (otalgia) can occur with ear infections, cerumen blockage, sinus infections, or teeth and gum problems.

Q Do you experience any ringing or crackling in your ears?

R Ringing in the ears (tinnitus) may be associated with excessive ear wax buildup, high blood pressure, or certain medications (such as streptomycin, gentamicin, kanamycin, neomycin, ethacrynic acid, furosemide, indomethacin, or aspirin).

Q Do you ever feel like you are spinning or that the room is spinning? Do you ever feel dizzy or unbalanced?

R Vertigo (true spinning motion) may be associated with an inner ear problem. It is termed *subjective vertigo* when the client feels that he is spinning around, and *objective vertigo* when the client feels that the room is spinning around him. It is important to distinguish vertigo from dizziness.

PAST HISTORY

Q Have you ever had any problems with your ears, such as infections, trauma, or earaches?

R A history of repeated infections can affect the tympanic membrane and hearing.

Q Describe any past treatments you have received for ear problems (medication, surgery, hearing aids). Were these successful? Were you satisfied?

R Client may be dissatisfied with past treatments for ear or hearing problems.

👓 The older client may have had a bad experience with certain hearing aids and may refuse to wear one. The client may also associate a negative self-image with a hearing aid.

FAMILY HISTORY

Q Is there a history of hearing loss in your family?

R In many cases, hearing loss is hereditary.

LIFESTYLE AND HEALTH PRACTICES

Q Do you work or live in an area with frequent or continuous loud noise? How do you protect your ears from the noise?

R Continuous loud noises (eg, machinery, music, explosives) can cause a hearing loss unless the ears are protected with ear guards (see Risk Factors—Hearing Loss).

Q Do you spend a lot of time swimming or in water? How do you protect your ears?

R Swimmer's ear (infection of the ear canal) may be seen when contaminated water is left in the ear. Earplugs may help to keep water out, and over-the-counter ear drops may be used to dry out the water in the ears.

Q Has your hearing loss affected your ability to care for yourself? To work?

R Hearing loss or ear pain may interfere with the client's ability to perform usual activities of daily living. Clients may not be able to drive, talk on the telephone, or operate machinery safely because of poor hearing ability. The ability to perform in occupations that rely heavily on hearing, such as a receptionist or telephone operator, may be affected.

Q Has your hearing loss affected your socializing with others?

R Clients who have decreased hearing may withdraw, isolate themselves, or become depressed because of the stress of verbal communication.

Q When was your last hearing examination?

R Yearly hearing tests are recommended for clients who are exposed to loud noises for long periods. Knowing the date of the examination helps determine recent changes.

Q How do you care for your ears?

R Use of cotton-tipped applicators inside the ear can cause ear wax to become impacted and cause ear damage.

Collecting Objective Data

The purpose of the ear and hearing examination is to evaluate the condition of the external ear, the condition and patency of the ear canal, the status of the tympanic membrane, bone and air conduction of sound vibrations, hearing acuity, and equilibrium. The external ear structures and ear canal are relatively easy to assess through inspection. Using the tuning fork to evaluate bone and air conduction is also a fairly simple procedure. However, more practice and expertise are needed to use the otoscope correctly to examine the condition of the structures of the tympanic membrane.

CLIENT PREPARATION

The client should be seated comfortably during the ear examination. This helps to promote the client's participation, which is very important in this examination. Therefore, the test should be explained thoroughly to guarantee accurate results. To ease any client anxiety, explain in detail what you will be doing. Also answer any questions the client may have. As you prepare the client for the ear examination, carefully note how he or she responds to your explanations. Does the client appear to hear you well, or does it seem he or she is straining to catch everything you say? Does the client respond to you verbally or nonverbally, or do you have to repeat what you say to get a response? This initial observation provides you with clues as to the status of the client's hearing.

EQUIPMENT AND SUPPLIES

- Watch with a second-hand for Romberg test
- Tuning fork (512 or 1,024 Hz)
- Otoscope (Display 12-1)

KEY ASSESSMENT POINTS

- Recognize the role of hearing in communication and adaptation to the environment particularly in regard to aging.
- Use the otoscope effectively when performing the ear examination.
- Understand the usefulness and significance of basic hearing tests.

(*text continues on page 218*)

RISK FACTORS
Hearing Loss

OVERVIEW

More than 70 million people in the world have a moderate to severe hearing loss. In the United States in 1995, there were 2 million deaf and 12 million hearing-impaired individuals (Cohen & Gorlin, 1995). About one third of the cases are hereditary, one third are acquired, and one third are of unknown cause. Genetic hearing loss occurs in about 1/1,000 births. Late-onset hearing loss (largely of genetic origin) occurs in nearly one half of the population older than age 80 years, with men more affected than women. In addition to heredity, presbycusis, infection (otitis media), and environmental noise are causes. Often, hearing loss or worsening of hearing loss could be prevented.

RISK FACTORS (BUPA FOUNDATION, 2000)

- Genetic predisposition
- Congenital anomalies
- Preauricular tag, if family history of sensori-neural hearing loss (Francois et al., 1995)
- Otitis media, especially if chronic or untreated
- Fluid in inner ear
- Loud noises
- Micronutrient deficiencies
- Ototoxic medications (eg, aspirin, quinine, some antibiotics)
- Age (presbycusis)
- Trauma to eardrum
- Otosclerosis or, rarely, rheumatoid arthritis affecting ossicles
- Viral infections of inner ear (eg, mumps, measles, chickenpox)
- Meniere's disease
- Impacted cerumen
- Acoustic neuroma of auditory nerve
- Brain diseases (eg, meningitis, encephalitis, multiple sclerosis, tumor, stroke)
- Child of mother who contracted rubella while pregnant
- In utero developmental problems that affect hearing

RISK REDUCTION TEACHING TIPS

- Avoid loud noises or sustained loud reverberations.
- Wear ear protection when exposed to loud noises.
- Obtain treatment for otitis media.
- Seek treatment for recurrent sinusitis, which can lead to otitis media.
- Eat a varied, well-balanced diet.
- Have any sudden hearing loss, dizziness, and tinnitus evaluated as soon as possible.
- Avoid medications associated with ototoxicity, if possible.

 ## CULTURAL CONSIDERATIONS

Only a few ethnic groups in developed countries are known to have a high rate of ear disease (Giles & Asher, 1991). High rates of otitis media (a major risk factor for hearing loss) are seen in populations with shorter, wider, and more horizontal eustachian tubes (Native Americans, Eskimos, New Zealand Maoris, a Nigerian population, and some aborigines) (Casselbrant et al., 1995). Blacks have lower rates of both otitis media and noise-induced or other forms of hearing loss (Overfield, 1995).

DISPLAY 12-1. How to Use the Otoscope

The otoscope is a flashlight-type viewer used to visualize the eardrum and external ear canal. Some guidelines for using it effectively follow.

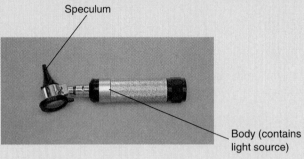

Speculum

Body (contains light source)

Otoscope.

1. Ask the client to sit comfortably with the back straight and the head tilted slightly away from you toward his or her opposite shoulder.
2. Choose the largest speculum that fits comfortably into the client's ear canal (usually 5 mm in the adult) and attach it to the otoscope. Holding the instrument in your dominant hand, turn the light on the otoscope to "on."
3. Use the thumb and fingers of your opposite hand to grasp the client's auricle firmly but gently. Pull out, up, and back to straighten the external auditory canal. Do not alter this positioning at any time during the otoscope examination.
4. Grasp the handle of the otoscope between your thumb and fingers and hold the instrument up or down, whichever is comfortable for you.
5. Position the hand holding the otoscope against the client's head or face. This position prevents forceful insertion of the instrument and helps to steady your hand throughout the examination, which is especially helpful if the client makes any unexpected movements.
6. Insert the speculum gently down and forward into the ear canal (approximately 0.5 inch). As you insert the otoscope, be careful not to touch either side of the inner portion of the canal wall. This area is bony and covered by a thin, sensitive layer of epithelium. Any pressure will cause the client pain.
7. Move your head in close to the otoscope and position your eye against the lens.

PHYSICAL ASSESSMENT

ASSESSMENT PROCEDURE	NORMAL FINDINGS	ABNORMAL FINDINGS

EXTERNAL EAR STRUCTURES

Inspect the auricle, tragus, and lobule, noting size, shape and position.

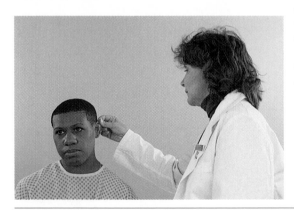

Inspecting the external ear. (© B. Proud.)

Ears are equal in size bilaterally (normally 4–10 cm). The auricle aligns with the corner of each eye and within a 10-degree angle of the vertical position. Earlobes may be free, attached, or soldered (tightly attached to adjacent skin with no apparent lobe).

Ears are smaller than 4 cm or larger than 10 cm.
   Malaligned or low-set ears may be seen with genitourinary disorders or chromosomal defects.

ASSESSMENT PROCEDURE	NORMAL FINDINGS	ABNORMAL FINDINGS
	Most blacks and whites have free lobes, whereas most Asians have attached or soldered lobes, although any type is possible in all cultural groups (Overfield, 1995).	
	The older client often has elongated earlobes with linear wrinkles.	
Continue inspecting the auricle, tragus, and lobule. Observe for lesions, discolorations, and discharge. 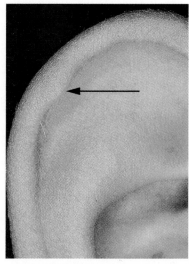 **Darwin's tubercle.**	The skin is smooth with no lesions, lumps, or nodules. Color is consistent with facial color. Darwin's tubercle, which is a clinically insignificant projection, may be seen on the auricle. No discharge should be present.	Some abnormal findings suggest various disorders, including: Enlarged preauricular and postauricular lymph nodes—infection Tophi (nontender, hard, cream-colored nodules on the helix or antihelix, containing uric acid crystals)—gout Blocked sebaceous glands—postauricular cysts Ulcerated, crusted nodules that bleed—cancer Redness, swelling, scaling, or itching—otitis externa Pale blue ear color—frostbite (Display 12-2).
Palpate the auricle and mastoid process.	Normally, the auricle, tragus, and mastoid process are not tender.	A painful auricle or tragus is associated with otitis externa or a postauricular cyst. Tenderness over the mastoid process suggests mastoiditis. Tenderness behind the ear may occur with otitis media.

(continued)

ASSESSMENT PROCEDURE	NORMAL FINDINGS	ABNORMAL FINDINGS

Otoscopic Examination

Inspect the external auditory canal. Following the guidelines provided in How to Use the Otoscope (see Display 12-1), note any discharge along with the color and consistency of cerumen (ear wax).

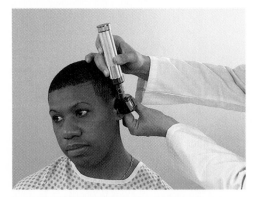

Inspecting the external canal and tympanic membrane. (© B. Proud.)

A small amount of odorless cerumen (ear wax) is the only discharge normally present. Cerumen may be yellow, orange, red, brown, gray, or black and soft, moist, dry, flaky, or even hard.

About 85% of Asians and Native Americans have dry ear wax whereas whites (97%) and blacks (99%) have wet ear wax (Overfield, 1995). Dry ear wax is more likely to become impacted.

Abnormal findings associated with specific disorders include:
    Foul-smelling, sticky, yellow discharge—otitis externa or impacted foreign body
    Bloody, purulent discharge—otitis media with ruptured tympanic membrane
    Blood or watery drainage (cerebrospinal fluid)—skull trauma (refer client to physician immediately)
    Impacted cerumen blocking the view of the external ear canal—conductive hearing loss

In some older clients, harder, drier cerumen tends to build as cilia in the ear canal become more rigid. Coarse, thick, wirelike hair may grow at the ear canal entrance as well. This is an abnormal finding if it impairs hearing.

Also observe the color and consistency of the ear canal walls and inspect the character of any nodules.

The canal walls should be pink and smooth and without nodules.

Abnormal findings in the ear canal may include:
    Reddened, swollen canals—otitis externa
    Exostoses (nonmalignant nodular swellings)
    Polyps (usually surrounded by purulent discharge and blocking the view of the eardrum (see Display 12-3)

Inspect the tympanic membrane (eardrum) using the guidelines provided in Display 12-1. Note color, shape, consistency, and landmarks.

The tympanic membrane should be pearly, gray, shiny, and translucent with no bulging or retraction. It is slightly concave, smooth and intact. A cone-shaped reflection of the otoscope light is normally seen at 5 o'clock in the right ear and at 7 o'clock in the left ear. The short process and handle of the malleus and the umbo are clearly visible (see Fig 12-2).

The older client's eardrum may appear cloudy. The landmarks may be more prominent because of atrophy of the tympanic membrane associated with the normal process of aging.

Abnormal findings in the tympanic membrane may include:
    Red, bulging eardrum and diminished or absent light reflex—acute otitis media
    Yellowish, bulging membrane with bubbles behind—serous otitis media
    Bluish or dark red color—blood behind the eardrum from skull trauma
    White spots—scarring from infections
    Perforations—trauma from infection
    Prominent landmarks—eardrum retraction from negative ear pressure resulting from an obstructed eustachian tube
    Obscured or absent landmarks—eardrum thickening from chronic otitis media (see Display 12-3)

(continued)

ASSESSMENT PROCEDURE	NORMAL FINDINGS	ABNORMAL FINDINGS

HEARING AND EQUILIBRIUM TESTS

The tests discussed below are performed to give the examiner a basic idea of whether the client has hearing loss, what type (conduction or sensorineural) of hearing loss it might be, and whether there is a problem with equilibrium. These tests present an opportunity to educate clients about risk factors for hearing loss.

Blacks have slightly better hearing at low and high frequencies (250 and 6000 Hz); Whites have better hearing at middle frequencies (2000 and 4000 Hz). Blacks are less susceptible to noise-induced hearing loss (Overfield, 1995).

These tests are not completely accurate and do not provide the examiner with any exact percentage of hearing loss. Therefore, the client should be referred to a hearing specialist for more accurate testing if a problem is suspected.

Whisper Test

Perform the whisper test to assess a client's "gross" hearing. Stand 1 to 2 feet behind the client so he or she cannot read your lips. Ask the client to place one finger on the tragus of the left ear and move it back and forth. This obscures the sound in that ear, making the test for the other ear more reliable. Whisper a word with two distinct syllables toward the client's right ear. Then ask the client to repeat the word back to you. Repeat the test for the left ear.

Client correctly repeats the two-syllable word.

Client cannot repeat the word or has difficulty repeating the word spoken by examiner.

Weber's Test

Perform Weber's test if the client reports diminished or lost hearing in one ear. The test helps evaluate the conduction of sound waves through bone to help distinguish between conductive hearing (sound waves transmitted by the external and middle ear) and sensorineural hearing (sound waves transmitted by the inner ear). Strike a tuning fork softly with the back of your hand and place it in the center of the client's head or forehead. Centering is the important part. Ask whether the client hears the sound better in one ear or the same in both ears.

Vibrations are heard equally well in both ears. No lateralization of sound to either ear.

With *conductive hearing loss,* the client reports lateralization of sound to the poor ear—that is, the client "hears" the vibrations in the poor ear. With *sensorineural hearing loss,* the client reports lateralization of sound to the good ear (Display 12-4).

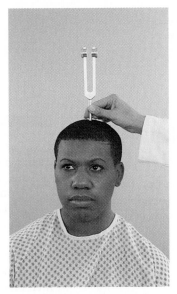

The Weber test assesses sound conducted via bone. (© B. Proud.)

(continued)

ASSESSMENT PROCEDURE	NORMAL FINDINGS	ABNORMAL FINDINGS

Rinne Test

To perform the Rinne test, which compares air and bone conduction sounds, strike a tuning fork and place the base of the fork on the client's mastoid process. Ask the client to tell you when the sound is no longer heard. Move the prongs of the tuning fork to the front of the external auditory canal. Ask the client to tell you when he or she no longer hears a sound.

Air conduction sound is normally heard longer than bone conduction sound (AC > BC).

With *conductive hearing loss,* bone conduction sound is heard longer than or equally as long as air conduction sound (BC≥AC). With *sensorineural hearing loss,* air conduction sound is heard longer than bone conduction sound (AC>BC) (see Display 12-4).

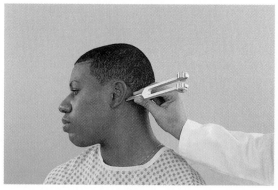
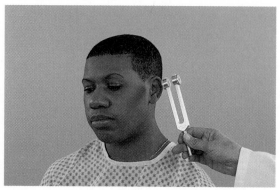

In the Rinne test the tuning fork base is placed first on the mastoid process (*left*), after which the prongs are moved to the front of the external auditory canal (*right*). (© B. Proud)

Romberg Test

The Romberg test is done to test the client's equilibrium. Ask the client to stand with feet together and arms at sides and eyes open and then with the eyes closed.

Client maintains position for 20 seconds without swaying or with minimal swaying.

Client moves feet apart to prevent falls or starts to fall from loss of balance. This may indicate a vestibular disorder.

 Tip From the Experts Put your arms around the client without touching him or her to prevent falls.

Validation and Documentation of Findings

Validate the ear assessment data that you have collected. This is necessary to verify that the data are reliable and accurate. Document the assessment data following the health care facility or agency policy.

EXAMPLE OF SUBJECTIVE DATA

Client denies recent changes in hearing. No drainage, pain, or ringing. Has not experienced any spinning sensations. States history of one ear infection several years ago. Has had no surgery, does not use a hearing aid device. Denies frequent exposure to loud noises. Last hearing examination was 3 years ago.

EXAMPLE OF OBJECTIVE DATA

Equal in size bilaterally, auricles aligned with the corner of each eye within a 10-degree angle of vertical position. Skin smooth, no lumps, lesions, nodules. No discharge. Non-tender on palpation. Small amount of moist yellow cerumen in external canal, no nodules present. Tympanic membrane pearly gray, shiny, transparent, no bulging or retraction, smooth, intact. Cone-shaped reflection at 5 o'clock position in right ear, 7 o'clock position in left ear. Short process, handle of malleus and umbo clearly visible. Center of tympanic membrane flutters during Valsalva maneuver. Whisper test: Client repeats two-syllable word. Weber's test: Hears vibration equally well in both ears. Rinne test: AC>BC. Romberg test: Maintains position for 20 seconds without swaying.

After you have collected your assessment data, you will need to analyze the data, using diagnostic reasoning skills. Refer to the discussion of diagnostic reasoning skills in Chapter 7.

DISPLAY 12-2. Abnormalities of the External Ear and Ear Canal

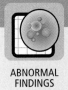

ABNORMAL
FINDINGS

All sorts of abnormalities may affect the external ear and ear canal; among them are infections and abnormal growths. Some are pictured below.

TOPHI

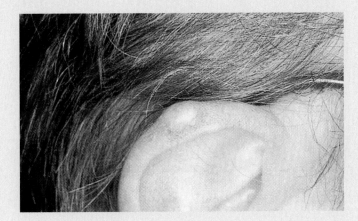

POSTAURICULAR CYST

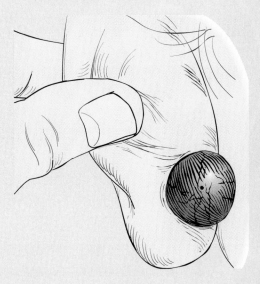

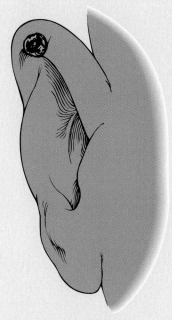

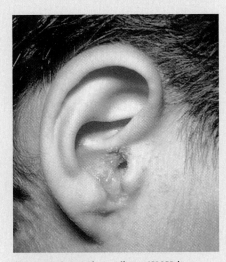

(© 1992 Science Photo Library/CMSP.)

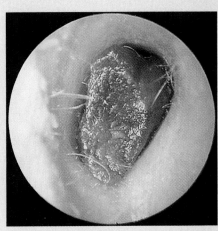

MALIGNANT LESION   OTITIS EXTERNA   BUILDUP OF CERUMEN IN EAR CANAL

(continued)

DISPLAY 12-2. Abnormalities of the External Ear and Ear Canal (Continued)

EXOTOSIS

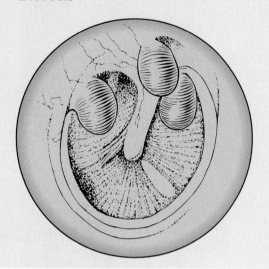

POLYP

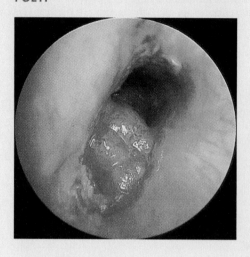

ABNORMAL
FINDINGS

DISPLAY 12-3. Abnormalities of the Tympanic Membrane

The thin, drumlike structure of the tympanic membrane is essential for hearing. It is also essential for promoting equilibrium and barring infection. Damage to the membrane may have grave and serious consequences.

ACUTE OTITIS MEDIA

Note the red, bulging membrane; decreased or absent light reflex.

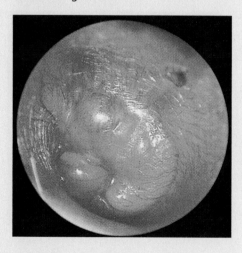

SEROUS OTITIS MEDIA

Note the yellowish, bulging membrane with bubbles behind it.

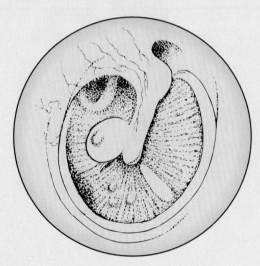

(continued)

DISPLAY 12-3. Abnormalities of the Tympanic Membrane (Continued)

BLUE/DARK RED TYMPANIC MEMBRANE

Indicates blood behind eardrum due to trauma.

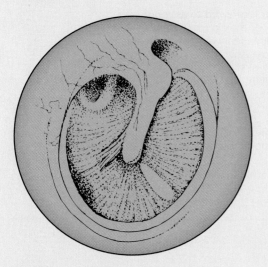

SCARRED TYMPANIC MEMBRANE

White spots and streaks indicate scarring from infections.

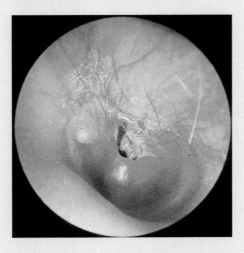

PERFORATED TYMPANIC MEMBRANE

Perforation results from rupture caused by increased pressure usually from untreated infection or trauma.

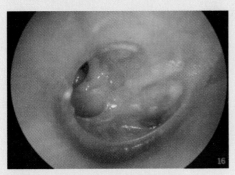

(© 1992 Science Photo Library/CMSP.)

RETRACTED TYMPANIC MEMBRANE

Prominent landmarks are caused by negative ear pressure due to obstructed eustachian tube or chronic otitis media.

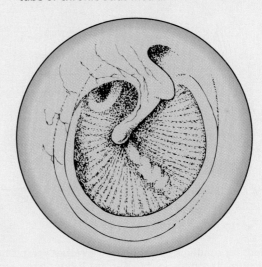

DISPLAY 12-4. Conductive and Sensorineural Hearing Loss

The various kinds of hearing loss have different causes and different treatments.

CONDUCTIVE HEARING LOSS AND WEBER'S TEST

The transmission of sound waves through the external and middle ear is referred to as *conductive hearing*. Therefore, with conductive hearing loss, there is dysfunction of the external or middle ear. Some of the causes of conductive hearing loss include impacted cerumen (ear wax), otitis media, perforated eardrum, otosclerosis, foreign objects, or drainage in middle ear.

Conductive hearing impairment is not uncommon in the older client because of the greater incidence of cerumen buildup and/or atrophy or sclerosis of the tympanic membrane.

With conductive loss, sound conducted by bone is heard for the same length of time or longer than sound conducted by air (BC≥AC). This occurs because air conduction is blocked in the external auditory canal or in the middle ear.

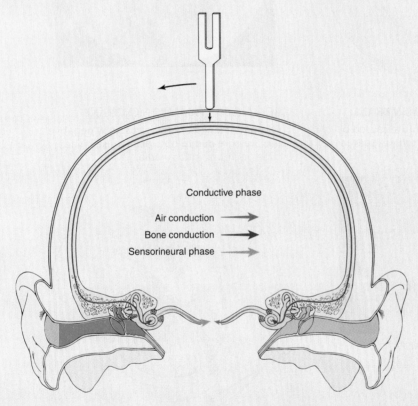

Conductive phase

Air conduction ⟶

Bone conduction ⟶

Sensorineural phase ⟶

A basic assessment for conductive hearing loss is Weber's test. During the performance of this test, the examiner suspects conductive hearing loss if the client reports lateralization of sound to the poor ear. The good ear is distracted by background noise, conducted by air, which the poor ear has trouble hearing. Thus, the poor ear receives most of the sound conducted by bone vibration.

(continued)

SENSORINEURAL HEARING LOSS AND THE RINNE TEST

The transmission of sound waves in the inner ear is referred to as *sensorineural hearing*. Therefore, a sensorineural hearing loss indicates a dysfunction of the inner ear. Sensorineural hearing loss is caused by damage to the cochlea or vestibulocochlear nerve.

A basic assessment for sensorineural hearing loss is the Rinne test. During the performance of this test, the examiner suspects sensorineural hearing loss if the client reports lateralization of sound to the good ear. This occurs because the inner ear of the poor ear cannot receive sound vibrations regardless of the type (bone or air).

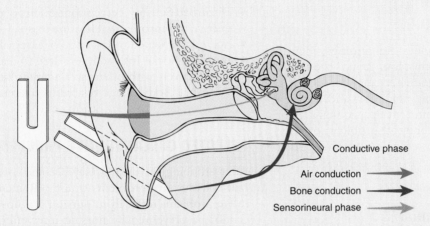

Conductive phase

Air conduction

Bone conduction

Sensorineural phase

Presbycusis, a gradual sensorineural hearing loss due to degeneration of the cochlea or vestibulocochlear nerve, is common in older (over age 50) clients. The client with presbycusis has difficulty hearing consonants and whispered words; this difficulty increases over time.

With sensorineural loss, air condition sound is heard for longer than bone conduction sound (AC>BC). The ratio is the same as the normal finding because no matter how sound travels to the inner ear (by bone or by air), the damaged inner ear is less able to transmit it. Although the ratio is the same, the length of time each sound is heard is much shorter than normal, which indicates a sensorineural disorder.

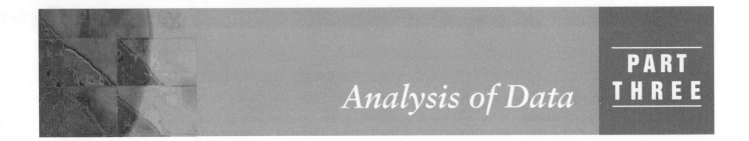

Diagnostic Reasoning: Possible Conclusions

To come to a conclusion about your findings, identify strengths and abnormal data, cluster or group the related cues, and write down what you think may be the problem. Generate possible nursing diagnoses and decide if nursing measures can treat or prevent the problem. If not, consider monitoring for collaborative problems or referring for medical problems. Listed below are some possible conclusions after assessment of the client's ears and hearing.

SELECTED NURSING DIAGNOSES

After collecting subjective and objective data pertaining to the ears, you will need to identify abnormal findings and cluster the data to reveal any significant patterns or abnormalities. These data will then be used to make clinical judgments (nursing diagnoses: wellness, risk, or actual) about the status of the client's ears. Following is a listing of selected nursing diagnoses that you may identify when analyzing data for this part of the assessment.

Nursing Diagnoses (Wellness)

- Opportunity to enhance auditory integrity

Nursing Diagnoses (Risk)

- Risk for Hearing Loss related to prolonged exposure to noise pollution
- Risk for Injury related to poor hearing ability
- Risk for Self-Care Deficit (specify) related to hearing loss

Nursing Diagnoses (Actual)

- Disturbed Sensory Perception: Auditory related to conductive or sensorineural hearing loss
- Acute Pain related to infection of external or middle ear
- Impaired Social Interaction related to inability to interact effectively with others secondary to hearing loss
- Disturbed Body Image related to concern over appearance and need to wear hearing aid

SELECTED COLLABORATIVE PROBLEMS

After grouping the data, it may become apparent that certain collaborative problems emerge. Remember, collaborative problems differ from nursing diagnoses in that they cannot be prevented by nursing interventions. However, these physiologic complications of medical conditions can be detected and monitored by the nurse. In addition, the nurse can use physician- and nurse-prescribed interventions to minimize the complications of these problems. The nurse may also have to refer the client in such situations for further treatment of the problem. The following is a list of collaborative problems that may be identified when assessing the ear. These problems are worded Potential Complications (or PC), followed by the problem.

- PC: Corneal ulceration/abrasion
- PC: Otitis media (acute, chronic, or serous)
- PC: Otitis externa
- PC: Perforated tympanic membrane

MEDICAL PROBLEMS

If after grouping the data, it becomes apparent that the client has signs and symptoms that may require medical diagnosis and treatment, referral to a primary care provider is necessary.

Diagnostic Reasoning: Case Study

The case study presents assessment data for a specific client. It is followed by an analysis of the data, working through the steps involved in diagnostic reasoning to arrive at specific conclusions.

Josephine Carmino is a 57-year-old woman who lives alone in a small urban apartment. She lives on a fixed income from her deceased husband's Social Security pension. She has come to the clinic for her routine checkup. During the initial interview, you notice that she does not always answer your questions appropriately and she talks very softly when she offers information spontaneously. When you check her hearing with the whisper test, she asks you to repeat the word several times, and finally tells you, with annoyance in her voice, "You just have to speak up if you expect people to hear you!" When you do the Rinne test, the results show BC>AC. When you question her about problems, she denies having any hearing loss. She says she has never had audiometric studies and she can't afford them now. She also tells you that she doesn't talk to friends on the telephone anymore, because they don't talk loudly enough.

1 Identify abnormal data and strengths (in both subjective and objective data).

SUBJECTIVE DATA

- Denies any hearing loss
- Never has had audiometry and can't afford it
- Doesn't talk to friends on telephone anymore
- Friends do not talk loud enough on the telephone

OBJECTIVE DATA

- Does not answer questions appropriately
- Speaks very softly
- Fails whisper test
- Rinne test: BC>AC

2 Cue Clusters	**3** Inferences	**4** Possible Nursing Diagnoses	**5** Defining Characteristics	**6** Confirm or Rule Out
A • Does not answer questions appropriately • Fails whisper test • Speaks very softly • Friends do not talk loud enough on the telephone • Rinne test: BC>AC	Data suggest a conduction hearing loss. Soft speaking voice indicates that she hears her own voice loudly, which also points to conductive loss in the middle ear	Impaired Verbal Communication related to lack of understanding of hearing deficit	*Major:* Inappropriate response does not answer nurse's questions appropriately *Minor:* Does not talk to friends on telephone because she cannot hear them (not understanding)	Confirm because it meets the major and minor defining characteristic
B • Denies hearing loss • Has never had audiometric studies and can't afford them	At risk for progression of hearing loss because she denies evident hearing problem, although it could just be lack of understanding if her voice sounds loud to her	Ineffective Health Maintenance related to denial of hearing problem and inadequate resources to get additional testing	*Major:* None specific, but implied because of denial of health problem and lack of financial resources for additional diagnostic measures *Minor:* None	Rule out at this time because not enough data to validate major defining characteristics. However, important to collect more information about this diagnosis because client may be at risk for deterioration of hearing without follow-up care.
C • Does not talk to friends on telephone anymore • Friends do not talk loud enough on the telephone	Limiting social contacts because she cannot hear well on the telephone	Impaired Social Interaction related to decreased ability to maintain contact with friends secondary to probable hearing deficit	*Major:* Reports insecurity in social situations (implied because refuses to talk with friends on phone because cannot hear them well enough) *Minor:* None specific	Accept diagnosis because it meets major defining characteristic

7 **Document conclusions.**

Two of the alternative diagnoses are appropriate for
Mrs. Carmino at this time:

- Impaired Communication related to lack of understanding of
  hearing deficit
- Impaired Social Interaction related to decreased ability to maintain contact with friends secondary to probable hearing deficit

No collaborative problems could be identified because there is no
medical diagnosis at this time. Mrs. Carmino should be referred
to a physician whose services she can afford and who can evaluate and recommend treatment for hearing loss. (In addition, it
would be useful also to refer her to a social worker for evaluation
of her financial status and to help her to locate resources to assist
with medical care.)

REFERENCES AND SELECTED READINGS

Anonymous. (1996). Clinical guidelines: Adult screening for hearing.
Nineteenth in a series of articles based on chapters excerpted from the
*Clinician's handbook for preventive services. Nurse Practitioner: American
Journal of Primary Health Care, 21*(6), 106–108.

Chanin, L. (2000). Management of acute infectious otitis externa . . .
recertification series. *Physician Assistant, 24*(6), 59–64.

Colizza, D. (1999). Otitis media in the pediatric patient. *Head and Neck
Nursing, 17*(1), 7–15.

Epstein, S. (2000). Sound advice. *Volta Voices, 7*(4), 17.

Estrem, S. (2000). Conductive hearing loss associated with pressure
equalization tubes. *Otolaryngology—Head and Neck Surgery, 122*(3),
349–351.

Facione, N. (1990). Otitis media: An overview of acute and chronic
disease. *Nurse Practitioner, 15*(10), 11–22.

Hebert, R. (2000). Tympanostomy tubes and otic suspensions. Do
they reach the middle ear space? *Otolaryngology—Head and Neck Surgery,
122*(3), 330–333.

Kacker, A. (1999). The otoscopic examination: What to look for—where
to search. *Consultant, 39*(9), 2397–2402, 2405–2406.

Kirkwood, D. (2000). "Stakeholders" identify hearing needs. *Hearing
Journal, 53*(9), 50.

Lynch, J. (2000). Patient education. Ear wax. *Lippincott's Primary
Care Practice, 4*(5), 542–543.

Pope, S. (2000). Functional status and hearing impairments in women
at midlife. *Journal of Gerontology, 55*(3), 109–194.

Rosenberg, M. (2000). Neuro-otologic history. *Otolaryngologic
Clinics of North America, 33*(3), 471–482.

Russell, J. (1995). Ear screening. *Community Nurse, 1*(4), 14–16.

Smeltzer, C. D. (1993). Primary care screening and evaluation of hearing loss. *Nurse Practitioner, 18*(8), 50–55.

Stone, C. (1999). Clinical outlook. Preventing cerumen impaction in
nursing facility residents. *Journal of Gerontological Nursing, 25*(5), 43–45.

Taylor, C. (2000). Screening for hearing loss and middle-ear disorders
in children using TEOAEs. *American Journal of Audiology, 9*(1), 50–55.

Thompson, F. (2000). Clinical update. Otitis media with effusion.
Community Practitioner, 73(9), 728–729.

Thompson, J. (2000). Otitis media. *Community Practitioner, 73*(7),
692–693.

Williams, D. (2000). Hearing loss from wax impaction. *Alternatives,
8*(12), 91–92.

Risk Factors—Hearing Loss

BUPA Foundation. (2000). Hearing loss. Health fact sheet from
BUPA [On-line]. Available: *http://hcd2.bupa.co.uk/fact_sheets/Mosby_
factsheet/hearing_loss.html.*

Casselbrant, M., Mandel, E., Kurs-Lasky, M., Rockette, H., &
Bluestone, C. (1995). Otitis media in a population of black American and
white American infants, 0–2 years of age. *International Journal of Pediatric
Otorhinolaryngology, 33*(1), 1–16.

Cohen, M., & Gorlin, R. (1995). Epidemiology, etiology, and genetic
patterns. In R. Gorlin, H. Toriello & M. Cohen. *Hereditary hearing loss
and its syndromes* (pp. 18–21). New York, NY: Oxford University Press.

Francois, M., Wiener-Vacher, S., Falala, M., & Narcy, P. (1995).
Audiological assessment of infants and children with preauricular tags.
Audiology, 34(1), 1–5.

Giles, M., & Asher, I. (1991). Prevalence and natural history of otitis
media with perforation in Maori school children. *Journal of Laryngology
and Otology, 105*(4), 257–260.

Overfield, T. (1995). *Biologic variation in health and illness* (2nd ed.).
Boca Raton, FL: CRC Press.

**For additional information on this book, be sure to
visit** http://connection.lww.com.

Mouth, Throat, Nose, and Sinus Assessment

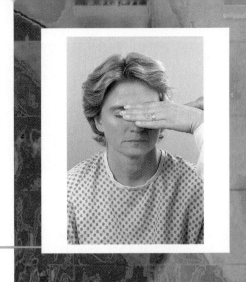

13

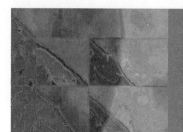

Structure and Function

The mouth and throat make up the first part of the digestive system and are responsible for receiving food (ingestion), taste, preparing food for digestion, and aiding in speech. Cranial nerves V (trigeminal), VII (facial), IX (glossopharyngeal), and XII (hypoglossal) assist with some of these functions (the cranial nerves are discussed in Chapter 23). The nose and paranasal sinuses constitute the first part of the respiratory system and are responsible for receiving, filtering, warming, and moistening air to be transported to the lungs. Receptors of cranial nerve I (olfactory) are also located in the nose. These receptors are related to the sense of smell.

Mouth

The mouth or oral cavity is formed by the lips, cheeks, hard and soft palates, uvula, and the tongue and its muscles (Fig. 13-1). The upper and lower lips form the entrance to the mouth and serve as a protective gateway to the digestive tract. The roof of the oral cavity is formed by the anterior hard palate and the posterior soft palate. An extension of the soft palate is the uvula, which hangs in the posterior midline of the oropharynx. The cheeks form the lateral walls of the mouth, whereas the tongue and its muscles form the floor of the mouth. The mandible (jaw bone) provides the structural support for the floor of the mouth.

Contained within the mouth are the tongue, teeth, gums, and the openings of the salivary glands (parotid, submandibular, and sublingual). The tongue is attached to the hyoid bone and styloid process of the temporal bone and is connected to the floor of the mouth by a fold of tissue called the frenulum. The tongue assists with moving food, swallowing, and speaking. The gums (gingiva) are covered by mucous membrane and normally hold 32 permanent teeth in the adult (Fig. 13-2). The top, visible, white enameled part of each tooth is the crown. The portion of the tooth that is embedded in the gums is the root. The crown and root are connected by the region of the tooth referred to as the neck.

The three pairs of salivary glands secrete saliva (watery, serous fluid containing salts, mucus, and salivary amylase) into the mouth (Fig. 13-3). The parotid glands, located below and in front of the ears, empty through Stensen's ducts, which are located inside the cheek across from the second upper molar. The submandibular glands, located in the lower jaw, open under the tongue on either side of the frenulum through openings called Wharton's ducts. The sublingual glands, located under the tongue, open through several ducts located on the floor of the mouth.

Throat

The throat (pharynx), located behind the mouth and nose, serves as a muscular passage for food and air. The upper part of the throat is the nasopharynx. Below the nasopharynx lies the oropharynx, and below the oropharynx lies the laryngopharynx. The soft palate, anterior and posterior pillars, and uvula connect behind the tongue to form arches. Masses of lymphoid tissue referred to as the palatine tonsils are located on both sides of the oropharynx at the end of the soft palate between the anterior and posterior pillars. The lingual tonsils lie at the base of the tongue. Pharyngeal tonsils or adenoids are found high in the nasopharynx. Because tonsils are masses of lymphoid tissue, they help protect against infection (Fig. 13-4).

Nose

The nose consists of an external portion covered with skin and an internal nasal cavity. It is composed of bone and cartilage and is lined with mucous membrane. The nasal cavity is located between the roof of the mouth and the cranium. It extends from the anterior nares (nostrils) to the posterior nares, which open into the nasopharynx. The nasal septum separates the cavity into two halves. The front of the nasal septum contains a rich supply of blood vessels and is known as Kiesselbach's area. This is a common site for nasal bleeding.

The superior, middle, and inferior turbinates are bony lobes, sometimes called conchae, that project from the lateral walls of the nasal cavity. These three turbinates serve to increase the surface area that is exposed to incoming air (see Fig. 13-4). As the person inspires air, nasal hairs (vibrissae) filter large particles from the air. Ciliated mucosal cells then capture and propel debris toward the throat, where it is swallowed. The rich blood supply of the nose warms the inspired air as it is moistened by the mucous membrane. A meatus underlies each turbinate and receives drainage from the paranasal sinuses and the nasolacrimal duct.

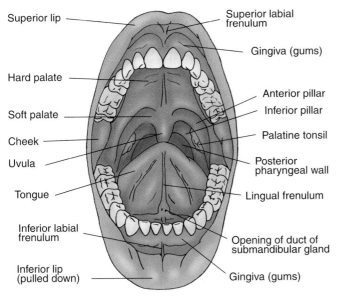

Superior lip

Superior labial frenulum

Gingiva (gums)

Hard palate

Anterior pillar

Inferior pillar

Soft palate

Palatine tonsil

Cheek

Posterior pharyngeal wall

Uvula

Tongue

Lingual frenulum

Inferior labial frenulum

Opening of duct of submandibular gland

Inferior lip (pulled down)

Gingiva (gums)

FIGURE 13-1. Structures of the mouth.

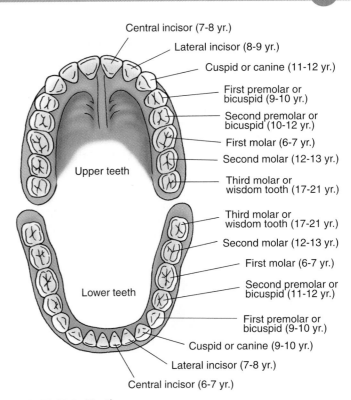

Central incisor (7-8 yr.)

Lateral incisor (8-9 yr.)

Cuspid or canine (11-12 yr.)

First premolar or bicuspid (9-10 yr.)

Second premolar or bicuspid (10-12 yr.)

First molar (6-7 yr.)

Second molar (12-13 yr.)

Third molar or wisdom tooth (17-21 yr.)

Upper teeth

Third molar or wisdom tooth (17-21 yr.)

Second molar (12-13 yr.)

First molar (6-7 yr.)

Second premolar or bicuspid (11-12 yr.)

Lower teeth

First premolar or bicuspid (9-10 yr.)

Cuspid or canine (9-10 yr.)

Lateral incisor (7-8 yr.)

Central incisor (6-7 yr.)

FIGURE 13-2. Teeth.

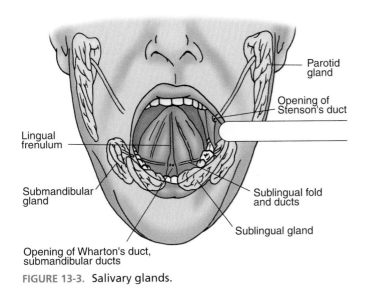

Parotid gland

Opening of Stenson's duct

Lingual frenulum

Submandibular gland

Sublingual fold and ducts

Sublingual gland

Opening of Wharton's duct, submandibular ducts

FIGURE 13-3. Salivary glands.

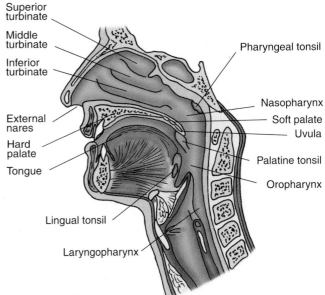

Superior turbinate

Middle turbinate

Inferior turbinate

Pharyngeal tonsil

Nasopharynx

Soft palate

Uvula

External nares

Hard palate

Tongue

Palatine tonsil

Oropharynx

Lingual tonsil

Laryngopharynx

FIGURE 13-4. Nasal cavity and throat structures.

Receptors for the first cranial nerve (olfactory) are located in the upper part of the nasal cavity and septum.

Sinuses

Four pairs of paranasal sinuses (frontal, maxillary, ethmoidal, and sphenoidal) are located in the skull (Fig. 13-5). These air-filled cavities decrease the weight of the skull and act as resonance chambers during speech. The paranasal sinuses are also lined with ciliated mucous membrane that traps debris and propels it toward the outside. The sinuses are often a primary site of infection because they can easily become blocked. The frontal sinuses (above the eyes) and the maxillary sinuses (in the upper jaw) are accessible to examination by the nurse. The ethmoidal and sphenoidal sinuses are smaller, located deeper in the skull, and are not accessible for examination.

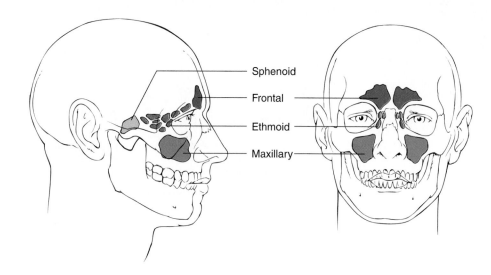

FIGURE 13-5. Paranasal sinuses.

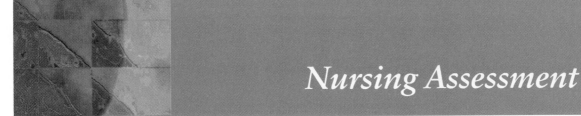

Collecting Subjective Data

Subjective data related to the mouth, throat, nose, and sinus can aid in detecting diseases and abnormalities that may affect the client's activities of daily living. Screening for cancer of the mouth, throat, nose, and sinuses is an important area of this assessment. These cancers are highly preventable (see Risk Factors—Cancers of the Oral Cavity). Data collected regarding the client's risk factors may form the basis for preventive teaching.

Other problems may cause discomfort and loss of function and can lead to serious systemic disorders. For example, malnutrition may develop in a client who cannot eat certain foods because of poorly fitting dentures. A client with frequent sinus infections and headaches may have impaired concentration, which affects job or school performance.

This examination also allows the nurse to evaluate the client's health practices. For example, improper use of nasal decongestants may explain recurrent sinus congestion, and infection and improper oral hygiene practices may cause tooth decay or gum disease. The nurse should provide teaching for a client with these health practices.

Nursing History
CURRENT SYMPTOMS

Question Do you experience tongue or mouth sores or lesions? Are they painful and do they recur?

Rationale Painful, recurrent ulcers in the mouth are seen with aphthous stomatitis (canker sores) and herpes simplex (cold sores). Mouth or tongue sores that do not heal; red or white patches that persist; a lump or thickening; or rough, crusty, or eroded areas are warning signs of cancer and need to be referred for further evaluation (see Risk Factors—Cancer of the Oral Cavity).

Q Do you experience redness, swelling, bleeding, or pain of the gums or mouth? Have you lost any permanent teeth?

R Red, swollen gums that bleed easily occur in early gum disease (gingivitis), whereas destruction of the gums with tooth loss occurs in more advanced gum disease (periodontitis). Pain can accompany inflammation and is a later sign of oral cancer.

The gums recede, become ischemic, and undergo fibrotic changes as a person ages. Tooth surfaces may be worn from prolonged use. These changes make the older client more susceptible to periodontal disease and tooth loss.

Q Do you have pain over your sinuses?

R Sinusitis may cause pressure and pain over the sinuses.

Q Do you experience nosebleeds?

R Nosebleeds may be seen with overuse of nasal sprays, excessively dry nasal mucosa, hypertension, leukemia, thrombocytopenia, and other blood disorders. A client who experiences frequent nosebleeds should be referred for further evaluation.

Q Do you experience frequent clear or mucous drainage from your nose?

R Thin, watery, clear nasal drainage (rhinorrhea) can indicate a chronic allergy or, in a person with a past head injury, a cerebrospinal fluid leak. Mucous drainage, especially yellow, is typical of a cold, rhinitis, or a sinus infection.

Q Can you breathe through both of your nostrils? Do you have a stuffy nose at times during the day or night?

R Inability to breathe through both nostrils may indicate sinus congestion, obstruction, or a deviated septum. Nasal congestion can interfere with daily activities or a restful sleep.

Q Have you experienced a change in your ability to smell or taste?

R A decrease in the ability to smell may occur with upper respiratory infections, smoking, cocaine use, or a neurologic lesion or tumor in the frontal lobe of the brain or in the olfactory bulb or tract. A decreased ability to taste may be reported by clients with upper respiratory infections or lesions of the facial nerve (VII). Changes in perception of smell also occur from a zinc deficiency and from menopause in some women.

The ability to smell and taste decreases with age. Medications can also decrease sense of smell and taste in older people.

Q Do you have difficulty chewing or swallowing food?

R Dysphagia (difficulty swallowing) may be seen in esophageal disorders, anxiety, poorly fitting dentures, or a

RISK FACTORS
Cancer of the Oral Cavity

OVERVIEW

More than 90% of oral cavity and oropharyngeal cancers are squamous cell cancers. Cancers develop in the lining, in the salivary glands, tonsils, or base of the tongue, but only squamous cell cancers of the oral and oropharyngeal cavity are discussed here. As of the year 2000, experts estimated that 30,200 new cases (20,000 in men and 10,000 in women) would be diagnosed in the United States with 7,800 deaths resulting. The incidence of oral cancer has slowly decreased in the United States since the early 1980s. Most cases (90%) occur in people who are heavy users of tobacco (smoking and smokeless) and alcohol and whose ages range in the fifties and sixties.

However, cases of oral cavity and tongue cancers are beginning to appear more frequently in people in their thirties and forties. Incidence is higher in men but is increasing in women. People with oral and oropharyngeal cancer often have another cancer or develop one at a later time. Follow-up examinations and avoidance of risk factors are extremely important for these clients (American Cancer Society [ACS], 2000).

RISK FACTORS (ACS, 2000)

- Tobacco use, smoking and smokeless
- Alcohol consumption
- Combined tobacco and alcohol use
- Alcohol dependence accompanied with nutritional deficiencies
- Age over 40
- Male gender (twice as likely to affect males as females, but incidence is rising in females)
- Genetic predisposition, family history
- Occupation related to nickel refining, woodworking, or textile fibers
- Vitamin A deficiency
- Ultraviolet light exposure (especially the lips)

POSSIBLE RISK FACTORS

- Chronic irritation
- Human papillomavirus (HPV) infection
- Immune system suppression
- Marijuana use
- Diet low in fruits and vegetables

RISK REDUCTION TEACHING TIPS (ACS, 2000)

- Stop smoking.
- Limit alcohol consumption.
- Eat a healthy, balanced diet.
- Take precautions when working in an environment where substances or particles could be inhaled.
- Avoid excessive exposure to ultraviolet light.
- Avoid sources of oral irritation.

 ### CULTURAL CONSIDERATIONS

The incidence for oral cancer is different for different countries. Scientists believe that environmental rather than genetic risk factors are responsible for the differences. Oral cancer is much more common in Hungary and France and less common in Mexico and Japan than in the United States (ACS, 2000). The rates of oral cavity and base-of-tongue cancers are high in Bombay, India, as are the rates of nasopharyngeal and hypopharyngeal cancers in Hong Kong and South China. Moreover, nasopharyngeal cancer rates are high in Sephardic Jews, especially of Moroccan origin (Nageris, Elidan, Hansen, Ankhol, & Veshler, 1994). The high rates in Southeast Asia are attributed to a combination of genetic and viral factors; those in India are attributed to chewing betel nut with lime. When teaching people about risks that are derived from ethnically accepted behaviors, such as betel nut chewing, the nurse first needs to understand what role the practice has in the life and beliefs of the cultural group and the individual.

neurologic disorder. Dysphagia increases the risk for aspiration, and clients with dysphagia may require consultation with a speech therapist. Difficulty chewing, swallowing, or moving the tongue or jaws may be a late sign of oral cancer. Malocclusion may also cause difficulty chewing or swallowing.

Q Do you have a sore throat? Describe.

R Throat irritation and soreness are common with sinus drainage and may also occur with a viral or bacterial infection. A sore throat that persists without healing may signal throat cancer.

Q Do you experience hoarseness?

R Hoarseness is associated with upper respiratory infections, allergies, hypothyroidism, overuse of the voice, smoking or inhaling other irritants, and cancer of the larynx. If hoarseness lasts 2 weeks or longer, refer the client for further evaluation.

PAST HISTORY

Q Have you ever had any oral, nasal, or sinus surgery?

R Present symptoms may be related to past problems.

Q Do you have a history of sinus infections? Describe your symptoms. Do you use nasal sprays? (What type? How much? How often?)

R Some clients are more susceptible to sinus infections, which tend to recur. Overuse of nasal sprays may cause nasal irritation, nosebleeds, and rebound swelling.

FAMILY HISTORY

Q Is there a history of mouth, throat, nose, or sinus cancer in your family?

R There is a genetic risk factor for mouth, throat, nose, and sinus cancer.

LIFESTYLE AND HEALTH PRACTICES

Q Do you smoke or use smokeless tobacco? If so, how much? Are you interested in quitting this habit?

R Cigarette, pipe, or cigar smoking and use of smokeless tobacco increase a person's risk for oral cancer. Cancer of the cheek is linked to chewing tobacco. Clients who want to quit using tobacco may benefit from a referral to a smoking cessation program (see Risk Factors—Cancer of the Oral Cavity).

Q Do you drink alcohol? How much and how often?

R Excessive use of alcohol increases a person's risk for oral cancer.

Q Do you grind your teeth?

R Grinding the teeth (bruxism) may be a sign of stress or of slight malocclusion. The practice may also precipitate temporomandibular joint (TMJ) problems and pain.

Q Describe how you care for your teeth or dentures. How often do you brush and use dental floss? When was your last dental examination? If the client wears braces: How do you care for your braces? Do you avoid any specific types of foods?

R Proper brushing, flossing, and oral hygiene can prevent dental caries and gum disease. Regular dental checkups and screening can help detect the early signs of gum disease and oral cancer, which promotes early treatment. Clients with braces should avoid crunchy, sticky, and chewy foods when wearing braces. These foods can damage the braces and the teeth.

Q Do you brush your tongue?

R Cleaning the tongue is a way to prevent bad breath resulting from bacteria that accumulates on the posterior tongue.

Q If the client wears dentures: How do your dentures fit?

Elderly and some disabled clients may have difficulty caring properly for teeth or dentures because of poor vision or impaired dexterity.

R Poorly fitting dentures may lead to poor eating habits, a reluctance to speak freely, and mouth sores or leukoplakia (thick white patches of cells). Leukoplakia is a precancerous condition.

Collecting Objective Data

Examination of the mouth and throat can help the nurse detect abnormalities of the lips, gums, teeth, oral mucosa, tonsils, and uvula. This examination also allows for early detection of oral cancer. Examination of the nose and sinuses assists the nurse with detection of a deviated septum, patency of the nose and nasopharynx, and detection of sinus infection. In addition, assessment of the mouth, throat, nose, and sinuses provides the nurse with clues to the client's nutritional and respiratory status.

The mouth and nose examination can be very useful to the nurse in many situations, both in the hospital and the home. Detection of impaired oral mucous membranes or a poor dental condition may require a change in the client's diet. Additional mouth care may be needed to facilitate ingestion of food or to prevent infection of the gums (gingivitis). Detection of nasal septal deviation may help the nurse determine which nostril to use to insert a nasogastric tube or how to suction a client. In addition, assessing for nasal obstruction may explain the reason for mouth breathing.

Assessment of the mouth, throat, nose, and sinuses usually follows the examination of the head and neck. Techniques for this examination are fairly simple to perform. However, the nurse develops proficiency in interpreting findings with continued practice. Interpretation of findings may be guided by using the COLDSPA mnemonic for a more thorough exploration of signs and symptoms.

COLDSPA

CHARACTER: Describe the sign or symptom. How does it feel, look, sound, smell, and so forth?
ONSET: When did it begin?
LOCATION: Where is it? Does it radiate?
DURATION: How long does it last? Does it recur?
SEVERITY: How bad is it?
PATTERN: What makes it better: What makes it worse?
ASSOCIATED FACTORS: What other symptoms occur with it?

CLIENT PREPARATION

Ask the client to assume a sitting position with the head erect. It is best if the client's head is at your eye level. Explain the specific structures you will be examining, and tell the client who wears dentures, a retainer, or rubber bands on braces that they will need to be removed for an adequate oral examination. The client wearing dentures may feel embarrassed and concerned about his or her appearance and over the possibility of breath odor on removing the dentures. A gentle, yet confident and matter-of-fact approach may help the client feel more at ease.

EQUIPMENT AND SUPPLIES

- Gloves (wear gloves when examining any mucous membrane)
- 4 × 4-inch gauze pad
- Penlight
- Short, wide-tipped speculum attached to the head of an otoscope (see How to Use the Otoscope in Chapter 12)
- Tongue depressor
- Nasal speculum

KEY ASSESSMENT POINTS

- Identify and understand the relationship among the structures of the mouth and throat, nose, and sinuses.
- Obtain an accurate and thorough history of oral and nasal health.
- Explain to clients risk factors and prevention strategies for oral cancer.
- Refine examination techniques.
- Describe age-related changes of the oral cavity and nasal and sinus structures.
- Identify ethnocultural phenomena related to oral and nasal health.

(*text continues on page 246*)

PHYSICAL ASSESSMENT

ASSESSMENT PROCEDURE	NORMAL FINDINGS	ABNORMAL FINDINGS
MOUTH		
Inspect the Lips		
Observe lip consistency and color.	Lips are smooth and moist without lesions or swelling. Pink lips are normal in light-skinned clients as are bluish or freckled lips in some dark-skinned clients, especially those of Mediterranean descent. Lip pits (up to 4 mm deep and looking like cheilosis) are seen in the crease between the upper and lower lip in about 20% of African Americans and less frequently in Asians and Caucasians (Overfield, 1995).	Pallor around the lips (circumoral pallor) is seen in anemia and shock. Bluish (cyanotic) lips may result from cold or hypoxia. Reddish lips are seen in clients with ketoacidosis, carbon monoxide poisoning, and COPD with polycythemia. Swelling of the lips (edema) is common in local or systemic allergic or anaphylactic reactions. Additional abnormal findings are pictured in Display 13-1.

ASSESSMENT PROCEDURE	NORMAL FINDINGS	ABNORMAL FINDINGS

Inspect the Teeth and Gums

Ask the client to open the mouth. Note the number, color, condition, and alignment of the teeth.

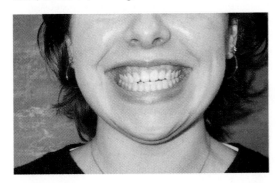

Retract the client's lips and cheeks to check gums for color and consistency.

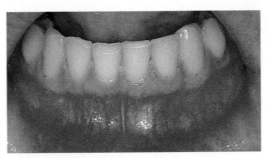

Lower gingiva (gums).

Inspect the Buccal Mucosa

Use a penlight and tongue depressor to retract the lips and cheeks to check color and consistency. Also note Stenson's ducts (parotid ducts) located on the buccal mucosa across from the second upper molars.

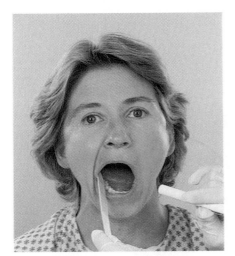

Inspecting the buccal mucosa.

Thirty-two pearly whitish teeth with smooth surfaces and edges. Upper molars should rest directly on the lower molars, and the front upper incisors should slightly override the lower incisors. Some clients normally have only 28 teeth if the four wisdom teeth do not erupt.

No repaired or decayed areas; no missing teeth or appliances.

Peg teeth (usually lateral incisors) occur in up to 8% of Asians, and occasionally in other cultural groups, especially those without third molars. Australian Aborigines and Melanesians may have four additional molars, totaling 36 teeth (Overfield, 1995).

Gums are pink, moist, and firm with tight margins to the tooth. No lesions or masses.

Pink in light-skinned clients, tissue pigmentation typically increases in dark-skinned clients. In both, tissue is smooth and moist without lesions. Stenson's ducts are visible with flow of saliva and with no redness, swelling, pain, or moistness in area. Fordyce spots or granules, yellowish-whitish raised spots, are normal ectopic sebaceous glands.

Oral mucosa is often drier and more fragile in the older client because the epithelial lining of the salivary glands degenerates.

Clients who smoke, drink large quantities of coffee or tea, or have an excessive intake of fluoride may have yellow or brownish teeth. Tooth decay (caries) may appear as brown dots or cover more extensive areas of chewing surfaces. Missing teeth can affect chewing as well as self-image A chalky white area in the tooth surface is a cavity that will turn darker with time. Malocclusion of teeth is seen when upper or lower incisors protrude. Poor occlusion of teeth can affect chewing, wearing down of teeth, speech, and self-image. White spots on teeth may result from antibiotic therapy.

Receding gums are abnormal in younger clients; in elderly clients, the teeth may appear longer because of age-related gingival recession, which is common.

Red, swollen gums that bleed easily are seen in gingivitis, scurvy (vitamin C deficiency), and leukemia. Receding red gums with loss of teeth are seen in periodontitis. Enlarged reddened gums (hyperplasia) that may cover some of the normally exposed teeth may be seen in pregnancy, puberty, leukemia, and use of some medications, such as phenytoin. A bluish-black or grey-white line along the gum line is seen in lead poisoning (see Display 13-1).

Leukoplakia may be seen in chronic irritation and smoking. Smokers may also have a yellow-brown coating on the tongue, which is not leukoplakia.

Leukoplakia is a precancerous lesion, and the client should be referred for evaluation. Whitish, curdlike patches that scrape off over reddened mucosa and bleed easily indicate "thrush" (Candida albicans) infection. Koplik's spots (tiny whitish spots that lie over reddened mucosa) are an early sign of the measles. Canker sores may be seen as may brown patches inside the cheeks of clients with adrenocortical insufficiency. See Display 13-1.

(continued)

ASSESSMENT PROCEDURE	NORMAL FINDINGS	ABNORMAL FINDINGS

Inspect and Palpate the Tongue

Ask client to stick out the tongue. Inspect for color, moisture, size, and texture. Observe for fasciculations (fine tremors), and check for midline protrusion. Palpate any lesions present for induration (hardness).

Tongue should be pink, moist, a moderate size, with papillae (little protuberances) present. A common variation is a fissured, topographic-map–like tongue, which is not unusual in older clients. No lesions are present.

Among possible abnormalities are deep longitudinal *fissures* seen in dehydration; a *black tongue* indicative of bismuth (PeptoBismol) toxicity: *black, hairy tongue*; a smooth, reddish, shiny tongue without papillae indicative of niacin or vitamin B_{12} deficiencies, certain anemias, and antineoplastic therapy (see Display 13-1). An enlarged tongue suggests hypothyroidism, acromegaly, or Down's syndrome, and angioneurotic edema of anaphylaxis. A very small tongue suggests malnutrition. An atrophied tongue or fasciculations point to cranial nerve (hypoglossal, CN 12) damage.

Fissured tongue. (Courtesy Dr. Michael Bennett.)

Ask the client to touch the tongue to the roof of mouth, and use a penlight to inspect ventral surface of tongue, frenulum, and the area under the tongue. Palpate the area if you see lesions, if the client is over age 50, or if the client uses tobacco or alcohol. Note any induration. Check also for a short frenulum that limits tongue motion (the origin of "tongue-tied").

The tongue's ventral surface is smooth, shiny, pink or slightly pale with visible veins and no lesions.

The older client may have varicose veins on the ventral surface of the tongue.

Leukoplakia, persistent lesions, ulcers, or nodules may indicate cancer and should be referred. Induration increases the likelihood of cancer.

Tip From the Experts   The area underneath the tongue is the most common site of oral cancer.

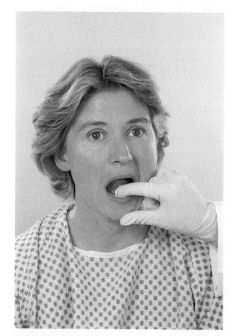

Palpating area under tongue.

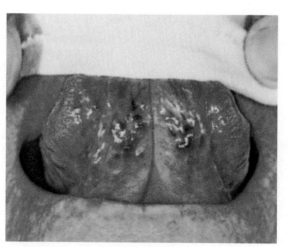

Varicose veins on ventral surface of tongue.

(continued)

ASSESSMENT PROCEDURE	NORMAL FINDINGS	ABNORMAL FINDINGS
Also inspect for Wharton's ducts—openings from the submandibular salivary glands—located on either side of the frenulum on the floor of the mouth.	The frenulum is midline; Wharton's ducts are visible with salivary flow or moistness in the area. The client has no swelling, redness, or pain.	Abnormal findings include lesions, ulcers, nodules, or hypertrophied duct openings on either side of frenulum.

To observe the sides of the tongue, use a square gauze pad to hold the client's tongue to each side. Palpate any lesions, ulcers, or nodules for induration.	No lesions, ulcers, or nodules are apparent.	Canker sores may be seen on the sides of the tongue in clients receiving certain kinds of chemotherapy. Leukoplakia, persistent lesions, ulcers, or nodules may indicate cancer and should be further evaluated medically. Induration increases the likelihood of cancer (see Display 13-1).

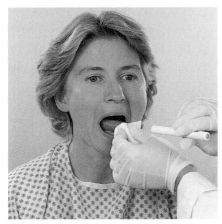

Inspecting side of tongue.

Tip From the Experts The side of the tongue is the most common site of tongue cancer.

Check the strength of the tongue. Place your fingers on the external surface of the client's cheek. Ask the client to press the tongue's tip against the inside of the cheek to resist pressure from your fingers. Repeat on the opposite cheek.	The tongue offers strong resistance.	Decreased tongue strength may occur with a defect of the twelfth cranial nerve — hypoglossal—or with a shortened frenulum that limits motion.
Check the anterior tongue's ability to taste by placing drops of sugar and salty water on the tip and sides of tongue with a tongue depressor.	The client can distinguish between sweet and salty.	Loss of taste discrimination occurs with zinc deficiency, a seventh cranial nerve (facial) defect, and certain medication use.

Inspect the Hard (Anterior) and Soft (Posterior) Palates and Uvula

Ask the client to open the mouth wide while you use a penlight to look at the roof. Observe color and integrity.	The hard palate is pale or whitish with firm, transverse rugae (wrinklelike folds).	A candidal infection may appear as thick white plaques on the hard palate. Deep purple, raised, or flat lesions may indicate a Kaposi's sarcoma (seen in clients with AIDS; see Display 13-1).
	A bony protuberance in the midline of the hard palate (called a torus palatinus) is a normal variation seen more often in females, Eskimos, Native Americans, and Asians. Palatine tissues are intact; the soft palate should be pinkish, movable, spongy, and smooth.	A yellow tint to the hard palate may indicate jaundice because bilirubin adheres to elastic tissue (collagen). An opening in the hard palate is known as a cleft palate.

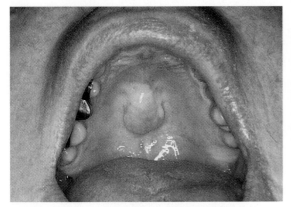

Torus palatinus. (Courtesy of Dr. Michael Bennett.)

(continued)

ASSESSMENT PROCEDURE	NORMAL FINDINGS	ABNORMAL FINDINGS

Note Odor

While the mouth is wide open, note any unusual or foul odor.

No unusual or foul odor is noted.

Fruity or acetone breath is associated with diabetic ketoacidosis. An ammonia odor is often associated with kidney disease. Foul odors may indicate an oral or respiratory infection, or tooth decay. Alcohol or tobacco use may be identified by breath odor. Fecal breath odor occurs in bowel obstruction; sulfur odor (fetor hepaticus) occurs in end-stage liver disease.

Inspect the Uvula

Apply a tongue depressor to the tongue (halfway between the tip and back of the tongue) and shine a penlight into the client's wide open mouth. Note the characteristics and positioning of the uvula. Ask the client to say "aaah" and watch for the uvula and soft palate to move.

The uvula is a fleshy, solid structure that hangs freely in the midline. No redness of or exudate from uvula or soft palate. Midline elevation of uvula and symmetric elevation of the soft palate.

A bifid uvula looks like it is split in two or partially severed. Clients with a bifid uvula may have a submucous cleft palate.

 A bifid uvula is common in Native Americans (see Display 13-1).

Unsymmetric movement or loss of movement may occur after a cerebrovascular accident (stroke) or with disruption of the vagus (glossopharyngeal) nerve, which can affect swallowing and result in choking.

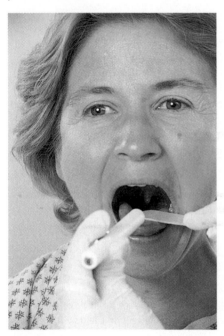

Inspecting the uvula.

Tip From the Experts Depress the tongue slightly off center to avoid eliciting the gag response.

(continued)

ASSESSMENT PROCEDURE	NORMAL FINDINGS	ABNORMAL FINDINGS
Inspect the Tonsils		
Using the tongue depressor to keep the mouth open wide, inspect the tonsils for color, size, and presence of exudate or lesions. Tonsils should be graded (Display 13-2).	Tonsils may be present or absent. They are normally pink and symmetric and may be enlarged to 1+ in healthy clients. No exudate, swelling, or lesions should be present.	Tonsils are red, enlarged (to 2+, 3+, or 4+), and covered with exudate in tonsillitis. They also may be indurated with patches of white or yellow exudate.
Inspect the Posterior Pharyngeal Wall		
Keeping the tongue depressor in place, shine the penlight on the back of the throat. Observe the color of the throat, and note any exudate or lesions.	Throat is normally pink without exudate or lesions.	A bright red throat with white or yellow exudate indicates pharyngitis. Yellowish mucus on throat may be seen with postnasal sinus drainage.

NOSE

ASSESSMENT PROCEDURE	NORMAL FINDINGS	ABNORMAL FINDINGS
Inspect and Palpate the External Nose		
Note nasal color, shape, consistency, and tenderness.	Color is the same as the rest of the face; the nasal structure is smooth and symmetric; the client reports no tenderness.	Nasal tenderness on palpation accompanies a local infection.
Check patency of air flow through the nostrils by occluding one nostril at a time and asking client to sniff.	Able to sniff through each nostril while other is occluded.	Client cannot sniff through a nostril that is not occluded, nor can he or she sniff or blow air through the nostrils. This may be a sign of swelling, rhinitis, or a foreign object obstructing the nostrils. A line across the tip of the nose just above the fleshy tip is common in clients with chronic allergies.
Inspect the Internal Nose		
To inspect the internal nose, use an otoscope with a short wide-tip attachment (or you can also use a nasal speculum and penlight). Use your nondominant hand to stabilize and gently tilt the client's head back. Insert the short wide tip of the otoscope into the client's nostril without touching the sensitive nasal septum. Slowly direct the otoscope back and up to view the nasal mucosa, nasal septum, the inferior and middle turbinates, and the nasal passage (the narrow space between the septum and the turbinates).	The nasal mucosa is dark pink, moist, and free of exudate. The nasal septum is intact and free of ulcers or perforations. Turbinates are dark pink (redder than oral mucosa), moist, and free of lesions. A deviated septum may appear to be an overgrowth of tissue. This is a normal finding as long as breathing is not obstructed.	Nasal mucosa is swollen and pale pink or bluish gray in clients with allergies. Nasal mucosa is red and swollen with upper respiratory infection. Exudate is common with infection and may range from large amounts of watery discharge to thick yellow-green purulent discharge. Bleeding (epistaxis) or crusting may be noted on lower anterior part of nasal septum with local irritation. Ulcers of the nasal mucosa or a perforated septum may be seen with use of cocaine, trauma, chronic infection, or chronic nose picking. Small, pale, round, firm overgrowths or masses on mucosa (polyps) are seen in clients with chronic allergies (see Display 13-1).

(continued)

ASSESSMENT PROCEDURE	NORMAL FINDINGS	ABNORMAL FINDINGS

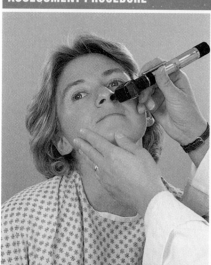

Inspecting the internal nose using an otoscope and wide-tipped attachment.

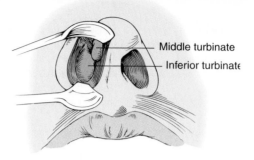

Middle turbinate
Inferior turbinate

Normal internal nose.

🎗 **Tip From the Experts** Position the otoscope's handle to the side to improve your view of the structures. If an otoscope is unavailable, use a penlight and hold the tip of the nose slightly up. A nasal speculum with a penlight also facilitates good visualization.

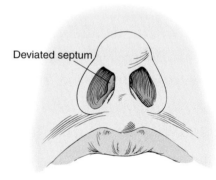

Deviated septum

Deviated septum.

SINUSES

Palpate the Sinuses

When an infection is suspected, the nurse can examine the sinuses through palpation, percussion, and transillumination. Palpate the frontal sinuses by using your thumbs to press up on the brow on each side of nose.

Frontal and maxillary sinuses are nontender to palpation, and no crepitus is evident.

Frontal or maxillary sinuses are tender to palpation in clients with allergies or sinus infection. If the client has a large amount of exudate, you may feel crepitus upon palpation over the maxillary sinuses.

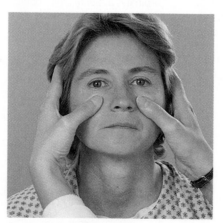

Palpating the frontal sinuses.

Palpating the maxillary sinuses.

Palpate the maxillary sinuses by pressing with thumbs up on the maxillary sinuses.

(continued)

ASSESSMENT PROCEDURE	NORMAL FINDINGS	ABNORMAL FINDINGS

Percuss the Sinuses

Lightly tap (percuss) over the frontal sinuses and over the maxillary sinuses for tenderness.

The sinuses are not tender on percussion.

The frontal and maxillary sinuses are tender upon percussion in clients with allergies or sinus infection.

Transilluminate the Sinuses

If sinus tenderness was detected during palpation and percussion, transillumination will let you see if the sinuses are filled with fluid or pus. Transilluminate the frontal sinuses by holding a strong, narrow light source snugly under the eyebrows (the room should be dark). Use your other hand to shield the light. Repeat this technique for the other frontal sinus.

A red glow transilluminates the frontal sinuses. This indicates a normal, air-filled sinus.

Absence of a red glow usually indicates a sinus filled with fluid or pus.

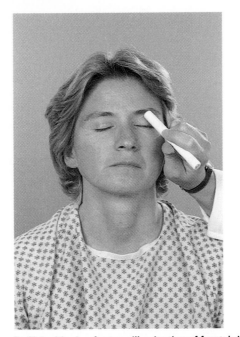 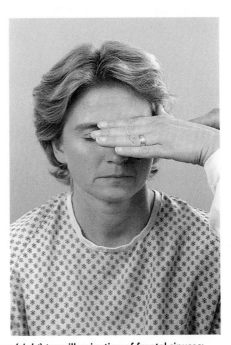

(*Left*) Positioning for transillumination of frontal sinuses; (*right*) transillumination of frontal sinuses; note the red glow. (This photograph shows a lighted room because of a special photographic technique. In practice, the room must be dark to see the red glow. © B. Proud).

(continued)

ASSESSMENT PROCEDURE	NORMAL FINDINGS	ABNORMAL FINDINGS

Transilluminate the maxillary sinuses by holding a strong, narrow light source over the maxillary sinus and asking the client to open his or her mouth. Repeat this technique for the other maxillary sinus.

A red glow transilluminates the maxillary sinuses. The red glow will be seen on the hard palate.

Absence of a red glow usually indicates a sinus filled with fluid, pus, or thick mucus (from chronic sinusitis).

 Tip From the Experts Upper dentures should be removed so the light is not blocked.

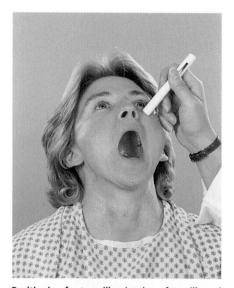

Positioning for transillumination of maxillary sinuses.

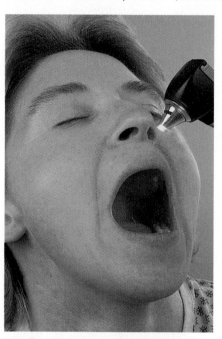

Transillumination of maxillary sinuses; note the red glow. (This photograph shows a lighted room because of a special photographic technique. In practice, the room must be dark for you to see the red glow.) (Photos © B. Proud.)

DISPLAY 13-1. Abnormalities of the Mouth, Throat, Nose, and Sinuses

ABNORMAL FINDINGS

Of the many abnormal findings associated with disorders of the mouth, throat, nose, and sinuses, the ones pictured below are some of the most common.

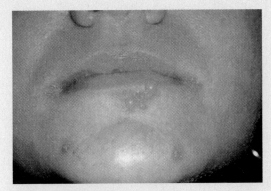

Herpes simplex type I.

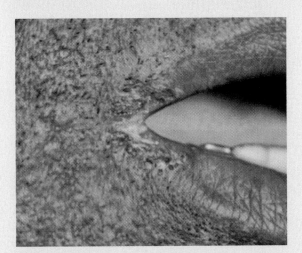

Cheilosis of lips.

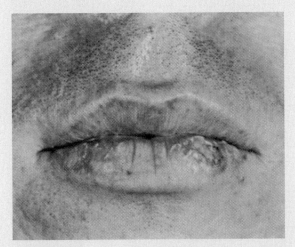

Carcinoma of lip.

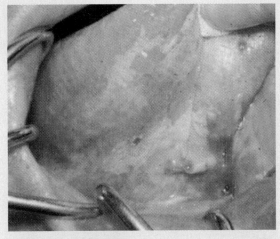

Leukoplakia (ventral surface.)

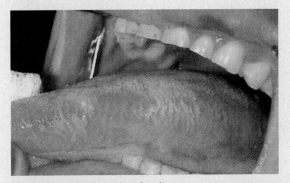

Hairy leukoplakia (lateral surface.)

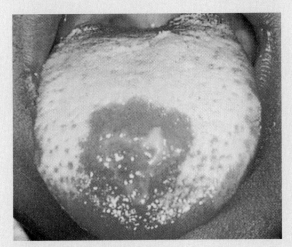

Candida albicans infection (thrush).

(continued)

DISPLAY 13-1. Abnormalities of the Mouth, Throat, Nose, and Sinuses (Continued)

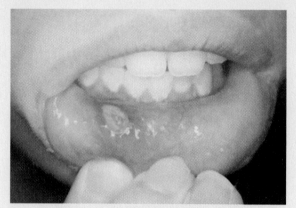

Canker sore.

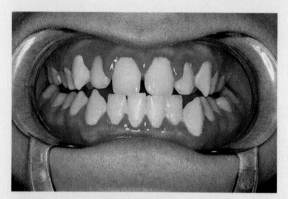

Gingivitis. (Dr. Michael Bennett.)

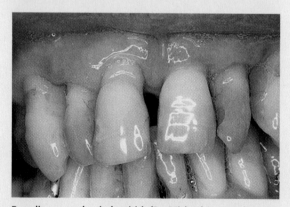

Receding gums (periodontitis). (Dr. Michael Bennett.)

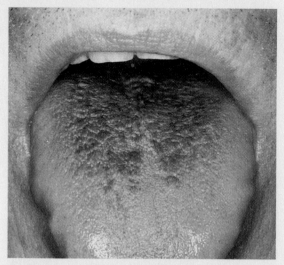

Black hairy tongue. (Dr. Michael Bennett.)

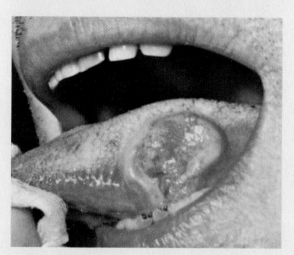

Carcinoma of tongue.

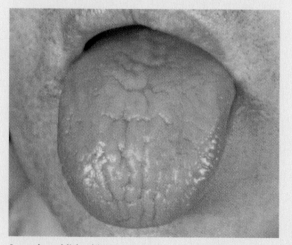

Smooth, reddish, shiny tongue without papillae due to vitamin B_{12} deficiency.

(continued)

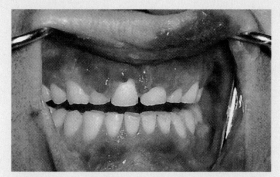

Kaposi's sarcoma lesions.

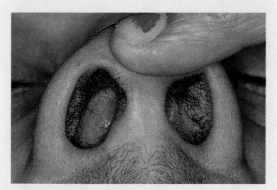

Nasal polyp. (© 1992 J. Barrabe.)

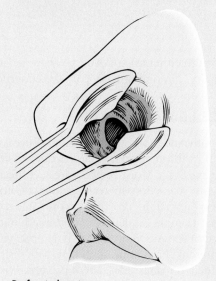

Perforated septum.

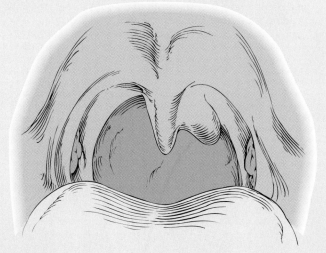

Bifid uvula.

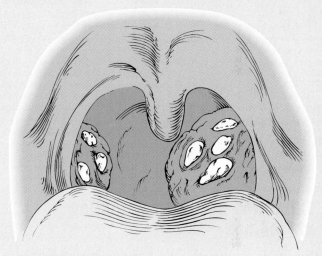

Acute tonsillitis and pharyngitis.

DISPLAY 13-2. Detecting and Grading Tonsillitis

In a client who has both tonsils and a sore throat, tonsilitis can be identified and ranked with a grading scale from 1 to 4 as follows:

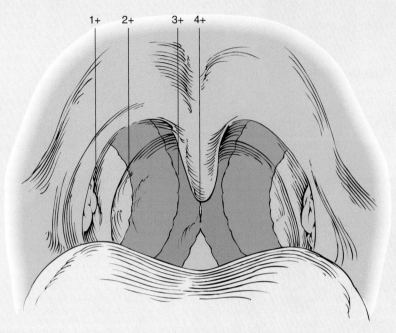

1+   Tonsils are visible.
2+   Tonsils are midway between tonsillar pillars and uvula.
3+   Tonsils touch the uvula.
4+   Tonsils touch each other.

Validation and Documentation of Findings

Validate the mouth, throat, nose, and sinus assessment data that you have collected. This is necessary to verify that the data are reliable and accurate. Document the assessment data following the health care facility or agency policy.

EXAMPLE OF SUBJECTIVE DATA

Client describes the condition of mouth, throat, and nose as "adequate." No history of past oral or nasal surgery. Has 32 permanent teeth. Had four teeth filled for cavities several years ago as a child. Brushes teeth twice a day and uses dental floss each evening. Occasional mild bleeding with flossing. Never needed braces. Receives regular dental checkups twice a year. Has occasional sinus headaches (one to two per year) and minor sore throats due to sinus drainage. Relieved with over-the-counter oral decongestants and acetaminophen (Tylenol). Nasal discharge clear to purulent occasionally. No oral or nasal lesions noted by client. Does not smoke or chew tobacco. No difficulty breathing through either nostril. Able to chew and swallow without difficulty. No oral or nasal pain or tenderness.

EXAMPLE OF OBJECTIVE DATA

Lips pink, smooth, and moist without lesions. Buccal mucosa pink, moist, and without exudate. Parotid ducts visible with no redness or swelling. Moist bubbles are seen near ducts. Thirty-two white to yellowish teeth present. Gums pink without redness or swelling. Protrudes geographic tongue in midline with no tremors. Equal bilateral strength in tongue. Ventral surface of tongue smooth and shiny pink with small visible veins present. Frenulum in midline with visible submandibular ducts on each side. Torus palatinus visible on whitish hard palate. Soft palate smooth and pink. Midline and symmetric elevation of uvula and soft palate with phonation. Tonsillar pillars pink and symmetric. Tonsils absent.

Nose somewhat large but smooth and symmetric. Able to sniff and blow through each nostril. Nasal septum slightly deviated to left, but does not obstruct air flow. Inferior and middle turbinates dark pink, moist, and free of lesions. No purulent drainage noted. Frontal and maxillary sinuses transilluminate and are nontender to palpation and percussion.

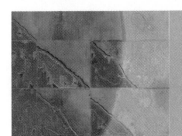

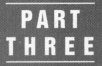

The text section Diagnostic Reasoning: Possible Conclusions provides an overview of common conclusions that you may reach after the peripheral vascular assessment, and the case study that follows shows how to analyze peripheral vascular assessment data for a specific client. Finally, you have an opportunity to analyze data in the critical thinking exercise that appears in Chapter 13 of the student laboratory manual.

Diagnostic Reasoning: Possible Conclusions

Write down your hunches about each cue cluster. Decide whether the problem can be treated with nursing interventions alone. If not, consider monitoring for collaborative problems or referring for medical problems.

SELECTED NURSING DIAGNOSES

After collecting subjective and objective data pertaining to the mouth, throat, nose, and sinuses, you will need to identify abnormal findings and cluster the data to reveal any significant patterns or abnormalities. These data will then be used to make clinical judgments (nursing diagnoses: wellness, risk, or actual) about the status of the client's mouth, throat, nose, and sinuses. The following is a listing of selected nursing diagnoses that you may identify when analyzing data for this part of the assessment.

Nursing Diagnoses (Wellness)

- Opportunity to enhance effective management of the teeth and gums
- Health-Seeking Behaviors: Requests information on how to quit smoking

Nursing Diagnoses (Risk)

- Risk for Aspiration related to decreased or absent gag reflex
- Risk for Imbalanced Nutrition: Less Than Body Requirements related to poorly fitting dentures or gum disease
- Risk for Infection of gums related to poor oral hygiene

- Risk for Injury to teeth and gums related to participation in active sports and lack of knowledge of protective mouth gear

Nursing Diagnoses (Actual)

- Ineffective Health Maintenance related to poor oral hygiene
- Bathing/Hygiene Self-Care Deficit: Oral mouth care related to paralysis or decreased cognitive functions
- Disturbed Sensory Perception: Olfactory related to local irritation of nasal mucosa, impairment of cranial nerve I, decrease in olfactory bulb function secondary to nasal obstruction
- Impaired Oral Mucous Membranes related to poor oral hygiene or dehydration
- Impaired Swallowing related to impaired neurologic or neuromuscular function (ie, CVA, damage to cranial nerves V, VII, IX, or X, cerebral palsy, myasthenia gravis, muscular dystrophy, cerebral palsy)
- Pain related to chronic sinusitis or inflammation of oral mucous membranes (gingivitis, peridontitis, canker sores)
- Disturbed Sensory Perception: Gustatory related to impairment of cranial nerve VII or IX, reduction of number of taste buds secondary to the aging process
- Imbalanced Nutrition: Less Than Body Requirements related to decreased appetite secondary to decreased sense of taste and smell and social isolation

SELECTED COLLABORATIVE PROBLEMS

After grouping the data, it may become apparent that certain collaborative problems emerge. Remember, collaborative problems differ from nursing diagnoses in that they cannot be prevented by nursing intervention. However, these physiologic complications of medical conditions can be detected and monitored by the nurse. In addition, the nurse can use physician- and nurse-prescribed interventions to minimize the complications of these problems. The nurse may also have to refer the client in such situations for further treatment of the problem. Following are a list of collaborative problems that may be identified when obtaining a general impression. These problems are worded as Potential Complications (or PC), followed by the problem.

- PC: Nosebleed
- PC: Sinus infection
- PC: Stomatitis
- PC: Gum infection (gingivitis, peridontitis)
- PC: Oral lesions
- PC: Laryngeal edema

MEDICAL PROBLEMS

After grouping the data, it may become apparent that the client has signs and symptoms that may require medical diagnosis and treatment. Referral to a primary care provider is necessary.

Diagnostic Reasoning: Case Study

The case study presents assessment data for a specific client. It is followed by an analysis of the data, working out the seven key steps to arrive at specific conclusions.

Jonathan Miller (JM), a 22-year-old college student, visits the student health service in mid-December complaining of severe throat pain ("like swallowing razor blades"), swollen lymph nodes, chills, fever, general fatigue, and anorexia. He admitted that he had been studying "day and night" for final exams and had "only one more to go." "This is the third time I've had this problem this year," he related. "I didn't even bother coming in the first or second time. I just stayed in bed between classes and treated myself."

Upon examination, you note that his face and neck are flushed, with dark circles underlining his eyes. His blood pressure is 126/72 rt. arm; pulse is 104; respirations are 24; and oral temperature reads 103.2°F/39.6°C. When inspecting his throat, you find erythema and edema of the pharynx and uvula with white, patchy exudate on the tonsilar areas. Tonsils are 3+ and injected. Cervical and retropharyngeal lymph nodes are grossly palpable and very tender.

1 Identify abnormal data and strengths (in both subjective and objective data).

SUBJECTIVE DATA

- Complains of severe throat pain ("like swallowing razor blades")
- Complains of swollen, tender lymph nodes; chills; fever; general fatigue; and anorexia
- Studying "day and night" for final exams
- ". . . third time I've had this problem this year"
- Did not seek health care with first two episodes of sore throat; treated self

OBJECTIVE DATA

- Flushed face and neck, dark circles under eyes
- BP 126/72, P 104, R 24
- Temp. 103.2°F
- Erythema and edema of the pharynx and uvula
- Tonsils are 3+ and injected
- White, patchy exudate on the tonsilar areas
- Cervical and retropharyngeal lymph nodes grossly palpable

2 Cue Clusters	**3** Inferences	**4** Possible Nursing Diagnoses	**5** Defining Characteristics	**6** Confirm or Rule Out
A • Complains of severe throat pain • Erythema/edema of pharynx/uvula • White, patchy exudate on tonsils • Tender, palpable lymph nodes • General fatigue and anorexia • BP 126/72, P 104, R 24	Signs and symptoms suggest pharyngeal and tonsillar inflammation. Client probably needs a medical referral. Pain upon swallowing can interfere with adequate nutrition.	Risk for Imbalanced Nutrition: Less Than Body Requirements related to anorexia and increased metabolic need secondary to throat pain and systemic response to possible infection	*Major:* Potential metabolic need in excess of intake *Minor:* None	Confirm because it meets the major defining characteristic and client validation. Collecting information about intake and output and weight loss could allow a change from a risk to an actual nursing diagnosis. Accept diagnosis because it meets both major and minor defining characteristics and has client validation. This information is needed to validate etiology and guide interventions.
		Pain related to possible knowledge deficit of appropriate pain management strategies	*Major:* Subjective communication of pain descriptors *Minor:* Increased pulse and respiration (although these may be related to hyperthermia)	

2 Cue Clusters	**3** Inferences	**4** Possible Nursing Diagnoses	**5** Defining Characteristics	**6** Confirm or Rule Out
B • Flushed face and neck, dark circles under eyes • Temp 103.2°F • P 100, R 24 • Chills, fever, fatigue	GAS—systemic response to possible throat infection	Hyperthermia	*Major:* Temperature greater than 100°F (103.6°F) *Minor:* Flushed skin, tachycardia, tachypnea, fatigue	This diagnosis meets the defining characteristics, but there is no condition that the nurse can treat; better placed as a collaborative problem.
C • Studying "day and night" for final exams • "... third time I've had this problem this year" • Did not seek health care with first two episodes of sore throat; treated self	Describing unhealthful behavior and not seeking treatment for illness appropriately	Ineffective Health Maintenance related to inadequate knowledge of practices to promote wellness during periods of stress	*Major:* Reports unhealthy practices (studying day and night and treating previous sore throats per self) *Minor:* None	Accept diagnosis because it meets major defining characteristics and is validated by client.
		Ineffective Management of Therapeutic Regimen related to attempting to self-treat illness		
		Ineffective Management of Therapeutic Regimen related to attempting to self-treat illness	*Major:* None *Minor:* Implied (verbalized not seeking medical treatment for previous illness)	Rule out this diagnosis because it does not meet defining characteristics. Ineffective Health Maintenance is the more appropriate diagnosis.

7 Document conclusions.

The following nursing diagnoses are appropriate for the client at this time:

• Risk for Imbalanced Nutrition: Less Than Body Requirements related to anorexia and increased metabolic need secondary to throat pain and systemic response to possible infection
• Acute Pain related to possible knowledge deficit of appropriate pain-management strategies
• Ineffective Health Maintenance related to inadequate knowledge of practices to promote wellness during periods of stress.

Collaborative problems related to the medical diagnosis could include:

• PC: Hyperthermia
• PC: Otitis media

JM needs an immediate referral to the primary care provider to diagnose and treat his throat condition.

REFERENCES AND SELECTED READINGS

Anonymous. (1995). Practice guidelines: Pharyngitis/tonsillitis. *ORL—Head & Neck Nursing, 13*(3), 26–27.

———. (1994). Chemosensory dysfunction (smell and taste disorders). *ORL—Head & Neck Nursing, 12*(3), 26–27.

Bartkiw, T. P., Pyrin, B. R., & Brown, D. H. (1995). Diagnosis and management of nasal fractures. *International Journal of Trauma Nursing, 1*(1), 11–18.

Bowsher, J. M., Boyle, S., & Griffith, J. (1999). Oral care. *Nursing Standard, 13*(37), 31.

Dibble, S. I., Shiba, G., MacPhail, L., & Dodd, M. J. (1996). MacDibbs mouth assessment. *Cancer Practice: A Multidisciplinary Journal of Cancer Care, 4*(3), 135–140.

Freer, S. K. (2000). Use of an oral assessment tool to improve practice. *Professional Nurse, 15*(10), 635–637.

Gilmurry, B. (2000). Wheezing, breathlessness, and cough—Is it really asthma? A look at vocal cord dysfunction. *Canadian Journal of Respiratory Therapy, 35*(4), 28–31.

Krejci, C. B., & Bissada, N. F. (2000). Periodontitis—The risks for its development. *General Dentistry, 48*(4), 430–436.

Krouse, J. H., & Krouse, H. J. (1999). Introduction to sinus disease—Part II. Diagnosis and treatment. *ORL—Head & Neck Nursing, 17*(3), 6–17.

Landry, S. T. (2000). Alternatives: Healthy teeth from the inside out. *Health (San Francisco), 14*(2), 82, 86, 89.

Leslie, M. L. (1995). Adolescent smokeless tobacco use: A health promotion issue for ORL nurses. *ORL—Head & Neck Nursing, 13*(3), 12–14.

McKennis, A. T., & Waddington, C. (1994). Unilateral vocal cord paralsis. *ORL—Head & Neck Nursing, 12*(1), 9–13.

Risk Factors—Cancer of the Oral Cavity

American Cancer Society (ACS). (2000). Oral Cavity and Oropharyngeal Cancer Resource Center. Available: www.cancer.org/cancerinfo/.

Nageris, B., Elidan, J., Hansen, M., Ankhol, O., & Veshler, Z. (1994). Nasopharyngeal carcinoma among the population in Jerusalem. *American Journal of Otolaryngology, 15*(3), 190–192.

For additional information on this book, be sure to visit http://connection.lww.com.

Thoracic and Lung Assessment

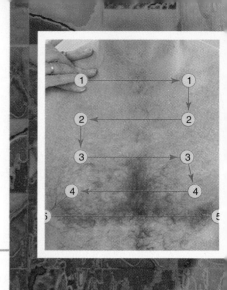

14

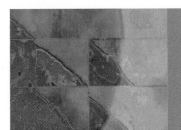

The lungs, along with the distal portion of the trachea and the bronchi, are contained in the thorax and constitute the lower respiratory system. The outer structure of the thorax is referred to as the *thoracic cage*, whereas the respiratory components are contained inside an area known as the *thoracic cavity*. A thorough assessment of the lower respiratory system must focus on the external chest as well as the respiratory components contained in the thorax.

Thorax

The term *thorax* identifies the portion of the body extending from the base of the neck superiorly to the level of the diaphragm inferiorly. This structure, also known as the thoracic cage, is constructed of the sternum, 12 pairs of ribs, 12 thoracic vertebrae, muscles, and cartilage. It provides support and protection for many important organs, including those of the lower respiratory system. The thorax consists of the anterior thoracic cage (Fig. 14-1) and the posterior thoracic cage (Fig. 14-2). The structures of the anterior and posterior thoracic cage, and several important landmarks that aid in examining thorax and lungs, are discussed in the following sections.

STERNUM

The sternum, or breastbone, lies in the center of the chest anteriorly and is divided into three parts: The manubrium, the body, and the xiphoid process. The clavicles (collar bones) extend from the manubrium to the acromion of the scapula. The manubrium connects laterally with the clavicles and the first two pairs of ribs.

A U-shaped indentation located on the superior border of the manubrium is an important landmark known as the *suprasternal notch*. A few centimeters below the suprasternal notch, a bony ridge can be palpated at the point where the manubrium articulates with the body of the sternum. This landmark, often referred to as the *sternal angle* (or angle of Louis), is also the location of the second pair of ribs and becomes a reference point for counting ribs and intercostal spaces.

RIBS AND THORACIC VERTEBRAE

The 12 pairs of ribs constitute the main structure of the thoracic cage. They are numbered superiorly to inferiorly,

the uppermost pair being number one. Each pair of ribs has a corresponding pair of intercostal spaces located immediately inferior to it. Anteriorly, the first seven pairs articulate with the sternum by way of costal cartilages. The first pair of ribs curve up immediately under the clavicles so only a small portion of these ribs and the first interspaces are palpable. The second ribs and intercostal spaces are easily located adjacent to the sternal angle. Ribs two through six are easy to count anteriorly because of their articulation with the sternal body.

The next four pairs of ribs (seven through ten) connect to the cartilages of the pair lying superior to them rather than to the sternum (see Fig. 14-1). This configuration forms an angle between the right and left costal margins meeting at the level of the xiphoid process. This angle, commonly referred to as the *costal angle*, is an important landmark for assessment. It is normally less than 90 degrees but may be increased in instances of long-standing hyperinflation of the lungs, as in emphysema. The 11th and 12th pairs of ribs are called "floating" ribs because they do not connect to either the sternum or another pair of ribs anteriorly. Instead, they are attached posteriorly to the vertebra, and their anterior tips are free and palpable (see Fig. 14-2).

The ribs are more difficult to palpate posteriorly. Each pair of ribs articulates with its respective thoracic vertebra. The spinous process of the seventh cervical vertebra (C7), also called the *vertebra prominens*, can be easily felt with the client's neck flexed. The process immediately inferior to the vertebra prominens is the first thoracic vertebra, which is adjacent to the posterior aspect of the first rib. When counting the spinous processes, it is helpful to know that they align with their corresponding ribs only to the fourth thoracic vertebra (T4). After this, the spinous processes angle downward from their own vertebral body and can be palpated over the vertebral body and rib below. The lower tip of each scapula is at the level of the seventh or eighth rib when the client's arms are at his or her side (see Fig. 14-2).

Vertical Reference Lines

By counting the ribs, an examiner can describe the location of a finding vertically. However, to describe a location around the circumference of the chest wall, imaginary lines running vertically on the chest wall are used. On the anterior chest,

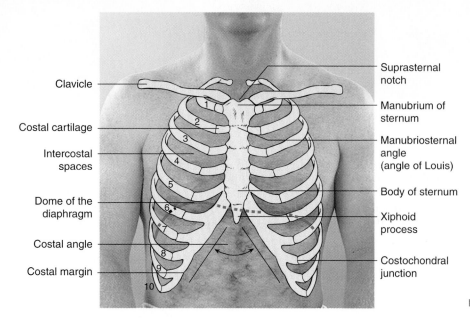

FIGURE 14-1. Anterior thoracic cage.

these lines are known as the *midsternal line* and the *right and left midclavicular lines* (Fig. 14-3).

The posterior thorax includes the vertebral (or spinal) line and the right and left scapular lines, which extend through the inferior angle of the scapulae when the arms are at the client's side (Fig. 14-4).

The lateral aspect of the thorax is divided into three parallel lines. The *midaxillary line* runs from the apex of the axillae to the level of the 12th rib. The *anterior axillary line* extends from the anterior axillary fold along the anterolateral aspect of the thorax, whereas the *posterior axillary line* runs from the posterior axillary fold down the posterolateral aspect of the chest wall (Fig. 14-5).

Thoracic Cavity

The thoracic cavity consists of the mediastinum and the lungs. The mediastinum refers to a central area in the thoracic cavity that contains the trachea, esophagus, heart, and great vessels. These structures are assessed in separate chapters. The lungs lie on each side of the mediastinum.

LUNGS

The lungs are two cone-shaped, elastic structures suspended within the thoracic cavity. The *apex* of each lung extends slightly above the clavicle, whereas the *base* is at the level of

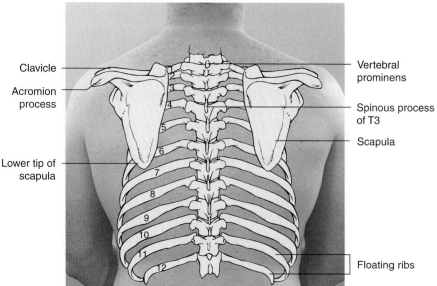

FIGURE 14-2. Posterior thoracic cage.

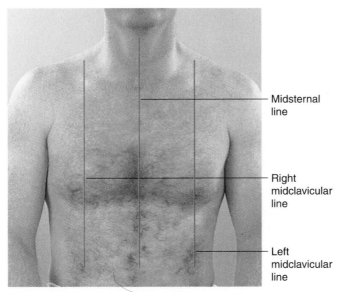

FIGURE 14-3. Anterior vertical lines, imaginary landmarks.

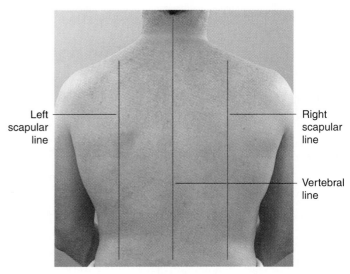

FIGURE 14-4. Posterior vertical lines, imaginary landmarks.

the diaphragm. At the point of the midclavicular line on the anterior surface of the thorax, the lung extends to approximately the sixth rib. Laterally, lung tissue reaches the level of the eighth rib, and, posteriorly, the lung base is at about the tenth rib (Fig. 14-6).

Although the lungs are paired, they are not completely symmetric. Both are divided into lobes by fissures. However, the right lung is made up of three lobes, whereas the left lung contains only two lobes. Fissures separating the lobes run obliquely through the chest, making the lobes appear as diagonal sloping segments. Anteriorly, the horizontal fissure separating the right upper lobe from the middle

lobe extends from the fifth rib in the right mid-axillary line to the third intercostal space or fourth rib at the right sternal border. Posteriorly, oblique fissures extend on both the right and left lungs from the level of T3 to the sixth rib at the midclavicular line.

In the healthy adult, during deep inspiration, the lungs move down to about the eighth intercostal space anteriorly and the twelfth intercostal space posteriorly. During expiration, the lungs rise to the fifth or sixth intercostal space anteriorly and tenth posteriorly.

It is important for the examiner to remember that most lung tissue in the upper lobes of both lungs is located on the

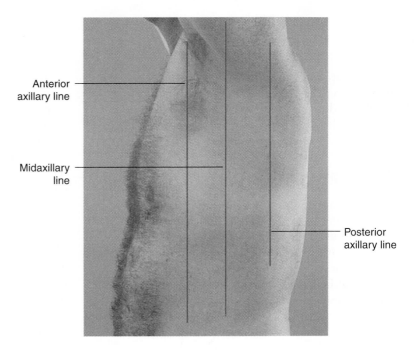

FIGURE 14-5. Lateral vertical lines, imaginary landmarks.

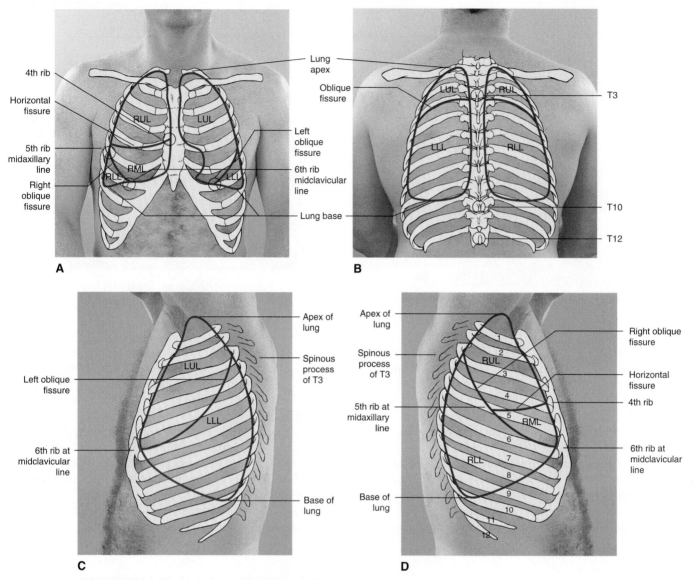

FIGURE 14-6. (**A**) Anterior view of lung position. (**B**) Posterior view of lung position. (**C**) Lateral view of left lung position. (**D**) Lateral view of right lung position.

anterior surface of the chest. Similarly, the lower lobes of both lungs are primarily located toward the posterior surface of the chest wall. In addition, the right middle lobe of the lung does not extend to the posterior side of the thoracic wall and, thus, must be assessed from the anterior surface alone.

PLEURAL MEMBRANES

The thoracic cavity is lined by a thin, double-layered serous membrane collectively referred to as the pleura (Fig. 14-7). The *parietal pleura* lines the chest cavity, whereas the *visceral pleura* covers the external surfaces of the lungs. The *pleural space* lies between the two pleural layers.

In the healthy adult, the two layers of pleura are moistened with a lubricating substance. Continual suction of excess fluid into lymph channels maintains a slight negative pressure between the parietal and visceral layers of the

pleura. This results in the lungs being held to the thoracic cavity.

However, the lubricating effect of the pleural fluid allows for free movement of the lungs during respiration. Because the pleural space is one of the physiologic third spaces for body fluid storage, severe dehydration will reduce the volume of pleural fluid, resulting in the increased transmission of lung sounds and a possible friction rub.

TRACHEA AND BRONCHI

The trachea lies anterior to the esophagus and is approximately 10 to 12 cm long in an adult (see Fig. 14-7). This flexible structure begins at the level of the cricoid cartilage in the neck and bifurcates at the level of the sternal angle. The trachea is made up of C-shaped rings of hyaline cartilage that help maintain its shape and prevent its collapse during respiration.

At the level of the sternal angle, the trachea bifurcates into the right and left main bronchi. Both bronchi are at an oblique position in the mediastinum and enter the lungs at the hilus. The right main bronchus is shorter and more vertical than the left main bronchus, making aspirated objects more likely to enter the right lung than he left.

The bronchi and trachea represent "dead space" in the respiratory system, where air is transported but no gas exchange takes place. They function primarily as a passageway for both inspired and expired air. In addition, the trachea and bronchi are lined with mucous membranes containing cilia. These hairlike projections help sweep dust, foreign bodies, and bacteria that have been trapped by the mucus toward the mouth for removal.

Inspired air travels through the trachea into the main bronchi and continues through the system as the bronchi repeatedly bifurcate into smaller passageways known as *bronchioles.* Eventually, the bronchioles terminate at the alveolar ducts, and air is channeled into the alveolar sacs, which contain the alveoli (see Fig. 14-7). Alveolar sacs contain a number of alveoli in a cluster formation (resembling grapes), creating millions of interalveolar walls that serve to increase the surface area available for gas exchange.

Mechanics of Breathing

The purpose of respiration is to maintain an adequate oxygen level in the blood to support cellular life. By providing oxygen and eliminating carbon dioxide, respiration assists in the rapid compensation for metabolic acid–base defects; however, changes in the respiratory pattern can cause acid–base imbalances.

External respiration, or ventilation, is the mechanical act of breathing and is accomplished by expansion of the chest, both vertically and horizontally. Vertical expansion is accomplished through contraction of the diaphragm. Horizontal expansion occurs as intercostal muscles lift the sternum and elevate the ribs, resulting in an increase in anteroposterior diameter.

As a result of this enlargement of the chest cavity, a slight negative pressure is created in the lungs in relation to the atmospheric pressure, resulting in an inflow of air into the lungs. This process, called *inspiration,* is shown in Figure 14-8. Expiration is mostly passive in nature and occurs with relaxation of the intercostal muscles and the diaphragm. As the diaphragm relaxes, forces within the abdomen and chest cage cause it to assume a domed shape. The resultant decrease in the size of the chest cavity creates a positive pressure, forcing air out of the lungs.

Breathing patterns change according to cellular demands—often without awareness on the part of the indi-

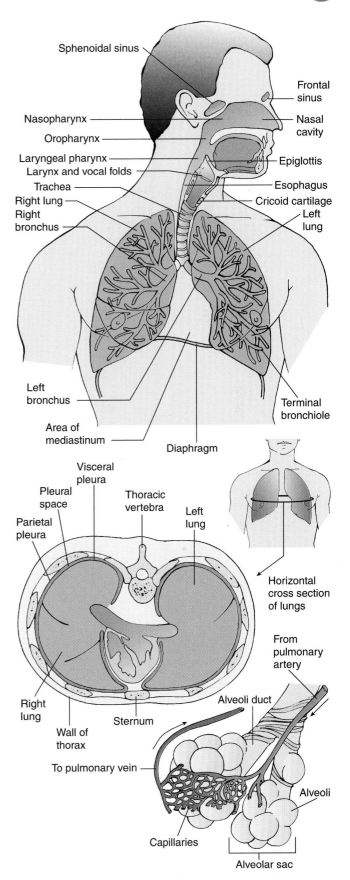

FIGURE 14-7. Major structures of the respiratory system.

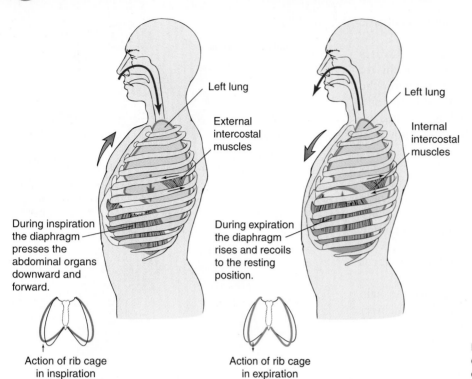

Left lung

External intercostal muscles

Left lung

Internal intercostal muscles

During inspiration the diaphragm presses the abdominal organs downward and forward.

During expiration the diaphragm rises and recoils to the resting position.

Action of rib cage in inspiration

Action of rib cage in expiration

FIGURE 14-8. Mechanics of normal—not deep, not shallow—inspiration (*left*) and expiration (*right*).

vidual. Such involuntary control of respiration is the work of the medulla and pons, located in the brain stem. The hypothalamus and the sympathetic nervous system also play a role in involuntary control of respiration in response to emotional changes, such as fear or excitement.

Changes in breathing patterns occur as a result of hormonal regulation, changes in oxygen or carbon dioxide levels in the blood, or changes in the hydrogen ion (pH) level. Under normal circumstances, the strongest stimulus to breathe is an increase of carbon dioxide in the blood (hypercapnia). A decrease in oxygen (hypoxemia) also increases respiration but is less effective than a rise in carbon dioxide levels.

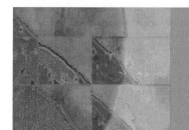

Collecting Subjective Data

Subjective data related to the thoracic and lung assessment provide many clues concerning risk for the development of lung disorders. Data concerning the client's level of functioning are also important because certain respiratory problems greatly impact a person's ability to perform activities of daily living.

When obtaining subjective data, the examiner must be careful to avoid judgmental approaches to poor health practices. Smoking, for example, has become a stigmatized addiction in our society. Health care providers should avoid conveying feelings of intolerance when caring for a smoker with respiratory complaints.

Nursing History

Also when collecting subjective data, the examiner must remember to follow up on the client's signs and symptoms. In addition to the following questions, a helpful resource to use as a guideline is the COLDSPA mnemonic.

COLDSPA

CHARACTER: Describe the sign or symptom. How does it feel, look, sound, smell, and so forth?
ONSET: When did it begin?
LOCATION: Where is it? Does it radiate?
DURATION: How long does it last? Does it recur?
SEVERITY: How bad is it?
PATTERN: What makes it better? What makes it worse?
ASSOCIATED FACTORS: What other symptoms occur with it?

CURRENT SYMPTOMS

Question Do you ever experience difficulty breathing? Describe. Do you have difficulty breathing when you are resting, or do any specific activities cause the difficulty breathing? Do you have any other symptoms when you have difficulty breathing?

Rationale Dyspnea (difficulty breathing) can indicate a number of health problems, most of which are respiratory

in nature. The presence of associated symptoms may indicate problems in other body systems. Edema or angina that occurs with dyspnea may indicate a cardiovascular problem. Gradual onset of dyspnea is usually indicative of lung changes such as emphysema, whereas sudden onset is associated with viral or bacterial infections.

 Keep in mind that older adults may experience dyspnea with certain activities related to aging changes of the lungs (loss of elasticity, fewer functional capillaries, and loss of lung resiliency).

Q Do you have difficulty breathing when you sleep? Do you use more than one pillow or elevate the head of the bed when you sleep?

R Orthopnea (difficulty breathing when lying supine) may be associated with congestive heart failure. Paroxysmal nocturnal dyspnea (severe dyspnea that awakens the person from sleep) also may be associated with congestive heart failure. Changes in sleep patterns may cause the client to feel fatigued during the day.

Q Do you snore when you sleep? Have you been told that you stop breathing at night when you snore?

R Sleep apnea (periods of breathing cessation during sleep) may be the source of snoring and gasping sounds. In general, sleep apnea diminishes the quality of sleep, which may account for fatigue or excessive tiredness, depression, irritability, loss of memory, lack of energy, and a risk for auto and workplace accidents.

Q Do you have chest pain? Is the pain associated with a cold, fever, or deep breathing?

R Pain-sensitive nerve endings are located in the parietal pleura, thoracic muscles, and tracheobronchial tree, but not in the lungs. Thus, chest pain associated with a pulmonary origin may be a late sign of pulmonary disease.

Chest pain related to pleuritis may be absent in older clients because of age-related alterations in pain perception.

Q Do you have a cough? When does it occur?

R Continuous coughs are usually associated with acute infections, whereas those occurring only early in the morning are often associated with chronic bronchial inflammation or smoking. Coughs late in the evening may be the result of exposure to irritant during the day. Coughs occurring at night are often related to postnasal drip or sinusitis. Non-productive coughs are often associated with upper respiratory irritations and early congestive heart failure.

The ability to cough effectively may be decreased in the older client because of weaker muscles and increased rigidity of the thoracic wall.

Q Do you produce any sputum when you cough? If so, what color is the sputum?

R White or mucoid sputum is often seen with common colds, viral infections, or bronchitis. Yellow or green sputum is often associated with bacterial infections. Blood in the sputum (hemoptysis) is seen with more serious respiratory conditions. Rust-colored sputum is associated with tuberculosis or pneumococcal pneumonia. Pink, frothy sputum may be indicative of pulmonary edema. Clients with excessive, tenacious secretions may need instruction on controlled coughing and measures to reduce viscosity of secretions.

Q Do you wheeze when you cough or when you are active?

R Wheezing indicates narrowing of the airways due to spasm or obstruction. Wheezing is associated with congestive heart failure (CHF), asthma (reactive airway disease), or excessive secretions.

PAST HISTORY

Q Have you had prior respiratory problems?

R A history of respiratory disease increases the risk for a recurrence. In addition, some respiratory diseases may imitate other disorders. For example, asthma symptoms may mimic symptoms commonly associated with emphysema or heart failure.

Q Have you ever had any thoracic surgery, biopsy, or trauma?

R Previous surgeries may alter the appearance of the thorax and cause changes in respiratory sounds. Trauma to the thorax can result in lung tissue changes.

Q Have you been tested for or diagnosed with allergies?

R Many allergic responses are manifested with respiratory symptoms such as dyspnea, cough, or hoarseness. Clients may need education on controlling the amount of allergens in their environment.

Q Have you ever had a chest x-ray, tuberculosis (TB) skin test, or influenza immunization? Have you had any other pulmonary studies in the past?

R Information on previous chest x-rays, TB skin tests, influenza immunizations, and so forth, is useful for comparison with current findings and gives information on self-care practices and possible teaching needs.

FAMILY HISTORY

Q Is there a history of lung disease in your family?

R The development of lung cancer is thought to be partially based on genetics. A history of certain respiratory diseases (asthma, emphysema) in a family may increase the risk for development of the disease. Exposure to viral or bacterial respiratory infections in the home increases the risk for development of these conditions.

Q Did any family members in your home smoke when you were growing up?

R Second-hand smoke puts individuals at risk for emphysema or lung cancer later in life.

LIFESTYLE AND HEALTH PRACTICES

Q Have you ever smoked cigarettes or other tobacco products? Do you currently smoke? At what age did you start? How much do you smoke and how much have you smoked in the past? What activities do you usually associate with smoking? Have you ever tried to quit?

R Smoking is linked to a number of respiratory conditions, including lung cancer (see Risk Factors—Lung Cancer). The number of years a person has smoked as well as the number of cigarettes per day also influence the risk for development of smoking-related respiratory problems. Clues to smoking behavior and previous efforts to quit may be helpful later in identifying measures to assist with smoking cessation.

Q Are you exposed to any environmental conditions that affect your breathing? Where do you work? Are you around smokers?

R Exposure to certain environmental inhalants can result in an increased incidence of certain respiratory conditions. Environmental irritants commonly associated with occupations include coal dust, insecticides, paint, pollution, asbestos fibers, and the like. Inhaling dust contaminated with *Histoplasma capsulatum* may cause histoplasmosis, a systemic fungal disease. This disease is common in the rural midwestern United States. Second-hand smoke is another irritant that can seriously affect a person's respiratory health.

Q Do you have difficulty performing your usual daily activities? Describe.

R Respiratory problems can negatively affect a person's ability to perform the usual activities of daily living.

Q What kind of stress are you experiencing at this time? How does it affect your breathing?

R Shortness of breath can be a manifestation of stress. Client may need education about relaxation techniques.

RISK FACTORS
Lung Cancer

Lung cancer is the leading cause of cancer death in the United States. Both incidence and mortality rates for lung cancer continue to increase despite decreasing mortality rates for most other cancers. However, the rates for men and women have changed: more women were estimated to die of lung cancer in 2000 than died in 1999, with fewer men dying in 2000 than in 1999, probably as a result of the drop in the numbers of young men who smoke.

Also by the year 2000, new cases of lung cancer increased by about 164,000 (89,500 among men and 74,500 among women), accounting for 13.4% of all new cancers. The average age of diagnosis is 60; a lung cancer diagnosis is unusual under age 40. For people whose cancer is found early and treated with surgery, the 5-year survival rate is about 42%, but only 15% of cases are diagnosed in the early stage (ACS, 2000).

RISK FACTORS

- Cigarette smoking
- Genetic predisposition, possibly associated with an interaction of genetics and smoking (Humphrey et al., 1995)
- Asbestos exposure
- Radon exposure
- Exposure to workplace pollutants: radioactive ores, mining chemicals (eg, arsenic, vinyl chloride, nickel, coal, mustard gas, chloromethyl esters, and fuels such as gasoline)
- Other environmental exposure: air pollution, passive tobacco smoke, marijuana smoking
- History of previous lung cancer, silicosis, berylliosis
- Recurring inflammation that leaves scars (eg, tuberculosis, some types of pneumonia)
- Diet low in vitamin E, lutein, high in cholesterol (LeMarchand, et al., 1995); low in fruits and vegetables, especially flavinoids (ACS, 2000)
- African American heritage, especially men
- Gender; women's lung cells may have a predisposition to lung cancer when exposed to tobacco smoke

RISK REDUCTION TEACHING TIPS

- Do not start smoking, and stop smoking if you do smoke.
- Join a smoking cessation program.
- Eat a healthy, low-cholesterol diet with adequate amounts of vitamin E and lutein.
- Limit exposure to air pollution and harmful substances.
- If your job requires frequent exposure to air pollution or dangerous substances, wear a mask for protection.

 ### CULTURAL CONSIDERATIONS

The variation in lung cancer rates among geographic and ethnic populations suggests the large influence of environmental risk factors, especially cigarette smoking. The lung cancer rate for nonsmokers has remained relatively constant over the last 26 years (Humphrey et al., 1995). Although 87% of lung cancers are attributed to smoking, only a fraction of individuals who smoke also develop lung cancer (Strom et al., 1995). Studies of genetics and smoking-related lung cancer suggest a genetic component (Caporaso & Landi, 1994). For example, lung cancer incidence is markedly lower in Fiji than in other South Pacific countries, despite similar smoking rates (Le Marchand et al., 1995). Compared to U.S. white men, African American men have higher incidence and mortality rates for lung cancer: 50% higher for African American men (American Lung Association, 2000). The difference may be due to increased smoking among black men. Lung cancer rates for U.S. Hispanics are approximately half of the rates observed for non-Hispanic whites (Davis et al., 1995; Strom et al., 1995).

Q Are you currently taking medications for breathing problems or other medications (prescription or OTC) that affect your breathing? Do you use any other treatments at home for your respiratory problems?

R All medications should be considered to determine if respiratory problems could be attributed to adverse reactions. Certain medications, for example, beta-adrenergic antagonists (beta blockers) such as atenolol (Tenormin) or metoprolol (Lopressor) and angiotensin-converting enzyme (ACE) inhibitors such as enalapril (Vasotec) or lisinopril (Zestril), are associated with the side effect of persistent cough. These medications are contraindicated with some respiratory problems (eg, asthma). If the client is using oxygen or other respiratory therapy at home, it is important to evaluate knowledge of proper use and precautions, as well as ability to afford the therapy.

Q Have you used any herbal medicines or alternative therapies to manage colds or other respiratory problems?

R Many people use herbal therapies, such as Echinacea, or alternative therapies, such as zinc lozenges, to decrease cold symptoms. Knowing what clients are using enables you to check for side effects or adverse interactions with prescribed medications.

Collecting Objective Data

Examination of the thorax and lungs begins when the nurse first meets the client and observes any obvious breathing difficulties. However, complete examination of the thorax and lungs consists of inspection, palpation, percussion, and auscultation of the posterior and anterior thorax to evaluate functioning of the lungs. Inspection and palpation are fairly simple skills to acquire; however practice and experience are the best ways to become proficient with percussion and auscultation.

CLIENT PREPARATION

Ask the client to sit in an upright position for the beginning of the examination, with arms relaxed at the sides. Also, have the client remove all clothing from the waist up and put on an examination gown or drape. The gown should open down the back and is used to limit exposure. Examination of a female client's chest may create anxiety because of embarrassment related to breast exposure. Explain that exposure of the entire chest is necessary during some parts of the examination and, to further ease client anxiety, explain the procedures before initiating the examination.

Also, provide explanations during the examination as you perform the various assessment techniques. The client should be encouraged to ask questions and to inform the examiner of any discomfort or fatigue he or she experiences during the examination. Try to make sure that the room temperature is comfortable for the client.

EQUIPMENT AND SUPPLIES

- Examination gown and drape
- Examination gloves
- Stethoscope (see How to Use the Stethoscope in Chapter 4, Collecting Objective Data)
- Examination light
- Mask
- Skin marker
- Metric ruler

KEY ASSESSMENT POINTS

- Provide privacy for the client and keep hands warm.
- Remain nonjudgmental regarding client's habits and lifestyle, particularly smoking. At the same time, educate and inform about risks, such as lung cancer and chronic obstructive pulmonary disease (COPD), related to habits.
- Learn and practice palpation, percussion, and auscultation sequences and techniques.

(*text continues on page 270*)

PHYSICAL ASSESSMENT

ASSESSMENT PROCEDURE	NORMAL FINDINGS	ABNORMAL FINDINGS
POSTERIOR THORAX		
Inspect Configuration		
While the client sits with arms at the sides, stand behind him or her and observe the position of scapulae and the shape and configuration of the chest wall.	Scapulae are symmetric and nonprotruding. Shoulders and scapulae are at equal horizontal positions. The ratio of anteroposterior to transverse diameter is 1:2.	Spinal processes that deviate laterally in the thoracic area may indicate scoliosis (see Display 14-1). Spinal configurations may have respiratory implications. Ribs appearing horizontal at an angle greater than 45 degrees with the spinal column are frequently the result of an increased

| ASSESSMENT PROCEDURE | NORMAL FINDINGS | ABNORMAL FINDINGS |

Tip From the Experts In general, some clinicians inspect the entire thorax first, followed by palpation of the anterior and posterior thorax, then percussion and auscultation of the anterior and posterior thorax.

Spinous processes appear straight, and thorax appears symmetric with ribs sloping downward at approximately a 45-degree angle in relation to the spine.

Kyphosis (an increased curve of the thoracic spine) is common in older clients (Display 14-1). It results from a loss of lung resiliency and a loss of skeletal muscle; it may be a normal finding.

The size of the thorax, which affects pulmonary function, differs by race. Compared with African Americans, Asians and Native Americans, adult Caucasians have a larger thorax and greater lung capacity (Overfield, 1995).

ratio between the anteroposterior–transverse diameter (barrel chest). This condition is commonly the result of emphysema due to hyperinflation of the lungs.

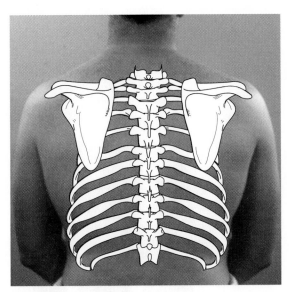

Observing the posterior thorax.

Observe Use of Accessory Muscles

Observe the client's use of accessory muscles when breathing.

The client does not use accessory (trapezius/shoulder) muscles to assist breathing. The diaphragm is the major muscle at work. This is evidenced by expansion of the lower chest during inspiration.

Trapezius, or shoulder, muscles are used to facilitate inspiration in cases of acute and chronic airway obstruction or atelectasis.

(continued)

ASSESSMENT PROCEDURE	NORMAL FINDINGS	ABNORMAL FINDINGS

Inspect Client's Positioning

Note the client's posture and the ability to support weight while breathing comfortably.

Client should be sitting up and relaxed, breathing easily, with arms at sides or in lap.

Client leans forward and uses arms to support weight and lift chest to increase breathing capacity in chronic obstructive pulmonary disease (COPD). This is referred to as the *tripod position* (see Display 14-1).

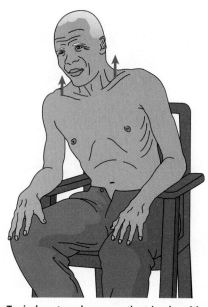

Typical posture, known as the tripod position, of client with COPD.

Palpate for Tenderness and Sensation

Follow the palpation sequence shown in Display 14-2, Guidelines for Palpating the Thorax. Use your fingers to palpate for tenderness, warmth, pain, or other sensations.

No tenderness, pain, or unusual sensations reported by client. Warmth should be equal bilaterally.

Tender or painful areas may indicate inflamed fibrous connective tissue. Pain over the intercostal spaces may be from inflamed pleurae. Pain over the ribs, especially at the costal condral junctions is a symptom of fractured ribs. Also, muscle soreness from exercise or the excessive work of breathing (as in COPD) may be palpated as tenderness. Increased warmth may be related to local infection.

Palpate for Crepitus

Palpate for possible crepitus, a crackling sensation (like bones or hairs rubbing against each other) that occurs when air passes through fluid or exudate. Crepitus, also called subcutaneous emphysema, can be palpated if air escapes from the lung or other airways into the subcutaneous tissue as occurs after an open thoracic injury, around a chest tube, or tracheostomy.

No palpable crepitus.

In areas of extreme congestion or consolidation, crepitus may be palpated. In such situations, margins should be marked and monitored to note any decrease or increase in the crepitant area.

(continued)

ASSESSMENT PROCEDURE	NORMAL FINDINGS	ABNORMAL FINDINGS

Palpate Surface Characteristics

Put on gloves and use your fingers to palpate any lesions that you noticed during inspection. Also, feel for any unusual masses.

Skin and subcutaneous tissue are free of lesions and masses.

Any unusual palpable mass, which should be evaluated further by a physician or other appropriate professional.

Palpate for Fremitus

Use the ball or ulnar edge of one hand to assess for fremitus (vibrations of air in the bronchial tubes transmitted to the chest wall, felt by the examiner when the client says "ninety-nine"). Refer to the guidelines for palpating the thorax (see Display 14-2).

🏵 **Tip From the Experts** The ball of the hand is best for assessing tactile fremitus because the area is especially sensitive to vibratory sensation. As you move your hand to each area, ask the client to say "ninety-nine." Assess all areas for symmetry and intensity of vibration.

Fremitus is symmetric and easily identified in the upper regions of the lungs. If fremitus is not palpable on either side, the client may need to speak louder. A decrease in the intensity of fremitus is normal as the examiner moves toward the base of the lungs. However, fremitus should remain symmetric for bilateral positions.

Unequal fremitus is usually the result of consolidation that increases fremitus or bronchial obstruction, air trapping in emphysema, pleural effusion, or pneumothorax that decreases fremitus. Diminished fremitus even with a loud spoken voice may indicate an obstruction of the tracheobronchial tree.

Palpate Chest Expansion

Place your hands on the posterior chest wall with your thumbs at the level of T9 or T10. As the client takes a deep breath, observe the movement of your thumbs.

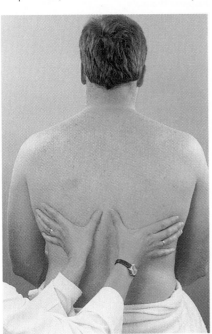

Palpating to assess symmetry of chest expansion.

When the client takes a deep breath, the examiner's thumbs should move 5 to 10 cm apart symmetrically.

👓 Because of calcification of the costal cartilages and loss of the accessory musculature, the older client's thoracic expansion may be decreased, although it should still be symmetric.

Unequal chest expansion can occur with severe atelectasis (collapse or incomplete expansion), pneumonia, chest trauma, or pneumothorax (air in the pleural space). Decreased chest excursion at the base of the lungs is characteristic of chronic obstructive pulmonary disease (COPD). This is due to decreased diaphragmatic function.

(continued)

ASSESSMENT PROCEDURE	NORMAL FINDINGS	ABNORMAL FINDINGS

Percuss for Tone

Starting at the apices above the scapulae, across the tops of both shoulders, percuss the intercostal spaces across and down, comparing sides. Percuss to the lateral aspects at the bases of the lungs and compare sides. Follow the sequence presented here.

Resonance is the percussion tone elicited over normal lung tissue.

Hyperresonance is elicited in cases of trapped air such as in emphysema or pneumothorax. Dullness is present when fluid or solid tissue replaces air in the lung or occupies the pleural space. Examples include lobar pneumonia, pleural effusion, or tumor.

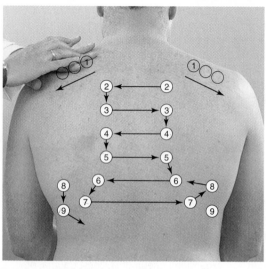

Sequence for percussing the posterior thorax.

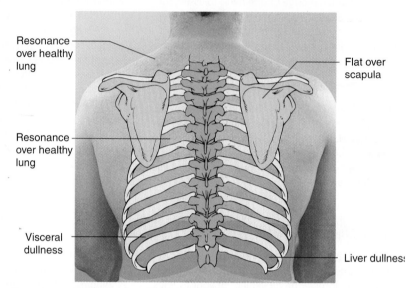

Resonance over healthy lung

Flat over scapula

Resonance over healthy lung

Visceral dullness

Liver dullness

Normal percussion tones heard from the posterior thorax.

(continued)

ASSESSMENT PROCEDURE	NORMAL FINDINGS	ABNORMAL FINDINGS

Percuss for Diaphragmatic Excursion

Ask the client to *exhale* forcefully and hold the breath. Beginning at the scapular line (T7), percuss the intercostal spaces of the right posterior chest wall. Percuss downward until the tone changes from resonance to dullness. Mark this level and allow the client to breathe. Next, ask the client to *inhale* deeply and hold it. Percuss the intercostal spaces from the mark downward until resonance changes to dullness. Mark the level and allow the client to breathe. Measure the distance between the two marks. Repeat the procedure on the left posterior thorax.

Excursion should be equal bilaterally and measure 3 to 5 cm in adults.

The level of the diaphragm may be higher on the right because of the position of the liver.

In well-conditioned clients, excursion can measure up to 7 or 8 cm.

Diaphragmatic descent may be limited by atelectasis of the lower lobes or by emphysema, in which diaphragmatic movement and air trapping are minimal. The diaphragm remains in a low position on inspiration and expiration.

Other possible causes for limited descent can be pain or abdominal changes such as extreme ascites, tumors, or pregnancy.

Uneven excursion may be seen with inflammation from unilateral pneumonia, damage to the phrenic nerve, or splenomegaly.

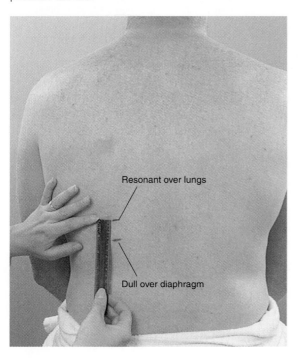

Resonant over lungs

Dull over diaphragm

Measuring diaphragmatic excursion.

(continued)

ASSESSMENT PROCEDURE	NORMAL FINDINGS	ABNORMAL FINDINGS

Auscultate for Breath Sounds

Follow the guidelines for auscultating the thorax (Display 14-3) and listen for normal breath sounds in the areas illustrated below.

🏵 **Tip From the Experts** Breath sounds are considered normal only in the area specified. Heard elsewhere, they are considered abnormal sounds. For example, bronchial breath sounds are abnormal if heard over the peripheral lung fields. (Display 14-4 describes normal breath sounds and their location.)

Three types of normal breath sounds may be auscultated—bronchial, bronchovesicular, and vesicular (see figures below).

Diminished or absent breath sounds often indicate that little or no air is moving in or out of the lung area being auscultated. This may indicate obstruction within the lungs as a result of secretions, mucus plug, or a foreign object. It may also indicate abnormalities of the pleural space. For example, pleural thickening, pleural effusion, or pneumothorax should be considered. In cases of emphysema, the hyperinflated nature of the lungs, together with a loss of elasticity of lung tissue, may result in diminished inspiratory breath sounds. Increased (louder) breath sounds often occur when consolidation or compression results in a denser lung area that enhances the transmission of sound.

Sometimes breath sounds may be hard to hear with obese or heavily muscled clients due to increased distance to underlying lung tissue.

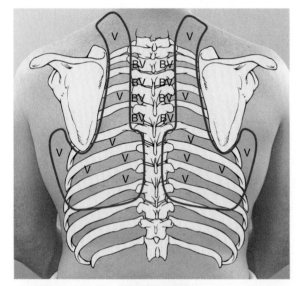

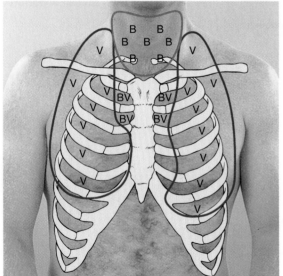

Location of breath sounds from (*top*) posterior thorax and (*bottom*) anterior thorax. B, bronchial sounds; V, vesicular sounds; BV, bronchovesicular sounds.

(continued)

ASSESSMENT PROCEDURE	NORMAL FINDINGS	ABNORMAL FINDINGS

Auscultate for Adventitious Sounds

Adventitious sounds are sounds that are added or superimposed over normal breath sounds and heard during auscultation. Be careful to note the location on the chest wall where adventitious sounds are heard as well as the location of such sounds within the respiratory cycle.

No adventitious sounds, such as crackles (discrete and discontinuous sounds) or wheezes (musical and continuous), are auscultated.

Adventitious lung sounds, such as crackles (formerly called rales) and wheezes (formerly called rhonchi) are evident. See Table 14-1 for a complete description of each type of adventitious breath sound.

Tip From the Experts If you hear an abnormal sound during auscultation, always have the client cough, then listen again and note any change.

Auscultate Voice Sounds

Bronchophony: Ask the client to repeat the phrase "ninety-nine" while you listen over the chest wall.

Voice transmission is soft, muffled, and indistinct. The sound of the voice may be heard, but the actual phrase cannot be distinguished.

The words will be easily understood and louder over areas of increased density. This may indicate consolidation from pneumonia, atelectasis, or tumor.

Egophony: Ask the client to repeat the letter "E" while you listen over the chest wall.

Voice transmission will be soft and muffled, but the letter "E" should be distinguishable.

Over areas of consolidation or compression, the sound will be louder and change to "A."

Whispered Pectoriloquy: Ask the client to whisper the phrase "one–two–three" while you listen over the chest wall.

Transmission of sound is very faint and muffled. It may be inaudible.

Over areas of consolidation or compression, the sound will be transmitted clearly and distinctly. In such areas, it will sound as if the client is whispering directly into the stethoscope.

ANTERIOR THORAX

Inspect Shape and Configuration

The client should be sitting with arms at his or her sides. Stand in front of the client and assess shape and configuration.

The anteroposterior diameter is less than the transverse diameter. The ratio of anteroposterior diameter to the transverse diameter is 1:2.

Anteroposterior equals transverse diameter, resulting in a barrel chest. This is often seen in emphysema because of hyperinflation of the lungs (see Display 14-1).

Inspect Position of Sternum

Observe the sternum from an anterior and lateral viewpoint.

Sternum midline and straight.

The sternum and ribs may be more prominent in the older client because of loss of subcutaneous fat.

Pectus excavatum is a markedly sunken sternum and adjacent cartilages (often referred to as funnel chest). *Pectus carinatum* is a forward protrusion of the sternum causing the adjacent ribs to slope backward. However, both of these conditions may restrict expansion of the lungs and decrease the lung capacity (see Display 14-1).

Watch for sternal retractions.

Retractions not observed.

Sternal retractions are noted with severe labored breathing.

(continued)

ASSESSMENT PROCEDURE	NORMAL FINDINGS	ABNORMAL FINDINGS
Inspect Slope of the Ribs		
Assess the ribs from an anterior and lateral viewpoint.	Ribs slope downward with symmetric intercostal spaces. Costal angle is within 90 degrees.	Barrel-chest configuration results in more horizontal position and costal angle of more than 90 degrees. This often results from long-standing emphysema.
Observe Quality and Pattern of Respiration		
Note breathing characteristics as well as rate, rhythm, and depth.	Respirations are relaxed, effortless, and quiet. They are of a regular rhythm and normal depth at a rate of 10 to 20 per minute in adults. Tachypnea and bradypnea may be normal in some clients (Table 14-2).	Labored and noisy breathing is often seen with severe asthma or chronic bronchitis. Tachypnea, bradypnea, hyperventilation, hypoventilation, Cheyne-Stokes respiration, and Biot's respiration are abnormal breathing patterns. Table 14-2 describes these patterns.

🎗️ **Tip From the Experts** When assessing respiratory patterns, it is more objective to describe the breathing pattern, rather than just labeling the pattern.

Inspect Intercostal Spaces		
Ask the client to breathe normally and observe the intercostal spaces.	No retractions or bulging of intercostal spaces noted.	Retraction of the intercostal spaces indicates an increased inspiratory effort. This may be the result of an obstruction of the respiratory tract or atelectasis. Bulging of the intercostal spaces indicates trapped air, such as is seen in emphysema or asthma.
Observe for Use of Accessory Muscles		
Ask the client to breathe normally and observe for use of accessory muscles.	Use of accessory muscles (sternomastoid and rectus abdominis) is not seen with normal respiratory effort. After strenuous exercise or activity, individuals with normal respiratory status may use neck muscles for a short time to enhance breathing.	Neck muscles (sternomastoid, scalene, and trapezius) are used to facilitate inspiration in cases of acute or chronic airway obstruction or atelectasis. The abdominal muscles and the internal intercostal muscles are used to facilitate expiration in COPD.
Inspect for nasal flaring.	Not observed. Normally, the diaphragm and the external intercostal muscles do most of the work of breathing. This is evidenced by outward expansion of the abdomen and lower ribs on inspiration and return to resting position on expiration.	Nasal flaring is seen with labored respirations (especially in small children) and is indicative of hypoxia. Pursed lip breathing may be seen in asthma, emphysema, or CHF as a physiologic response to help slow down expiration and keep alveoli open longer.
Observe color of face, lips, chest. Also inspect color and shape of nails.	Ambient skin color with pink undertones.	Cyanosis may be seen if client is cold or hypoxic; ruddy to purple complexion may be seen in clients with COPD or CHF as a result of polycythemia.

(continued)

ASSESSMENT PROCEDURE	NORMAL FINDINGS	ABNORMAL FINDINGS

Palpate for Tenderness, Sensation, Surface Problems

Follow the guidelines for palpating the thorax (see Display 14-1) and use your fingers to palpate for tenderness and sensation. Palpate for tenderness at costachondral junctions of ribs. Assess for crepitus as you would on the posterior thorax (described previously). Also palpate any surface masses or lesions.

No tenderness or pain palpated over the lung area with respirations.

   No crepitus palpated and no unusual surface masses or lesions.

In areas of extreme congestion or consolidation, crepitus may be palpated, particularly in clients with lung disease. Tenderness over thoracic muscles can result from exercising (eg, push ups and the like) especially in a previously sedentary client. Tenderness or pain at the costachondral junction of the ribs is seen with fractures, especially in older clients with osteoporosis.

Palpate for Fremitus

Follow the guidelines presented in Display 14-1 and the instructions stated previously in the text. Assess for symmetry and intensity of the vibrations.

Tip From the Experts When you assess for fremitus on the female client, avoid palpating the breast. Breast tissue damps the vibrations.

Fremitus symmetric and easily identified in the upper regions of the lungs. A decreased intensity of fremitus is expected toward the base of the lungs; however, fremitus should be symmetric bilaterally.

Diminished vibrations, even with a loud spoken voice, may indicate an obstruction of the tracheobronchial tree.

   Clients with emphysema may have considerably decreased fremitus as a result of air trapping.

Palpate Anterior Chest Expansion

Place your hands on the anterolateral wall with the thumbs along the costal margins and pointing toward the xiphoid process. As the client takes a deep breath, observe the movement of your thumbs.

Thumbs move outward in a symmetric fashion from the midline.

Unequal chest expansion can occur with severe atelectasis, pneumonia, chest trauma, pleural effusion, or pneumothorax. Decreased chest excursion at the bases of the lungs is seen with COPD.

Palpating anterior chest expansion.
(© B. Proud.)

(continued)

ASSESSMENT PROCEDURE	NORMAL FINDINGS	ABNORMAL FINDINGS

Percuss for Tone

Percuss the apices above the clavicles. Then percuss the intercostal spaces across and down, comparing sides.

> **Tip From the Experts** Percussion elicits dullness over breast tissue, the heart, and the liver. Tympany is detected over the stomach, and flatness is detected over the muscles and bones.

Resonance is the percussion tone elicited over normal lung tissue.

Hyperresonance is elicited in cases of trapped air, such as in emphysema or pneumothorax. Dullness may characterize areas of increased density such as consolidation, pleural effusion, or tumor.

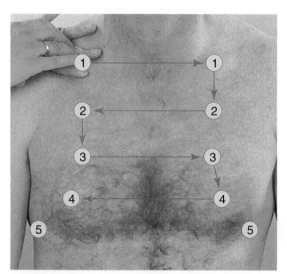

Sequence for percussing anterior thorax.

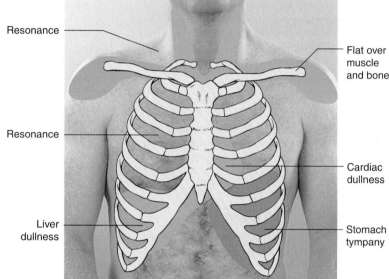

Normal percussion tones heard from anterior thorax.

Auscultate Anterior Breath Sounds, Adventitious Sounds, and Voice Sounds

Follow the auscultation guidelines in Display 14-3. Listen for breath, adventitious, and voice sounds.

See Display 14-4, which describes breath sounds. Normal adventitious and vocal vibrations were discussed previously.

See the posterior thorax text material and Table 14-1.

Validation and Documentation of Findings

Validate the thorax and lung assessment data that you have collected. This is necessary to verify that the data are reliable and accurate. Document the assessment data following the health care facility or agency policy.

EXAMPLE OF SUBJECTIVE DATA

No dyspnea, cough, or chest pain with breathing at rest or with activity. No past history or family history of respiratory diseases. Has never smoked and works in well-ventilated factory. Reports "one or two" colds per year. No known allergies. Last TB skin test performed 5 months ago with negative results. Last chest x-ray 4 years ago after "minor" car accident. X-ray report at that time was normal.

EXAMPLE OF OBJECTIVE DATA

Respirations 18/minute, relaxed and even. Anteroposterior less than transverse diameter. Chest expansion symmetric. No retracting or bulging of intercostal spaces. No pain or tenderness noted on palpation. Tactile fremitus symmetric. Percussion tones resonant over all lung fields. Diaphragmatic excursion 4 cm and equal bilaterally. Vesicular breath sounds auscultated over lung fields. No adventitious sounds present.

After you have collected your assessment data, you will need to analyze the data, using diagnostic reasoning skills.

DISPLAY 14-1. Thoracic Deformities and Configurations

ABNORMAL
FINDINGS

Some of the different sizes and shapes of the human thorax are displayed here, with the shape considered most normal presented first for comparison.

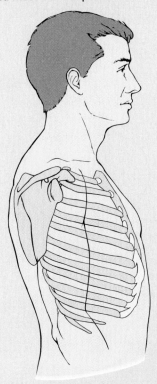

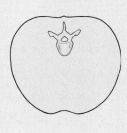

Cross section
of thorax

Normal thoracic configuration and cross-section.

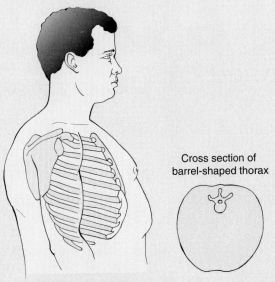

Cross section of
barrel-shaped thorax

The barrel chest configuration typically results from emphysema. Note the barrel shape of the cross section.

(continued)

DISPLAY 14-1. Thoracic Deformities and Configurations (Continued)

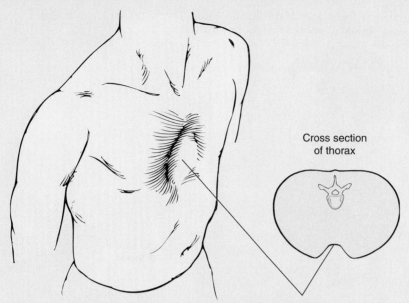

Cross section
of thorax

Pectus excavatum (funnel chest) is a congenital malformation characterized by a sunken sternum and seldom causing symptoms other than self-consciousness.

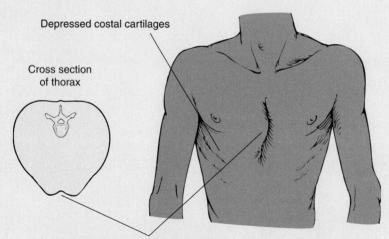

Depressed costal cartilages

Cross section
of thorax

Anteriorly displaced sternum

Pectus carinatum (pigeon chest) is a minor deformity in which the sternum protrudes but requires no treatment.

(continued)

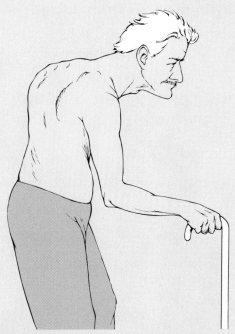
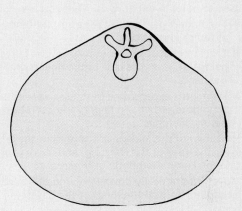

Kyphosis, a pronounced forward curvature of the thoracic spine, is most common in older adults.

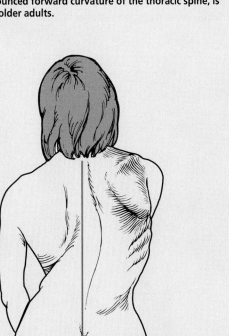
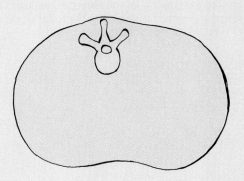

Scoliosis imparts an S shape to the spine. The spinal deformity is commonly detected in young people—primarily females—by school nurses.

DISPLAY 14-2. Palpating the Thorax

GUIDELINES

Palpating the thorax helps you evaluate the client's level of sensation, degree of fremitus (vocal vibration), and efficiency of thoracic expansion. Palpation may be performed with one or both hands, whereas the sequence of palpation is established—starting near the neck and proceeding from side to side areas just above the waist as shown below.

POSTERIOR THORAX

1. As a beginning examiner, palpate the posterior (and anterior) thorax with one hand. (Two hands may be used as you gain experience. A two-handed method enables the simultaneous comparison of palpation findings and speeds up the assessment.) The part of the hand that is used to palpate depends on what you are assessing.

   - The fingers may be best for assessing sensation as well as lumps and lesions.
   - Tactile fremitus, however, may best be felt with the palm—either at the base of the fingers or the heel of the hand.
   - Symmetric expansion is best assessed with two hands—thumbs together and fingers apart on the client's back below the lungs.

2. Start toward the midline at the level of the left scapula (over the apex of the left lung) and move your hand left to right, comparing findings bilaterally.

3. Move systematically downward and out to cover the lateral portions of the lungs at the bases.

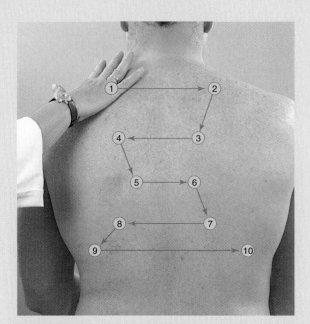

Sequence for palpating posterior thorax.

ANTERIOR THORAX

The sequence for palpating the anterior thorax is similar to that for the posterior thorax. And, again, the part of the hand that you use depends on what characteristic you are assessing (sensation, vibration, or expansion).

 Tip From the Experts Anterior thoracic palpation is best for assessing the lung's right middle lobe.

The technique to use is described below.

1. Start with your hand positioned over the left clavicle (over the apex of the left lung) and move your hand left to right, comparing findings bilaterally.

2. Move your hand systematically downward, toward the midline at the level of the breasts and outward at the base to include the lateral aspect of the lung. The established sequence for palpating the anterior thorax serves as a guide for positioning your hands.

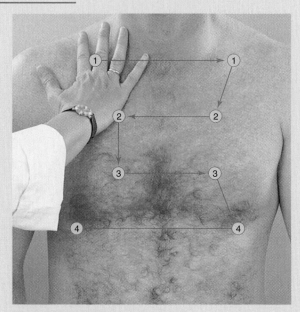

Sequence for palpating anterior thorax.

DISPLAY 14-3. Auscultating the Thorax

GUIDELINES

To best assess lung sounds, you will need to hear the sounds as directly as possible. Do not attempt to listen through clothing or a drape, which may produce additional sound or muffle lung sounds that exist.

POSTERIOR THORAX

1. To begin, place the diaphragm of the stethoscope firmly and directly on the posterior chest wall at the apex of the lung at C7.
2. Ask the client to breathe deeply through his or her mouth for each area of auscultation (each placement of the stethoscope) in the auscultation sequence so you can best hear inspiratory and expiratory sounds. Be alert to the client's comfort and offer times for rest and normal breathing if fatigue is becoming a problem.

   Deep mouth breathing may be especially difficult for the older client, who may fatigue easily. Thus, offer rest as needed.

3. Auscultate from the apices of the lungs at C7 to the bases of the lungs at T10 and laterally from the axilla down to the seventh or eighth rib.
4. Listen at each site for at least one complete respiratory cycle. Follow the auscultating sequence shown here.

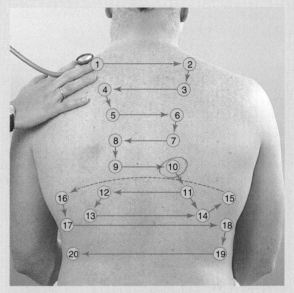

Sequence for auscultating posterior thorax.

ANTERIOR THORAX

1. Place the diaphragm of the stethoscope firmly and directly on the anterior chest wall. Again, do not attempt to listen through clothing or other materials. However, if the client has a large amount of hair on the chest, listening through a thin T-shirt can decrease extraneous sounds that may be misinterpreted as crackles.
2. Auscultate from the apices of the lungs slightly above the clavicles to the bases of the lungs at the sixth rib.
3. Ask the client to breathe deeply through his or her mouth in an effort to avoid transmission of sounds that may occur with nasal breathing. Be alert to the client's comfort and offer times for rest and normal breathing if fatigue is becoming a problem, particularly for the older client.
4. Listen at each site for at least one complete respiratory cycle. Follow the sequence for anterior auscultation shown here.

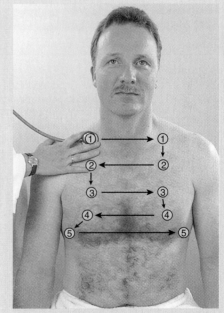

Sequence for auscultating anterior thorax.

DISPLAY 14-4. **Normal Breath Sounds**

BRONCHIAL BREATH SOUNDS

Pitch: High
Quality: Harsh or hollow
Amplitude: Loud
Duration: Short during inspiration, long in expiration
Location: Trachea and larynx

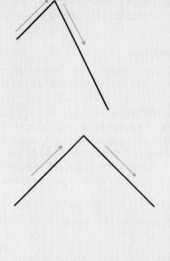

BRONCHOVESICULAR BREATH SOUNDS

Pitch: Moderate
Quality: Mixed
Amplitude: Moderate
Duration: Same in inspiration and expiration
Location: Over the major bronchi—*posterior:* between the scapulae; *anterior:* around the upper sternum in the first and second intercostal spaces

VESICULAR BREATH SOUNDS

Pitch: Low
Quality: Breezy
Amplitude: Soft
Duration: Long in inspiration, short in expiration
Location: Peripheral lung fields

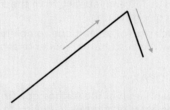

TABLE 14-1. **Adventitious Breath Sounds**

Abnormal Sound	Characteristics	Source	Conditions
Discontinuous Sounds			
Crackles (fine) 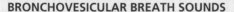	High-pitched, short, popping sounds heard during inspiration and not cleared with coughing; sounds are discontinuous and can be simulated by rolling a strand of hair between your fingers near your ear.	Inhaled air suddenly opens the small deflated air passages that are coated and sticky with exudate.	Crackles occurring late in inspiration are associated with restrictive diseases such as pneumonia and congestive heart failure. Crackles occurring early in inspiration are associated with obstructive disorders such as bronchitis, asthma, or emphysema.
Crackles (coarse)	Low-pitched, bubbling, moist sounds that may persist from early inspiration to early expiration; also described as softly separating Velcro.	Inhaled air comes into contact with secretions in the large bronchi and trachea.	Can indicate such things as pneumonia, pulmonary edema, and pulmonary fibrosis. "Velcro rales" of pulmonary fibrosis are heard louder and closer to stethoscope, usually do not change location, and are more common in clients with long-term COPD.
Continuous Sounds			
Pleural friction rub	Low-pitched, dry, grating sound. Sound is much like crackles, only more superficial and occurs during both inspiration and expiration.	Sound is the result of rubbing of two inflamed pleural surfaces.	Pleuritis

(continued)

TABLE 14-1. Adventitious Breath Sounds (Continued)

Abnormal Sound	Characteristics	Source	Conditions
Wheeze (sibilant)	High-pitched, musical sounds heard primarily during expiration but may also be heard on inspiration.	Air passing through constricted passages caused by swelling, secretions, or tumor.	Sibilant wheezes are often heard in cases of acute asthma or chronic emphysema.
Wheeze (sonorous)	Low-pitched snoring or moaning sounds heard primarily during expiration but may be heard throughout the respiratory cycle. These wheezes may clear with coughing.	Same as sibilant wheeze. The pitch of the wheeze cannot be correlated to the size of the passageway that generates it.	Sonorous wheezes are often heard in cases of bronchitis or single obstructions and snoring before an episode of sleep apnea. *Stridor* is a harsh honking wheeze with severe broncholaryngospasm, such as occurs with croup.

TABLE 14-2. Respiration Patterns

Type	Description	Pattern	Clinical Indication
Normal	12 to 20/min and regular		Normal breathing pattern
Tachypnea	>24/min and shallow		May be a normal response to fever, anxiety, or exercise Can occur with respiratory insufficiency, alkalosis, pneumonia, or pleurisy
Bradypnea	<10/min and regular		May be normal in well-conditioned athletes Can occur with medication-induced depression of the respiratory center, diabetic coma, neurologic damage
Hyperventilation	Increased rate and increased depth		Usually occurs with extreme exercise, fear, or anxiety Kussmaul's respirations are a type of hyperventilation associated with diabetic ketoacidosis. Other causes of hyperventilation include disorders of the central nervous system, an overdose of the drug salicylate, or severe anxiety.
Hypoventilation	Decreased rate, decreased depth, irregular pattern		Usually associated with overdose of narcotics or anesthetics
Cheyne-Stokes respiration	Regular pattern characterized by alternating periods of deep, rapid breathing followed by periods of apnea		May result from severe congestive heart failure, drug overdose, increased intracranial pressure, or renal failure May be noted in elderly persons during sleep, not related to any disease process
Biol's respiration	Irregular pattern characterized by varying depth and rate of respirations followed by periods of apnea		May be seen with meningitis or severe brain damage

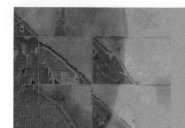

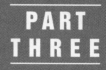
Diagnostic Reasoning: Possible Conclusions

The case study presented on these pages shows you how to analyze thoracic and lung assessment data for a specific client. The critical thinking exercise included in the study guide/lab manual that complements this text also offers opportunities to analyze assessment data.

SELECTED NURSING DIAGNOSES

After collecting subjective and objective data pertaining to the thorax and lung assessment, you will need to identify abnormal findings and cluster the data to reveal any significant patterns or abnormalities. These data may then be used to make clinical judgments (nursing diagnoses: wellness, risk, or actual) about the status of the client's thorax and lungs. Following is a listing of selected nursing diagnoses that you may identify when analyzing data for this part of the assessment.

Nursing Diagnoses (Wellness)

- Opportunity to Enhance Breathing Patterns
- Health-Seeking Behaviors: Requests information on TB skin testing, how to quit smoking, or on exercises to improve respiratory status

Nursing Diagnoses (Risk)

- Risk for Respiratory Infection related to exposure to environmental pollutants and lack of knowledge of precautionary measures
- Risk for Activity Intolerance related to imbalance between oxygen supply and demand
- Risk for Imbalanced Nutrition: Less Than Body Requirements related to fatigue secondary to dyspnea
- Risk for Ineffective Health Maintenance related to lack of knowledge of condition, infection transmission, and prevention of recurrence
- Risk for Impaired Oral Mucous Membranes related to mouth breathing

Nursing Diagnoses (Actual)

- Anxiety related to dyspnea and fear of suffocation
- Activity Intolerance related to fatigue secondary to inadequate oxygenation
- Ineffective Airway Clearance related to inability to clear thick, mucous secretions secondary to pain and fatigue
- Impaired Gas Exchange related to chronic lung tissue damage secondary to chronic smoking
- Ineffective Airway Clearance related to bronchospasm and increased pulmonary secretions
- Ineffective Breathing Pattern: Hyperventilation related to hypoxia and lack of knowledge of controlled breathing techniques
- Disturbed Sleep Pattern related to excessive coughing
- Impaired Gas Exchange related to poor muscle tone and decreased ability to remove secretions secondary to the aging process

SELECTED COLLABORATIVE PROBLEMS

After grouping the data, certain collaborative problems may become apparent. Remember, collaborative problems differ from nursing diagnoses in that they cannot be prevented by nursing intervention. However, these physiologic complications of medical conditions can be detected and monitored by the nurse. In addition, the nurse can use physician- and nurse-prescribed interventions to minimize the complications of these problems. The nurse may also have to refer the client in such situations for further treatment of the problem. Following is a list of collaborative problems that may be identified when obtaining a general impression. These problems are worded as Potential Complications (or PC), followed by the problem.

- PC: Atelectasis
- PC: Pneumonia
- PC: Chronic obstructive pulmonary disease
- PC: Asthma
- PC: Bronchitis
- PC: Pleural effusion
- PC: Pneumothorax
- PC: Pulmonary edema
- PC: Tuberculosis

MEDICAL PROBLEMS

After grouping the data, the client's signs and symptoms may clearly require medical diagnosis and treatment. Referral to a primary care provider is necessary.

Diagnostic Reasoning: Case Study

The case study presents assessment data for a specific client. It is followed by an analysis of the data, working out the key steps presented in Chapters 6 and 7 to arrive at conclusions.

This is your third weekly home visit with George Burney, a 60-year-old white man who was discharged after being hospitalized for 10 days with acute respiratory failure secondary to chronic obstructive pulmonary disease (COPD). His eyes sparkling, he tells you he is feeling great and that he was able to walk outside on his patio for a few minutes today without his oxygen. He uses oxygen at 2 L/min when he exercises and prn for shortness of breath. He reports a "chronic cough, as usual" but denies sputum production. He says he still has difficulty "getting off a good cough" because "I just don't have the energy anymore."

His facial color and lips are ruddy, but nail beds are pink. Breathing pattern is regular, unlabored, but tachypneic at 28 respirations per minute, which is his usual rate. Examining his thorax, you note he is barrel-chested with a transverse-to-lateral ratio of about 2.5 to 3. Although he is not using accessory muscles to breathe, you do note slight intercostal bulging and rigidly upright posture in the chair. While auscultating his lungs, you note diminished breath sounds bilaterally in most of lower lobes and a small, discrete area of coarse crackles in the upper portion of the left lower lobe. You also note the odor of cigarettes on his breath, and, when you confront him with this information, he says, "I didn't think one would hurt when I was outside."

1 Identify abnormal data and strengths (in both subjective and objective data).

SUBJECTIVE DATA

- "Chronic cough, as usual" but denies sputum production
- Difficulty coughing effectively R/T decreased energy
- Didn't think having one cigarette while outside would hurt him
- Feels great today
- Walked on patio for a few minutes without oxygen

OBJECTIVE DATA

- Recent hospitalization for respiratory failure
- Ruddy facial and lip color, pink nail beds
- Tachypnea, but regular and unlabored
- Barrel chest, intercostal bulging, rigid posture
- Diminished breath sounds in lower lobes
- Discrete, coarse crackles in upper segment of LLL

2 Cue Clusters	**3** Inferences	**4** Possible Nursing Diagnoses	**5** Defining Characteristics	**6** Confirm or Rule Out
A • Ruddy coloring • Intercostal bulging • Barrel chest	Signs consistent with COPD diagnosis			
B • Chronic cough • No sputum • Discrete crackles • Diminished breath sounds • Tachypnea • Verbalizes decreased energy	Airway clearance impaired due to ineffective cough May need instruction in energy-conserving cough techniques	Ineffective Airway Clearance related to knowledge deficit of energy-conserving and possibly appropriate coughing techniques	*Major:* Ineffective cough (no sputum produced) and inability to remove airway secretions *Minor:* Abnormal breath sounds (crackles) and abnormal respiratory rate tachypnea)	Accept diagnosis because it was validated by the client and because it meets all the defining characteristics.
		Activity Intolerance related to decreased energy secondary to compromised gas exchange from COPD	*Major:* None identified (dyspnea implied) *Minor:* Weakness (verbalized decreased energy)	Rule out diagnosis because it does not meet the major defining characteristic. Because of the client's limited physical activity, this diagnosis is implied, but needs further data for validation.

2 Cue Clusters	**3** Inferences	**4** Possible Nursing Diagnoses	**5** Defining Characteristics	**6** Confirm or Rule Out
C • Odor of cigarettes on breath • "Didn't think one (cigarette) would hurt when I was outside." • Chronic cough	Denying hazardous effects of smoking on current health status	Ineffective Health Maintenance related to denial of effects of cigarette smoking on current health status	*Major:* Reports smoking cigarettes; denies significance *Minor:* Chronic cough	Accept diagnosis because it meets major and minor defining characteristics.
		Ineffective Management of Therapeutic Regimen related to denial of effect of smoking on current health status	*Major:* None *Minor:* Verbalized did not take action (in this case, did forbidden action—smoking) to reduce risk factor	Rule out because it does not meet major defining characteristics even though does meet a minor characteristic. It could be easy to confuse which diagnosis would be appropriate, but, after examining the defining characteristics, a fit can be made.

7 Document conclusions.

Nursing diagnoses that are appropriate for this client include:

- Ineffective Airway Clearance related to knowledge deficit of energy-conserving and possibly appropriate coughing techniques
- Ineffective Health Maintenance related to denial of effects of cigarette smoking on current health status

Potential collaborative problems include the following:

- PC: Respiratory failure
- PC: Hypoxemia
- PC: Upper respiratory infection
- PC: Right-sided heart failure

REFERENCES AND SELECTED READINGS

Ailani, R. K., Ravakhah, K., DiGiovine, B., Jacobsen, G., Tun, T., Epstein, D., & West, B. C. (1999). Dyspnea Differentiation Index: A new method for the rapid separation of cardiac vs pulmonary dyspnea. *Chest, 116*(4), 1100–1104.

Basfield-Holland, E. S. (1997). Home health: Assessing pulmonary status: It's more than listening to breath sounds. *Nursing97, 27*(8), 32hh 1–2, 4–9.

Boutotte, J. M. (1999). Keeping TB in check. . . tuberculosis. *Nursing99, 29*(3), 34–40.

Boyars, M. C. (1997). Chest auscultation: How to maximize its diagnostic value in lung disease. *Consultant, 37*(2), 415–419, 423, 427.

Camp-Sorrell, D. (1999). Surviving the cancer, surviving the treatment: Acute cardiac and pulmonary toxicity. *Oncology Nursing Forum, 26*(6), 983–990.

Carroll, P. (1999). Trauma! Chest injuries. *RN, 62*(1), 36–40, 42–43.

Conway, A. (1998). Respiratory care. Breathing life into an idea. *Nursing Times, 94*(39), 72, 74.

Cox, C. L., & McGrath, A. (1999). Respiratory assessment in critical care units. *Intensive and Critical Care Nursing, 15*(4), 226–234.

Dunlap, N. E., Bass, J., Fujiwara, P., Hopewell, P., Horsburgh, C. R., Jr., Salfinger, M. M., & Simone, P. M. (2000). American Thoracic Society. Diagnostic standards and classification of tuberculosis in adults and children. *American Journal of Respiratory and Critical Care Medicine, 161*(4), 1376–1395.

Edmonds, P., Higginson, I., Altmann, D., Sen-Gupta, G. M., & McDonnell, M. (2000). Is the presence of dyspnea a risk factor for morbidity in cancer patients? *Journal of Pain and Symptom Management, 19*(1), 15–22.

Eid, N., Yandell, B., Howell, L., Eddy, M., & Sheikh, S. (2000). Can peak expiratory flow predict airflow obstruction in children with asthma? *Pediatrics, 105*(2), 354–358.

Gift, A. G., & Narsavage, G. (1998). Validity of the numeric rating scale as a measure of dyspnea. *American Journal of Critical Care, 7*(3), 200–204.

Lewis, A. M. (1999). Respiratory emergency! *Nursing99, 29*(8), 62–64.

McManus, T. (1999). Chronic cough: A common but treatable condition. *PMA, 32*(6), 20–22.

Moloney-Harmon, P. A. (1999). When the lung fails: Acute respiratory distress syndrome in children. *Critical Care Nursing Clinics of North America, 11*(4), 519–528.

O'Hanlon-Nichols, T. (1998). Basic assessment series: The adult pulmonary system. *American Journal of Nursing, 98*(2), 39–45.

Owen, A. (1998). Respiratory assessment revisited. *Nursing 98, 28*(4), 48–49.

Reinke, L. F., & Hoffman, L. (2000). Asthma education: Creating a partnership. *Heart & Lung, 29*(3), 225–236.

Salzman, S. (1999). Pulmonary function testing: Tips on how to interpret the results. *Journal of Respiratory Diseases, 21*(2), 101–106, 111–113.

Sharma, S. K., & Chan, E. D.. (2000). Lung disease in the elderly: Diagnosing asthma. *Journal of Respiratory Diseases, 21*(2), 101–106, 111–113.

Shelton, B. K. (1998). Mounting an offense against lobar pneumonia. *Nursing98, 28*(12), 42–47.

Shortall, S. P., & Perkins, L. A. (1999). Interpreting the ins and outs of pulmonary function tests. *Nursing99, 29*(12), 41–47.

Trudeau, M. E., & Solano-McGuire, S. M. (1999). Evaluating the quality of COPD care. . . chronic obstructive pulmonary care. *American Journal of Nursing, 99*(3), 47–50.

Van Orden-Wallace, C. (1998). Emergency! Acute pulmonary edema. *RN, 61*(1), 36–41.

Risk Factors—Lung Cancer

American Cancer Society (ACS). (2000). Lung Cancer Resource Center [On-line]. Available: http://www.cancer.org/cancerinfo/.

American Lung Association. (2000). Facts about lung cancer [On-line]. Available: http://lungusa.org/diseases/lungcanc.html.

Caporaso, N., & Landi, M. (1994). Molecular epidemiology: A new perspective for the study of toxic exposures in man. A consideration of the influence of genetic susceptibility factors on risk in different lung cancer histologies. *Medicina del Lavoro, 85*(1), 68–77.

Davis, F., Persky, V., Ferre, C., Howe, H., Barrett, R., & Haenszel, W. (1995). Cancer incidence of Hispanics and non-Hispanic whites in Cook County. *Cancer, 75*(12), 2939–2945.

Humphrey, E., Ward, H., & Perri, R. (1995). Lung cancer. In G. Murphy, W. Lawrence, & R. Lenhard. *American Cancer Society textbook of clinical oncology* (2nd ed., pp. 220–235). Atlanta, GA: American Cancer Society.

Le Marchand, L., Hankin, J., Bach, F., Kolonel, L., et al. (1995). An ecological study of diet and lung cancer in the South Pacific. *International Journal of Cancer, 63*(1), 18–23.

Strom, S., Wu, S., Sigurdson, A., Hsu, T., et al. (1995). Lung cancer, smoking patterns, and mutagen sensitivity in Mexican-Americans. *Monographs—National Cancer Institute,* (18), 29–33.

For additional information on this book, be sure to visit http://connection.lww.com.

Breast and Lymphatic Assessment

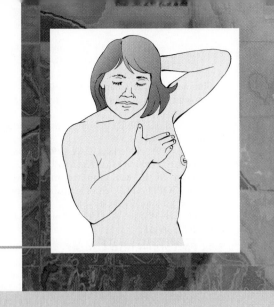

15

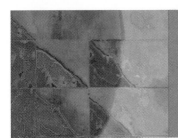

Structure and Function

PART ONE

The breasts are paired mammary glands that lie over the muscles of the anterior chest wall, anterior to the pectoralis major and serratus anterior muscles. Depending on their size and shape, the breasts extend vertically from the second to the sixth rib and horizontally from the sternum to the midaxillary line (Fig. 15-1).

The male and female breasts are similar until puberty, when female breast tissue enlarges in response to hormones—estrogen and progesterone—released from the ovaries. The female breast is an accessory reproductive organ with two functions: to produce and store milk, providing nourishment for newborns, and to aid in sexual stimulation. The male breasts have no functional capability.

For purposes of describing the location of assessment findings, the breasts are divided into four quadrants by drawing horizontal and vertical imaginary lines that intersect at the nipple.

The upper outer quadrant, which extends into the axillary area, is referred to as the tail of Spence. Most breast tumors occur in this quadrant (Fig. 15-2).

Lymph nodes are present in both male and female breasts. These structures drain lymph from the breasts to filter out microorganisms and return water and protein to the blood.

External Anatomy

The skin of the breasts is smooth and varies in color depending on the client's skin tones. The nipple, which is located in the center of the breast, contains the tiny openings of the lactiferous ducts through which milk passes. The areola surrounds the nipple and contains elevated sebaceous glands (Montgomery glands), which secrete a protective lipid substance during lactation. Hair follicles commonly appear around the areola. Smooth muscle fibers in the areola cause the nipple to become more erectile during stimulation.

The nipple and areola typically have darker pigment than the surrounding breast. Their color ranges from dark pink to dark brown, depending on the person's skin color. The amount of pigmentation increases with pregnancy and then decreases after lactation. It does not, however, entirely return to its original coloration.

In some clients, supernumerary nipples or other breast tissue may appear along an area called the "milk line" (Fig. 15-3). This milk line or ridge extends from each axilla to

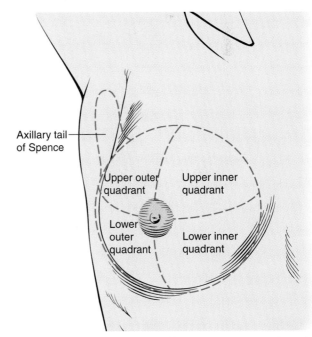

FIGURE 15-1. Anatomic breast landmarks and their position in the thorax.

FIGURE 15-2. Breast quadrants. The upper outer quadrant is the area most targeted by breast cancer.

283

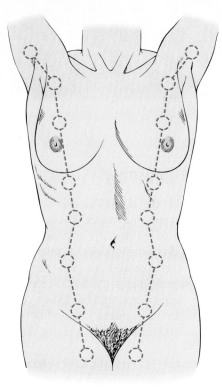

FIGURE 15-3. Supernumerary nipples may appear along the "milk line," which extends bilaterally from the axilla to the groin.

the groin area and appears during embryonic development. It gradually atrophies and disappears as the person grows and develops.

Internal Anatomy

Female breasts consist of three types of tissue: glandular, fibrous, and fatty (adipose; Fig. 15-4). Glandular tissue constitutes the functional part of the breast, allowing for milk production. Glandular tissue is arranged in 15 to 20 lobes that radiate in a circular fashion from the nipple. Each lobe contains several lobules in which the secreting alveoli (acini cells) are embedded in grapelike clusters.

Mammary ducts from the alveoli converge into a single lactiferous duct that leaves each lobe and conveys milk to the nipple. The slight enlargement in each duct before it reaches the nipple is called the lactiferous sinus. The milk can be stored in the lactiferous sinus until stimulated to be released from the nipple.

The fibrous tissue provides support for the glandular tissue largely by way of bands called Cooper's ligaments. These ligaments run from the skin through the breast and attach to the deep fascia of the muscles of the anterior chest wall.

Fatty tissue is the third component of the breast. It is in the fatty tissue that the glandular tissue is embedded. This subcutaneous and retromammary fat provides most of the substance to the breast and thus determines the size and shape of the breasts. The functional capability of the breast is not related to size but rather to the glandular tissue present.

The amount of glandular, fibrous, and fatty tissue varies according to various factors including the client's age, body build, nutritional status, hormonal cycle, and whether she is pregnant or lactating.

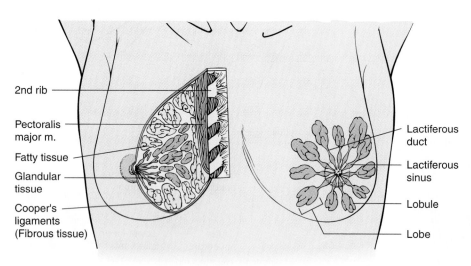

2nd rib

Pectoralis major m.

Fatty tissue

Glandular tissue

Cooper's ligaments (Fibrous tissue)

Lactiferous duct

Lactiferous sinus

Lobule

Lobe

FIGURE 15-4. Internal anatomy of the breast.

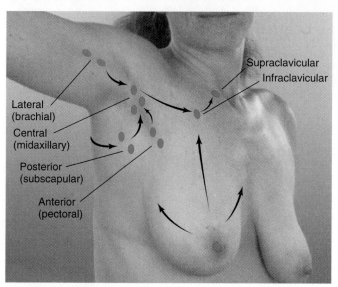

FIGURE 15-5. The lymph nodes drain impurities from the breasts (arrows show direction).

Lymph Nodes

The major axillary lymph nodes consist of the anterior (pectoral), posterior (subscapular), lateral (brachial), and central (midaxillary) nodes (Fig. 15-5). The anterior nodes drain the anterior chest wall and breasts. The posterior chest wall and part of the arms are drained by the posterior nodes.

The lateral nodes drain most of the arms, and the central nodes receive drainage from the anterior, posterior, and lateral lymph nodes. A small proportion of the lymph also flows into the infraclavicular or supraclavicular lymph nodes or deeper into nodes within the chest or abdomen.

Collecting Subjective Data

When interviewing clients, especially female clients, about the breasts, keep in mind that this topic may evoke a spate of emotions from the client. Explore your own feelings regarding body image, fear of breast cancer, and the influence of the breasts on self-esteem. Western culture emphasizes the breasts for femininity and beauty as well as lactation. Fear, anxiety, or embarrassment may influence the client's ability to discuss the condition of the breasts and breast self-examination (BSE). Men with gynecomastia or cancer of the breast may be embarrassed to have what they consider a "female condition."

This chapter covers the examination of the nonpregnant woman's breasts. Subjective data related to breast changes associated with pregnancy are covered in Chapter 25. Remember, if the client reports any symptom, you need to explore it further by performing a symptom analysis using the following guide:

COLDSPA

CHARACTER: Describe the sign or symptom. How does it feel, look, sound, smell, and so forth?

ONSET: When did it begin?

LOCATION: Where is it? Does it radiate?

DURATION: How long does it last? Does it recur?

SEVERITY: How bad is it?

PATTERN: What makes it better: What makes it worse?

ASSOCIATED FACTORS: What other symptoms occur with it?

Nursing History

You will compile the health history data early in the physical assessment. Interview questions (Q) regarding breast health and the rationale (R) for the questions follow.

CURRENT SYMPTOMS

Question Have you noticed any lumps or swelling in your breasts? If so, does the lump or swelling change during your menstrual cycle?

Rationale Lumps may be present with benign breast disease (fibrocystic breast disease), fibroadenomas, or malignant tumors (see Risk Factors—Breast Cancer). Any lumps should be assessed further, and the client should be referred to a physician. Premenstrual breast lumpiness and soreness that subside after the end of the menstrual cycle may indicate benign breast disease (fibrocystic breast disease).

Q Have you noticed any redness, warmth, or dimpling of your breasts?

R Redness and warmth indicate inflammation. A dimpling or retraction of the nipple or fibrous tissue may indicate breast cancer.

Q Have you noticed any change in the size or firmness of your breasts?

R A recent increase in the size of one breast may indicate inflammation or abnormal growth.

The older client may notice a decrease in the size and firmness of the breast as she ages because of a decrease in estrogen levels. Glandular tissue decreases whereas fatty tissue increases. A well-fitting supportive bra can reduce breast discomfort related to sagging breasts.

Q Do you experience any pain in your breasts? If so, does it occur at any specific time during your menstrual cycle?

R Pain and tenderness of the breasts are common in benign breast disease and just before and during menstruation. This is especially true for clients taking oral contraceptives. Breast pain can also be a late sign of breast cancer.

Q Do you have any discharge from the nipples? If so, describe its color, consistency, and odor, if any. Which nipple has the discharge?

R If the client reports any blood or blood-tinged discharge, she should be referred to a physician for further evaluation. Sometimes, a clear benign discharge may be manually expressed from a breast that is frequently stimulated. Certain medications (oral contraceptives, phenothiazines, steroids, digitalis, and diuretics) are also associated with a clear discharge.

RISK FACTORS
Breast Cancer

OVERVIEW

Breast cancer is the most common cancer among women, and the incidence is rising. Breast cancer is the second leading cause of cancer death among white American women and the number one cause of death among African-American women (Brown & Williams, 1994). However, early detection and treatment have resulted in increased survival rates. A 2% yearly increase since the 1980s has now leveled off at about 110 diagnosed cases per 100,000 women (American Cancer Society, 2000).

RISK FACTORS

- Gender (100 times more common in women)
- Age (risk increases with increasing age)
- Genetics (In 10% of breast cancers, mutations of BRCA1 and BRCA2 genes are identified. In addition, a p53 tumor suppressor gene has been identified in some breast cancers.)
- Family history of breast cancer
- Personal history of breast cancer
- Early menarche and late menopause
- No natural children
- First child born to mother older than age 30
- Oral contraceptive use (slight risk)
- Regular alcohol intake, especially with two to five drinks daily
- Higher education and socioeconomic status
- Previous breast irradiation
- Hormone replacement therapy with progesterone
- Wet ear wax

POSSIBLE RISK FACTORS FOR BREAST CANCER

- Taller height (Albanes & Taylor, 1992)
- High waist-to-hip ratio (ACS, 2000; Sellers, 1992); obesity beginning as adult or after menopause

- High-fat diet (ambivalent findings; see Kushi et al., 1992; ACS, 2000)
- Low number of births
- No breast-feeding (ACS, 2000)
- Low level of physical activity

POSSIBLE RISK FACTORS FOR MORTALITY

- No (or poor) breast self-examination
- Poor screening (physical examination or mammography)

RISK REDUCTION TEACHING TIPS

- Not delaying pregnancy until after 30 years of age
- Breast-feeding
- Performing monthly breast self-examination (BSE)
- Following the American Cancer Society Guidelines for clinical evaluation and mammography
- Strenuous exercise, especially in youth but also in adulthood
- Nonsteroidal anti-inflammatory drug (NSAID) therapy (may have protective effect)

 ### CULTURAL CONSIDERATIONS

The highest incidence of breast cancer occurs in the United States and Europe, and the rate continues to increase in Europe. There is a low incidence of breast cancer in the rest of the world, especially in Native Americans and in Saudi Arabia, Japan, and Singapore. However, some areas of Brazil have breast cancer rates similar to the United States (Azevedo & Mendonca, 1993). This pattern may relate to the lower incidence of breast cancer in women with dry ear wax (glands in ear canal and breast are apocrine glands; Overfield, 1995). In the United States, African Americans have the highest age-adjusted death rates from breast cancer followed by non-Hispanic whites (Overfield, 1995).

Cultural beliefs about what causes breast cancer do not always agree with medical findings. Hispanic Americans may associate breast cancer with physical stress, trauma, and behavior or lifestyle choices, such as use of alcohol or illegal drugs (Chavez, Hubbell, McMullin, Martinez & Mishra, 1995a, b). Health teaching by breast cancer patients of the same race and cultural background and use of settings, such as local churches, community centers, and beauty salons, has significantly increased the use of screening methods such as breast self-examination and mammography (Erwin, Spatz & Turturro, 1992; Forte, 1995).

PAST HISTORY

Q Have you had any prior breast disease? Have you ever had breast surgery, a breast biopsy, breast implants, or breast trauma? What was the result?

R A personal history of breast cancer increases the risk for recurrence of cancer. Previous surgeries may alter the appearance of the breasts. Breast problems may occur with silicone breast implants. Trauma to the breasts from sports, accidents, or physical abuse can result in breast tissue changes.

Q How old were you when you began to menstruate? Have you experienced menopause?

R Early menses (before age 13) or delayed menopause (after age 52) increases the risk for breast cancer.

Q Have you given birth to any children? At what age did you have your first child?

R The risk of breast cancer is greater for women who have never given birth or for those who had their first child after age 30.

Q When was the first and last day of your menstrual cycle?

R This information will inform you if this is the optimal time to examine the breasts. Hormone-related swelling, breast tenderness, and generalized lumpiness are reduced right after menstruation.

FAMILY HISTORY

Q Is there a history of breast cancer in your family?

R A history of breast cancer in one's family increases one's risk for breast cancer.

LIFESTYLE AND HEALTH PRACTICES

Q Are you taking any hormones, contraceptives, or antipsychotic agents?

R Hormones and some antipsychotic agents can cause breast engorgement in women. Hormones and oral contraceptives also increase the risk of breast cancer. Haloperidol (Haldol), an antipsychotic drug, can cause galactorrhea (persistent milk secretion whether the woman is breast-feeding or not) and lactation. This is also a side effect of medroxyprogesterone (Depo-Provera) injections.

Q Do you live or work in an area where you have excessive exposure to radiation, benzene, or asbestos?

R Exposure to these environmental hazards can increase the risk of breast cancer.

Q What is your typical daily diet?

R A high-fat diet may increase the risk for breast cancer.

Q How much alcohol do you drink each day?

R Alcohol intake exceeding two drinks per day has been associated with a higher risk for breast cancer.

Q How much coffee, tea, cola (or other forms of caffeine) do you consume each day?

R Caffeine can aggravate fibrocystic breast disease.

Q Do you engage in any type of regular exercise? If so, what type of bra do you wear when you exercise?

R Breast tissue can lose its elasticity if vigorous exercise (ie, running, aerobics) is performed without support for the breast. A well-fitting, supportive bra can also reduce discomfort in the breasts during exercise.

Q How important are your breasts to you in relation to a positive feeling about yourself and your physical appearance? Do you have any fears regarding breast disease?

R The condition of the breasts may significantly influence how a woman feels about herself. Alterations in the breasts may threaten a woman's body image and feelings of self-worth, and men may be embarrassed to have enlarged breasts.

Q Do you examine your own breasts? Describe when you do this. (The client should demonstrate BSE during the physical assessment.)

Tip From the Experts Older clients and others who no longer menstruate may find it helpful to pick a set day of the month for BSE—one they will remember each month, such as the day of the month they were born.

R The American Cancer Society (ACS) recommends that BSE be performed monthly for all women age 20 years and older. The best time is right after menstruation, or between the fourth and seventh day of the cycle if the cycle is regular. If the client is on cyclic estrogen therapy, she should examine her breasts on the last day that the medicine is not being taken. Women who have had a breast lumpectomy, augmentation, or breast reconstruction also should perform BSE.

Q Have you ever had your breasts examined by a physician? When was your last examination?

R The ACS recommends a clinical breast examination by a health care professional every 3 years for women ages 20 to 39 and every year for women age 40 and older (ACS, 2000).

Q Have you ever had a mammogram? If so, when was your last one?

R The ACS recommends an annual mammogram for women age 40 and older (ACS, 2000).

Collecting Objective Data

The purpose of breast assessment is to identify signs of breast disease and then to initiate early treatment. The incidence of breast cancer in women is rising, but early detection and treatment have resulted in increased survival rates.

It is often convenient to assess the breasts immediately after assessment of the thorax and lungs. Female breast examinations are also performed by the nurse before a mammogram or by the gynecologist or nurse practitioner before a routine pelvic examination. A breast examination should also be a routine part of the complete male assessment. However, the male breast examination is not as detailed as the female breast examination.

Keep in mind that breast palpation requires practice and skill because the consistency of the breasts varies widely from client to client. Some breasts are more difficult to palpate than others. For example, it is more difficult to palpate and inspect large, pendulous breasts to ensure adequate evaluation of all breast tissue. It may also be difficult to detect new lumps in women who have fibrocystic breast disease and who have granular, singular, or multiple mobile, tender lumps in their breasts.

The actual hands-on physical examination of the breast may create client anxiety. The client may be embarrassed about exposing his or her breasts and may be anxious about what the assessment will reveal. Explain in detail what is happening throughout the assessment and answer any questions the client might have. In addition, attempt to provide the client with as much privacy as possible during the examination.

This chapter covers the examination of the nonpregnant woman's breasts. Objective data related to breast changes associated with pregnancy are covered in Chapter 25.

CLIENT PREPARATION

Prepare for the breast examination by having the client sit in an upright position. Explain that it will be necessary to expose both breasts to compare for symmetry during inspection. One breast may be draped while the other breast is palpated. Be sensitive to the fact that many women may feel embarrassed to have their breasts examined.

The breasts are first inspected in the sitting position while the client is asked to hold arms in different positions. The breasts are then palpated while the client assumes a supine position.

The final part of the examination involves teaching clients how to perform BSE and asking them to demonstrate what they have learned. If the client states that she or he already knows how to perform BSE, then ask the client to demonstrate how this is done. See the printed client information sheet on BSE in the study guide/laboratory manual for this book.

EQUIPMENT AND SUPPLIES

- Centimeter ruler
- Small pillow
- Gloves
- Client handout: Breast Self-Examination (which is in the study guide for this book)
- Slide for specimen

KEY ASSESSMENT POINTS

- Explain to the client what the steps of the examination are and the rationale for them.
- Warm hands.
- Observe and inspect breast skin, areolas, and nipples for size, shape, rashes, dimpling, swelling, discoloration, retraction, asymmetry and other unusual findings.
- Palpate breasts and axillary lymph nodes for swelling, lumps, masses, warmth or inflammation, tenderness, and other abnormalities.
- Perform the physical assessment just as carefully on male clients.

(*text continues on page 295*)

PHYSICAL ASSESSMENT

ASSESSMENT PROCEDURE	NORMAL FINDINGS	ABNORMAL FINDINGS

FEMALE BREASTS

Inspect Size and Symmetry

Have the client disrobe and sit with arms hanging freely. Explain what you are observing to help ease client anxiety.

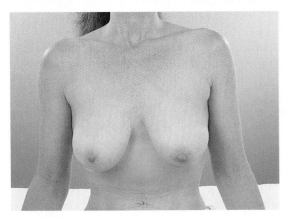

Client should sit with arms hanging freely at sides during assessment of breast size and symmetry.

Breasts can be a variety of sizes and are somewhat round and pendulous. One breast may normally be larger than the other.

The older client often has more pendulous, less firm, and saggy breasts.

A recent increase in the size of one breast may indicate inflammation or an abnormal growth.

A pigskin-like or orange-peel (peau d'orange) appearance results from edema, which is seen in metastatic breast disease. The edema is caused by blocked lymphatic drainage.

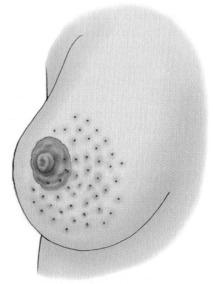

Resulting from edema, an orange peal (peau d'orange) appearance of the breast is associated with cancer.

Inspect Color and Texture

Be sure to note client's overall skin tone when inspecting the breast skin.

Color varies depending on the client's skin tone. Texture is smooth with no edema.

Linear stretch marks may be seen during and after pregnancy or with significant weight gain or loss.

Redness is associated with breast inflammation.

Inspect Superficial Venous Pattern

Observe visibility and pattern of breast veins.

Veins radiate either horizontally and toward the axilla (transverse) or vertically with a lateral flare (longitudinal).

These two patterns are seen in varying proportions among different cultural groups. However, both patterns are normal, and the transverse pattern predominates.

A prominent venous pattern may occur as a result of increased circulation due to a malignancy. An asymmetric venous pattern may be due to malignancy.

(continued)

ASSESSMENT PROCEDURE	NORMAL FINDINGS	ABNORMAL FINDINGS

Inspect the Areolas

Note the color, size, shape, and texture of the areolas of both breasts.

Areolas vary from dark pink to dark brown, depending on the client's skin tones. They are round and may vary in size. Small Montgomery tubercles are present.

Peau d'orange skin, associated with carcinoma, may be first seen in the areola, whereas red, scaly, crusty areas are indicative of Paget's disease.

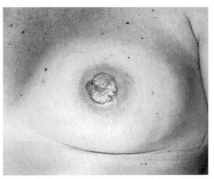

Paget's disease is typified by a crusty, red scaliness of the nipple.

Inspect the Nipples

Note the size and direction of the nipples of both breasts.

Nipples are nearly equal bilaterally in size and are in the same location on each breast. Nipples are usually everted, but they may be inverted or flat. Supernumerary nipples may appear along the embryonic "milk line." No discharge should be present.

The older client may have smaller, flatter nipples that are less erectile on stimulation.

A recently retracted nipple that was previously everted suggests malignancy. Any type of spontaneous discharge should be referred for cytologic study and further evaluation.

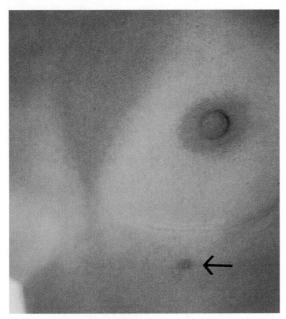

Supernumerary nipple. (Logan-Young, W., & Hoffman, N. Y. [1994]. *Breast cancer: A practical guide to diagnosis.* Rochester, NY: Mt. Hope Publishing.)

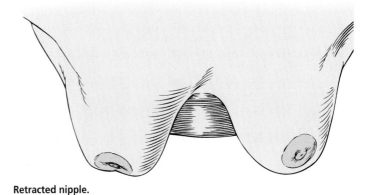

Retracted nipple.

(continued)

ASSESSMENT PROCEDURE	NORMAL FINDINGS	ABNORMAL FINDINGS

Inspect for Retraction and Dimpling

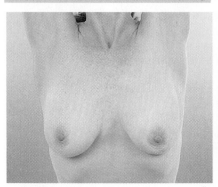 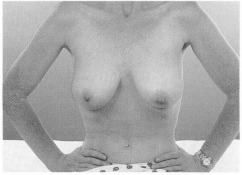 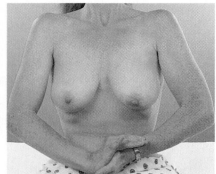

During assessment for retraction and dimpling, the client first (left) raises her arms over her head, (center) lowers them and presses them against the hips, then (right) presses the hands together with fingers of the one hand pointing opposite to the fingers of the other hand.

To inspect the breasts accurately for retraction and dimpling, ask the client to remain seated while performing several different maneuvers. Ask the client to raise her arms overhead; then, press her hands against her hips. Next, ask her to press her hands together. These actions contract the pectoral muscles.

The client's breasts should rise symmetrically with no sign of dimpling or retraction.

Dimpling or retraction is usually caused by a malignant tumor that has fibrous strands attached to the breast tissue and the fascia of the muscles. As the muscle contracts, it draws the breast tissue and skin with it, causing dimpling or retraction

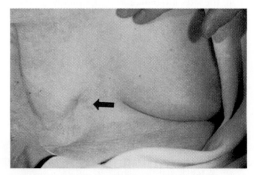

Dimpling of the breast nipple. Logan-Young, W., & Hoffman, N.Y. [1994] *Breast cancer: A practical guide to diagnosis*, Rochester, NY: Mt. Hope Publishing).

Finally, ask the client to lean forward from the waist. This is a good position to use in women who have large, pendulous breasts.

Breasts should hang freely and symmetrically.

Restricted movement of breast or retraction of the skin or nipple indicates fibrosis and fixation of the underlying tissues. This is usually due to an underlying malignant tumor.

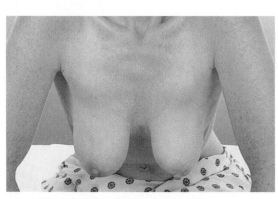

Forward-leaning position for breast inspection.

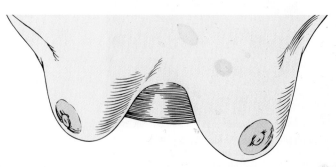

Retracted breast tissue.

(continued)

ASSESSMENT PROCEDURE	NORMAL FINDINGS	ABNORMAL FINDINGS

Palpate Texture and Elasticity

See Display 15-1.

Smooth, firm, elastic tissue.

The older client's breasts may feel more granular, and the inframammary ridge may be more easily palpated as it thickens.

Thickening of the tissues may occur with an underlying malignant tumor.

PALPATE TENDERNESS AND TEMPERATURE

See Display 15-1.

A generalized increase in nodularity and tenderness may be a normal finding associated with the menstrual cycle or hormonal medications. Breasts should be a normal body temperature.

Painful breasts may be indicative of benign breast disease but can also occur with a malignant tumor. The client should be referred for further evaluation. Heat in the breasts of women who have not just given birth or who are not lactating indicates inflammation.

Palpate for Masses

Note location, size in centimeters, shape, mobility, consistency, and tenderness (see Display 15-1).

If you detect any lump, refer the client for further evaluation.

No masses should be palpated. However, a firm inframammary transverse ridge may normally be palpated at the lower base of the breasts.

Malignant tumors are most often found in the upper outer quadrant of the breast. They are usually unilateral, with irregular, poorly delineated borders. They are hard and nontender and fixed to underlying tissues.

Fibroadenomas are usually 1- to 5-cm, round or oval, mobile, firm, solid, elastic, nontender, single or multiple benign masses that are found in one or both breasts.

Benign breast disease consists of bilateral, multiple, firm, regular, rubbery, mobile nodules with well-demarcated borders. Pain and fullness occurs just before menses (Display 15-2).

Palpate the Nipples

Wear gloves to compress the nipple gently with your thumb and index finger. Note any discharge.

If spontaneous discharge occurs from the nipples, a specimen must be applied to a slide and the smear sent to the laboratory for cytologic evaluation.

The nipple may become erect and the areola may pucker in response to stimulation. A milky discharge is usually normal only during pregnancy and lactation. However, some women may normally have a clear discharge.

Discharge may be seen in endocrine disorders and with certain medications (ie, antihypertensives, tricyclic antidepressants, and estrogen). Discharge from one breast may indicate benign intraductal papilloma, fibrocystic disease, or cancer of the breast.

Palpating nipples for masses and discharge.

(continued)

ASSESSMENT PROCEDURE	NORMAL FINDINGS	ABNORMAL FINDINGS

Palpate Mastectomy or Lumpectomy Site

If the client has had a mastectomy or lumpectomy, it is still important to perform a thorough examination. Palpate the scar and any remaining breast or axillary tissue for redness, lesions, lumps, swelling, or tenderness.

Scar is whitish with no redness or swelling. No lesions, lumps, or tenderness noted.

Redness and inflammation of the scar area may indicate infection. Any lesions, lumps, or tenderness should be referred for further evaluation.

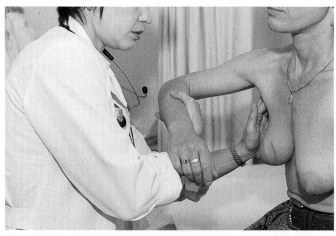

Palpating surgical site. (©Dorothy Littell Greco 1993, Stock Boston.)

THE AXILLAE

Inspect and Palpate the Axillae

Ask the client to sit up. Inspect the axillary skin for rashes or infection.

No rash or infection noted.

Redness and inflammation may be seen with infection of the sweat gland. Dark, velvety pigmentation of the axillae (acanthosis nigricans) may indicate an underlying malignancy.

Hold the client's elbow with one hand, and use the three fingerpads of your other hand to palpate firmly the axillary lymph nodes.

No palpable nodes or one to two small (less than 1 cm), discrete, nontender, movable nodes in the central area.

Enlarged (greater than 1 cm) lymph nodes may indicate infection of the hand or arm. Large nodes that are hard and fixed to the skin may indicate an underlying malignancy.

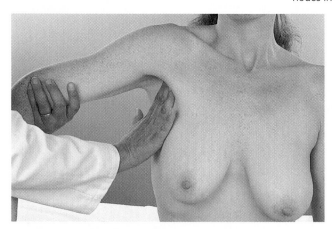

Palpating the axillary lymph nodes.

First, palpate high into the axillae, moving downward against the ribs to feel for the central nodes. Continue to move down the posterior axillae to feel for the posterior nodes. Use bimanual palpation to feel for the anterior axillary nodes. Finally, palpate down the inner aspect of the upper arm.

(continued)

ASSESSMENT PROCEDURE	NORMAL FINDINGS	ABNORMAL FINDINGS

THE MALE BREASTS

Inspect and Palpate the Breasts, Areolas, Nipples, and Axillae

Note any swelling, nodules, or ulceration. Palpate the flat disc of undeveloped breast tissue under the nipple.	No swelling, nodules, or ulceration should be detected.	Soft, fatty enlargement of breast tissue is seen in obesity. Gynecomastia, a smooth, firm, movable disc of glandular tissue, may be seen in one breast in males during puberty for a temporary time. However, it may also be seen in hormonal imbalances, drug abuse, cirrhosis, leukemia, and thyrotoxicosis. Irregularly shaped, hard nodules occur in breast cancer.

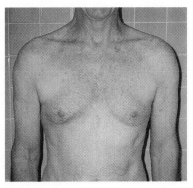

Gynecomastia.

Validation and Documentation of Findings

Validate the breast and lymph node assessment data that you have collected. This is necessary to verify that the data are reliable and accurate. Document the assessment data following the health care facility or agency policy.

EXAMPLE OF SUBJECTIVE DATA

Forty-year-old woman. No history of breast disease, biopsies, or surgery in self or family. Takes hormone replacement therapy for early onset of menopause. Performs monthly BSE. Reports no breast lesions, lumps, swelling, pain, rashes, or discharge. Has yearly mammogram and breast examination by gynecologist. Eats a low-fat diet. Does not drink alcohol. Exercises four times a week wearing supportive, firm bra. Menstruation started at age 14.

Has one adopted child. Comfortable with discussing condition of breasts.

EXAMPLE OF OBJECTIVE DATA

Inspection

Bilateral breasts moderate in size, pendulant, and symmetric. Breast skin pale pink with light brown areola. Montgomery tubercles present. Nipples everted bilaterally. Free movement of breasts with position changes of arms and hands. No dimpling, retraction, lesions, or inflammation noted. Axillae free of rashes or inflammation.

Palpation

No masses or tenderness palpated. Bilateral mammary ridge present. No discharge from nipples. Axillary (central, anterior, or posterior) and lateral arm lymph nodes nonpalpable. Demonstrates appropriate technique for BSE.

DISPLAY 15-1. Guidelines for Palpating the Breasts

1. Ask the client to lie down and to place overhead the arm on the same side as the breast being palpated. Place a small pillow or rolled towel under the breast being palpated.

2. Use the flat pads of three fingers to palpate the client's breasts.

3. Palpate the breasts using one of three different patterns. Choose one that is most comfortable for you, but be consistent and thorough with the method chosen.

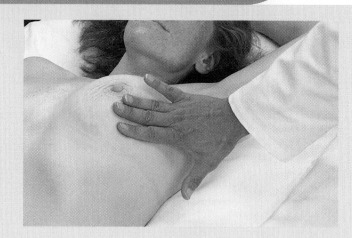

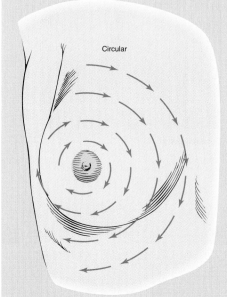

Circular or clockwise.

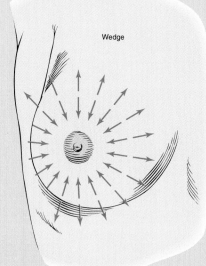

Wedged.

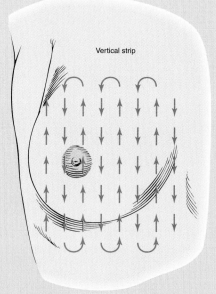

Vertical strip.

4. Be sure to palpate every square inch of the breast, from the nipple and areola to the periphery of the breast tissue and up into the tail of Spence. Vary the levels of pressure as you palpate.

   Light—superficial
   Medium—mid-level tissue
   Firm—to the ribs

5. Use the bimanual technique if the client has large breasts. Support the breast with your nondominant hand, and use your dominant hand to palpate.

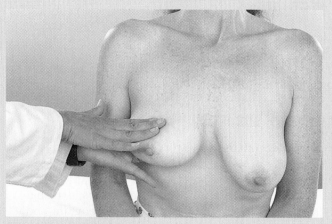

Bimanual palpation.

DISPLAY 15-2. Abnormalities of the Breasts

Whereas some abnormalities of the breast are readily apparent, such as peau d' orange and Paget's disease, some breast internal changes are detected only by palpation and mammography. The following illustrations represent breast abnormalities characteristic of tumors, fibroadenomas, and benign disease (fibrocystic breasts).

CANCEROUS TUMORS

These are irregular, firm, hard, not defined masses, which may be fixed or mobile. They are not usually tender and usually occur after age 50.

FIBROADENOMAS

These lesions are lobular, ovid, or round. They are firm, well defined, seldom tender, and usually singular and mobile. They occur more commonly between puberty and menopause.

BENIGN BREAST DISEASE

Also called fibrocystic breast disease, benign breast disease is marked by round, elastic, defined, tender, and mobile cysts. The condition is most common from age 30 to menopause, after which it decreases.

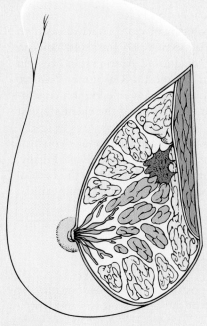

Tumor.

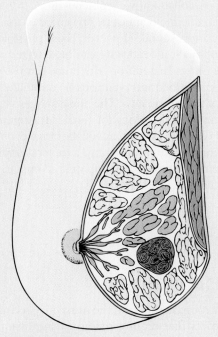

Fibroadenoma.

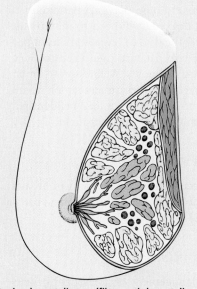

Benign breast disease (fibrocystic breast disease).

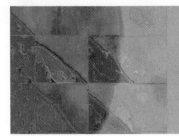

After you collect your assessment data, you will need to analyze the data, using diagnostic reasoning skills. You can review key steps of the diagnostic reasoning process in Chapter 7. After that, in Diagnostic Reasoning: Possible Conclusions, you will see an overview of common conclusions that you may reach after assessing the client's breast and lymph nodes.

Next, Diagnostic Reasoning: Case Study shows you how to analyze the assessment data for a specific client. Finally, you will have an opportunity to analyze data in the Critical Thinking Exercise in your laboratory manual/study guide.

Diagnostic Reasoning: Possible Conclusions

Listed below are some possible conclusions that may be reached after assessment of the client's breasts and lymph nodes.

SELECTED NURSING DIAGNOSES

After collecting subjective and objective data pertaining to the breasts and lymph nodes, you will need to identify abnormal findings and cluster the data to reveal significant patterns or abnormalities. These data are then used to make clinical judgments (nursing diagnoses: wellness, risk, or actual) about the status of the client's breasts and lymph nodes. The following selected nursing diagnoses may be identified when analyzing data for this part of the assessment.

Nursing Diagnoses (Wellness)

- Opportunity to enhance health management of breasts
- Health-Seeking Behavior: Requests information on breast self-examination (BSE)

Nursing Diagnoses (Risk)

- Risk for Ineffective Management of Therapeutic Regimen related to busy lifestyle and lack of knowledge of monthly BSE

Nursing Diagnoses (Actual)

- Fear of breast cancer related to increased risk factors
- Ineffective Individual Coping related to diagnoses of breast cancer
- Body Image Disturbance related to mastectomy
- Anticipatory Grieving related to anticipation of poor outcome of breast biopsy
- Ineffective Management of Therapeutic Regimen related to lack of knowledge of BSE

SELECTED COLLABORATIVE PROBLEMS

After grouping the data related to the breasts and lymph nodes, certain collaborative problems may emerge. Remember, collaborative problems differ from nursing diagnoses in that they cannot be prevented or treated by nursing interventions alone. However, these physiologic complications of medical conditions can be detected and monitored by the nurse. In addition, the nurse can use physician- and nurse-prescribed interventions to minimize the complications of these problems. The nurse may also have to refer the client in such situations for further treatment of the problem. Following is a list of collaborative problems that may be identified when obtaining a general impression. These problems are worded as Potential Complications (or PC), followed by the problem.

- PC: Infection (abscess)
- PC: Hematoma
- PC: Benign breast disease

MEDICAL PROBLEMS

After grouping the data, the nurse may recognize signs and symptoms that require medical diagnosis and treatment. Referral to a primary care provider is necessary.

Diagnostic Reasoning: Case Study

The case study presents assessment data for a specific client. It is followed by an analysis of the data, working out the seven key diagnostic reasoning steps to arrive at specific conclusions.

During her routine physical examination ("I schedule one every year now because I want to live to a healthy old age"), Mrs. Nicole Barnes, a 42-year-old African American, tells you that she is concerned with the lumps and tenderness that occur in her breasts each month, just a few days before her menstrual period. In response to questioning, she relates that she is a "heavy coffee drinker" and is under a great deal of stress in her job. She reports that a maternal aunt died of breast cancer. She wants to know if the lumps could be cancerous or what can be done to eliminate this breast problem. On examination, you note that her breasts feel nodular but without discrete masses. Other findings include no evidence of inflammation, no axillary node enlargement, and no lesions or nipple drainage. You suspect that she has fibrocystic changes characteristic of benign breast disease.

1 Identify abnormal data and strengths (in both subjective and objective data).

SUBJECTIVE DATA

- Schedules yearly physical examinations to promote health
- Complains of breast lumps and tenderness that occur shortly before menses
- Drinks excessive amount of coffee—experiencing much stress
- Says maternal aunt died of cancer
- Fears that she might have cancer
- Wants information about managing breast problem

OBJECTIVE DATA

- Nodular breasts without discrete masses
- No inflammation, lesions, nipple drainage, or enlarged axillary lymph nodes

2 Cue Clusters	**3** Inferences	**4** Possible Nursing Diagnoses	**5** Defining Characteristics	**6** Confirm or Rule Out
A • Verbalizes breast tenderness and lumps • Maternal aunt died from breast cancer • Negative for other findings of breast disease • Premenopausal symptoms related to menstrual cycle • Excessive coffee consumption and increased stress	May have fibrocystic breast syndrome but can be at risk for cancer due to family history Has risk factors for polycystic breast syndrome	Altered Health Maintenance related to knowledge deficit regarding cause and management of breast problem Ineffective Individual Coping	*Major:* Reports an unhealthy practice (excessive coffee intake and unmanaged stress) *Minor:* None *Major:* None *Minor:* Reported increased stress with job but did not state difficulty in managing stress (although implied)	Confirm because it meets the major defining characteristic and is validated by client. Rule out because not enough data to validate major defining characteristic. However, important to collect more information because it is a risk factor for presenting signs and symptoms.
B • Schedules regular yearly physical examinations • Wants information to manage breast problems	Interested in promoting health into old age and preventing disease	Health-Seeking Behaviors	*Major:* Expressed desire to seek information for health promotion *Minor:* Expressed desire for increased help with health events	Accept diagnosis because it meets both major and minor defining characteristics.
C • Expresses concern that she might have cancer • Lumps and tenderness in breasts • Maternal aunt died of breast cancer	Cancer anxiety because of family history	Anxiety related to inadequate knowledge regarding cause of present breast symptoms and presence of family history of breast cancer	*Major:* Admits to feelings of apprehension (concern) about having cancer. No physiologic or cognitive characteristics noted *Minor:* None tested for this diagnosis	Confirm because it meets one area of defining characteristics (emotional), but need to collect additional information to identify the degree of anxiety and its effect on client's well-

②	③	④	⑤	⑥
Cue Clusters	Inferences	Possible Nursing Diagnoses	Defining Characteristics	Confirm or Rule Out
		Fear related to consequences of possible cancer diagnosis	*Major:* None *Minor:* None	being and to determine helpful nursing interventions. Rule out—does not meet defining characteristics. Anxiety is the more appropriate diagnosis.

⑦ Document conclusions.

Three of the proposed diagnoses are appropriate for Mrs. Barnes at this time:

- Altered Health Maintenance related to knowledge deficit regarding cause and management of breast problem
- Health-Seeking Behaviors
- Anxiety related to inadequate knowledge regarding cause of present breast symptoms and presence of family history of breast cancer

No collaborative problems could be identified because there is no medical diagnosis at this time.

Mrs. Barnes needs a referral to her physician for evaluation, diagnosis, and possible biopsy of her breast lumps. There are also medications that the physician may recommend if the problem cannot be managed by reducing the risk factors. Mrs. Barnes should also be referred for yearly mammography because of her family history and her age.

REFERENCES AND SELECTED READINGS

Ali, N. S. (1991). Teaching early breast cancer detection strategies. *Advancing Clinical Care, 6*(4), 21–23.

American Cancer Society. (2000). *Cancer facts and figures—2000.* Atlanta: Author.

Briggs, F. E. (1996). Newly diagnosed women with breast cancer: The nurse's role. *Nurse Practitioner: American Journal of Primary Health Care, 21*(4), 153–155.

Brown, E. W. (1999). Are you at risk for breast cancer? *Medical Update, 23*(2), 6.

"Buddy system" gets word out on breast examinations: Reminder system increases use of self-exams. (1999). *Patient Education Management, 6*(12), 142–144.

D'Epiro, N. W. (1999). Breast cancer prevention: Are we making progress? *Patient Care, 33*(17), 30–40.

Dienger, M. J., & Llewellyn, J. (1995). Increasing compliance with breast self-examination. *MedSurg Nursing, 4*(5), 359–366.

Feldman, E. B. (1999). Breast cancer risk and intake of fat. *Nutrition Reviews, 57*(11), 353–356.

George, S. A. (2000). Barriers to breast cancer screening: An integrative review. *Health Care for Women International, 21*(1), 53–65.

Hindel, W. H. (1998). Palpable breast mass: The physical examination. *Hospital Medicine, 34*(3), 42–45.

Houfek, J. F., & Barron, C. R. (1993). Research corner: Psychological factors related to the practice of breast self-examination. *Nebraska Nurse, 26*(4), 27.

Houfek, J. F., Waltman, N. L., & Kile, M. A. (1999). Special continuing education section: A nurse's guide to breast cancer. The nurse's role in promoting breast cancer screening... Adapted from article [sic] in the *Nebraska Nurse*, vol 30, no 3, August 1997. *Georgia Nursing, 59*(1), 11–14, 25–27.

Lauver, D. R., Kane, J., Bodden, J., McNeel, J., & Smith, L. (1999). Engagement in breast cancer screening behaviors. *Oncology Nursing Forum, 26*(3), 545–554.

Maurer, F. (1997). A peer education model for teaching breast self-examination to undergraduate college women. *Cancer Nursing, 20*(1), 49–61.

McCool, W. F., Stone-Condry, M., & Bradfor, H. M. (1998). Breast health care: A review. *Journal of Nurse-Midwifery, 43*(6), 406–430.

Northouse, L. (1990). A longitudinal study of the adjustment of patients and husbands to breast cancer. *Oncology Nursing Forum, 17*(3), 39–43.

O'Connor, A. M., & Perrault, D. J. (1995). Importance of physician's role highlighted in survey of women's breast screening practices. *Canadian Journal of Public Health, 86*(1), 42–45.

Pasacreta, J. V. (1999). Psychosocial issues associated with increased breast and ovarian cancer risk: Findings from focus groups. *Archives of Psychiatric Nursing, 13*(3), 127–136.

Pennypacker, H. S., Naylor, L., Sander, A. A., & Goldstein, M. K. (1999). Why can't we do better breast examinations? *Nurse Practitioner Forum, 10*(3), 122–128.

Prescott, B. (1999). Breast self-examination: How important is it? *Pulse, 36*(2), 5.

Salazar, M. K. (1994). Breast self-examination beliefs: A descriptive study. *Public Health Nursing, 11*(1), 49–56.

Sloand, E. (1998). Pediatric and adolescent breast health. *Lippincott's Primary Care Practice, 2*(2), 170–175.

Sternberger, C. (1994). Breast self-examination: How nurses can influence performance. *MedSurg Nursing, 3*(5), 367–371.

Taylor, P. (1999). Protocols in practice. Case management program for breast cancer education. *Nursing Case Management, 4*(3), 135–144.

Underwood, P. W. (1998). Vital signs. Breast cancer awareness begins with you. *American Journal of Nursing, 98*(10), 80.

Weber, P. A., Fos, P., Zhang, X., & Pond, M. (1996). An examination of differential follow-up rates in breast cancer screening. *Journal of Community Health, 21*(2), 123–132.

Wheaton, P. (1992). One nurse's blueprint for change . . . breast health specialist Amy Chou, R.N., M.A. *Revolution, 2*(2), 104–112.

Winslow, M. N. B. (1993). Commentary on self-esteem and the practice of breast self-examination . . . including commentary by Olson K. and Humenick S. S. with author response. *ONS Nursing Scan in Oncology, 2*(3), 3.

Zook, E. G., & Grado, C. E. (1991). Poland's syndrome. *Plastic Surgical Nursing, 11*(3), 113–118.

Risk Factors—Breast Cancer

Albanes, D., & Taylor, P. (1992). The international differences in body height and weight and their relationships to cancer incidence. *Nutrition and Cancer, 14*(1), 69–77.

American Cancer Society. (2000). *ACS Breast Cancer Resource Center.* Available: www.cancer.org.

———. (2000). *Cancer facts and figures—2000.* Atlanta: Author.

Azevedo, G., & Mendonca, S. (1993). Cancer in the female population in Brazil. *Rev Saude Publica, 27*(1), 68–75.

Brown, L. W., & Williams, R. (1994). Culturally sensitive breast cancer screening programs for older black women. *Nurse Practitioner 19*(3), 21–26.

Chavez, L., Hubbell, F., McMullin, J., Martinez, R., & Mishra, S. (1995a). Structure and meaning in models of breast and cervical risk factors: A comparison of perceptions among Latinas, Anglo women, and physicians. *Medical Anthropology Quarterly, 9*(1), 40–74.

———. (1995b). Understanding knowledge and attitudes about breast cancer. A cultural analysis. *Archives of Family Medicine, 4*(2), 145–152.

Erwin D., Spatz, T., & Turturro, C. (1992). Development of an African-American role model intervention to increase breast self-examination and mammography. *Journal of Cancer Education, 7*(4), 311–319.

Forte, D. (1995). Community-based breast cancer intervention program for older African-American women in beauty salons. *Public Health Reports, 110*(2), 179–183.

Kushi, L., Sellers, T., Potter, J., Nelson, C., et al. (1992). Dietary fat and postmenopausal breast cancer. *Journal of the National Cancer Institute, 84*(14), 1092–1099.

Mahon, S. M. (1998). Cancer risk assessment: Conceptual considerations for clinical practice. *Oncology Nursing Forum, 25*(9), 1535–1547.

Overfield, T. (1995). *Biologic variation in health and illness: Race, age, and sex differences* (2nd ed.). Boca Raton, FL: CRC Press.

Sellers, T., Kushi, L., Potter, J., Kaye, S., Nelson, C., McGovern, P., & Folsom, A. (1992). The effect of family history, body-fat distribution, and reproductive factors on the risk of postmenopausal breast cancer. *New England Journal of Medicine, 326*(20), 1323–1329.

Short, R. (1994). What the breast does for the baby, and what the baby does for the breast. *Australian–New Zealand Journal of Obstetrics and Gynecology, 34*(3), 262–264.

For additional information on this book, be sure to visit http://connection.lww.com.

Heart and Neck Vessel Assessment

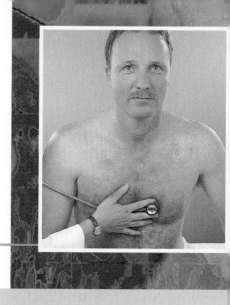

16

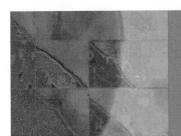

The cardiovascular system is a highly complex system comprising the heart and a closed system of blood vessels. The examiner must have appropriate knowledge regarding the structure and function of the heart, great vessels, the electrical conduction system of the heart, the cardiac cycle, production of heart sounds, cardiac output, and neck vessels. This information assists the examiner to differentiate between normal and abnormal findings as they relate to the cardiovascular system.

◆ Heart and Great Vessels

The heart is a hollow, muscular, four-chambered organ located in the middle of the thoracic cavity between the lungs in the space called the *mediastinum*. It is about the size of a clenched fist and weighs approximately 255 g (9 oz) in women and 310 g (10.9 oz) in men. The heart extends vertically from the second to the fifth intercostal space (ICS) and horizontally from the right edge of the sternum to the left midclavicular line (MCL). The heart can be described as an inverted cone. The upper portion, near the second ICS, is the base, and the lower portion, near the fifth ICS and the left MCL, is the apex. The anterior chest area that overlies the heart and great vessels is called the *precordium* (Fig. 16-1). The heart pumps blood. The right side of the heart pumps blood to the lungs for gas exchange (pulmonary circulation); the left side of the heart pumps blood to all other parts of the body (systemic circulation).

The large veins and arteries leading directly to and away from the heart are referred to as the *great vessels*. The *superior and inferior vena cava* return blood to the right atrium from the upper and lower torso, respectively. The *pulmonary artery* exits the right ventricle, bifurcates, and carries blood to the lungs. The *pulmonary veins* (two from each lung) return oxygenated blood to the left atrium. The *aorta* transports oxygenated blood from the ventricle to the body (Fig. 16-2).

HEART CHAMBERS, VALVES, AND CIRCULATION

The heart consists of four chambers or cavities: two upper chambers, the *right and left atria*, and two lower chambers, the *right and left ventricles*. The right and left sides of the heart are separated by a partition called the *septum*. The thin-walled atria receive blood returning to the heart and pump blood into the ventricles. The thicker-walled ventri-cles pump blood out of the heart. The left ventricle is thicker than the right ventricle because the left side of the heart has a greater workload.

The entrance and exit of each ventricle are protected by one-way valves that direct the flow of blood through the heart. The *atrioventricular* (AV) valves are located at the entrance into the ventricles. There are two AV valves: the tricuspid valve and the bicuspid, which is also called the *mitral valve*. The tricuspid valve is composed of three cusps or flaps and is located between the right atrium and the right ventricle; the bicuspid (mitral) valve is composed of two cusps or flaps and is located between the left atrium and the left ventricle. Collagen fibers, called *chordae tendineae*, anchor the AV valve flaps to papillary muscles within the ventricles.

Open AV valves allow blood to flow from the atria into the ventricles. However, as the ventricles begin to contract, the AV valves snap shut, preventing the regurgitation of blood into the atria. The valves are prevented from blowing open in the reverse direction (ie, toward the atria) by their secure anchors to the papillary muscles of the ventricular wall. The *semilunar valves* are located at the exit of each ventricle at the beginning of the great vessels. Each valve has three cusps or flaps that look like half-moons, hence the name "semilunar." There are two semilunar valves: the pulmonic valve is located at the entrance of the pulmonary artery as it exits the right ventricle, and the aortic valve is located at the beginning of the ascending aorta. These valves are open during ventricular contraction and close from the pressure of blood when the ventricles relax. Blood is thus prevented from flowing backward into the relaxed ventricles (see Fig. 16-2).

HEART COVERING AND WALLS

The *pericardium* is a tough, inextensible, loose-fitting, fibroserous sac that attaches to the great vessels and thereby surrounds the heart. A serous membrane lining, the *parietal pericardium*, secretes a small amount of pericardial fluid that allows for smooth, friction-free movement of the heart. This same type of serous membrane covers the outer surface of the heart and is known as the *epicardium*. The *myocardium* is the thickest layer of the heart and is made up of contractile cardiac muscle cells. The *endocardium* is a thin layer of endothelial tissue that forms the innermost layer of the heart and is continuous with the endothelial lining of blood vessels (see Fig. 16-2).

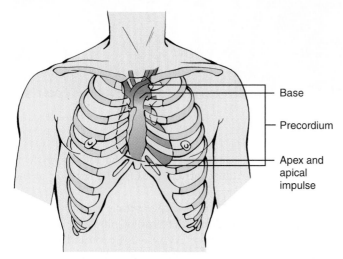

FIGURE 16-1. The heart and major blood vessels lie centrally in the chest behind the protective sternum.

Electrical Conduction of the Heart

Cardiac muscle cells have a unique inherent ability. They can spontaneously generate an electrical impulse and conduct it through the heart. The generation and conduction of electrical impulses by specialized sections of the myocardium regulate the events associated with the filling and emptying of the cardiac chambers. The process is called the *cardiac cycle*.

PATHWAYS

The *sinoatrial (SA) node* (or sinus node) is located on the posterior wall of the right atrium, near the superior vena cava. The SA node, with inherent rhythmicity, generates impulses (at a rate of 70 to 80 per minute) that are conducted over both atria, causing them to contract simultaneously and send blood into the ventricles. The current, initiated by the SA node, is conducted across the atria to the *AV node*, located in the lower interatrial septum (Fig. 16-3). The AV node slightly delays incoming electrical impulses from the atria and then relays the impulses to the AV bundle (bundle of His) in the upper interventricular septum. The electrical impulse then travels down the right and left bundle branches and the Purkinje fibers in the myocardium of both ventricles, causing them to contract almost simultaneously. Although the SA node functions as the "pacemaker of the heart," this activity shifts to other areas of the conduction system, such as the AV node (with an inherent discharge of 40 to 60 per minute), if the SA node cannot function.

ELECTRICAL ACTIVITY

Electrical impulses, which are generated by the SA node and travel throughout the cardiac conduction circuit, can

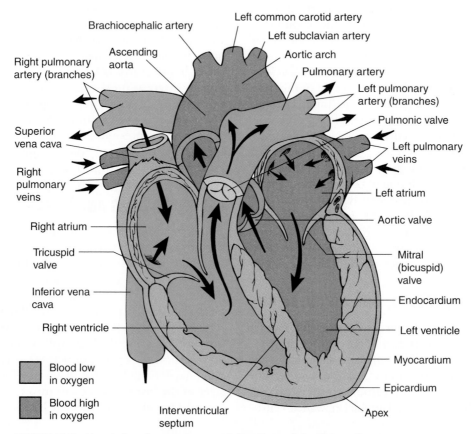

Right pulmonary artery (branches)

Ascending aorta

Brachiocephalic artery

Left common carotid artery

Left subclavian artery

Aortic arch

Pulmonary artery

Left pulmonary artery (branches)

Pulmonic valve

Left pulmonary veins

Superior vena cava

Right pulmonary veins

Right atrium

Tricuspid valve

Inferior vena cava

Right ventricle

Left atrium

Aortic valve

Mitral (bicuspid) valve

Endocardium

Left ventricle

Myocardium

Epicardium

Apex

Blood low in oxygen

Blood high in oxygen

Interventricular septum

FIGURE 16-2. Heart chambers, valves, and direction of circulatory flow.

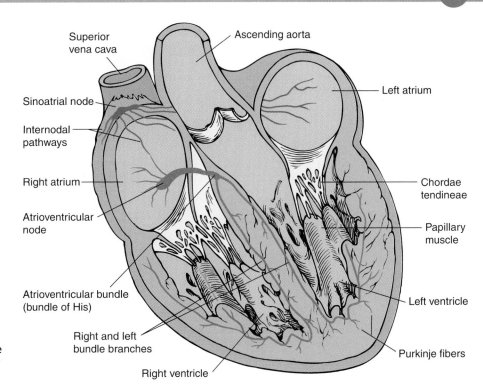

Superior vena cava

Ascending aorta

Sinoatrial node

Left atrium

Internodal pathways

Right atrium

Chordae tendineae

Atrioventricular node

Papillary muscle

Atrioventricular bundle (bundle of His)

Left ventricle

Right and left bundle branches

Purkinje fibers

Right ventricle

FIGURE 16-3. The electrical conduction system of the heart begins with impulses generated by the sinoatrial node (*green*) and circuited continuously over the heart.

be detected on the surface of the skin. This electrical activity can be measured and recorded by electrocardiography (ECG, aka EKG), which records the depolarization and repolarization of the cardiac muscle. The phases of the ECG are known as P, Q, R, S, and T. Display 16-1 describes the phases of the ECG.

The Cardiac Cycle

The cardiac cycle consists of the filling and emptying of the heart's chambers. The cardiac cycle has two phases: diastole (relaxation of the ventricles, known as filling) and systole (contraction of the ventricles, known as emptying). Diastole endures for approximately two thirds of the cardiac cycle, and systole is the remaining one third (Fig. 16-4).

DIASTOLE

During ventricular diastole, the AV valves are open and the ventricles are relaxed. This causes higher pressure in the atria than in the ventricles. Therefore, blood rushes through the atria into the ventricles. This early, rapid, passive filling is called *early or protodiastolic filling.* This is followed by a period of slow passive filling. Finally, near the end of ventricular diastole, the atria contract and complete the emptying of blood out of the upper chambers by propelling it into the ventricles. This final active filling phase is called *presystole, atrial systole,* or sometimes the *"atrial kick."* This action raises left ventricular pressure.

SYSTOLE

The filling phases during diastole result in a large amount of blood in the ventricles, causing the pressure in the ventricles to be higher than in the atria. This causes the AV valves (mitral and tricuspid) to shut. Closure of the AV valves produces the first heart sound (S_1), which is the beginning of systole. This valve closure also prevents blood from flowing backward (a process known as *regurgitation*) into the atria during ventricular contraction.

At this point in systole, all four valves are closed and the ventricles contract (isometric contraction). There is now high pressure inside the ventricles, causing the aortic valve to open on the left side of the heart and the pulmonic valve to open on the right side of the heart. Blood is ejected rapidly through these valves. With ventricular emptying, the ventricular pressure falls and the semilunar valves close. This closure produces the second heart sound (S_2), which signals the end of systole. After closure of the semilunar valves, the ventricles relax. Atrial pressure is now higher than the ventricular pressure, causing the AV valves to open and diastolic filling to begin again.

Production of Heart Sounds

Heart sounds are produced by valve closure. The opening of valves is silent. Normal heart sounds, characterized as "lub dubb" (S_1 and S_2), and, occasionally, extra heart sounds and murmurs can be auscultated with a stethoscope

DISPLAY 16-1. Phases of the Electrocardiogram

The phases of the electrocardiogram (ECG), which records depolarization and repolarization of the heart, are assigned letters: P, Q, R, S, and T.

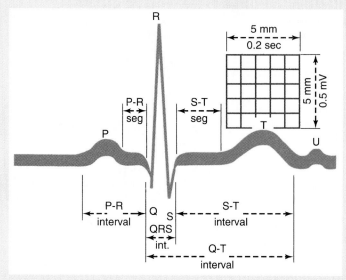

Phases of the electrocardiogram (ECG).

- **P wave:** Atrial depolarization; conduction of the impulse throughout the atria.
- **PR interval:** The time from the beginning of atrial depolarization to the beginning of ventricular depolarization, that is, from the beginning of the P wave to the beginning of the QRS complex.
- **QRS complex:** Ventricular depolarization (also atrial repolarization); conduction of the impulse throughout the ventricles, which then triggers contraction of the ventricles; measured from the beginning of the Q wave to the end of the S wave.
- **ST segment:** Period between ventricular depolarization and the beginning of ventricular repolarization.
- **T wave:** Ventricular repolarization; the ventricles return to a resting state.
- **QT interval:** Total time for ventricular depolarization and repolarization, that is, from the beginning of the Q wave to the end of the T wave; the QT interval varies with heart rate.
- **U wave:** May or may not be present; if it is present, it follows the T wave and represents the final phase of ventricular repolarization.

over the precordium, the area of the anterior chest overlying the heart and great vessels. The sections dealing with auscultation for heart sounds in the Physical Assessment section of this chapter provide detail of where and how to assess for heart sounds on the precordium.

NORMAL HEART SOUNDS

The first heart sound (S_1) is the result of closure of the AV valves—the mitral and tricuspid valves. As mentioned previously, S_1 correlates with the beginning of systole (see Display 16-2 for more information about S_1 and variations of S_1). S_1 ("lub") is usually heard as one sound, but may be heard as two sounds (see also Figure 16-4). If heard as two sounds, the first component represents mitral valve closure

(M_1), and the second component represents tricuspid closure (T_1). M_1 occurs first because of increased pressure on the left side of the heart and because of the route of myocardial depolarization. S_1 may be heard over the entire precordium but is heard best at the apex (left MCL, fifth ICS).

The second heart sound (S_2) results from closure of the semilunar valves (aortic and pulmonic) and correlates with the beginning of diastole (Fig. 16-5). S_2 ("dubb") is also usually heard as one sound but may be heard as two sounds. If S_2 is heard as two sounds, the first component represents aortic valve closure (A_2) and the second component represents pulmonic valve closure (P_2). A_2 occurs first because of increased pressure on the left side of the heart and because of the route of myocardial depolarization. If S_2 is heard as two distinct sounds, it is called a *split*

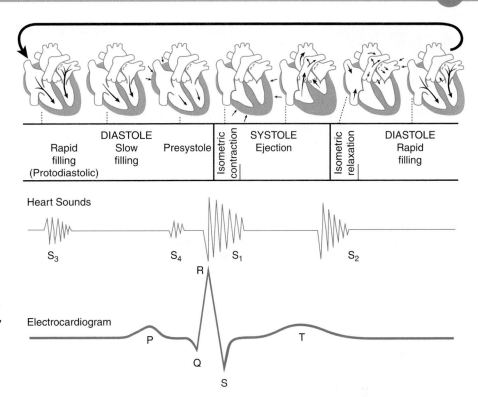

FIGURE 16-4. The cardiac cycle consists of filling and ejection. Heart sounds S_2, S_3, and S_4 are associated with diastole, while S_1 is associated with systole. The electrical activity of the heart is measured throughout diastole and systole by electrocardiography.

S_2. A splitting of S_2 may be exaggerated during inspiration and disappear during expiration. S_2 is heard best at the base of the heart. See Display 16-3 for more information about variations of S_2.

EXTRA HEART SOUNDS

S_3 and S_4 are referred to as diastolic filling sounds or extra heart sounds, which result from ventricular vibration secondary to rapid ventricular filling. If present, S_3 can be heard early in diastole, after S_2 (see Fig. 16-4). S_4 also results from ventricular vibration, but, contrary to S_3, the vibration is secondary to ventricular resistance (noncompliance) during atrial contraction. If present, S_4 can be heard late in diastole, just before S_1 (see Fig. 16-4). S_3 is often termed *ventricular gallop*, and S_4 is called *atrial gallop*. Extra heart sounds are described further in the Physical Assessment section of the text and in Display 16-4.

MURMURS

Blood normally flows silently through the heart. There are conditions, however, that can create turbulent blood flow. In this situation, a swooshing or blowing sound may be auscultated over the precordium. Conditions that contribute to turbulent blood flow include (1) increased blood velocity, (2) structural valve defects, (3) valve malfunction, and (4) abnormal chamber openings (eg, septal defect). See Display 16-5 for a detailed description of heart murmurs.

Cardiac Output

Cardiac output (CO) is the amount of blood pumped by the ventricles during a given period of time (usually 1 min) and is determined by the stroke volume (SV) multiplied by the heart rate (HR): $SV \times HR = CO$. The normal adult cardiac output is 5 to 6 L/min.

STROKE VOLUME

Stroke volume is the amount of blood pumped from the heart with each contraction (stroke volume from the left ventricle is usually 70 mL). Stroke volume is influenced by several factors:

- The degree of stretch of the heart muscle up to a critical length before contraction (preload); the greater the preload, the greater the stroke volume. This holds true unless the heart muscle is stretched so much that it cannot contract effectively.
- The pressure against which the heart muscle has to eject blood during contraction (afterload); increased afterload results in decreased stroke volume.
- Synergy of contraction (ie, the uniform, synchronized contraction of the myocardium); conditions that cause an asynchronous contraction decrease stroke volume.
- Compliance or distensibility of the ventricles; decreased compliance decreases stroke volume.
- Contractility or the force of contractions of the myocardium under given loading conditions; increased contractility increases stroke volume.

COMMON VARIATIONS

DISPLAY 16-2. Understanding Normal S₁ Sounds and Variations

S_1, which is the first heart sound, is produced by the atrioventricular (AV) closing. S_1 (the "lub" portion of "lub dubb") correlates with the beginning of systole.

The intensity of S_1 depends on the position of the mitral valve at the start of systole, the structure of the valve leaflets, and how quickly pressure rises in the ventricle. All of these factors influence the speed and amount of closure the valve experiences, which, in turn, determine the amount of sound produced.

Normal variations in S_1 are heard at the base and the apex of the heart. S_1 is softer at the base and louder at the apex of the heart. An S_1 may be split along the lower left sternal border, where the tricuspid component of the sound, usually too faint to be heard, can be auscultated. A split S_1 heard over the apex may be an S_4.

ACCENTUATED S₁

An accentuated S_1 sound is louder than an S_2. This occurs when the mitral valve is wide open and closes quickly. Examples include:

- Hyperkinetic states in which blood velocity increases, such as fever, anemia, and hyperthyroidism
- Mitral stenosis, in which the leaflets are still mobile but increased ventricular pressure is needed to close the valve

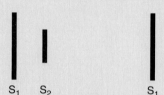

DIMINISHED S₁

Sometimes, the S_1 sound is softer than the S_2 sound. This occurs when the mitral valve is not fully open at the time of ventricular contraction and valve closing. Examples include:

- Delayed conduction from the atria to the ventricles, as in first-degree heart block, which allows the mitral valve to drift closed before ventricular contraction closes it
- Mitral insufficiency, in which extreme calcification of the valve limits mobility
- Delayed or diminished ventricular contraction arises from forceful atrial contraction into a noncompliant ventricle, as in severe pulmonary or systemic hypertension

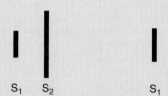

SPLIT S₁

As named, a split S_1 occurs as a split sound. This occurs when the left and right ventricles contract at different times (asynchronous ventricular contraction). Examples include:

- Conduction delaying the cardiac impulse to one of the ventricles, as in bundle branch block
- Ventricular ectopy, in which the impulse starts in one ventricle, contracting it first, and then spreads to the second ventricle

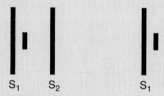

VARYING S₁

This occurs when the mitral valve is in different positions when contraction occurs. Examples include:

- Rhythms in which the atria and ventricles are beating independently of each other
- Totally irregular rhythms, such as atrial fibrillation

Although cardiac muscle has an innate pattern of contractility, cardiac activity is also mediated by the autonomic nervous system to respond to changing needs. The sympathetic impulses increase heart rate and, therefore, cardiac output. The parasympathetic impulses, which travel to the heart by the vagus nerve, decrease the heart rate and, therefore, decrease cardiac output.

Neck Vessels

Assessment of the cardiovascular system includes evaluation of the vessels of the neck—the carotid artery and the jugular veins. Assessment of the pulses of these vessels reflects the integrity of the heart muscle (see Fig. 16-5).

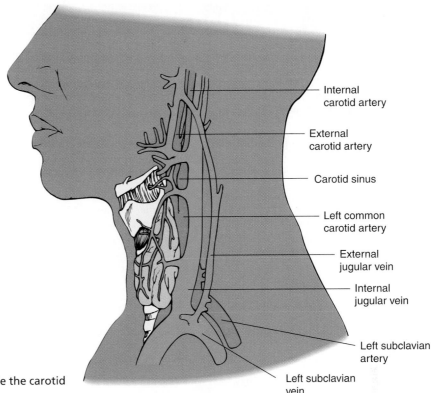

FIGURE 16-5. Major neck vessels include the carotid arteries and the jugular veins.

CAROTID ARTERY PULSE

The right and left common carotid arteries extend from the brachiocephalic trunk and the aortic arch and are located in the groove between the trachea and the right and left sternocleidomastoid muscles. Slightly below the mandible, each bifurcates into an internal and external carotid artery. They supply the neck and head, including the brain, with oxygenated blood. The carotid artery pulse is a centrally located arterial pulse. Because it is close to the heart, the pressure wave pulsation coincides closely with ventricular systole. The carotid arterial pulse is good for assessing amplitude and contour of the pulse wave. The pulse should normally have a smooth, rapid upstroke that occurs in early systole, and a more gradual downstroke.

JUGULAR VENOUS PULSE AND PRESSURE

There are two sets of jugular veins, internal and external. The internal jugular veins lie deep and medial to the sternocleidomastoid muscle. The external jugular veins are more superficial; they lie lateral to the sternocleidomastoid muscle and above the clavicle. The jugular veins return blood to the heart from the head and neck by way of the superior vena cava.

Assessment of the jugular venous pulse is important for determining the hemodynamics of the right side of the heart. The level of the jugular venous pressure reflects right atrial (central venous) pressure and, usually, right ventricular diastolic filling pressure (Fig. 16-6). Right-sided heart

failure raises pressure and volume, thus raising jugular venous pressure.

Decreased jugular venous pressure occurs with reduced left ventricular output or reduced blood volume. The right internal jugular vein is most directly connected to the right atrium and provides the best assessment of pressure changes. Components of the jugular venous pulse follow:

a wave—reflects rise in atrial pressure that occurs with atrial contraction

x descent—reflects right atrial relaxation and descent of the atrial floor during ventricular systole

v wave—reflects right atrial filling, increased volume, and increased atrial pressure

y descent—reflects right atrial emptying into the right ventricle and decreased atrial pressure

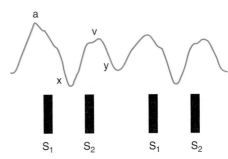

FIGURE 16-6. Jugular venous pulse wave reflects pressure levels in the heart.

DISPLAY 16-3. Variations in S₂

COMMON
VARIATIONS

The S_2 sound depends on the closure of the aortic and pulmonic valves. Closure of the pulmonic valve is delayed by inspiration, resulting in a split S_2 sound. The components of the split sound are referred to as A_2 (aortic valve sound) and P_2 (pulmonic valve sound). If either sound is absent, no split sounds are heard. The A_2 sound is heard best over the second right intercostal space. P_2 is normally softer than A_2.

ACCENTUATED S₂

An accentuated S_2 means that S_2 is louder than S_1. This occurs in conditions in which the aortic or pulmonic valve has a higher closing pressure. Examples include:

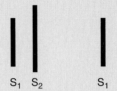

- Increased pressure in the aorta from exercise, excitement, or systemic hypertension (a booming S_2 is heard with systemic hypertension)
- Increased pressure in the pulmonary vasculature, which may occur with mitral stenosis or congestive heart failure
- Calcification of the semilunar valve, in which the valve is still mobile, as in pulmonic or aortic stenosis

DIMINISHED S₂

A diminished S_2 means that S_2 is softer than S_1. This occurs in conditions in which the aortic or pulmonic valves have decreased mobility. Examples include:

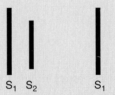

- Decreased systemic blood pressure, which weakens the valves, as in shock
- Aortic or pulmonic stenosis, in which the valves are thickened and calcified, with decreased mobility

NORMAL (PHYSIOLOGIC) SPLIT S₂

A normal split S_2 can be heard over the second or third left intercostal space. It is usually heard best during inspiration and disappears during expiration. Over the aortic area and apex, the pulmonic component of S_2 is usually too faint to be heard, and S_2 is a single sound resulting from aortic valve closure. In some patients, S_2 may not become single on expiration unless the patient sits up. Splitting that does not disappear during expiration is suggestive of heart disease.

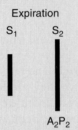
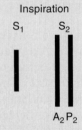

WIDE SPLIT S₂

This is an increase in the usual splitting that persists throughout the entire respiratory cycle and widens on expiration. It occurs when there is delayed electrical activation of the right ventricle. Example includes:

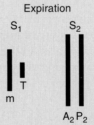
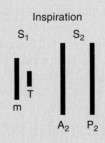

- Right bundle branch block, which delays pulmonic valve closing

FIXED SPLIT S₂

This is a wide splitting that does not vary with respiration. It occurs when there is delayed closure of one of the valves. Example includes:

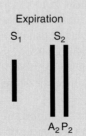
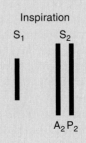

- Atrial septal defect and right ventricular failure, which delay pulmonic valve closing

(continued)

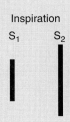

DISPLAY 16-3. Variations in S₂ (Continued)

REVERSED SPLIT S₂

This is a split S₂ that appears on expiration and disappears on in-spiration—also known as paradoxical split. It occurs when closure of the aortic valve is abnormally delayed, causing A₂ to follow P₂ in expiration. Normal inspiratory delay of P₂ makes the split disappear during inspiration. Example includes:

- Left bundle branch block

ACCENTUATED A₂

An accentuated A₂ is loud over the right, second intercostal space. This occurs with increased pressure, as in systemic hypertension and aortic root dilation, because of the closer position of the aortic valve to the chest wall.

DIMINISHED A₂

A diminished A₂ is soft or absent over the right, second intercostal space. This occurs with immobility of the aortic valve in calcific aortic stenosis.

ACCENTUATED P₂

An accentuated P₂ is louder than or equal to an A₂ sound. This occurs with pulmonary hypertension, dilated pulmonary artery, and atrial septal defect. A wide split S₂, heard even at the apex, indicates an accentuated P₂.

DIMINISHED P₂

A soft or absent P₂ sound occurs with an increased anteroposterior diameter of the chest, which is associated with aging or pulmonic stenosis.

DISPLAY 16-4. Extra Heart Sounds

Additional heart sounds can be classified by their timing in the cardiac cycle. The presence of the sound during systole or diastole helps in its identification. Some sounds extend into both systole and diastole.

EXTRA HEART SOUNDS DURING SYSTOLE—CLICKS

High-frequency sounds heard just after S₁ (ejection clicks) are produced by a functioning but diseased valve. Clicks can occur in early or mid-to-late systole and are best heard through the diaphragm of the stethoscope.

AORTIC EJECTION CLICK

Heard during early systole at the second right intercostal space and apex, the aortic ejection click occurs with the opening of the aortic valve and does not change with respiration.

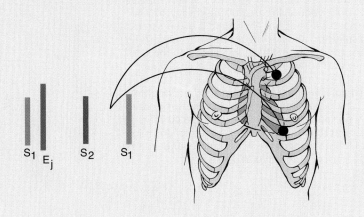

(continued)

DISPLAY 16-4. Extra Heart Sounds (Continued)

PULMONIC EJECTION CLICK

Best heard at the second left intercostal space during early systole, the pulmonic ejection click often becomes softer with inspiration.

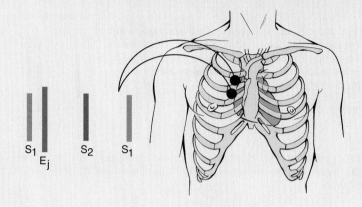

MIDSYSTOLIC CLICK

Heard in middle or late systole, a midsystolic click can be heard over the mitral or apical area and is the result of mitral valve leaflet prolapse during left ventricular emptying. A late systolic murmur typically follows, indicating mild mitral regurgitation.

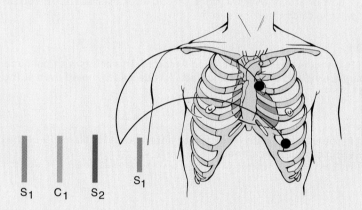

EXTRA HEART SOUNDS DURING DIASTOLE

Opening Snap

Occurring in early diastole, an opening snap (OS) is heard with the opening of a stenotic or stiff mitral valve. Heard throughout the whole precordium, it does not vary with respirations. Often mistaken for a split S_2 or an S_3, the opening snap occurs earlier in diastole and has a higher pitch than an S_3.

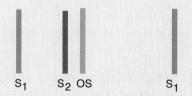

S_3 (Third Heart Sound)

Also called a ventricular gallop, the S_3 has a low frequency and is heard best using the bell of the stethoscope at the apical area or lower right ventricular area of the chest with the patient in the left lateral position. The sound is often accentuated during inspiration and has the rhythm of the word "Ken-tuc-ky." S_3 is the result of vibrations caused by the blood hitting the ventricular wall during rapid ventricular filling.

The S_3 can be a normal finding in young children, people with a high cardiac output, and in the third trimester of pregnancy. It is rarely normal in people older than age 40 years and is usually associated with decreased myocardial contractility, myocardial failure, congestive heart failure, and volume overload of the ventricle from valvular disease.

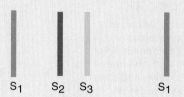

(continued)

S₄ (Fourth Heart Sound)

Also called an atrial gallop, S_4 is a low-frequency sound occurring at the end of diastole when the atria contract. It is caused by vibrations from blood flowing rapidly into the ventricles after atrial contraction. S_4 has the rhythm of the word "Ten-nes-see" and may increase during inspiration. It is best heard with the bell of the stethoscope over the apical area with the patient in a supine or left lateral position and is never heard in the absence of atrial contraction.

The S_4 can be a normal sound in trained athletes and some older patients, especially after exercise. However, it is usually an abnormal finding and is associated with coronary artery disease, hypertension, aortic and pulmonic stenosis, and acute myocardial infarction.

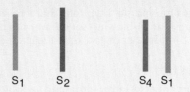

Summation Gallop

The simultaneous occurrence of S_3 and S_4 is called a summation gallop. It is brought about by rapid heart rates in which diastolic filling time is shortened, moving S_3 and S_4 closer together, resulting in one prolonged sound. Summation gallop is associated with severe congestive heart disease.

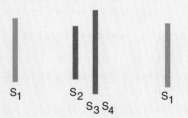

EXTRA HEART SOUNDS IN BOTH SYSTOLE AND DIASTOLE

Pericardial Friction Rub

Usually heard best in the third intercostal space to the left of the sternum, a pericardial friction rub is caused by inflammation of the pericardial sac. A high-pitched, scratchy, scraping sound, the rub may increase with exhalation and when the patient leans forward. For best results, use the diaphragm of the stethoscope and have the patient sit up, lean forward, exhale, and hold his or her breath.

The pericardial friction rub can have up to three components: atrial systole, ventricular systole, and ventricular diastole. These components are associated with cardiac movement. The first two components are usually present. If only one component is present, the rub may be confused with a murmur. Friction rubs are commonly heard during the first week after a myocardial infarction. If a significant pericardial effusion is present, S_1 and S_2 sounds will be distant.

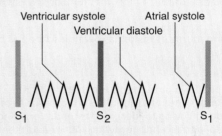

Patent Ductus Arteriosus

Patent ductus arteriosus (PDA) is a congenital anomaly that leaves an open channel between the aorta and pulmonary artery. Found over the second left intercostal space, the murmur of PDA may radiate to the left clavicle. It is classified as a continuous murmur because it extends through systole and into part of diastole. It has a medium pitch and a harsh, machinery-like sound. The murmur is loudest in late systole, obscures S_2, fades in diastole, and often has a silent interval in late diastole.

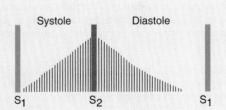

Venous Hum

Common in children, a venous hum is a benign sound caused by turbulence of blood in the jugular veins. It is heard above the medial third of the clavicles, especially on the right, and may radiate to the first and second intercostal spaces. A low-pitched sound, it is often described as a humming or roaring continuous murmur without a silent interval, and is loudest in diastole. A venous hum can be obliterated by putting pressure on the jugular veins.

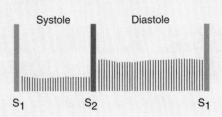

ABNORMAL FINDINGS

DISPLAY 16-5. Identifying Heart Murmurs

Heart murmurs are typically characterized by turbulent blood flow, which creates a swooshing or blowing sound over the precordium. When listening to the heart, be alert for this turbulence and keep the characteristics of heart murmurs in mind.

CHARACTERISTICS

Heart murmurs are assessed according to various characteristics, which include timing, intensity, pitch, quality, shape or pattern, location, transmission, and ventilation and position.

Timing

A murmur can occur during systole or diastole. In addition to determining when it occurs, it is important to determine where it occurs, because a systolic murmur can be present in a healthy heart whereas a diastolic murmur always indicates heart disease. Systolic murmurs can be divided into three categories: midsystolic, pansystolic, and late systolic. Diastolic murmurs can be divided into three categories: early diastolic, mid-diastolic, and late diastolic.

Intensity

Six grades describe the intensity of a murmur:

Grade 1: Very faint, heard only after the listener has "tuned in"; may not be heard in all positions
Grade 2: Quiet, but heard immediately on placing the stethoscope on the chest
Grade 3: Moderately loud
Grade 4: Loud*
Grade 5: Very loud, may be heard with a stethoscope partly off the chest*
Grade 6: May be heard with the stethoscope entirely off the chest*

Pitch

Murmurs can assume a high, medium, or low pitch.

Quality

The sound murmurs make has been described as blowing, rushing, roaring, rumbling, harsh, or musical.

Shape or Pattern

The shape of a murmur is determined by its intensity from beginning to end. There are four different categories of shape: crescendo (growing louder), decrescendo (growing softer), crescendo–decrescendo (growing louder and then growing softer), and plateau (staying the same throughout).

Location

Determine where you can best hear the murmur; this is the point where the murmur originates. Try to be as exact as possible in describing its location. Use the heart landmarks in your description (eg, the second interspace at the left sternal border).

Transmission

The murmur may be felt in areas other than the point of origination. If you determine where the murmur transmits, you can determine the direction of blood flow and the intensity of the murmur.

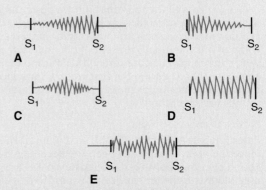

Shape or pattern of murmurs: (A) crescendo, (B) decrescendo, (C) crescendo-decrescendo (diamond), (D) plateau (even), (E) variable (uneven).

Ventilation and Position

Determine if the murmur is affected by inspiration, expiration, or a change in body position.

MIDSYSTOLIC MURMURS

The most common type of heart murmurs, midsystolic murmurs occur during ventricular ejection and can be innocent, physiologic, or pathologic. They have a crescendo–decrescendo shape and usually peak near midsystole and stop before S_2.

(continued)

* Palpable thrills are associated with murmurs of grades 4–6.

Innocent Murmur

Not associated with any physical abnormality, innocent murmurs occur when the ejection of blood into the aorta is turbulent. Very common in children and young adults, they may also be heard in older people with no evidence of cardiovascular disease. A patient may have an innocent murmur and another kind of murmur.

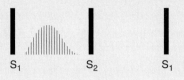

Location: Second to fourth left intercostal spaces between the left sternal border and the apex
Radiation: Little radiation
Intensity: Grade 1 to 2
Pitch: Medium
Quality: Variable
Position: Usually disappear when the patient sits

Physiologic Murmur

Caused by a temporary increase in blood flow, a physiologic murmur can occur with anemia, pregnancy, fever, and hyperthyroidism.

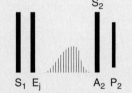

Location: Second to fourth left intercostal spaces between the left sternal border and the apex
Radiation: Little radiation
Intensity: Grade 1 to 2
Pitch: Medium
Quality: Harsh

Murmur of Pulmonic Stenosis

A pathologic murmur, the murmur of pulmonic stenosis occurs from impeded flow across the pulmonic valve and increased right ventricular afterload. Often occurring as a congenital anomaly, the murmur is commonly found in children. Pathologic changes in flow across the valve, as in an atrial septal defect, may also mimic this condition.

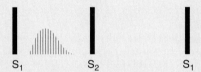

With severe pulmonic stenosis, the S_2 is widely split and P_2 is diminished. An early pulmonic ejection sound is also common. A right-sided S_4 may also be present, and the right ventricular impulse is often stronger and may be prolonged.

Location: Second and third intercostal spaces
Radiation: Toward the left shoulder and neck
Intensity: Soft to loud (may be associated with a thrill if loud)
Pitch: Medium
Quality: Harsh
Position: Loudest during inspiration

Murmur of Aortic Stenosis

The murmur of aortic stenosis occurs when stenosis of the aortic valve impedes blood flow across the valve and increases left ventricular afterload. Aortic stenosis may result from a congenital anomaly, rheumatic disease, or a degenerative process. Conditions that may mimic this murmur include aortic sclerosis, a bicuspid aortic valve, a dilated aorta, or any condition that mimics the flow across the valve, such as aortic regurgitation.

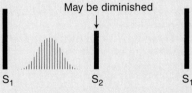

If valvular disease is severe, A_2 may be delayed, resulting in an unsplit S_2 or a paradoxical split S_2. An S_4 may occur as a result of decreased left ventricular compliance. An aortic ejection sound, if present, suggests a congenital cause.

Location: Right second intercostal space
Radiation: May radiate to the neck and down the left sternal border to the apex
Intensity: Usually loud, with a thrill
Pitch: Medium
Quality: Harsh, may be musical at the apex
Position: Heard best with the patient sitting and leaning forward, loudest during expiration

(continued)

DISPLAY 16-5. Identifying Heart Murmurs (Continued)

Murmur of Hypertrophic Cardiomyopathy

Caused by unusually rapid ejection of blood from the left ventricle during systole, the murmur of cardiac hypertrophy results from massive hypertrophy of the ventricular muscle. There may be a coexisting obstruction to blood flow. If there is an accompanying distortion of the mitral valve, mitral regurgitation may result. The patient may also have an S_3 and an S_4. There may be a sustained apical impulse with two palpable components.

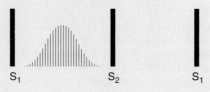

Location: Third and fourth left interspace, decreases with squatting, increases with straining down
Intensity: Variable
Pitch: Medium
Quality: Harsh

PANSYSTOLIC MURMURS

Occurring when blood flows from a chamber with high pressure to a chamber of low pressure through an orifice that should be closed, pansystolic murmurs are pathologic. Also called *holosystolic murmurs,* these murmurs, begin with S_1 and continue through systole to S_2.

Murmur of Mitral Regurgitation

Occurring when the mitral valve fails to close fully in systole, the murmur of mitral regurgitation is the result of blood flowing from the left ventricle back into the left atrium. Volume overload occurs in the left ventricle, causing dilatation and hypertrophy.

The S_1 sound is often decreased, and the apical impulse is stronger and may be prolonged. Left ventricular volume overload should be suspected if an apical S_3 is heard.

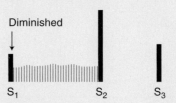

Location: Apex
Radiation: To the left axilla, less often to the left sternal border
Intensity: Soft to loud, an apical thrill is associated with loud murmurs
Pitch: Medium to high
Quality: Blowing
Position: Heard best with patient in the left lateral decubitus position, does not become louder with inspiration

Murmur of Tricuspid Regurgitation

Blood flowing from the right ventricle back into the right atrium over a tricuspid valve that has not fully closed causes the murmur of tricuspid regurgitation. Right ventricular failure with dilatation is the most common cause, and usually results from pulmonary hypertension or left ventricular failure.

With this murmur, the right ventricular impulse is stronger and may be prolonged. There may be an S_3 along the lower left sternal border, and the jugular venous pressure is often elevated, with visible *v* waves.

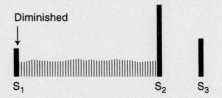

Location: Lower left sternal border
Radiation: To the right of the sternum, to the xiphoid area, and sometimes to the midclavicular line; there is no radiation to the axilla
Intensity: Variable
Pitch: Medium to high
Quality: Blowing
Position: May increase slightly with inspiration

(continued)

DISPLAY 16-5. **Identifying Heart Murmurs** (Continued)

Ventricular Septal Defect

A congenital abnormality in which blood flows from the left ventricle into the right ventricle through a hole in the septum, a ventricular septal defect causes a loud murmur that obscures the A_2 sound. Other findings vary depending on the severity of the defect and any associated lesions.

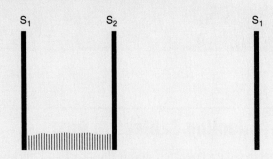

Location: Third, fourth, and fifth left intercostal space
Radiation: Often wide
Intensity: Very loud, with a thrill
Pitch: High
Quality: Harsh
Position: Increases with exercise

DIASTOLIC MURMURS

Usually indicative of heart disease, diastolic murmurs occur in two types. Early decrescendo diastolic murmurs indicate flow through an incompetent semilunar valve, commonly the aortic valve. Rumbling diastolic murmurs in mid- or late diastole indicate valve stenosis, usually of the mitral valve.

Aortic Regurgitation

Occurring when the leaflets of the aortic valve fail to close completely, the murmur of aortic regurgitation is the result of blood flowing from the aorta back into the left ventricle. This results in left ventricular volume overload. An ejection sound also may be present. Severe regurgitation should be suspected if an S_3 or S_4 is also present. The apical impulse becomes displaced downward and laterally with a widened diameter and increased duration. As the pulse pressure increases, the arterial pulses are often large and bounding.

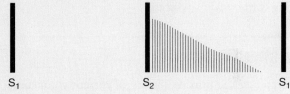

Location: Second to fourth left intercostal spaces
Radiation: May radiate to the apex or left sternal border
Intensity: Grade 1 to 3
Pitch: High
Quality: Blowing, sometimes mistaken for breath sounds
Position: Heard best with the patient sitting, leaning forward. Have the patient exhale and then hold his or her breath.

Murmur of Mitral Stenosis

The murmur of mitral stenosis is the result of blood flow across a diseased mitral valve. Thickened, stiff, distorted leaflets are usually the result of rheumatic fever. The murmur is loud during mid-diastole as the ventricle fills rapidly, grows quiet, and becomes loud again immediately before systole, as the atria contract. In patients with atrial fibrillation, the second half of the murmur is absent because of the lack of atrial contraction.

The patient also has a loud S_1, which may be palpable at the apex. There is often an opening snap (OS) after S_2. P_2 becomes loud and the right ventricular impulse becomes palpable if pulmonary hypertension develops.

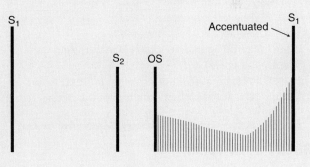

Location: Apex
Radiation: Little or none
Intensity: Grade 1 to 4
Pitch: Low
Quality: Rumbling
Position: Best heard with the bell exactly on the apex, and the patient turned to a left lateral position. Mild exercise and listening during exhalation also make the murmur easier to hear.

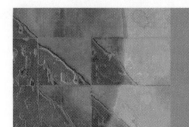

Collecting Subjective Data

Subjective data collected about the heart and neck vessels can help the nurse identify abnormal conditions that may affect the client's ability to perform activities of daily living and to fulfill his or her role and responsibilities. Data collection also provides information on the client's risk for cardiovascular disease and helps to identify area where health education is needed. The client may not be aware of the significant role that health promotion activities can play in preventing cardiovascular disease.

Nursing History

When compiling the nursing history of current complaints or symptoms, personal and family history, and lifestyle and health practices, remember to thoroughly explore signs and symptoms that the client brings to your attention either intentionally or inadvertently. Use the COLDSPA mnemonic as a guide.

COLDSPA

CHARACTER: Describe the sign or symptom. How does it feel, look, sound, smell, and so forth?
ONSET: When did it begin?
LOCATION: Where is it? Does it radiate?
DURATION: How long does it last? Does it recur?
SEVERITY: How bad is it?
PATTERN: What makes it better? What makes it worse?
ASSOCIATED FACTORS: What other symptoms occur with it?

CURRENT SYMPTOMS

Question Do you experience chest pain? Describe the type of pain, location, radiation, duration, and how often you experience the pain. Rate the pain on a scale of 0 to 10, with 10 being the worst possible pain.

Rationale Chest pain can be cardiac, pulmonary, muscular, or gastrointestinal in origin. Angina (cardiac chest pain) is usually described as a sensation of squeezing around the heart; a steady, severe pain; and a sense of pressure. It may radiate to the left shoulder and down the left arm, or to the jaw.

Q Do you tire easily? Do you experience fatigue? Describe when the fatigue started. Was it sudden or gradual? Do you notice it at any particular time of day?

R Fatigue may result from compromised cardiac output. Fatigue related to decreased cardiac output is worse in the evening or as the day progresses.

Q Do you have dyspnea, difficulty breathing, or shortness of breath?

R Dyspnea may result from congestive heart failure, pulmonary disorders, coronary artery disease, myocardial ischemia, and myocardial infarction. Dyspnea may occur at rest, during sleep, or with mild, moderate, or extreme exertion.

Q Do you experience nocturia?

R Enhanced renal perfusion during periods of rest or recumbency may promote nocturia.

Q Do you experience palpitations?

R Palpitations may occur with an abnormality of the heart's conduction system or during the heart's attempt to increase cardiac output by increasing the heart rate. Palpitations may cause the client to feel anxious.

Q Do you experience dizziness?

R Dizziness may indicate decreased blood flow to the brain, although there are several other causes. Dizziness may put the client at risk for falls.

Q Do you experience swelling in your feet, ankles, or legs?

R Swelling in the lower extremities usually occurs as a result of heart failure.

PAST HISTORY

Q Have you been diagnosed with a heart defect or a murmur?

R Congenital or acquired defects affect the heart's ability to pump, decreasing the oxygen supply to the tissues.

Q Have you ever had rheumatic fever?

R Approximately 40% of people with rheumatic fever develop rheumatic carditis. Rheumatic carditis develops after exposure to group A beta-hemolytic streptococci and results in inflammation of all layers of the heart, impairing contraction and valvular function.

Q Have you ever had heart surgery or cardiac balloon interventions?

R Previous heart surgery may change the heart sounds heard during auscultation. Surgery and cardiac balloon interventions indicate prior cardiac compromise.

FAMILY HISTORY

Q Is there a history of hypertension, myocardial infarction (MI), coronary heart disease (CHD), elevated cholesterol levels, or diabetes mellitus (DM) in your family?

R A genetic predisposition to these risk factors increases a client's chance for development of heart disease.

LIFESTYLE AND HEALTH PRACTICES

Q Do you smoke? How many packs of cigarettes per day and for how many years?

R Cigarette smoking greatly increases the risk of heart disease (see Risk Factors—Coronary Heart Disease).

Q What type of stress do you have in your life? How do you cope with it?

R Stress has been identified as a possible risk factor for heart disease.

Q Describe what you usually eat in a 24-hour period. How much alcohol do you consume each day?

R An elevated cholesterol level increases the chance of fatty plaque formation in the coronary vessels. Excessive intake of alcohol has been linked to hypertension.

Q Do you exercise? What type of exercise and how often?

R A sedentary lifestyle is a known modifiable risk factor contributing to heart disease. Aerobic exercise three times per week for 30 min is more beneficial than anaerobic exercise or sporadic exercise in preventing heart disease.

Q Describe your daily activities. How are they different from your routine 5 or 10 years ago? Does fatigue, chest pain, or shortness of breath limit your ability to perform daily activities? Describe. Are you able to care for yourself?

R Heart disease may impede the ability to perform daily activities. Exertional dyspnea or fatigue may indicate heart failure. An inability to complete activities of daily living may necessitate a referral for home care.

Q Has your heart disease had any effect on your sexual activity?

R Many clients with heart disease are afraid that sexual activity will precipitate chest pain. If the client can walk one block or climb two flights of stairs without experiencing symptoms, it is generally acceptable for the client to engage in sexual intercourse. Nitroglycerin can be taken before intercourse as a prophylactic for chest pain. In addition, the side-lying position for sexual intercourse may reduce the workload on the heart.

Q How many pillows do you use to sleep at night? Do you get up to urinate during the night? Do you feel rested in the morning?

R If heart function is compromised, cardiac output to the kidneys is reduced during episodes of activity. At rest, cardiac output increases, as does glomerular filtration and urinary output. Orthopnea (the inability to breathe while supine) and nocturia may indicate heart failure. In addition, these two conditions may also impede the ability to get adequate rest.

Q How important is having a healthy heart to your ability to feel good about yourself and your appearance? What fears about heart disease do you have?

R A person's feeling of self-worth may depend on his or her ability to perform usual daily activities and fulfill his or her usual roles.

Q Have you ever had an electrocardiogram (ECG)? When was the last one performed?

R A prior ECG allows the health care team to evaluate for any changes in cardiac conduction.

Q Have you ever had a blood test called a lipid profile? Do you know your cholesterol level?

R Dyslipidemia presents the greatest risk for the developing coronary artery disease. Elevated cholesterol levels are linked to the development of atherosclerosis (Libby, Schoenbeck, Mach, Selwyn & Ganz, 1998).

Q Do you take medications or use other treatments for heart disease? How often do you take them? Why do you take them?

R Clients may have medications prescribed for heart disease but may not take them regularly. Clients may skip taking their diuretics because of having to urinate frequently. Beta-blockers may be omitted because of the adverse effects on sexual energy. Education about medications may be needed.

Q Do you monitor your own heart rate or blood pressure?

R Self-monitoring of heart rate or blood pressure is recommended if the client is taking cardiotonic or antihypertensive medications, respectively. A demonstration is necessary to ensure appropriate technique.

RISK FACTORS
Coronary Heart Disease

OVERVIEW

According to the American Heart Association (2001), coronary heart disease (CHD) is the single largest killer of Americans, both male and female. In 1998, a total of 459,841 deaths in the United States were from CHD. Moreover, about 12.4 million people alive today have a history of heart attack, chest pain, or both. The rates are declining, however. There was a 28.4% decline in CHD deaths between 1988 and 1998. However, in 2001, about 1.1 million Americans had a new or recurrent coronary attack with more than 40% dying as a result. Of those who died, 85% were age 65 or older, and 80% of deaths in those under age 65 occurred during the first attack. The lifetime risk of developing CHD after age 40 is 49% for men and 32% for women. About 25% of men and 38% of women will die within 1 year after an initial recognized heart attack.

RISK FACTORS (AHA, 1999 AND 2001, EXCEPT AS NOTED)

- Age: Male over age 45; female over age 55 (post-menopausal or ovaries removed and not on estrogen replacement therapy)
- Family history: Father or brother had heart attack before age 55; mother or sister before age 65; close relative had stroke
- Cigarette smoking or exposure to second-hand smoke
- Cholesterol or high-density lipoprotein (HDL) levels: Total cholesterol greater than 240 mg/dL; HDL less than 35 mg/dL
- Blood pressure above 140/90
- Limited physical activity: Fewer than 30 min of moderate activity most days
- Body weight: 20 or more pounds overweight; upper body adiposity (Azevedo, Ramos, vonHafe & Barros, 1999)
- Diabetes or fasting blood glucose level at or greater than 126 mg/dL
- Dietary intake low in antioxidants, especially fruit (Eichholzer, Luthy, Gutzwiller & Stahelin, 2001)
- Low-grade systemic infection/inflammation (elevated C-reactive protein; Rifai & Ridker, 2001)
- Low birth weight (Leeson, Kattenhorn, Morley, Lucas & Deanfield, 2001)
- Stress: Psychological/emotional or physical stress; family relationship stresses; burnout; and daily hassles, especially in women (Hallmen, Burell, Setterlind, Oden & Lisspirs, 2001)

RISK REDUCTION TEACHING TIPS

Young Clients (Misra, 2000)
- Learn about heart and related diseases.
- Maintain ideal body weight.
- Exercise regularly.
- Avoid smoking and chewing tobacco.
- Eat a balanced diet.

Adult Clients
- Have blood pressure checked regularly.
- Exercise regularly (three to five times per week for 20–30 min.)
- Avoid smoking or stop smoking cigarettes; avoid second-hand smoke.
- Eat a well-balanced diet: Low in cholesterol and saturated fats, high in fruits and vegetables; moderate amounts of salt.
- Have regular medical checkups.
- Maintain a healthy weight; lose weight if overweight or obese.
- Learn about heart disease and the signs of heart attack.
  - Uncomfortable pressure, fullness, squeezing, or pain in the center of the chest that lasts for more than a few minutes
  - Pain spreading to the shoulders, neck, or arms
  - Chest discomfort with lightheadedness, fainting, sweating, nausea, or shortness of breath

Postmenopausal Clients
- Learn about estrogen replacement therapy.
- Maintain controlled blood glucose levels.
- Take antihypertensive medications if prescribed.
- Minimize stress levels whenever possible.

CULTURAL CONSIDERATIONS

According to the AHA (2001), among American adults age 20 and older, the estimated age-adjusted (2000 standard) prevalence of CHD is 69% for non-Hispanic white men and 5.4% for women; 7.1% for non-Hispanic black men and 9% for women; 7.2% for Mexican-American men and 6.8% for women. For heart attack (myocardial infarction), the prevalence is 5.2% for non-Hispanic white men

(continued)

and 2% for women; 4.3% for non-Hispanic black men and 3.3% for women; and 4.1% for Mexican-American men and 1.9% for women.

Racial differences in incidence of CHD have both genetic and environmental components. For example, African Americans have higher HDL levels but higher lifestyle risk factors than white Americans. However, both groups have a similar CHD frequency. Blacks also have been noted to have higher rates of hypertension than whites, and Hispanics have lower rates than either of the other two groups in the United States. How much of the variation is due to genetic and how much to cultural and lifestyle differences is not known. Overfield (1995) notes that hypertension in blacks is clinically and biochemically different from that in whites. Blood pressure correlates with darker skin color, which may be due to the role of melanin as a reservoir for heavy metals like sodium. Comparisons of blacks and whites of higher education and socioeconomic levels indicate little difference in hypertension rates (Overfield, 1995). However, rates for blacks remain high, and for black women the rates are rising. Compared with US white women, hypertension in US black women has a higher incidence, earlier onset, and longer duration, and results in higher mortality, which remains among the highest rate in the industrialized world (Gillum, 1996).

Teaching is needed for individuals, families, and communities because of the widespread nature of CHD in developed countries. Immigrants need instruction on avoiding lifestyle changes that can increase their risks. It has been suggested that the best method for preventing CHD in the United States is a population-based approach, especially educating children to adopt and maintain healthy lifestyles (Berenson & Pickoff, 1995).

Collecting Objective Data

A major purpose of this examination is to identify any sign of heart disease and thereby initiate early referral and treatment. Since 1900, cardiovascular disease (CVD) has been the number one killer in the United States every year except 1918, and more than 2,600 Americans die of CVD every day, for an average of one death every 33 seconds (AHA, 2000). Some 60.8 million Americans have one or more types of CVD (AHA, 2001). The National Cholesterol Education Project (NCEP) recommends that all adults age 20 years or older have their total cholesterol and HDL cholesterol levels checked at least once every 5 years.

Assessment of the heart and neck vessels is an essential part of the total cardiovascular examination. It is important to remember that additional data gathered during assessment of the blood pressure, skin, nails, head, thorax and lungs, and peripheral pulses all play a part in the complete cardiovascular assessment. These additional assessment areas are covered in Chapters 7, 8, 9, 12, and 19.

The part of the cardiovascular assessment covered in this chapter involves inspection, palpation, and auscultation of the neck and anterior chest area (precordium). Inspection is a fairly easy skill to acquire. However, auscultation requires many hours of practice to develop expert proficiency (Display 16-6). Novice practitioners may be able to recognize an abnormal heart sound but may have difficulty determining what and where it is exactly. Continued exposure and experience increase the practitioner's ability

to determine the exact nature and characteristics of abnormal heart sounds. In addition, it may be difficult to palpate the apical impulse in clients who are obese or barrel chested because these conditions increase the distance from the apex of the heart to the precordium.

Heart and neck vessel assessment skills are useful to the nurse in all types of health care settings, including acute, clinical, and home health care. When performing a total body system examination, it is often convenient to assess the heart and neck vessels immediately after assessment of the thorax and lungs.

CLIENT PREPARATION

Prepare clients for the examination by explaining that they will need to expose the anterior chest. Female clients may keep their breasts covered and may simply hold the left breast out of the way when necessary. Explain to the client that he or she will need to assume several different positions for this examination. Auscultation and palpation of the neck vessels and inspection, palpation, and auscultation of the precordium are performed with the client in the supine position with the head elevated to about 30 degrees. The client will be asked to assume a left lateral position for palpation of the apical impulse if the examiner is having trouble locating the pulse with the client in the supine position. In addition, the client will be asked to assume a left lateral and a sitting-up and leaning-forward position so the examiner can auscultate for the presence of any abnormal heart

DISPLAY 16-6. **Auscultating Heart Sounds**

Most nurses need many hours of practice in auscultating heart sounds to assess a client's health status and interpret findings proficiently and confidently. Practitioners may be able to recognize an abnormal heart sound but may have difficulty determining what and where it is exactly. Continued exposure and experience increase one's ability to determine the exact nature and characteristics of abnormal heart sounds. An added difficulty involves palpation, particularly of the apical impulse in clients who are obese or barrel chested. These conditions increase the distance from the apex of the heart to the precordium.

WHERE TO AUSCULTATE

Heart sounds can be auscultated in the traditional five areas on the precordium, which is the anterior surface of the body overlying the heart and great vessels. The traditional areas include the aortic area, the pulmonic area, Erb's point, the tricuspid area, and the mitral or apical area. The four valve areas do not reflect the anatomic location of the valves. Rather, they reflect the way in which heart sounds radiate to the chest wall. Sounds always travel in the direction of blood flow. For example, sounds that originate in the tricuspid valve are usually best heard along the left lower sternal border at the fourth or fifth intercostal space.

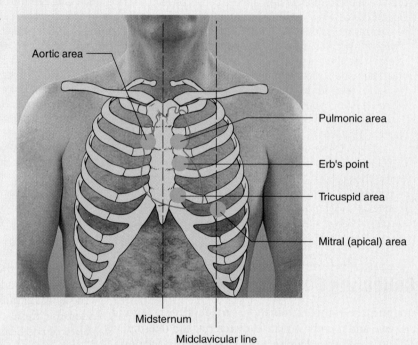

Aortic area

Pulmonic area

Erb's point

Tricuspid area

Mitral (apical) area

Midsternum

Midclavicular line

Traditional areas of auscultation.

In reality, the areas described above overlap extensively, and sounds produced by the valves can be heard all over the precordium. Therefore, it is important to listen to more than just five specific points on the precordium. Keep the fact of overlap in mind and use the names of the chambers instead of Erb's point, mitral, and tricuspid areas when auscultating over the precordium. "Alternative" (versus the traditional) areas of auscultation overlap and are not as discrete as the traditional areas. The alternative areas are the aortic area, pulmonic area, left atrial area, right atrial area, left ventricular area, and right ventricular area.

Cover the entire precordium. As you auscultate in all areas, concentrate on systematically moving the stethoscope from left to right across the entire heart area from the base to the apex (top to bottom) or from the apex to the base (bottom to top).

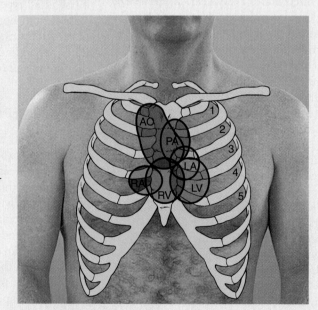

Alternative areas of auscultation.

(continued)

DISPLAY 16-6. Auscultating Heart Sounds (Continued)

Traditional Areas of Auscultation

- Aortic area: Second intercostal space at the right sternal border—the base of the heart
- Pulmonic area: Second or third intercostal space at the left sternal border—the base of the heart
- Erb's point: Third to fifth intercostal space at the left sternal border
- Mitral (apical): Fifth intercostal space near the left midclavicular line—the apex of the heart
- Tricuspid area: Fourth or fifth intercostal space at the left lower sternal border

Alternative Areas of Auscultation

- Aortic area: Right second intercostal space to apex of heart
- Pulmonic area: second and third left intercostal spaces close to sternum, but may be higher or lower
- Left atrial area: Second to fourth intercostal space at the left sternal border
- Right atrial area: Third to fifth intercostal space at the right sternal border
- Left ventricular area: Second to fifth intercostal spaces, extending from the left sternal border to the left midclavicular line
- Right ventricular area: Second to fifth intercostal spaces, centered over the sternum

HOW TO AUSCULTATE

Position yourself on the client's right side. The client should be supine with the upper trunk elevated 30 degrees. Use the diaphragm of the stethoscope to auscultate all areas of the precordium for high-pitched sounds. Use the bell of the stethoscope to detect (differentiate) low-pitched sounds or gallops. The diaphragm should be applied firmly to the chest, whereas the bell should be applied lightly.

Focus on one sound at a time as you auscultate each area of the precordium. Start by listening to the heart's rate and rhythm. Then identify the first and second heart sounds, concentrate on each heart sound individually, listen for extra heart sounds, listen for murmurs, and finally listen with the client in different positions.

 Tip From the Experts Closing your eyes reduces visual stimuli and distractions and may enhance your ability to concentrate on auditory stimuli.

---

sounds. These positions may bring out an abnormal sound that was not detected with the client in the supine position. Make sure you explain to the client that you will be listening to the heart in a number of places and that this does not necessarily mean that anything is wrong. Provide the client with as much modesty as possible during the examination, describe the steps of the examination, and answer any questions the client may have. These actions will help to ease any client anxiety.

EQUIPMENT AND SUPPLIES

- Stethoscope with a bell and diaphragm
- Small pillow
- Penlight or movable examination light
- Watch with second hand
- Centimeter rulers (two)

KEY ASSESSMENT POINTS

- Understand the anatomy and function of the heart and major coronary vessels to identify and interpret heart sounds and electrocardiograms accurately.
- Collect health history data related to heart health and disease thoroughly and efficiently.
- Prepare the client for cardiac examination, and educate the client about risk factors of coronary heart disease.
- Describe normal variations of the cardiovascular system in the elderly client.

(text continues on page 330)

PHYSICAL ASSESSMENT

ASSESSMENT PROCEDURE	NORMAL FINDINGS	ABNORMAL FINDINGS

NECK VESSELS

Auscultate the Carotid Arteries

Auscultate the carotid arteries if the client is middle-aged or older or if you suspect cardiovascular disease. Place the bell of the stethoscope over the carotid artery and ask the client to hold his or her breath for a moment so breath sounds do not conceal any vascular sounds.

No blowing or swishing or other sounds heard

A bruit, a blowing or swishing sound caused by turbulent blood flow through a narrowed vessel, is indicative of occlusive arterial disease. However, if the artery is more than two thirds occluded, a bruit may not be heard.

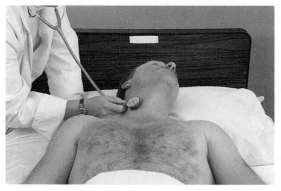

Auscultating the carotid artery. (© B. Proud.)

 Tip From the Experts Always auscultate the carotid arteries before palpating.

Palpate the Carotid Arteries

Palpate each carotid artery alternately by placing the pads of the index and middle fingers medial to the sternocleidomastoid muscle on the neck. Note amplitude and contour of the pulse, elasticity of the artery, and any thrills.

Pulses equally strong; a 2+ or normal with no variation in strength from beat to beat. Contour is normally smooth and rapid on the upstroke and slower and less abrupt on the downstroke. Arteries are elastic and no thrills are noted. The strength of the pulse is evaluated on a scale from 0 to 4 as follows:

Pulse inequality may indicate arterial constriction or occlusion in one carotid.

Weak pulses may indicate hypovolemia, shock, or decreased cardiac output.

A bounding, firm pulse may indicate hypervolemia or increased cardiac output.

Variations in strength from beat to beat or with respiration are abnormal and may indicate a variety of problems (Display 16-7).

A delayed upstroke may indicate aortic stenosis.

Loss of elasticity may indicate arteriosclerosis. Thrills may indicate a narrowing of the artery.

Pulse Amplitude Scale
0 = Absent
1+ = Weak
2+ = Normal
3+ = Increased
4+ = Bounding

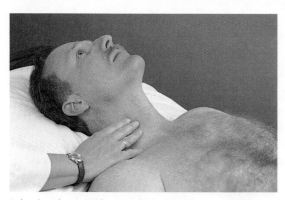

Palpating the carotid artery. (© B. Proud.)

(continued)

ASSESSMENT PROCEDURE	NORMAL FINDINGS	ABNORMAL FINDINGS

Tip From the Experts If you detect occlusion during auscultation, palpate very lightly to avoid blocking circulation or triggering vagal stimulation and bradycardia, hypotension, or even cardiac arrest. Palpate the carotid arteries individually because bilateral palpation could result in reduced cerebral blood flow. Be cautious with older clients because atherosclerosis may have caused obstruction and compression may easily block circulation.

Observe the Jugular Venous Pulse

Inspect the jugular venous pulse by standing on the right side of the client. The client should be in a supine position with the torso elevated 30 to 45 degrees. Make sure the head and torso are on the same plane. Ask the client to turn the head slightly to the left. Shine a tangential light source onto the neck to increase visualization of pulsations as well as shadows. Next, inspect the suprasternal notch or the area around the clavicles for pulsations of the internal jugular veins.

The jugular venous pulse is not normally visible with the client sitting upright. This position fully distends the vein, and pulsations may or may not be discernible.

Fully distended jugular veins with the client's torso elevated more than 45 degrees indicate increased central venous pressure that may be the result of right ventricular failure, pulmonary hypertension, pulmonary emboli, or cardiac tamponade.

Tip From the Experts Be careful not to confuse pulsations of the carotid arteries with pulsations of the internal jugular veins.

Evaluate Jugular Venous Pressure

Evaluate jugular venous pressure by watching for distention of the jugular vein. It is normal for the jugular veins to be visible when the client is supine so to evaluate jugular vein distention, position the client in a supine position with the head of the bed elevated 30, 45, 60, and 90 degrees. At each increase of the elevation, have the client's head turned slightly away from the side being evaluated. Using tangential lighting, observe for distention, protrusion, or bulging.

The jugular vein should not be distended, bulging, or protruding at 45 degrees.

Distention, bulging, or protrusion at 45, 60, or 90 degrees may indicate right-sided heart failure. Document at which positions (45, 60, and/or 90) you observe distention.

Clients with obstructive pulmonary disease may have elevated venous pressure only during expiration.

An inspiratory increase in venous pressure, called Kussmaul's sign, may occur in clients with severe constrictive pericarditis.

Note: In acute care settings, invasive cardiac monitors (pulmonary artery catheters) are used for precisely measuring pressures.

(continued)

ASSESSMENT PROCEDURE	NORMAL FINDINGS	ABNORMAL FINDINGS

HEART (PRECORDIUM)

Inspect Pulsations

Assist the client into supine position with the head of the bed elevated between 30 and 45 degrees. Stand on the client's right side and look for the apical impulse and any abnormal pulsations.

Tip From the Experts The apical impulse was originally called the point of maximal impulse (PMI). However, this term is not used any more because a maximal impulse may occur in other areas of the precordium as a result of abnormal conditions.

The apical impulse may or may not be visible. If apparent, it would be in the mitral area (left midclavicular line, fourth or fifth intercostal space). The apical impulse is a result of the left ventricle moving outward during systole.

Pulsations, which may also be called heaves or lifts, other than the apical pulsation are considered abnormal and should be evaluated. A heave or lift may occur as the result of an enlarged ventricle from an overload of work (Display 16-8).

Palpate the Apical Impulse

Remain on the client's right side and ask the client to remain supine. Use the palmar surfaces of your hand to palpate the apical impulse in the mitral area (fourth or fifth intercostal space at the midclavicular line). After locating the pulse, use one finger pad for more accurate palpation.

Tip From the Experts If this pulsation cannot be palpated, have the client assume a left lateral position. This displaces the heart toward the left chest wall and relocates the apical impulse farther to the left.

The apical impulse is palpated in the mitral area and may be the size of a nickel (1–2 cm). Amplitude is usually small—like a gentle tap. The duration is brief, lasting through the first two thirds of systole and often less. In obese clients the apical impulse may be unpalpable.

The apical impulse may be impossible to palpate in clients with pulmonary emphysema. If the apical impulse is larger than 1 to 2 cm, displaced, more forceful, or of longer duration, suspect cardiac enlargement.

In older clients the apical impulse may be difficult to palpate because of increased anteroposterior chest diameter.

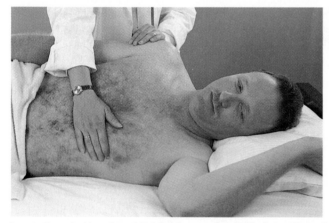 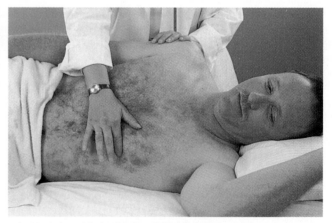

Locate the apical impulse with the palmar surface (*left*), then palpate the apical impulse with the fingerpad (*right*). (© B. Proud.)

(continued)

ASSESSMENT PROCEDURE	NORMAL FINDINGS	ABNORMAL FINDINGS

Palpate for Abnormal Pulsations

Use your palmar surfaces to palpate the apex, left sternal border, and base.

No pulsations or vibrations palpated in the areas of the apex, left sternal border, or base.

A thrill, which feels similar to a purring cat, or a pulsation is usually associated with a grade IV or higher murmur.

Auscultate Heart Rate and Rhythm

Follow the guidelines given in Display 16-6, place the diaphragm of the stethoscope at the apex and listen closely to the rate and rhythm of the apical impulse.

Rate: 60 to 100 beats per minute with regular rhythm. A regularly irregular rhythm, such as sinus arrhythmia when the heart rate increases with inspiration and decreases with expiration, may be normal in young adults (Display 16-9). Normally, the pulse rate in females is 5 to 10 beats per minute faster than in males. Pulse rates do not differ by race or age in adults (Overfield, 1995).

Bradycardia (less than 60 beats/min) or tachycardia (more than 100 beats/min) may result in decreased cardiac output. Clients with regular irregular rhythms (ie, premature atrial contraction or premature ventricular contractions) and irregular irregular rhythms (ie, atrial fibrillation and atrial flutter with varying block) should be referred for further evaluation. These types of irregular patterns may predispose the client to decreased cardiac output, heart failure, or emboli (see Display 16-9).

If you detect an irregular rhythm, auscultate for a pulse rate deficit. This is done by palpating the radial pulse while you auscultate the apical pulse. Count for a full minute.

The radial and apical pulse rates should be identical.

A pulse deficit (difference between the apical and peripheral/radial pulses) may indicate atrial fibrillation, atrial flutter, premature ventricular contractions, and varying degrees of heart block.

Auscultate to Identify S_1 and S_2

Auscultate the first heart sound (S_1 or "lub") and the second heart sound (S_2 or "dubb"). These two sounds make up the cardiac cycle of systole and diastole. S_1 starts systole, and S_2 starts diastole. The space, or systolic pause, between S_1 and S_2 is of short duration (thus, S_1 and S_2 occur very close together), whereas the space, or diastolic pause, between S_2 and the start of another S_1 is of longer duration.

S_1 corresponds with each carotid pulsation and is loudest at the apex of the heart. S_2 immediately follows after S_1 and is loudest at the base of the heart.

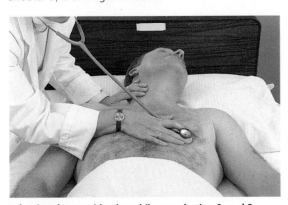

Palpating the carotid pulse while auscultating S_1 and S_2.
© B. Proud.)

(continued)

ASSESSMENT PROCEDURE	NORMAL FINDINGS	ABNORMAL FINDINGS

🌸 **Tip From the Experts** If you are experiencing difficulty differentiating S_1 from S_2, palpate the carotid pulse: the harsh sound that occurs with the carotid pulse is S_1.

Listen to S_1

Use the diaphragm of the stethoscope to best hear S_1.

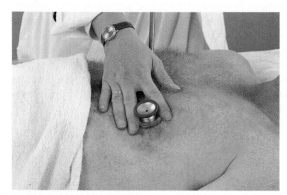

Auscultating S_1. (© B. Proud.)

Distinct sound heard in each area but loudest at the apex. May become softer with inspiration. A split S_1 may be heard normally in young adults at the left lateral sternal border.

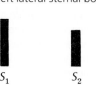

S_1 S_2

Normal S_1.

Accentuated, diminished, varying, or split.

Listen to S_2

Use the diaphragm of the stethoscope. Ask the client to breath regularly.

🌸 **Tip From the Experts** Do not ask the client to hold his or her breath. Breath holding will cause any normal or abnormal split to subside.

Distinct sound heard in each area, but loudest at the base. A split S_2 (into two distinct sounds of its components—A_2 and P_2) is normal and termed *physiologic splitting*. It is usually heard late in inspiration at the second or third left interspaces (see Display 16-3).

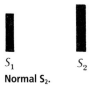

S_1 S_2

Normal S_2.

Any split S_2 heard in expiration is abnormal. The abnormal split can be one of three types: wide, fixed, or reversed.

(continued)

ASSESSMENT PROCEDURE	NORMAL FINDINGS	ABNORMAL FINDINGS
Auscultate for Extra Heart Sounds		
Use the diaphragm first and then the bell to auscultate over the entire heart area. Note the characteristics (eg, location, timing) of any extra sound heard. Display 16-4 provides a full description of the extra heart sounds (normal and abnormal) of systole and diastole. Auscultate during the systolic pause (space heard between S_1 and S_2).	Normally, no sounds are heard.	Ejection sounds or clicks (eg, a mid-systolic click associated with mitral valve prolapse). A friction rub may also be heard during the systolic pause.
Auscultate during the diastolic pause (space heard between end of S_2 and the next S_1).	Normally, no sounds are heard. A physiologic S_3 heart sound is a benign finding commonly heard at the beginning of the diastolic pause in children, adolescents, and young adults. It is rare after age 40. The physiologic S_3 usually subsides upon standing or sitting up. A physiologic S_4 heart sound may be heard near the end of diastole in well-conditioned athletes and in adults older than age 40 or 50 with no evidence of heart disease, especially after exercise.	A pathologic S_3 (ventricular gallop) may be heard with ischemic heart disease, hyperkinetic states (eg, anemia), or restrictive myocardial disease. A pathologic S_4 (atrial gallop) toward the left side of the precordium may be heard with coronary artery disease, hypertensive heart disease, cardiomyopathy, and aortic stenosis. A pathologic S_4 toward the right side of the precordium may be heard with pulmonary hypertension and pulmonic stenosis. S_3 and S_4 pathologic sounds together create a quadruple rhythm, which is called a *summation gallop*. Opening snaps occur early in diastole and indicate mitral valve stenosis. A friction rub may also be heard during the diastolic pause (see Display 16-4).

Tip From the Experts While auscultating, keep in mind that development of a pathologic S_3 may be the earliest sign of heart failure.

ASSESSMENT PROCEDURE	NORMAL FINDINGS	ABNORMAL FINDINGS
Auscultate for Murmurs		
A murmur is a swishing sound caused by turbulent blood flow through the heart valves or great vessels. Auscultate for murmurs across the entire heart area. Use the diaphragm and the bell of the stethoscope in all areas of auscultation because murmurs have a variety of pitches. Also, auscultate with the client in different positions because some murmurs occur or subside according to the client's position (see "Position Changes for Auscultation," immediately below).	Normally, no murmurs are heard. However, innocent and physiologic midsystolic murmurs may be present in a healthy heart.	Pathologic midsystolic, pansystolic, and diastolic murmurs. Display 16-5 describes pathologic murmurs.

(continued)

ASSESSMENT PROCEDURE	NORMAL FINDINGS	ABNORMAL FINDINGS

Position Changes for Auscultation

Ask the client to assume a left lateral position. Use the bell of the stethoscope and listen at the apex of the heart.	S_1 and S_2 heart sounds are normally present.	An S_3 or S_4 heart sound or a murmur of mitral stenosis that was not detected with the client in the supine position may be revealed when the client assumes the left lateral position.
Ask the client to sit up, lean forward, and exhale. Use the diaphragm of the stethoscope and listen over the apex and along the left sternal border.	S_1 and S_2 heart sounds are normally present.	Murmur of aortic regurgitation may be detected when the client assumes this position.

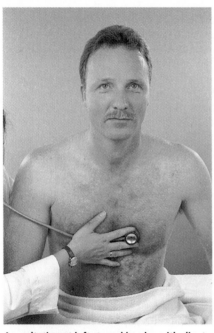

Auscultating at left sternal border with client sitting up, leaning forward, and exhaling. (© B. Proud.)

Validation and Documentation of Findings

Validate the heart and neck vessel assessment data that you have collected. This is necessary to verify that the data are reliable and accurate. Document the assessment data following the health care facility or agency policy.

EXAMPLE OF SUBJECTIVE DATA

No chest pain, dyspnea, dizziness, or palpitations. No previous history of cardiovascular disease. Denies rheumatic fever. No current medications or treatments. Denies family history of hypertension, myocardial infarction, coronary heart disease, high cholesterol levels, or diabetes mellitus. Client has never had an ECG. States he needs to exercise more and consume less fat. Client does not monitor own pulse or blood pressure. Denies the use of tobacco. Sleeps 6 to 8 h per night. Feels rested after sleep. States that job can be somewhat stressful.

EXAMPLE OF OBJECTIVE DATA

Carotid pulse equal bilaterally, 2+, elastic. No bruits auscultated over carotids. Jugular venous pulsation disappears when upright. Jugular venous pressure × 2 cm. No visible pulsations, heaves, or lifts on precordium. Apical impulse palpated in the fifth ICS at the left MCL, approximately the size of a nickel, with no thrill. Apical heart rate auscultated, 70 beats/min, regular rhythm, S_1 heard best at apex, S_2 heard best at base. No S_3 or S_4 auscultated. No splitting of heart sounds, snaps, clicks, or murmurs noted.

ABNORMAL FINDINGS

DISPLAY 16-7. Abnormal Arterial Pulse and Pressure Waves

A normal pulse, represented below, has a smooth, rounded wave with a notch on the descending slope. The pulse should feel strong and regular. The notch is not palpable. The pulse pressure (the difference between the systolic and diastolic pressure) is 30 to 40 mmHg. Pulse pressure may be measured in waveforms, which are produced when a pulmonary artery catheter is used to evaluate arterial pressure.

mm Hg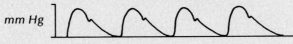

Normal pulse and pressure wave.

The arterial pressure waveform consists of five parts: Anacrotic limb, systolic peak, dicrotic limb, dicrotic notch, and end diastole. The initial upstroke, or anacrotic limb, occurs as blood is rapidly ejected from the ventricle through the open aortic valve into the aorta. The anacrotic limb ends at the systolic peak, the waveform's highest point. Arterial pressure falls as the blood continues into the peripheral vessels, and the waveform turns downward, forming the dicrotic limb. When the pressure in the ventricle is less than the pressure in the aortic root, the aortic valve closes, and a small notch (dicrotic notch) appears on the waveform. The closing of the aortic notch is the beginning of diastole. The pressure continues to fall in the aortic root until it reaches its lowest point, seen on the waveform as the diastolic peak.

Changes in circulation and heart rhythm affect the pulse and its waveform. Listed below are some of the variations you may find.

SMALL, WEAK PULSE

Characteristics

- Diminished pulse pressure
- Weak and small on palpation
- Slow upstroke
- Prolonged systolic peak

Causes

- Conditions causing a decreased stroke volume
- Heart failure
- Hypovolemia
- Severe aortic stenosis
- Conditions causing increased peripheral resistance
- Hypothermia
- Severe congestive heart failure

LARGE, BOUNDING PULSE

Characteristics

- Increased pulse pressure
- Strong and bounding on palpation
- Rapid rise and fall with a brief systolic peak

Causes

- Conditions that cause an increased stroke volume or decreased peripheral resistance
- Fever
- Anemia
- Hyperthyroidism
- Aortic regurgitation
- Arteriovenous fistulas
- Patent ductus arteriosus
- Conditions resulting in increased stroke volume due to decreased heart rate
- Bradycardia
- Complete heart block

DISPLAY 16-7. Abnormal Arterial Pulse and Pressure Waves (Continued)

- Conditions resulting in decreased compliance of the aortic walls
- Aging
- Atherosclerosis

BISFERIENS PULSE

Characteristics

- Double systolic peak

Causes

- Pure aortic regurgitation
- Combined aortic stenosis and regurgitation
- Hypertrophic cardiomyopathy

PULSUS ALTERNANS

Characteristics

- Regular rhythm
- Changes in amplitude (or strength) from beat to beat (you may need a sphygmomanometer to detect the difference)

Causes

- Left ventricular failure (usually accompanied by an S₃ sound on the left)

BIGEMINAL PULSE

Characteristics

- Regular, irregular rhythm (one normal beat followed by a premature contraction)
- Alternates in amplitude (one strong pulse followed by a quick, weaker one)

Causes

- Premature ventricular contractions

Premature contractions

PARADOXICAL PULSE

Characteristics

- Palpable decrease in pulse amplitude on quiet inspiration
- Pulse becomes stronger with expiration
- You may need a sphygmomanometer to detect the change (the systolic pressure will decrease by more than 10 mmHg during inspiration)

Causes

- Pericardial tamponade
- Constrictive pericarditis
- Obstructive lung disease

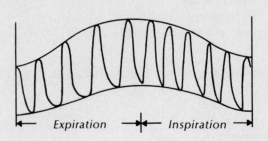

Expiration ←→ *Inspiration*

DISPLAY 16-8. Ventricular Impulses

ABNORMAL FINDINGS

Assessment of the chest may reveal abnormalities or variations of the ventricular impulse, signs of hypertension, hypertrophy, volume overload, and pressure overload. Some of the abnormalities or variations include the following:

LIFT

A diffuse lifting left during systole at the left lower sternal border, a lift or heave is associated with right ventricular hypertrophy caused by pulmonic valve disease, pulmonic hypertension, and chronic lung disease. You may also see retraction at the apex, from the posterior rotation of the left ventricle caused by the oversized right ventricle.

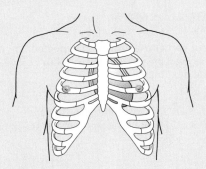

THRILL

A thrill is palpated over the second and third intercostal space; a thrill may indicate severe aortic stenosis and systemic hypertension. A thrill palpated over the second and third left intercostal spaces may indicate pulmonic stenosis and pulmonic hypertension.

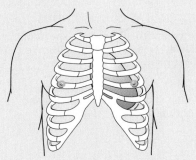

ACCENTUATED APICAL IMPULSE

A sign of pressure overload, the accentuated apical impulse has increased force and duration but is not usually displaced in left ventricular hypertrophy without dilatation associated with aortic stenosis or systemic hypertension.

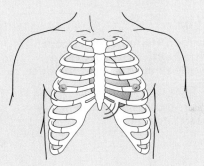

LATERALLY DISPLACED APICAL IMPULSE

A sign of volume overload, an apical impulse displaced laterally and found over a wider area is the result of ventricular hypertrophy and dilatation associated with mitral regurgitation, aortic regurgitation, or left-to-right shunts.

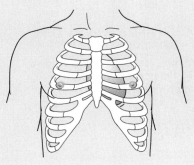

DISPLAY 16-9. Abnormal Heart Rhythms

ABNORMAL
FINDINGS

Changes in the heart rhythm alter the sounds heard on auscultation.

PREMATURE ATRIAL OR NODAL CONTRACTIONS

These beats occur earlier than the next expected beat and are followed by a pause. The rhythm resumes with the next beat.

Auscultation

The early beat has an S_1 of different intensity and a diminished S_2. S_1 and S_2 are otherwise similar to normal beats.

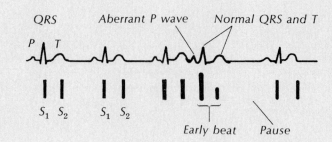

PREMATURE VENTRICULAR CONTRACTIONS

These beats occur earlier than the next expected beat and are followed by a pause. The rhythm resumes with the next beat.

Auscultation

The early beat has an S_1 of different intensity and a diminished S_2. Both sounds are usually split.

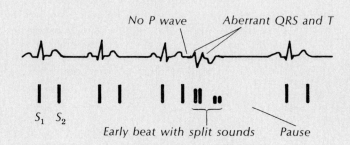

SINUS ARRHYTHMIA

With this dysrhythmia, the heart rate speeds up and slows down in a cycle, usually becoming faster with expiration and slower with expiration.

Auscultation

S_1 and S_2 sounds are usually normal. The S_1 may vary with the heart rate.

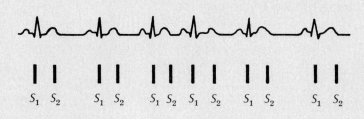

ATRIAL FIBRILLATION AND ATRIAL FLUTTER WITH VARYING VENTRICULAR RESPONSE

With this dysrhythmia, ventricular contraction occurs irregularly. At times, short runs of the irregular rhythm may appear regularly.

Auscultation

S_1 varies in intensity.

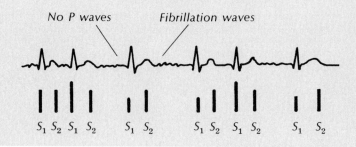

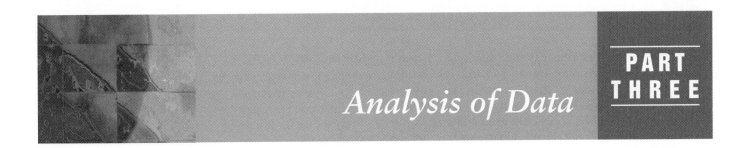

After you have collected your assessment data, you will need to analyze the data, using diagnostic reasoning skills (refer to Chapter 7). Use the case study on the following pages as a guide to analyzing the assessment data for a *specific* client. In the same way, practice diagnostic reasoning skill in the critical thinking exercise included in the lab manual/study guide that is available for this textbook.

Diagnostic Reasoning: Possible Conclusions

SELECTED NURSING DIAGNOSES

After collecting subjective and objective data pertaining to the heart and neck vessels, you will need to identify abnormals and cluster the data to reveal any significant patterns or abnormalities. These data will then be used to make clinical judgments (nursing diagnoses: wellness, risk, or actual) about the status of the client's heart and neck vessels. The following is a listing of selected nursing diagnoses that you may identify when analyzing data for this part of the assessment.

Nursing Diagnoses (Wellness)

- Opportunity to enhance cardiac output
- Health-Seeking Behavior: desired information on exercise and low-fat diet

Nursing Diagnoses (Risk)

- Risk for Sexual Dysfunction related to misinformation or lack of knowledge regarding sexual activity and heart disease
- Risk for Ineffective Denial related to smoking and obesity

Nursing Diagnoses (Actual)

- Fatigue related to decreased cardiac output

- Activity Intolerance related to compromised oxygen transport secondary to heart failure
- Acute Pain: Cardiac related to an inequality between oxygen supply and demand
- Anxiety
- Ineffective Tissue Perfusion: Cardiac related to impaired circulation

SELECTED COLLABORATIVE PROBLEMS

After grouping the data, you may see various collaborative problems emerge. Remember, collaborative problems differ from nursing diagnoses in that they cannot be prevented by nursing interventions. However, these physiologic complications of medical conditions can be detected and monitored by the nurse. In addition, the nurse can use physician- and nurse-prescribed interventions to minimize the complications of these problems. The nurse may also have to refer the client in such situations for further treatment of the problem. Following is a list of collaborative problems that may be identified when assessing the heart and neck vessels. These problems are worded as Potential Complications (or PC), followed by the problem.

- PC: Decreased cardiac output
- PC: Dysrhythmias
- PC: Hypertension
- PC: Congestive heart failure
- PC: Angina
- PC: Cerebrovascular accident
- PC: Cerebral hemorrhage
- PC: Renal failure

MEDICAL PROBLEMS

Once the data are grouped, certain signs and symptoms may become evident and may require medical diagnosis and treatment. Referral to a primary care provider is necessary.

Diagnostic Reasoning: Case Study

The case study presents assessment data for a specific client. It is followed by an analysis of the data, working out the seven key steps to arrive at specific conclusions.

Malcolm Winchester is being admitted to the coronary care unit (CCU) with a diagnosis of hypertension, angina, R/O MI (myocardial infarction). He is a tall, slender black man who looks younger than his stated age of 45. He is in no acute distress. Mr. Winchester says, "I don't know why they brought me here—I guess my wife panicked and called 911. I have these pains all of the time, but my doc said they were from my high blood pressure. I don't hurt now."

His wife arrives, looking pale and anxious. "I don't know what to do with him. I work so hard to keep him healthy, but he goes out to that fast food place and eats burgers and fries. I'm so tired of dealing with him when he won't help himself." Mr. Winchester grins and says, "I just got to have my junk food! That low-fat, low-salt diet my doctor put me on is impossible."

Physical assessment reveals BP 210/110 right arm reclining and 200/108 left arm reclining, pulse 88 regular and strong, respirations 16 regular and moderately shallow, temperature 36.5°C (97.7°F). His apical beat is also 88 and strong; heart sounds: S_1 and S_2 with no murmurs and clicks, but an S_4 is noted. Evaluation of the thorax reveals no heaves or visible pulsation. Neck veins are flat at >45 degrees and no carotid bruits noted. Skin is warm and dry, dark brown with pink nail beds, palms, and oral mucous membranes. Pedal pulses strong; 1 + ankle edema present.

SUBJECTIVE DATA

- "I don't know why they brought me here."
- "I have these pains all of the time"—physical said due to high blood pressure.
- Denies pain at this time
- Has to have junk food—low fat, low-salt diet "impossible"
- Wife: "Don't know what to do with him"—works hard to keep client healthy
- Wife: "He eats hamburgers and french fries and forgets to take medication"
- Wife: "Tired of dealing with him when he won't help himself"

OBJECTIVE DATA

- Admitted with angina, R/O MI
- BP 210/110 right arm reclining and 200/108 left arm reclining
- S_4 heart sound
- 1 + pedal edema

1 Identify abnormal data and strengths (in both subjective and objective data).

2 Cue Clusters	**3** Inferences	**4** Possible Nursing Diagnoses	**5** Defining Characteristics	**6** Confirm or Rule Out
A • BP 210/110 and 200/108 • S_4 heart sound	Dangerously high blood pressure with concurrent atrial gallop seen with hypertension			
B • Confirms eating junk food • Finds low-fat, low-salt diet "impossible"	Chooses not to follow special diet Unable to tolerate special diet	Impaired Health Maintenance related to choice not to follow prescribed dietary treatment of hypertension	*Major:* Reports unhealthful practices (eg, high-fat, high-salt diet) *Minor:* None, except possibly compulsive behavior regarding diet ("have to have my junk food")	Accept diagnosis because it meets defining characteristics and is validated by client although it may not be the best diagnosis on which to focus because it deals with noncompliance etiology, which needs a reason to plan appropriate interventions. Confirm, because diagnosis meets both major and minor defining characteristics. However, also important to collect more data regarding what other treatment regimens would be acceptable to him to control this dangerous condition.
		Ineffective Therapeutic Regimen Management related to intolerance of therapeutic diet and knowledge deficit of alternative strategies for managing hypertension*	*Major:* Verbalizes dislike of and difficulty with integration of prescribed regimen (diet) for treatment of illness *Minor:* Verbalizes he did not take action to include treatment into daily routine	

* Ineffective Therapeutic Regimen Management refers to therapeutic noncompliance. Noncompliance usually is diagnosed when it is a nurse problem rather than a client problem, and even as a client problem is limited to circumstances in which the client wants to comply but has difficulty doing so.

2 Cue Clusters	3 Inferences	4 Possible Nursing Diagnoses	5 Defining Characteristics	6 Confirm or Rule Out
C • "I have pains all the time" • Denies pain at this time	Not experiencing pain currently but has history of pain related to hypertension	Risk for Acute Pain: Acute pain (angina) related to knowledge deficit of management strategies	*Major:* Reports pain "all the time" but not at this time *Minor:* None	Can accept this diagnosis because it meets the major defining characteristics and is validated by client, although it is a risk diagnosis because not currently present. Need to collect additional data.
D • Wife: "Don't know what to do with him . . . tired of dealing with him when he won't help himself" • Called 911 when he had pain	Wife, who perceives herself as a caregiver is frustrated and anxious about client's ill health and noncompliance—possibly burned out	Caregiver Role Strain related to frustration with client's noncompliant behavior and possible anxiety over seriousness of symptoms Ineffective Family Coping related to strain on family from client's illness	Possibly implied apprehension about the future for care receiver's health. Also possibly depressed feelings and anger. *Subjective:* None specific *Objective:* None specific	Data are insufficient to accept this diagnosis, although it is certainly a risk diagnosis given the wife's verbalization of frustration. Need to collect more specific subjective and objective data to validate this diagnosis. Rule out diagnosis because it does not meet the major defining characteristic. More data are needed to identify how his family functions in the face of the client's illness and to validate or rule out this diagnosis.

7 Document conclusions.

The following diagnoses are appropriate for Mr. Winchester at this time:

- Ineffective Health Maintenance related to choice not to follow dietary treatment of hypertension
- Ineffective Therapeutic Regimen Management* related to intolerance of therapeutic diet and knowledge deficit of alternative strategies for managing hypertension
- Risk for Acute Pain: acute pain (angina) related to knowledge deficit of management strategies

Collaborative problems related to Mr. Winchester's medical diagnoses could include:

- PC: Cerebrovascular accident
- PC: Retinal hemorrhage
- PC: Myocardial infarction
- PC: Congestive heart failure
- PC: Renal failure

REFERENCES AND SELECTED READINGS

Appel, L. J., Moore, T. J., et al. (1997). A clinical trial of the effects of dietary patterns on blood pressure. *New England Journal of Medicine, 336,* 1–17.

Carabello, B. A., & Crawford, J. (1997). Valvular heart disease. *New England Journal of Medicine, 337,* 32.

Fabius, D. B. (2000). Solving the mystery of heart murmurs. *Nursing 2000, 30*(7), 39–44.

Geyer, N., & Naude, S. (1996). Continuing education—clinical. Diagnostic skills: Assessment of the cardiovascular system. *Nursing News (South Africa), 20*(6), 46–48.

Kirton, C. A. (2000). Physical assessment. Assessing normal heart sounds. *Nursing2000, 30*(2), 52–54.

Marshall, K. G. (1998). More techniques of auscultation: General principles of murmurs. *Patient Care, 9*(2), S1–S5.

Pflieger, K. L., & Strong, W. B. (1992). Screening for heart murmurs: What's normal and what's not. *Physician and Sportsmedicine, 20*(10), 71–74.

Talbot, L., & Curtis, I. (1996). Cardiovascular assessment of the patient with renal problems. *ANNA Journal, 23*(5), 445–456.

Wasserman, A. (2000). Chest pain. Is it life-threatening—or benign? *Consultant, 40*(7), 1204–1208.

Risk Factors—Coronary Heart Disease

American Heart Association (AHA). (2001). Coronary heart disease. Available online. Author.

————. (1999). Risk factor assessment for heart attack or stroke. Available online. Author.

Azevedo, A., Ramos, E., vonHafe, P., & Barros, H. (1999). Upper-body adiposity and risk of myocardial infarction. *Journal of Cardiovascular Risk, 6*(5), 321–325.

Berenson, G., & Pickoff, A. (1995). Preventive cardiology and its potential influence on the early natural history of adult heart diseases: The Bogalusa Heart Study and the Heart Smart Program. *American Journal of the Medical Sciences, 310*(Suppl 1), S1333–S138.

Eichholzer, M., Luthy, J., Gutzwiller, F., & Stahelin, H. (2001). The role of folate, antioxidant vitamins and other constituents in fruit and vegetables in the prevention of cardiovascular disease: The epidemiological evidence. *International Journal for Vitamin and Nutrition Research, 71*(1), 5–17.

Gillum, R. (1996). Epidemiology of hypertension in African American women. *American Heart Journal, 131*, 385–395.

Hallmen, T., Burell, G., Setterlind, S., Oden, A., & Lisspers, J. (2001). Psychosocial risk factors for coronary heart disease, their importance compared with other risk factors and gender differences in sensitivity. *Journal of Cardiovascular Risk, 8*(1), 39–49.

Leeson, C.P., Kattenhorn, M., Morley, R., Lucas, A, & Deanfield, J. (2001). Impact of low birth weight and cardiovascular risk factors on endothelial function in early adult life. *Circulation, 103*(9), 1264–1268.

Libby, P., Schoenbeck, V., Mach, F., Selwyn, A., & Ganz, P. (1998). Current concepts in cardiovascular pathology: The role of LDL cholesterol in plaque rupture and stabilization. *American Journal of Medicine, 104*(24), 145–185.

Misra, A. (2000). Risk factors for atherosclerosis in young individuals. *Journal of Cardiovascular Risk, 7*(3), 215–219.

Overfield, T. (1995). *Biological variation in health and illness: Race, age, and sex differences* (2nd ed.). Boca Raton, FL: CRC Press.

Rifai, N. M., & Ridker, P. M. (2001). High sensitivity C-reactive protein: A novel and promising marker of coronary heart disease. *Clinical Chemistry, 47*(3), 403–411.

For additional information on this book, be sure to visit http://connection.lww.com.

Peripheral Vascular Assessment

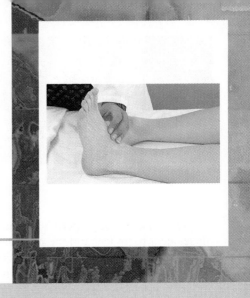

17

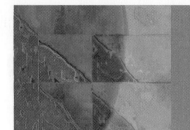

Structure and Function

To perform a thorough peripheral vascular assessment, the nurse needs to understand the structure and function of the arteries and veins of the arms and legs, the lymphatic system, and the capillaries. Equally important is an understanding of fluid exchange. The information provided on these pages can help you compile subjective and objective data related to the peripheral vascular system and differentiate normal vascular findings from normal variations and abnormalities.

Arteries

Arteries are the blood vessels that carry oxygenated, nutrient-rich blood from the heart to the capillaries. The arterial system is a high-pressure system. Blood is propelled under pressure from the left ventricle of the heart. Because of this high pressure, arterial walls must be thick and strong. Figure 17-1 illustrates the layers and the relative thickness of arterial walls. Each heartbeat forces blood through the arterial vessels under high pressure, creating a surge. This surge of blood is the arterial pulse. The pulse can be felt only by lightly compressing a superficial artery against an underlying bone. Many arteries are located in protected areas, far from the surface of the skin. Therefore, the arteries discussed in this chapter include only major arteries of the arms and legs—the peripheral arteries—that are accessible to examination. The other major arteries accessible to examination—temporal, carotid, and aorta—are discussed in Chapters 10, 16, and 18, respectively.

MAJOR ARTERIES OF THE ARM

The brachial artery is the major artery that supplies the arm. The brachial pulse can be palpated medial to the biceps tendon in and above the bend of the elbow. The brachial artery divides near the elbow to become the radial artery (extending down the thumb side of the arm) and the ulnar artery (extending down the little finger side of the arm). Both of these arteries provide blood to the hand. The radial pulse can be palpated on the lateral aspect of the wrist. The ulnar pulse, located on the medial aspect of the wrist, is a deeper pulse and may not be easily palpated. The radial and ulnar arteries join to form two arches just below their pulse sites. The superficial and deep palmar arches provide extra protection against arterial occlusion to the hands and fingers (Fig. 17-2).

MAJOR ARTERIES OF THE LEG

The femoral artery is the major supplier of blood to the legs. Its pulse can be palpated just under the inguinal ligament. This artery travels down the front of the thigh and then crosses to the back of the thigh, where it is termed the popliteal artery. The popliteal pulse can be palpated behind the knee. The popliteal artery divides below the knee into anterior and posterior branches. The anterior branch descends down the top of the foot, where it becomes the dorsalis pedis artery. Its pulse can be palpated on the great toe side of the top of the foot. The posterior branch is called the posterior tibial artery. The posterior tibial pulse can be palpated behind the medial malleolus of the ankle. The dorsalis pedis artery and posterior tibial artery form the dorsal arch, which, like the superficial and deep palmar arches of the hands, provides the feet and toes with extra protection from arterial occlusion (see Fig. 17-2). For a discussion of pulse measurement, see Display 17-1.

Veins

Veins are the blood vessels that carry deoxygenated, nutrient-depleted, waste-laden blood from the tissues back to the heart. The veins of the arms, upper trunk, head, and neck carry blood to the superior vena cava, where it passes into the right atrium. Blood from the lower trunk and legs drains upward into the inferior vena cava. The veins contain nearly 70% of the body's blood volume. Because blood in the veins is carried under much lower pressure than in the arteries, the vein walls are much thinner (see Fig. 17-1). In addition, veins are larger in diameter than arteries and can expand if blood volume increases. This helps to reduce the workload on the heart.

This chapter focuses on those veins that are most susceptible to dysfunction: the three types of veins in the legs. Two other major veins that are important to assess—the internal and external jugular veins—are discussed in Chapter 16.

There are three types of veins: deep veins, superficial veins, and perforator (or communicator) veins. The two deep veins in the leg are the femoral vein in the upper thigh and the popliteal vein located behind the knee. These veins account for about 90% of venous return from the lower extremities. The superficial veins are the great and small saphenous veins. The great saphenous vein is the longest of

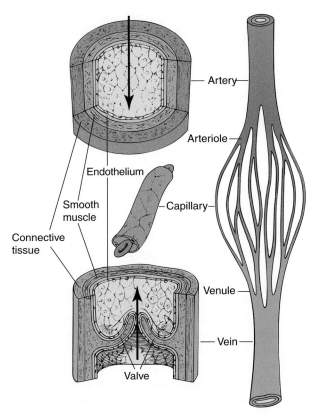

FIGURE 17-1. Blood vessel walls. Arterial walls are constructed to accommodate the high pulsing pressure of blood transported by the pumping heart, whereas venous walls are constructed with valves that promote the return of blood and prevent backflow.

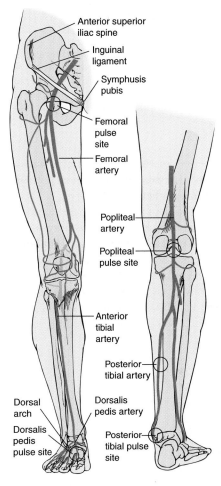

FIGURE 17-2. Major arteries of the arms and legs.

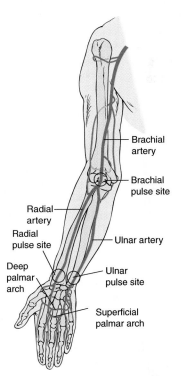

all veins and extends from the medial dorsal aspect of the foot, crosses over the medial malleolus, and continues across the thigh to the medial aspect of the groin, where it joins the femoral vein. The small saphenous vein begins at the lateral dorsal aspect of the foot, travels up behind the lateral malleolus on the back of the leg, and joins the popliteal vein. The perforator veins connect the superficial veins with the deep veins (Fig. 17-3).

Veins differ from arteries in that there is no force that propels forward blood flow; the venous system is a low-pressure system. This fact is of special concern in the veins of the leg. Blood from the legs and lower trunk must flow upward with no help from the pumping action of the heart. Three mechanisms of venous function help to propel blood back to the heart. The first mechanism has to do with the structure of the veins. Deep, superficial, and perforator veins all contain one-way valves. These valves permit blood to pass through them on the way to the heart, and they prevent blood from returning through them in the opposite direction. The second mechanism is muscular contraction. Skeletal muscles contract with movement and, in effect, squeeze blood toward the heart through the one-way valves. The third mechanism is the creation of a pressure gradient

Palpation of the pulses in the peripheral vascular examination is typically to assess amplitude or strength. Pulse amplitude is graded on a 0 to 4+ scale, with 4+ being the strongest. Elasticity of the artery wall may also be noted during the peripheral vascular examination, by palpating for a resilient (bouncy) quality rather than a more rigid arterial tone, whereas pulse rate and rhythm are best assessed during examination of the heart and neck vessels (see Chapter 14).

through the act of breathing. Inspiration decreases intrathoracic pressure while increasing abdominal pressure, thus producing a pressure gradient.

If there is a problem with any of these mechanisms, venous return is impeded and venous stasis results. Risk factors for venous stasis include long periods of standing still, sitting, or lying down. Lack of muscular activity causes blood to pool in the legs, which, in turn, increases pressure in the veins. Other causes of venous stasis include varicose (tortuous and dilated) veins, which increase venous pressure. Damage to the vein wall can also contribute to venous stasis.

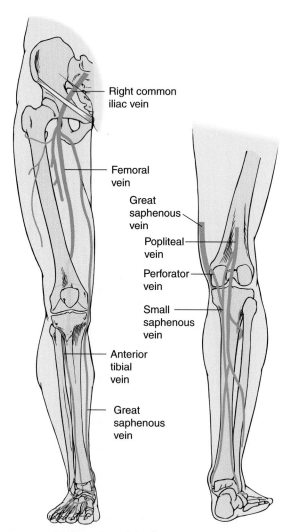

FIGURE 17-3. Major veins of the legs.

Lymphatic System

The lymphatic system, an integral and complementary component of the circulatory system, is a complex vascular system composed of lymphatic capillaries, lymphatic vessels, and lymph nodes. Its primary function is to drain excess fluid and plasma proteins from bodily tissues and return them to the venous system. This action prevents edema, which is a buildup of fluid in the interstitial spaces. The fluids and proteins absorbed into the lymphatic vessels by the microscopic lymphatic capillaries become lymph. These capillaries join to form larger vessels that pass through filters known as lymph nodes, where microorganisms, foreign materials, dead blood cells, and abnormal cells are trapped and destroyed. After the lymph is filtered, it travels to either the right lymphatic duct (which drains the upper right side of the body) or the thoracic duct (which drains the rest of the body) and then back into the venous system through the subclavian veins.

This unique filtering feature of the lymph nodes allows the lymphatic system to perform a second function as a major part of the immune system defending the body against microorganisms. A third function of the lymphatic system is to absorb fats (lipids) from the small intestine into the bloodstream.

Lymph nodes are somewhat circular or oval. Normally, they vary from very small and nonpalpable to 1 to 2 cm in diameter. Lymph nodes tend to be grouped together. They are both deep and superficial, and many are located near major joints. The superficial lymph nodes are the only lymph nodes accessible to examination. The cervical and axillary superficial lymph nodes are discussed in Chapters 10 and 15, respectively. The superficial lymph nodes of the arms and legs that are assessed in this chapter include the epitrochlear nodes and the superficial inguinal nodes.

The epitrochlear nodes are located approximately 3 cm above the elbow on the inner (medial) aspect of the arm. These lymph nodes drain the lower arm and hand. Lymph from the remainder of the arm and hand drains to the axillary lymph nodes. The superficial inguinal nodes consist of two groups, a horizontal and vertical chain of nodes. The horizontal chain is located on the anterior thigh, just under the inguinal ligament, and the vertical chain is located close to the great saphenous vein. These nodes drain the legs, external genitalia, and lower abdomen and buttocks (Fig. 17-4).

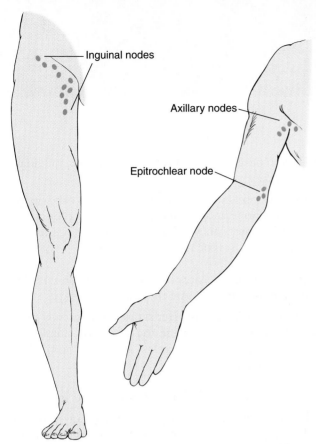

FIGURE 17-4. Superficial lymph nodes of the arms and legs.

Capillaries and Fluid Exchange

Capillaries are small blood vessels that form the connection between the arterioles and venules and allow the circulatory system to maintain the vital equilibrium between the vascular and interstitial spaces. Oxygen, water, and nutrients in the interstitial fluid are delivered by the arterial vessels to the microscopic capillaries (Fig. 17-5). Hydrostatic force (generated by the blood pressure) is the primary mechanism by which the interstitial fluid diffuses out of the capillaries and enters the tissue space. The interstitial fluid releases the oxygen, water, and nutrients and picks up waste products such as carbon dioxide and other by-products of cellular metabolism. The fluid then reenters the capillaries by osmotic pressure and is transported away from the tissues and interstitial spaces by venous circulation. As mentioned previously, the lymphatic capillaries function to remove any excess fluid left behind in the interstitial spaces. Thus, the capillary bed is very important in maintaining the equilibrium of interstitial fluid and preventing edema.

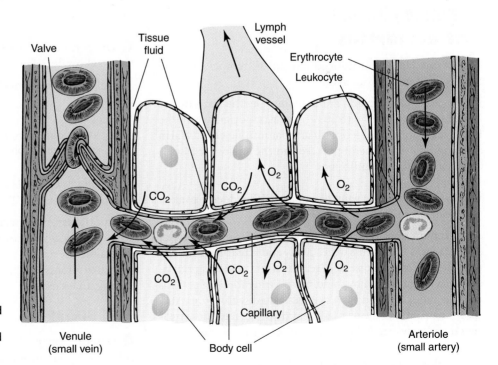

FIGURE 17-5. Normal capillary circulation ensures removal of excess fluid (edema) from the interstitial spaces as well as delivery of oxygen (O_2) and removal of carbon dioxide (CO_2).

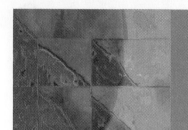

Collecting Subjective Data

Disorders of the peripheral vascular system may develop gradually. Severe symptoms may not occur until there is extensive damage. Therefore, it is important for the nurse to ask questions about symptoms that the client may consider inconsequential. It is also important for the nurse to ask about personal and family history of vascular disease. This information provides insight into the client's risk for a recurrence or development of problems with the peripheral vascular system. It is especially important to evaluate aspects of the client's lifestyle and health factors that may impair peripheral vascular health. These questions provide the nurse with an avenue for discussing healthy lifestyles that can prevent or minimize peripheral vascular disease. Some of the history questions may overlap those asked when assessing the heart and the skin because of the close relationship between systems.

Nursing History

CURRENT SYMPTOMS

Question Have you noticed any color, temperature, or texture changes in your skin?

Rationale Cold, pale, clammy skin on the extremities and thin, shiny skin with loss of hair, especially over the lower legs, are associated with arterial insufficiency. Warm skin and brown pigmentation around the ankles are associated with venous insufficiency.

Q Do you experience pain in your legs? If so, does it awaken you from sleep?

R Intermittent claudication characterized by pain, tension, and weakness that occurs with activity and is relieved with rest may indicate arterial disease. Heaviness and an aching sensation that is aggravated by standing or sitting for long periods of time and is relieved by rest is associated with venous disease. Leg pain that awakens a client from sleep is often associated with advanced chronic arterial occlusive disease.

Older clients with arterial disease may not have the classic symptoms of intermittent claudication, but may experience coldness, color change, numbness, and abnormal sensations.

Q Do you have any leg veins that are ropelike, bulging, or contorted?

R Varicose veins are hereditary but may also develop from increased venous pressure and venous pooling (eg, as happens during pregnancy). Standing in one place for long times also increases the risk for varicosities.

Q Do you have any sores or open wounds on your legs? Where are they located? Are they painful?

R Ulcers associated with arterial disease are usually painful and are often located on the toes, foot, or lateral ankle. Venous ulcers are usually painless and occur on the lower leg or medial ankle.

Q Do you have any swelling (edema) in your legs or feet?

R Peripheral edema (swelling) results from an obstruction of the lymphatic flow or from venous insufficiency from such conditions as incompetent valves or decreased osmotic pressure in the capillaries. It may also occur with deep vein thrombosis.

Q Do you have any swollen glands or lymph nodes? Do they feel tender?

R Enlarged lymph nodes may indicate a local or systemic infection.

With aging, lymphatic tissue is lost, resulting in smaller and fewer lymph nodes.

Q *For male clients:* Have you experienced a change in your usual sexual activity? Describe.

R Impotence may occur in clients with decreased blood flow or an occlusion of the blood vessels such as aortoiliac occlusion (Leriche's syndrome). Men may be reluctant to report or discuss difficulties they have achieving or maintaining an erection.

PAST HISTORY

Q Describe any problems you had in the past with the circulation in your arms and legs (eg, blood clots, ulcers, coldness, hair loss, numbness, swelling, or poor healing).

R A history of prior peripheral vascular disease increases a person's risk for a recurrence.

Q Have you had any heart or blood vessel surgeries or treatments, such as coronary artery bypass grafting, repair of an aneurysm, or vein stripping?

R Previous surgeries may alter the appearance of the skin and underlying tissues surrounding the blood vessels. Grafts for bypass surgeries are often taken from veins in the legs.

FAMILY HISTORY

Q Do you have a family history of diabetes, hypertension, coronary heart disease, or elevated cholesterol or triglyceride levels?

R These disorders tend to be hereditary and cause damage to blood vessels.

LIFESTYLE AND HEALTH PRACTICES

Q Do you (or did you in the past) smoke cigarettes or use any other form of tobacco? How much and for how long?

R Smoking cigarettes (and using other forms of tobacco) significantly increases a person's risk for chronic arterial insufficiency. The risk increases according to the length of time a person smokes and the amount of tobacco smoked (see Risk Factors—Peripheral Vascular Disease).

Q Do you exercise regularly?

R Regular exercise improves peripheral vascular circulation and decreases stress, pulse, and blood pressure, thereby decreasing the risk for developing peripheral vascular disease.

Q *For female clients:* Do you take oral contraceptives?

R Oral contraceptives increase the risk for thrombophlebitis, Raynaud's disease, hypertension, and edema.

Q Describe the degree of stress you normally have.

R Stress increases the heart rate and blood pressure and can contribute to vascular disease.

Q How have problems with your circulation (ie, peripheral vascular system) affected your ability to function?

R Pain associated with chronic arterial disease and the aching heaviness associated with venous disease may limit a client's ability to stand or walk for long periods. This, in turn, may affect job performance and the ability to care for a home and family or participate in social events.

Q Do leg ulcers or varicose veins affect how you feel about yourself?

R If clients perceive the appearance of their legs as disfiguring, their body image or feelings of self-worth may be negatively influenced.

Q Do you regularly take medications prescribed by your physician to improve your circulation?

R Drugs that inhibit platelet aggregation, such as clopidogrel (Plavix) or pentoxifylline (Trental), may be prescribed to increase blood flow. Aspirin also prevents blood clotting and is used to reduce the risks associated with peripheral vascular disease. Clients who fail to take their medications regularly are at risk for developing peripheral vascular problems. These clients require teaching about their medication and the importance of taking it regularly.

Q Do you wear support hose to treat varicose veins?

R Support stockings help to reduce venous pooling and increase blood return to the heart.

Collecting Objective Data

The purpose of the peripheral vascular assessment is to identify any signs or symptoms of peripheral vascular disease, including arterial insufficiency, venous insufficiency, or lymphatic involvement. This is accomplished by performing an assessment of first the arms and then the legs, concentrating on skin color and temperature, major pulse sites, and major groups of lymph nodes.

Examination of the peripheral vascular system is very useful in acute care, extended care, and home health care settings. Early detection of peripheral vascular disease can prevent long-term complications. A complete peripheral vascular examination involves inspection, palpation, and auscultation. In addition, there are several special assessment techniques that are necessary to perform on clients with suspected peripheral vascular problems.

The arms and legs should be closely compared bilaterally. Better objective data can be gained by assessing a particular feature on one extremity and then the other. For example, evaluate the strength of the dorsalis pedis pulse on the right foot and compare your findings with those of the left foot.

Whenever the client reports a symptom or has a complaint related to peripheral circulation and whenever you detect a sign or symptom that is unusual, explore it further with a symptom analysis. Use the COLDSPA mnemonic as a guide.

COLDSPA

CHARACTER: Describe the sign or symptom. How does it feel, look, sound, smell, and so forth?
ONSET: When did it begin?
LOCATION: Where is it? Does it radiate?
DURATION: How long does it last? Does it recur?
SEVERITY: How bad is it?
PATTERN: What makes it better: What makes it worse?
ASSOCIATED FACTORS: What other symptoms occur with it?

RISK FACTORS
Peripheral Vascular Disease

OVERVIEW

Peripheral vascular disease (PVD) includes five common vascular disorders (aortic aneurysms, cerebrovascular disease, deep vein thrombosis and pulmonary embolism, peripheral arterial occlusive disease [PAOD], and varicose veins). However, PVD usually refers to diseases of the arteries and veins of the lower extremities. The lower extremity chronic peripheral Diseases (PAOD and varicose veins) have differences in prevalence as well as in risk factors. At least 12% of community-dwelling adults age 65 and older have PAOD, most without classic intermittent claudication (Newman, 2000).

Venous disease (varicose veins and venous insufficiency) have a much higher incidence and prevalence than arterial disease. One 2-year study showed a yearly varicose vein incidence of 51.9 women and 39.4 men per 1000 subjects. Other studies show prevalence of any venous disease to be as high as 55% for women and 40% for men (Barnes, 1995). Other studies report a varicose vein prevalence of between 10% and 18% (Overfield, 1995).

MAJOR RISK FACTORS FOR ARTERIAL DISEASE (CRIQUI, DENENBERG, LANGER & FRONEK, 1997)

- Age—older adults (especially over 50)
- Diabetes mellitus
- Tobacco smoking
- Hypertension
- Elevated blood lipid levels (high level of low-density lipoproteins and low level of high-density lipoproteins)
- Coronary or cerebral vascular disease
- Male sex (somewhat higher)
- Family history

(handwritten note: high good low bad)

POSSIBLE RISK FACTORS FOR ARTERIAL DISEASE

- Elevated cholesterol
- Obesity (especially android-central fat pattern)
- High-fat diet
- Heavy alcohol intake
- Coagulation abnormalities
- Physical inactivity (Balkau, Vray & Eschwege, 1994)

RISK REDUCTION TEACHING TIPS FOR ARTERIAL DISEASE

- Stop smoking
- Control hypertension
- Eat a low-fat diet
- Control high blood sugars of diabetes mellitus
- Limit alcohol intake
- Get regular exercise

RISK FACTORS FOR VENOUS DISEASE

- Pregnancy
- Job with prolonged standing or sitting (*Note:* This is also a risk factor for the varicose veins known as hemorrhoids)
- Limited physical activity and /or poor physical fitness
- Congenital or acquired vein wall or valve weakness or anatomic structure
- Female sex
- Increasing age
- Genetics—non-African American
- Obesity
- Family history
- Lack of dietary fiber
- Use of constrictive clothing

RISK REDUCTION TEACHING TIPS FOR VENOUS DISEASE

- Get regular exercise.
- Avoid prolonged standing or sitting; modify work and leisure habits to vary position (eg, to reduce risk for hemorrhoids, use squatting position when toileting).
- Increase physical activity to moderate level.
- Maintain weight within ideal range for height and body structure.
- Increase dietary fiber intake.
- Avoid constrictive clothing, including girdles, garters for stockings or tightly cuffed knee-high hose, or any items that compress vessels.

CULTURAL CONSIDERATIONS

Prevalence of PAOD varies by geographic location. The highest prevalence has been found in elderly Italians, the lowest prevalence in 40- to 59-year-old Danes, and an intermediate prevalence in Americans age 65 and older (Balkau, Vray & Eschwege, 1994). An important variation in prevalence of varicose veins relates to race. Black Africans have fewer valves in the external iliac veins but considerably more valves lower in the leg than do Caucasians, which may account for a lower prevalence of varicose veins in blacks (1% to 3%) than in whites (10% to 18%; Overfield, 1995).

CLIENT PREPARATION

Have the client wear an examination gown and sit upright on an examination table. Make sure the room is a comfortable temperature (about 72°F) without drafts. This helps prevent vasodilation or vasoconstriction. Before you begin the assessment, inform the client that it will be necessary to inspect and palpate all four extremities and that the groin will also need to be exposed for palpation of the inguinal lymph nodes and palpation and auscultation of the femoral arteries. Explain that the client can sit for examination of the arms but will need to lie down for examination of the legs and groin, and will need to follow your directions for several special assessment techniques toward the end of the examination. As you perform the examination, explain in detail what you are doing and answer any questions the client may have. This helps to ease any client anxiety.

EQUIPMENT AND SUPPLIES

- Centimeter tape
- Stethoscope
- Doppler ultrasound device (Display 17-2)
- Conductivity gel

GUIDELINES

DISPLAY 17-2. How to Use the Doppler Ultrasound Device

The Doppler ultrasound device with a vascular probe (also called a *transducer*) transmits and receives ultrasound waves to evaluate blood flow. The device works by transmitting ultra high frequency sound waves in such a way that they strike red blood cells (RBCs) in an artery (primarily) or vein. The rebounding ultrasound waves produce a whooshing sound when echoing from an artery and a nonpulsating rush when echoing from a vein. The strength of the sound is determined by the velocity of the RBCs. In partially occluded vessels, RBCs pass more slowly through the vessel, thus decreasing the sound. Fully occluded vessels produce no sound. The battery-operated hand-held Doppler device is used to

- Assess unpalpable pulses in the extremities
- Determine the patency of arterial bypass grafts
- Assess the adequacy of tissue perfusion in an extremity (eg, by determining systolic BP)

OPERATING THE DEVICE

When assessing peripheral circulation with a Doppler ultrasound device, first inform the patient that the assessment is painless and noninvasive. Then, the test can proceed as follows:

- Apply a fingertip-sized mound of lukewarm gel over the blood vessel to be assessed.
- At a 45- to 60-degree angle, lightly place the vascular probe at the top of the mound of gel.
- Listen for a whooshing (artery) or nonpulsating rushing (vein) sound.
- Clean the skin with gauze or tissue.
- Clean the probe as recommended by the manufacturer.
- Mark the site with a waterproof pen if repeated assessments will be needed.
- Document your findings.

OBTAINING THE BEST RESULTS

- A warm extremity will increase the likelihood of a stronger signal.
- Use conductivity gel that is compatible with the Doppler device being used.
- Place the tube or packet of gel in warm water before use because cold gel will promote vasoconstriction and make it more difficult to detect a signal.
- Avoid holding the probe straight or pressing it snugly against the skin because this may result in the signal being obliterated.

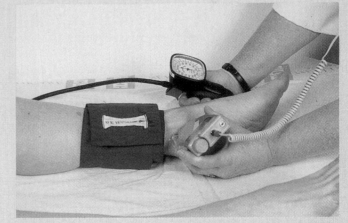

Using the Doppler ultrasound instrument to detect the character of blood flow in peripheral vessels helps the health care team to understand the nature of peripheral vascular disease. (© B. Proud.)

(Adapted with permission from Rice, K. L. [1998]. Sounding out blood flow with a Doppler device. *Nursing 98, 28* [9], 56–57.)

- Tourniquet
- Gauze or tissue
- Waterproof pen
- Blood pressure cuff

KEY ASSESSMENT POINTS

- Discuss risk factors for peripheral vascular disease with client

- Accurately inspect arms and legs for edema and venous patterning.
- Observe carefully for signs of arterial and venous insufficiency (skin color, venous pattern, hair distribution, lesions or ulcers) and inadequate lymphatic drainage.
- Recognize characteristic clubbing.
- Palpate pulse points correctly.
- Use the Doppler ultrasound instrument correctly.

(*text continues on page 359*)

PHYSICAL ASSESSMENT

ASSESSMENT PROCEDURE	NORMAL FINDINGS	ABNORMAL FINDINGS

INSPECT THE ARMS

Observe arm size and venous pattern; also look for edema.	Arms are bilaterally symmetric with minimal variation in size and shape. No edema or prominent venous patterning.	Lymphedema results from blocked lymphatic circulation, which may be caused by breast surgery. It usually affects one extremity, causing induration and nonpitting edema. Prominent venous patterning with edema may indicate venous obstruction.
Observe coloration of the hands and arms.	Color varies depending on the client's skin tone, although color should be the same bilaterally (see Chapter 9 for more information).	Raynaud's disease, a vascular disorder caused by vasoconstriction or vasospasm of the fingers or toes, is characterized by rapid changes of color (pallor, cyanosis, and redness), swelling, pain, numbness, tingling, burning, throbbing, and coldness. The disorder commonly occurs bilaterally; symptoms last minutes to hours.

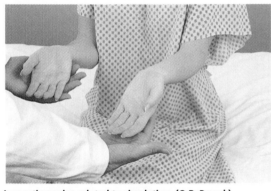

Inspecting color related to circulation. (© B. Proud.)

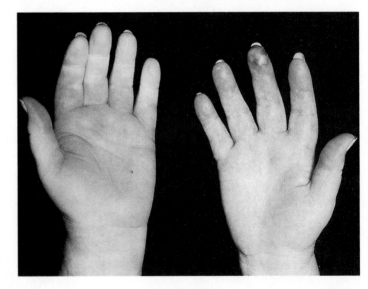

Hallmarks of Raynaud's disease are color changes. (With permission from Effeney, D. J., & Stoney, R. J. [1993]. *Wylie's atlas of vascular surgery: Disorders of the extremities.* Philadelphia: Lippincott Williams & Wilkins.)

Inspect fingertips for clubbing (discussed in Chapter 9).	No clubbing noted.	Clubbing, or enlargement of fingertips and flattening of the angle between the fingernail and nailbed, occurs with circulatory problems resulting from disorders, such as heart disease and lung disease.

(continued)

ASSESSMENT PROCEDURE	NORMAL FINDINGS	ABNORMAL FINDINGS

PALPATE PERIPHERAL VESSELS AND PULSES

Palpate the client's fingers, hands, and arms, and note the *temperature*.	Skin is warm to the touch bilaterally from fingertips to upper arms.	A cool extremity may be a sign of arterial insufficiency. Cold fingers and hands, for example, are common findings with Raynaud's disease.
Palpate to assess *capillary refill time*. Compress the nailbed until it blanches. Release the pressure, and calculate the time it takes for color to return. This test indicates peripheral perfusion and reflects cardiac output.	Capillary beds refill (and therefore color returns) in 2 seconds or less. *Note:* Some authorities consider normal capillary refill time to be 3 seconds or less.	Capillary refill time exceeding 2 seconds may indicate vasoconstriction, decreased cardiac output, shock, arterial occlusion, or hypothermia.

🎗 **Tip From the Experts** Inaccurate findings may result if the room is cool, if the client has edema, or if the client recently smoked a cigarette.

Palpate the *radial pulse* by gently pressing the radial artery against the radius.	Radial pulses have equal strength bilaterally (2+). Artery walls have a resilient quality (bounce).	Increased radial pulse volume indicates a hyperkinetic state. Diminished or absent pulse suggests partial or complete arterial occlusion (which is more common in the legs than the arms). The pulse could also be decreased from Buerger's disease or scleroderma. Obliteration of the pulse may result from compression by external sources, as in compartment syndrome.

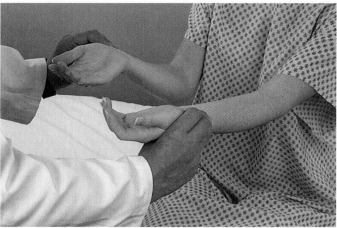

Palpating the radial pulse. (© B. Proud.)

🎗 **Tip From the Experts** For difficult-to-palpate pulses, apply more pressure on the most distal palpating finger to magnify the pulse wave against the other two fingers; or use a Doppler ultrasound device. (see Display 17-2).

(continued)

ASSESSMENT PROCEDURE	NORMAL FINDINGS	ABNORMAL FINDINGS

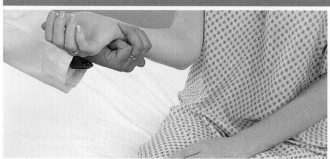

Palpating the ulnar pulse. (© B. Proud.)

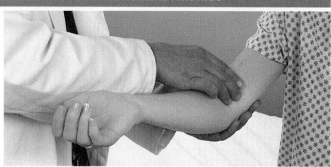

Palpating the brachial pulse. (© B. Proud.)

To palpate the *ulnar pulses,* apply pressure with your first three fingertips to the medial aspects of the inner wrists. The ulnar pulses are not routinely assessed because they are located deeper than the radial pulses and are difficult to detect. Palpate the ulnar arteries if you suspect arterial insufficiency.

The ulnar pulses may not be detectable.

Lack of resilience or inelasticity of the artery wall may indicate arteriosclerosis.

You can also palpate the *brachial pulses* if you suspect arterial insufficiency. Do this by placing the first three fingertips of each hand at the client's right and left medial antecubital creases. Alternatively, palpate the brachial pulse in the groove between the biceps and triceps.

Brachial pulses have equal strength bilaterally.

Brachial pulses are increased, diminished, or absent.

PALPATE THE EPITROCHLEAR LYMPH NODES

Take the client's left hand in your right hand as if you were shaking hands. Flex the client's elbow about 90 degrees. Use your left hand to palpate behind the elbow in the groove between the biceps and triceps muscles.

Normally, epitrochlear lymph nodes are not palpable.

Enlarged epitrochlear lymph nodes may indicate an infection in the hand or forearm, or they may occur with generalized lymphadenopathy. Enlarged lymph nodes may also occur because of a lesion in the area.

If nodes are detected, evaluate for size, tenderness, and consistency. Repeat palpation on the opposite arm.

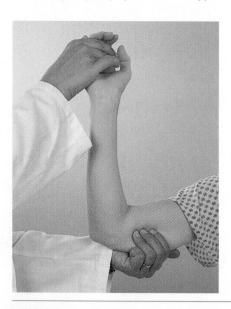

Palpating the epitrochlear lymph nodes located in the upper inside of the arm. (© B. Proud.)

(continued)

PERFORM THE ALLEN TEST

The Allen test evaluates patency of the radial or ulnar arteries. It is implemented when patency is questionable or before such procedures as a radial artery puncture. The test begins by assessing ulnar patency.

Pink coloration returns to the palms within 3 to 5 seconds if the ulnar artery is patent.

Pink coloration returns within 3 to 5 seconds if the radial artery is patent.

With arterial insufficiency or occlusion of the ulnar artery, pallor persists.

With arterial insufficiency or occlusion of the radial artery, pallor persists.

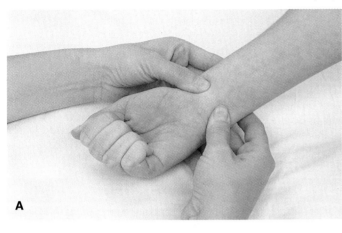

A

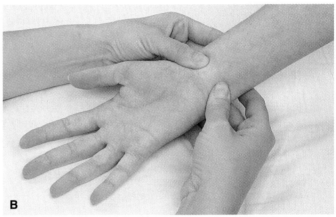

(A) Have the client rest the hand palm side up on the examination table and then make a fist. Use your thumbs to occlude the radial and ulnar arteries.

B

(B) Continue pressure to keep both arteries occluded, and have the client release the fist. Note that the palm remains pale.

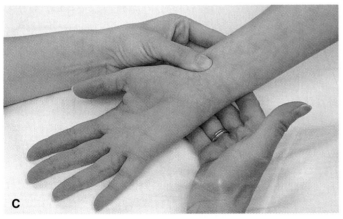

C

(C) Release the pressure on the ulnar artery and watch for color to return to the hand. To assess radial patency, repeat the procedure as before, but at the last step, release pressure on the radial artery. (© B. Proud.)

> **Tip From the Experts** Opening the hand into exaggerated extension may cause persistent pallor (false-positive Allen's test).

(continued)

ASSESSMENT PROCEDURE	NORMAL FINDINGS	ABNORMAL FINDINGS

INSPECT THE LEGS

ASSESSMENT PROCEDURE	NORMAL FINDINGS	ABNORMAL FINDINGS
Ask the client to lie supine. Then, drape the groin area and place a pillow under the client's head for comfort. Observe *skin color* while inspecting both legs from the toes to the groin.	Pink color for lighter-skinned clients and pink or red tones visible under darker-pigmented skin. There should be no changes in pigmentation.	Pallor, especially when elevated, and rubor, when dependent, suggests arterial insufficiency. Cyanosis when dependent suggests venous insufficiency. A rusty or brownish pigmentation around the ankles indicates venous insufficiency.
Inspect *distribution of hair.*	Hair covers the skin on the legs and appears on the dorsal surface of the toes. Hair loss on the lower extremities occurs with aging and is, therefore, not an absolute sign of arterial insufficiency in the older client.	Loss of hair on the legs suggests arterial insufficiency. Often, thin, shiny skin is noted as well.

ASSESSMENT PROCEDURE	NORMAL FINDINGS	ABNORMAL FINDINGS
Inspect for *lesions or ulcers.*	Legs are free of lesions or ulcerations.	Ulcers with smooth, even margins that occur at pressure areas, such as the toes and lateral ankle, result from arterial insufficiency. Ulcers with irregular edges, bleeding, and possible bacterial infection that occur on the medial ankle, result from venous insufficiency (Table 17-1).
Inspect for *edema.* Inspect the legs for unilateral or bilateral edema. Note veins, tendons, and bony prominences. If the legs appear asymmetric, use a centimeter tape to measure in four different areas: circumference at midthigh, largest circumference at the calf, smallest circumference above the ankle, and across the forefoot. Compare both extremities at the same locations.	Identical size and shape bilaterally; no swelling or atrophy.	Bilateral edema may be detected by the absence of visible veins, tendons, or bony prominences. Bilateral edema usually indicates a systemic problem, such as congestive heart failure, or a local problem, such as lymphedema (abnormal or blocked lymph vessels) or prolonged standing or sitting (orthostatic edema). Unilateral edema is characterized by a 1-cm difference in measurement at the ankles, or a 2-cm difference at the calf, and a swollen extremity. It is usually caused by venous stasis due to insufficiency or an obstruction. It may also be caused by lymphedema (Display 17-3). A difference in measurement between legs may also be due to muscular atrophy. Muscular atrophy usually results from disuse due to stroke or from being in a cast for a prolonged time.

Tip From the Experts Taking a measurement in centimeters from patella to the location to be measured can aid in getting the exact location on both legs. If additional readings are necessary, use a felt-tipped pen to ensure exact placement of the measuring tape.

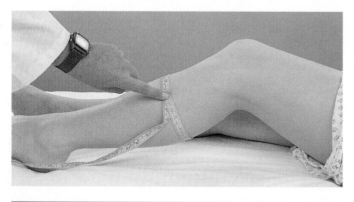

Measuring the calf circumference. (© B. Proud.)

(continued)

ASSESSMENT PROCEDURE	NORMAL FINDINGS	ABNORMAL FINDINGS

PALPATE EDEMA

If edema is noted during inspection, palpate the area to determine if it is pitting or nonpitting (Display 17-3). Press the edematous area with the tips of your fingers, hold for a few seconds, and then release. If the depression does not rapidly refill and the skin remains indented on release, pitting edema is present.

No edema (pitting or nonpitting) present in the legs.

Pitting edema is associated with systemic problems, such as congestive heart failure or hepatic cirrhosis, and local causes, such as venous stasis due to insufficiency or obstruction or prolonged standing or sitting (orthostatic edema). A 1+ to 4+ scale is used to grade the severity of the pitting edema.

PALPATE SKIN AND BLOOD AND LYMPHATIC VESSELS

Palpate bilaterally for *temperature* of the feet and legs by using the backs of your fingers. Compare your findings in the same areas bilaterally. Note location of any changes in temperature.

Toes, feet, and legs are equally warm bilaterally.

Generalized coolness in one leg or change in temperature from warm to cool as you move down the leg suggests arterial insufficiency. Increased warmth in the leg may be caused by superficial thrombophlebitis resulting from a secondary inflammation in the tissue around the vein.

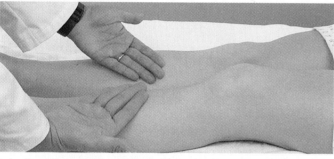

Palpating skin temperature. (© B. Proud.)

🏵 **Tip From the Experts** Bilateral coolness of the feet and legs suggests one of the following: The room is too cool, the client may have recently smoked a cigarette, or the client is anxious. All of these factors cause vasoconstriction, resulting in cool skin.

Palpate the superficial inguinal lymph nodes. First, expose the client's inguinal area, keeping the genitals draped. Feel over the upper medial thigh for the vertical and horizontal groups of superficial inguinal lymph nodes. If detected, determine size, mobility, or tenderness. Repeat palpation on the opposite thigh.

Nontender, movable lymph nodes up to 1 or even 2 cm are commonly palpated.

Lymph nodes larger than 2 cm with or without tenderness (lymphadenopathy) may be from a local infection or generalized lymphadenopathy. Fixed nodes may indicate malignancy.

PALPATE THE FEMORAL PULSES

Ask the client to bend the knee and move it out to the side. Press deeply and slowly below and medial to the inguinal ligament. Use two hands if necessary. Release pressure until you feel the pulse. Repeat palpation on the opposite leg. Compare amplitude bilaterally.

Femoral pulses strong and equal bilaterally.

Weak or absent femoral pulses indicate partial or complete arterial occlusion.

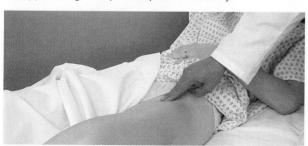

Palpating the femoral pulses. (© B. Proud.)

(continued)

ASSESSMENT PROCEDURE	NORMAL FINDINGS	ABNORMAL FINDINGS

AUSCULTATE THE FEMORAL PULSES

If arterial occlusion is suspected in the femoral pulse, position the stethoscope over the femoral artery and listen for bruits. Repeat for other artery.

No sounds auscultated over the femoral arteries.

Bruits over one or both femoral arteries suggest partial obstruction of the vessel and diminished blood flow to the lower extremities.

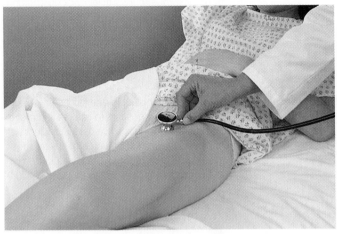

Auscultating the femoral pulse to detect bruits. (© B. Proud.)

PALPATE THE POPLITEAL PULSES

Ask the client to raise (flex) the knee partially. Place your thumbs on the knee while positioning your fingers deep in the bend of the knee. Apply pressure to locate the pulse. It is usually detected lateral to the medial tendon.

It is not unusual for the popliteal pulse to be difficult or impossible to detect, and yet for circulation to be normal.

Although normal popliteal arteries may be nonpalpable, an absent pulse may also be the result of an occluded artery. Further circulatory assessment (temperature and color) distal to the popliteal artery assists in determining the significance of an absent pulse.

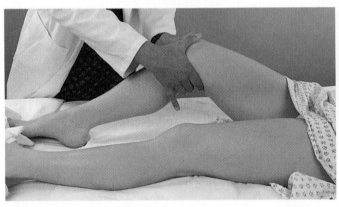 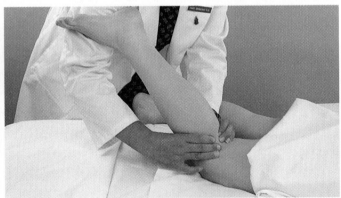

Palpating the popliteal pulse with the client (*left*) supine and (*right*) prone. (© B. Proud.)

If you cannot detect a pulse, try palpating with the client in a prone position. Partially raise the leg, and place your fingers deep in the bend of the knee. Repeat palpation in opposite leg, and note amplitude bilaterally.

(continued)

ASSESSMENT PROCEDURE	NORMAL FINDINGS	ABNORMAL FINDINGS

PALPATE THE DORSALIS PEDIS PULSES

Dorsiflex the client's foot, and apply light pressure lateral to and along the side of the extensor tendon of the big toe. The pulses of both feet may be assessed at the same time to aid in making comparisons. Assess amplitude bilaterally.

Dorsalis pedis pulses are bilaterally strong. This pulse is congenitally absent in 5% to 10% of the population.

A weak or absent pulse may indicate impaired arterial circulation. Further circulatory assessments (temperature and color) are warranted to determine the significance of an absent pulse.

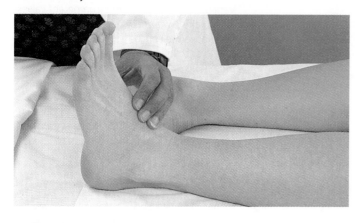

Palpating the dorsalis pedis pulse. (© B. Proud.)

Tip From the Experts It may be difficult or impossible to palpate a pulse in an edematous foot. A Doppler ultrasound device may be useful in this situation.

PALPATE THE POSTERIOR TIBIAL PULSES

Palpate behind and just below the medial malleolus (in the groove between the ankle and the Achilles tendon). Palpating both posterior tibial pulses at the same time aids in making comparisons. Assess amplitude bilaterally.

The posterior tibial pulses should be strong bilaterally. However, in about 15% of healthy clients, the posterior tibial pulses are absent.

A weak or absent pulse indicates partial or complete arterial occlusion.

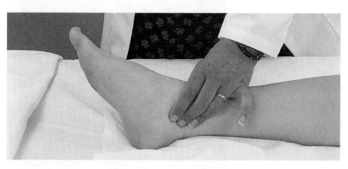

Palpating the posterior tibial pulse. (© B. Proud.)

Tip From the Experts Edema in the ankles may make it difficult or impossible to palpate a posterior tibial pulse. In this case, Doppler ultrasound may be used to assess the pulse.

(continued)

ASSESSMENT PROCEDURE	NORMAL FINDINGS	ABNORMAL FINDINGS

INSPECT FOR VARICOSITIES AND THROMBOPHLEBITIS

Ask the client to stand because varicose veins may not be visible when the client is supine and not as pronounced when the client is sitting. As the client is standing, inspect for superficial vein thrombophlebitis. To fully assess for a suspected phlebitis, palpate for tenderness. If superficial vein thrombophlebitis is present, note redness or discoloration on the skin surface over the vein.

Veins are flat and barely seen under the surface of the skin

👓 Varicosities are common in the older client.

Varicose veins may appear as distended, nodular, bulging, and tortuous, depending on severity. Varicosities are common in the anterior lateral thigh and lower leg, the posterior lateral calf, or anus (known as hemorrhoids). Varicose veins result from incompetent valves in the veins, weak vein walls, or an obstruction above the varicosity. Despite venous dilation, blood flow is decreased and venous pressure is increased. Superficial vein thrombophlebitis is marked by redness, thickening, and tenderness along the vein. Aching or cramping may occur with walking or dorsiflexion of the foot (positive Homans' sign). Swelling and inflammation are often noted.

Check for Homans' Sign

You can use two methods to elicit Homans' sign. The client should be supine for both methods. First, flex the client's knee about 5 degrees, place your hands under the client's calf muscle, and quickly squeeze the muscle against the tibia. Ask the client to report any pain or tenderness. Repeat procedure on opposite leg.

No pain or tenderness elicited with these maneuvers. Homans' sign is negative.

Calf pain and tenderness elicited with these maneuvers are a positive Homans' sign. A positive sign may indicate deep vein thrombosis (blood clot in deep vein) or superficial thrombophlebitis (inflammation of a superficial vein). However, further diagnostic testing (ie, venogram) and referral are indicated for a definitive diagnosis.

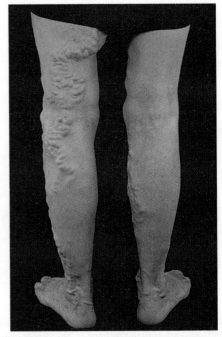

Varicose veins. (© 1995 Science Photo Library.)

(continued)

| ASSESSMENT PROCEDURE | NORMAL FINDINGS | ABNORMAL FINDINGS |

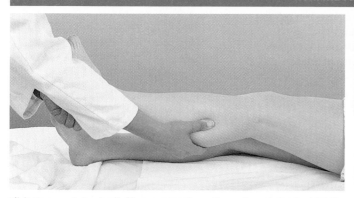 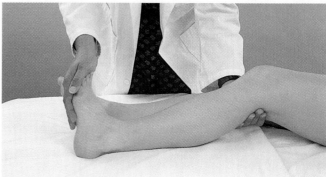

Elicit Hormans' sign by (*left*) squeezing the calf muscle and also by (*right*) passive dorsiflexion of the foot. (© B. Proud.)

Tip From the Experts Flexing the knee helps eliminate confusion between calf pain and Achilles tendon pain. A second method calls for putting your hand under the knee, slightly flexing it, and sharply dorsiflexing the foot. Ask the client to report pain or tenderness. Repeat this on the opposite leg.

SPECIAL TESTS FOR ARTERIAL OR VENOUS INSUFFICIENCY

Position Change Test for Arterial Insufficiency

If pulses in the legs are weak, further assessment for arterial insufficiency is warranted. The client should be in a supine position. Place both of your hands under both of the client's ankles. Raise the legs about 12 inches above the level of the heart. As you support the client's legs, ask the client to pump the feet up and down for about a minute to drain the legs of venous blood, leaving only arterial blood to color the legs.

Feet pink to slightly pale in color in the light-skinned client with elevation. Inspect the soles in the dark-skinned client, although it is more difficult to see subtle color changes in darker skin. When the client sits up and dangles the legs, a pinkish color returns to the tips of the toes in 10 seconds or less. The superficial veins on top of the feet fill in 15 seconds or less.

Marked pallor with legs elevated is an indication of arterial insufficiency. Return of pink color that takes longer than 10 seconds and superficial veins that take longer than 15 seconds to fill suggest arterial insufficiency. Persistent rubor (dusky redness) of toes and feet with legs dependent also suggests arterial insufficiency.

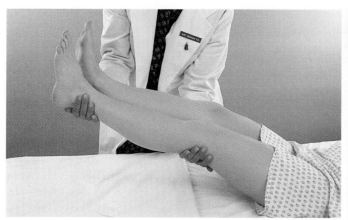 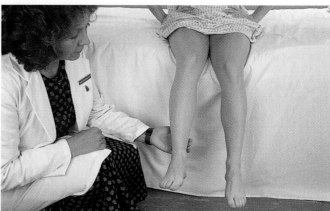

Testing for arterial insufficiency by (*left*) elevating the legs and then (*right*) having client dangle the legs. (© B. Proud.)

(continued)

ASSESSMENT PROCEDURE	NORMAL FINDINGS	ABNORMAL FINDINGS

Then, ask the client to sit up and dangle the legs off the side of the examination table. Note the color of both feet and the time it takes for color to return.

Normal responses with absent pulses suggest that an adequate collateral circulation has developed around an arterial occlusion.

> 🎗 **Tip From the Experts** This assessment maneuver will not be accurate if the client has peripheral vascular disease of the veins with incompetent valves.

Manual Compression Test

If the client has varicose veins, perform manual compression to assess the competence of the vein's valves. Ask the client to stand. Firmly compress the lower portion of the varicose vein with one hand. Place your other hand 6 to 8 inches above your first hand. Feel for a pulsation to your fingers in the upper hand. Repeat this test in the other leg if varicosities are present.

No pulsation is palpated if the client has competent valves.

You will feel a pulsation with your upper fingers if the valves in the veins are incompetent.

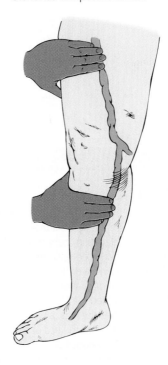

Performing manual compression to assess competence of venous valves in clients with varicose veins. (© B. Proud.)

Trendelenburg Test

If the client has varicose veins, perform the Trendelenburg test to determine the competence of the saphenous vein valves and the retrograde (backward) filling of the superficial veins. The client should lie supine. Elevate the client's leg 90 degrees for about 15 seconds or until the veins empty. With the leg elevated, apply a tourniquet to the upper thigh.

Saphenous vein fills from below in 30 seconds. No rapid filling of the varicose veins from above (retrograde filling) after removal of tourniquet if valves are competent.

Filling from above with the tourniquet in place and the client standing suggests incompetent valves in the saphenous vein. Rapid filling of the superficial varicose veins from above after the tourniquet has been removed also indicates retrograde filling past incompetent valves in the veins.

> 🎗 **Tip From the Experts** Arterial blood flow is not occluded if there are arterial pulses distal to the tourniquet.

Assist the client to a standing position, and observe for venous filling. Remove the tourniquet after 30 seconds, and watch for sudden filling of the varicose veins from above.

TABLE 17-1. Characteristics of Venous and Arterial Leg Ulcers

Characteristics	Venous Ulcer	Arterial Ulcer
Pulses	Present	Diminished or absent
Capillary refill	<3 seconds	>3 seconds
Skin temperature	Warm no temperature gradient	Cool/temperature gradient
Ankle-brachial index	.90 to 1.0	<.75
Ulcer location	Typically near medial malleolus	Tips of toes, foot or lateral malleolus
Ulcer margin	Irregular	Rounded and smooth
Ulcer tissue	Dark red granulation tissue	Black eschar or pale pink granulation tissue
Ulcer drainage	Moderate to large amount	Minimal
Periulcer skin	Bronzy-brown pigmentation, thick, hardened, and indurated	Pale, thin, friable, and shiny, thick toe nails, elevation pallor; dependency rubor
Dermatitis	Frequently occurs	Rarely occurs
Pruritis	Frequently occurs	Rarely occurs
Edema	Moderate to severe	Minimal unless leg constantly in dependent position
Pain	Ulcer often painful, especially if infected	Intermittent claudication or rest pain in foot; ulcer not painful

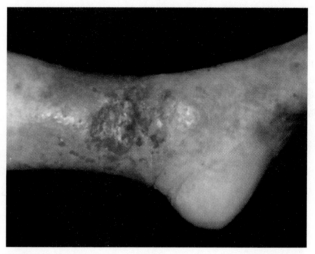

Characteristic ulcer of arterial insufficiency. (© 1994 Michael English, M.D.)

Characteristic ulcer of venous insufficiency. (Courtesy of Dermik Laboratories, Inc.)

(Used with permission from Wipke-Tevis, D. D. [1999]. Caring for vascular leg ulcers. *Home Healthcare Nurse* 17[2], 87–95.)

Validation and Documentation of Findings

Validate the peripheral vascular assessment data that you have collected. This is necessary to verify that the data are reliable and accurate. Document the assessment data following the health care facility or agency policy.

EXAMPLE OF SUBJECTIVE DATA

A 43-year-old man reports no color or temperature changes in arms or legs, no pain in legs, no open sores on legs, no swelling of arms or legs. States no bulging veins, no swollen glands, no problems with sexual activity, no history of circulatory problems, no previous surgery on the veins or arteries. Explains that his mother has hypertension and his father's brother died from complications of diabetes. Client states he does not smoke, manages his stress well, and exercises regularly.

EXAMPLE OF OBJECTIVE DATA

Arms are equal in size, no swelling, pinkish skin tone, no clubbing of fingertips, warm bilaterally. Capillary refill time less than 2 seconds, radial and brachial pulses strong bilaterally, no epitrochlear lymph nodes palpated. Legs are pink from toes to groin bilaterally, normal distribution of hair, no ulcers or edema. Legs are warm bilaterally, 1-cm nontender inguinal lymph nodes palpated, femoral, popliteal, dorsalis pedis, and posterior tibial pulses strongly palpated bilaterally. No apparent varicosities or superficial thrombophlebitis.

DISPLAY 17-3. Types of Peripheral Edema

EDEMA ASSOCIATED WITH LYMPHEDEMA

- Caused by abnormal or blocked lymph vessels
- Nonpitting
- Usually bilateral; may be unilateral
- No skin ulceration or pigmentation

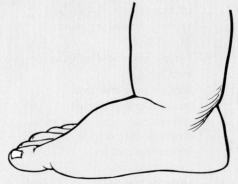

Swelling associated with lymphatic abnormality.

EDEMA ASSOCIATED WITH CHRONIC VENOUS INSUFFICIENCY

- Caused by obstruction or insufficiency of deep veins
- Pitting, documented as:
    - 1+ = slight pitting
    - 2+ = deeper than 1+
    - 3+ = noticeably deep pit; extremity looks larger
    - 4+ = very deep pit; gross edema in extremity
- Usually unilateral; may be bilateral
- Skin ulceration and pigmentation may be present

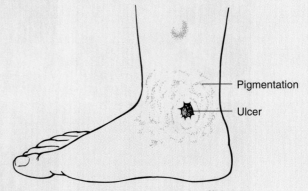

Edema associated with chronic venous insufficiency.

DISPLAY 17-4. Calculating the Ankle-Brachial Index (ABI)

The ankle-brachial index (ABI) is the ratio of the ankle systolic blood pressure to the arm (brachial) systolic blood pressure. The ABI is considered an accurate objective assessment for determining the degree of peripheral arterial disease. It detects decreased systolic pressure distal to the area of stenosis or arterial narrowing and allows the nurse to quantify this measurement (Cantwell-Gab, 1996). Use the following steps to measure ABI:

- Have the client rest in a supine position for at least 5 minutes.
- Apply the blood pressure (BP) cuff to first one arm and then the other to determine the brachial pressure using the Doppler. First, palpate the pulse and use the Doppler to hear the pulse. The "whooshing" sound indicates the brachial pulse. Pressures in both arms are assessed because asymptomatic stenosis in the subclavian artery can produce an abnormally low reading and should not be used in the calculations (Cantwell-Gab, 1996). Record the *higher* reading.
- Apply the BP cuff to the right ankle and then palpate the posterior tibial pulse at the medial aspect of the ankle and the dorsalis pedis pulse on the dorsal aspect of the foot. Using the same Doppler technique as in the arms, determine and record *both* systolic pressures. Repeat this procedure on the left ankle. If you are unable to assess these pulses, use the popliteal artery.

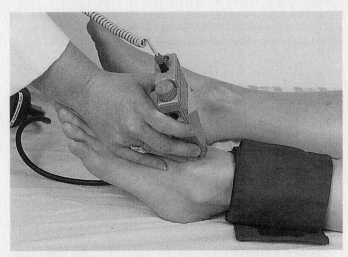

When measuring systolic pressure from the dorsalis pedis artery, apply the blood pressure cuff above the malleolus and the Doppler device at a 45- to 60-degree angle over the anterior tibial artery. Then move the device downward along the length of the vessel. (With permission from Cantwell-Gab, K. [1996]. Identifying chronic peripheral arterial disease. *AJN,96* [7], 40–47.)

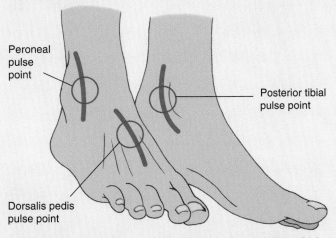

If you cannot measure pressure in the dorsalis pedis or posterior tibial artery, measure it in the peroneal artery. The blood pressure cuff can remain in place.

(continued)

DISPLAY 17-4. Calculating the Ankle-Branchial Index (ABI) (Continued)

- ABI calculation: Divide the higher ankle pressure for each foot by the higher brachial pressure. For example, you may have measured the highest brachial pulse as 160, the highest pulse in the right ankle as 80, and the highest pulse in the left ankle as 94. Dividing each by 160 (80/160 and 94/160) will result in a right ABI of 0.5 and a left ABI of 0.59.

Tips From the Experts to Ensure Accurate ABI Calculations

- Make sure to use a correctly sized blood pressure cuff. The bladder of the cuff should be 20% wider than the diameter of the client's limb.

- Document blood pressure cuff sizes used on the nursing plan of care (eg, "12-cm BP cuff used for brachial pressure: 10-cm BP cuff used for ankle pressure"). This minimizes the risk of shift-to-shift discrepancies in ABIs.

- Inflate the blood pressure cuff enough to ensure complete closure of the artery. Inflation should be 20 to 30 mmHg beyond the point at which the last arterial signal was detected.

- Avoid deflating the blood pressure cuff too rapidly. Instead, try to maintain a deflation rate of 2 to 4 mmHg/s for clients without arrhythmias and 2 mmHg/s or slower for clients with arrhythmias. Deflating the cuff more rapidly than that may cause you to miss the client's highest pressure and record an erroneous (low) blood pressure measurement.

- Be suspicious of arterial pressure recorded at less than 40 mmHg. This may mean that the venous signal was mistaken for the arterial signal. If you measure arterial pressure, which is normally 120 mmHg at below 40 mmHg, ask a colleague to double-check your findings before you record the arterial pressure.

- Suspect medial calcific sclerosis any time you calculate an ABI of 1.3 or greater or measure ankle pressure at more than 300 mmHg. This condition is associated with diabetes mellitus, chronic renal failure, and hyperparathyroidism. Medial calcific sclerosis produces falsely elevated ankle pressure by making the vessels noncompressible.

NORMAL FINDINGS

Generally, the ankle pressure in a healthy person is the same or slightly higher than the brachial pressure, resulting in an ABI of approximately 1, or no arterial insufficiency.

ABNORMAL FINDINGS

An ABI of 0.5 to 0.95 indicates mild to moderate arterial insufficiency whereas an ABI of 0.25 or lower indicates severe ischemia (Cantwell-Gab, 1996).

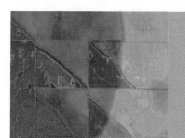

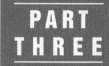

After collecting the assessment data, you will need to analyze it, using the diagnostic reasoning skills outlined in Chapter 7. In this chapter, the text section, Diagnostic Reasoning: Possible Conclusions, provides an overview of common conclusions that you may reach after the peripheral vascular assessment, and the case study that follows shows how to analyze peripheral vascular assessment data for a specific client. Finally, you are given an opportunity to analyze data in the Critical Thinking Exercise that appears in Chapter 17 of the laboratory manual.

Diagnostic Reasoning: Possible Conclusions

Listed below are some possible conclusions following an assessment of the client's peripheral vascular system.

SELECTED NURSING DIAGNOSES

After collecting subjective and objective data pertaining to the peripheral vascular system, you will need to identify abnormal findings and cluster the data to reveal any significant patterns or abnormalities. These data will then be used to make clinical judgments (nursing diagnoses: wellness, risk, or actual) about the status of the client's peripheral vascular system. Following is a list of selected nursing diagnoses that you may identify when analyzing data for this part of the assessment.

Nursing Diagnoses (Wellness)

- Opportunity to enhance circulation to extremities
- Health-Seeking Behavior: Requests information on regular monitoring of pulse, blood pressure, cholesterol and triglyceride levels, regular exercise, and smoking cessation

Nursing Diagnoses (Risk)

- Risk for Ineffective Individual Therapeutic Regimen Management (monitoring of pulse, blood pressure, cholesterol and triglyceride levels, regular exercise, and smoking

cessation) related to a busy lifestyle, lack of knowledge and resources to follow healthy lifestyle
- Risk for Infection related to poor circulation to and impaired skin integrity of lower extremities
- Risk for Injury related to decreased sensation in lower extremities secondary to edema and/or neuropathies
- Risk for Impaired Skin Integrity related to poor circulation to extremities secondary to arterial or venous insufficiency
- Risk for Activity Intolerance related to leg pain on walking
- Risk for Peripheral Neurovascular Dysfunction related to venous or arterial occlusion secondary to trauma, surgery, or mechanical compression

Nursing Diagnoses (Actual)

- Ineffective Tissue Perfusion related to arterial insufficiency
- Impaired Skin Integrity related to arterial or venous insufficiency
- Pain related to arterial or venous insufficiency
- Fear of loss of extremities related to arterial insufficiency
- Disturbed Body Image related to leg ulcerations, edema, or varicosities

SELECTED COLLABORATIVE PROBLEMS

After grouping the data, it may become apparent that certain collaborative problems emerge. Remember, collaborative problems differ from nursing diagnoses in that they cannot be prevented through nursing interventions. However, these physiologic complications of medical conditions can be detected and monitored by the nurse. In addition, the nurse can use physician- and nurse-prescribed interventions to minimize the complications of these problems. The nurse may also have to refer the client in such situations for further treatment of the problem. Following is a list of collaborative problems that may be identified when assessing the peripheral vascular system. These problems are worded as Potential Complications (or PC), followed by the problem.

- PC: Thromboembolic/deep vein thrombosis
- PC: Arterial occlusion
- PC: Peripheral vascular (arterial or venous) insufficiency
- PC: Hypertension
- PC: Ischemic ulcers
- PC: Gangrene

MEDICAL PROBLEMS

After grouping the data, it may become apparent that the client has signs and symptoms that may require medical diagnosis and treatment. Referral to a primary care provider is necessary.

Diagnostic Reasoning: Case Study

The case study presents assessment data for a specific client. It is followed by an analysis of the data, working through the seven key steps to arrive at specific conclusions.

Mr. Lee is a 40-year-old, previously healthy but obese (250 lb at 5 feet, 9 inches tall) man who comes to see the nurse practitioner with the complaint, "I must have pulled something in my right leg. I was walking along and I heard a pop, and now, 3 days later, my right leg is very sore. It really hurts to walk." He states that he is self-employed, developing software programs for computers. He says that he usually sits at his computer for about 4 hours at a stretch, then he walks two blocks to his favorite coffee shop for lunch (a sandwich or a salad with cheese and fruit, and usually a piece of cake or pie). After lunch, he goes back to work for another 5 to 6 hours. At night, he eats dinner and watches television for a few hours. His medical history includes a coronary artery bypass graft (CABG) 5 years ago for angina, complicated postoperatively by a pulmonary embolus. However, he has not had any problems since then. The nurse's physical assessment reveals his right calf to be swollen, slightly flushed, red, warm, and tender to palpation. His right calf measures 42 cm at 20 cm above the ankle (medial malleolus); his left calf is 34.5 cm at the same location. Homans' sign is positive for pain in the right calf only. He denies numbness, tingling, or loss of mobility in either extremity.

1 **Identify abnormal data and strengths (in both subjective and objective data).**

SUBJECTIVE DATA

- "I must have pulled something in my right leg."
- "I heard a pop when I was walking."
- Three days later, "right leg is very sore."
- Pain in right calf with walking
- Sits at computer 9 to 10 hours a day with only short lunch break
- Walks about four blocks a day
- Watches television in evening for several hours
- Eats sandwich or salad with cheese and fruit for lunch
- Eats pie or cake at lunch daily
- History of CABG for angina with complication of pulmonary embolus

OBJECTIVE DATA

- Obese (250 lb at 5 feet, 9 inches tall)
- Right calf swollen, slightly flushed red, warm, and tender to palpation
- Right calf 42 cm at 20 cm above the ankle
- Left calf is 34.5 cm at the same location
- Positive Homans' sign in right calf only

2 Cue Clusters	**3** Inferences	**4** Possible Nursing Diagnoses	**5** Defining Characteristics	**6** Confirm or Rule Out
A • Right calf swollen, slightly flushed red, warm, and tender to palpation • Right calf 42 cm at 20 cm above the ankle • Left calf is 34.5 cm at the same location • Positive Homans' sign in right calf only	Although the "popping" sound Mr. Lee perceived when walking implies a possible musculoskeletal problem, the rest of the signs and symptoms with his lifestyle and medical history point to the possibility of a deep vein thrombosis.	Ineffective Health Maintenance related to lack of knowledge of behaviors necessary to promote wellness and prevent recurring vascular problems	*Major:* Reports unhealthful practices, such as excessive sitting and lack of exercise *Minor:* None	Confirm because it meets the major defining characteristics.

2 Cue Clusters	3 Inferences	4 Possible Nursing Diagnoses	5 Defining Characteristics	6 Confirm or Rule Out
• "I must have pulled something in my right leg" • Heard a pop when walking • Three days later "right leg is very sore"	Therefore, Mr. Lee needs an immediate referral to the clinic physician. Collaborative problems should also be identified.			
• Eats pie or cake daily—obese • Sits at computer 9 to 10 hours a day with only short lunch break • Walks only about 4 blocks a day • Watches TV at night • History of CABG for angina with complication of pulmonary embolus	Mr. Lee's sedentary lifestyle, obesity, and dietary habits can continue to affect his health status.			
B • Obese (250 lb at 5 feet, 9 inches tall) • Eats sandwich or cheese and fruit for lunch • Eats pie or cake at lunch daily • Walks about 4 blocks a day • Watches TV in evening for several hours	Dietary habit of cake and pie daily and insufficient exercise are suggestive of inadequate balance of intake and energy output, which his obesity may verify.	Altered Nutrition: More Than Body Requirements related to decreased activity and inappropriate food choices	*Major:* Obese (>20% over ideal body weight) *Minor:* Sedentary activity patterns	Confirm because it meets the major and minor defining characteristics. More data collection is needed to determine his actual dietary patterns.

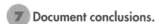

7 Document conclusions.

Two diagnoses are appropriate for Mr. Lee at this time:

- Imbalanced Nutrition: More Than Body Requirements related to decreased activity and possibly inappropriate food choices
- Ineffective Health Maintenance related to lack of knowledge of behaviors necessary to promote wellness and prevent recurring vascular problems

Collaborative problems related to the medical diagnoses could include:

- PC: Pulmonary embolism
- PC: Cellulitis

Mr. Lee should not be allowed to leave the clinic without seeing a physician for evaluation related to possible deep vein thrombosis.

REFERENCES AND SELECTED READINGS

Armstrong, D. G., & Lavery, L. A. (1998). Diabetic foot ulcers: Prevention, diagnosis and classification. *American Family Physician, 57*(6), 1325–1332.

Cantwell-Gab, K. (1996). Identifying chronic peripheral arterial disease. *American Journal of Nursing, 96*(7), 40–46.

Chase, S. K., Whittemore, R., Crosby, N., Freney, D., Howes, P., & Phillips, T. J. (2000). Living with chronic venous leg ulcers: A descriptive study of knowledge and functional health status. *Journal of Community Health Nursing, 17*(1), 1–13.

Church, V. (2000). Staying on guard for DVT & PE. *Nursing 2000, 30*(2), 35–42.

Hauser, D. E. (1999). Promotion of foot health in diabetes. *Clinical Excellence for Nurse Practitioners, 3*(4), 210–213.

Marinella, M. A., Kathula, S. K., & Markert, R. J. (2000). Spectrum of upper-extremity deep venous thrombosis in a community teaching hospital. *Heart & Lung, 29*(2), 113–117.

Rice, K. L. (1998). Sounding out blood flow with a Doppler device. *Nursing98, 28*(9), 56–57.

Sloan, H., & Wills, E. M. (1999). Ankle-brachial index. Calculating your patient's vascular risks. *Nursing99, 29*(10), 58–59.

Smeltzer, S. C., & Bare, B. G. (2000). Assessment and management of patients with vascular disorders. In *Brunner & Suddarth's Medical Surgical Nursing* (9th ed.). Philadelphia: Lippincott Williams & Wilkins.

Wipke-Tevis, D. D. (1999). Caring for vascular leg ulcers: Essential knowledge for the home health nurse. *Home Healthcare Nurse, 17*(2), 87–95.

Risk Factors—Peripheral Vascular Disease

Balkau, B., Vray, M., & Eschwege, E. (1994). Epidemiology of peripheral arterial disease. *Journal of Cardiovascular Pharmacology, 23*(Suppl. 3), S8–S16.

Barnes, R. (1995). Vascular holism: The epidemiology of vascular disease. *Annals of Vascular Surgery, 9*(6), 576–582.

Criqui, M. H., Denenberg, J., Langer, R., & Fronek, A. (1997). The epidemiology of peripheral arterial disease: Importance of identifying the population at risk. *Vascular Medicine, 2*(3), 221–226.

Newman, A. (2000). Peripheral arterial disease: Insights from population studies of older adults. *Journal of the American Geriatric Society, 48*(9), 1157–1162.

Overfield, T. (1995). *Biologic variation in health and illness: Race, age, and sex differences* (2nd ed.). Boca Raton, FL: CRC Press.

For additional information on this book, be sure to visit http://connection.lww.com.

Abdominal Assessment

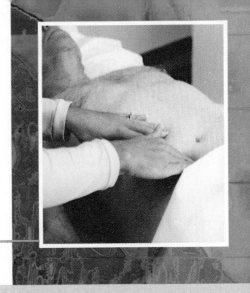

18

The abdomen is bordered superiorly by the costal margins, inferiorly by the symphysis pubis and inguinal canals, and laterally by the flanks (Fig. 18-1). To perform an adequate assessment of the abdomen, the nurse needs to understand the anatomic divisions known as the abdominal quadrants, the abdominal wall muscles, and the internal anatomy of the abdominal cavity.

Abdominal Quadrants

The abdomen is divided into four quadrants for purposes of physical examination. These are termed the right upper quadrant (RUQ), right lower quadrant (RLQ), left lower quadrant (LLQ), and left upper quadrant (LUQ). The quadrants are determined by an imaginary vertical line (midline) extending from the tip of the sternum (xiphoid), through the umbilicus to the symphysis pubis. This line is bisected perpendicularly by the lateral line, which runs through the umbilicus across the abdomen. Familiarization with the organs and structures in each quadrant is essential to accurate data collection, interpretation, and documentation of findings (Display 18-1). Another, older method divides the abdomen into nine regions. Three of these regions are still commonly used to describe abdominal findings—epigastric, umbilical, and hypogastric or suprapubic.

Abdominal Wall Muscles

The abdominal contents are enclosed externally by the abdominal wall musculature, which includes three layers of muscle extending from the back, around the flanks, to the front. The outermost layer is the external abdominal oblique; the middle layer is the internal abdominal oblique; and the innermost layer is the transverse abdominis. Connective tissue from these muscles extends forward to encase a vertical muscle of the anterior abdominal wall called the rectus abdominis. The fibers and connective tissue extensions of these muscles (aponeuroses) diverge in a characteristic plywood-like pattern (several thin layers arranged at right angles to each other), which provides strength to the abdominal wall. The joining of these muscle fibers and aponeuroses at the midline of the abdomen forms a white line called the linea alba, which extends vertically from the

xiphoid process of the sternum to the symphysis pubis (Fig. 18-2). The abdominal wall muscles protect the internal organs and allow normal compression during functional activities such as coughing, sneezing, urination, defecation, and childbirth.

Internal Anatomy

A thin, shiny, serous membrane called the peritoneum lines the abdominal cavity (parietal peritoneum) and also provides a protective covering for most of the internal abdominal organs (visceral peritoneum). Within the abdominal cavity are structures of several different body systems—gastrointestinal, reproductive (female), lymphatic, and urinary. These structures are typically referred to as the abdominal viscera and can be divided into two types—solid viscera and hollow viscera. Solid viscera are those organs that maintain their shape consistently—the liver, pancreas, spleen, adrenal glands, kidneys, ovaries, and uterus. The hollow viscera consist of structures that change shape depending on their contents. These include the stomach, gallbladder, small intestine, colon, and bladder. Palpation of the abdominal viscera depends on location, structural consistency, and size.

SOLID VISCERA

The liver is the largest solid organ in the body. It is located below the diaphragm in the RUQ of the abdomen. It is composed of four lobes that fill most of the RUQ and extend to the left midclavicular line. In many people, the liver extends just below the right costal margin, where it may be palpated. If palpable, the liver has a soft consistency. The liver functions as an accessory digestive organ and has a variety of metabolic and regulatory functions as well (Fig. 18-3).

The pancreas, located mostly behind the stomach, deep in the upper abdomen, is normally not palpable. It is a long gland, extending across the abdomen from the RUQ to the LUQ. The pancreas has two functions. It is an accessory organ of digestion and an endocrine gland.

The spleen is approximately 7 cm wide and is located above the left kidney, just below the diaphragm at the level of the ninth, tenth, and eleventh ribs. It is posterior to the left midaxillary line and posterior and lateral to the stomach.

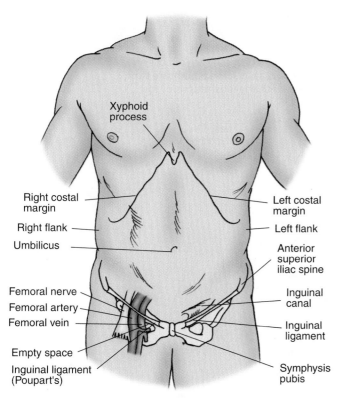

Xyphoid
process

Right costal
margin

Right flank

Umbilicus

Femoral nerve
Femoral artery
Femoral vein

Empty space

Inguinal ligament
(Poupart's)

Left costal
margin

Left flank

Anterior
superior
iliac spine

Inguinal
canal

Inguinal
ligament

Symphysis
pubis

FIGURE 18-1. Landmarks of the abdomen.

This soft, flat structure is normally not palpable. In some healthy clients, the lower tip can be felt below the left costal margin. When the spleen enlarges, the lower tip extends down and toward the midline. The spleen functions primarily to filter the blood of cellular debris, to digest microorganisms, and to return the breakdown products to the liver.

The kidneys are located high and deep under the diaphragm. These glandular, bean-shaped organs, measuring approximately $10 \times 5 \times 2.5$ cm, are considered posterior organs and approximate with the level of the T12 to L3 vertebrae. The tops of both kidneys are protected by the posterior rib cage. Kidney tenderness is best assessed at the costovertebral angle (Fig. 18-4). The right kidney is positioned slightly lower because of the position of the liver. Therefore, in some thin clients, the bottom portion of the right kidney may be palpated anteriorly. The primary function of the kidneys is filtration and elimination of metabolic waste products. However, the kidneys also play a role in blood pressure control and maintenance of water, salt, and electrolyte balance. In addition, they function as endocrine glands by secreting hormones.

The pregnant uterus may be palpated above the level of the symphysis pubis in the midline. The ovaries are located in the RLQ and LLQ and are normally palpated only during a bimanual examination of the internal genitalia (see Chapter 20).

HOLLOW VISCERA

The abdominal cavity begins with the stomach. It is a distensible, flasklike organ located in the LUQ, just below the diaphragm and in between the liver and spleen. The stomach is not usually palpable. The stomach's main function is to store, churn, and digest food.

The gallbladder, a muscular sac approximately 10 cm long, functions primarily to concentrate and store the bile needed to digest fat. It is located near the posterior surface of the liver lateral to the midclavicular line. It is not normally palpated because it is difficult to distinguish between the gallbladder and the liver.

The small intestine is actually the longest portion of the digestive tract (approximately 7.0 m long) but is named for its small diameter (approximately 2.5 cm). Two major functions of the small intestine are digestion and absorption of nutrients through millions of mucosal projections lining its walls. The small intestine, which lies coiled in all four quadrants of the abdomen, is not normally palpated.

The colon, or large intestine, has a wider diameter than the small intestine (approximately 6.0 cm) and is approximately 1.4 m long. It originates in the RLQ, where it attaches to the small intestine at the ileocecal valve. The colon is composed of three major sections: ascending, transverse, and descending. The ascending colon extends up along the right side of the abdomen. At the junction of the liver in the RUQ, it flexes at a right angle and becomes the transverse colon. The transverse colon runs across the upper abdomen. In the LUQ near the spleen, the colon forms another right angle and then extends downward along the left side of the abdomen as the descending colon. At this point, it curves in toward the midline to form the sigmoid colon in the LLQ. The sigmoid colon is often felt as a firm structure on palpation, whereas the cecum and ascending colon may feel softer. The transverse and descending colon may also be felt on palpation.

The colon functions primarily to secrete large amounts of alkaline mucus to lubricate the intestine and neutralize acids formed by the intestinal bacteria. Water is also absorbed through the large intestine, leaving waste products to be eliminated in stool.

The urinary bladder, a distensible muscular sac located behind the pubic bone in the midline of the abdomen, functions as a temporary receptacle for urine. A bladder filled with urine may be palpated in the abdomen above the symphysis pubis.

VASCULAR STRUCTURES

The abdominal organs are supplied with arterial blood by the abdominal aorta and its major branches. Pulsations of the aorta are frequently visible and palpable midline in the upper abdomen. The aorta branches into the right and left iliac arteries just below the umbilicus. Pulsations of the right and left iliac arteries may be felt in the RLQ and LLQ (Fig. 18-5).

DISPLAY 18-1. Locating Abdominal Structures by Quadrants

Abdominal assessment findings are commonly allocated to the quadrant in which they are discovered, or their location may be described according to the nine abdominal regions that some healthcare staff may still use as reference marks. Quadrants and contents are listed here with the illustrations of the quadrants and the nine abdominal regions.

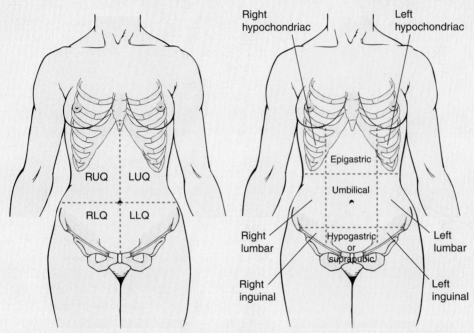

Abdominal quadrants (*left*) and abdominal regions (*right*).

RIGHT UPPER QUADRANT (RUQ)

Ascending and transverse colon
Duodenum
Gallbladder
Hepatic flexure of colon
Liver
Pancreas (head)
Pylorus (the small bowel—or ileum—traverses all quadrants)
Right adrenal gland
Right kidney (upper pole)
Right ureter

RIGHT LOWER QUADRANT (RLQ)

Appendix
Ascending colon
Cecum
Right kidney (lower pole)
Right ovary and tube
Right ureter
Right spermatic cord

LEFT UPPER QUADRANT (LUQ)

Left adrenal gland
Left kidney (upper pole)
Left ureter
Pancreas (body and tail)
Spleen
Splenic flexure of colon
Stomach
Transverse ascending colon

LEFT LOWER QUADRANT (LLQ)

Left kidney (lower pole)
Left ovary and tube
Left ureter
Left spermatic cord
Sigmoid colon

MIDLINE

Bladder
Uterus
Prostate gland

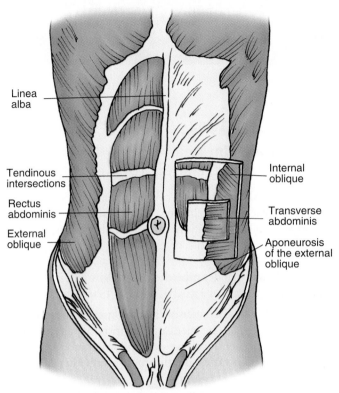

FIGURE 18-2. Abdominal wall muscles.

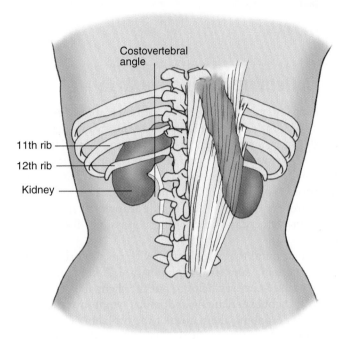

FIGURE 18-4. Position of the kidneys.

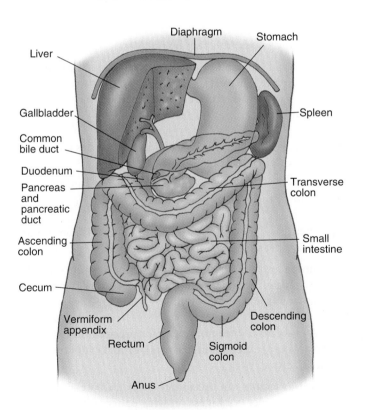

FIGURE 18-3. Abdominal viscera.

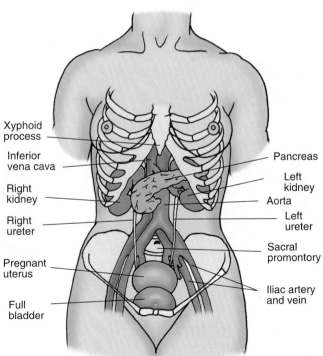

FIGURE 18-5. Abdominal and vascular structures (aorta and iliac artery and vein).

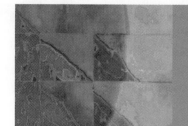

Nursing Assessment

PART TWO

Collecting Subjective Data

Subjective data concerning the abdomen are collected as part of a client's overall health history interview or as a focused history for a current abdominal complaint. The data focus on symptoms of particular abdominal organs and the function of the digestive system, along with aspects of nutrition, usual bowel habits, and lifestyle. The nurse aims to assure the client that all the questions are important tools for detecting and treating a possible disorder or disease.

Keep in mind that the client may be uncomfortable discussing certain issues such as elimination. Asking questions in a matter-of-fact way helps to put the client at ease. In addition, a client experiencing abdominal symptoms may have difficulty describing the nature of the problem. Therefore, the nurse may need to facilitate client responses and quantitative answers by encouraging descriptive terms and examples (ie, pain as sharp or knifelike, headache as throbbing, or back pain as searing), rating scales, and accounts of effects on activities of daily living.

COLDSPA

CHARACTER: Describe the sign or symptom. How does it feel, look, sound, smell, and so forth?

ONSET: When did it begin?

LOCATION: Where is it? Does it radiate?

DURATION: How long does it last? Does it recur?

SEVERITY: How bad is it?

PATTERN: What makes it better: What makes it worse?

ASSOCIATED FACTORS: What other symptoms occur with it?

Nursing History

During the interview, you will ask the client many questions (Q), examples of which appear below along with the reason (R for rationale) for the question.

CURRENT SYMPTOMS

Abdominal Pain

Question Are you experiencing abdominal pain?

Rationale Abdominal pain occurs when specific digestive organs or structures are affected by chemical or mechanical factors such as inflammation, infection, distention, stretching, pressure, obstruction, or trauma.

Q How would you describe the pain? How bad is the pain (severity) on a scale of 1 to 10, with 10 being the worst?

R The quality or character of the pain may suggest its origin (Display 18-2). The client's perception of pain provides data on his or her response to, and tolerance of, pain. Sensitivity to pain varies greatly among individuals.

> Sensitivity to pain may diminish with aging. Therefore, elderly patients must be carefully assessed for acute abdominal conditions.

Q How did (does) the pain begin?

R The onset of pain is a diagnostic clue to its origin. For example, acute pancreatitis produces sudden onset of pain, whereas the pain of pancreatic cancer may be gradual or recurrent.

Q Where is the pain located? Does it move or has it changed from the original location?

R Location helps determine the pain source and whether it is primary or referred (see Display 18-2).

Q When does the pain occur (timing and relation to particular events, such as eating, exercise, bedtime)?

R Timing and the relationship of particular events may be a clue to origin of pain (eg, the pain of a duodenal ulcer may awaken the client at night).

Q What seems to bring on the pain (precipitating factors), make it worse (exacerbating factors), or make it better (alleviating factors)?

R Various factors can precipitate or exacerbate abdominal pain, such as alcohol ingestion with pancreatitis or supine position with gastroesophageal reflux disease. Lifestyle and stress factors may be implicated in certain digestive disorders

DISPLAY 18-2. Mechanisms and Sources of Abdominal Pain

Abdominal pain may be formally described as visceral, parietal, or referred.

KINDS OF PAIN

- *Visceral pain* occurs when hollow abdominal organs, such as the intestines, become distended or contract forcefully or when the capsules of solid organs such as the liver and spleen are stretched. Poorly defined or localized and intermittently timed, this type of pain is often characterized as dull, aching, burning, cramping, or colicky.
- *Parietal pain* occurs when the parietal peritoneum becomes inflamed, as in appendicitis or peritonitis. This type of pain tends to localize more to the source and is characterized as a more severe and steady pain.
- *Referred pain* occurs at distant sites that are innervated at approximately the same levels as the disrupted abdominal organ. This type of pain travels, or refers, from the primary site and becomes highly localized at the distant site. The accompanying illustrations show common clinical patterns and referents of pain.

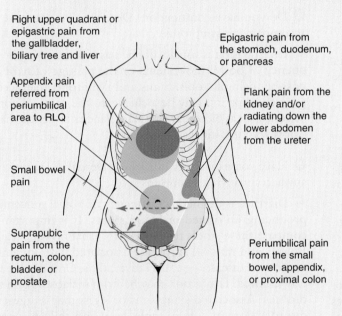

Right upper quadrant or epigastric pain from the gallbladder, biliary tree and liver

Appendix pain referred from periumbilical area to RLQ

Small bowel pain

Suprapubic pain from the rectum, colon, bladder or prostate

Epigastric pain from the stomach, duodenum, or pancreas

Flank pain from the kidney and/or radiating down the lower abdomen from the ureter

Periumbilical pain from the small bowel, appendix, or proximal colon

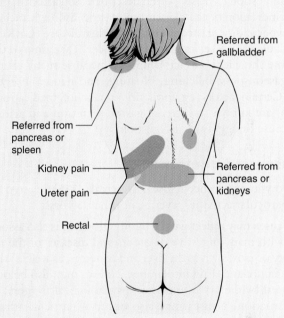

Referred from gallbladder

Referred from pancreas or spleen

Kidney pain

Ureter pain

Referred from pancreas or kidneys

Rectal

Patterns and referents of abdominal pain.

CHARACTER OF ABDOMINAL PAIN AND IMPLICATIONS

Dull, Aching
Appendicitis
Acute hepatitis
Biliary colic
Cholecystitis
Cystitis
Dyspepsia
Glomerulonephritis
Incarcerated or strangulated hernia
Irritable bowel syndrome
Hepatocellular cancer
Pancreatitis
Pancreatic cancer
Perforated gastric or duodenal ulcer
Peritonitis

Peptic ulcer disease
Prostatitis

Burning, Gnawing
Dyspepsia
Peptic ulcer disease
Cramping ("crampy")
Acute gastritis
Acute mechanical obstruction
Appendicitis
Colitis
Diverticulitis
Gastroesophageal reflux disease (GERD)

Pressure
Benign prostatic hypertrophy
Prostate cancer

Prostatitis
Urinary retention

Colicky
Colon cancer

Sharp, Knifelike
Splenic abscess
Splenic rupture
Renal colic
Renal tumor
Ureteral colic
Vascular liver tumor

Variable
Stomach cancer

such as peptic ulcer disease. Alleviating factors, such as using antacids or histamine blockers, may be a clue to origin.

Q Is the pain associated with any of the following symptoms: nausea, vomiting, diarrhea, constipation, gas, fever, weight loss, fatigue, or yellowing of the eyes or skin?

R Associated signs and symptoms may provide diagnostic evidence to support or rule out a particular origin of pain. For example, epigastric pain accompanied by tarry stools suggests a gastric or duodenal ulcer.

Indigestion

Q Do you experience indigestion? Describe. Does anything in particular seem to cause or aggravate this condition?

R Indigestion (pyrosis), often described as heartburn, may be an indication of acute or chronic gastric disorders, including hyperacidity, gastroesophageal reflux disease (GERD), peptic ulcer disease, and stomach cancer. Take time to determine the client's exact symptoms because many clients call gaseousness, belching, bloating, and nausea indigestion. Certain factors (eg, food, drinks, alcohol, medications, stress) are known to increase gastric secretion and acidity and cause or aggravate indigestion.

Nausea and Vomiting

Q Do you experience nausea? Describe. Is it triggered by any particular activities, events, or other factors?

R Nausea may reflect gastric dysfunction and is also associated with many digestive disorders and diseases of the accessory organs, such as the liver and pancreas, as well as with renal failure and drug intolerance. Nausea may also be precipitated by dietary intolerance, psychological triggers, or menstruation. Nausea may also occur at particular times such as early in the day with some pregnant clients ("morning sickness"), after meals with gastric disorders, or between meals with changes in blood glucose levels.

Q Have you been vomiting? Describe the vomitus. Is it associated with any particular trigger factors?

R Vomiting is associated with impaired gastric motility or reflex mechanisms. Description of vomitus (emesis) is a clue to the source. For example, bright hematemesis is seen with bleeding esophageal varices and ulcers of the stomach or duodenum. Elderly or neuromuscular- or consciousness-impaired clients are at risk for lung aspiration with vomiting.

Q Have you noticed a change in your appetite? Has this change affected how much you eat or your normal weight?

R Loss of appetite (anorexia) is a general complaint often associated with digestive disorders, chronic syndromes, cancers, and psychological disorders. Appetite changes should be carefully correlated with dietary history and weight monitoring.

Significant appetite changes and food intake may adversely affect the client's weight and put the client at additional risk.

Older clients may experience a decline in appetite from various factors, such as altered metabolism, decreased taste sensation, decreased mobility, and possibly depression. If appetite declines, the client's risk for nutritional imbalance increases.

Bowel Elimination

Q Have you experienced a change in bowel elimination patterns? Describe.

R Changes in bowel patterns must be compared to usual patterns for the client. Normal frequency varies from two to three times per day to three times per week.

Q Do you have constipation? Describe. Do you have any accompanying symptoms?

R Constipation is usually defined as a decrease in the frequency of bowel movements or the passage of hard and possibly painful stools. Signs and symptoms that accompany constipation may be a clue as to the cause of constipation, such as bleeding with malignancies or pencil-shaped stools with intestinal obstruction.

Q Have you experienced diarrhea? Describe. Do you have any accompanying symptoms?

R Diarrhea is defined as frequency of bowel movements producing unformed or liquid stools. It is important to compare these stools to the client's usual bowel patterns. Bloody and mucoid stools are associated with inflammatory bowel diseases (eg, ulcerative colitis, Crohn's disease); clay-colored, fatty stools may be from malabsorption syndromes. Associated symptoms or signs may suggest the disorder's origin. For example, fever and chills may result from an infection, or weight loss and fatigue may result from a chronic intestinal disorder or a cancer.

Older clients are especially at risk for potential complications with diarrhea, such as fluid volume deficit, dehydration, electrolyte, and acid–base imbalances, because they have a higher fat-to-lean muscle ratio.

Q Have you experienced any yellowing of your skin or whites of your eyes, itchy skin, dark urine (yellow-brown or tea colored), or clay-colored stools?

R These symptoms should be evaluated to rule out possible liver disease.

PAST HISTORY

Q Have you ever had any of the following gastrointestinal disorders: Ulcers, gastroesophageal reflux, inflammatory or obstructive bowel disease, pancreatitis, gallbladder or liver disease, diverticulosis, or appendicitis?

R Presenting the client with a list of the more common disorders may help the client identify any that he or she has or has had.

Q Have you had any urinary tract disease such as infections, kidney disease or nephritis, or kidney stones?

R Urinary tract infections may become recurrent and chronic. Moreover, resistance to drugs used to treat infection must be evaluated. Chronic kidney infection may lead to permanent kidney damage.

Older clients are prone to urinary tract infections because the activity of protective bacteria in the urinary tract declines with age.

Q Have you ever had viral hepatitis (type A, B, or C)? Have you ever been exposed to viral hepatitis?

R Various populations (eg, school and health care personnel) are at increased risk for exposure to hepatitis viruses. Any type of viral hepatitis may cause liver damage.

Q Have you ever had abdominal surgery or other trauma to the abdomen?

R Prior abdominal surgery or trauma may cause abdominal adhesions, thereby predisposing the client to future complications or disorders.

Q What prescription or over-the-counter medications do you take?

R Medications may produce side effects that adversely affect the gastrointestinal tract. For example, aspirin, ibuprofen, and steroids may cause gastric bleeding. Chronic use of antacids or histamine-2 blockers may mask the symptoms of more serious stomach disorders. Overuse of laxatives may decrease intestinal tone and promote dependency. High iron intake may lead to chronic constipation.

FAMILY HISTORY

Q Is there a history of any of the following diseases or disorders in your family: colon, stomach, pancreatic, liver, kidney, or bladder cancer; liver disease; gallbladder disease; kidney disease?

R Family history of certain disorders increases the client's risk for those disorders. Genetic testing can now identify the risk for certain cancers (colon, pancreatic, and prostate) and other diseases. Client awareness of family history can serve as a motivation for health screening and positive health promotion behaviors.

LIFESTYLE AND HEALTH PRACTICES

Q Do you drink alcohol? How much? How often?

R Alcohol ingestion can affect the gastrointestinal tract through immediate and long-term effects on such organs as the stomach, pancreas, and liver. Alcohol-related disorders include gastritis, esophageal varices, pancreatitis, and liver cirrhosis.

Q What types of foods and how much food do you typically consume each day? How much noncaffeinated fluid do you consume each day? How much caffeine do you think you consume each day (eg, in tea, coffee, chocolate, and soft drinks)?

R A baseline dietary and fluid survey helps determine nutritional and fluid adequacy and risk factors for altered nutrition, constipation, diarrhea, and diseases such as cancer.

Q How much and how often do you exercise? Describe your activities during the day.

R Regular exercise promotes peristalsis and thus regular bowel movements. In addition, exercise may help reduce risk factors for various diseases, such as cancer and hypertension (see Risk Factors—Gallbladder Cancer).

Q What kind of stress do you have in your life? How does it affect your eating or elimination habits?

R Lifestyle and associated stress and psychological factors can affect gastrointestinal function through effects on secretion, tone, and motility.

Q If you have a gastrointestinal disorder, how does it affect your lifestyle and how you feel about yourself?

R Certain gastrointestinal disorders and their effects (eg, weight loss) or treatment (eg, drugs, surgery) may produce physiologic or anatomic effects that affect the client's perception of self, body image, social interaction and intimacy, and life goals and expectations.

Collecting Objective Data

The abdominal examination is performed for a variety of different reasons: as part of a comprehensive health examination; to explore gastrointestinal complaints; to assess abdominal pain, tenderness, or masses; or to monitor the client postoperatively. Assessing the abdomen can be challenging, considering the number of organs of the digestive system and the need to distinguish the source of clinical signs and symptoms.

The sequence for assessment of the abdomen differs from the typical order of assessment. Auscultate after you inspect so as not to alter the client's pattern of bowel sounds. Percussion and then palpation follow auscultation. Adjust the bed level as necessary throughout the examination, and approach the client from the right side. Use tangential lighting, if available, for optimal visualization of the abdomen.

The nurse needs to understand and anticipate various concerns of the client by listening and observing closely for

RISK FACTORS
Gallbladder Cancer

OVERVIEW

Of the several types of tumors that affect the gallbladder, about 80% are adenocarcinomas (ACS, 2000). The American Cancer Society reports that gallbladder cancer is the fifth most common gastrointestinal cancer and that between 5000 and 7000 new cases are diagnosed each year in the United States. Only 10% of patients survive 5 years due to late discovery after the cancer has advanced. Gallbladder cancer is described as "an age-dependent malignancy that is present mostly in women and that may be intimately associated with long-standing benign gall stone disease of the gall bladder" (Vitetta, Sali, Little & Mrazeh, 2000).

Women are affected two and one half times as often as men. Gallstones are the most common risk factor, especially when onset is at or before middle age or when there is one large stone. Many risk factors for gallbladder cancer are associated with gallstones, including high parity, obesity, and abnormalities of the biliary system promoting chronic inflammation.

RISK FACTORS

Age (over 70 years)
Female Sex
  After menopause (Khan et al., 1999),
  Increased parity (Lowenfels et al., 1999)
Ethnicity
  Native American (United States; North, Central,
    and South America)
  New Zealand Maori (Lowenfels et al., 1999)
Health and Habit History
  Gallstones, especially early onset or large gallstone
  Chronic inflammation of gallbladder
  Porcelain gallbladder (calcium deposits)
  Gallbladder polyps
  Common bile duct abnormalities
  Typhoid carrier
  Obesity
  Diet high in carbohydrates and fats and low in fiber
  Cigarette smoking
  Environmental exposure to industrial chemicals
    used in rubber and metal manufacturing

RISK REDUCTION TEACHING TIPS

- Stop smoking.
- Avoid obesity. Follow ACS diet and exercise suggestions. Diet consists of five servings of fruits and vegetables; six servings of bread, grains, and legumes; and fewer fatty foods. Exercise consists of 30 minutes most days.
- Avoid industrial chemical exposure.
- Schedule periodic medical examinations to assess gallbladder and general status, especially if a history of risk factors is identified.

 ## CULTURAL CONSIDERATIONS

Gallbladder disease and cancer rates differ among ethnic groups. Native American populations have much higher rates than most world populations. Reports form the mid 1980s note that the risk for gallbladder cancer in African American women was 3 per 100,000; for white women, 11.5; and for Native American women 46.4 (Overfield, 1995, p. 110). The pattern for gallbladder disease has been noted to be similar, with 36% of Pima Indians being admitted to the hospital with gallbladder disease as compared to 6% of whites in Massachusetts (Comess, Bennet, & Burch, 1967; quoted in Overfield, 1995, p. 112). In addition to Native Americans in North Central and South America, the New Zealand Maori have a high rate as well (Lowenfels et al., 1999).

verbal and nonverbal cues. Commonly, clients feel anxious and modest during the examination, possibly from anticipated discomfort or fear that the examiner will find something seriously wrong. As a result, the client may tense the abdominal muscles, voluntarily guarding the area. (Tips for minimizing voluntary guarding appear in Display 18-3.) Explaining each aspect of the examination, answering the client's questions, and draping the client's genital area and breasts (in women) when these are not being examined all help to ease anxiety.

Another potential factor to deal with is ticklishness. A ticklish client has trouble lying still and relaxing during the hands-on parts of the examination. Try to combat this using a controlled hands-on technique and by placing the client's hand under your own for a few moments at the beginning of palpation. Finally, warm hands are essential for the abdominal examination. Cold hands cause the client to tense the abdominal muscles. Rubbing them together or holding them under warm water just before the hands-on examination may be helpful.

CLIENT PREPARATION

Ask the client to empty the bladder before beginning the examination to eliminate bladder distention and interference with an accurate examination. Instruct the client to remove clothes and to put on a gown if desired. Help the client to lie supine with the arms folded across the chest or resting by the sides (Fig. 18-6).

Raising arms above the head or folding them behind the head will tense the abdominal muscles. A flat pillow may be placed under the client's head for comfort. Slightly flex the client's legs by placing a pillow or rolled blanket under the client's knees to help relax the abdominal muscles. Drape the client with sheets so the abdomen is visible from the lower rib cage to the pubic area.

Instruct the client to breathe through the mouth and to take slow, deep breaths; this promotes relaxation. Before touching the abdomen, ask the client about painful or tender areas. These areas should always be assessed at the end of the examination. Reassure the client that you will forewarn him or her when you will examine these areas. Approach the client with slow, gentle, and fluid movements.

EQUIPMENT AND SUPPLIES

- Small pillow or rolled blanket
- Centimeter ruler
- Stethoscope (with a warm diaphragm and bell)
- Marking pen

KEY ASSESSMENT POINTS

- Observe and inspect abdominal skin and overall contour and symmetry.
- Auscultate after inspection and before percussion, and, finally, palpate.
- Assessment examination evaluates the following abdominal structures in the abdominal quadrants: skin, stomach, bowel, spleen, liver, kidneys, aorta, and bladder.
- Common abnormal findings include abdominal edema, or swelling, signifying ascites; abdominal masses signifying abnormal growths or constipation; unusual pulsations, such as those seen with an aneurysm of the abdominal aorta; and pain associated with appendicitis.

(*text continues on page 396*)

DISPLAY 18-3. **Palpating the Abdomen**

GUIDELINES

1. Avoid touching tender or painful areas until last, and reassure the client of your intentions.
2. Perform light palpation before deep palpation to detect tenderness and superficial masses.
3. Keep in mind that the normal abdomen may be tender, especially in the areas over the xiphoid process, liver, aorta, lower pole of the kidney, gas-filled cecum, sigmoid colon, and ovaries.
4. Overcome ticklishness and minimize voluntary guarding by asking the client to perform self-palpation. Place your hands over the client's. After a while, let your fingers glide slowly onto the abdomen while still resting mostly on the client's fingers. The same can be done by using a warm stethoscope as a palpating instrument, again letting your fingers drift over the edge of the diaphragm and palpate without promoting a ticklish response.
5. Work with the client to promote relaxation and minimize voluntary guarding. Use the following techniques:
   - Place a pillow under the client's knees.
   - Ask the client to take slow, deep breaths through the mouth.
   - Apply light pressure over the client's sternum with your left hand while palpating with the right. This encourages the client to relax the abdominal muscles during breathing against sternal resistance.

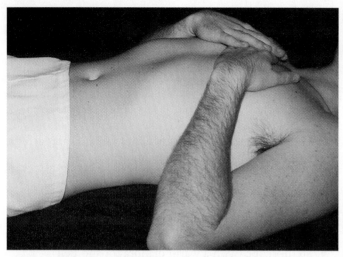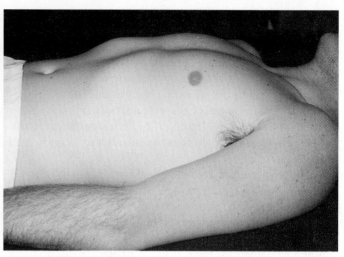

FIGURE 18-6. Two positions are appropriate for the abdominal assessment. The client may lie supine with hands resting on the center of the chest (*left*) or with arms resting comfortably at the sides (*right*). These positions best promote relaxation of the abdominal muscles. (Photos courtesy of M. B. Cunningham.)

PHYSICAL ASSESSMENT

ASSESSMENT PROCEDURE	NORMAL FINDINGS	ABNORMAL FINDINGS

ABDOMEN

Inspect the Skin

Observe the coloration of the skin.	Abdominal skin may be paler than the general skin tone because this skin is so seldom exposed to the natural elements.	Purple discoloration at the flanks (Grey Turner sign) indicates bleeding within the abdominal wall, possibly from trauma to the kidneys, pancreas, or duodenum or from pancreatitis. The yellow hue of jaundice may be more apparent on the abdomen. Pale, taut skin may be seen with ascites (significant abdominal swelling indicating fluid accumulation in the abdominal cavity). Redness may indicate inflammation. Bruises or areas of local discoloration are also abnormal.
Note the vascularity of the abdominal skin.	Scattered fine veins may be visible. Blood in the veins located above the umbilicus flows toward the head; blood in the veins located below the umbilicus flows toward the lower body. Dilated superficial capillaries without a pattern may be seen in older clients. They are more visible in sunlight.	Dilated veins may be seen with cirrhosis of the liver, obstruction of the inferior vena cava, portal hypertension, or ascites. Dilated surface arterioles and capillaries with a central star (spider angioma) may be seen with liver disease or portal hypertension.

(continued)

ASSESSMENT PROCEDURE	NORMAL FINDINGS	ABNORMAL FINDINGS
Note any striae.	Old, silvery, white striae or stretch marks from past pregnancies or weight gain are normal.	Dark bluish-pink striae are associated with Cushing's syndrome. Striae may also be caused by ascites, which stretches the skin. Ascites usually results from liver failure or liver disease.
Inspect for scars. Ask about the source of a scar, and use a centimeter ruler to measure the scar's length. Document the location by quadrant and reference lines, shape, length, and any specific characteristics (eg, 3-cm vertical scar in RLQ 4 cm below the umbilicus and 5 cm left of the midline). With experience, many examiners can estimate the length of a scar visually without a ruler.	Pale, smooth, minimally raised old scars may be seen.	Nonhealing scars, redness, inflammation. Deep, irregular scars may result from burns. Keloids (excess scar tissue) result from trauma or surgery and are more common in blacks and Asians.

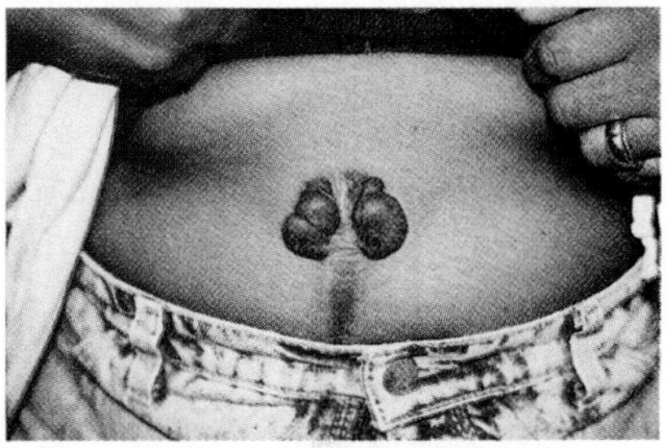

Tip From the Experts
Scarring should be an alert for possible internal adhesions.

Keloid beyond border of surgical scar.

ASSESSMENT PROCEDURE	NORMAL FINDINGS	ABNORMAL FINDINGS
Look for lesions and rashes.	Abdomen is free of lesions or rashes. Flat or raised brown moles, however, are normal and may be apparent.	Changes in moles including size, color, and border symmetry. Any bleeding moles or petechiae (reddish or purple lesions) may also be abnormal (see Chapter 9).

Inspect the Umbilicus

Note the color of the umbilical area.	Umbilical skin tones are similar to surrounding abdominal skin tones or even pinkish.	Bluish or purple discoloration around the umbilicus (Cullen's sign) indicates intra-abdominal bleeding.
Observe umbilical location.	Midline at lateral line	A deviated umbilicus may be caused by pressure from a mass, enlarged organs, hernia, fluid, or scar tissue.

(continued)

ASSESSMENT PROCEDURE	NORMAL FINDINGS	ABNORMAL FINDINGS
Assess contour of umbilicus.	Recessed (inverted) or protruding no more than 0.5 cm; round or conical	An everted umbilicus is seen with abdominal distention (see Display 18-5). An enlarged, everted umbilicus suggests umbilical hernia (see Display 18-6).

Inspect Contour, Symmetry, Movement

To inspect abdominal contour, look across the abdomen at eye level from the client's right side, from behind the client's head, and from the foot of the bed.

Abdomen is flat, rounded, or scaphoid (usually seen in thin adults). Abdomen should be evenly rounded.

A generalized protuberant or distended abdomen may be due to air (gas) or fluid accumulation (see Display 18-5).

Distention below the umbilicus may be due to a full bladder, uterine enlargement, or an ovarian tumor or cyst.

Distention of the upper abdomen may be seen with masses of the pancreas or gastric dilation.

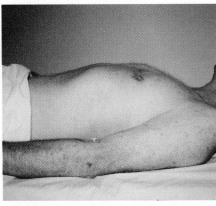

View abdominal contour from the client's side. Many abdomens are more or less flat; and many are round, scaphoid, or distended. (© B. Proud.)

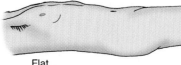

Flat

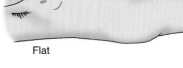

Rounded

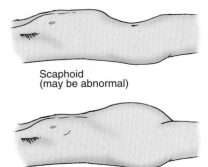

Scaphoid (may be abnormal)

Distended/protuberant (usually abnormal)

To assess abdominal symmetry, look at the client's abdomen as he or she lies in a relaxed supine position.

Abdomen is symmetric.

🏵 **Tip From the Experts** The major causes of abdominal distention are sometimes referred to as the "6 Fs": Fat, feces, fetus, fibroids, flatulence, and fluid (Display 18-5).

To further assess the abdomen for herniation or diastasis recti, or to differentiate a mass within the abdominal wall from one below it, ask the client to raise the head.

Abdomen does not bulge when client raises head.

A scaphoid (sunken) abdomen may be seen with severe weight loss or cachexia related to starvation or terminal illness.

Asymmetry may be seen with organ enlargement, large masses, hernia, diastasis recti, or bowel obstruction.

A hernia (protrusion of the bowel through the abdominal wall) is seen as a bulging in the abdominal wall.

Diastasis recti appears as a bulging between a vertical midline separation of the abdominis rectus muscles. This condition is of little significance. An incisional hernia may occur when a defect develops in the abdominal muscles because of a surgical incision. A mass within the abdominal wall is more prominent when the head is raised, whereas a mass below the abdominal wall is obscured (Display 18-6).

(continued)

ASSESSMENT PROCEDURE	NORMAL FINDINGS	ABNORMAL FINDINGS
Inspect abdominal movement when the client breathes (respiratory movements).	Abdominal respiratory movement may be seen, especially in male clients.	Diminished abdominal respiration or change to thoracic breathing in male clients may reflect peritoneal irritation.
Observe aortic pulsations.	A slight pulsation of the abdominal aorta, which is visible in the epigastrium, extends full length in thin people.	Vigorous, wide, exaggerated pulsations may be seen with abdominal aortic aneurysm.
Watch for peristaltic waves.	Normally, peristaltic waves are not seen, although they may be visible in very thin people as slight ripples on the abdominal wall.	Peristaltic waves are increased and progress in a ripple-like fashion from the LUQ to the RLQ with intestinal obstruction (especially small intestine). In addition, abdominal distention typically is present with intestinal wall obstruction.

Auscultate for Bowel Sounds

Follow the guidelines for auscultating bowel sounds in Display 18-7. Note the intensity, pitch, and frequency of the sounds.	A series of intermittent, soft clicks and gurgles are heard at a rate of 5 to 30 per minute. Hyperactive bowel sounds that may be heard normally are the loud, prolonged gurgles characteristic of stomach growling. These hyperactive bowel sounds are called "borborygmi."	Hypoactive bowel sounds indicate diminished bowel motility. Common causes include abdominal surgery or late bowel obstruction.

Tip From the Experts Postoperatively, bowel sounds resume gradually depending on the type of surgery. The small intestine functions normally in the first few hours postoperatively; stomach emptying takes 24 to 48 hours to recover; and the colon requires 3 to 5 days to recover propulsive activity.

Hyperactive bowel sounds indicate increased bowel motility. Common causes include diarrhea, gastroenteritis, or early bowel obstruction.

Decreased or absent bowel sounds signify the absence of bowel motility, which constitutes an emergency requiring immediate referral.

Absent bowel sounds may be associated with peritonitis or paralytic ileus. High-pitched tinkling and rushes of high-pitched sounds with abdominal cramping usually indicate obstruction.

Tip From the Experts The increasing pitch of bowel sounds is most diagnostic of obstruction because it signifies intestinal distention.

(continued)

ASSESSMENT PROCEDURE	NORMAL FINDINGS	ABNORMAL FINDINGS

Auscultate for Vascular Sounds and Friction Rubs

Use the bell of the stethoscope to listen for bruits (low-pitched, murmurlike sound) over the abdominal aorta and renal, iliac, and femoral arteries.

🎗 **Tip From the Experts** Auscultating for vascular sounds is especially important if the client has hypertension or if you suspect arterial insufficiency to the legs.

Bruits are not normally heard over abdominal aorta or renal, iliac, or femoral arteries. However, bruits confined to systole may be normal in some clients depending on other differentiating factors.

A bruit with both systolic and diastolic components occurs when blood flow in an artery is turbulent or obstructed. This usually indicates aneurysm or arterial stenosis. If the client has hypertension and you auscultate a renal artery bruit with both systolic and diastolic components, suspect renal artery stenosis as the cause.

Using the bell of the stethoscope, listen for a venous hum in the epigastric and umbilical areas.

Venous hum is not normally heard over the epigastric and umbilical areas.

Venous hums are rare. However, an accentuated venous hum heard in the epigastric or umbilical areas suggests increased collateral circulation between the portal and systemic venous systems, as in cirrhosis of the liver.

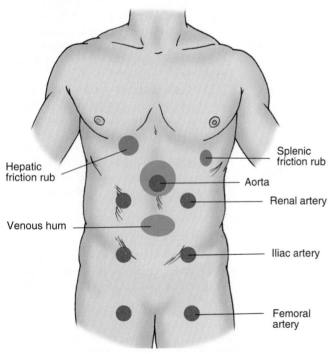

Hepatic friction rub

Venous hum

Splenic friction rub

Aorta

Renal artery

Iliac artery

Femoral artery

Vascular sounds and friction rubs can best be heard over these areas.

Auscultate for a friction rub over the liver and spleen by listening over the right and left lower rib cage with the diaphragm of the stethoscope.

No friction rub over liver or spleen.

Friction rubs are rare. If heard, they have a high-pitched, rough, grating sound produced when the large surface area of the liver or spleen rubs the peritoneum. They are heard in association with respiration.

A friction rub heard over the lower right costal area is associated with hepatic abscess or metastases.

A rub heard at the anterior axillary line in the lower left costal area is associated with splenic infarction, abscess, infection, or tumor.

(continued)

ASSESSMENT PROCEDURE	NORMAL FINDINGS	ABNORMAL FINDINGS

Percuss for Tone

Lightly and systematically percuss all quadrants. Two sequences are illustrated below.

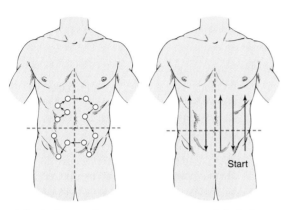

Abdominal percussion sequences may proceed clockwise or up and down over the abdomen.

Generalized tympany predominates over the abdomen because of air in the stomach and intestines. Normal dullness is heard over the liver and spleen.

Dullness may also be elicited over a nonevacuated descending colon.

Accentuated tympany or hyperresonance is heard over a gaseous distended abdomen.

An enlarged area of dullness is heard over an enlarged liver or spleen.

Abnormal dullness is heard over a distended bladder, large masses, or ascites.

If you suspect ascites, perform the shifting dullness and fluid wave tests. These special techniques are described later.

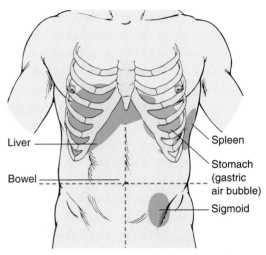

Document normal findings after percussing the liver, bowel, sigmoid colon, stomach, and spleen.

Percuss the Liver

Percuss the span or height of the liver by determining its lower and upper borders.

To assess the lower border, begin in the RLQ at the mid-clavicular line (MCL) and percuss upward. Note the change from tympany to dullness. Mark this point—it is the lower border of liver dullness.

The lower border of liver dullness is located at the costal margin to 1 to 2 cm below.

Tip From the Experts If you cannot find the lower border of the liver, keep in mind that the lower border of liver dullness may be difficult to estimate when obscured by intestinal gas.

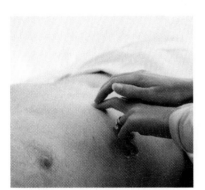

Begin liver percussion in the RLQ and percuss upward toward the chest. (© B. Proud.)

(continued)

ASSESSMENT PROCEDURE	NORMAL FINDINGS	ABNORMAL FINDINGS

To assess the descent of the liver, ask the client to take a deep breath, then repeat the procedure. To assess the upper border, percuss over the upper right chest at the MCL and percuss downward, noting the change from lung resonance to liver dullness. Mark this point—it is the upper border of liver dullness.

On deep inspiration, the lower border of liver dullness may descend from 1 to 4 cm below the costal margin. The upper border of liver dullness is located between the left fifth and seventh intercostal spaces.

Tip From the Experts The upper border of liver dullness may be difficult to estimate if obscured by pleural fluid or lung consolidation.

Measure the distance between the two marks—this is the span of the liver.

The normal liver span at the MCL is 6 to 12 cm (greater in men and taller clients, less in shorter clients).

Normally, liver size decreases after age 50.

Hepatomegaly, a liver span that exceeds normal limits (enlarged), is characteristic of liver tumors, cirrhosis, abscess, and vascular engorgement.

Atrophy of the liver is indicated by a decreased span.

A liver in a lower position than normal may be caused by emphysema, whereas a liver in a higher position than normal may be caused by an abdominal mass, ascites, or a paralyzed diaphragm. A liver in a lower or higher position should have a normal span (Display 18-8).

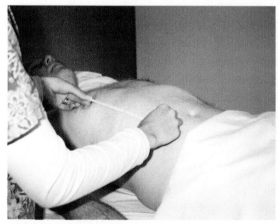

The distance between the liver's lower and upper border is denoted by a span of percussed dullness. (*Left*) Determine this by marking the distance from beginning to end of percussion and measuring with a ruler. (*Right*) Normal liver span.

Repeat percussion of the liver at the midsternal line (MSL).

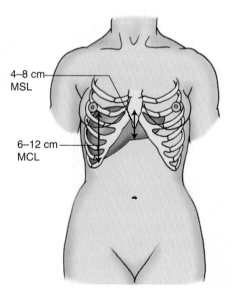

4–8 cm
MSL

6–12 cm
MCL

The normal liver span at the MSL is 4 to 8 cm.

(continued)

ASSESSMENT PROCEDURE	NORMAL FINDINGS	ABNORMAL FINDINGS

Perform the Scratch Test

If you cannot accurately percuss the liver borders, perform the scratch test. Auscultate over the liver and, starting in the RLQ, scratch lightly over the abdomen, progressing upward toward the liver.

The sound produced by scratching becomes more intense over the liver.

An enlarged liver may be roughly estimated (not accurately) when more intense sounds outline a liver span or borders outside the normal range.

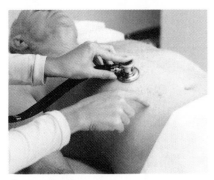

The scratch test.

Percuss the Spleen

Begin posterior to the left mid-axillary line (MAL), and percuss downward, noting the change from lung resonance to splenic dullness.

The spleen is an oval area of dullness approximately 7 cm wide near the left tenth rib, and slightly posterior to the MAL.

Splenomegaly is characterized by an area of dullness greater than 7 cm wide. The enlargement may result from traumatic injury, portal hypertension, and mononucleosis.

 Tip From the Experts Results of splenic percussion may be obscured by air in the stomach or bowel.

A second method for detecting splenic enlargement is to percuss the last left interspace at the anterior axillary line (AAL) while the client takes a deep breath.

Normally, tympany (or resonance) is heard at the last left interspace.

On inspiration, dullness at the last left interspace at the AAL suggests an enlarged spleen (see Display 18-8).

 Tip From the Experts Other sources of dullness (eg, full stomach or feces in the colon) must be ruled out before confirming splenomegaly.

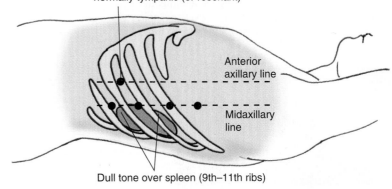

Percuss last interspace:
normally tympanic (or resonant)

Anterior axillary line

Midaxillary line

Dull tone over spleen (9th–11th ribs)

Last left interspace at the anterior axillary line.

(continued)

ASSESSMENT PROCEDURE	NORMAL FINDINGS	ABNORMAL FINDINGS

Perform Blunt Percussion on the Liver and Kidneys

To assess for tenderness in difficult-to-palpate structures, perform blunt (indirect fist) percussion. Percuss the liver by placing your left hand flat against the lower right rib cage. Use the ulnar side of your right fist to strike your left hand.	Normally, no tenderness is elicited.	Tenderness elicited over the liver may be associated with inflammation or infection (eg, hepatitis or cholecystitis).
Perform blunt percussion on the kidneys at the costovertebral angles (CVA) over the twelfth rib.	Normally, no tenderness or pain is elicited or reported by the client. The examiner senses only a dull thud.	Tenderness or sharp pain elicited over the CVA suggests kidney infection (pyelonephritis), renal calculi, or hydronephrosis.

🎗 **Tip From the Experts** This technique requires that the client is sitting with his or her back to you. Therefore, it may be best to incorporate blunt percussion of the kidneys with your thoracic assessment because the client will already be in this position.

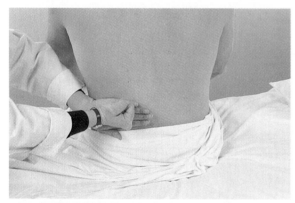

Performing blunt percussion over the kidney. (© B. Proud.)

Perform Light Palpation

Follow the guidelines for palpating the abdomen (see Display 18-3), and palpate lightly in all quadrants. Light palpation is used to identify areas of tenderness and muscular resistance. Using the fingertips, begin palpation in a nontender quadrant, and compress to a depth of 1 cm in a dipping motion. Then, gently lift the fingers and move to the next area.	Nontender	

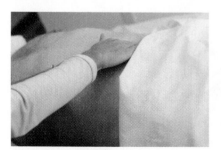

Performing light palpation. (© B. Proud.)

(continued)

ASSESSMENT PROCEDURE	NORMAL FINDINGS	ABNORMAL FINDINGS
To minimize the client's voluntary guarding (a tensing or rigidity of the abdominal muscles, usually involving the entire abdomen), see Display 18-3. Keep in mind that the rectus abdominis muscle relaxes on expiration.	No guarding; abdomen is soft.	Involuntary reflex guarding is serious and reflects peritoneal irritation. The abdomen is rigid and the rectus muscle fails to relax with palpation when the client exhales. It can involve all or part of the abdomen but is usually seen on the side (ie, right vs left, rather than upper or lower) because of nerve tract patterns. Right-sided guarding may be due to cholecystitis.

Perform Deep Palpation

Deeply palpate all quadrants to delineate abdominal organs and detect subtle masses. Using the palmar surface of the fingers, compress to a maximum depth, (5 to 6 cm). Perform bimanual palpation if you encounter resistance or to assess deeper structures.	Normal (mild) tenderness is possible over the xiphoid, aorta, cecum, sigmoid colon, and ovaries with deep palpation.	Severe tenderness or pain may be related to trauma, peritonitis, infection, tumors, or enlarged or diseased organs.

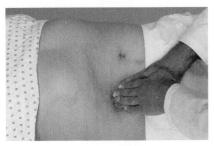

Performing deep bimanual palpation.

Palpate for masses and their location, size (cm), shape, consistency, demarcation, pulsatility, tenderness, and mobility. Do not confuse a mass with a normally palpated organ or structure.	No palpable masses	A mass detected in any quadrant may be due to a tumor, cyst, abscess, enlarged organ, aneurysm, or adhesions.

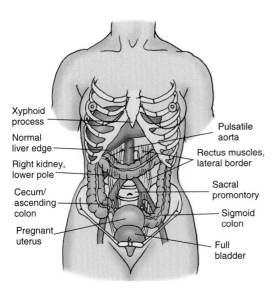

Xyphoid process
Normal liver edge
Right kidney, lower pole
Cecum/ascending colon
Pregnant uterus
Pulsatile aorta
Rectus muscles, lateral border
Sacral promontory
Sigmoid colon
Full bladder

Normally palpable structures in the abdomen.

(continued)

ASSESSMENT PROCEDURE	NORMAL FINDINGS	ABNORMAL FINDINGS

Palpate the Umbilicus

Palpate the umbilicus and surrounding area for swellings, bulges, or masses.

Umbilicus and surrounding area are free of swellings, bulges, or masses.

A soft center of the umbilicus can be a potential for herniation. Palpation of a hard nodule in or around the umbilicus may indicate metastatic nodes from an occult gastrointestinal cancer.

Palpate the Aorta

Use your thumb and first finger or use two hands and palpate deeply in the epigastrium, slightly to the left of midline.

Assess the pulsation of the abdominal aorta. If the client is older than age 50 or has hypertension, assess the width of the aorta.

The normal aorta is approximately 2.5 to 3.0 cm wide with a moderately strong and regular pulse. Possibly, mild tenderness may be elicited.

A wide, bounding pulse may be felt with an abdominal aortic aneurysm. A prominent, laterally pulsating mass above the umbilicus, with an accompanying audible bruit, strongly suggests an aortic aneurysm (see Display 18-8).

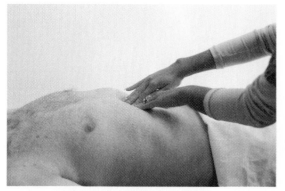

Palpating the aorta. (© B. Proud.)

Tip From the Experts Do not palpate a pulsating midline mass; it may be a dissecting aneurysm that can rupture from the pressure of palpation. Also avoid deep palpation over tender organs as in the case of polycystic kidneys, Wilms' tumor, transplantation, or suspected splenic trauma.

(continued)

.ASSESSMENT PROCEDURE	NORMAL FINDINGS	ABNORMAL FINDINGS

Palpate the Liver

Palpate to note consistency and tenderness. To palpate *bimanually,* stand at the client's right side and place your left hand under the client's back at the level of the eleventh to twelfth ribs. Lay your right hand parallel to the right costal margin (your fingertips should point toward the client's head). Ask the client to inhale, then compress upward and inward with your fingers.

To palpate by *hooking,* stand to the right of the client's chest. Curl (hook) the fingers of both hands over the edge of the right costal margin. Ask the client to take a deep breath, and gently, but firmly, pull inward and upward with your fingers.

The liver is usually not palpable, although it may be felt in some thin clients. If the lower edge is felt, it should be firm, smooth, and even. Mild tenderness may be normal.

A hard, firm liver may indicate cancer. Nodularity may occur with tumors, metastatic cancer, late cirrhosis, or syphilis. Tenderness may be from vascular engorgement (eg, congestive heart failure), acute hepatitis, or abscess.

A liver more than 1 to 3 cm below the costal margin is considered enlarged (unless pressed down by the diaphragm). Enlargement may be due to hepatitis, liver tumors, cirrhosis, and vascular engorgement.

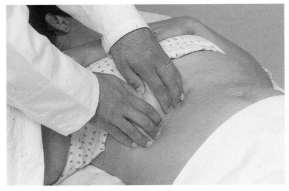

Hooking technique for liver palpation.

Palpate the Spleen

Stand at the client's right side, reach over the abdomen with your left arm and place your hand under the posterior lower ribs. Pull up gently. Place your right hand below the left costal margin with the fingers pointing toward the client's head. Ask the client to inhale, and press inward and upward as you provide support with your other hand.

The spleen is seldom palpable at the left costal margin; rarely, the tip is palpable in the presence of a low, flat diaphragm (eg, chronic obstructive lung disease) or with deep diaphragmatic descent on inspiration.

A palpable spleen suggests enlargement (up to three times the normal size), which may result from trauma, mononucleosis, chronic blood disorders, and cancers. The splenic notch may be felt, which is an indication of splenic enlargement.

Tip From the Experts *Caution:* To avoid traumatizing and possibly rupturing the organ, be gentle when palpating an enlarged spleen.

Palpating the spleen.

(continued)

ASSESSMENT PROCEDURE	NORMAL FINDINGS	ABNORMAL FINDINGS

Alternatively, asking the client to turn onto the right side may facilitate splenic palpation by moving the spleen downward and forward. Document the size of the spleen in centimeters below the left costal margin. Also note consistency and tenderness.

If the edge of the spleen can be palpated, it should be soft and nontender.

The spleen feels soft with a rounded edge when it is enlarged from infection. It feels firm with a sharp edge when it is enlarged from chronic disease.

Tenderness accompanied by peritoneal inflammation or capsular stretching is associated with splenic enlargement.

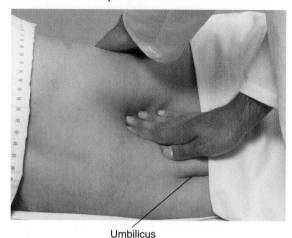

Umbilicus

Palpating the spleen with the client in side-lying position.

> **Tip From the Experts** Be sure to palpate with your fingers below the costal margin so you do not miss the lower edge of an enlarged spleen

Palpate the Kidneys

To palpate the right kidney, support the right posterior flank with your left hand, and place your right hand in the RUQ just below the costal margin at the MCL.

To capture the kidney, ask the client to inhale. Then, compress your fingers deeply during peak inspiration. Ask the client to exhale and hold the breath briefly. Gradually release the pressure of your right hand. If you have captured the kidney, you will feel it slip beneath your fingers. To palpate the left kidney, reverse the procedure.

The kidneys are normally not palpable. Sometimes, the lower pole of the right kidney may be palpable by the capture method because of its lower position. If palpated, it should feel firm, smooth, and rounded. The kidney may or may not be slightly tender.

An enlarged kidney may be due to a cyst, tumor, or hydronephrosis. It can be differentiated from splenomegaly by its smooth rather than sharp edge, absence of a notch, and overlying tympany on percussion (see Display 18-8).

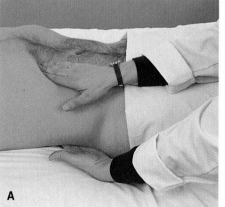

A

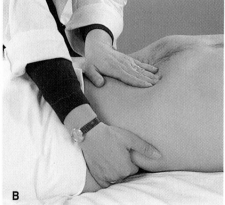

B

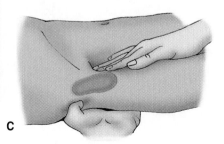

C

Palpating (A) the right kidney and (B, C) the left kidney.

(continued)

ASSESSMENT PROCEDURE	NORMAL FINDINGS	ABNORMAL FINDINGS

Palpate the Urinary Bladder

Palpate for a distended bladder when the client's history or other findings warrant (eg, dull percussion noted over the symphysis pubis). Begin at the symphysis pubis, and move upward and outward to estimate bladder borders.

Normally not palpable

A distended bladder is palpated as a smooth, round, and somewhat firm mass, extending as far as the umbilicus. It may be further validated by dull percussion tones.

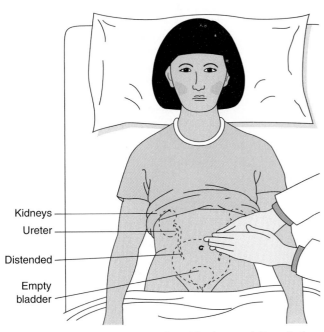

Kidneys
Ureter
Distended
Empty bladder

Palpating distended bladder (*larger dotted line* is area of distention).

(continued)

ASSESSMENT PROCEDURE	NORMAL FINDINGS	ABNORMAL FINDINGS

SPECIAL ABDOMINAL TESTS

Test for Shifting Dullness

If you suspect that the client has ascites because of a distended abdomen or bulging flanks, perform this special percussion technique. The client should remain supine. Percuss the flanks from the bed upward toward the umbilicus. Note the change from dullness to tympany, and mark this point. Now, help the client turn onto his or her side. Percuss the abdomen from the bed upward. Mark the level where dullness changes to tympany.

The borders between tympany and dullness remain relatively constant throughout position changes.

When ascites is present and the client is supine, the fluid assumes a dependent position and produces a dull percussion tone around the flanks. Air rises to the top, and tympany is percussed around the umbilicus. When the client turns onto one side and ascites is present, the fluid assumes a dependent position and air rises to the top. There is a marked increase in the height of the dullness. This test is not always reliable, and definitive testing by ultrasound is necessary.

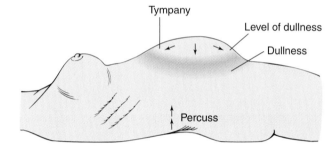

A

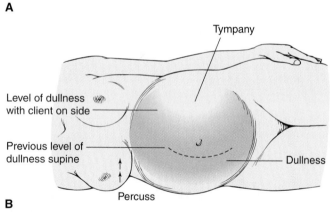

B

Percussing for level of dullness with (A) client supine and (B) lying on the side.

(continued)

ASSESSMENT PROCEDURE	NORMAL FINDINGS	ABNORMAL FINDINGS

Ascites and the Fluid Wave Test

A second special technique to detect ascites is the fluid wave test. The client should remain supine. You will need assistance with this test. Ask the client or an assistant to place the ulnar side of the hand and the lateral side of the forearm firmly along the midline of the abdomen. Firmly place the palmar surface of your fingers and hand against one side of the client's abdomen. Use your other hand to tap the opposite side of the abdominal wall.

No fluid wave is transmitted.

Movement of a fluid wave against the resting hand suggests large amounts of fluid are present (ascites). Because this test is not completely reliable, definitive testing by ultrasound is needed.

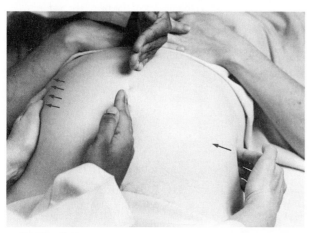

Performing fluid wave test.

Ballottement Technique for Masses

Ballottement is a palpation technique performed to identify a mass or enlarged organ within an ascitic abdomen. Ballottement can be performed two different ways: Single-handed or bimanually.

No palpable mass or masses

In the client with ascites, you can feel a freely movable mass moving upward (floats). It can be felt at the fingertips. A floating mass can be palpated for size.

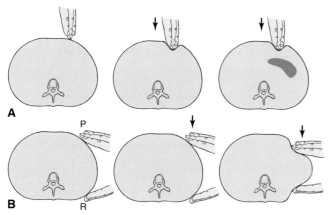

Performing ballottement with one hand (A) and bimanually (B).

Single-Hand Method
Using a tapping or bouncing motion of the fingerpads over the abdominal wall, feel for a floating mass.

Bimanual Method
Place one hand under the flank (receiving/feeling hand), and push the anterior abdominal wall with the other hand.

(continued)

ASSESSMENT PROCEDURE	NORMAL FINDINGS	ABNORMAL FINDINGS

Tests for Appendicitis

Rebound Tenderness and Rovsing's Sign

Abdominal pain and tenderness may indicate peritoneal irritation. To assess this possibility, test for rebound tenderness. Palpate deeply in the abdomen where the client has pain, and then suddenly release pressure. Listen and watch for the client's expression of pain. Ask the client to describe which hurt more—the pressing in or the releasing—and where on the abdomen the pain occurred.

No rebound tenderness

Tip From the Experts
The test for rebound tenderness should always be performed at the end of the examination because a positive response produces pain and muscle spasm that can interfere with the remaining examination.

The client has rebound tenderness when he or she perceives sharp, stabbing pain as the examiner releases pressure from the abdomen (Blumberg's sign). It suggests peritoneal irritation (as from appendicitis). If the client feels pain at an area other than where you were assessing for rebound tenderness, consider that area as the source of the pain (see test for referred rebound tenderness, below).

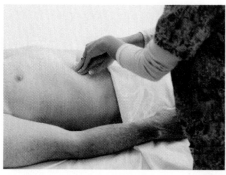 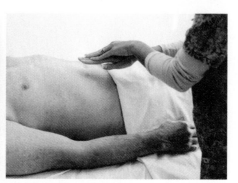

Assessing for rebound tenderness: (*left*) palpating deeply; (*right*) releasing pressure rapidly.

Palpate deeply in the LLQ.

No pain

Pain in the RLQ during pressure in the LLQ is a positive Rovsing's sign. It suggests acute appendicitis.

Referred Rebound Tenderness

Palpate deeply in the LLQ and, quickly release pressure.

No rebound pain

Pain in the RLQ during pressure in the LLQ (referred rebound tenderness) suggests appendicitis.

Tip From the Experts *Caution:* Avoid continued palpation when test findings are positive for appendicitis because of the danger of rupturing the appendix.

(continued)

ASSESSMENT PROCEDURE	NORMAL FINDINGS	ABNORMAL FINDINGS
Psoas Sign Raise the client's right leg from the hip, and place your hand on the lower thigh. Ask the client to try to keep the leg elevated as you apply pressure downward against the lower thigh.	No abdominal pain	Pain in the RLQ is associated with irritation of the iliopsoas muscle due to an appendicitis (an inflamed appendix).

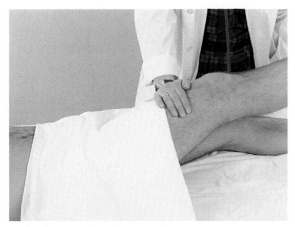

Testing for psoas sign. (© B. Proud.)

Obturator Sign Support the client's right knee and ankle. Flex the hip and knee, and rotate the leg internally and externally.	No abdominal pain	Pain in the RLQ indicates irritation of the obturator muscle due to appendicitis or a perforated appendix.

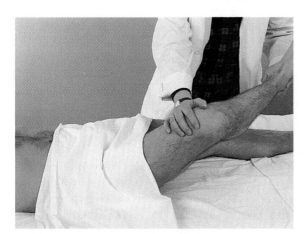

Testing for obturator sign. (© B. Proud.)

Hypersensitivity Test Stroke the abdomen with a sharp object (eg, broken cottontip applicator or tongue blade), or grasp a fold of skin with your thumb and index finger and quickly let go. Do this several times along the abdominal wall.	The client feels no pain and no exaggerated sensation.	Pain or an exaggerated sensation felt in the RLQ is a positive skin hypersensitivity test and may indicate appendicitis.
Test for Cholecystitis To assess RUQ pain or tenderness, which may signal cholecystitis (inflammation of the gallbladder), press your fingertips under the liver border at the right costal margin and ask the client to inhale deeply.	No increase in pain	Accentuated sharp pain that causes the client to hold his or her breath (inspiratory arrest) is a positive Murphy's sign and is associated with acute cholecystitis (see Display 18-8).

GUIDELINES

In clients with abdominal distention, abdominal girth (circumference) should be assessed periodically (eg, daily in hospital, or during a doctor's office visit, or in home nursing visits) to evaluate the progress or treatment of distention. To facilitate accurate assessment and interpretation, certain guidelines are recommended:

1. Measure abdominal girth at the same time of day, ideally in the morning just after voiding, or at a designated time for bedridden clients or those with indwelling catheters.
2. The ideal position for the client is standing; otherwise, the client should be in the supine position. The client's head may be slightly elevated (for orthopneic clients). The client should be in the same position for all measurements.
3. Use a disposable or easily cleaned tape measure. If a tape measure is not available, use a strip of cloth or gauze, then measure the gauze with a cloth tape measure or yardstick.
4. Place the tape measure behind the client and measure at the umbilicus.

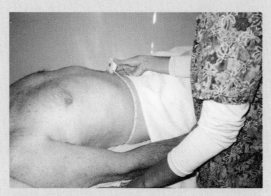

Use the umbilicus as a starting point when measuring abdominal girth, especially when distention is apparent.

5. Record the distance in designated units (inches or centimeters).
6. Take all future measurements from the same location. Marking the abdomen with a ballpoint pen can help you identify the measuring site. As a courtesy, the nurse needs to explain the purpose of the marking pen and ask the patient not to wash the mark off until it is no longer needed.

Validation and Documentation of Findings

Validate the abdominal assessment data that you have collected. This is necessary to verify that the data are reliable and accurate. Document the assessment data following the health care facility or agency policy.

EXAMPLE OF SUBJECTIVE DATA

A 44-year-old male client denies pain in abdomen, indigestion, nausea, vomiting, constipation, and diarrhea. He says that he has had no change in his usual bowel habits and denies yellowing of skin, itching, dark urine, or clay-colored stools. Client states he has never had ulcers, gastroesophageal reflux, inflammatory or obstructive bowel disease, pancreatitis, gallbladder or liver disease, diverticulosis, or appendicitis. He did have one urinary tract infection 3 years ago but has had no other problems since that time. He never had viral hepatitis and denies known exposure. Client denies abdominal surgery or trauma to the abdomen. He does not take prescribed or over-the-counter medications except for an occasional ibuprofen for headache. He denies any family history of colon, stomach, pancreatic, liver, kidney, or bladder cancer; liver disease; gallbladder disease; or kidney disease. Client tries to follow a low-fat, high-carbohydrate, moderated protein diet and drinks a lot of fluids daily. He has approximately two alcoholic drinks per week, runs 3 days a week, and bikes 2 days a week. He reports a moderate amount of stress from work but copes with it through exercise and spending time with his wife and children.

EXAMPLE OF OBJECTIVE DATA

Skin of abdomen is free of striae, scars, lesions, or rashes. Umbilicus is midline and recessed with no bulging. Abdomen is flat and symmetric with no bulges or lumps. No

(*text continues on page 405*)

ABNORMAL FINDINGS

DISPLAY 18-5. Abdominal Distention

With the exception of pregnancy (which causes a generalized protuberant abdomen, protruberant umbilicus, a fetal heart beat that can be heard on auscultation, percussable tympany over the intestines, and dullness over the uterus), abdominal distention is usually considered an abnormal finding. However, fat, feces, masses, flatus, and fluid (ascites) are somewhat common and may sometimes be disclosed by percussion.

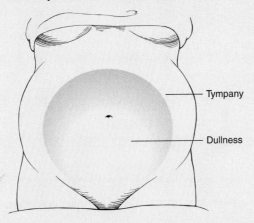

Tympany

Dullness

Pregnancy.

FAT

Obesity accounts for most uniformly protuberant abdomens. The abdominal wall is thick and tympany is the percussion tone elicited. The umbilicus usually appears sunken.

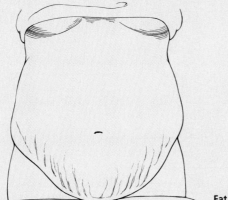

Fat.

FECES

Hard stools in the colon appear as a localized distention. Percussion over the area discloses dullness.

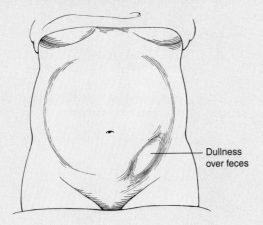

Dullness over feces

Feces.

(continued)

FIBROIDS AND OTHER MASSES

A large ovarian cyst or fibroid tumor appears as generalized distention in the lower abdomen. The mass displaces bowel, and, thus, the percussion tone over the distended area is dullness with tympany at the periphery. The umbilicus may be everted.

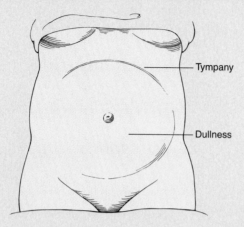

Tympany

Dullness

Fibroids and masses.

FLATUS

The abdomen distended with gas may appear as a generalized protuberance (as shown), or it may appear more localized. Tympany is the percussion tone over the area.

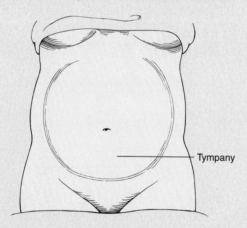

Tympany

Flatus.

ASCITIC FLUID

Fluid in the abdomen causes generalized protuberance, bulging flanks, and an everted umbilicus. Percussion reveals dullness over fluid (bottom of abdomen and flanks) and tympany over intestines (top of abdomen).

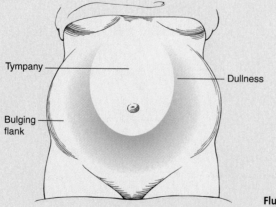

Tympany

Dullness

Bulging flank

Fluid.

ABNORMAL FINDINGS

DISPLAY 18-6. Abdominal Bulges

UMBILICAL HERNIA

An umbilical hernia results from the bowel protruding through a weakness in the umbilical ring. This condition occurs more frequently in infants, but it also occurs in adults.

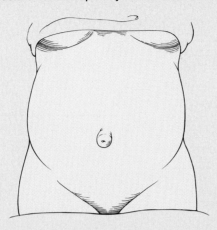

Umbilical hernia.

EPIGASTRIC HERNIA

An epigastric hernia occurs when bowel protrudes through a weakness in the linea alba. The small bulge appears midline between the xiphoid process and the umbilicus. It may be discovered only on palpation.

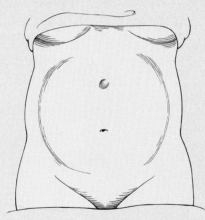

Epigastric hernia.

DIASTASIS RECTI

Diastasis recti occurs when bowel protrudes through a separation between the two rectus abdominis muscles. It appears as a midline ridge. The bulge may appear only when client raises head or coughs. The condition is of little significance.

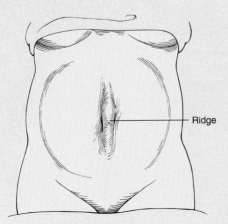

Ridge

Diastasis recti.

(continued)

DISPLAY 18-6. Abdominal Bulges (Continued)

INCISIONAL HERNIA

An incisional hernia occurs when bowel protrudes through a defect or weakness resulting from a surgical incision. It appears as a bulge near a surgical scar on the abdomen.

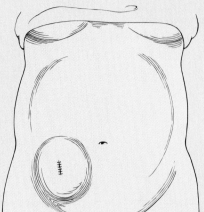

Incisional hernia.

GUIDELINES

DISPLAY 18-7. Auscultating Bowel Sounds

Always auscultate bowel sounds before touching the abdomen. This prevents alteration of bowel sounds.

1. Use the diaphragm of the stethoscope, and make sure that it is warm before you place it on the client's abdomen.
2. Apply light pressure or simply rest the stethoscope on a tender abdomen.
3. Begin in the RLQ and proceed clockwise, covering all quadrants.

 Tip From the Experts Bowel sounds may be more active over the ileocecal valve in the RLQ.

4. Confirm bowel sounds in each quadrant. Listen for up to 5 minutes (minimum of 1 minute per quadrant) to confirm the absence of bowel sounds.

 Tip From the Experts Bowel sounds normally occur every 5 to 15 seconds. An easy way to remember is to equate one bowel sound to one breath sound.

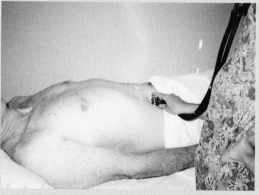

Be sure the diaphragm of the stethoscope is warm before placing it on the abdomen.

ABNORMAL
FINDINGS

DISPLAY 18-8. **Enlarged Abdominal Organs and Other Abnormalities**

ENLARGED LIVER

An enlarged liver (hepatomegaly) is defined as a span greater than 12 cm at the midclavicular (MCL) and greater than 8 cm at the midsternal line (MSL). An enlarged nontender liver suggests cirrhosis. An enlarged tender liver suggests congestive heart failure, acute hepatitis, or abscess.

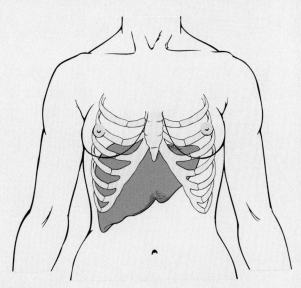

Enlarged liver.

ENLARGED NODULAR LIVER

An enlarged firm, hard, nodular liver suggests cancer. Other causes may be late cirrhosis or syphilis.

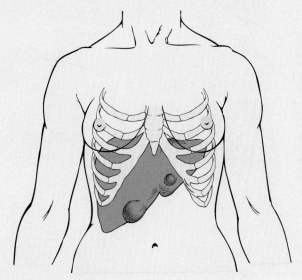

Enlarged nodular liver.

(continued)

DISPLAY 18-8. Enlarged Abdominal Organs and Other Abnormalities (Continued)

LIVER HIGHER THAN NORMAL

A liver that is in a higher position than normal with a normal span may be caused by an abdominal mass, ascites, or a paralyzed diaphragm.

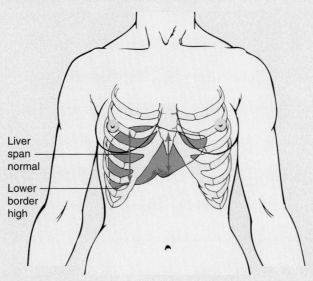

Liver span normal

Lower border high

Liver higher than normal.

LIVER LOWER THAN NORMAL

A liver in a lower position than normal with a normal span may be caused by emphysema because the diaphragm is low.

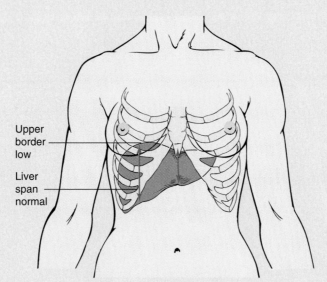

Upper border low

Liver span normal

Liver lower than normal.

(continued)

ENLARGED SPLEEN

An enlarged spleen (splenomegaly) is defined by an area of dullness exceeding 7 cm. When enlarged, the spleen progresses downward and in toward the midline.

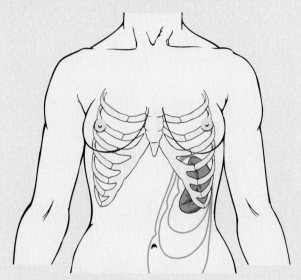

Enlarged spleen.

AORTIC ANEURYSM

A prominent, laterally pulsating mass above the umbilicus strongly suggests an aortic aneurysm. It is accompanied by a bruit and a wide, bounding pulse.

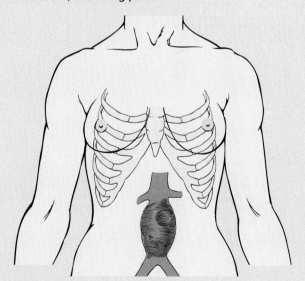

Aortic aneurysm.

(continued)

ENLARGED KIDNEY

An enlarged kidney may be due to a cyst, tumor, or hydronephrosis. It may be differentiated from an enlarged spleen by its smooth rather than sharp edge, the absence of a notch, and tympany on percussion.

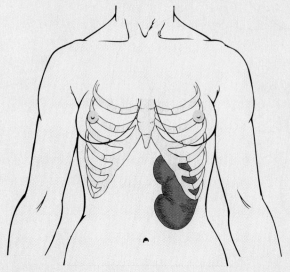

Enlarged kidney.

ENLARGED GALLBLADDER

An extremely tender, enlarged gallbladder suggests acute cholecystitis. A positive finding is Murphy's sign (sharp pain that causes the client to hold the breath).

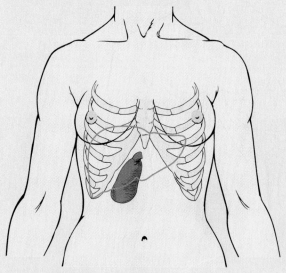

Enlarged gallbladder.

bulges noted when client raises head. Slight respiratory movements and aortic pulsations noted. No peristaltic waves seen. Soft clicks and gurgles heard at a rate of 15 per minute. No bruits, venous hums, or friction rubs auscultated.

Percussion reveals generalized tympany over all four quadrants, with dullness over the liver, spleen, and descending colon. Percussion of liver span reveals MCL = 8 cm and MSL = 6 cm. Percussion over spleen discloses a dull oval area approximately 7 cm wide near left tenth rib posterior to MAL. No tenderness elicited with blunt percussion over liver and kidneys. No tenderness or guarding in any quadrant with light palpation. Mild tenderness elicited over xiphoid, aorta, cecum, and sigmoid colon with deep palpation.

No masses palpated. Umbilicus and surrounding area free of masses, swelling, and bulges. Aortic pulsation moderately strong, regular, and approximately 3.0 cm wide. Liver, spleen, kidneys, and urinary bladder not palpable. Test for shifting dullness reveals constant borders between tympany and dullness throughout position changes. No fluid wave transmitted during fluid wave test. No mass palpated during ballottement test. All test findings for appendicitis are negative as is test finding for cholecystitis.

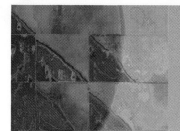

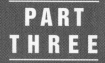

After collecting assessment data, you will need to analyze the data using diagnostic reasoning skills. In Chapter 7 you can review the general steps of the diagnostic reasoning process. After that, in Diagnostic Reasoning: Possible Conclusions, you will see an overview of common conclusions that you may reach after abdominal assessment. Next, the case study presents an opportunity to analyze abdominal assessment data for a specific client.

Diagnostic Reasoning: Possible Conclusions

Listed below are some possible conclusions that may be drawn after assessment of the client's abdomen.

SELECTED NURSING DIAGNOSES

After collecting subjective and objective data pertaining to the abdomen, you will need to identify abnormals and cluster the data to reveal any significant patterns or abnormalities. These data will then be used to make clinical judgments (nursing diagnoses: wellness, risk, or actual) about the status of the client's abdomen. Following is a listing of selected nursing diagnoses that you may identify when analyzing data for this part of the assessment.

Nursing Diagnoses (Wellness)

- Opportunity to enhance nutritional status
- Opportunity to enhance bowel elimination pattern
- Opportunity to enhance bladder elimination pattern
- Health-Seeking Behavior: Requests information on ways to improve nutritional status

Nursing Diagnoses (Risk)

- Risk for Fluid Volume Deficit related to excessive nausea and vomiting or diarrhea
- Risk for Impaired Skin Integrity related to fluid volume deficit secondary to decreased fluid intake, nausea, vomiting, diarrhea, fecal or urinary incontinence, or ostomy drainage
- Risk for Altered Oral Mucous Membranes related to fluid volume deficit secondary to nausea, vomiting, diarrhea, or gastrointestinal intubation

- Risk for Urinary Infection related to urinary stasis and decreased fluid intake
- Risk for Altered Nutrition: Less Than Body Requirements related to lack of dietary information or inadequate intake of nutrients secondary to values or religious beliefs or eating disorders.

Nursing Diagnoses (Actual)

- Altered Nutrition: Less Than Body Requirements related to malabsorption, decreased appetite, frequent nausea, and vomiting
- Altered Nutrition: More Than Body Requirements related to intake that exceeds caloric needs
- Altered Sexuality Patterns related to fear of rejection by partner secondary to offensive odor and drainage from colostomy or ileostomy
- Grieving related to change in manner of bowel elimination
- Altered Body Image related to change in abdominal appearance secondary to presence of stoma
- Diarrhea related to malabsorption and chronic irritable bowel syndrome or medications
- Constipation related to decreased fluid intake, decreased dietary fiber, decreased physical activity, bedrest, or medications
- Perceived Constipation related to decrease in usual pattern and frequency of bowel elimination
- Bowel Incontinence related to muscular or neurologic dysfunction secondary to age, disease, or trauma
- Altered Health Maintenance related to chronic or inappropriate use of laxatives or enemas
- Self-Concept Disturbance related to obesity and difficulty losing weight
- Self-Concept Disturbance related to loss of bowel or bladder control
- Activity Intolerance related to fecal or urinary incontinence
- Anxiety related to fear of fecal or urinary incontinence
- Social Isolation related to anxiety and fear of fecal or urinary incontinence
- Pain: Abdominal (referred, distention, or surgical incision)
- Altered Urinary Elimination related to catheterization secondary to obstruction, trauma, infection, neurologic disorders, or surgical intervention

- Urinary Retention related to obstruction of part of the urinary tract or malfunctioning of drainage devices (catheters) and need to learn bladder emptying techniques
- Altered Patterns of Urinary Elimination related to bladder infection
- Functional Incontinence related to age-related urgency and inability to reach toilet in time secondary to decreased bladder tone and inability to recognize "need-to-void cues"
- Reflex Incontinence related to lack of knowledge of ways to trigger a more predictable voiding schedule
- Stress Incontinence related to knowledge deficit of pelvic floor muscle exercises
- Total Incontinence related to need for bladder retraining program
- Urge Incontinence related to need for knowledge of preventive measures secondary to infection, trauma, or neurogenic problems

SELECTED COLLABORATIVE PROBLEMS

After grouping the data, certain collaborative problems may emerge. Remember, collaborative problems differ from nursing diagnoses in that they cannot be prevented by nursing interventions. However, these physiologic complications of medical conditions can be detected and monitored by the nurse. In addition, the nurse can use physician- and nurse-prescribed interventions to minimize the complications of these problems. The nurse may also have to refer the client in such situations for further treatment of the problem. Following is a list of collaborative problems that may be identified when assessing the abdomen. These problems are worded as Potential Complications (or PC), followed by the problem.

- PC: Peritonitis
- PC: Ileus
- PC: Afferent loop syndrome
- PC: Early dumping syndrome
- PC: Late dumping syndrome
- PC: Malabsorption syndrome
- PC: Intestinal bleeding
- PC: Renal calculi
- PC: Abscess formation
- PC: Bowel obstruction
- PC: Toxic megacolon
- PC: Mesenteric thrombosis
- PC: Obstruction of bile flow
- PC: Fistula formation
- PC: Hyponatremia/hypernatremia
- PC: Hypokalemia/hyperkalemia
- PC: Hypoglycemia/hyperglycemia
- PC: Hypocalcemia/hypercalcemia
- PC: Metabolic acidosis
- PC: Uremic syndrome
- PC: Stomal changes
- PC: Urinary obstruction
- PC: Hypertension
- PC: Gastroesophageal reflux disease
- PC: Peptic ulcer disease
- PC: Hepatic failure
- PC: Pancreatitis

MEDICAL PROBLEMS

After grouping the data, it may become apparent that the client has signs and symptoms that may require medical diagnosis and treatment. Referral to a primary care provider is necessary.

Diagnostic Reasoning: Case Study

The case study presents assessment data for a specific client. It is followed by an analysis of the data, working out the seven key steps (see Chapter 7) to arrive at specific conclusions.

Nikki Chen, a 32-year-old graduate student, comes into the clinic complaining of undifferentiated abdominal discomfort. She states that she has been "constipated for the last 4 days." She appears nervous and fidgety and, when asked, confesses that she is very anxious about her upcoming final comprehensive examinations. "Sometimes I get so tense and upset I can't calm down. I really would like some help to learn new ways to handle my stress and to be more healthy. I'm concerned that, if I don't do something soon, I will have high blood pressure like my father does." She indicates that her father took up smoking in his native China before coming to America, so she doesn't

know if his high blood pressure is something she could inherit or if it's the result of his smoking. "I never got involved with that bad habit!" she says. During the interview, she describes her dietary habits as terrible: She eats salty, high-fat junk food and doesn't drink water, just "lots of regular sodas with caffeine." She comments that her mother cooks healthful meals of rice and vegetables at home, but Nikki doesn't get home very often any more. "Exercise? What graduate student has time for that?"

An examination of the client's abdomen reveals a moderately rounded, slightly firm, nontender abdomen with several small (quarter-sized), round, firm masses in the LLQ (sigmoid colon). Bowel sounds are active, moderate-pitched gurgles in all four quadrants. The abdomen is mostly tympanic upon percussion with scattered dullness in the LUQ. McBurney's and Rovsing's signs are both negative for rebound tenderness. A rectal examination reveals hard stool in the ampulla.

1 Identify abnormal data and strengths (in both subjective and objective data).

SUBJECTIVE DATA

- Complains of undifferentiated abdominal discomfort
- Reports constipation for the last 4 days
- Feels very anxious about upcoming final comprehensive examinations
- Gets tense and upset and cannot calm self
- Wants help learning new ways to handle stress and to be more healthy
- Voices concern that she will have high blood pressure like father who smokes
- Denies a smoking habit
- Describes diet as terrible: salty, high-fat junk food
- Doesn't drink water, just lots of sugary sodas with caffeine
- Says mother prepares healthful meals, but client rarely eats at home
- Has no time for exercise

OBJECTIVE DATA

- Nervous and fidgety
- Moderately rounded, slightly firm, nontender abdomen
- Several small, quarter-sized, round, firm masses palpated in the sigmoid colon
- Bowel sound active with moderately pitched gurgles in all quadrants
- Abdomen mostly tympanic on percussion, scattered dullness in the LUQ
- Examination discloses no McBurney's or Rovsing's signs
- Rectal examination findings include hard stool in the ampulla

2 Cue Clusters	**3** Inferences	**4** Possible Nursing Diagnoses	**5** Defining Characteristics	**6** Confirm or Rule Out
A Complains of undifferentiated abdominal discomfort • Constipated for the last 4 days • Very anxious about examinations • Gets tense and upset • Eats salty, high-fat junk food • Doesn't drink water; does drink lots of sugary, caffeinated sodas • No time for exercise • Moderately rounded, slightly firm abdomen, not tender to palpation • Several small, round, firm masses in sigmoid colon • Abdomen tympanic on percussion • Negative McBurney's and Rovsing's signs • Hard stool in the ampulla	Nikki has diagnosed her own problem. The data strongly suggest constipation, probably as a result of poorly managed stress, lack of exercise, inadequate water intake.	Colonic Constipation related to body tension, poor dietary habits, lack of exercise, and inadequate water intake	*Major:* Decreased frequency, dry stool, abdominal distention *Minor:* Abdominal discomfort	Confirm because it meets the major and minor defining characteristics.
B Anxious about final examinations • Gets tense and upset; unable to calm self • Wants to learn new ways to handle stress and to be healthier	Able to identify unhealthful behaviors and inadequate coping strategies, but does not verbalize that she knows how to manage her stressors.	Ineffective Individual Coping related to increased life stress and lack of knowledge of appropriate management strategies	*Major:* Verbalization of inability to cope *Minor:* Reported difficulty with life stressors	Confirm because it meets the major and minor defining characteristics.

② Cue Clusters	③ Inferences	④ Possible Nursing Diagnoses	⑤ Defining Characteristics	⑥ Confirm or Rule Out
• Describes dietary habits as terrible: high-fat junk food • Doesn't drink water, just "lots of sugary, caffeinated sodas" • No time for exercise	Client appears to be seeking help for her current problems of constipation and unmanaged stress, but she is also taking this opportunity to get more information about possible risk factors and ways to promote health.	Altered Health Maintenance related to knowledge deficit and, possibly, lack of motivation to change unhealthful behaviors	*Major:* Reports unhealthful practices *Minor:* None	Confirm because it meets the major defining characteristic. More data needed to determine whether the etiology is knowledge deficit or lack of motivation
		Health-Seeking Behaviors	*Major:* Expressed desire to seek information for health promotion *Minor:* None	Confirm

⑦ Document conclusions.

The following diagnoses are appropriate for Ms. Chen at this time:

* Colonic Constipation related to body tension, lack of exercise, and inadequate water intake
* Ineffective Individual Coping related to increased life stress and lack of knowledge of appropriate management strategies
* Altered Health Maintenance related to knowledge deficit and possibly lack of motivation to change unhealthful behaviors
* Health-Seeking Behaviors

Because there is no medical diagnosis, there are no collaborative problems at this time.

REFERENCES AND SELECTED READINGS

Allison, O. C., Porter, M. E., & Briggs, G. C. (1994). Chronic constipation: Assessment and management in the elderly. *Journal of the American Academy of Nursing Practice, 6*(7), 311–317.

Ambrose, M., & Drecker, H. M. (1996). Pancreatitis: Managing a flare-up. *Nursing96, 26*(4), 33–39.

Breitfeller, J. (1999). Peritonitis. *American Journal of Nursing, 99*(4), 33.

Goldsmith, C. (1998). Gastroesophageal reflux disease. *American Journal of Nursing, 98*(9), 44–45.

Greenberg, L. (1994). Fast action for splenic rupture. *American Journal of Nursing, 94*(2), 51.

Heslin, J. (1997). Peptic ulcer disease. *Nursing97, 27*(3), 34–39.

Johnson, S. T. (2000). From incontinence to confidence. *American Journal of Nursing, 100*(2), 69–74, 76.

Kamen, B. J. (1999). Combating upper G.I. bleeding. *Nursing99, 29*(7), 32hn1–hn6.

Katz, S. K., Gordon, K. B., & Roenigk, H. H. (1996). The cutaneous manifestations of gastrointestinal disease. *Primary Care: Gastroenterology, 23*(3), 455–475.

Kirton, C. (1997). Assessing bowel sounds. *Nursing97, 27*(3), 64.

———. (1997). Assessing for bladder distention. *Nursing97, 27*(5), 52–57.

———. (1996). Assessing for ascites. *Nursing96, 26*(4), 53.

Lane-Reticker, A. (1993). Assessment of the injured abdomen. *Topics in Emergency Medicine, 15*(1), 1–7.

Langan, J. C. (1998). Abdominal assessment in the home: From A to Zzz. *Home Health Nurse, 16*(1), 50–57.

McConnell, E. (1994). Loosening the grip of intestinal obstructions. *Nursing94, 24*(3), 34–41.

Muscari, M. E., & Milks, C. J. (1995). Assessing acute abdominal pain in adolescent females. *Pediatric Nursing, 21*(3), 215–220.

Nebelkopf, H. (1998). Abdominal compartment syndrome. *American Journal of Nursing, 99*(11), 53–60.

O'Hanlon-Nichols, T. (1998). Basic assessment series: Gastrointestinal system. *American Journal of Nursing, 98*(4), 48–53.

O'Toole, M. (1992). Advanced assessment of the abdomen and gastrointestinal problems. *Nursing Clinics of North America, 25*(4), 771–776.

Stone, R. (1998). Acute abdominal pain. *Lippincott's Primary Care Practice, 2*(4), 341–357.

———. (1996). Primary care diagnosis of acute abdominal pain. *Nurse Practitioner, 21*(12, Part 1), 19–20, 23–30, 35–39.

Town, J. (1997). Bringing acute abdomen into focus. *Nursing97, 27*(5), 52–57.

Wachtel, T. C. (1994). Critical care concepts in the management of abdominal trauma. *Critical Care Nursing Quarterly, 17*(2), 34–50.

Wiener, S. L. (1993). *Differential diagnosis of acute pain by body region.* New York: McGraw-Hill.

Wright, J. A. (1997). Seven abdominal signs every emergency nurse should know. *Journal of Emergency Nursing, 23*(5), 446–450.

Risk Factors

American Cancer Society (ACS). (2000). *Gallbladder cancer: Prevention and risk factors.* ACS Gallbladder Cancer Resource Center. Available: www3.cancer.org/cancerinfo/load_cont.asp?st=pr&ct=68&language=english. Accessed 12/20/2000.

Comess, L., Bennet, P., & Burch, T. (1967). Clinical gallbladder disease in Pima Indians: Its high incidence in contrast to Framingham, Massachusetts. *New England Journal of Medicine, 277*(17), 894.

Khan, Z. R., Neugut, A., Ahsan, H., & Chabot, J. (1999). Risk factors for biliary tract cancers. *American Journal of Gastroenterology, 94*(1), 149–154.

Lowenfels, A. B., & Maisonneuve, P. (1999). Pancreatic biliary malignancy: Prevalence and risk factors. *Annals of Oncology, 10*(Suppl 4), 1–3.

Lowenfels, A. B., Maisonneuve, P., Boyle, P., & Zatonski, W. (1999). Epidemiology of gallbladder cancer. *Hepatogastroenterology, 46*(27), 1529–1532.

Overfield, T. (1995). *Biological variation in health and illness: Race, age, and sex differences* (2nd ed.). Boca Raton, FL: CRC Press.

Sheth, S., Bedfore, A., & Chopra S. (2000). Primary gallbladder cancer: Recognition of risk factors and the role of prophylactic cholestectomy. *American Journal of Gastroenterology, 95*(6), 1402–1410.

Vitetta, L., Sali, A., Little, P. M., & Mrazek, L. (2000). Gallstones and gallbladder carcinoma. *Australian and New Zealand Journal of Surgery, 70*(9), 667–673.

For additional information on this book, be sure to visit http://connection.lww.com.

Male Genitalia Assessment

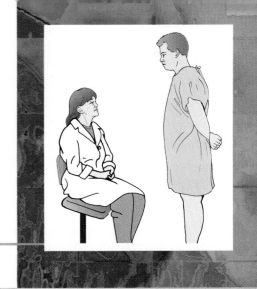

19

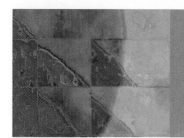

To assess the male genitalia, a basic understanding of normal structure and function is necessary; it helps guide the physical examination and readily assists the examiner in identifying abnormalities. Male genitalia are classified as external structures and internal structures. (*Note:* Glandular structures accessory to the male genital organs—the prostate, the seminal vesicles, and Cowper's [bulbourethral] glands—are discussed in Chapter 21.) In addition to an understanding of the male genital structures, the nurse needs to be familiar with the inguinal (or groin) structures because hernias are common in this area.

External Genitalia

The external genitalia consist of the penis and the scrotum (Fig. 19-1). The penis is the male reproductive organ. Attached to the pubic arch by ligaments, the penis is freely movable. The shaft of the penis is composed of three cylindrical masses of vascular erectile tissue that are bound together by fibrous tissue—two corpora cavernosa on the dorsal side and the corpus spongiosum on the ventral side. The corpus spongiosum extends distally to form the acorn-shaped glans. The base of the glans, or corona, is somewhat enlarged. If the man has not been circumcised, the glans is covered by a hoodlike fold of skin called the foreskin. In the center of the corpus spongiosum is the urethra, which travels through the shaft and opens as a slit at the tip of the glans as the urethral meatus. A fold of foreskin that extends ventrally from the urethral meatus is called the frenulum. The penis has a role in both reproduction and urination.

The scrotum is a thin-walled sac that is suspended below the pubic bone, posterior to the penis. This darkly pigmented structure contains sweat and sebaceous glands and consists of folds of skin (rugae) and the cremaster muscle. The scrotum functions as a protective covering for the testes, epididymis, and vas deferens and helps to maintain the cooler-than-body temperature necessary for production of sperm. The scrotum can maintain temperature control because the cremaster muscle is sensitive to changes in temperature. The muscle contracts when too cold, raising the scrotum and testes upward toward the body for warmth (cremasteric reflex). This accounts for the wrinkled appearance of the scrotal skin. When the temperature is warm, the muscle relaxes, lowering the scrotum and testes away from the heat of the body. When the cremaster muscle relaxes, the scrotal skin appears smooth.

Internal Genitalia

Internally, the scrotal sac is divided into two portions, each portion containing one testis (testicle; see Fig. 19-1). The testes are a pair of ovoid-shaped organs, similar to the ovaries in the woman, that are approximately 3.7 to 5 cm long, 2.5 cm wide, and 2.5 cm deep. Each testis is covered by a serous membrane called the tunica vaginalis, which separates the testis from the scrotal wall. The function of the testis is to produce spermatozoa and the male sex hormone testosterone.

The testes are suspended in the scrotum by a spermatic cord. The spermatic cord contains blood vessels, lymphatic vessels, nerves, and the vas deferens (or ductus deferens), which transports spermatozoa away from the testis. The spermatic cord on the left side is usually longer; thus, the left testis hangs lower than the right testis.

The epididymis is a comma-shaped, coiled tubular structure that curves up over the upper and posterior surface of the testis. In some men, it may be located anteriorly. It is within the epididymis that the spermatozoa mature.

The vas deferens is a firm, muscular tube that is continuous with the lower portion of the epididymis (see Fig. 19-1). It travels up within the spermatic cord through the inguinal canal into the abdominal cavity. At this point, it separates from the spermatic cord and curves behind the bladder. It joins with the duct of the seminal vesicle and forms the ejaculatory duct. Finally, the ejaculatory duct empties into the urethra within the prostate gland.

The tubular structures just described make up the route for transporting sperm from the testes to the urethra for ejaculation. Along the way, secretions from the vas deferens, seminal vesicles, prostate gland, and Cowper's or bulbourethral glands mix with the sperm and form semen.

Inguinal Area

When assessing the male genitalia, the nurse needs to be familiar with structures of the inguinal or groin area because hernias (protrusion of loops of bowel through weak areas of the musculature) are common in this location (Fig. 19-2).

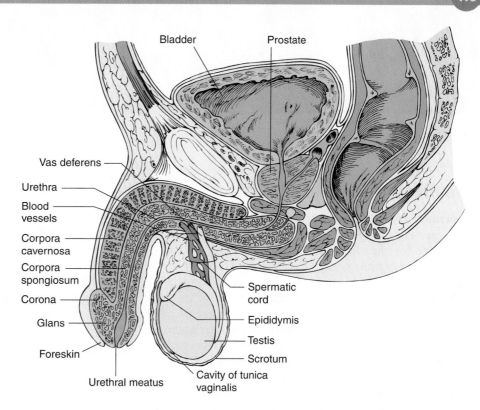

FIGURE 19-1. External and internal male genitalia.

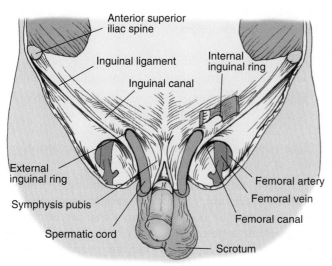

FIGURE 19-2. Inguinal area.

The inguinal area is contained between the anterior superior iliac spine laterally and the symphysis pubis medially.

Running diagonally between these two landmarks, just above and parallel with the inguinal ligament, is the inguinal canal. The inguinal canal is a tubelike structure through which the vas deferens travels as it passes through the lower abdomen.

The external inguinal ring is the exterior opening of the inguinal canal and can be palpated above and lateral to the symphysis pubis. It feels triangular and slitlike. The internal inguinal ring is the internal opening of the inguinal canal. It is located 1 to 2 cm above the midpoint of the inguinal ligament and cannot be palpated. The femoral canal is another potential spot for a hernia. The femoral canal is located posterior to the inguinal canal and medial to and running parallel with the femoral artery and vein.

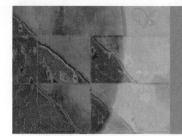
Collecting Subjective Data

When interviewing the male client for information regarding his genitalia, keep in mind that this may be a very sensitive topic for the client and for the examiner as well. Moreover, the examiner should be aware of his or her own feelings regarding body image, fear of cancer, and sexuality. Western culture emphasizes the importance of the male sex role function. Self-esteem and body image are entwined with the male sex role. Anxiety, embarrassment, and fear may influence the client's ability to discuss problems and ask questions. A trusting relationship is key to a successful interview. Keep in mind that serious or life-threatening problems may be present. Testicular cancer, for example, carries a high mortality rate, especially if not detected early. The information gathered during this portion of the health history interview provides a basis for teaching about important health screening issues, such as testicular self-examination. Additionally, symptoms that the client reports, or hints at, need to be explored in some depth with a symptom analysis. Use the COLDSPA mnemonic as a guide:

COLDSPA

CHARACTER: Describe the sign or symptom. How does it feel, look, sound, smell, and so forth?

ONSET: When did it begin?

LOCATION: Where is it? Does it radiate?

DURATION: How long does it last? Does it recur?

SEVERITY: How bad is it?

PATTERN: What makes it better: What makes it worse?

ASSOCIATED FACTORS: What other symptoms occur with it?

Nursing History

CURRENT SYMPTOMS

Question Do you have pain in your penis, scrotum, testes, or groin?

Rationale Complaints of pain in these areas may indicate a hernia or an inflammatory process, such as epididymitis.

Q Have you noticed any lesions on your penis or genital area?

R Lesions may be a sign of a sexually transmitted disease (STD) or cancer.

Q Have you noticed any discharge from your penis? If so, what color is it? What type of odor does it have?

R Discharge may indicate an infection.

Q Do you have any lumps, swelling, or masses in your scrotum, genital, or groin area?

R These findings may indicate infection, hernia, or cancer.

Q Do you have a heavy, dragging feeling in your scrotum?

R A testicular tumor or scrotal hernia may cause a feeling of heaviness in the scrotum.

Q Do you experience difficulty urinating (ie, hesitancy, frequency, or difficulty starting or maintaining a stream)?

R Difficulty urinating may indicate an infection or blockage, including prostatic enlargement.

Q Have you noticed any change in the color, odor, or amount of your urine?

R Changes in urine color or odor may indicate an infection. Blood in the urine (hematuria) should be referred for medical investigation because this may indicate infection, benign prostatic hypertrophy (BPH), or cancer. A decrease in amount of voided urine may indicate prostate enlargement or kidney problems.

Q Do you experience any pain or burning when you urinate?

R Painful urination may be a sign of urinary tract infection, prostatitis, or an STD, also called sexually transmitted infection (STI).

Q Do you ever experience urinary incontinence or dribbling?

R Incontinence may occur after prostatectomy. Dribbling may be a sign of overflow incontinence.

Q Have you recently had a change in your pattern of sexual activity or sexual desire?

R A change in sexual activity or sexual desire (libido) needs to be investigated to determine the cause.

Q Do you have difficulty attaining or maintaining an erection? Do you have any problem with ejaculation?

R Erectile dysfunction occurs frequently in adult males and may be attributed to various factors or disorders (eg, alcohol use, diabetes, depression, antihypertensive medications).

 Erectile dysfunction increases in frequency with age.

Q Do you have or have you had any trouble with fertility?

R About 30% of all infertility experienced by couples is due to male infertility.

PAST HISTORY

Q Describe any prior medical problems you have had, how they were treated, and the results.

R Prior problems directly affect the physical assessment findings. For example, if cancer was present in the past, it may recur. Diabetes may cause impotence.

Q When was the last time you had a testicular examination by a physician? What was the result?

R The American Cancer Society recommends testicular examination by a physician every 3 years for asymptomatic men ages 20 to 39 and every year for asymptomatic men age 40 years and older.

Q Have you ever been tested for human immunodeficiency virus (HIV)? What was the result? Why were you tested?

R HIV increases the client's risk for other infections. A high-risk exposure may require serial testing.

FAMILY HISTORY

Q Is there a history of cancer in your family? What type and which family member(s)?

R Cancers of the prostate and testes have a familial tendency.

LIFESTYLE AND HEALTH PRACTICES

Q How many sexual partners do you have?

R A client with multiple sexual partners increases his risk of contracting an STD or HIV (see Risk Factors for Adults—HIV/AIDS).

Q What kind of birth control method do you use, if any?

R Vasectomy for permanent birth control results in a decreased amount of ejaculate, which concerns some men. Vasectomy affords no protection from STDs. The only type of temporary birth control method for men is the male condom. Failure to use condoms increases the client's risk for contracting and transmitting STDs and HIV and increases the female partner's risk of becoming pregnant.

Q Are you currently exposed to chemicals or radiation? Have you been exposed in the past?

R Exposure to radiation and certain chemicals increases the risk of developing cancer.

Q Describe the activity you perform in a typical day. Do you do any heavy lifting?

R Strenuous activity and heavy lifting may predispose the client to development of an inguinal hernia.

Q Are you satisfied with your current level of activity and sexual functioning?

R Pain or heaviness due to hernias may limit the ability to work or perform regular exercise. Infection may limit a client's ability to engage in sexual activity. An erectile dysfunction impedes sexual intercourse. Incontinence may affect the client's ability to work or engage in social activities.

Q Do you have concerns about fertility? If you experience fertility troubles, how has this affected your relationship?

R Concerns about fertility can increase stress and can have a negative impact on relationships.

Q What is your sexual preference?

R An awareness of the client's sexual preference allows the examiner to focus the examination. Acceptance of a client's sexual preference helps to put the client at ease. Therefore, the client will be more likely to talk about his special health issues or fears.

Q Do you have any fears related to sex? Can you identify any stress in your current relationship that relates to sex?

R Fear can cause inhibition and decrease sexual satisfaction. Stress can prevent satisfactory sexual performance.

Q Do you feel comfortable communicating with your partner about your sexual likes and dislikes?

R Lack of open communication can cause problems with relationships and lead to feelings of guilt and depression.

Q What do you know about STDs and their prevention?

R The client's knowledge of STDs and their prevention provides a basis for health education in this area.

RISK FACTORS
Adults—HIV/AIDS

OVERVIEW

The World Health Organization (WHO, 2000) reports that, by the end of 1999, 34.3 million adults and children are living with HIV/AIDS; in 1999, there were 5.4 million people infected with HIV, and 2.8 million deaths from AIDS. Since the epidemic began, there have been 18.8 million AIDS deaths worldwide.

In the United States, the Centers for Disease Control and Prevention (CDC, 2000) notes that the highest incidence of HIV occurs in men who have sex with men (MSM). The next highest group affected are intravenous drug users, especially in the Northeast. However, incidence patterns are changing as more heterosexuals, women, and children are affected.

The CDC (2000) reports some slowing of the rate of increase in the incidence of HIV infection throughout the United States. The rate dropped in males by 8% between 1995 and 1996, mostly due to a slowing of the rate for white gay men. The rate for women increased steadily until 1994, but has slowed to a 1% increase from 1995 to 1996. The rates of increase for intravenous drug users and for heterosexuals have slowed as well. Education and treatment are credited with the slowing rates in the United States.

According to microbiologist Dr. Christina Frazier (Southeast Missouri State University), the reduced incidence of HIV infection in older homosexual males is attributed to a combination of education on risk factors and safer sexual practices and personal experience of at least three friends' deaths due to AIDS. Younger homosexual men who have not had the experience of so many friends dying are not following the safer practices, and a serious increase in infection is expected to begin.

RISK FACTORS

- Anal intercourse (especially men having sex with men—MSM)
- Intravenous drug use (especially among people who share needles)
- Heterosexual transmission: having multiple sexual partners, bisexual partners, or partner who uses intravenous drugs (sex with any infected partner)

RISK REDUCTION TEACHING TIPS

Use precautions to decrease transfer of bodily fluids:
- Practice sexual abstinence
- Use condoms
- Double glove when handling sharp objects
- Single glove when handling bodily secretions or objects that touch bodily secretions
- Follow guidelines for safe handling of contaminated items

Avoid other high-risk behaviors, such as:
- Intravenous drug use (especially sharing needles)
- Sex with multiple partners
- Mixing sex and alcohol or drugs
- Anal intercourse

Openly discuss HIV risk behavior history with partner and use above precautions.

 ## CULTURAL CONSIDERATIONS

As in the United States, heterosexual transmission of HIV is increasing steadily and is the predominant mode of transmission throughout the developing world (Chin, 2000). Sub-Saharan Africa has continued to have the highest levels of HIV infection and AIDS cases with 24.5 million persons living with HIV/AIDS at the end of 1999 (WHO, 2000). Only a few other areas of the world have high HIV prevalence rates, defined as more than 1% of the population between ages 15 and 49, including a few countries of the Caribbean and southern and southeastern Asia (Chin, 2000).

Mukhopadhyay (1996) noted that a majority of AIDS cases in the United States were in Caucasians, except in the Northeast and Mid-Atlantic, where the largest percentage was in African Americans. Hispanic cases accounted for over one fifth of the cases in the Northeast and South. According to the CDC (2000), in the United States, the highest overall rates are in the South, followed by the Northeast, Midwest, and West. The highest rates are in males between ages 25 and 44 years of age. The rate is increasing in African Americans partially due to a decrease in the rate for Caucasian gay males. By 1996, however, the rate increase leveled off to 0% rate of increase in African Americans, 5% decline in Hispanics, and 4% decline in Asians and Native Americans.

Q Do you perform testicular self-examinations?

R Male clients who do not perform testicular self-examinations need to be informed about the connection between self-examination and early interventions for abnormalities.

Q When was the last time you performed this examination?

R Male clients should be aware of the need for a monthly testicular self-examination and its importance in the early diagnosis and treatment of testicular cancer.

Collecting Objective Data

The purpose of examining the male genitalia is to detect abnormalities that may range from life-threatening diseases to painful conditions that interfere with normal function. Abnormalities should be detected as early as possible so the client can be referred for further testing or treatment. The physical assessment is also a good time to allow the client to demonstrate the proper techniques for testicular self-examination and to provide teaching if necessary.

The hands-on physical examination of the male genitalia may create anxiety, embarrassment, and nervousness about exposing the genitals and about what might be discovered. Ease client anxiety by explaining in detail what is going to occur and by explaining the significance of each portion of the examination while you are performing it. Also, attempt to expose only those areas necessary at that point in the examination. This will help preserve the client's modesty. It is also helpful to encourage the client to ask questions during the examination.

 Tip From the Experts Examiners and the client are often worried that the male client will have an erection during the hands-on examination. Usually, the client is too nervous for this to occur. If it does occur, reassure the client that it is not unusual and continue the examination in an unhurried and unflappable manner.

CLIENT PREPARATION

Before the examination, instruct the client to empty his bladder so he will be comfortable. If a urine specimen is necessary, provide the client with a container. If the client is not wearing an examination gown for a total physical examination, provide a drape and ask him to lower his pants and underwear. Explain to the client that he will be asked to stand (if able) for most of the examination.

EQUIPMENT AND SUPPLIES

* Stool
* Gown
* Disposable gloves

Tip From the Experts Wear gloves for every step of the male genitalia examination.

* Flashlight (for possible transillumination)
* Stethoscope (for possible auscultation)

KEY ASSESSMENT POINTS

* Wear disposable gloves.
* Preserve client's privacy.
* Inspect and palpate penis, scrotum, and inguinal area for inflammation, infestations, rashes, lesions, and lumps.
* If helpful, distract the client during the examination by describing the importance of testicular self-examination and explaining how to perform the examination as you are performing it.

(text continues on page 423)

PHYSICAL ASSESSMENT

ASSESSMENT PROCEDURE	NORMAL FINDINGS	ABNORMAL FINDINGS

PENIS

Inspect the Base and Pubic Hair

Sit on a stool with the client facing you and standing. Ask the client to raise his gown or drape. Note pubic hair growth pattern and any excoriation, erythema, or infestation at the base of the penis and within the pubic hair.

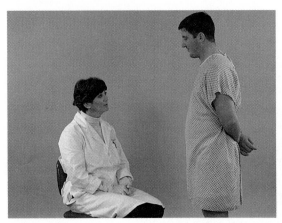

In positioning the male client for a genital examination, the examiner sits and the client stands. (© B. Proud.)

The normal pubic hair pattern in adults is hair covering the entire groin area, extending to the medial thighs and up the abdomen toward the umbilicus. The base of the penis and the pubic hair are free of excoriation, erythema, and infestation (Table 19-1).

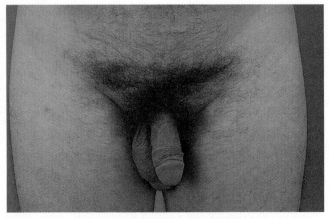

Normal appearance of external male genitalia. (© B. Proud.)

Absence or scarcity of pubic hair may be seen in clients receiving chemotherapy. Lice or nit (eggs) infestation at the base of the penis or pubic hair is known as pediculosis pubis. This is commonly referred to as "crabs."

👓 Pubic hair may be gray and sparse in elderly clients. In addition, the penis becomes smaller and the testes hang lower in the scrotum in elderly clients.

Inspect the Skin of the Shaft

Observe for rashes, lesions, or lumps.

The skin of the penis is normally free of rashes, lesions, or lumps.

👥 Pubertal rites in some cultures include slitting the penile shaft, leaving an opening that may extend the entire length of the shaft (DeMeo, 1989).

Rashes, lesions, or lumps may indicate STD or cancer (Display 19-1).

Palpate the Shaft

Palpate any abnormalities noted during inspection. Also note any hardened or tender areas.

The penis in a nonerect state is usually soft, flaccid, and nontender.

Hardness along the ventral surface may indicate cancer or a urethral stricture. Tenderness may indicate inflammation or infection.

(continued)

ASSESSMENT PROCEDURE	NORMAL FINDINGS	ABNORMAL FINDINGS
Inspect the Foreskin		
Observe for color, location, and integrity of the foreskin in uncircumcised men.	The foreskin, which covers the glans in an uncircumcised male client, is intact and uniform in color with the penis.	Discoloration of the foreskin may indicate scarring or infection.
Inspect the Glans		
Observe for size, shape, and lesions or redness.	The glans size and shape vary, appearing rounded, broad, or even pointed. It is normally free of lesions and redness.	Chancres (red, oval ulcerations) from syphilis, venereal warts, and pimplelike lesions from herpes are sometimes detected on the glans.

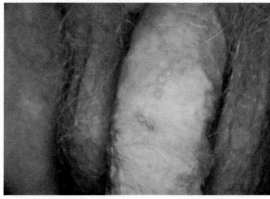

Genital herpes. (Courtesy of Dermik Laboratories, Inc.)

If the client is not circumcised, ask him to retract his foreskin to allow observation of the glans.	The foreskin retracts easily. A small amount of whitish material, called smegma, normally accumulates under the foreskin.	A tight foreskin that cannot be retracted is called *phimosis*. A foreskin that once retracted cannot be returned to cover the glans is called *paraphimosis*. Chancres (red, oval ulcerations) from syphilis and venereal warts are sometimes detected under the foreskin (see Display 19-1).
Note the location of the urinary meatus on the glans	The urinary meatus is normally found in the center of the glans.

👪 If pubertal mutilation has occurred, actual discharge of urine and semen will occur at the location of the shaft opening. | *Hypospadias* is displacement of the urinary meatus to the ventral surface of the penis. *Epispadias* is displacement of the urinary meatus to the dorsal surface of the penis (see Display 19-1). |

(continued)

ASSESSMENT PROCEDURE	NORMAL FINDINGS	ABNORMAL FINDINGS

Palpate for Urethral Discharge

Gently squeeze the glans between the index finger and thumb.

The urinary meatus is normally free of discharge.

A yellow discharge is usually associated with gonorrhea. A clear or white discharge is usually associated with urethritis. All discharge should be cultured.

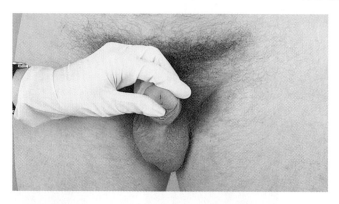

Palpating for urethral discharge. (© B. Proud.)

SCROTUM

Inspect the Size, Shape, and Position

Ask the client to hold his penis out of the way. Observe for swelling, lumps, or bulges.

The scrotum varies in size (according to temperature) and shape. The scrotal sac hangs below or at the level of the penis. The left side of the scrotal sac usually hangs lower than the right side.

An enlarged scrotal sac may result from fluid (hydrocele), blood (hematocele), bowel (hernia), or tumor (cancer) (Display 19-2).

Inspect the Scrotal Skin

Observe color, integrity, and lesions or rashes. To perform an accurate inspection, you must spread out the scrotal folds (rugae) of skin. Lift the scrotal sac to inspect the posterior skin.

Scrotal skin is thin and rugated (crinkled) with little hair dispersion. Its color is slightly darker than that of the penis. Lesions and rashes are not normally present. However, sebaceous cysts (small, yellowish, firm, nontender, benign nodules) are a normal finding.

Rashes, lesions, and inflammation are abnormal findings.

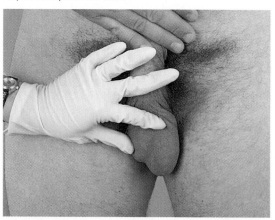

When inspecting the scrotal skin, have the client hold the penis aside while the examiner inspects. (© B. Proud.)

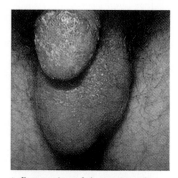

Inflammation of the penis and scrotum may be seen in Reiter's syndrome, an idiopathic inflammatory disorder affecting the skin, joints, and mucous membranes. (With permission from Goodheart, H. P. [1999]. *A photoguide of common skin disorders.* **Baltimore: Lippincott Williams & Wilkins.)**

(continued)

ASSESSMENT PROCEDURE	NORMAL FINDINGS	ABNORMAL FINDINGS

Palpate the Scrotal Contents

Palpate each *testis* and *epididymis* between your thumb and first two fingers. Note size, shape, consistency, nodules, and tenderness.

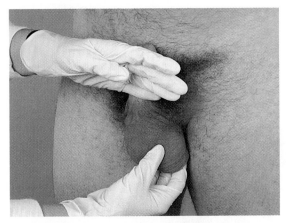

Palpating the scrotal contents. (© B Proud.)

Testes are ovoid, approximately 3.5 to 5 cm long, 2.5 cm wide, and 2.5 cm deep, and equal bilaterally in size and shape. They are smooth, firm, rubbery, mobile, free of nodules, and rather tender to pressure. The epididymis is nontender, smooth, and softer than the testes.

 Testes do not get smaller with normal aging although they may decrease in size with long-term illness.

Absence of a testis suggests *cryptorchidism* (an undescended testicle). Painless nodules may indicate cancer. Tenderness and swelling may indicate acute orchitis, torsion of the spermatic cord, a strangulated hernia, or epididymitis (see Display 19-2). If the client has epididymitis, passive elevation of the testes may relieve the scrotal pain (Prehn's sign). If the client has a strangulated hernia, the client should be referred immediately to the physician and prepared for surgery.

Tip From the Experts   Do not apply too much pressure to the testes because this will cause pain.

Palpate each *spermatic cord* and vas deferens from the epididymis to the inguinal ring. The spermatic cord will lie between your thumb and finger. Note any nodules, swelling, or tenderness.

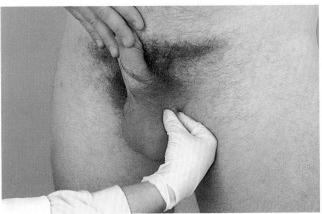

When palpating the spermatic cord, have the client continue to hold the penis aside while the examiner palpates. (© B. Proud.)

The spermatic cord and vas deferens should feel uniform on both sides. The cord is smooth, nontender, and ropelike.

Palpable, tortuous veins suggest varicocele. A beaded or thickened cord indicates infection or cysts. If you palpate a scrotal mass, have the client lie down. The mass may return to the abdomen by itself. If it does not, place your fingers above the scrotal mass. If you can get your fingers above the mass, suspect hydrocele (see Display 19-2). Cyst suggests hydrocele of the spermatic cord.

Continue the examination of a scrotal mass by auscultating with a stethoscope.

Normal findings are not expected.

Bowel sounds may be auscultated over a hernia, but will not be heard over a hydrocele.

Transilluminate the Scrotal Contents

If an abnormal mass or swelling was noted in the scrotum, transillumination should be performed. Darken the room and shine a light from the back of the scrotum through the mass. Look for a red glow.

Normally, scrotal contents do not transilluminate.

Swellings or masses that contain serous fluid—hydrocele, spermatocele—light up with a red glow. Swellings or masses that are solid or filled with blood—tumor, hernias, or varicocele—do not light up with a red glow.

(continued)

ASSESSMENT PROCEDURE	NORMAL FINDINGS	ABNORMAL FINDINGS

INGUINAL AREA

Inspect for Inguinal and Femoral Hernia

Inspect the inguinal and femoral areas for bulges. Ask the client to bear down, and continue to inspect the areas.

The inguinal and femoral areas are normally free from bulges.

Bulges that appear at the external inguinal ring or at the femoral canal when the client bears down may signal a hernia (Display 19-3).

Palpate for Inguinal Hernia and Inguinal Nodes

Ask the client to shift his weight to the left for palpation of the right inguinal canal and vice versa. Place your right index finger into the client's right scrotum and press upward, invaginating the loose folds of skin. Palpate up the spermatic cord until you reach the triangular-shaped, slitlike opening of the external inguinal ring. Try to push your finger through the opening and, if possible, continue palpating up the inguinal canal. When your finger is in the canal or at the external inguinal ring, ask the client to bear down or cough. Feel for any bulges against your finger. Then, repeat the procedure on the opposite side.

Bulging or masses are not normally palpated.

A bulge or mass may indicate a hernia.

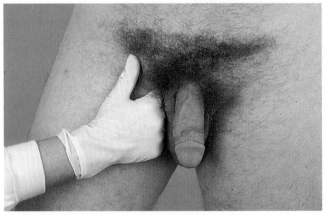

Palpating for an inguinal hernia. (© B. Proud.)

Palpate inguinal lymph nodes.

No enlargement or tenderness is normal.

Enlarged or tender nodes may indicate an inflammatory process or lesion on the penis or scrotum.

Palpate for Femoral Hernia

Palpate on the front of the thigh in the femoral canal area. Ask the client to bear down or cough. Feel for bulges. Repeat on the opposite thigh.

Bulges or masses are not normally palpated.

A bulge or mass may be from a hernia.

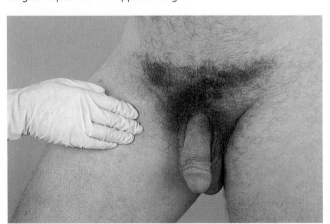

Palpating for a femoral hernia. (© B. Proud.)

(continued)

ASSESSMENT PROCEDURE	NORMAL FINDINGS	ABNORMAL FINDINGS

Inspect and Palpate for Scrotal Hernia

If you discovered a mass during inspection and palpation of the scrotum and you suspect it may be a hernia, ask the client to lie down; note whether the bulge disappears. If the bulge remains, auscultate it for bowel sounds. Finally, gently palpate the mass and try to push it upward into the abdomen.

If the bulge disappears, no scrotal hernia is present, but the mass may result from something else and the client should be referred for further evaluation.

If the bulge disappears when the client lies down, a scrotal hernia is present. Bowel sounds auscultated over the mass indicate the presence of bowel and thus a scrotal hernia. If you cannot push the mass into the abdomen, suspect an *incarcerated hernia*. A hernia is *strangulated* when its blood supply is cut off. The client typically complains of extreme tenderness and nausea (see Display 19-3).

Tip From the Experts If the client complains of extreme tenderness or nausea, do not try to push the mass up into the abdomen.

Validation and Documentation of Findings

Validate the male genitalia assessment data that you have collected. This is necessary to verify that the data are reliable and accurate. Document the assessment data in accord with the health care facility or agency policy.

EXAMPLE OF SUBJECTIVE DATA

A 35-year-old male military officer reports no current pain, lesions, discharge from penis, swelling, lumps, or heavy feeling in scrotum. States no difficulty urinating; no change in color, amount, or odor of urine; no pain when urinating; no urinary incontinence. Reports no change in sexual activity or desire, no current difficulty in attaining or maintaining an erection, and no difficulty ejaculating. Is not aware of any fertility problem. Client reports history of a right inguinal hernia 4 years ago that was surgically repaired with no complications. Last testicular examination was 3 years ago. Is tested for HIV annually as part of his military physical requirements. Reports negative results.

No family history of cancer. Client states he is currently sexually monogamous with his fiancée and he uses condoms as a backup birth control method. Denies exposure to chemicals and is very careful when he has to lift heavy items. He reports he is sexually satisfied and can talk to his fiancée about anything. He performs monthly testicular self-examinations.

EXAMPLE OF OBJECTIVE DATA

Pubic hair growth pattern is normal for adult male; pubic hair and base of penis are free of excoriation and infestation. Circumcised penis is free of rashes, lesions, and lumps and is soft, flaccid, and nontender on palpation. Glans is rounded and free of lesions; urinary meatus is centrally located on glans; no discharge is palpated from urinary meatus. No masses or swelling noted in scrotum, and left side hangs slightly lower than right side. Skin is free of lesions and appears rugated and darkly pigmented. Two descended testes palpated. No swelling, tenderness, or masses palpated along the testicle, epididymis, or spermatic cord on either side. No bulges or masses palpated in inguinal or femoral canal.

TABLE 19-1. **Tanner's Sexual Maturity Rating for Boys**			
Stage	**Pubic Hair**	**Penis**	**Testes and Scrotum**
1 (preadolescent)	None, except for fine body hair	Same size and proportions as in childhood	
2	Sparse growth, slightly curly	Slight or no enlargement	Both larger, reddened, exhibiting textural changes
3	Darker, coarse, curly, sparse hair over symphysis pubis	Larger, longer	Further enlargement
4	Coarse, curly hair that does not extend to medial thighs	Increased length and width	Further enlargement and scrotal skin darkens
5	Adult hair in texture and quantity extends to medial aspect of thighs	Adult size and shape	

Adapted from Tanner, 1962. *Growth at adolescence.* [2nd ed.]. Oxford: Blackwell Scientific Publications.

DISPLAY 19-1. Abnormalities of the Penis

ABNORMAL
FINDINGS

Some of the most common abnormalities detected during a penile assessment are those
that are featured below.

SYPHILITIC CHANCRE

- Initially, a small, silvery-white papule that develops
  a red oval ulceration
- Painless
- This chancre, which is the sign of primary syphilis, a sexually transmitted disease (STD), spontaneously regresses.

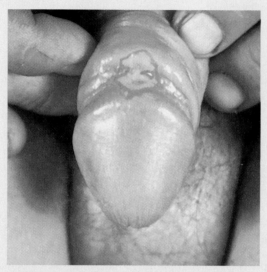

Syphilitic chancre. (Courtesy of UpJohn Co.)

HERPES PROGENITALIS

- Pictured in "Inspect the Glans"
- Clusters of pimplelike, clear vesicles that erupt and become ulcers
- Painful
- The initial lesions of this STD, typically caused by HSV-1 or HSV-2, disappear, and the infection
  remains dormant for varying periods of time. Recurrences can be frequent or minimally
  episodic.

GENITAL WARTS

- Single or multiple, moist, fleshy papules
- Painless
- STD caused by the human papillomavirus.

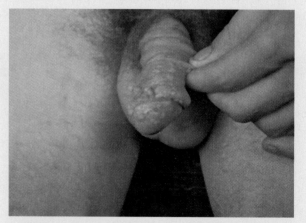

Genital warts. (Courtesy of Reed & Carnick Pharmaceuticals.)

(continued)

CANCER OF THE GLANS PENIS

- Appears as hardened nodule or ulcer on the glans
- Painless
- Occurs primarily in noncircumcised men

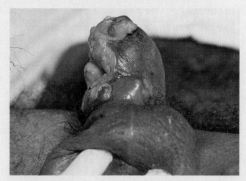

Penile carcinoma. (© 1993. Jennifer Watson-Holton/ Custom Medical Stock Photo.)

PHIMOSIS

Foreskin is so tight that it cannot be retracted over the glans.

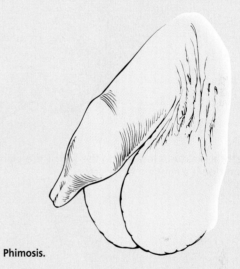

Phimosis.

PARAPHIMOSIS

Foreskin is so tight that, once retracted, it cannot be returned back over the glans.

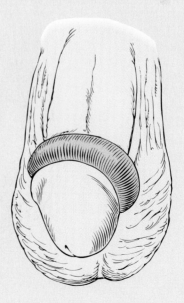

Paraphimosis.

(continued)

DISPLAY 19-1. Abnormalities of the Penis (Continued)

HYPOSPADIAS

- The urethral meatus is located underneath the glans (ventral side).
- This condition is a congenital defect.
- A groove extends from the meatus to the normal location of the urethral meatus.

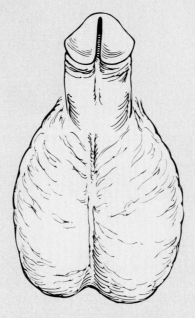

Hypospadias.

EPISPADIAS

- The urethral meatus is located on the top of the glans (dorsal side); occurs rarely.
- This condition is a congenital defect.

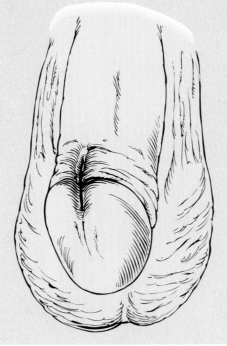

Epispadias.

DISPLAY 19-2. Abnormalities in the Scrotum

ABNORMAL
FINDINGS

Although some scrotal abnormalities can be seen by visual inspection, most must be palpated. Some common abnormalities are described below.

HYDROCELE

Collection of serous fluid in the scrotum, outside the testes within the tunica vaginalis. It appears as swelling in the scrotum and is usually painless. Usually, the examiner can get fingers above this mass during palpation.

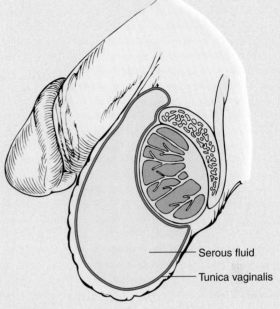

Serous fluid

Tunica vaginalis

Hydrocele.

SCROTAL HERNIA

In scrotal hernia, a loop of bowel protrudes into the scrotum to create what is known as an indirect inguinal hernia. The hernia appears as swelling in the scrotum, it is palpable as a soft mass, and fingers cannot get above the mass.

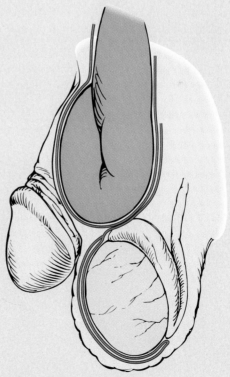

Scrotal hernia.

(continued)

TESTICULAR TUMOR

Initially, this is a small, firm, nontender nodule on the testis. As the tumor grows, the scrotum appears enlarged and the client complains of a heavy feeling. When palpated, the testis feels enlarged and smooth—tumor replaces testis.

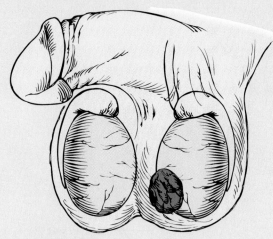

Early testicular tumor.

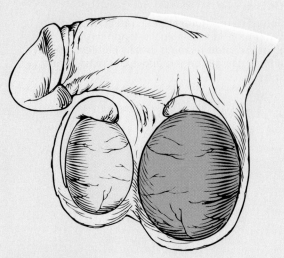

Late testicular tumor.

CRYPTORCHIDISM

Failure of one or both testicles to descend into scrotum. Scrotum appears undeveloped, and testis cannot be palpated.

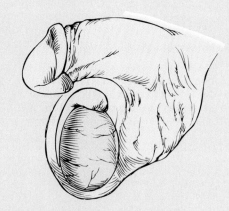

Cryptorchidism.

EPIDIDYMITIS

Infection of the epididymis. Client usually complains of sudden pain. Scrotum appears enlarged, reddened, and swollen; tender epididymis is palpated. Usually associated with prostatitis or bacterial infection.

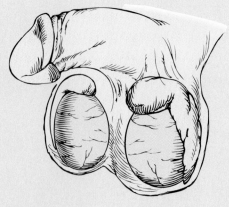

Epididymitis.

(continued)

ORCHITIS

Inflammation of the testes, associated frequently with mumps. Client complains of pain, heaviness, and fever. Scrotum appears enlarged and reddened. Swollen, tender testis is palpated. The examiner may have difficulty differentiating between testis and epididymis.

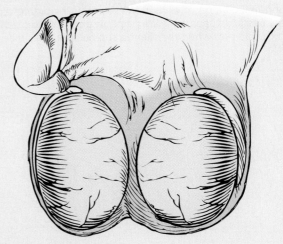

Orchitis.

SMALL TESTES

Small, soft testes (less than 3.5 cm long) indicate atrophy. Atrophy may result from cirrhosis, hypopituitarism, estrogen administration, extended illness, or the disorder may occur after orchitis. Small, firm testes may indicate Klinefelter's syndrome.

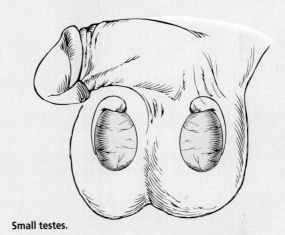

Small testes.

TORSION OF SPERMATIC CORD

This very painful condition is caused by twisting of spermatic cord. Scrotum appears enlarged and reddened. Palpation reveals thickened cord and swollen, tender testis that may be higher in scrotum than normal. This condition requires immediate referral for surgery because circulation is obstructed.

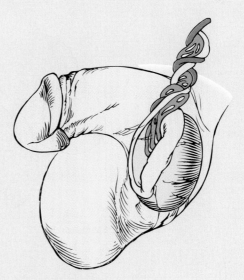

Torsion of spermatic cord.

(continued)

VARICOCELE

Abnormal dilation of veins in the spermatic cord. Client may complain of discomfort and testicular heaviness. Tortuous veins are palpable and feel like a soft, irregular mass or "a bag of worms," which collapses when the client is supine. Infertility may be associated with this condition.

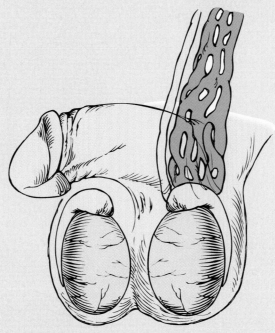

Varicocele.

SPERMATOCELE

Sperm-filled cystic mass located on epididymis. Palpable as small and nontender, and movable above the testis. This mass will appear on transillumination.

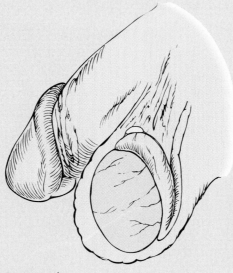

Spermatocele.

DISPLAY 19-3. Inguinal and Femoral Hernias

ABNORMAL
FINDINGS

INDIRECT INGUINAL HERNIA

Bowel herniates through internal inguinal ring and remains in the inguinal canal or travels down into the scrotum (scrotal hernia). This is the most common type of hernia. It may occur in adults but is more frequent in children.

DIRECT INGUINAL HERNIA

Bowel herniates from behind and through the external inguinal ring. It rarely travels down into the scrotum. This type of hernia is less common than an indirect hernia. It occurs mostly in adult men older than age 40.

FEMORAL HERNIA

Bowel herniates through the femoral ring and canal. It never travels into the scrotum, and the inguinal canal is empty. This is the least common type of hernia. It occurs mostly in women.

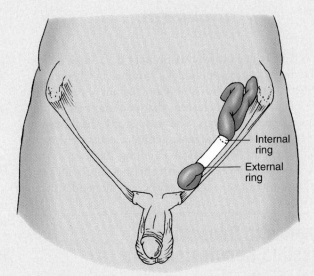

Indirect inguinal hernia.

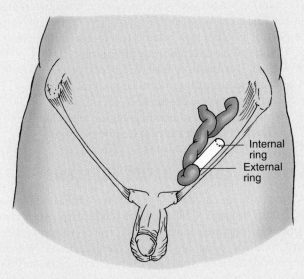

Direct inguinal hernia.

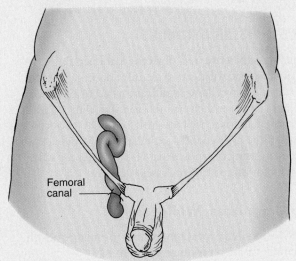

Femoral hernia.

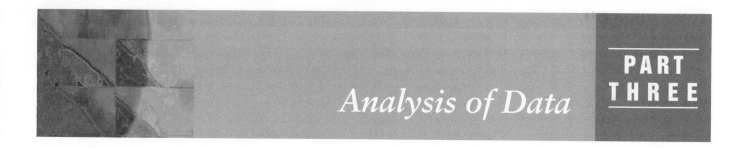

After you have collected your assessment data, analyze the data using diagnostic reasoning skills (outlined in Chapter 7). Diagnostic Reasoning: Possible Conclusions presents an overview of common conclusions that you may reach after a male genitalia assessment. The case study that follows teaches you how to analyze male genitalia assessment data for a specific client. The Critical Thinking Exercise in the laboratory manual developed with this book provides an opportunity to work through the process independently.

Diagnostic Reasoning: Possible Conclusions

Listed below are some possible conclusions after assessment of the male client's genitalia.

SELECTED NURSING DIAGNOSES

After collecting subjective and objective data pertaining to the male genitalia, you will need to identify abnormalities and cluster the data to reveal any significant patterns or abnormalities. These data can then be used to make clinical judgments (nursing diagnoses: wellness, risk, or actual) about the health status of the male client's genitalia. Following is a listing of selected nursing diagnoses that you may identify when analyzing data for this part of the assessment.

Nursing Diagnoses (Wellness)

- Health-Seeking Behavior: Opportunity to enhance health management of the reproductive system
- Health-Seeking Behavior: Requests information on testicular self-examination (TSE)
- Health-Seeking Behavior: Requests information on ways to prevent an STD
- Health-Seeking Behavior: Requests information on birth control
- Health-Seeking Behavior: Requests information on proper lifting techniques to prevent hernia formation

Nursing Diagnoses (Risk)

- Risk for Ineffective Therapeutic Regimen Management (monthly testicular self-examination, TSE) related to lack of knowledge of the importance of TSE
- Risk for Injury related to poor lifting techniques
- Risk for Infection related to unprotected sexual intercourse
- Risk for Ineffective Sexuality Patterns related to impending surgery

Nursing Diagnoses (Actual)

- Fear of testicular cancer related to existing risk factors
- Disturbed Body Image related to hernia repair
- Pain: Dysuria related to gonorrhea, infection, or genital reproductive surgery
- Ineffective Therapeutic Regimen Management related to lack of knowledge of testicular self-examination
- Sexual Dysfunction related to decreased libido secondary to fear of urinary incontinence, pain in surgical site, anxiety, or fear
- Sexual Dysfunction related to erectile dysfunction secondary to psychological or physiologic factors
- Sexual Dysfunction related to lack of ejaculation secondary to surgical removal of seminal vesicles and transection of the vas deferens
- Anxiety related to impending genital reproductive surgery and lack of knowledge of outcome of surgery

SELECTED COLLABORATIVE PROBLEMS

After grouping the data, you may see certain collaborative problems emerge. Collaborative problems cannot be prevented by nursing interventions. However, you can detect and monitor these physiologic complications of medical conditions. In addition, you can use physician- and nurse-prescribed interventions to minimize the complications of these problems. You may also have to refer the client in such situations for further treatment of the problem. Following is a list of collaborative problems that may be identified when assessing the male genitalia. These problems are worded as Potential Complications (PC), followed by the problem.

- PC: Gonorrhea
- PC: Syphilis
- PC: Genital warts
- PC: Erectile dysfunction
- PC: Inability to ejaculate
- PC: Hernia
- PC: Hemorrhage

- PC: Urinary incontinence
- PC: Urinary retention

MEDICAL PROBLEMS

After grouping the data, you may realize that the client has signs and symptoms that may require medical diagnosis and

treatment. In such cases, referral to a primary care provider is necessary.

- Fear of erectile dysfunction related to upcoming surgery
- Grieving related to erectile dysfunction
- Disturbed Body Image related to impaired sexual functioning

Diagnostic Reasoning: Case Study

The case study presents assessment data for a specific client. It is followed by an analysis of the data, working out the seven key steps to arrive at specific conclusions.

Carl Weeks is a 72-year-old man who has been receiving follow-up care by the home care nurse since his discharge from the hospital 3 weeks ago, during which he was treated for a diabetic coma. His diabetic status is currently stable, but he complains to the home health nurse that he is having problems with urination. He states that he is "peeing often in little dribbles," has difficulty maintaining his urinary stream, and wakes up three or four times a night to void. His wife, Marie, states that neither of them is getting much sleep. She asks how she can help her husband with this problem. Mr. Weeks also reports that for the last 2 days he has had discomfort in his bladder and burning with urination. Mrs. Weeks tells the nurse that he won't drink water and he can't have fruit juice because of his diabetes (she has heard that cranberry juice may help prevent urinary problems). On physical examination, distention is noted in the suprapubic area about 5 cm above the symphysis pubis, which is slightly tender to palpation, and a distinct area of dullness is noted in the same area. Mr. Weeks' vital signs and blood glucose level are within normal limits, but his temperature is 99.2°F.

1 Identify abnormal data and strengths (in both subjective and objective data).

SUBJECTIVE DATA

- Problems with urination
- "Peeing in little dribbles"
- Has difficulty maintaining urinary stream
- Discomfort in bladder
- Burning with urination
- Up three and four times a night to void
- Neither he nor wife is getting much sleep
- Wife asks how to help her husband with this problem
- Mr. Weeks won't drink water
- Can't have fruit juice because of diabetes
- Wife believes that cranberry juice may prevent urinary problems

OBJECTIVE DATA

- Diabetes stable at this time
- Suprapubic distention 5 cm above the symphysis pubis
- Slight suprapubic tenderness to palpation
- Distinct suprapubic dullness on percussion
- Vital signs, blood glucose level within normal limits
- Temperature 99.2°F

2 Cue Clusters	**3** Inferences	**4** Possible Nursing Diagnoses	**5** Defining Characteristics	**6** Confirm or Rule Out
A • "Peeing often in little dribbles" • Has difficulty maintaining his stream • Up three and four times a night to void • Suprapubic distention 5 cm above the symphysis pubis • Distinct suprapubic dullness on percussion	Not emptying bladder with each void; just voiding the overflow. Could be secondary to diabetic autonomic neuropathy. Monitor for collaborative problems. Could also be enlarged prostate—further assessment needed, and referral to physician.			

2 Cue Clusters	3 Inferences	4 Possible Nursing Diagnoses	5 Defining Characteristics	6 Confirm or Rule Out
B • Discomfort in bladder • Burning with urination • Slight suprapubic tenderness to palpation • Temperature 99.2°F • Does not drink water or cranberry juice	Beginning infection due to retained urine. Unhealthy habit of not drinking water to decrease risk factors	Risk for Infection related to inadequate fluid intake and inability to empty bladder with each void secondary to possible diabetic autonomic neuropathy or possible prostate enlargement.	*Major:* risk factors such as diabetes (increased sugar in urine), retaining urine in bladder, not drinking water or acidic-ash fruit juices	Confirm
		Ineffective Health Maintenance related to lack of behaviors to protect against bladder infection	*Major:* Demonstrates unhealthful practices *Minor:* None	Confirm
C • Up three and four times a night to void • Neither he nor wife is getting much sleep	Bladder problem is interfering with a full night's rest, which could further impair immune response and increase infection risk.	Disturbed Sleep Pattern related to frequent awakenings secondary to frequency of voiding and bladder discomfort	*Major:* Difficulty remaining asleep *Minor:* Not verbalized, but implied fatigue of both client and wife	Confirm because it meets the major and minor defining characteristics.
D • Wife asks how she can help her husband with this problem • Wife knows that cranberry juice could prevent urinary problems • Diabetes stable at this time	Wife seeking additional information to manage/prevent client's health problems and promote improved health.	Health-Seeking Behaviors: wife requesting information to help promote husband's health.	*Major:* Expressed desire to seek information for health promotion *Minor:* Expressed concern about current conditions or health status	Confirm because it meets the major and minor defining characteristics.

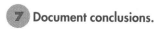

7 Document conclusions.

Four diagnoses are appropriate for Mr. and Mrs. Weeks at this time:

- Risk for Infection related to inadequate fluid intake and inability to empty bladder with each void secondary to possible diabetic autonomic neuropathy or prostate enlargement
- Ineffective Health Maintenance related to lack of behaviors to protect against bladder infection
- Disturbed Sleep Pattern related to frequent awakenings secondary to frequency of voiding and discomfort
- Health-Seeking Behaviors: Wife seeks information regarding urinary problem interfering with sleep

Collaborative problems related to the medical diagnoses could include:

- PC: Kidney infection
- PC: Hydronephrosis
- PC: Ruptured bladder
- PC: Renal failure
- PC: Sepsis
- PC: Urethral obstruction

Mr. Weeks should be referred to his physician for evaluation and management of causes of urinary retention and of infection.

REFERENCES AND SELECTED READINGS

Adelman, W. P., & Joffe, A. (1999). The adolescent male genital examination: What's normal and what's not. *Contemporary Pediatrics, 16*(7), 76–78, 80, 85–86.

Altman, C. E., Hamill, R., & Pujals, J. (1999). Multiple cutaneous granular cell tumors of the scrotum. *Cutis, 63*(2), 77–80.

Cline, K. J., Mata, J. A., Venable, D. D., & Eastham, J. A. (1998). Penetrating trauma to the male external genitalia. *Journal of Trauma: Injury, Infection, and Critical Care, 44*(3), 492–494.

Coley, C. M., Barry, M. J., Fleming, C., Fahs, M. C., & Mulley, A. G. (1997). Early detection of prostate cancer. Part II: Estimating the risks, benefits, and costs. *Annals of Internal Medicine, 126*(6), 468–479.

DeMeo, J. (1989). *The geography of genital mutilation.* Paper presented at the First Symposium on Circumcision. Available: www. NOHAMM.ORG/geography.htm.

Dorey, G. (2000). Clinical. Male patients with lower urinary tract symptoms 1: Assessment. *British Journal of Nursing, 9*(8), 497–501.

Galejs, L. E., & Kass, E. J. (1999). Diagnosis and treatment of the acute scrotum. *American Family Physician, 59*(4), 817–824.

Geyer, N., & Laude, S. (1997). Continuing education—clinical. Genital assessment: Male. *Nursing News (South Africa), 21*(5), 46–47.

———. (1997). Genital self-examination for men. *Nursing News (South Africa), 21*(9), 54.

Junnila, J., & Lassen, P. (1998). Testicular masses. *American Family Physician, 57*(4), 685–692.

Karakiewicz, P. I., & Aprikian, A. G. (1998). Prostate cancer: 5. Diagnostic tools for early detection. *Canadian Medical Association Journal, 159*(9), 1139–1146.

Klingman, L. (1999). Assessing the male genitalia. *American Journal of Nursing, 99*(7), 47–50.

Nehal, K. S., Levine, V. J., & Ashinoff, R. (1998). Basal cell carcinoma of the genitalia. *Dermatologic Surgery, 24*(12), 1361–1363.

Peate, I. (1998). Clinical. Cancer of the prostate 2: The nursing role in health promotion. *British Journal of Nursing, 7*(4), 196, 198–200.

Ross, J. H., Kay, R., Yetman, R. J., & Angermeier, K. (1998). Primary lymphedema of the genitalia in children and adolescents. *Journal of Urology, 160*(4), 1485–1489.

Schleicher, S. M. (2000). Diagnosis at a glance . . . red scrotum syndrome . . . molluscum contagiosum. *Emergency Medicine, 32*(2), 101–102.

Tanner, J. M. (1962). *Growth at adolescence* (2nd ed.). Oxford: Blackwell Scientific Publications.

Risk Factors—HIV/AIDS

Centers for Disease Control and Prevention (CDC). (2000). HIV/AIDS surveillance report. Available: www.cdc.gov/hiv/stats/hasrlink.htm.

Chin, J. (Ed.). (2000). *Control of communicable diseases manual* (17th ed.). Washington, DC: American Public Health Association.

World Health Organization (WHO). (2000, June). Report on the global HIV/AIDS epidemic. Available: www.unaids.org/epidemic_update/report/glo_estim.pdf.

For additional information on this book, be sure to visit http://connection.lww.com.

Female Genitalia Assessment

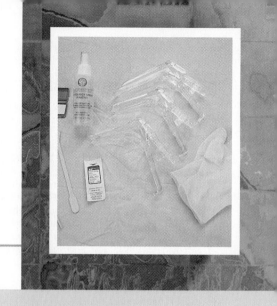

20

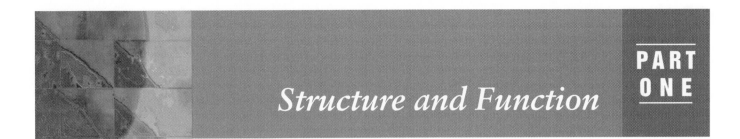

To perform an adequate assessment of the female genitalia, the nurse needs to have a basic understanding of the structure and function of the female reproductive system. This will guide the physical examination and readily assist in identifying abnormalities. The female genitalia consist of external structures and internal structures.

External Genitalia

The external genitalia include those structures that can be readily identified through inspection (Fig. 20-1). The area is sometimes referred to as the *vulva* or *pudendum* and extends from the mons pubis to the anal opening. The *mons pubis* is the fat pad located over the symphysis pubis. The normal adult mons pubis is covered with pubic hair in a triangular pattern. It functions to absorb force and to protect the symphysis pubis during coitus. The *labia majora* are two folds of skin that extend posteriorly and inferiorly from the mons pubis to the perineum. The skin folds are composed of adipose tissue, sebaceous glands, and sweat glands. The outer surface of the labia majora is covered with pubic hair in the adult, whereas the inner surface is pink, smooth, and moist.

Inside the labia majora are the thinner skin folds of the *labia minora*. These folds join anteriorly at the clitoris and form a *prepuce* or hood; posteriorly the two folds join to form the *frenulum*. Compared with the labia majora, the labia minora are usually darker pink. They contain numerous sebaceous glands that promote lubrication and maintain a moist environment in the vaginal area. The *clitoris* is located at the anterior end of the labia minora. It is a small, cylindrical mass of erectile tissue and nerves with three parts: the *glans*, the *corpus*, and the *crura*. The glans is the visible rounded portion of the clitoris. The corpus is the body, and the crura are two bands of fibrous tissue that attach the clitoris to the pelvic bone. The clitoris is similar to the male penis and contains many blood vessels that become engorged during sexual arousal.

The skin folds of the labia majora and labia minora form a boat-shaped area or fossa called the *vestibule*. Located between the clitoris and the vaginal orifice is the *urethral meatus*. The openings of *Skene's glands* are located on either side of the urethral opening. They are usually not visible. These small glands are often referred to as the *lesser vestibular glands*. Skene's glands secrete mucus that lubricates and maintains a moist vaginal environment.

Below the urethral meatus is the *vaginal orifice*. This is the external opening of the vagina and has either a slitlike or irregular circular structure, depending on the presence of a *hymen*. If the hymen is intact, it is a fold of membranous tissue that covers part of the vagina. On either side of the vaginal orifice and slightly posterior (between the vaginal orifice and the labia minora) are the openings to *Bartholin's glands*. Through the openings, the glands secrete mucus, which lubricates the area during sexual intercourse. These small glands are often referred to as the *greater vestibular glands*. The glands and the openings are not visible to the naked eye.

Internal Genitalia

The internal genital structures function as the female reproductive organs (Fig. 20-2). They include the vagina, the uterus, the cervix, the fallopian tubes, and the ovaries. The *vagina*, a muscular, tubular organ, extends up and slightly back toward the rectum from the vaginal orifice (external opening) to the cervix. It lies between the rectum posteriorly and the urethra and bladder anteriorly and is approximately 10 cm long. The vagina performs many functions. It allows the passage of menstrual flow, it receives the penis during sexual intercourse, and it serves as the lower portion of the birth canal during delivery.

The vaginal wall comprises four layers. The outer layer is composed of pink squamous epithelium and connective tissue. It is under the direct influence of the hormone estrogen and contains many mucus-producing cells. This outer layer of epithelium lies in transverse folds called *rugae*. These transverse folds allow the vagina to expand during intercourse; they also facilitate vaginal delivery of a fetus. The second layer is the submucosal layer. It contains the blood vessels, nerves, and lymphatic channels. The third layer is composed of smooth muscle, and the fourth layer consists of connective tissue and the vascular network. The normal vaginal environment is acidic (pH of 3.8 to 4.2). This environment is maintained because the vaginal flora is composed of Doderlein's bacilli, and the bacilli act on glycogen to produce lactic acid. This acidic environment helps prevent vaginal infection.

In the upper end of the vagina, the cervix dips down and forms a circular recess that gives rise to areas known as the anterior and posterior fornices. The *cervix* (or neck of the

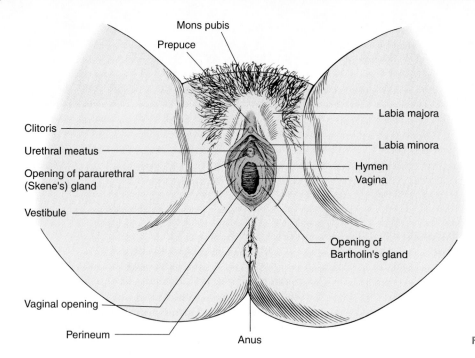

FIGURE 20-1. External genitalia.

uterus) separates the upper end of the vagina from the isthmus of the uterus. The junction of the isthmus and the cervix forms the *internal os*, and the junction of the cervix and the vagina forms the *external os* or ectocervix. The "os" refers to the opening in the center of the cervix. A woman who is nulliparous (having borne no offspring) has a small, round opening that appears as a depression on examination. A woman who has had her cervix dilated during childbirth has a slitlike external os.

The cervix is composed of smooth muscle, muscle fibers, and connective tissue. Two types of epithelium may cover the external os or ectocervix—pink squamous epithelium (which lines the vaginal walls) and red, rough-looking columnar epithelium (which lines the endocervical canal). The columnar epithelium may be visible around the os. The point where the two types of epithelium meet is called the *squamocolumnar junction*. The cervix functions to allow the entrance of sperm into the uterus and to allow

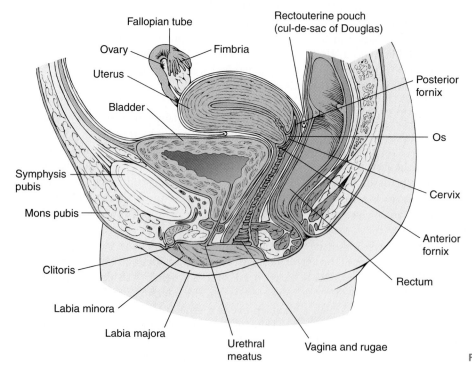

FIGURE 20-2. Internal genitalia.

the passage of menstrual flow. It also secretes mucus and prevents the entrance of vaginal bacteria. During childbirth, the cervix can stretch to allow the passage of the fetus. The cervical cells are scraped for analysis during a Papanicolaou smear (Pap test).

The *uterus* is a pear-shaped muscular organ that has two components—the *corpus*, or body, and the *cervix*, or neck (discussed previously). The corpus of the uterus is divided into the fundus (upper portion), the body (central portion), and the isthmus (narrow lower portion). The uterus is usually situated in a forward position above the bladder at approximately a 45-degree angle to the vagina when standing (anteverted and anteflexed position). The normal-sized uterus is approximately 7.5 cm long, 5 cm wide, and 2.5 cm thick.

The *endometrium*, the *myometrium*, and the *peritoneum* are the three layers of the uterine wall. The endometrium is the inner mucosal layer. The endometrium is composed of epithelium, connective tissue, and a vascular network; the thickness of this tissue is influenced by estrogen and progesterone. Uterine glands contained within the endometrium secrete an alkaline substance that keeps the uterine cavity moist. A portion of the endometrium sheds during menses and childbirth. The myometrium is the middle layer of the uterus. It is composed of three layers of smooth muscle fibers that surround blood vessels. This layer functions to expel the products of conception. The peritoneum is the outer uterine layer that separates it from the abdominal cavity. The peritoneum forms an anterior and posterior pouch around the uterus. The posterior pouch is called the *recto-uterine pouch* or the *cul-de-sac of Douglas.*

The *ovaries* are a pair of small, oval-shaped organs. Each is approximately 3 cm long, 2 cm wide, and 1 cm deep, and each is situated on a lateral aspect of the pelvic cavity. The ovaries are connected to the uterus by the ovarian ligament. The ovary functions to develop and release ova and to produce hormones such as estrogen, progesterone, and testosterone. The ovum travels from the ovary to the uterus through the fallopian tubes. These 8- to 12-cm long tubes begin near the ovaries and enter the uterus just beneath the fundus. The end of the tube near the ovary has fringelike extensions called *fimbriae*. The ovaries, fallopian tubes, and supporting ovarian ligaments are referred to as the *adnexa* (Latin for appendages).

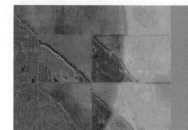

Collecting Subjective Data

When interview topics turn to the reproductive system and female genitalia, keep in mind the sensitivities of the client as well as your own feelings regarding body image, fear of cancer, sexuality, and the like. Western culture tends to emphasize the importance of a woman's reproductive ability, thereby entwining self-esteem and body image with the female sex role. Anxiety, embarrassment, and fear may affect the client's ability to discuss problems and ask questions. Because some problems can be serious or even life-threatening, it is important to establish a trusting relationship with the client because the information gathered during the subjective examination may suggest a problem or point to the possibility of a problem developing. Cancer of the cervix, for example, is associated with a high mortality rate but related risk factors are highly modifiable and, in disease that is discovered early, cure rates are high as well. Keep the COLDSPA memory help in mind as you proceed with the nursing health history.

COLDSPA

CHARACTER: Describe the sign or symptom. How does it feel, look, sound, smell, and so forth?

ONSET: When did it begin?

LOCATION: Where is it? Does it radiate?

DURATION: How long does it last? Does it recur?

SEVERITY: How bad is it?

PATTERN: What makes it better? What makes it worse?

ASSOCIATED FACTORS: What other symptoms occur with it?

Nursing History

Before proceeding with the interview, keep both the topic of the health history and the client's culture clearly in mind. In some cases, your gender may interfere with accurate results.

Clients from some cultures (eg, Islam) may accept subjective or physical assessment only by a female nurse, especially when genital and/or sexual issues are being addressed.

CURRENT SYMPTOMS

Question What was the date of your last menstrual period? Do your menstrual cycles occur on a regular schedule? How long do they last? Describe the typical amount of blood flow you have with your periods.

Rationale A normal menstrual cycle usually occurs approximately every 18 to 45 days. The average length of menstrual blood flow is 3 to 7 days. The absence of menstruation, excessive bleeding, or a marked change in menstrual pattern indicates a need to collect more information.

Q What other symptoms do you experience before or during your period?

R Headache, weight gain, mood swings, abdominal cramping, and bloating are common complaints before or during the menstrual period. Some women experience premenstrual syndrome (PMS), in which the symptoms become severe enough to impair the women's ability to function.

Q How old were you when you started your period?

R In North America, the average age is 12.5 years. Menstruation usually begins when the woman reaches 48 kg (106 lb).

Note: Menarche (beginning of menstruation) tends to begin earlier in women living in developed countries and later in women who live in undeveloped countries. Ages of menarche range from 10 to 16 years of age, with earlier onset in shorter and fatter girls (Overfield, 1995). Women who are poor or from less developed countries have earlier menopause.

Q Have you stopped menstruating or have your periods become irregular? What symptoms have you experienced?

R Irregularities or amenorrhea may be due to pregnancy, depression, ovarian tumors, ovarian cysts, autoimmune disease, and hormonal imbalances. Cessation of menstruation is termed *menopause*.

Menopause is a normal physiologic process that occurs in women between the ages of 40 to 58 years, with a mean age of 50. Menopause occurring before age 30 is termed *premature menopause;* menopause between ages 31 and 40 is considered early; menopause occurring in women older than age 58 years is termed *delayed menopause*. Premature and delayed menopause may be due to genetic predisposition, an endocrine disorder, or gynecologic dysfunction. Artificial or surgical menopause occurs in women who have dysfunctional ovaries or who have had their ovaries removed surgically. About 60% of menopausal women experience hot flashes and night sweats. Mood swings, decreased appetite, vaginal dryness, spotting, and irregular vaginal bleeding may also occur.

Q Are you experiencing vaginal discharge that is unusual in terms of color, amount, or odor?

R Vaginal discharge may be from an infection.

Q Do you experience pain or itching in your genital or groin area?

R Complaints of pain in the area of the vulva, vagina, uterus, cervix, or ovaries may indicate infection. Itching may indicate infection or infestation.

The older client is more susceptible to vaginal infection because of atrophy of the vaginal mucosa associated with aging.

Q Do you have any lumps, swelling, or masses in your genital area?

R These findings may indicate infection, lymphedema, or cancer. Past occurrences should be monitored for recurrence.

Q Do you have any difficulty urinating? Has your urine changed color or developed an odor?

R Urinary frequency, burning, or pain (dysuria) are signs of infection (urinary tract or sexually transmitted disease), whereas hesitancy or straining could indicate blockage. Change in color and development of an abnormal odor could indicate infection.

Q Do you have difficulty controlling your urine?

R Difficulty controlling urine (incontinence) may indicate urgency or stress incontinence. During sneezing or coughing, increased abdominal pressure causes spontaneous urination.

Urinary incontinence may develop in older women from muscle weakness or loss of urethral elasticity.

Q Do you have any problems with your sexual performance?

R A broad opening question about sex allows the client to focus the interview to areas where she has concerns. Some women have difficulty achieving orgasm and may believe there is something wrong with them.

Q Have you recently had a change in your sexual activity pattern or libido?

R A change in sexual activity or libido needs to be investigated for the cause. A woman who is dissatisfied with her sexual performance may experience a decreased libido.

As women age, their estrogen production decreases, causing atrophy of the vaginal mucosa. These women may need to use lubrication to increase comfort during intercourse. Women experiencing surgical menopause, symptoms of which occur more abruptly, may also benefit from lubrication.

Q Do you experience (or have you experienced) problems with fertility?

R Infertility is defined as unprotected sex for 1 year without pregnancy. Approximately 35% of infertility cases are related to female fertility factors from a variety of causes.

PAST HISTORY

Q Describe any prior gynecologic problems you have had and the results of any treatment.

R Some problems, such as cancer, may recur. Prior problems directly affect the physical assessment.

Q When was your last pelvic examination by a health care provider? Was a Pap test performed? What was the result?

R Pelvic and rectal examinations are used to detect masses, ovarian tenderness, or organ enlargement. The Pap smear is a screening test for cervical cancer. The American Cancer Society recommends an annual Pap test and pelvic examination for all women who are or who have been sexually active, or who have reached age 18 years. Once a woman has had four or more consecutive satisfactory normal annual examinations, the Pap test may be performed less frequently at the discretion of the health care provider (see Risk Factors—Cervical Cancer).

Q Have you ever been diagnosed with a sexually transmitted disease (STD)? How was it treated?

R Sexually transmitted diseases, also called sexually transmitted infections (STIs), can increase the client's risk of pelvic inflammatory disease, which leads to scarring and adhesions on the fallopian tubes. Scarred fallopian tubes increase the risk for infertility and ectopic pregnancy.

Q Have you ever been pregnant? How many times? How many children do you have? Is there any chance that you might be pregnant now?

R The female client's ability to become impregnated and carry a fetus to term is important baseline information. It is important to know if the client is pregnant in case medications or x-ray tests need to be prescribed.

Q Have you ever been diagnosed with diabetes?

R Diabetes predisposes women to vaginal yeast infections.

FAMILY HISTORY

Q Is there a history of reproductive or genital cancer in your family? What type? How is the family member related to you?

RISK FACTORS
Cervical Cancer

OVERVIEW

The American Cancer Society (ACS, 2000) describes cervical cancer as a slowly progressing condition beginning in the lining of the cervix wherein gradual changes lead to a precancerous state and then possibly to cancer. The cancer may be squamous cell carcinoma (85%–90%) or adenocarcinoma (10%–15%), or a few rarer types. Because early cervical cancers can usually be found by Pap test and are nearly 100% curable, routine screening is recommended. The ACS recommends that all women begin yearly Pap tests at age 18 or when they become sexually active, whichever occurs earlier. If a woman has had three normal annual Pap test results in a row, the test may be done less often at the judgment of the woman's health care provider. After hysterectomy, more frequent Pap tests may be recommended.

According to the ACS, the vast majority of cervical cancers can be prevented. First, to prevent pre-cancers, women can avoid risk factors (see risk factors and risk reduction measures below). Second, to prevent invasive cancers, women should have a Pap test to detect human papillomavirus (HPV) infection and precancers and thereby treat disease in the earliest stage possible. Even so, and after a 74% decline in the disease between 1955 and 1992, about 4,400 women will die from cervical cancer in the United States during the year 2001. The 5-year survival rate for cervical precancer is nearly 100%, and for cervical cancer diagnosis is between 70% and 91%.

RISK FACTORS

- HPV infection, the most important risk factor
- Female between ages 50 and 55; females from the late teens to age 50 are also at risk but less so
- Failure to have regular Pap tests
- Cigarette smoking
- Human immunodeficiency virus (HIV) infection
- Diet low in fruits and vegetables
- Multiple sexual partners, especially unprotected sex and especially beginning at young age
- Use of oral contraceptives for 5 or more years (possible risk factor)
- Low socioeconomic status associated with low level of preventive care
- African American, Hispanic, Native American heritage

RISK REDUCTION TEACHING TIPS

- Practice sexual monogamy.
- Use barrier-type contraceptive to prevent HPV and other sexually transmitted diseases.
- Limit number of lifetime sexual partners.
- Follow ACS guidelines for annual Pap testing and any recommended follow-up treatment.
- Learn and practice good genital hygiene.
- Do not smoke cigarettes.
- Eat a diet rich in fruits and vegetables, especially vitamins A, C, and folate.

 ## CULTURAL CONSIDERATIONS

The ACS (2000) notes that several racial and ethnic groups have cervical cancer death rates that are higher than the US average. The death rate for African Americans is over twice the national average, and the rates for Hispanics and Native Americans are above the national average. Murphy et al. (1995) found that cervical cancer is a major form of neoplasia in developing countries, with an inverse relation-ship to socioeconomic status in industrialized countries. This pattern of occurrence may be associated with early sexual intercourse under conditions of poor hygiene, including sex with uncircumcised males. Other factors that may increase risk in the developing world are cigarette smoking and nutritional deficiencies, especially of vitamins A and C and folate.

R Cancer has a tendency to occur in families. In such clients, the examination can focus on areas in which risk may be present.

LIFESTYLE AND HEALTH PRACTICES

Q Do you smoke?

R Smoking and taking oral contraceptives increase the risk of cardiovascular problems. In addition, the risk for cervical cancer increases in clients who have the human papillomavirus (a type of STD) and who smoke.

Q How many sexual partners do you have?

R A client who has multiple sexual partners increases her risk of contracting STDs.

Q Do you use contraceptives? What kind? How often?

R Minor side effects (eg, weight gain, breast tenderness, headaches, nausea) might develop from oral contraceptives but usually subside after the third cycle. Major side effects include thromboembolic disorders, cerebrovascular accident (CVA), and myocardial infarction (MI). Failure to use a barrier type of contraceptive (male or female condom) may increase the risk of STDs and human immunodeficiency virus (HIV) infection. Failure to use any type of contraceptive increases the risk of becoming pregnant.

Q Have genital problems affected the way in which you normally function?

R Diseases or disorders of the genitalia may cause pain and discomfort that affect a client's ability to work, to perform normal household duties, or to care for family. In addition, normal sexual activity may be affected because of pain, embarrassment, or decreased libido. Oral contraceptives increase the glycogen content of vaginal secretions, which increases the risk of vaginal yeast infections.

Q What is your sexual preference?

R An awareness of the client's sexual preference allows the examiner to focus the examination. If the client is homosexual, she may not have the same concerns as a heterosexual woman. If she engages in oral sex, she will need to take precautions to prevent orovaginal transmission of infection.

Q Do you feel comfortable communicating with your partner about your sexual likes and dislikes?

R Sexual relationships are enhanced through open communication. Lack of open communication can cause problems with relationships and lead to feelings of guilt and depression.

Q Do you have any fears related to sex? Can you identify any stress in your current relationship that relates to stress?

R Fear can inhibit performance and decrease sexual satisfaction. Stress can prevent satisfactory sex role performance.

Q Do you have concerns about fertility? If you have trouble with fertility, how has this affected your relationship with your partner or family?

R Women often feel responsible for infertility and need to discuss their feelings. Concerns about fertility can increase stress. Problems with fertility can have a negative impact on relationships with the partner and can cause tension within a family, especially when other women in the family have children.

Q Do you perform monthly genital self-examinations?

R Each female client should be aware of the need for monthly genital self-examination and its importance in early diagnosis and treatment of problems.

Q How do you feel about going through menopause?

R Menopause is a normal development of aging. However, in some women the process induces fear, anxiety, or even grief. The nurse can assist the client to resolve some of these feelings.

Q Do you take estrogen replacement therapy?

R Estrogen sometimes alleviates the symptoms of menopause. However, estrogen has been linked to some types of cancer (ie, breast, endometrial) and, in increasing the glycogen content in vaginal secretions, predisposes clients to yeast infections.

Q Have you ever been tested for HIV? What was the result? Why were you tested?

R HIV increases the client's risk for any other infection. A high-risk exposure may require serial testing.

Q What do you know about toxic shock syndrome?

R Toxic shock syndrome is a life-threatening infection that can be prevented by frequently changing tampons.

Q What do you know about STDs and their prevention?

R The client's knowledge of STDs and prevention provides a basis for health education in this area.

Q Do you wear cotton underwear and avoid tight jeans?

R Cotton allows air to circulate. Nylon and tight-fitting jeans create a moist environment, which promotes vaginal yeast infections.

Q After a bowel movement or urination, do you wipe from front to back?

R The vaginal and urethral openings are close to the anus and are easily contaminated by *Escherichia coli* and other bacteria if care is not taken to wipe from front to back.

Q Do you douche frequently?

R Frequent douching changes the natural flora of the vagina, predisposing the vagina to yeast infections.

Collecting Objective Data

The physical examination of the female genitalia may create client anxiety. The client may be very embarrassed about exposing her genitalia and nervous that an infection or disorder will be discovered. Be sure to explain in detail what you will be doing throughout the examination and to explain the significance of each portion of the examination. Encourage the client to ask questions. Begin by sitting on a stool at the end of the examination table and draping the client so only the vulva is exposed. This helps to preserve the client's modesty. Shine your light source so it illuminates the genital area, allowing you to see all structures clearly.

CLIENT PREPARATION

The client should be told ahead of time not to douche for 48 hours before a gynecologic examination. When the client arrives for the examination, ask her to urinate before the examination so she does not experience bladder discomfort. If a clean-catch urine specimen is needed, provide a container and vaginal wipes. When the client is back in the examining room, ask her to remove her underwear and bra and to put on a gown with the opening in the back. If she is also having a breast examination at this time, suggest that she leave the opening in the front—a sheet can be used for draping. Tell her that she can leave her socks on if desired because the stirrups on the examination table are metal and may be cool. You should leave the room while she changes.

After the client has changed and you have returned to the room, help her into the dorsal lithotomy position. This is a supine position with the feet in stirrups. The client's hips should be positioned toward the bottom of the examination table so the feet can rest comfortably in the stirrups. Ask the client not to put her hands over her head because this tightens the abdominal muscles. She should relax her arms at her sides. If possible, elevate the client's head and shoulders. This allows you to maintain eye contact with her during the examination and enables her to see what you are doing. Another technique is to offer the client a mirror so she can view the examination (Fig. 20-3). This is a good way to teach normal anatomy and to get the client more involved and interested in maintaining or improving her genital health.

EQUIPMENT AND SUPPLIES

- Stool
- Light
- Speculum (see Display 20-1, How to Use the Speculum, and Fig. 20-4)
- Water-soluble lubricant

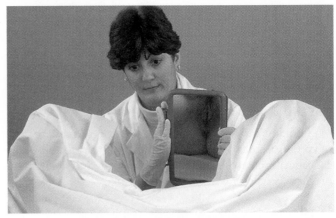

FIGURE 20-3. Mirror image of the examination promotes interest in gynecologic health. (© B. **Proud.**)

- Cotton-tipped applicators
- *Chlamydia* culture tube
- Culturette
- Test tube with water
- Sterile disposable gloves
- Ayre spatula (plastic)
- Endocervical broom
- pH paper
- Feminine napkins
- Mirror

KEY ASSESSMENT POINTS

- Respect the client's privacy.
- Wash hands, wear gloves, be sure equipment is between room and body temperature.
- Inspect and palpate female external and internal structures correctly.
- Use examination and laboratory equipment properly.
- Recognize the difference between common variations and abnormal findings.

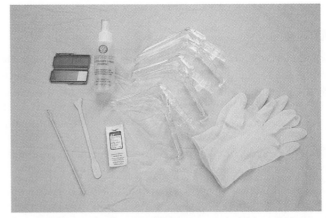

FIGURE 20-4. Some of the equipment needed for examining female genitalia includes disposable gloves, speculums, slides and special solutions, spatulas, endocervical brooms, and other devices.

(*text continues on page 453*)

DISPLAY 20-1. How to Use the Speculum

GUIDELINES

1. Before using the speculum, choose the instrument that is the correct size for the client. Vaginal speculums come in two basic types:
   - *Graves speculum*—appropriate for most adult women and available in various lengths and widths.
   - *Pederson speculum*—appropriate for virgins and some postmenopausal women who have a narrow vaginal orifice. Speculums can be metal with a thumb screw that is tightened to lock the blades in place or plastic with a clip that is locked to keep the blades in place. (Plastic speculums are shown.)

2. Encourage the client to take deep breaths and to maintain her feet in the stirrups with her knees resting in an open, relaxed fashion.

3. Place two fingers of your nondominant hand against the posterior vaginal wall and wait for relaxation to occur.

4. Insert the fingers of your nondominant hand about 2.5 cm into the vagina and spread them slightly while pushing down against the posterior vagina.

5. Lubricate the blades of the speculum with vaginal secretions from the client. Do not use commercial lubricants on the speculum. Lubricants are typically bacteriostatic and will alter vaginal pH and the cell specimens collected for cytologic, bacterial, and viral analysis.

6. Hold the speculum with two fingers around the blades and the thumb under the screw or lock. This is important for keeping the blades closed. Position the speculum so the blades are vertical.

7. Insert the speculum between your fingers into the posterior portion of the vaginal orifice at a 45-degree angle downward. When the blades pass your fingers inside the vagina, rotate the closed speculum so the blades are in a horizontal position.

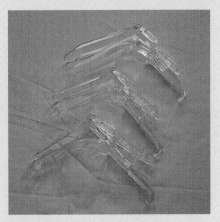

Speculums.

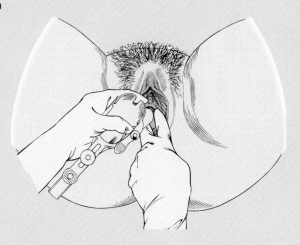

Tip From the Experts Be careful during the speculum insertion not to pinch the labia or pull the pubic hair. If the vaginal orifice seems tight or you are having trouble inserting the speculum, ask the client to bear down. This may help relax the muscles of the perineum and promote opening.

---

8. Continue inserting the speculum until the base touches the fingertips inside the vagina.

9. Remove the fingers of your nondominant hand from the client's posterior vagina.

DISPLAY 20-1. How to Use the Speculum (Continued)

10. Press handles together to open blades and allow visualization of the cervix.

11. Secure the speculum in place by tightening the thumb screw or locking the plastic clip.

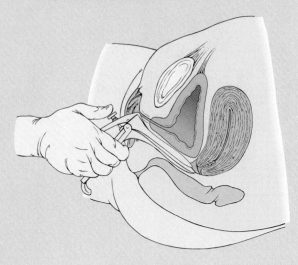

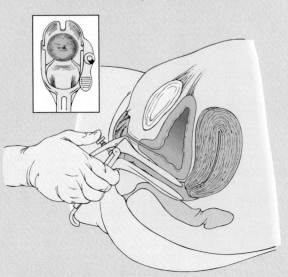

PHYSICAL ASSESSMENT

ASSESSMENT PROCEDURE	NORMAL FINDINGS	ABNORMAL FINDINGS

EXTERNAL GENITALIA

Inspect the Mons Pubis

Wash your hands and put on gloves. As you begin the examination, note the distribution of pubic hair. Also be alert for signs of infestation.

Normally, pubic hair is distributed in a triangular pattern and there are no signs of infestation.

Older clients may have gray, thinning pubic hair.

Some clients, particularly younger ones, shave (photo at left) or pluck the pubic hair, and it is increasingly common to find clitoral rings or studs implanted to enhance sexual pleasure.

Absence of pubic hair in the adult client is abnormal.

Lice or nits (eggs) at the base of the pubic hairs indicates infestation with pediculosis pubis. This condition, commonly referred to as "crabs," is most often transmitted by sexual contact.

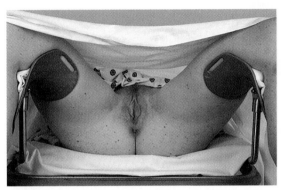

Inspecting the pubic hair, labia majora, and perineum. (© B. Proud.)

Inspect the Labia Majora and Perineum

Observe the labia majora and perineum for lesions, swelling, excoriation.

Keep in mind the woman's childbearing status during inspection. For example, the labia of a woman who has not delivered offspring vaginally will meet in the middle. The labia of a woman who has delivered vaginally will not meet in the middle and may appear shriveled.

The labia majora are equal in size and free of lesions, swelling, and excoriation. A healed tear or episiotomy scar may be visible on the perineum if the client has given birth.

Lesions may be from an infectious disease, such as herpes or syphilis (Display 20-2). Excoriation and swelling may be from scratching or self-treatment of the lesions. All lesions must be evaluated and the client referred for treatment.

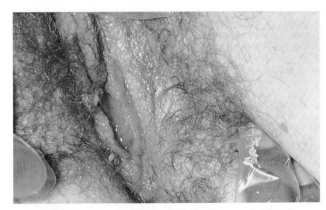

Small, painful, red-based, ulcer-like lesions of herpes simplex virus, type 2. (© 1992. Science Photo Library/CMSP.)

In pubertal rites in some cultures, the clitoris is surgically removed and the labia are sutured, leaving only a small opening for menstrual flow. Once married, the woman undergoes surgery to reopen the labia.

(continued)

ASSESSMENT PROCEDURE	NORMAL FINDINGS	ABNORMAL FINDINGS

Inspect the Labia Minora, Clitoris, Urethral Meatus, and Vaginal Opening

Use your gloved hand to separate the labia majora and inspect for lesions, excoriation, swelling, and/or discharge.

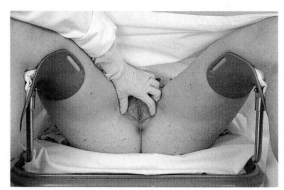

Inspecting the labia minora, clitoris, urethral orifice, and vaginal opening.

The labia minora appear symmetric, dark pink, and moist. The urethral meatus is small and slitlike. The vaginal opening is positioned below the urethral meatus. Its size depends on sexual activity or vaginal delivery, and it may be covered partially or completely by a hymen.

Asymmetric labia may indicate abscess. Lesions, swelling, bulging in the vaginal opening, and discharge are abnormal findings (see Display 20-2). Excoriation may result from the client scratching or self-treating a perineal irritation.

Palpate Bartholin's Glands

If the client has labial swelling or a history of it, palpate Bartholin's glands for swelling, tenderness, and discharge. Place your index finger in the vaginal opening and your thumb on the labia majora. With a gentle pinching motion, palpate from the inferior portion of the posterior labia majora to the anterior portion. Repeat on the opposite side.

Technique for palpating Bartholin's glands.

Bartholin's glands are usually soft, nontender, and drainage free.

Swelling, pain, and discharge may result from infection and abscess. If you detect a discharge, obtain a specimen to send to the laboratory for culture (Display 20-3).

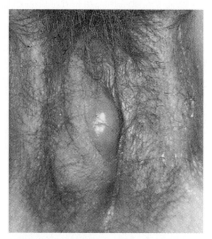

Abscess of Bartholin's gland, a painful condition and common sign of *Neisseria gonorrhoeae* infection. (© 1992, National Medical Slide Bureau/CMSP.)

(continued)

ASSESSMENT PROCEDURE	NORMAL FINDINGS	ABNORMAL FINDINGS

Palpate the Urethra

If the client reports urethral symptoms or urethritis, or if you suspect inflammation of Skene's glands, insert your gloved index finger into the superior portion of the vagina and milk the urethra from the inside, pushing up and out.

No drainage should be noted from the urethral meatus. The area is normally soft and non-tender.

Drainage from the urethra indicates possible urethritis. Any discharge should be cultured. Urethritis may occur with infection with *Neisseria gonorrhoeae* or *Chlamydia trachomatis*.

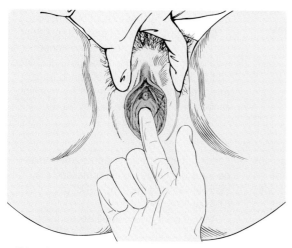

Milking the urethra.

INTERNAL GENITALIA

Inspect the Size of the Vaginal Opening and the Angle of the Vagina

Insert your gloved index finger into the vagina, noting the size of the opening. Then attempt to touch the cervix. This will help you establish the size of the speculum you need to use for the examination and the angle at which to insert it.

Next, gently, while maintaining tension, pull the labia majora outward. Note hymenal configuration and transections.

The normal vaginal opening varies in size according to the client's age, sexual history, and whether she has given birth vaginally. The vagina is typically tilted posteriorly at a 45-degree angle.

Any loss of hymenal tissue between the 3 o'clock position and the 9 o'clock position indicates trauma (penetration by digits, penis or foreign objects) in children. See Chapter 24 for more information about sexual abuse in children. This finding is not as relevant in adults.

Inspect the Vaginal Musculature

Keep your index finger inserted in the client's vaginal opening. Ask the client to squeeze around your finger.

The client should be able to squeeze around the examiner's finger. Typically, the nulliparous woman can squeeze tighter than the multiparous woman.

Absent or decreased ability to squeeze the examiner's finger indicates decreased muscle tone. Decreased tone may decrease sexual satisfaction.

Use your middle and index fingers to separate the labia minora. Ask the client to bear down.

No bulging and no urinary discharge.

Bulging of the anterior wall may indicate a cystocele. Bulging of the posterior wall may indicate a rectocele. If the cervix or uterus protrudes down, the client may have uterine prolapse (see Display 20-2). If urine leaks out, the client may have stress incontinence.

(continued)

ASSESSMENT PROCEDURE	NORMAL FINDINGS	ABNORMAL FINDINGS

Inspect the Cervix

Follow the guidelines in Display 20-1. With the speculum inserted in position to visualize the cervix, observe cervical color, size, and position. Also observe the surface and the appearance of the os. Look for discharge and lesions as well.

After inspecting the cervix, obtain specimens for the Pap smear and, if indicated, specimens for culture and sensitivity testing to identify possible STDs. Follow the procedure presented in Display 20-3.

The surface of the cervix is normally smooth, pink, and even (Display 20-4).

In pregnant clients, the cervix appears blue (Chadwick's sign).

In older women, the cervix appears pale after menopause.

In a nonpregnant woman, a bluish cervix may indicate cyanosis, and, in a nonmenopausal woman, a pale cervix may indicate anemia. Redness may be from inflammation.

Cervical enlargement or projection into the vagina more than 3 cm may be from prolapse or tumor, and further evaluation is needed.

Asymmetric, reddened areas, strawberry spots, and white patches are also abnormal as is colored, malodorous, or irritating discharge, and a specimen should be obtained for culture. Cervical lesions may result from polyps, cancer, or infection (see Display 20-3).

Inspect the Vagina

Unlock the speculum and slowly rotate and remove it. Inspect the vagina as you remove the speculum. Note the vaginal color, surface, consistency, and any discharge.

If you are preparing a wet mount slide, collect the specimen of vaginal secretions from the anterior vaginal fornix or the lateral vaginal walls before you collect the specimens for the Pap or other test. Avoid the posterior fornix, which is contaminated with cervical secretions. Use part of the wet mount sample to test the pH of the vaginal secretions.

The vagina should appear pink, moist, smooth, and free of lesions and irritation. It should also be free of any colored, malodorous discharge.

Reddened areas, lesions, and colored, malodorous discharge are abnormal and may indicate vaginal infections, STDs, or cancer (Display 20-5).

Altered pH may indicate infection.

BEGIN THE BIMANUAL EXAMINATION: PALPATE THE VAGINAL WALL

Tell the client that you are going to do a manual examination and explain its purpose. Apply water-soluble lubricant to the gloved index and middle fingers of your dominant hand. Then stand and approach the client at the correct angle. Placing your nondominant hand on the client's lower abdomen, insert your index and middle fingers into the vaginal opening. Apply pressure to the posterior wall, and wait for the vaginal opening to relax before palpating the vaginal walls for texture and tenderness.

The vaginal wall should feel smooth, and the client should not report any tenderness.

Tenderness or lesions may indicate infection.

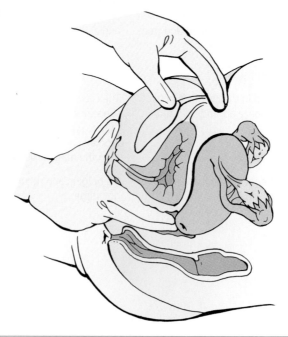

Hands positioned for palpating the vaginal wall.

(continued)

ASSESSMENT PROCEDURE	NORMAL FINDINGS	ABNORMAL FINDINGS

Palpate the Cervix

Advance your fingers until they touch the cervix. Palpate for:
- Contour
- Consistency
- Mobility
- Tenderness

The cervix should feel firm and soft (like the tip of your nose). It is rounded, and can be moved somewhat from side to side without eliciting tenderness.

A hard, immobile cervix may indicate cancer. Pain with movement of the cervix may indicate infection.

Palpate the Uterus

Move your fingers intravaginally into the opening above the cervix and gently press the hand resting on the abdomen downward, squeezing the uterus between the two hands. Note uterine size, position, shape, and consistency.

The fundus, the large upper end of the uterus, is normally round, firm, and smooth. In most women, it is at the level of the pubis, and the cervix is aimed posteriorly (anteverted position). However, several other positions are considered normal (Display 20-6).

An enlarged uterus above the level of the pubis is abnormal, and an irregular shape suggests abnormalities, such as myomas (fibroid tumors) or endometriosis (Display 20-7).

Attempt to bounce the uterus between your two hands to assess mobility and tenderness.

The normal uterus moves freely and is not tender.

A fixed or tender uterus may indicate fibroids, infection, or masses (see Display 20-7).

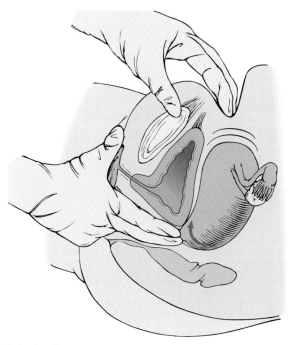

Palpating the uterus.

(continued)

ASSESSMENT PROCEDURE	NORMAL FINDINGS	ABNORMAL FINDINGS

Palpate the Ovaries

Slide your intravaginal fingers toward the left ovary in the left lateral fornix and place your abdominal hand on the left lower abdominal quadrant. Press your abdominal hand toward your intravaginal fingers and attempt to palpate the ovary.

Slide your intravaginal fingers to the right lateral fornix and attempt to palpate the right ovary. Note size, shape, consistency, mobility, and tenderness.

   Withdraw your intravaginal hand and inspect the glove for secretions.

Ovaries are approximately 3 × 2 × 1 cm (or the size of a walnut) and almond shaped.

Ovaries are firm, smooth, mobile, and somewhat tender on palpation.

   A clear, minimal amount of drainage appearing on the glove from the vagina is normal.

Enlarged size, masses, immobility, and extreme tenderness are abnormal and should be evaluated (Displays 20-8 and 20-9).

Large amounts of colorful, frothy, or malodorous secretions are abnormal. Ovaries that are palpable 3 to 5 years after menopause are also abnormal.

> **Tip From the Experts** It is normal for the ovaries to be difficult or impossible to palpate in obese women, in postmenopausal women because the ovaries atrophy, or in women who are tense during the examination.

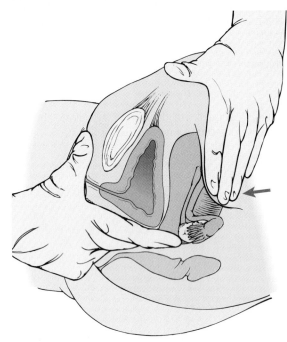

Palpating the ovaries.

(continued)

ASSESSMENT PROCEDURE	NORMAL FINDINGS	ABNORMAL FINDINGS

PERFORM THE RECTOVAGINAL EXAMINATION

Explain that you are going to perform a rectovaginal examination and explain its purpose. Forewarn the client that she may feel uncomfortable as if she wants to move her bowels, but that she will not. Encourage her to relax. Change the glove on your dominant hand and lubricate your index and middle fingers with a water-soluble lubricant.

Ask the client to bear down to promote relaxation of the sphincter and insert your index finger into the vaginal orifice and your middle finger into the rectum. While pushing down on the abdominal wall with your other hand, palpate the internal reproductive structures through the anterior rectal wall. Pay particular attention to the area behind the cervix, the rectovaginal septum, the cul-de-sac, and the posterior uterine wall. Withdraw your vaginal finger and continue with the rectal examination (see Chapter 21, Anus, Rectum, and Prostate Assessment).

The rectovaginal septum is normally smooth, thin, movable, and firm. The posterior uterine wall is normally smooth, firm, round, movable, and nontender.

Masses, thickened structures, immobility, and tenderness are abnormal.

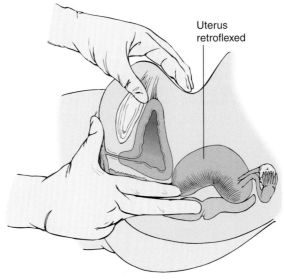

Uterus retroflexed

Hands positioned for rectovaginal examination.

Validation and Documentation of Findings

Validate the female genitalia assessment data that you have collected. This is necessary to verify that the data are reliable and accurate. Document the assessment data following the health care facility or agency policy.

EXAMPLE OF SUBJECTIVE DATA

Client states regular menstrual cycle. Last menstrual period occurred 2 weeks ago, beginning on the 10th and ending on the 13th. Experiences bloating and mild cramping with period. No vaginal discharge, pain, itching in genitalia, lumps, swelling, or masses. No difficulty urinating or controlling urine. Denies problems with sexual performance, change in sexual patterns, and decrease in sexual desire. No problems with fertility. No prior gynecologic problems.

Last pelvic examination and Pap smear 1 year ago with normal results. Denies history of sexually transmitted diseases. Gravida 2, para 1. No family history of reproductive or gynecologic cancer. Client states she does not smoke, she is married and monogamous and uses female condom for birth control. She states she is comfortable discussing sexual issues with husband. Performs monthly vulvar self-examination and is aware of risks for toxic shock syndrome. She wears tampons only during heavy flow and changes them every few hours.

EXAMPLE OF OBJECTIVE DATA

Inspection discloses normal hair distribution, no lesions, masses, or swelling. Labia majora pink, smooth, and free of lesions, excoriation, and swelling. Labia minora dark pink, moist, and free of lesions, excoriation, swelling, and discharge. No bulging at vaginal orifice. No discharge from urethral opening.

Cervix slightly anterior, pink, smooth, slitlike os, mobile, nontender, and firm without lesions or discharge. Vaginal walls smooth and pink.

Palpation indicates firm fundus located anteriorly at level of symphysis pubis, without tenderness, lesions, or nodules. Smooth, firm, almond-shaped, mobile ovaries

(text continue on page 466)

ABNORMAL
FINDINGS

DISPLAY 20-2. Identifying Abnormalities of the External Genitalia and Vaginal Opening

When assessing the female genitalia, the nurse will see various abnormal lesions on the external genitalia as well as abnormal bulging in the vaginal opening. Besides the lesions caused by herpes simplex virus (type 2) pictured earlier in the physical assessment section of the text, some common findings appear below.

SYPHILITIC CHANCRE

Syphilitic chancres often first appear on the perianal area as silvery white papules that become superficial red ulcers. Syphilitic chancres are painless. They are sexually transmitted and usually develop at the site of initial contact with the infecting organism.

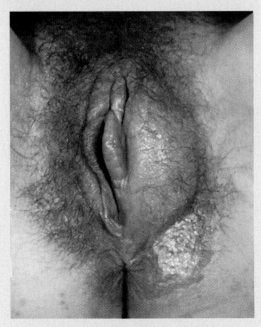

Chancre typical of syphilis. (Courtesy of Upjohn Co.)

GENITAL WARTS

Genital warts, caused by the human papilloma virus (HPV), are moist, fleshy lesions on the labia and within the vestibule. They are painless and believed to be sexually transmitted.

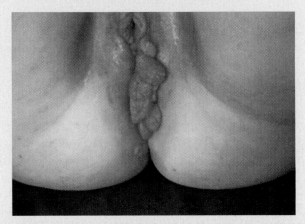

Genital warts. (Courtesy Reed & Carnrick Pharmaceuticals.)

CYSTOCELE

A cystocele is a bulging in the anterior vaginal wall caused by thickening of the pelvic musculature. As a result, the bladder, covered by vaginal mucosa, prolapses into the vagina.

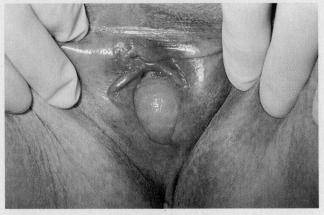

Cystocele. (© 1995 Science Photo Library/CMSP.)

RECTOCELE

A rectocele is a bulging in the posterior vaginal wall caused by weakening of the pelvic musculature. Part of the rectum covered by the vaginal mucosa protrudes into the vagina.

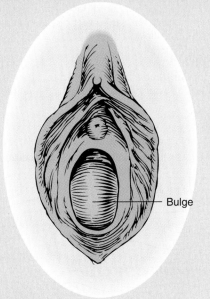

Rectocele.

UTERINE PROLAPSE

Uterine prolapse occurs when the uterus protrudes into the vagina. It is graded according to how far it protrudes into the vagina. In first-degree prolapse, the cervix is seen at the vaginal opening; in second-degree prolapse the uterus bulges outside of vaginal openings; in third-degree prolapse, the uterus bulges completely out of the vagina.

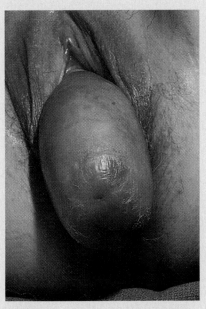

Prolapsed uterus. (© 1991, Michael English, MD/CMSP.)

(continued)

DISPLAY 20-3. Obtaining Tissue Specimens for Analysis

GUIDELINES

Various laboratory tests are based on an analysis of cells obtained from tissue specimens and prepared on culture media or on slides for microscopic examination. For women especially, such tests are life-saving tools that can detect disease in early treatable stages. Some methods for obtaining tissue specimens follow:

PAPANICOLAOU SMEAR

The Papanicolaou (or Pap) smear is a screening test for cervical cancer. The procedure for gathering the specimens consists of three parts: Obtaining a specimen of ectocervical cells, endocervical cells, and vaginal cells.

Obtaining an Ectocervical Specimen

1. Insert one end of a plastic spatula (that is longer on the ends than in the middle) into the cervical os.
2. Press down and rotate the spatula, scraping the cervix and the transformation zone (squamo-columnar junction), in a full circle.

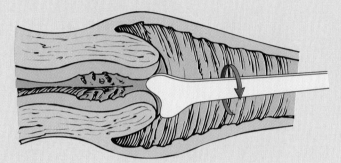

3. Withdraw the spatula.
4. Smear the specimen from both sides of the spatula onto the glass slide. Use one motion and spread the specimen thinly.
5. Spray the slide immediately with a special fixative to prevent drying.

Obtaining an Endocervical Specimen

1. Insert the endocervical brush into the cervical os. Use the endocervical brush to increase the number of cells obtained for analysis.
2. Rotate the brush in a full circle very gently to minimize possible bleeding.

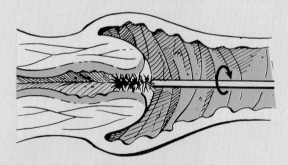

3. Withdraw the brush.
4. Rotate the brush gently onto a glass slide, spreading the specimen thinly in one motion.
5. Spray the slide immediately with a special fixative to prevent drying.

Tip From the Experts Do not apply great pressure when transferring the specimens onto the glass slides. Too much pressure may alter or destroy the cell structure. In addition, if you will be obtaining a specimen with the endocervical brush, do so after you obtain a tissue specimen with a spatula because bleeding may follow use of the brush.

(continued)

Obtaining a Combined Specimen

An alternative one-step procedure for gathering the endocervical and ectocervical specimens is sometimes performed on nonpregnant clients. This combined procedure uses a special cytobroom to collect both endocervical and ectocervical cells.

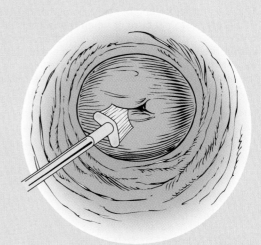

1. Insert the cytobroom into the cervical os.
2. Rotate the cytobroom in a full circle one or two times, collecting cell specimens from the squamocolumnar junction and the cervical surface.
3. Withdraw the cytobroom.
4. Swish in preservative solution.

Vaginal Specimen

1. Moisten a cotton-tipped applicator with saline.
2. Insert the applicator into the vagina and rotate it against the vaginal wall, anterior and lateral to the cervix.

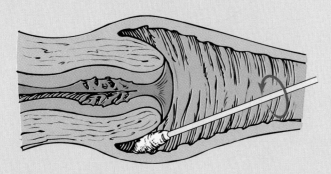

3. Withdraw the applicator.
4. Wipe the applicator gently onto a glass slide.
5. Spray the slide with a special fixative to prevent drying.

CULTURE SPECIMENS: GONORRHEA AND CHLAMYDIA

Specimens for gonorrhea or *Chlamydia* cultures are obtained if you suspect the client has these sexually transmitted diseases. The exact procedures for gathering and preparing the specimens vary according to each laboratory's policy. General guidelines are provided below.

1. Insert a cotton-tipped applicator into the cervical os and rotate it in a full circle.
2. Leave the applicator in place for approximately 20 seconds to make sure it becomes saturated with specimen.
3. Withdraw the applicator.
4. For *Neisseria gonorrhoeae* cultures: Spread the specimen onto a special culture plate (Thayer-Martin) in a "Z" pattern while rotating the applicator, or put in a liquid medium for transport and send to the laboratory.

   For *Chlamydia trachomatis* cultures: Immerse a special swab (provided with test medium) in a liquid medium and refrigerate the sample until it is transported to the laboratory.

DISPLAY 20-4. **Variations of the Cervix**

Certain cervical variations are common. Such variations include cervical eversion, Nabothian cysts, differently shaped cervical os (in nulliparous women and parous women), and various lacerations.

CERVICAL EVERSION

This is a normal finding in many women and usually occurs after vaginal birth or when the woman takes oral contraceptives. The columnar epithelium from within the endocervical canal is everted and appears as a deep red, rough ring around the cervical os, surrounded by the normal pink color of the cervix.

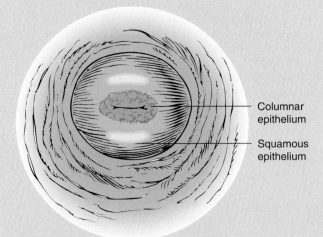

Columnar epithelium

Squamous epithelium

NABOTHIAN (RETENTION) CYSTS

Nabothian (retention) cysts are normal findings after childbirth. These cysts are small (less than 1 cm), yellow, translucent nodules on the cervical surface. Normal odorless and nonirritating secretions may be present on pink, healthy tissue. (Irritating secretions would appear on reddened tissue.) The viscosity of these secretions ranges from thin to thick; their appearance ranges from clear to cloudy, depending on the phase of the menstrual cycle.

Additionally, Nabothian cysts may occur when the everted columnar epithelium spontaneously transforms into squamous epithelium, a process called *squamous metaplasia*. Occasionally, the tissue blocks endocervical glands and the cysts develop.

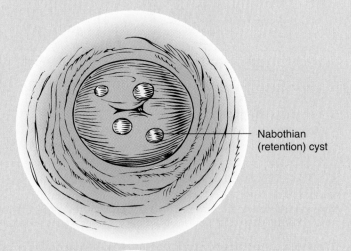

Nabothian (retention) cyst

CERVICAL OS (NULLIPAROUS WOMEN)

The cervical os in nulliparous women appears as a small round or oval opening.

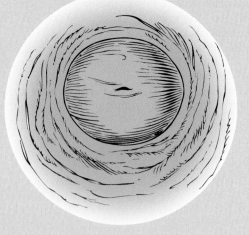

(continued)

CERVICAL OS (PAROUS WOMEN)

The cervical os in parous women appears slitlike.

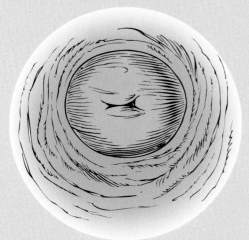

BILATERAL TRANSVERSE LACERATION

This drawing illustrates a type of healed laceration that may be seen in a woman who has given birth vaginally.

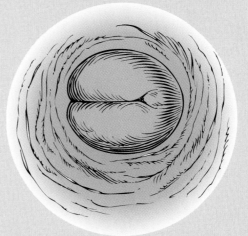

UNILATERAL TRANSVERSE LACERATION

Vaginal birth may cause trauma to the cervix and produce tears or lacerations. Therefore, healed lacerations may be seen as a normal variation. This drawing illustrates a unilateral transverse laceration.

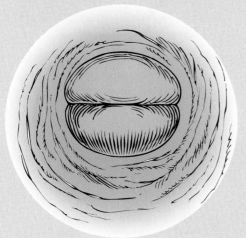

STELLATE LACERATION

This drawing illustrates a type of healed laceration that may be seen in a woman who has given birth vaginally.

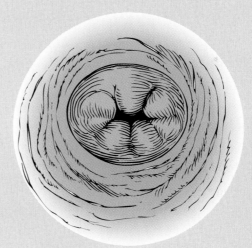

DISPLAY 20-5. Abnormalities of the Cervix

CYANOSIS OF THE CERVIX

The cervix normally appears bluish in the client who is in her first trimester of pregnancy. However, if the client is not pregnant, a bluish color to the cervix indicates venous congestion or a diminished oxygen supply to the tissues.

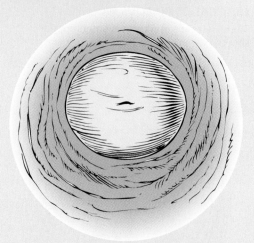

CANCER OF THE CERVIX

A hardened ulcer is usually the first indication of cervical cancer, but it may not be visible on the ectocervix. In later stages, the lesion may develop into a large cauliflowerlike growth. A Pap smear is essential for diagnosis.

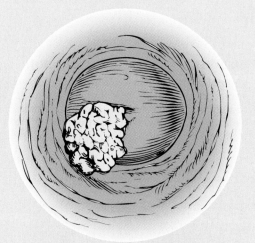

CERVICAL POLYP

A polyp typically develops in the endocervical canal and may protrude visibly at the cervical os. It is soft, red, and rather fragile. Cervical polyps are benign.

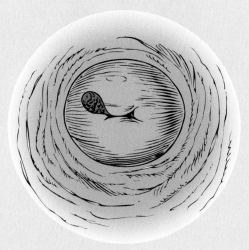

(continued)

CERVICAL EROSION

This condition differs from cervical eversion in that normal tissue around the external os is inflamed and eroded, appearing reddened and rough. Erosion usually occurs with mucopurulent cervical discharge.

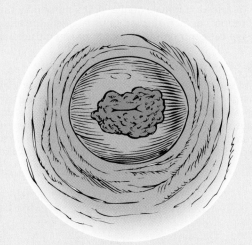

MALFORMATIONS FROM EXPOSURE TO DIETHYLSTILBESTROL (DES)

DES, a drug used more than 50 years ago to prevent spontaneous abortion and premature labor, was learned to be teratogenic (capable of causing malformations in the fetus). Women who were exposed to this drug as fetuses may have cervical abnormalities that may progress to cancer. Some abnormalities associated with maternal DES use include columnar epithelium that covers most or all of the ectocervix; columnar epithelium that extends onto the vaginal wall; a circular column of tissue that separates the cervix from the vaginal wall; transverse ridge; and enlarged upper ectocervical lip.

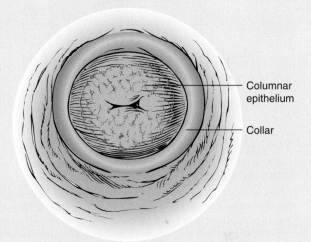

Columnar epithelium

Collar

MUCOPURULENT CERVICITIS

This condition produces a mucopurulent yellowish discharge from the external os. It usually indicates infection with *Chlamydia* or gonorrhea. However, these sexually transmitted diseases may also occur with no visible signs although the discharge may change the cervical pH (3.8–4.2).

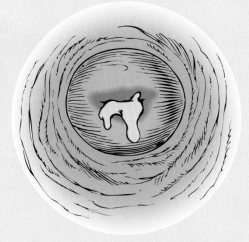

DISPLAY 20-6. **Vaginitis**

ABNORMAL
FINDINGS

In assessing female genitalia, the nurse may suspect vaginal infection from signs such as redness or lack of color, unusual discharge and secretions, reported itching, and other typical symptoms of the kinds of vaginitis discussed below.

TRICHOMONAS VAGINITIS (TRICHOMONIASIS)

This type of vaginal infection is caused by a protozoan organism and is usually sexually transmitted. The discharge is typically yellow-green, frothy, and foul smelling. The labia may appear swollen and red, and the vaginal walls may be red, rough, and covered with small red spots or petechiae. This infection causes itching and urinary frequency in the client. Upon testing, the pH of vaginal secretion will be greater than 4.5 (usually 7.0 or more). If a sample of vaginal secretions are stirred into a potassium hydroxide solution (KOH prep), a foul odor (typically known as a "+" amine) may be noted.

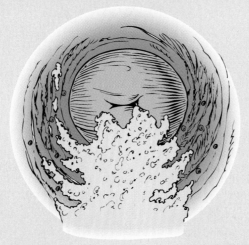

ATROPHIC VAGINITIS

Atrophic vaginitis occurs after menopause when estrogen production is low. The discharge produced may be blood-tinged and is usually minimal. The labia and vaginal mucosa appear atrophic. The vaginal mucosa is typically pale, dry, and contains areas of abrasion that bleed easily. Atrophic vaginitis causes itching, burning, dryness, and painful urination.

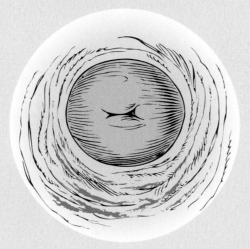

(continued)

CANDIDAL VAGINITIS (MONILIASIS)

This infection is caused by the overgrowth of yeast in the vagina. It causes a thick, white, cheesy discharge. The labia may be inflamed and swollen. The vaginal mucosa may be reddened and typically contains patches of the discharge. This infection causes intense itching and discomfort.

The pH of vaginal secretions will be <4.5 amine (vaginal secretions in KOH) is negative.

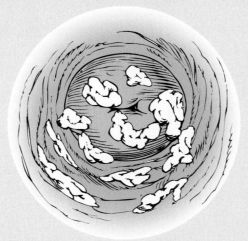

BACTERIAL VAGINOSIS

The cause of bacterial vaginosis is unknown (possibly anaerobic bacteria), but it is thought to be sexually transmitted. The discharge is thin and gray-white, has a positive amine (fishy smell), and coats the vaginal walls and ectocervix. The labia and vaginal walls usually appear normal and pH is greater than 4.5 (5.5–6.0).

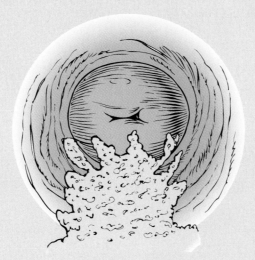

DISPLAY 20-7. Positions of the Uterus

ANTEVERTED

This is the most typical position of the uterus. The cervix is pointed posteriorly, and the body of the uterus is at the level of the pubis over the bladder.

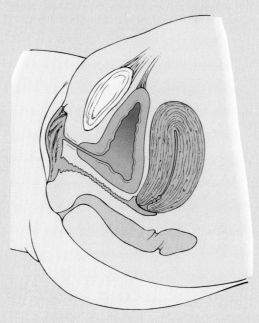

MIDPOSITION

This is a normal variation. The cervix is pointed slightly more anterior (compared with the anteverted position), and the body of the uterus is positioned more posterior than the anteverted position, midway between the bladder and the rectum. It may be difficult to palpate the body through the abdominal and rectal walls with the uterus in this position.

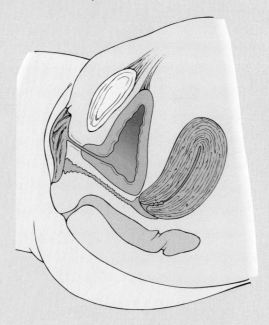

(continued)

ANTEFLEXED

Anteflexion is a normal variation that consists of the uterine body flexed anteriorly in relation to the cervix. The position of the cervix remains normal.

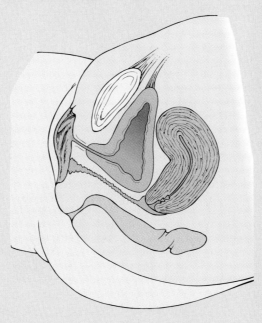

RETROVERTED UTERUS

Retroversion is a normal variation that consists of the cervix and body of the uterus tilting backward. The uterine wall may not be palpable through the abdominal wall or the rectal wall in moderate retroversion. However, if the uterus is prominently retroverted, the wall may be felt through the posterior fornix or the rectal wall.

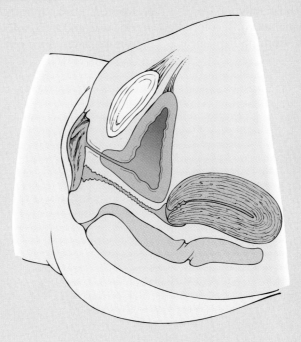

DISPLAY 20-7. Positions of the Uterus (Continued)

RETROFLEXED UTERUS

Retroflexion is a normal variation that consists of the uterine body being flexed posteriorly in relation to the cervix. The position of the cervix remains normal. The body of the uterus may be felt through the posterior fornix or the rectal wall.

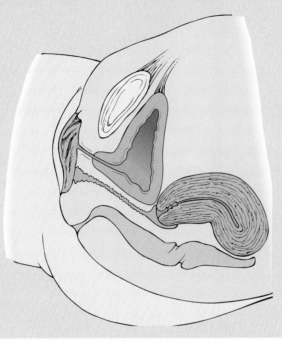

approximately 3 cm in size palpated bilaterally, no excessive tenderness or masses noted. No malodorous, colored vaginal discharge on gloved fingers. Routine Pap smear performed. Firm, smooth, nontender, movable posterior uterine wall and firm, smooth, thin, movable rectovaginal septum palpated during rectovaginal examination.

ABNORMAL
FINDINGS

DISPLAY 20-8. Uterine Enlargement

The only uterine enlargement that is normal results from pregnancy and fetal growth. In such cases, the isthmus feels soft (Hegar's sign) on palpation, and the fundus and isthmus are compressible at between 10 and 12 weeks of pregnancy.

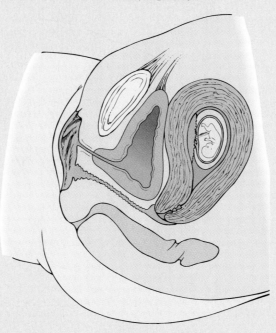

UTERINE FIBROIDS (MYOMAS)

Uterine fibroid tumors are common and benign. They are irregular, firm nodules that are continuous with the uterine surface. They may occur as one or many and may grow quite large. The uterus will be irregularly enlarged, firm, and mobile.

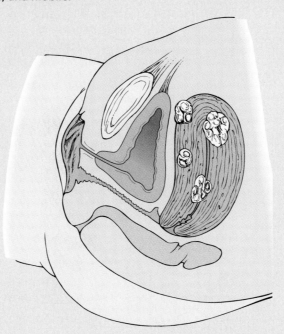

(continued)

UTERINE CANCER (CANCER OF THE ENDOMETRIUM)

The uterus may be enlarged with a malignant mass. Irregular bleeding, bleeding between periods, or postmenopausal bleeding may be the first sign of a problem.

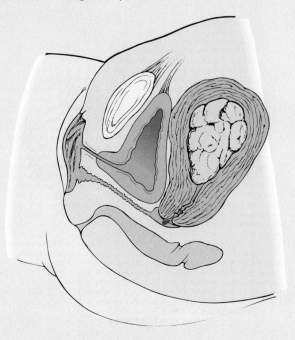

ENDOMETRIOSIS

In endometriosis, the uterus is fixed and tender. Growths of endometrial tissue are usually present throughout the pelvic area and may be felt as firm, nodular masses. Pelvic pain and irregular bleeding are common.

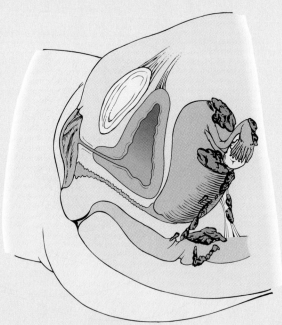

DISPLAY 20-9. Adnexal Masses

PELVIC INFLAMMATORY DISEASE (PID)

PID is typically caused by infection of the fallopian tubes (salpingitis) or fallopian tubes and ovaries (salpingo-oophoritis) with a sexually transmitted disease (ie, gonorrhea, *Chlamydia*). It causes extremely tender and painful bilateral adnexal masses (positive chandelier sign).

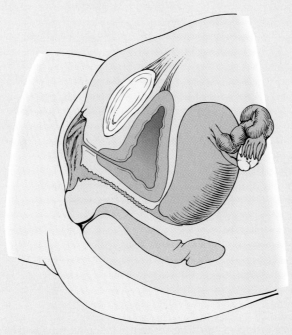

OVARIAN CYST

Ovarian cysts are benign masses on the ovary. They are usually smooth, mobile, round, compressible, and nontender.

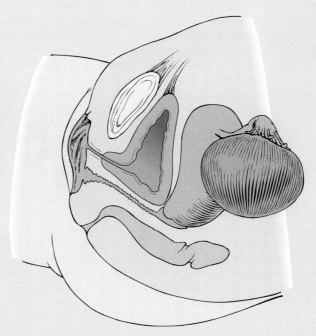

(continued)

OVARIAN CANCER

Masses that are cancerous are usually solid, irregular, nontender, and fixed.

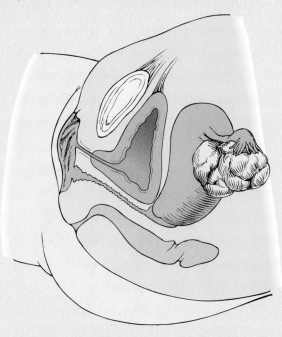

ECTOPIC PREGNANCY

Ectopic pregnancy occurs when a fertilized egg attaches to the fallopian tube and begins developing instead of continuing its journey to the uterus for development. A solid, mobile, tender, and unilateral adnexal mass may be palpated if tenderness allows. The cervix and uterus will be softened, and movement of these structures will cause pain.

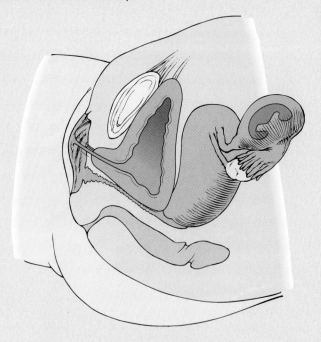

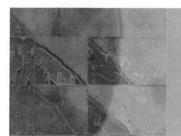

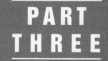

After you have collected your assessment data, you will need to analyze the data, using diagnostic reasoning skills (refer to Chapters 6 and 7). Use the Diagnostic Reasoning: Case Study (below) as a guide or model to analyzing female genitalia assessment data for a *specific* client. Use the critical thinking exercise provided in the study guide/lab manual as an additional opportunity to hone your analytical skills.

Diagnostic Reasoning: Possible Conclusions

Listed below are some possible conclusions that follow an assessment of female genitalia.

SELECTED NURSING DIAGNOSES

After collecting subjective and objective data pertaining to the female genitalia, you will need to identify abnormal findings and cluster the data to reveal any significant patterns or abnormalities. These data will then be used to make clinical judgments (nursing diagnoses: wellness, risk, or actual) about the status of the client's genitalia. Following is a listing of selected nursing diagnoses that you may identify when analyzing data for this part of the assessment.

Nursing Diagnoses (Wellness)

- Opportunity to enhance health management of the genitalia
- Health-Seeking Behavior: requests information on external genitalia examination
- Health-Seeking Behavior: requests information on ways to prevent sexually transmitted diseases
- Health-Seeking Behavior: requests information on ways to prevent yeast infections
- Health-Seeking Behavior: requests information on birth control
- Health-Seeking Behavior: requests information on cessation of menses and hormone replacement therapy

Nursing Diagnoses (Risk)

- Risk of Ineffective Therapeutic Regimen Management (monthly external genitalia examination) related to lack of knowledge of the importance of the examination
- Risk for Infection related to unprotected sexual intercourse
- Risk for Disturbed Body Image related to perceived effects on feminine role and sexuality

Nursing Diagnoses (Actual)

- Fear of ovarian cancer related to high incidence of risk factors
- Ineffective Sexuality Patterns related to decreased libido
- Ineffective Therapeutic Regimen Management related to lack of knowledge of external genitalia self-examination
- Acute Pain: dysuria related to infection
- Anticipatory Grieving related to impending loss of reproductive organs secondary to gynecologic surgery
- Ineffective Sexuality Patterns related to perceptions of effects of surgery on sexual functioning and attractiveness
- Acute Pain related to surgical incision
- Acute Pain: dyspareunia (painful intercourse) related to inadequate vaginal lubrication

SELECTED COLLABORATIVE PROBLEMS

After grouping the data, you may discover that certain collaborative problems emerge. Remember, collaborative problems differ from nursing diagnoses in that they cannot be prevented by nursing interventions. However, these physiologic complications of medical conditions can be detected and monitored by the nurse. In addition, the nurse can use physician- and nurse-prescribed interventions to minimize the complications posed by these problems. The nurse may also have to refer the client in such situations for further treatment of the problem. The following list of collaborative problems may be identified when assessing the female genitalia. These problems are worded as Potential Complication (PC), followed by the problem.

- PC: Gonorrhea
- PC: Syphilis
- PC: *Chlamydia*
- PC: Infertility
- PC: Pregnancy
- PC: Urinary incontinence
- PC: Ovarian nodule
- PC: Abnormal Pap smear result
- PC: Vaginal bleeding

MEDICAL PROBLEMS

After grouping the data, you may see that the client has signs and symptoms that may require medical diagnosis and treatment. Referral to a primary care provider is necessary.

Diagnostic Reasoning: Case Study

The case study presents assessment data for a specific client. It is followed by an analysis of the data arrived at by a diagnostic reasoning process to arrive at specific conclusions.

Melinda is a 22-year-old college student who comes into the college nurse-managed clinic. She complains, "I feel like I have the flu—no energy, a headache, and fever." She reports a recent outbreak of genital lesions after a sexual encounter 10 days ago ("first and only") with a fellow student she only recently met. She denies the use of any protection or birth control, stating, "He refused to use anything and I didn't insist." She denies any problems with her menstrual cycle, no previous sexual activity, and no vaginal infections. "I have always been healthy—I don't know why I behaved so stupidly and put my health at risk." The lesions are present as vesicles and ulcerations on the external genitalia, labia, and mons, with a few vesicles extending into the perianal area. The rest of the perineal and pelvic examination is negative. Some enlarged, tender lymph nodes are noted in the inguinal areas bilaterally. Melinda's temperature by oral route is 100.6°F. When questioned, she confirms that she has a great deal of pain in the vaginal area and "urinating hurts a lot."

1 Identify abnormal data and strengths (in both subjective and objective data).

SUBJECTIVE DATA

- Flulike symptoms: fatigue, headache, fever
- Recent outbreak of genital lesions after unprotected sex
- "First and only"
- "He refused to use anything, and I didn't insist"
- Denies previous sexual activity or gynecologic problems
- "Always been healthy"
- "I don't know why I behaved so stupidly and put my health at risk"
- Much pain in vaginal area
- "Urinating hurts a lot"

OBJECTIVE DATA

- Came to nurse-managed clinic for help
- Vesicles and ulcerations on the external genitalia, labia, and mons
- Few vesicles extending into the perianal area
- Rest of perineal and pelvic examination negative
- Enlarged, tender inguinal lymph nodes
- Oral temperature 100.6°F

2 Cue Clusters	**3** Inferences	**4** Possible Nursing Diagnoses	**5** Defining Characteristics	**6** Confirm or Rule Out
A • Flulike symptoms: fatigue, headache, fever • Recent outbreak of genital lesions after unprotected sex • Much pain in vaginal area • "Urinating hurts a lot" • Vesicles and ulcerations on the external genitalia, labia, and mons • Few vesicles extending into the perianal area • Rest of perineal and pelvic examination normal • Enlarged, tender inguinal lymph nodes • Oral temperature 100.6°F	The history of client's chief complaint coupled with the information gleaned from the interview and examination strongly suggests an STD. The nurse should obtain a specimen for culture of the lesions to assist in the medical diagnosis and refer the client to the clinic physician. Collaborative problems should also be identified.			

2	3	4	5	6
Cue Clusters	**Inferences**	**Possible Nursing Diagnoses**	**Defining Characteristics**	**Confirm or Rule Out**
B • Vesicles and ulcerative lesions on labia, mons, and perianal area • Reports much pain in vaginal area • "Urinating hurts a lot" • "I don't know why I behaved so stupidly and put my health at risk"	Open, ulcerated lesions in a highly sensitive area of the body can result in severe pain that can persist for weeks until lesions heal. The client will need to learn strategies to decrease discomfort. In addition, the client's statement indicates some degree of self-anger and blame, which can increase the pain because of increased emotional response to the situation.	Acute Pain related to knowledge deficit of pain management strategies	*Major, Subjective:* Communication of pain descriptors *Major, Objective:* None specific other than the lesions that conventionally are considered to be pain producing, but this is not listed under defining characteristics	Confirm because it meets the major defining characteristics.
		Acute Pain related to possible excessive emotional response secondary to self-anger or blame	*Major, Subjective:* Communication of pain descriptors *Major, Objective:* Self-focusing statement	This also meets the defining characteristics; however, the care for this client might be better focused under a different diagnosis, such as Situational Low Self-Esteem.
C • Came to nurse-managed clinic for help • Recent outbreak of genital lesions after unprotected sex • "First and only" • "He refused to use anything and I didn't insist" • Denies previous sexual activity or gynecologic problems • "Always been healthy" • "I don't know why I behaved so stupidly and put my health at risk"	Because this was the client's first sexual experience and it resulted in a probable STD, she appears to be experiencing negative feelings about her judgment and lack of assertiveness in insisting on protection. Her statement implies self-blame for her illness. She did seek help as soon as symptoms became apparent. It should also be noted that she did not know her partner very well, so other factors may be present that are not identified.	Situational Low Self-Esteem related to perceived lack of assertiveness in protecting health	*Major:* None identified	Rule out, not specific enough.
		Situational Low Self-Esteem related to unknown factors or changes occurring in present life situation	*Major:* Episodic occurrence of negative self-appraisal *Minor:* Self-negating verbalizations; expressions of shame/guilt (implied)	Confirm, but collect more data as to why the client chose a relative stranger for a first sexual experience and why behavior was non-assertive regarding health protection.
		Health-Seeking Behaviors	*Major:* None—sought help for symptoms of illness *Minor:* Inferred desire for increased control of health	Rule out because client sought illness management rather than health promotion at this time. However, the nurse has a great opportunity for health teaching while this client is undergoing treatment.

7 **Document conclusions.**

Three diagnoses are appropriate for Melinda at this time:

- Acute Pain related to knowledge deficit of pain management strategies
- Acute Pain related to possible excessive emotional response secondary to self-anger or blame

- Situational Low Self-Esteem related to unknown factors or changes occurring in present life situation

In addition, an identified potential complication could be urinary retention (secondary to dysuria). Melinda should be referred to a physician for diagnosis and treatment of her genital lesions.

REFERENCES AND SELECTED READINGS

Ashfaq, R., Gibbons, D., Vela, C., Saboorian, M. H., & Iliya, F. (1999). Thin Prep Pap test accuracy for glandular disease. *Acta Cytologica, 43*(1).

Association of Reproductive Health Professionals. (2000, September). Mature sexuality: Patient realities and provider challenges. *Clinical Proceedings.*

Centers for Disease Control and Prevention. (1999). Achievements in public health, 1900–1999: Family planning. *Morbidity & Mortality Weekly Report, 48*, 1073–1080.

———. (1998). 1998 guidelines for treatment of sexually transmitted diseases. *Morbidity & Mortality Weekly Report, 47*(RR-1), 88–94.

Change, R. J., & Katz, S. E. (1999). Diagnosis of polycystic ovary syndrome. *Endocrinology & Metabolism Clinics of North America, 28*(2), 397–408.

Cullins, V. E., Dominguez, L., Guberski, T., Secor, R. M., & Wysocki, S. J. Treating vaginitis. *Nurse Practitioner, 24*, 1046–1060.

Daley, E. (1998). Diagnosis and management of the adnexal mass. *American Family Physician, 57*(10).

Drake, J. (1998). Diagnosis and management of the adnexal mass. *American Family Physician, 57*(10).

Ellerbrock, T., Chiasson, M., Bush, T. M., Sun, X., Sawo, D., Brudney, D. M., & Wright T. (2000). Incidence of cervical squamous intraepithelial lesions in HIV-infected women. *Journal of the American Medical Association 283*, 1031–1037.

Koeckeritz, J. L. (1983). Assessing the genitalia. *RN, 46*(1), 52–59.

Machia, J. (2001). Breast cancer: Risk, prevention and tamoxifen. *American Journal of Nursing, 101*(4), 26–34.

Markle, M. E. (2001). Polycystic ovary syndrome: Implications for the advanced practice nurse in primary care. *Journal of the American Academy of Nurse Practitioners, 13*(4), 160–163.

McFadden, S. E., & Schumann, L. (2001). The role of human papillomavirus in screening for cervical cancer. *Journal of the American Academy of Nurse Practitioners, 13*(3), 113–115.

McGregor, H. F. (2001). Postmenopausal bleeding: A practical approach. *Journal of the American Academy of Nurse Practitioners 13*(3), 113–115.

Moller, L. A., & Lose, G. (2000, July). The outcome of pelvic examinations in women 40–60 years of age with lower urinary tract symptoms. *Journal of Obstetrics and Gynecology, 20*(4), 414.

Moore, A. A., & Noonan, M. D. (1996). A nurse's guide to hormone replacement therapy. *Journal of Obstetric, Gynecologic and Neonatal Nursing, 25*, 24–31.

Oddens, B. J. (1999). Women's satisfaction with birth control: A population survey of physical and psychological effects of oral contraceptive, intrauterine devices, condoms, natural family planning and sterilization among 1466 women. *Contraception, 59*, 277–286.

Scott, P. M. (1996). Abnormal Pap smears: When is colposcopy needed? *JAAPA/Journal of the American Academy of Physician Assistants, 9*(1), 71–72, 74, 76.

Sellers, J. W., Mahony, J. B., Kaczorowski, J., Lytwyn, A., Bangura, H., Chong, S., Lorincz, A., Dalby, D. M., Janjusevic, V., & Keller, J. L. (2000). Prevalence and predictors of human papilloma virus infection in women in Ontario, Canada. *Canadian Medical Association Journal, 163*(5), 503.

Vizcaino, A. P., Moreno, V., & Bosch, F. X. (1998). International trends in the incidence of cervical cancer: I. Adenocarcinoma and adenosquamous cell carcinomas. *International Journal of Cancer, 75.*

Youngkin, E. Q., & Davis, M. S. (1998). *Women's health: A primary care clinical guide* (2nd ed.). Stamford, CT: Appleton & Lange.

Risk Factors—Cervical Cancer

American Cancer Society (ACS). (2000). Cervical cancer [On-line]. Available: ACS: Cervical Cancer Resource Center, *http://www.cancer.org.*

Averette, H., & Nguyen, H. (1995). Gynecologic cancer. In G. Murphy, W. Lawrence, & R. Lenhard. *American Cancer Society textbook of clinical oncology* (2nd ed.). Atlanta, GA: American Cancer Society.

Brinton, L., Herrero, R., Reeves, W., de Britton, R., Gaitan, E., & Tenorio, F. (1993). Risk factors for cervical cancer by histology. *Gynecologic Oncology, 51*(3), 299–300.

Murphy, G., Lawrence, W., & Lenhard, R. (1995). *American Cancer Society textbook of clinical oncology* (2nd ed.). Atlanta, GA: American Cancer Society.

For additional information on this book, be sure to visit http://connection.lww.com.

Anus, Rectum, and Prostate Assessment

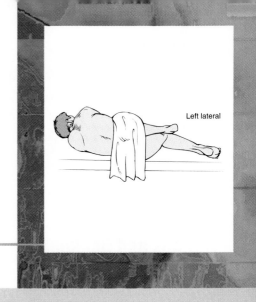

Left lateral

21

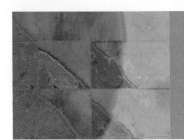

Anus and Rectum

The anal canal is the final segment of the digestive system. It measures from 2.5 cm to 4 cm long. It is lined with skin that contains no hair or sebaceous glands but does contain many somatic sensory nerves, making it very sensitive to touch. The anal opening or anal verge can be distinguished from the perianal skin by its hairless moist appearance. The anal verge extends interiorly, overlying the external anal sphincter.

Within the anus are the two sphincters that normally hold the anal canal closed. The external sphincter is composed of skeletal muscle and is under voluntary control. The internal sphincter is composed of smooth muscle and is under involuntary control by the autonomic nervous system. Dividing the two sphincters is the palpable intersphincteric groove. The anal canal proceeds upward toward the umbilicus. Just above the internal sphincter is the anorectal junction, the dividing point of the anal canal and the rectum. The rectum is lined with folds of mucosa that contain a network of arteries, veins, and visceral nerves. If the veins in these folds undergo chronic pressure, they may become engorged with blood, forming hemorrhoids (Fig. 21-1).

The rectum is the lowest portion of the large intestine and is approximately 12 cm long, extending from the end of the sigmoid colon to the anorectal junction. It enlarges above the anorectal junction and proceeds in a posterior direction toward the hollow of the sacrum and coccyx. (Therefore, the anal canal and rectum are at approximately right angles to each other.) The inside of the rectum contains three inward foldings called the valves of Houston. The lowest valve may be felt, usually on the client's left side.

The peritoneum lines the upper two thirds of the anterior rectum and dips down enough so that it may be palpated where it forms the rectovesical pouch in men and the rectouterine pouch in women.

Prostate

The prostate gland surrounds the neck of the bladder and urethra and lies between these structures and the rectum in male clients. It consists of two lobes separated by a shallow groove called the median sulcus (Fig. 21-2). It secretes a thin, milky substance that promotes sperm motility and neutralizes female acidic vaginal secretions. This chestnut- or heart-shaped organ can be palpated through the anterior wall of the rectum.

Prostatic hyperplasia, enlargement of the prostate gland, has become increasingly common in men over age 40.

Located on either side of, and above, the prostate gland are the seminal vesicles. These are rabbit-ear–shaped structures that produce the ejaculate that nourishes and protects sperm. They are not normally palpable. The Cowper's or bulbourethral glands are mucus-producing, pea-sized organs located posterior to the prostate gland. These glands surround and empty into the urethra. They are not normally palpable either.

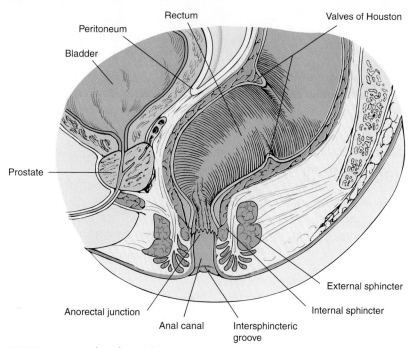

Peritoneum
Bladder
Rectum
Valves of Houston
Prostate
External sphincter
Internal sphincter
Anorectal junction
Anal canal
Intersphincteric groove

FIGURE 21-1. Anal and rectal structures.

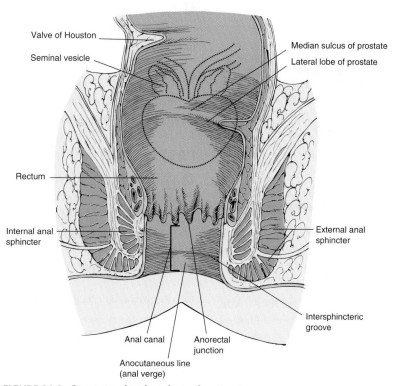

Valve of Houston
Seminal vesicle
Median sulcus of prostate
Lateral lobe of prostate
Rectum
Internal anal sphincter
External anal sphincter
Intersphincteric groove
Anal canal
Anorectal junction
Anocutaneous line (anal verge)

FIGURE 21-2. Prostate gland and nearby structures.

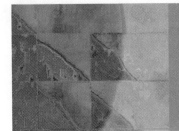

Nursing Assessment

Collecting Subjective Data

The data gathered during subjective assessment provide clues to the client's overall health and whether he or she is at risk for diseases and disorders of the anus, rectum, or prostate. The subjective assessment is a good time to teach the client about risk factors related to diseases, such as colorectal or prostate cancer, and about ways to decrease those risk factors.

Collecting data about the anus, rectum, and prostate can be embarrassing for both the examiner and the client. Some questions are very personal. Therefore, it is important to ease the client's anxiety as much as possible. Ask the questions in a straightforward manner, and let the client voice any concerns throughout the assessment. In some cultural groups, only nurses of the same gender will be considered acceptable assessors of intimate body areas.

COLDSPA

CHARACTER: Describe the sign or symptom. How does it feel, look, sound, smell, and so forth?
ONSET: When did it begin?
LOCATION: Where is it? Does it radiate?
DURATION: How long does it last? Does it recur?
SEVERITY: How bad is it?
PATTERN: What makes it better: What makes it worse?
ASSOCIATED FACTORS: What other symptoms occur with it?

Nursing History
CURRENT SYMPTOMS

Question What is your usual bowel pattern? Have you noticed any recent change in the pattern?

Rationale A change in bowel pattern is associated with many disorders and is one of the warning signs of cancer. A more thorough evaluation, including laboratory tests and proctosigmoidoscopy, may be necessary.

Q Do you experience constipation?

R Constipation may indicate a bowel obstruction or the need for dietary counseling.

Q Do you experience diarrhea?

R Diarrhea may signal impaction or indicate the need for dietary counseling.

Q Do you have trouble controlling your bowels?

R Fecal incontinence occurs with neurologic disorders and some gastrointestinal infections.

Q What is the color of your stool? Have you noticed any blood on or in your stool?

R Black stools may indicate gastrointestinal bleeding or the use of iron supplements or Pepto-Bismol. Red blood in the stool is found with hemorrhoids, polyps, cancer, or colitis. Clay-colored stools result from a lack of bile pigment.

Q Have you noticed any mucus in your stool?

R Mucus in the stool may indicate steatorrhea (excessive fat in the stool).

Q Do you experience any itching or pain in the rectal area?

R Sexually transmitted diseases, hemorrhoids, pinworms, or anal trauma may cause itching or pain.

PAST HISTORY

Q Have you ever had anal or rectal trauma or surgery? Were you born with any congenital deformities of the anus or rectum? Have you had prostate surgery?

R Past conditions influence the findings of physical assessment. Congenital deformities, such as imperforate anus, are often surgically repaired when the client is very young.

Q When was the last time you had a stool test to detect blood?

R The American Cancer Society recommends a stool test every year after age 50 to detect occult blood. Clinical trials have determined that the fecal occult blood test has increased detection of both adenomatous polyps and colorectal cancer and is associated with a 15% to 33% decline in the death rate from these conditions (http://cancernet.nci.nih.gov/).

Q Have you ever had proctosigmoidoscopy?

R A proctosigmoidoscopic examination is recommended every 3 to 5 years after age 50 based on the advice of a physician.

Q When was the last time you had a digital rectal examination (DRE) by a physician?

R A DRE may reveal rectal masses, prostate enlargement, or prostate nodules. The American Cancer Society recommends a DRE every year after age 40.

Q Have you ever had blood taken for a prostate screening, which measures the level of prostate-specific antigen (PSA) in your blood? When was the test and what was the result?

R PSA is a biologic marker for prostate cancer. The American Cancer Society recommends a PSA measurement yearly for men age 50 years and older (see Risk Factors—Prostate Cancer).

FAMILY HISTORY

Q Is there a history of polyps, colon or rectal cancer, or prostate cancer in your family?

R Colorectal and prostate cancer have a tendency to affect members of the same family.

LIFESTYLE AND HEALTH PRACTICES

Q Do you use any laxatives, stool softeners, enemas, or other bowel movement-enhancing medications?

R Long-term use of these agents can alter the body's ability to regulate bowel function. Short-term use may indicate the need for dietary counseling.

Q Do you engage in anal sex?

R Anal sex increases the risk for sexually transmitted disease, infection by human immunodeficiency virus (HIV), fissures, rectal prolapse, and hemorrhoid formation.

Q Do you take any medications for your prostate?

R Men with benign prostatic hypertrophy (BPH) with "voiding symptoms," such as urinary urgency, may take an alpha-adrenergic blocker, such as terazosin (Hytrin) or an androgen hormone inhibitor, such as finasteride (Proscar).

Q How much high-fiber food and roughage do you consume every day? Do you eat foods high in saturated fat?

R Although high-fat diets have been implicated in colon cancer (see Risk Factors—Colorectal Cancer), the role of dietary fat continues to be controversial. The Nurses' Health Study indicates that the risk of colon cancer increases with the consumption of red meat and saturated and monounsaturated fats. But the Iowa Women's Health Study and a National Cancer Institute study found no such relationship. The role of dietary fiber, which was once thought to offer protection against colon cancer is also in question. Although a majority of studies conducted over the last 20 years suggest dietary fiber offers protection against colon cancer, several studies—including the Nurses' Health Study—do not support these benefits of fiber.

Q Do you engage in regular exercise?

R Sedentary lifestyle has been linked to the development of colorectal cancer, and physical activity has been associated with a reduction in risk. The amount of exercise needed has not been established.

Q Do you use calcium supplements?

R Some observational studies indicate that the colon cancer risk drops as calcium intake increases; others do not reflect any effect.

Q For postmenopausal women: Do you use hormone replacement therapy?

R Studies, including a retrospective study of 400,000 women conducted by the American Cancer Society and the Nurses' Health Study, a prospective study of 120,000 women, have indicated that postmenopausal estrogen use reduces the risk of colon cancer. Further studies are needed.

Q Has any anal or rectal problem affected your normal activities of daily living (working or engaging in recreation)?

R Some problems, such as hemorrhoids or bowel incontinence, may affect a client's ability to work or interact socially.

Collecting Objective Data

A physical examination of the anus and rectum should be performed on all adult men and women. It should be performed regardless of whether the client complains of symptoms because some conditions, such as cancerous tumors, may be asymptomatic. A DRE is recommended for both men and women every year after age 40, and a stool blood test is recommended every year after age 50. In addition, a proctosigmoidoscopic examination is recommended every 3 to 5 years after age 50 (American Cancer Society, 1996). Detecting problems with the anus, rectum, or prostate is the primary objective of this examination. Early detection of a problem is one way to promote early treatment and a more positive outcome. The examiner may also use this time (especially if the examination is a well examination) to integrate teaching about ways to reduce risk factors for diseases and disorders of the anus, rectum, and prostate.

The hands-on physical examination of the anus, rectum, and prostate can cause most clients anxiety and embarrassment. It is important to proceed slowly and to explain all

(*text continues on page 482*)

RISK FACTORS
Colorectal Cancer

OVERVIEW

Cancer of the colon and rectum is the third most common type of cancer in men and women in Western industrialized societies. About 93,800 new cases of colon cancer and 36,400 new cases of rectal cancer were expected to be diagnosed in the United States in 2000, and about 47,700 persons were expected to die from colorectal cancer in 2000. The death rate has been dropping for the last 20 years, possibly due to earlier detection and improved treatment. The 5-year survival rate for colorectal cancers that have not spread is 90%, but only 37% of such cancers are found at that early stage (American Cancer Society, 2000).

RISK FACTORS (AMERICAN CANCER SOCIETY, 2000)

- Age over 40 years (90% occur over age 50)
- Personal history of rectal or colon polyps or cancer
- Inflammatory bowel diseases
- Genetics: Family history of cancer or familial colorectal cancer syndromes
- Ashkenazi Jewish descent (Eastern European)
- Diet mostly from animal sources (high in fat and animal protein; low in fruits, vegetables, and fiber)
- Physical inactivity
- Obesity

RISK REDUCTION TEACHING TIPS (AMERICAN CANCER SOCIETY, 2000)

- For people at average risk: Beginning at age 50, have a fecal occult blood test (FOBT) every year and a sigmoidoscopic examination every 5 years, or a colonoscopic examination every 10 years, or a double contrast barium enema every 5 to 10 years.
- For people at moderate risk, with polyps or previous cancer: Follow ACS guidelines for screening.
- For people with a personal history of polyps or with first-degree relatives who are cancer patients: Have colonoscopy at age 40 and every 5 to 10 years thereafter.

- Eat a diet high in fiber, fruit, and vegetables and low in fat and animal protein.
- Eat a half cup of raisins or three-quarters cup of grapes daily (tartaric acid and fiber reduce bile acids and speed food through system; Spiller, 2001)
- Get regular exercise for at least 30 minutes most days.
- Talk to physician about advisability of taking aspirin or nonsteroidal antiinflammatory drugs (NSAIDs) or postmenopausal estrogen replacement therapy (ERT), both shown to be associated with decreased incidence of colorectal cancer.
- Be aware of colorectal cancer symptoms, and, if they develop, check with your physician. Symptoms include:
  - A change in bowel habits, such as diarrhea, constipation, or narrowing of the stool (pencil thin) that lasts for more than a few days; the feeling that you need to have a bowel movement that is not relieved by doing so
  - Rectal bleeding or blood in the stool
  - Cramping or steady abdominal pain
  - Decreased appetite
  - Weakness and fatigue
  - Jaundice (American Cancer Society, 2000)

 ## CULTURAL CONSIDERATIONS

Recent research has found an inherited tendency to develop colorectal cancer among some Jews of Eastern European descent. An inherited mutation is present in about 6% of American Jews. The risk for cancer development appears to be relatively small, but more research is being done (American Cancer Society, 2000). Outside the United States, colorectal cancer is increasing in Western countries (Crutti et al., 1995). Although the disease is predominantly one of Western industrialized societies, as other societies adopt a more Western-style diet (eg, high fat, low fiber), the incidence of colorectal cancer increases. The role of environmental factors, especially dietary practices, in colon cancer development has been so strongly supported that racial variation is believed to be of little importance (Overfield, 1995).

RISK FACTORS
Prostate Cancer

OVERVIEW

Prostate cancer is the most common cancer besides skin cancer, and the second leading cause of cancer death (after lung cancer) in American men. The American Cancer Society estimated that 180,400 new cases of prostate cancer would be diagnosed in the United States during the year 2000 and that 31,900 men would die of the disease. About 92% of men diagnosed with prostate cancer survive at least 5 years. About 58% of prostate cancers are detected while they are still localized (confined to the prostate). Of the 11% of men whose cancer has spread to distant body parts at the time of diagnosis, about 31% survive 5 years (American Cancer Society, 2000)

RISK FACTORS (AMERICAN CANCER SOCIETY, 2000)

- Advanced age (incidence increases each decade over age 50)
- Nationality or ethnic group (higher in African-American males in the United States)
- Diet high in fat, animal products, and calcium; low in fruits, vegetables, fructose (fruit sugar), lycopenes (in tomatoes, grapefruit, and watermelon), and selenium
- Limited or low levels of physical activity

POSSIBLE RISK FACTORS

- Exposure to cadmium (Murphy et al., 1995)
- High-risk occupations: tire and rubber manufacturing, farming, mechanics, sheet metal work (Murphy et al., 1995)
- History of sexually transmitted diseases (Overfield, 1995)
- Lack of circumcision (Overfield, 1995)
- Vasectomy, especially before age 35 (American Cancer Society, 2000)
- Vitamin A supplements (American Cancer Society, 2000)
- Depression (Gallo, 2001)

RISK REDUCTION TEACHING TIPS

- Eat a diet low in fat (especially animal food sources) and high in vegetables, fruits, grains; include tomatoes, grapefruit (if compatible with medications taken), and watermelon.
- Take vitamin E, 50 mg daily (possibly associated with reduced risk); avoid vitamin A supplements.
- Limit exposure to cadmium.
- Follow all Occupational Safety and Health Administration (OSHA) safety measures if employed in a high-risk occupation.
- Avoid giving or getting sexually transmitted disease (STD), and seek treatment as soon as possible if STD symptoms arise.
- If culturally acceptable, circumcise males; uncircumcised men need to carefully clean the area beneath the penile foreskin (Murphy et al., 1995).
- Get treatment for depression (Gallo, 2001).

 ### CULTURAL CONSIDERATIONS

Prostate cancer is most common in North America and northwestern Europe. It is less common in Asia, Africa, Central and South America. However, prostate cancer is about twice as common in African-American men as it is in Caucasian American men (American Cancer Society, 2000). Worldwide, cancer of the prostate occurs considerably less frequently in Japan and the Arctic countries and at intermediate rates in Italy, Greece, and Finland; Japanese men who migrate to the United States have higher prostate cancer rates, but Cuban men who migrate to the United States have lower rates than in their home countries (Overfield, 1995).

steps of the examination as you proceed. Use gentle movements with your finger and make sure you use adequate lubrication. Listen to and watch the client for signs of discomfort or tensing muscles. Encourage relaxation and explain each step of the examination as you proceed. If the examination is being performed as part of the comprehensive physical examination, it is best to perform the examination of the anus, rectum, and prostate at the end of the genitalia examination.

CLIENT PREPARATION

Client positioning is important for this examination, and several different positions can be assumed (Fig. 21-3). It is most logical for the female client to stay in the lithotomy position after the vaginal examination for the anus and rectum examination. Some examiners find it easiest to perform the male anus, rectum, and prostate examination while the client stands and bends over the examining table with his hips flexed. Whichever position you decide would be best for the particular client and examination, it is important to determine if the client is as comfortable as possible in that position.

The most frequently used position is the left lateral position. This position allows adequate inspection and palpation of the anus, rectum, and prostate (in men) and is usually more comfortable for the client. The client's torso and legs can be draped during the examination, which helps to lessen the feeling of vulnerability. To help the client into this position, ask him or her to lie on the left side, with the buttocks as close to the edge of the examining table as possible, and to bend the right knee. No matter which position is chosen, the examiner must realize that he or she will only be able to examine to a certain point up in the rectum using the finger. If an examination of the upper rectum and sigmoid colon is necessary, a proctosigmoidoscopy should be performed.

EQUIPMENT AND SUPPLIES

- Gloves
- Water-soluble lubricant

KEY ASSESSMENT POINTS

- Obtain an accurate and complete health history.
- Alert clients to risk factors for colorectal cancer and prostate cancer and healthful practices to help prevent these diseases.
- Understand the structures and functions of the anorectal region.
- Prepare the client thoroughly for the physical examination to put the client at the greatest ease.
- Perform the examination professionally and preserve the client's modesty.

(*text continues on page 486*)

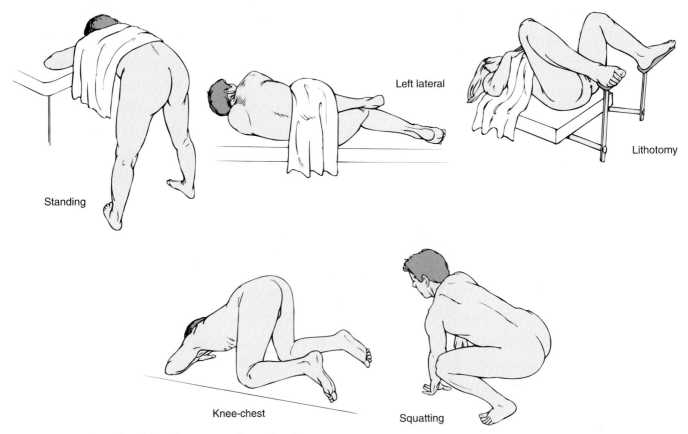

FIGURE 21-3. Selected positions for anorectal examination.

PHYSICAL ASSESSMENT

ASSESSMENT PROCEDURE	NORMAL FINDINGS	ABNORMAL FINDINGS

ANUS AND RECTUM

Inspect the Perianal Area

Spread the client's buttocks and inspect the anal opening and surrounding area for the following:
- Lumps
- Ulcers
- Lesions
- Rashes
- Redness
- Fissures
- Thickening of the epithelium

The anal opening should appear hairless, moist, and tightly closed. The surrounding perianal area should be free of redness, lumps, ulcers, lesions, and rashes.

Lesions may indicate sexually transmitted diseases, cancer, or hemorrhoids. A thrombosed external hemorrhoid appears swollen. It is itchy, painful, and bleeds when the client passes stool. A previously thrombosed hemorrhoid appears as a skin tag that protrudes from the anus.

A painful mass that is hardened and reddened suggests a perianal abscess. A swollen skin tag on the anal margin may indicate a fissure in the anal canal. Redness and excoriation may be from scratching an area infected by fungi or pinworms. A small opening in the skin that surrounds the anal opening may be an anorectal fistula (Display 21-1).

Thickening of the epithelium suggests repeated trauma from anal intercourse.

Inspecting the perianal area.

Ask the client to perform Valsalva's maneuver by straining or bearing down. Inspect the anal opening for any bulges or lesions.

No bulging or lesions appear.

Bulges of red mucous membrane may indicate a rectal prolapse. Hemorrhoids or an anal fissure may also be seen (see Display 21-1).

Inspect the Sacrococcygeal Area

Inspect this area for any signs of swelling, redness, dimpling, or hair.

Area is normally smooth, and free of redness and hair.

A reddened, swollen, or dimpled area covered by a small tuft of hair located midline on the lower sacrum suggests a pilonidal cyst (see Display 21-1).

Palpate the Anus

Inform the client that you are going to perform the internal examination at this point. Explain that it may feel like his or her bowels are going to move but that this will not happen. Lubricate your gloved index finger, and ask the client to bear down. As the client bears down, place the pad of your index finger on the anal opening.

Client's sphincter relaxes, permitting entry.

Sphincter tightens, making further examination unrealistic.

> **Tip From the Experts** Never use your fingertip—this causes the sphincter to tighten and, if forced into the rectum, may cause pain.

(continued)

ASSESSMENT PROCEDURE	NORMAL FINDINGS	ABNORMAL FINDINGS

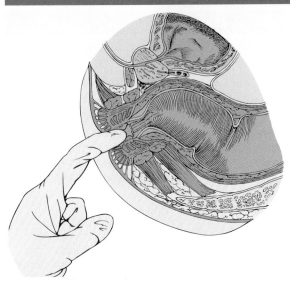

Palpating the anus.

When you feel the sphincter relax, insert your finger gently with the pad facing down.

If the sphincter does not relax and the client reports severe pain, spread the gluteal folds with your hands in close approximation to the anus and attempt to visualize a lesion that may be causing the pain. If tension is maintained on the gluteal folds for 60 seconds, the anus will dilate normally.

Examination finger enters anus.

Examination finger cannot enter the anus.

Tip From the Experts If severe pain prevents your entrance to the anus, do not force the examination.

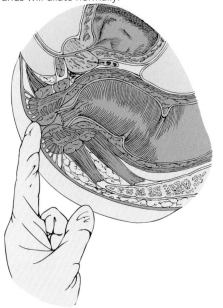

Relaxing the anal sphincter.

Ask the client to tighten the external sphincter, and note the tone.

The client can normally close the sphincter around the gloved finger.

Poor sphincter tone may be the result of a spinal cord injury, previous surgery, trauma, or a prolapsed rectum. Tightened sphincter tone may indicate anxiety, scarring, or inflammation.

(continued)

ASSESSMENT PROCEDURE	NORMAL FINDINGS	ABNORMAL FINDINGS
Palpate for tenderness, nodules, and hardness.	The anus is normally smooth, nontender, and free of nodules and hardness.	Tenderness may indicate hemorrhoids, fistula, or fissure. Nodules may indicate polyps or cancer. Hardness may indicate scarring or cancer.

Palpate the Rectum

Insert your finger further into the rectum as far as possible. Next, turn your hand clockwise and then counterclockwise. This allows palpation of as much rectal surface as possible. Note tenderness, irregularities, nodules, and hardness.	The rectal mucosa is normally soft, smooth, nontender, and free of nodules.	Hardness and irregularities may be from scarring or cancer. Nodules may indicate polyps or cancer (see Display 21-1).

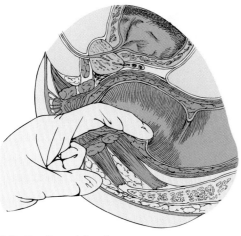

Palpating the rectal wall.

Palpate the Peritoneal Cavity

This area may be palpated in men above the prostate gland in the area of the seminal vesicles on the anterior surface of the rectum. In women, this area may be palpated on the anterior rectal surface in the area of the rectouterine pouch (behind the cervix and the uterus). Note tenderness or nodules.	This area is normally smooth and nontender.	A peritoneal protrusion into the rectum (called a *rectal shelf*) may indicate a cancerous lesion or peritoneal metastasis. Tenderness may indicate peritoneal inflammation.

Inspect the Stool

Withdraw your gloved finger. Inspect any fecal matter on your glove. Assess the color, and test the feces for occult blood. Provide the client with a towel to wipe the anorectal area.	Stool is normally semi-solid, brown, and free of blood.	Black stool may indicate upper gastrointestinal bleeding, gray or tan stool results from the lack of bile pigment, and yellow stool suggests steatorrhea (increased fat content). Blood detected in the stool may indicate cancer of the rectum or colon. An endoscopic examination of the colon should be performed.

(continued)

ASSESSMENT PROCEDURE	NORMAL FINDINGS	ABNORMAL FINDINGS

PROSTATE GLAND

Palpate the Prostate

The prostate can be palpated on the anterior surface of the rectum by turning the hand fully counterclockwise so the pad of your index finger faces toward the client's umbilicus. Tell the client that he may feel an urge to urinate but that he will not. Move the pad of your index finger over the prostate gland, trying to feel the sulcus between the lateral lobes. Note the size, shape, and consistency of the prostate, and identify any nodules or tenderness.

The prostate is normally non-tender and rubbery. It has two lateral lobes that are divided by a median sulcus. The lobes are normally smooth, 2.5 cm long, and heart-shaped.

A swollen, tender prostate may indicate acute prostatitis. An enlarged smooth, firm, slightly elastic prostate that may not have a median sulcus suggests benign prostatic hypertrophy (BPH). A hard area on the prostate or hard, fixed, irregular nodules on the prostate suggest cancer (Display 21-2).

🏵 **Tip From the Experts** You may need to move your body away from the client to achieve the proper angle for examination.

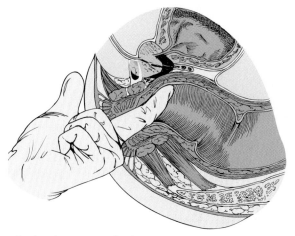

Palpating the prostate gland.

Validation and Documentation of Findings

Validate the anus, rectum, and prostate assessment data that you have collected. This is necessary to verify that the data are reliable and accurate. Document the assessment data following the health care facility or agency policy.

EXAMPLE OF SUBJECTIVE DATA

A 52-year-old client reports no recent change in bowel patterns, no constipation, diarrhea, or blood in stool. He has no trouble controlling his bowels and denies pain and itching in anal area. He has no history of anal or rectal surgery or trauma and no congenital deformities. He states that his last DRE, test for occult blood, and PSA screening were 1 year ago. No significant findings were reported. He says he had a proctosigmoidoscopic examination 2 years ago and the results were normal. He has no knowledge of polyps or cancer (colon, rectal, or prostate) in his family. The client explains that he seldom uses laxatives and has never used an enema. He denies engaging in anal sexual intercourse. He does not know exactly how much water and bulk he consumes, but would guess a moderate to high amount.

EXAMPLE OF OBJECTIVE DATA

Client's anal opening is hairless, moist, and closed tightly. Perianal area is free of redness, lumps, ulcers, lesions, and rashes. No bulging or lesions appear when client performs Valsalva's maneuver. The sacrococcygeal area is smooth, free of redness and hair. Client can close external sphincter around gloved finger. Anus is smooth, nontender, and free of nodules and hardness. Rectal mucosa is soft, smooth, nontender, and free of nodules. Peritoneal cavity area is smooth and nontender. Prostate gland palpated as two smooth, nontender, rubbery lobes approximately 2.5 cm long. The median sulcus is palpated between the two lobes.

After you have collected the assessment data, you will analyze the data, using diagnostic reasoning skills (refer to Chapters 6 and 7). The following section, entitled "Diagnostic Reasoning: Possible Conclusions," presents an overview of common conclusions that you may reach after assessing the anus, rectum, and prostate. The subsequent case study shows you how to analyze your assessment data for a specific client. Finally, you can work through the analysis from beginning to end in the critical thinking exercise that appears in the accompanying study guide/laboratory manual.

(*text continues on page 493*)

DISPLAY 21-1. Abnormalities of the Anus and Rectum

ABNORMAL FINDINGS

Although the anorectal examination is possibly the one examination that produces the greatest discomfort for both the client and the nurse, it is one of the most important for detecting serious problems early in their development.

EXTERNAL HEMORRHOID

Hemorrhoids are usually painless papules caused by varicose veins. They can be internal or external (above or below the anorectal junction). This external hemorrhoid has become thrombosed—it contains clotted blood, is very painful and swollen, and itches and bleeds with bowel movements.

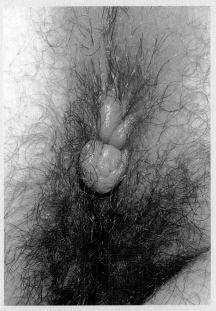

External hemorrhoid. (© 1995 Dr. P. Marazzi/ Science Photo Library/CMSP.)

PERIANAL ABSCESS

Perianal abscess is a cavity of pus, caused by infection in the skin around the anal opening. It causes throbbing pain and is red, swollen, hard, and tender.

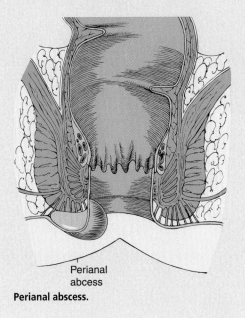

Perianal abcess

Perianal abscess.

(continued)

ANAL FISSURE

These splits in the tissue of the anal canal are caused by trauma. A swollen skin tag ("sentinel tag") is often present below the fissure on the anal margin. They cause intense pain, itching, and bleeding.

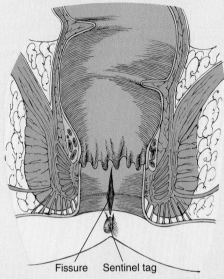

Fissure   Sentinel tag

Anal fissure.

ANORECTAL FISTULA

This is evidenced by a small, round opening in the skin that surrounds the anal opening. It suggests an inflammatory tract from the anus or rectum out to the skin. A previous abscess may have preceded the fistula.

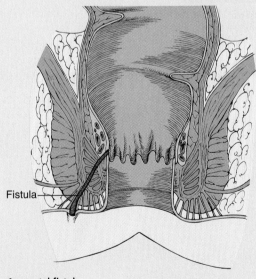

Fistula

Anorectal fistula.

RECTAL PROLAPSE

This occurs when the mucosa of the rectum protrudes out through the anal opening. It may involve only the mucosa or the mucosa and the rectal wall. It appears as a red, doughnutlike mass with radiating folds.

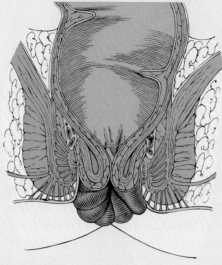

Rectal prolapse.

PILONIDAL CYST

This congenital disorder is characterized by a small dimple or cyst/sinus that contains hair. It is located midline in the sacrococcygeal area and has a palpable sinus tract.

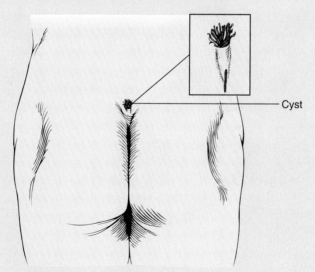

Pilonidal cyst.

(continued)

RECTAL POLYPS

These soft structures are rather common and occur in varying size and number. There are two types: Pedunculated (on a stalk) and sessile (on the mucosal surface).

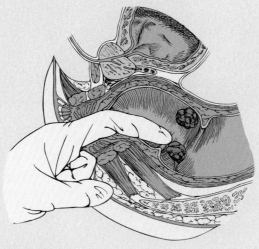

Rectal polyps.

RECTAL CANCER

A rectal carcinoma is usually asymptomatic until it is quite advanced. Thus, routine rectal palpation is essential. A cancer of the rectum may feel like a firm nodule, an ulcerated nodule with rolled edges, or, as it grows, a large, irregularly shaped, fixed, hard nodule.

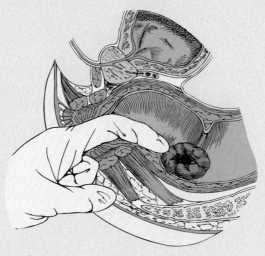

Rectal cancer.

(continued)

RECTAL SHELF

If cancer metastasizes to the peritoneal cavity, it may be felt as a nodular, hard, shelflike structure that protrudes onto the anterior surface of the rectum in the area of the seminal vesicles in men and in the area of the rectouterine pouch in women.

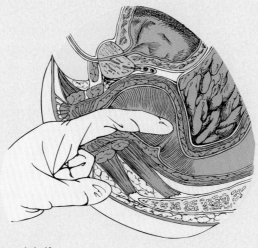

Rectal shelf.

ABNORMAL
FINDINGS

DISPLAY 21-2. **Abnormalities of the Prostate Gland**

ACUTE PROSTATITIS

The prostate is swollen, tender, firm, and warm to the touch. Prostatitis is caused by a bacterial infection.

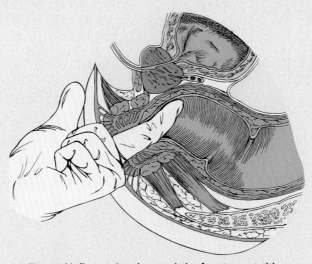

Swelling and inflammation characteristic of acute prostatitis.

(continued)

DISPLAY 21-2. Abnormalities of the Prostate Gland (Continued)

BENIGN PROSTATIC HYPERTROPHY

The prostate is enlarged, smooth, firm, and slightly elastic. The median sulcus may not be palpable. It is common in men older than age 50 years.

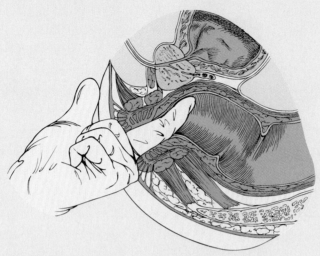

Enlargement characteristic of benign prostatic hypertrophy.

CANCER OF THE PROSTATE

A hard area on the prostate or hard, fixed, irregular nodules on the prostate suggest cancer. The median sulcus may not be palpable.

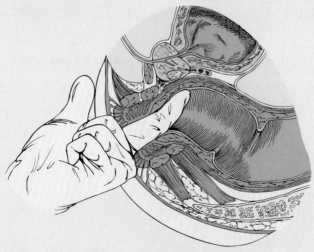

Mass characteristic of prostate cancer.

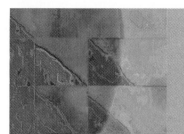

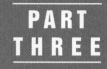

Diagnostic Reasoning: Possible Conclusions

Listed below are some possible conclusions drawn from assessment of the client's anus, rectum, and prostate.

SELECTED NURSING DIAGNOSES

After collecting subjective and objective information pertaining to the anus, rectum, and prostate, you can identify abnormal data and cluster the data to reveal significant patterns or abnormalities. These data form the basis for formulating clinical judgments (nursing diagnoses: wellness, risk, or actual) about the status of the client's anal, rectal, and prostatic health. You may identify some of the following nursing diagnoses when you analyze data collected from your own client.

Nursing Diagnoses (Wellness)

- Opportunity to enhance bowel elimination pattern
- Health-Seeking Behaviors: Requests information on purpose and need for colorectal examination

Nursing Diagnoses (Risk)

- Risk for Ineffective Health Maintenance related to lack of knowledge of need for recommended colorectal and prostate examinations
- Risk for Impaired Skin Integrity in rectal area related to chronic irritation secondary to diarrhea

Nursing Diagnoses (Actual)

- Acute Pain: Rectal
- Diarrhea related to chronic inflammatory bowel disease

- Ineffective Sexuality Patterns related to feelings of loss of femininity/masculinity and sexual attractiveness secondary to chronic diarrhea or pain
- Situational Low Self-Esteem related to loss of control over bowel elimination

SELECTED COLLABORATIVE PROBLEMS

After grouping the data, you may find that certain collaborative problems emerge. Remember, collaborative problems differ from nursing diagnoses in that they cannot be prevented by nursing interventions. However, the nurse can detect and monitor these physiologic complications of medical conditions. In addition, physician- and nurse-prescribed interventions can be implemented to minimize these complications. The nurse may also have to refer the client in such situations for further treatment of the problem. Following is a list of collaborative problems that may be identified when assessing the anus, rectum, and prostate. These problems are worded as Potential Complications (or PC), followed by the problem.

- PC: Prostatic hypertrophy
- PC: Fistula
- PC: Fissure
- PC: Hemorrhoids
- PC: Rectal bleeding
- PC: Rectal abscess

MEDICAL PROBLEMS

In your analysis, you may discover that the client's signs and symptoms appear to require medical diagnosis and treatment, in which case referral to a primary care provider is necessary.

Diagnostic Reasoning: Case Study

The case study presents assessment data for a specific client. It is followed by an analysis of the data by which seven key steps are used to derive specific conclusions.

George Kowalsky, 42 years old, seeks advice from the company nurse because he has been "bleeding from his rectum" and has pain and pressure in the rectal area. Mr. Kowalsky is the head ac-

countant and tax consultant for the company. He is currently preparing for the annual audit and reports to the nurse that he is "very uptight." When questioned, he reports that he has observed small amounts of bright red blood on his stool for the last 2 days and his bowel movements have been quite painful—"like passing ground glass"—for about the last week.

He states he has had hard bowel movements for many years. He reports drinking mostly coffee—10 to 12 cups a day. He says his meals are traditional eggs and bacon for breakfast and meat and potatoes for dinner. He doesn't much like vegetables and fruit. He doesn't eat excessively and has maintained his weight "within the chart norms" for over 20 years. He states he has used Preparation H for his "piles" for years with relief—until lately. When the anorectal area is inspected, several bluish, rounded swellings are present external to the anal sphincter and a small fissure is noted in the lining of the anus. A small amount of light red blood is visible near the anal fissure.

1 Identify abnormal data and strengths (in both subjective and objective data).

SUBJECTIVE DATA

- "Bleeding from his rectum"
- Pain and pressure in the rectal area
- Observed small amounts of bright red blood on his stool for the last 2 days

- Bowel movements have been quite painful, "like passing ground glass," for about the last week
- Hard bowel movements for many years
- "Very uptight"—preparing for annual audit
- Drinks 10 to 12 cups of coffee daily
- Traditional eggs and bacon for breakfast and meat and potatoes for dinner
- Has maintained his weight "within the chart norms" for over 20 years
- Used Preparation H for relief for many years until recently

OBJECTIVE DATA

- Bluish, rounded swellings noted external to the anal sphincter
- Small fissure in the anal lining
- Small amount of light red blood visible near the anal fissure

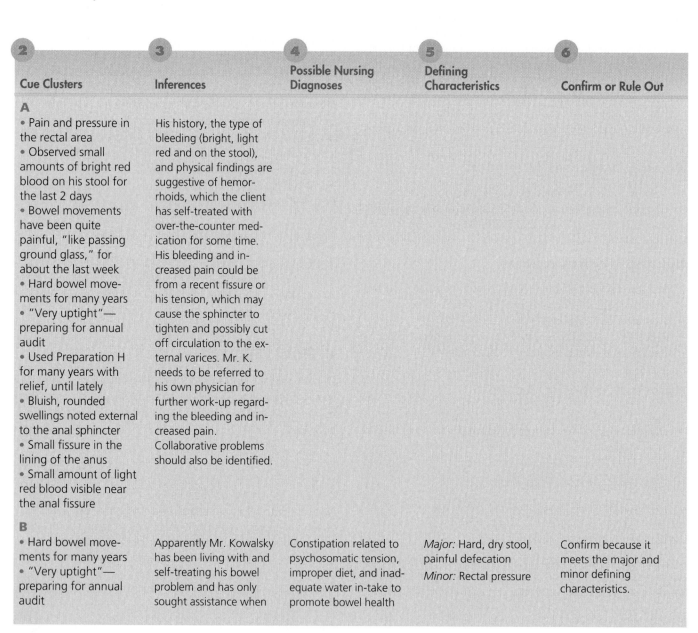

2 Cue Clusters	**3** Inferences	**4** Possible Nursing Diagnoses	**5** Defining Characteristics	**6** Confirm or Rule Out
A • Pain and pressure in the rectal area • Observed small amounts of bright red blood on his stool for the last 2 days • Bowel movements have been quite painful, "like passing ground glass," for about the last week • Hard bowel movements for many years • "Very uptight"—preparing for annual audit • Used Preparation H for many years with relief, until lately • Bluish, rounded swellings noted external to the anal sphincter • Small fissure in the lining of the anus • Small amount of light red blood visible near the anal fissure	His history, the type of bleeding (bright, light red and on the stool), and physical findings are suggestive of hemorrhoids, which the client has self-treated with over-the-counter medication for some time. His bleeding and increased pain could be from a recent fissure or his tension, which may cause the sphincter to tighten and possibly cut off circulation to the external varices. Mr. K. needs to be referred to his own physician for further work-up regarding the bleeding and increased pain. Collaborative problems should also be identified.			
B • Hard bowel movements for many years • "Very uptight"—preparing for annual audit	Apparently Mr. Kowalsky has been living with and self-treating his bowel problem and has only sought assistance when	Constipation related to psychosomatic tension, improper diet, and inadequate water in-take to promote bowel health	*Major:* Hard, dry stool, painful defecation *Minor:* Rectal pressure	Confirm because it meets the major and minor defining characteristics.

2 Cue Clusters	**3** Inferences	**4** Possible Nursing Diagnoses	**5** Defining Characteristics	**6** Confirm or Rule Out
• Drinks 10 to 12 cups of coffee daily • Traditional eggs and bacon for breakfast and meat and potatoes for dinner	he noted bleeding. His occupational stress and dietary habits tend to promote continuation of this problem. He does not indicate a desire to change his habits at this time.	Ineffective Health Maintenance related to insufficient knowledge of stress management and other health-promoting behaviors Ineffective Health Maintenance related to lack of motivation to change lifestyle and not seeking treatment for chronic problem	*Major:* Demonstrates unhealthful practices and lifestyle *Minor:* None *Major:* Demonstrates unhealthful practices and lifestyle *Minor:* None	Either or both may be confirmed because they meet the major defining characteristics. However, additional data must be collected to determine the correct cause of the disorder so proper nursing orders can be implemented.

7 **Document conclusions.**

Three diagnoses are appropriate for George Kowalsky at this time:

- Constipation related to psychosomatic tension, and improper diet and inadequate water intake to promote bowel health
- Ineffective Health Maintenance related to insufficient knowledge of stress management and other health-promoting behaviors

- Ineffective Health Maintenance related to lack of motivation to change lifestyle and not seeking treatment for chronic problem

Collaborative problems related to the medical diagnosis could include:

- PC: Hemorrhage
- PC: Variceal thrombosis
- PC: Variceal strangulation

Mr. Kowalsky should be referred to a physician for evaluation and treatment of rectal bleeding and pain.

REFERENCES AND SELECTED READINGS

Berger, N. S. (1993). Prostate cancer: Screening and early detection update. *Seminars in Oncology Nursing, 9*(3), 180–183.

Conrad, G. L. (1994). Prostatic evaluation: Benign versus cancerous. *Physician Assistant, 18*(12), 39–40, 42–44, 47.

Entrekin, N. M., & McMillan, S. C. (1993). Nurses' knowledge, beliefs, and practices related to cancer prevention and detection. *Cancer Nursing, 16*(6), 431–439.

Gelfand, D. E., Parzuchowski, J., Cort, M., & Powell, I. (1995). Digital rectal examinations and prostate cancer screening: Attitudes of African American men. *Oncology Nursing Forum, 22*(8), 1253–1255.

Motley, C., Crump, W. J., & Pierce, P. J. (1992). Health maintenance for adults. Screening for colorectal and breast cancer: Practical applications of the USPSTF recommendations. *Consultant, 32*(7), 59–62, 67.

Pearce, K. L. (1994). Levels I and II: Care in the outpatient setting. *Nurse Practitioner Forum, 5*(3), 146–151.

Pienta, K. J., & Esper, P. S. (1993). Risk factors for prostate cancer. *Annals of Internal Medicine, 118,* 793–803.

Pobursky, J. (1995). Prostate cancer: Detection and treatment options. *Today's OR Nurse, 17*(3), 5–9.

Small, E. J. (1993). Prostate cancer: Who to screen, and what the results mean. *Geriatrics, 48*(12), 28–38.

Trump, D. L. (1992). Prostate cancer: How to screen—and what the results mean. *Consultant, 32*(8), 27–30, 33, 36.

U. S. Department of Health and Human Services. (1994). Benign prostatic hyperplasia: Diagnosis and treatment. *Journal of the American Academy of Nursing Practice, 6*(4), 167–174.

Waldman, A. R., & Osborne, D. M. (1994). Screening for prostate cancer. *Oncology Nursing Forum, 21*(9), 1512–1517.

Risk Factors—Colorectal Cancer

American Cancer Society. (2000). *Cancer facts & figures—2000.* Atlanta, GA: American Cancer Society.

Crucitti, F., Sofo, L., Ratto, C., Merica, M., Ippoliti, M., Crucitti, P., & Doglietto, G. (1995). Colorectal cancer: Epidemiology, etiology, pathogenesis and prevention. *Rays, 20,* 121–131.

Levin, B. (2000). *Colorectal cancer: A thorough and compassionate resource for patients and their families.* Atlanta, GA: American Cancer Society.

Overfield, T. (1995). *Biologic variation in health and illness: Race, age, and sex differences* (2nd ed.). Boca Raton, FL: CRC Press.

Steele, G. (1995). Colorectal cancer. In G. Murphy, W. Lawrence, & R. Lenhard (Eds.), *American Cancer Society textbook of clinical oncology* (2nd ed., pp. 236–250). Atlanta, GA: American Cancer Society.

Risk Factors—Prostate Cancer

American Cancer Society. (2000). *Cancer facts & figures—2000.* Atlanta, GA: American Cancer Society.

Bostwick, D. G., MacLennan, G. T., & Larson, T. R. (1999). *Prostate cancer* (Revised ed.). Atlanta, GA: American Cancer Society.

Coley, C. M., Barry, M. J., Fleming, C., Fahs, M. C., & Mulley, A. G. (1997). Early detection of prostate cancer. Part II: Estimating the risks, benefits and costs. *Annals of Internal Medicine, 126*(6), 468–479.

Karakiewicz, P. I., & Aprikian, A. G. (1998). Prostate cancer: 5. Diagnostic tools for early detection. *Canadian Medical Association Journal, 159*(9), 1139–1146.

Overfield, T. (1995). *Biologic variation in health and illness: Race, age, and sex differences* (2nd ed.). Boca Raton, FL: CRC Press.

Peate, I. (1998). Clinical. Cancer of the prostate 2: The nursing role in health promotion. *British Journal of Nursing, 7*(4), 196, 198–200.

For additional information on this book, be sure to visit http://connection.lww.com.

Musculoskeletal Assessment

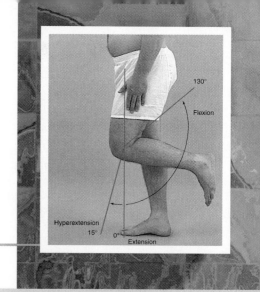

22

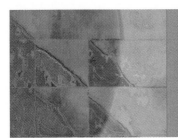

The body's bones, muscles, and joints compose the musculoskeletal system. Controlled and innervated by the nervous system, the musculoskeletal system's overall purpose is to provide structure and movement for body parts.

Bones

Bones provide structure, give protection, serve as levers, store calcium, and produce blood cells. Two hundred and six (206) bones make up the axial skeleton (head and trunk) and the appendicular skeleton (extremities, shoulders, and hips; Fig. 22-1).

Composed of osseous tissue, bones can be divided into two types: Compact bone, which is hard and dense and makes up the shaft and outer layers; and spongy bone, which contains numerous spaces and makes up the ends and centers of the bones. Bone tissue is formed by active cells called *osteoblasts* and broken down by cells referred to as *osteoclasts*. Bones contain red marrow that produces blood cells and yellow marrow that is composed mostly of fat.

The periosteum covers the bones and contains osteoblasts and blood vessels that promote nourishment and formation of new bone tissues. Bone shapes vary and include short bones (eg, carpals), long bones (eg, humerus, femur), flat bones (eg, sternum, ribs), and bones with an irregular shape (eg, hips, vertebrae).

Skeletal Muscles

The body consists of three types of muscles: skeletal, smooth, and cardiac. The musculoskeletal system is made up of 650 skeletal (voluntary) muscles, which are under conscious control (Fig. 22-2). Made up of long muscle fibers (fasciculi) that are arranged together in bundles and joined by connective tissue, skeletal muscles attach to bones by way of strong, fibrous cords called *tendons*. Skeletal muscles assist with posture, produce body heat, and allow the body to move. Skeletal muscle movements are illustrated in Display 22-1.

Joints

The joint (or articulation) is the place where two or more bones meet. Joints provide a variety of ranges of motion (ROM) for the body parts and may be classified as fibrous, cartilaginous, or synovial.

Fibrous joints (eg, sutures between skull bones) are joined by fibrous connective tissue. Cartilaginous joints (eg, joints between vertebrae) are joined by cartilage. Synovial joints (eg, shoulders, wrists, hips, knees, ankles; Fig. 22-3) contain a space between the bones that is filled with synovial fluid, a lubricant that promotes a sliding movement of the ends of the bones. Bones in synovial joints are joined by ligaments, which are strong, dense bands of fibrous connective tissue. Synovial joints are enclosed by a fibrous capsule made of connective tissue and connected to the periosteum of the bone. Articular cartilage smooths and protects the bones that articulate with each other.

Some synovial joints contain bursae, which are small sacs filled with synovial fluid that serve to cushion the joint. Table 22-1 reviews the appearance, characteristics, and motion of major joints.

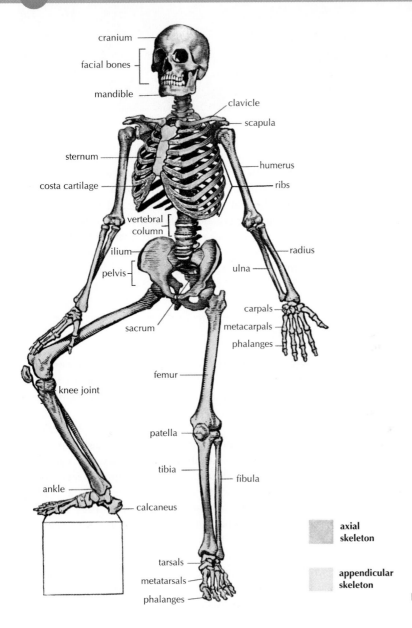

cranium

facial bones

mandible

clavicle

scapula

sternum

humerus

costa cartilage

ribs

vertebral column

ilium

radius

pelvis

ulna

sacrum

carpals

metacarpals

phalanges

femur

knee joint

patella

tibia

fibula

ankle

calcaneus

tarsals

metatarsals

phalanges

axial skeleton

appendicular skeleton

FIGURE 22-1. Major bones of the skeleton.

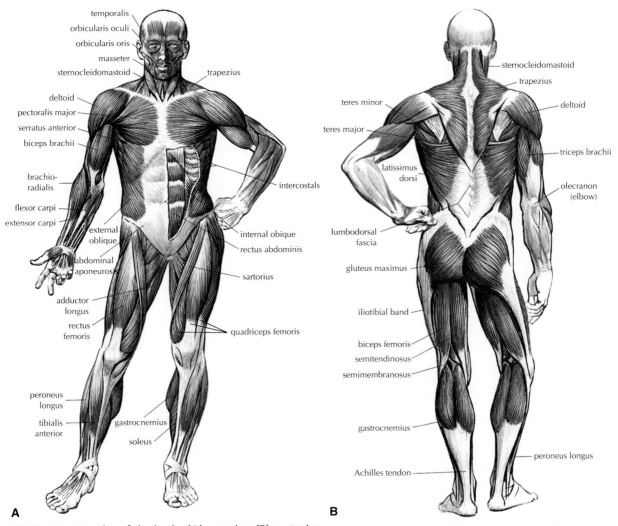

temporalis
orbicularis oculi
orbicularis oris
masseter
sternocleidomastoid
deltoid
pectoralis major
serratus anterior
biceps brachii
brachio-radialis
flexor carpi
extensor carpi
external oblique
abdominal aponeurosis
adductor longus
rectus femoris
peroneus longus
tibialis anterior
trapezius
intercostals
internal obique
rectus abdominis
sartorius
quadriceps femoris
gastrocnemius
soleus

sternocleidomastoid
trapezius
teres minor
teres major
deltoid
triceps brachii
latissimus dorsi
olecranon (elbow)
lumbodorsal fascia
gluteus maximus
iliotibial band
biceps femoris
semitendinosus
semimembranosus
gastrocnemius
peroneus longus
Achilles tendon

A   B

FIGURE 22-2.   Muscles of the body: (**A**) anterior; (**B**) posterior.

DISPLAY 22-1.   Illustrated Glossary of Musculoskeletal Motion

Abduction—Moving away from the midline of the body
Adduction—Moving toward the midline of the body

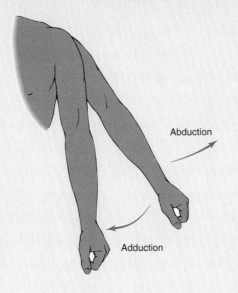

Abduction

Adduction

(continued)

DISPLAY 22-1. Illustrated Glossary of Musculoskeletal Motion (Continued)

Circumduction—Circular motion

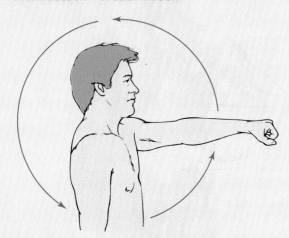

Eversion—Moving outward
Inversion—Moving inward

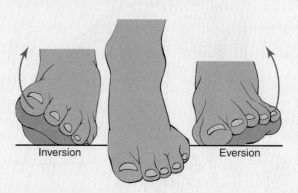

Inversion   Eversion

Extension—Straightening the extremity at the joint and increasing the angle of the joint
Flexion—Bending the extremity at the joint and decreasing the angle of the joint

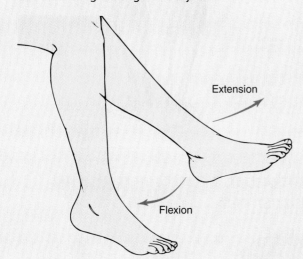

Extension

Flexion

Pronation—Turning or facing downward
Supination—Turning or facing upward

Pronation

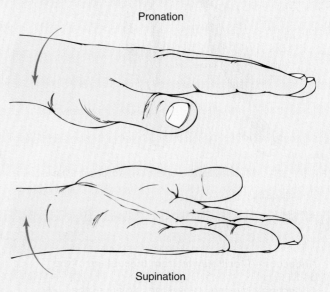

Supination

(continued)

DISPLAY 22-1. Illustrated Glossary of Musculoskeletal Motion (Continued)

Protraction—Moving forward
Retraction—Moving backward

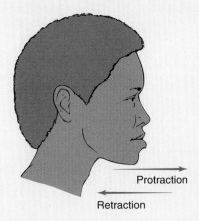

Protraction

Retraction

Rotation—Turning
    External: Turning toward the midline of the body
    Internal: Turning away from the midline of the body

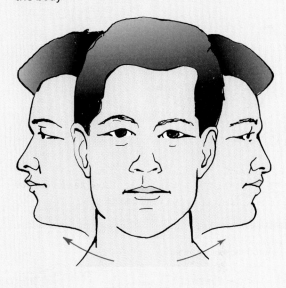

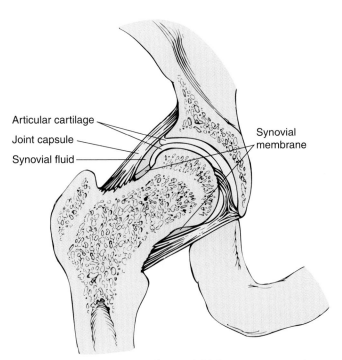

Articular cartilage
Joint capsule
Synovial fluid
Synovial membrane

FIGURE 22-3. Components of synovial joints.

TABLE 22-1. Understanding Major Joints

Joint	Characteristics	Motion
Temporomandibular 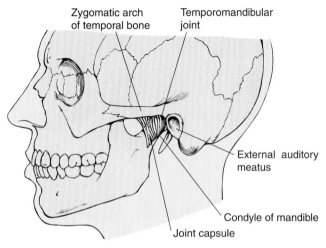	Articulation between the temporal bone and mandible	• Opens and closes mouth • Projects and retracts jaw • Moves jaw from side to side
Sternoclavicular 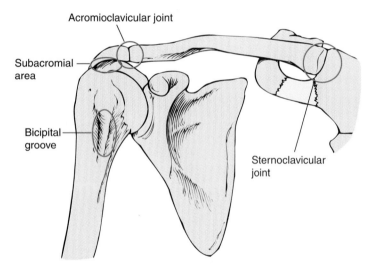	Junction between the manubrium of the sternum and the clavicle	No obvious movements
Shoulder (right anterior view) 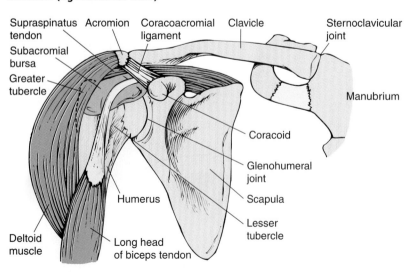	Articulation of the head of the humerus in the glenoid cavity of the scapula. The acromioclavicular joint includes the clavicle and acromion process of the scapula. It contains the subacromial and subscapular bursae.	• Flexion and extension • Abduction and adduction • Circumduction • Rotation (internal and external)

Temporomandibular diagram labels: Zygomatic arch of temporal bone; Temporomandibular joint; External auditory meatus; Condyle of mandible; Joint capsule

Sternoclavicular diagram labels: Acromioclavicular joint; Subacromial area; Bicipital groove; Sternoclavicular joint

Shoulder diagram labels: Supraspinatus tendon; Acromion; Coracoacromial ligament; Clavicle; Sternoclavicular joint; Subacromial bursa; Greater tubercle; Manubrium; Coracoid; Glenohumeral joint; Humerus; Scapula; Lesser tubercle; Deltoid muscle; Long head of biceps tendon

(continued)

TABLE 22-1. **Understanding Major Joints** (Continued)

Joint	Characteristics	Motion
Elbow (left posterior view) 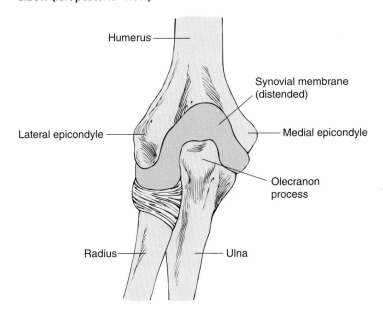	Articulation between the ulna and radius of the lower arm and the humerus of the upper arm; contains a synovial membrane and several bursae	• Flexion and extension of the forearm • Supination and pronation of the forearm
Wrist, fingers, thumb (right anterior view) 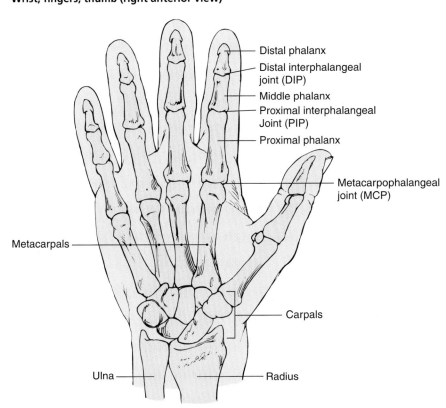	Articulation between the distal radius, ulnar bone, carpals, and metacarpals. Contains ligaments and is lined with a synovial membrane.	• Wrists: Flexion, extension, hyperextension, radial and ulnar deviation • Fingers: Flexion, extension, hyperextension, abduction, and circumduction • Thumb: Flexion, extension, and opposition

Elbow labels: Humerus; Synovial membrane (distended); Lateral epicondyle; Medial epicondyle; Olecranon process; Radius; Ulna

Wrist labels: Distal phalanx; Distal interphalangeal joint (DIP); Middle phalanx; Proximal interphalangeal Joint (PIP); Proximal phalanx; Metacarpophalangeal joint (MCP); Metacarpals; Carpals; Ulna; Radius

(continued)

TABLE 22-1. Understanding Major Joints (Continued)

Joint	Characteristics	Motion
Vertebrae (lateral view) 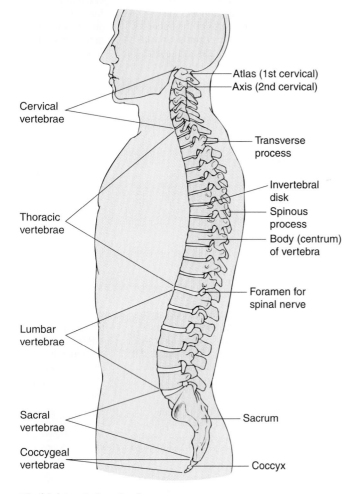	Thirty-three bones: 7 con-cave-shaped cervical (C), 12 convex-shaped thoracic (T), 5 concave-shaped lumbar (L), 5 sacral (S), and 3 to 4 coccygeal, connected in a vertical column. Bones are cushioned by elastic fibrocartilaginous plates (intervertebral discs) that provide flexibility and posture to the spine. Paravertebral muscles are positioned on both sides of vertebrae.	• Flexion • Hyperextension • Lateral bending • Rotation
Hip (right anterior view) 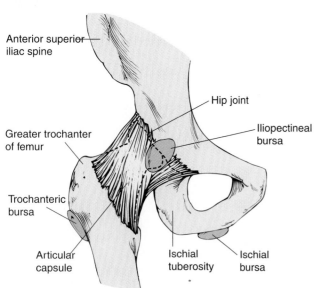	Articulation between the head of the femur and the acetabulum. Contains a fibrous capsule, ligaments, and three bursae to reduce friction produced by motion.	• Flexion with knee flexed and with knee extended • Extension and hyperextension • Circumduction • Rotation (internal and external)

Labels for Vertebrae (lateral view): Cervical vertebrae; Atlas (1st cervical); Axis (2nd cervical); Transverse process; Invertebral disk; Spinous process; Body (centrum) of vertebra; Foramen for spinal nerve; Thoracic vertebrae; Lumbar vertebrae; Sacral vertebrae; Sacrum; Coccygeal vertebrae; Coccyx

Labels for Hip (right anterior view): Anterior superior iliac spine; Hip joint; Iliopectineal bursa; Greater trochanter of femur; Trochanteric bursa; Articular capsule; Ischial tuberosity; Ischial bursa

(continued)

TABLE 22-1. **Understanding Major Joints** (Continued)

Joint	Characteristics	Motion
Knee (left anterior view) 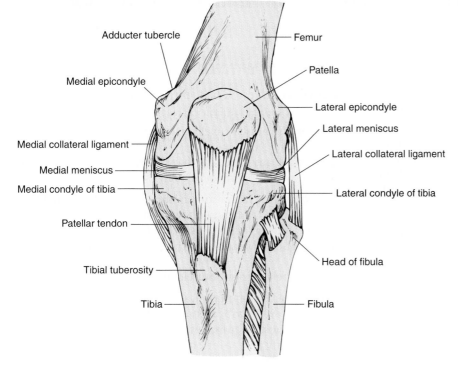	Articulation of the femur, tibia, and patella; contains fibrocartilaginous discs (medial and lateral menisci) and many bursae	• Flexion • Extension
Ankle and foot (right lateral view) 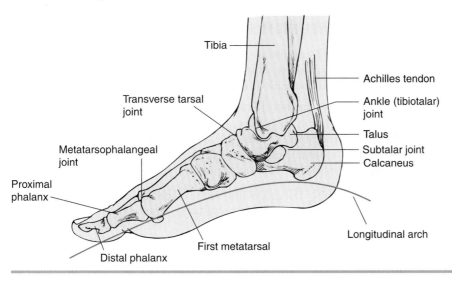	Articulation between the talus (large posterior foot tarsal), tibia, and fibula. The talus also articulates with the navicular bones. The heel (calcaneus bone) is connected to the tibia and fibula by ligaments.	**Ankle:** Plantar flexion and dorsiflexion **Foot:** Inversion and eversion **Toes:** Flexion, extension, abduction, adduction

Knee labels:
- Adducter tubercle
- Medial epicondyle
- Medial collateral ligament
- Medial meniscus
- Medial condyle of tibia
- Patellar tendon
- Tibial tuberosity
- Tibia
- Femur
- Patella
- Lateral epicondyle
- Lateral meniscus
- Lateral collateral ligament
- Lateral condyle of tibia
- Head of fibula
- Fibula

Ankle and foot labels:
- Tibia
- Transverse tarsal joint
- Metatarsophalangeal joint
- Proximal phalanx
- Distal phalanx
- First metatarsal
- Achilles tendon
- Ankle (tibiotalar) joint
- Talus
- Subtalar joint
- Calcaneus
- Longitudinal arch

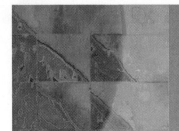
Collecting Subjective Data

Assessment of the musculoskeletal system helps evaluate the client's level of functioning with activities of daily living. This system affects the entire body, from head to toe, and greatly influences what physical activities a client can and cannot do. Only the client can give you data regarding pain, stiffness, and levels of movement and how his or her activities of daily living are affected. In addition, information regarding the client's nutrition, activities, and exercise is a significant part of the musculoskeletal assessment. Pain or stiffness is often a chief concern with musculoskeletal problems; therefore, a pain assessment may also be needed. Always, the nurse needs to remember to investigate signs and symptoms reported by the client. Using the mnemonic COLDSPA can help in this regard.

COLDSPA

CHARACTER: Describe the sign or symptom. How does it feel, look, sound, smell, and so forth?

ONSET: When did it begin?

LOCATION: Where is it? Does it radiate?

DURATION: How long does it last? Does it recur?

SEVERITY: How bad is it?

PATTERN: What makes it better? What makes it worse?

ASSOCIATED FACTORS: What other symptoms occur with it?

Remember, too, that the neurologic system is responsible for coordinating the functions of the skeleton and muscles. Therefore, it is important to understand how these systems relate to each other and ask questions accordingly. From this assessment, the nurse can learn the client's daily activity and exercise patterns that promote either healthy or unhealthy functioning of the musculoskeletal system. Hence, client teaching regarding exercise, diet, positioning, posture, and safety habits to promote health also becomes an essential part of this examination.

Nursing History

During the interview, you will ask the client many questions (Q), examples of which appear below along with the rationale (R) for the question.

CURRENT SYMPTOMS

Question Have you had any recent weight gain?

Rationale Weight gain can increase physical stress and strain on the musculoskeletal system.

Q Describe any difficulty that you have chewing. Is it associated with tenderness or pain?

R Clients with temporomandibular joint (TMJ) dysfunction may have difficulty chewing and may describe their jaws as "getting locked or stuck." Jaw tenderness, pain, or a clicking sound may also be present with ROM.

Q Describe any joint, muscle, or bone pain you have.

R Bone pain is often dull, deep, and throbbing. Joint or muscle pain is described as aching. Sharp, knifelike pain occurs with most fractures and increases with motion of the affected body part. Motion increases pain associated with many joint problems, but decreases pain associated with rheumatoid arthritis.

PAST HISTORY

Q Describe any past problems or injuries you have had to your joints, muscles, or bones. What treatment was given? Do you have any after-effects from the injury or problem?

R This information provides baseline data for the physical examination. Past injuries may affect the client's current range of motion (ROM) and level of function in affected joints and extremities. A history of recurrent fractures should raise the question of possible physical abuse.

Bones lose their density with age, putting the older client at risk for bone fractures, especially of the wrists, hips, and vertebrae. Older clients who have osteomalacia or osteoporosis are at an even greater risk for fractures.

Q When were your last tetanus and polio immunizations?

R Joint stiffening and other musculoskeletal symptoms may be a transient effect of the tetanus or polio vaccines.

Joint-stiffening conditions may be misdiagnosed as arthritis, especially in the older adult.

Q Have you ever been diagnosed with diabetes mellitus, sickle cell anemia, systemic lupus erythematosus (SLE), or osteoporosis?

R Having diabetes mellitus, sickle cell anemia, or SLE places the client at risk for development of musculoskeletal problems, such as osteoporosis and osteomyelitis. Clients who are immobile or have a reduced intake of calcium and vitamin D are especially prone to development of osteoporosis.

Osteoporosis is more common as a person ages because that is a time when bone resorption increases, calcium absorption decreases, and production of osteoblasts decreases as well.

Q For middle-aged women: Have you started menopause? Are you receiving estrogen replacement therapy?

R Women who begin menarche late or begin menopause early are at greater risk for development of osteoporosis because of decreased estrogen levels, which tend to decrease the density of bone mass.

FAMILY HISTORY

Q Do you have a family history of rheumatoid arthritis, gout, or osteoporosis?

R These conditions tend to be familial and can increase the client's risk for development of these diseases.

LIFESTYLE AND HEALTH PRACTICES

Q What activities do you engage in to promote the health of your muscles and bones (eg, exercise, diet, weight reduction)?

R This question provides the examiner with knowledge of how much the client understands and actively participates in trying to promote the health of the musculoskeletal system.

Q What medications are you taking?

R Some medications can affect musculoskeletal function. Diuretics, for example, can alter electrolyte levels leading to muscle weakness. Steroids can deplete bone mass, thereby contributing to osteoporosis. Adverse reactions to HMG-CoA reductase inhibitors (statins) can include myopathy, which can cause muscle aches or weakness.

Q Do you smoke tobacco? How much and how often?

R Smoking increases the risk of osteoporosis (see Risk Factors—Osteoporosis).

Q Do you drink alcohol or caffeinated beverages? How much and how often?

R Excessive consumption of alcohol or caffeine can increase the risk of osteoporosis.

Q Describe your typical 24-hour diet. Are you able to consume milk or milk-containing products? Do you take any calcium supplements?

R Adequate protein in the diet promotes muscle tone and bone growth; vitamin C promotes healing of tissues and bones. A calcium deficiency increases the risk of osteoporosis. A diet high in purine (eg, liver, sardines) can trigger gouty arthritis.

Between 80% and 90% of all people except Caucasians, and 10% to 15% of Caucasians, are lactose intolerant as adults (Overfield, 1995).

Q Describe your activities during a typical day. How much time do you spend in the sunlight?

R A sedentary lifestyle increases the risk of osteoporosis. Prolonged immobility leads to muscle atrophy. Exposure to 20 minutes of sunlight per day promotes the production of vitamin D in the body. Vitamin D deficiency can cause osteomalacia.

Q Describe any routine exercise that you do.

R Regular exercise promotes flexibility, bone density, and muscle tone and strength, and can help slow the usual musculoskeletal changes (progressive loss of total bone mass and degeneration of skeletal muscle fibers) that occur with aging. Improper body positioning in contact sports results in injury to the bones, joints, or muscles.

Q Describe your occupation.

R Certain job-related activities increase the risk for development of musculoskeletal problems. For example, incorrect body mechanics, heavy lifting, or poor posture can contribute to back problems; consistent, repetitive wrist and hand movements can lead to the development of carpal tunnel syndrome.

Q Describe your posture at work and at leisure. What type of shoes do you usually wear?

R Poor posture, prolonged forward bending (as in sitting) or backward leaning (as in working overhead), or long-term carrying of heavy objects on the shoulders can result in back problems. Contracture of the Achilles tendon can occur with prolonged use of high-heeled shoes.

Q Do you have difficulty performing normal activities of daily living? Do you use assistive devices (eg, walker, cane, braces) to promote your mobility?

R Impairment of the musculoskeletal system may impair the client's ability to perform normal activities of daily living. Correct use of assistive devices can promote safety and independence. Some clients may feel embarrassed and not use their prescribed or needed assistive device.

Q How have your musculoskeletal problems interfered with your ability to interact or socialize with others? Have they interfered with your usual sexual activity?

R Musculoskeletal problems, especially chronic ones, can disable and cripple the client, which may impair socialization

RISK FACTORS
Osteoporosis

OVERVIEW

One of the major health problems facing the aging world populace, osteoporosis occurs when bone-forming cells cannot keep pace with bone-destroying cells (low bone density). Bone fractures are the most important consequences of osteoporosis. Worldwide, lifetime risk for osteoporotic fractures is 30% to 40% in women and 13% in men (IOF, 2001). A major public health threat in the United States, osteoporosis affects about 28 million Americans, 80% of them women. About 10 million have actual osteoporosis and about 15 million have the forerunner of low bone mass. Approximately 1.5 million fractures are attributed to osteoporosis annually in the United States, with the major fracture sites being the proximal femur (hip), distal forearm (wrist), and vertebrae.

The high costs in pain, disability, and money support a strong need for prevention programs. Moderate to strenuous exercise and moderate to high calcium intake during the skeletal bone-building years and throughout life tend to increase bone density and provide a protective effect against osteoporosis.

UNCONTROLLABLE RISK FACTORS

- Gender: 80% women
- Age: 70 years or older (female); 80 years or older (male)
- Body size: Small-boned, thin
- Ethnicity: Caucasian and Asian at highest risk; African American and Latino, at lower, but significant, risk
- Family history or personal history of bone fractures as an adult (IOF, 2001; NIH, 2001; NOF, 2001)

MODIFIABLE RISK FACTORS

- Little or no physical exercise or activity; bed rest
- Low calcium intake
- For women: Low estrogen levels; post-menopausal woman not on estrogen replacement therapy
- Smoking
- Excessive caffeine or alcohol consumption
- Medication intake (corticosteroids particularly) for chronic disorders such as rheumatoid arthritis, endocrine disorders (eg, underactive thyroid), seizures, gastrointestinal diseases (IOF, 2001; NIH, 2001; NOF, 2001)

RISK-REDUCTION TEACHING TIPS

- Increase physical exercise or activity, especially weight bearing (regular moderate exercise three times a week for 20 to 45 minutes each time).
- Increase calcium intake to recommended daily allowances through diet or supplements (NIH recommends 1000–1500 mg/day for adults).
- Get adequate vitamin D to absorb calcium (sun exposure; dietary sources include fortified milk, oily fish, liver, egg yolk).
- Avoid excessive caffeine or alcohol consumption.
- Avoid or stop smoking.
- Avoid use of steroids.
- Consider estrogen replacement therapy if post-menopausal or approaching menopause.
- Discuss with primary health care provider how steroids or other medications taken for chronic disorders can affect bones.
- Also discuss advisability of taking bone protective medications and tests for bone density.
- If diagnosed with osteoporosis, explore ways to prevent falls.

 ### CULTURAL CONSIDERATIONS

After peak bone mass is achieved (age 35 to 40 in both sexes), bone density decreases with age in both sexes and across races at a relatively uniform and parallel rate (Overfield, 1995). However, men have denser bones than women after puberty, and blacks have denser bones than whites (Overfield, 1995). Early studies of eastern populations noted that bone density of Chinese, Japanese, and Eskimo individuals is below that of Caucasians, but that of Polynesian women is 20% higher than Caucasian women (Overfield, 1995). The increase in the aged populace worldwide is expected to increase the number of persons with osteoporosis and hip fractures. The Middle East, Latin America, and Asia are expecting dramatic increases in the next 20 years (IOF, 2001).

and prevent the client from performing the same roles as in the past. Back problems, joint pain, or muscle stiffness may interfere with sexual activities.

Q How did you view yourself before you had this musculoskeletal problem, and how do you view yourself now?

R Body image disturbances and chronic low self-esteem may occur with a disabling or crippling problem.

Q Has your musculoskeletal problem added stress to your life? Describe.

R Musculoskeletal problems often greatly affect activities of daily living and role performance, resulting in changed relationships and increased stress.

Collecting Objective Data

Physical assessment of the musculoskeletal system provides data regarding the client's posture, gait, bone structure, muscle strength, and joint mobility, as well as the client's ability to perform activities of daily living.

The physical assessment includes inspecting and palpating the joints, muscles, and bones, testing ROM, and assessing muscle strength. See Display 22-2 for guidelines to use when performing the musculoskeletal assessment.

CLIENT PREPARATION

Because this examination is lengthy, be sure the room is at a comfortable temperature and provide rest periods as necessary. Provide adequate draping to avoid unnecessary exposure of the client, yet adequate visualization of the part being examined. Explain that you will ask the client frequently to change positions and to move various body parts against resistance and gravity. Clear, simple directions need to be given throughout the examination to help the client understand how to move body parts to allow you to assess the musculoskeletal system. Demonstrating to the client how to move the various body parts and providing verbal directions facilitate examination.

Some positions required for this examination may be very uncomfortable for the older client, who may have decreased flexibility. Be sensitive to the client's needs and adapt your technique as necessary.

EQUIPMENT AND SUPPLIES

- Tape measure
- Goniometer (optional)

KEY ASSESSMENT POINTS

- Observe gait and posture.
- Inspect joints, muscles, and extremities for size, symmetry, and color.
- Palpate joints, muscles, and extremities for tenderness, edema, heat, nodules, or crepitus.
- Test muscle strength and ROM of joints.
- Compare bilateral findings of joints and muscles.
- Perform special tests for carpal tunnel syndrome.
- Perform the "bulge," "ballottement," and McMurray's knee tests.

(*text continues on page 535*)

DISPLAY 22-2. Guidelines for Assessing Joints and Muscles

The following are guidelines for assessing joints and muscle strength:

GUIDELINES **JOINTS**

1. Inspect size, shape, color, and symmetry. Note any masses, deformities, or muscle atrophy. Compare bilateral joint findings.
2. Palpate for edema, heat, tenderness, pain, nodules, or crepitus. Compare bilateral joint findings.
3. Test each joint's range of motion (ROM). Demonstrate how to move each joint through its normal ROM, then ask the client actively to move the joint through the same motions. Compare bilateral joint findings.

Older clients usually have slower movements, reduced flexibility, and decreased muscle strength because of age-related muscle fiber and joint degeneration, reduced elasticity of the tendons, and joint capsule calcification.

(continued)

DISPLAY 22-2. Guidelines for Assessing Joints and Muscles (Continued)

If you identify a limitation in the ROM, measure ROM with a goniometer (a device that measures movement in degrees). To do so, move the arms of the goniometer to match the angle of the joint being assessed. Then describe the limited motion of the joint in degrees: for example, "elbow flexes from 45 degrees to 90 degrees."

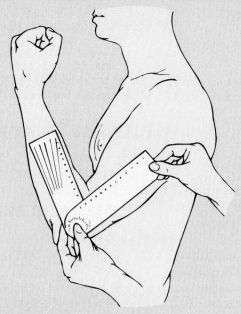

Goniometer.

MUSCLES

1. Test muscle strength by asking the client to move each extremity through its full ROM against resistance. Do this by applying some resistance against the part being moved. Document muscle strength by using a standard scale (see Rating Scale for Muscle Strength, below). If the client cannot move the part against your resistance, ask the client to move the part against gravity. If this is not possible, then attempt passively to move the part through its full ROM. If this is not possible, then inspect and feel for a palpable contraction of the muscle while the client attempts to move it. Compare bilateral joint findings.

🏵 **Tip From the Experts** Do not force the part beyond its normal range. Stop passive motion if the client expresses discomfort or pain. Be especially cautious with the older client when testing ROM. When comparing bilateral strength, keep in mind that the client's dominant side will tend to be the stronger side.

---

2. Rate muscle strength in accord with the strength table below.

Rating	Explanation	Strength Classification
5	Active motion against full resistance	Normal
4	Active motion against some resistance	Slight weakness
3	Active motion against gravity	Average weakness
2	Passive ROM (gravity removed and assisted by examiner)	Poor ROM
1	Slight flicker of contraction	Severe weakness
0	No muscular contraction	Paralysis

PHYSICAL ASSESSMENT

ASSESSMENT PROCEDURE	NORMAL FINDINGS	ABNORMAL FINDINGS

GAIT

Observe Gait

Observe the client's gait as the client enters and walks around the room. Note:
- Base of support
- Weight-bearing stability
- Foot position
- Stride and length and cadence of stride
- Arm swing
- Posture

Evenly distributed weight. Client able to stand on heels and toes. Toes point straight ahead. Equal on both sides. Posture erect, movements coordinated and rhythmic, arms swing in opposition, stride length appropriate. have a slower gait, wide-based stance, and smaller arm swing, and the head and trunk may be flexed.

Uneven weight bearing is evident. Client cannot stand on heels or toes. Toes point in or out. Client limps, shuffles, propels forward, or has wide-based gait. (See Chapter 23, Neurologic Assessment, for specific abnormal gait findings.)

Assess for the risk of falling backward in the older or handicapped client by performing the "nudge test." Stand behind the client and put your arms around the client while you gently nudge the sternum.

Client does not fall backward.

Some older clients have an impaired sense of position in space, which may contribute to the risks of falling.

Falling backward easily is seen with cervical spondylosis and Parkinson's disease.

TEMPOROMANDIBULAR JOINT (TMJ)

Inspect, Palpate, and Test ROM

With the client sitting, inspect and palpate the TMJ by putting your index and middle fingers just anterior to the external ear opening. Ask the client to
- Open the mouth as widely as possible. (The tips of your fingers should drop into the joint spaces as the mouth opens.)
- Move the jaw from side to side.
- Protrude (push out) and retract (pull in) jaw.

The client's mouth opens and closes smoothly. Mouth opens 1 to 2 inches.

Jaw moves laterally 1 to 2 cm. Snapping and clicking may be felt and heard in the normal client.

Jaw protrudes and retracts easily.

Decreased ROM, swelling, tenderness, or crepitus may be seen in arthritis. Pain, tenderness, decreased ROM, and a clicking, popping, or grating sound may be noted with TMJ dysfunction.

Decreased muscle strength with muscle and joint disease.

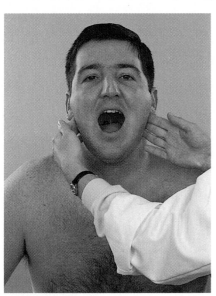

Palpating the temporomandibular joint. (© B. Proud.)

(continued)

ASSESSMENT PROCEDURE	NORMAL FINDINGS	ABNORMAL FINDINGS
Ask the client to open the mouth and move the jaw laterally against resistance. Next, feel for the contraction of the temporal and masseter muscles to test the integrity of cranial nerve V (trigeminal nerve).	Jaw has full ROM against resistance. Contraction palpated with no pain or spasms.	Lack of full contraction with cranial nerve V lesion. Pain or spasms occur with myofacial pain syndrome.

STERNOCLAVICULAR JOINT

Inspect and Palpate

With client sitting, inspect the sternoclavicular joint for location in midline, color, swelling, and masses. Then palpate for tenderness or pain.	No visible bony overgrowth, swelling, or redness; joint is nontender.	Swollen, red, or enlarged joint or tender, painful joint is seen with inflammation of the joint.

CERVICAL, THORACIC, AND LUMBAR SPINE

Inspect and Palpate

With the client standing erect and with the gown positioned to allow an adequate view of the spine, observe the cervical, thoracic, and lumbar curves from the side and then from behind.	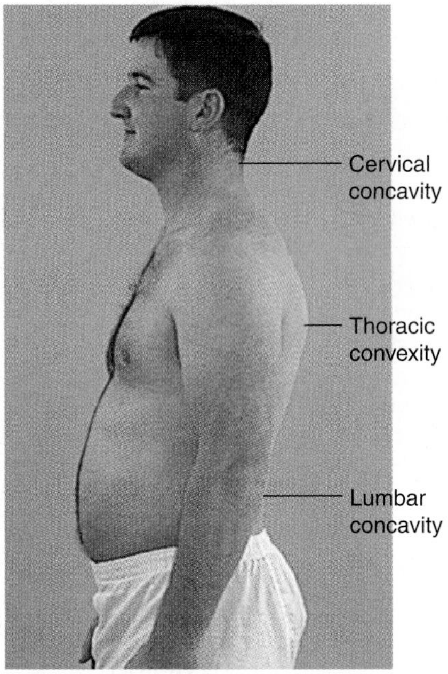 Cervical and lumbar spines are concave; thoracic spine is convex. Spine is straight (when observed from behind). An exaggerated thoracic curve (kyphosis) is common with aging.	A flattened lumbar curvature may be seen with a herniated lumbar disc or ankylosing spondylitis. Lateral curvature of the thoracic spine with an increase in the convexity on the side that is curved is seen in scoliosis. An exaggerated lumbar curve (lordosis) is often seen in pregnancy or obesity (Display 22-3). Some findings that appear to be abnormalities are, in fact, variations related to culture or sex. For example, some blacks have a large gluteal prominence, making the spine appear to have lumbar lordosis. In addition, the number of vertebrae may differ. Frequent variations from the usual 24 include women, especially black women, who may have 23 vertebrae; and men, especially Eskimo and Indian men, with 25.

Cervical concavity
Thoracic convexity
Lumbar concavity

Normal curve of the spine. (© B. Proud.)

Palpate the spinous processes and the paravertebral muscles on both sides of the spine for tenderness or pain.	Nontender spinous processes; well-developed, firm and smooth, nontender paravertebral muscles.	Tenderness and pain at the spinous processes and paravertebral muscles are abnormal findings.

(continued)

ASSESSMENT PROCEDURE	NORMAL FINDINGS	ABNORMAL FINDINGS

Test ROM of the Cervical Spine

Test ROM of the cervical spine by asking the client to touch the chin to the chest (flexion) and to look up at the ceiling (hyperextension).

A full 45 degrees of flexion and 55 degrees of hyperextension are considered normal.

Cervical strain is the most common cause of neck pain. It is characterized by impaired ROM and neck pain from abnormalities of the soft tissue (muscles, ligaments, and nerves) due to straining or injuring the neck. Causes of strains can include sleeping in the wrong position, carrying a heavy suitcase, or being in an automobile crash.

Cervical disc degenerative disease or spinal cord tumor are associated with impaired ROM and pain that radiates to the back, shoulder, or arms. Neck pain with a loss of sensation in the legs may occur with cervical spinal cord compression.

Impaired ROM and neck pain associated with fever, chills, and headache could be indicative of a serious infection such as meningitis.

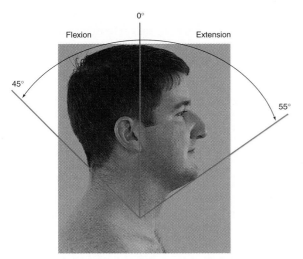

Normal range of motion of cervical spine: (*A*) flexion-hyperextension. (© B. Proud.)

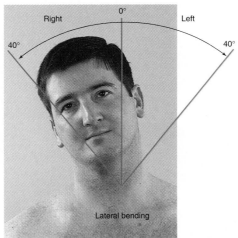

Normal range of motion of cervical spine: (*B*) lateral bending. (© B. Proud.)

(continued)

ASSESSMENT PROCEDURE	NORMAL FINDINGS	ABNORMAL FINDINGS
Next, ask the client to touch each ear to the shoulder on that side (lateral bending).	Normally, the client can bend 40 degrees to the left and 40 degrees to the right sides (see above).	
Ask the client to turn head to right and left (rotation).	About 70 degrees degrees of rotation is normal.	

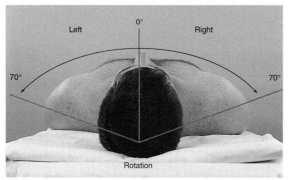

Normal range of motion of cervical spine: (C) rotation. (© B. Proud.)

ASSESSMENT PROCEDURE	NORMAL FINDINGS	ABNORMAL FINDINGS
Ask the client to repeat the cervical ROM movements against resistance.	Client has full ROM against resistance.	Decreased ROM against resistance is seen with joint or muscle disease.

Test ROM of the Thoracic and Lumbar Spine

ASSESSMENT PROCEDURE	NORMAL FINDINGS	ABNORMAL FINDINGS
Ask the client to bend forward and touch the toes (flexion).	Flexion of 75 degrees to 90 degrees, smooth movement, lumbar concavity flattens out.	Lateral curvature disappears in functional scoliosis; unilateral exaggerated thoracic convexity increases in structural scoliosis.

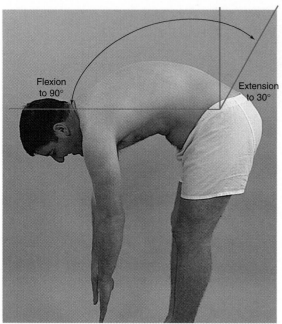

Thoracic and lumbar spines: flexion. (© B. Proud.)

Similarly, ask an older client to bend forward, but do not insist that he or she touch toes unless the client is comfortable with the movement.

(continued)

ASSESSMENT PROCEDURE	NORMAL FINDINGS	ABNORMAL FINDINGS
Sit down behind the client, stabilize the client's pelvis with your hands, and ask the client to bend sideways (lateral bending), bend backward toward you (hyperextension), and twist the shoulders one way, then the other (rotation).	Lateral bending capacity of the thoracic and lumbar should be about 35 degrees; hyperextension about 30 degrees; and rotation about 30 degrees.	Low back strain from injury to soft tissues is a common cause of impaired ROM and pain in the lumbar and thoracic regions. Other causes of impaired ROM in the lumbar and thoracic areas include osteoarthritis, ankylosing spondylitis, and congenital abnormalities that may affect the spinal vertebral spacing and mobility.

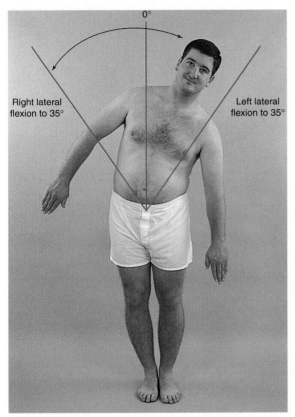

Thoracic and lumbar spines: lateral bending. (© B. Proud.)

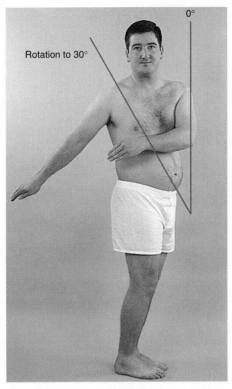

Thoracic and lumbar spines: rotation. (© B. Proud.)

(continued)

ASSESSMENT PROCEDURE	NORMAL FINDINGS	ABNORMAL FINDINGS

Test for Back and Leg Pain

If the client has low back pain that radiates down the back, perform Lasègue's test (straight leg raising) to check a herniated nucleus pulposus. Ask the client to lie flat and raise the affected leg to the point of pain. At the point, dorsiflex the client's foot.

Pain not reproduced.

Pain is reproduced. Pain that shoots and radiates down one or both legs (sciatica) below the knees may be due to a herniated intervertebral disc. Continuous, aching pain at night not relieved by rest may be from metastases. Lower back pain with tenderness and limited ROM is common in osteoporosis.

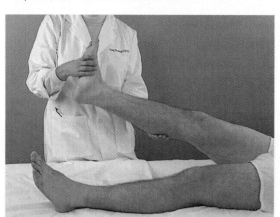

Performing Lasègue's test. (© B. Proud.)

MEASURE LEG LENGTH

If you suspect that the client has one leg longer than the other, measure them. Ask the client to lie down with legs extended. With a tape, measure the distance between the anterior superior iliac spine and the medial malleolus, crossing the tape on the medial side of the knee (true leg length).

Measurements are equal or within 1 cm. If the legs still look unequal, assess the apparent leg length by measuring from a nonfixed point (the umbilicus) to a fixed point (medial malleolus) on each leg.

Unequal leg lengths are associated with scoliosis. Equal true leg lengths but unequal apparent leg lengths are seen with abnormalities in the structure or position of the hips and pelvis.

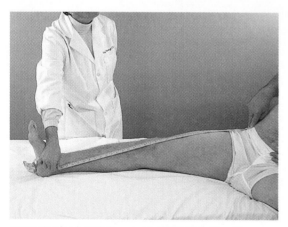

Measuring leg length (true leg length). (© B. Proud.)

(continued)

ASSESSMENT PROCEDURE	NORMAL FINDINGS	ABNORMAL FINDINGS

SHOULDERS, ARMS, AND ELBOWS

Inspect and Palpate Shoulders and Arms

With the client standing or sitting, inspect for symmetry, color, swelling, and masses. Palpate for tenderness, swelling, or heat.

Shoulders are symmetrically round, no redness, swelling, or deformity or heat. Muscles are fully developed. Clavicles and scapulae are even and symmetric. The client reports no tenderness.

Flat, hollow, or less wounded shoulders are seen with dislocation. Muscle atrophy is seen with nerve or muscle damage or lack of use. Tenderness, swelling, and heat may be noted with shoulder strains, sprains, arthritis, bursitis, and degenerative joint disease.

Test ROM

Explain to the client that you will be assessing his or her range of motion (consisting of flexion, extension, adduction abduction, and motion against resistance). Ask client to stand with both arms straight down at sides. Next, ask him to move the arms forward (flexion), then backward with elbows straight.

Then, have the client bring both hands together overhead, elbows straight, followed by moving both hands in front of the body past the midline with elbows straight (this tests adduction and abduction).

Extent of forward flexion should be 180 degrees; extension, 50 degrees; adduction, 50 degrees; and abduction 180 degrees.

Painful and limited abduction accompanied by muscle weakness and atrophy are seen with a rotator cuff tear. Client has sharp catches of pain when bringing hands overhead when he or she has rotator cuff tendinitis. Chronic pain and severe limitation of all shoulder motions are seen with calcified tendinitis.

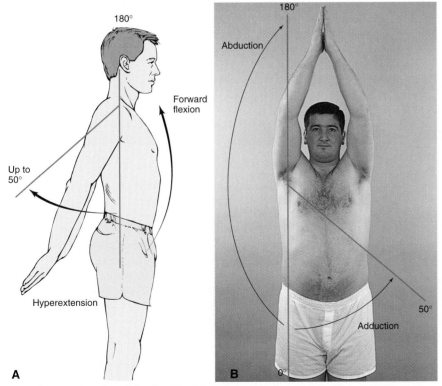

Normal range of motion of the shoulder: (*A*) flexion-extension; (*B*) adduction-abduction.

(continued)

ASSESSMENT PROCEDURE	NORMAL FINDINGS	ABNORMAL FINDINGS

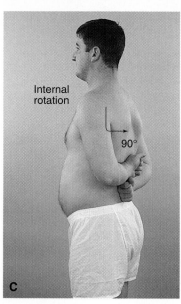 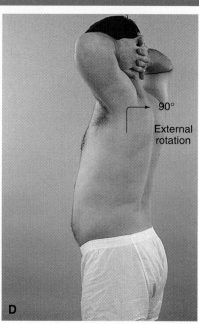

Normal range of motion of the shoulder: (C) internal rotation; (D) external rotation. (© B. Proud.)

In a continuous motion, have the client bring the hands together behind the head with elbows flexed (this tests external rotation) and behind the back (internal rotation). Repeat these maneuvers against resistance.	Extent of external and internal rotation should be about 90 degrees, respectively. The client can flex, extend, adduct, abduct, rotate, and shrug shoulders against resistance.	Inability to shrug shoulders against resistance is seen with a lesion of cranial nerve XI (spinal accessory). Decreased muscle strength is seen with muscle or joint disease.

ELBOWS

Inspect and Palpate

Inspect for size, shape, deformities, redness, or swelling.	Elbows are symmetric without deformities, redness, or swelling.	Redness, heat, and swelling may be seen with bursitis of the olecranon process due to trauma or arthritis.
With the elbow relaxed and flexed about 70 degrees, use your thumb and middle fingers to palpate the olecranon process and epicondyles.	Nontender; without nodules.	Firm, nontender, subcutaneous nodules may be palpated in rheumatoid arthritis or rheumatic fever. Tenderness or pain over the epicondyles may be palpated in epicondylitis (tennis elbow) due to repetitive movements of the forearm or wrists.

(continued)

ASSESSMENT PROCEDURE	NORMAL FINDINGS	ABNORMAL FINDINGS

Test ROM

Ask the client to perform the following movements to test flexion, extension, pronation, supination, and ROM against resistance:

    Flex the elbow and bring the hand to the forehead.

    Straighten the elbow.

    Then hold arm out, turn the palm down, then turn the palm up.

    Last, have the client repeat the movements against your resistance.

Normal ranges of motion are 160 degrees of flexion; 180 degrees of extension. 90 degrees of pronation. 90 degrees of supination.

    The client should have full ROM against resistance.

Decreased ROM against resistance is seen with joint or muscle disease.

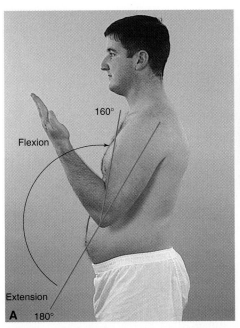 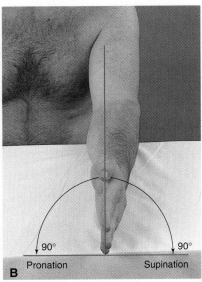

Normal range of motion of the elbow: (*A*) flexion-extension; (*B*) pronation-supination. (© B. Proud.)

WRISTS

Inspect and Palpate

Inspect wrist size, shape, symmetry, color, and swelling. Then palpate for tenderness and nodules.

Wrists are symmetric without redness, or swelling. They are nontender and free of nodules.

Swelling is seen with rheumatoid arthritis. Tenderness and nodules may be seen with rheumatoid arthritis. A nontender, round, enlarged, swollen, fluid-filled cyst (ganglion) may be noted on the wrists (Display 22-4).

Palpating the wrists. (© B. Proud.)

(continued)

ASSESSMENT PROCEDURE	NORMAL FINDINGS	ABNORMAL FINDINGS

TEST ROM

Ask the client to bend wrist down and back (flexion and extension). Next, have the client hold the wrist straight and move the hand outward and inward (deviation). Repeat these maneuvers against resistance.

Normal ranges of motion are 90 degrees, flexion; 70 degrees, hyperextension; 55 degrees, ulnar deviation; and 20 degrees, radial deviation. Client should have full ROM against resistance.

Ulnar deviation of the wrist and fingers with limited ROM is often seen in rheumatoid arthritis.

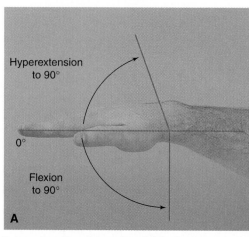

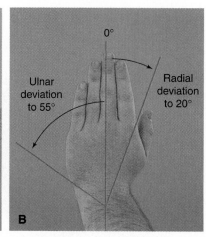

Range of motion of the wrists: (*A*) flexion-hyperextension; (*B*) radial-ulnar deviation. (© B. Proud.)

Unequal lengths of the ulna and radius have been found in some ethnic groups (eg, Swedes and Chinese) (Overfield, 1995).

Increased pain with extension of the wrist against resistance is seen in epicondylitis of the lateral side of the elbow. Increased pain with flexion of the wrist against resistance is seen in epicondylitis of the medial side of the elbow. Decreased muscle strength is noted with muscle and joint disease.

(continued)

ASSESSMENT PROCEDURE	NORMAL FINDINGS	ABNORMAL FINDINGS

Test for Carpal Tunnel Syndrome

Perform Phalen's test. Ask the client to place the backs of both hands against each other while flexing the wrists 90 degrees downward. Have the client hold this position for 60 seconds.

Optionally, test for Tinel's sign. With your finger, percuss lightly over the median nerve (located on the inner aspect of the wrist).

No tingling, numbness, or pain result from Phalen's test or from Tinel's test.

After either test, client may report tingling, numbness, and pain with carpal tunnel syndrome.

Median nerve entrapped in the carpal tunnel results in pain, numbness, and impaired function of the hand and fingers.

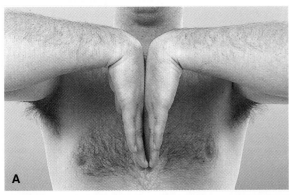
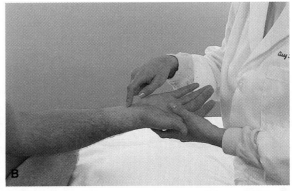

Tests for carpal tunnel syndrome: (*A*) Phalen's test; (*B*) Tinel's test. (© B. Proud.)

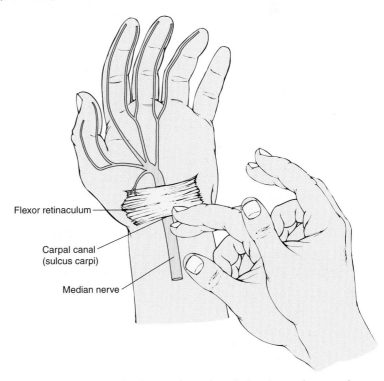

Median nerve entrapped in the carpal tunnel results in pain, numbness, and impaired function of the hand and fingers.

(continued)

ASSESSMENT PROCEDURE	NORMAL FINDINGS	ABNORMAL FINDINGS

HANDS AND FINGERS

Inspect and Palpate

Inspect size, shape, symmetry, swelling, and color. Palpate for tenderness and nodules.

Hands and fingers are symmetric, nontender, and without nodules. Fingers lie in straight line. No swelling or deformities. Rounded protuberance noted next to the thumb over the thenar prominence. Smaller protuberance seen adjacent to the small finger.

Swollen, stiff, tender finger joints are seen in acute rheumatoid arthritis. Boutonnière deformity and swan-neck deformity are seen in long-term rheumatoid arthritis (see Display 22-4). Atrophy of the thenar prominence is evident in carpal tunnel syndrome.

In osteoarthritis, hard, painless nodules may be seen over the distal interphalangeal joints (Heberden's nodes) and over the proximal interphalangeal joints (Bouchard's nodes).

Test ROM

Ask the client to (A) spread the fingers apart (abduction), (B) make a fist (adduction), (C) bend the fingers down (flexion) and then up (hyperextension), (D) move the thumb away from other fingers and then (E) touch the thumb to the base of the small finger. Repeat these maneuvers against resistance.

Normal ranges are 20 degrees of abduction, full adduction of fingers (touching), 90 degrees of flexion, and 30 degrees of hyperextension. The thumb should easily move away from other fingers and 50 degrees of thumb flexion is normal.

The client normally has full ROM against resistance.

Inability to extend the ring and little fingers is seen in Dupuytren's contracture. Painful extension of a finger may be seen in tenosynovitis (infection of the flexor tendon sheathes; see Display 22-4). Decreased muscle strength against resistance is associated with muscle and joint disease.

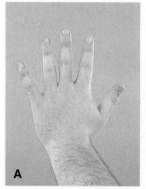
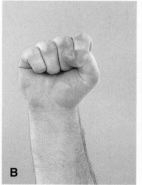
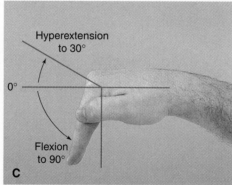
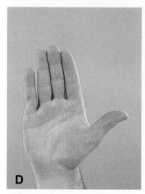
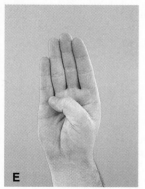

Normal range of motion of the fingers: (A) abduction, (B) adduction, (C) flexion-hyperextension, (D) thumb away from fingers, (E) thumb touching base of small finger. (© B. Proud.)

(continued)

ASSESSMENT PROCEDURE	NORMAL FINDINGS	ABNORMAL FINDINGS

HIPS

Inspect and Palpate

With the client standing, inspect symmetry and shape of hips. Palpate for stability, tenderness, and crepitus.

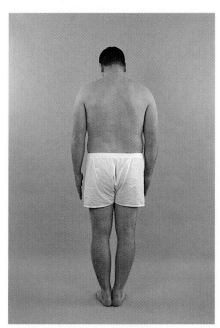

Inspecting the hips and buttocks.
(© B. Proud.)

Buttocks are equally sized, iliac crests are symmetric in height. Hips are stable, nontender, and without crepitus.

Instability, inability to stand, and/or a deformed hip area are indicative of a fractured hip. Tenderness, edema, decreased ROM, and crepitus are seen in hip inflammation and degenerative joint disease.

(continued)

ASSESSMENT PROCEDURE	NORMAL FINDINGS	ABNORMAL FINDINGS

Test ROM

With the client supine, ask the client to
  Raise extended leg.
  Flex knee up to chest while keeping other leg extended.

Normal ROM: 90 degrees of flexion and 120 degrees of flexion with other leg remaining straight.

Inability to abduct hip is a common sign of hip disease.

Tip From the Experts If the client has had a total hip replacement, do not test ROM unless the physician gives permission to do so. This is done to reduce the risk of dislocating the hip prosthesis.

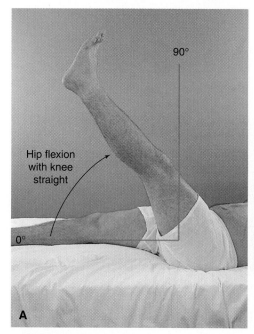
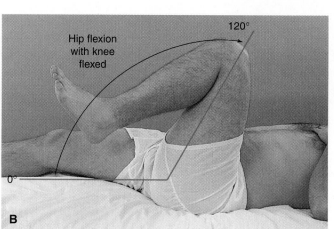

Normal range of motion of the hips: (*A*) hip flexion with extended knee straight and (*B*) hip flexion with knee bent (© B. Proud.)

(continued)

ASSESSMENT PROCEDURE	NORMAL FINDINGS	ABNORMAL FINDINGS
Move extended leg (*A*) away from midline of body as far as possible and then toward midline of body as far as possible (abduction and adduction). Bend knee and turn leg (*B*) inward (rotation) and then outward (rotation). Ask the client to lie prone (*C*) and lift extended leg off table. Alternatively, ask the client to stand and swing extended leg backward. Repeat these maneuvers against resistance.	Normal ROM: 45 degrees to 50 degrees of abduction; 20 degrees to 30 degrees of adduction. 40 degrees internal hip rotation, 45 degrees external hip rotation. 15 degrees hip hyperextension. Full ROM against resistance.	A decrease in internal hip rotation may be an early sign of hip disease. Decreased muscle strength against resistance is seen in muscle and joint disease.

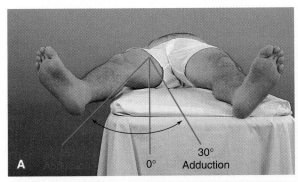

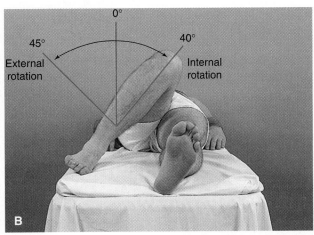

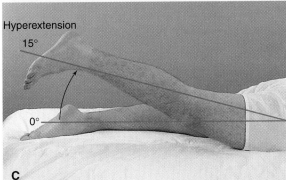

Normal range of hip motion: (*A*) abduction-adduction, (*B*) internal and external rotation, (*C*) hyperextension. (© B. Proud.)

(continued)

ASSESSMENT PROCEDURE	NORMAL FINDINGS	ABNORMAL FINDINGS

KNEES

Inspect and Palpate

With the client supine and then sitting with knees dangling, inspect for size, shape, symmetry, swelling, deformities, and alignment.

Palpate for tenderness, warmth, consistency, and nodules. Begin palpation 10 cm above the patella, using your fingers and thumb to move downward toward the knee.

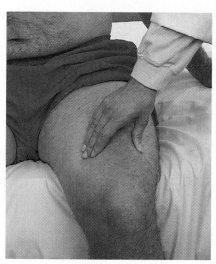

Palpating the knee area. (© B. Proud.)

Knees symmetric, hollows present on both sides of the patella, no swelling or deformities. Lower leg in alignment with upper leg.

Some older clients may have a bowlegged appearance because of decreased muscle control.

Nontender and cool. Muscles firm. No nodules.

Knees turn in with knock knees (genu valgum) and turn out with bowed legs (genu varum). Swelling above or next to the patella may indicate fluid in the knee joint or thickening of the synovial membrane.

Tenderness and warmth with a boggy consistency may be symptoms of synovitis.

(continued)

ASSESSMENT PROCEDURE	NORMAL FINDINGS	ABNORMAL FINDINGS

Tests for Swelling

If you notice swelling, perform the bulge test to determine if the swelling is due to accumulation of fluid or soft tissue swelling. The bulge test helps detect small amounts of fluid in the knee. With the client in a supine position, use the ball of your hand firmly to stroke the medial side of the knee upward, three to four times, to displace any accumulated fluid. Then, press on the lateral side of the knee and look for a bulge on the medial side of the knee.

No bulge of fluid appears on medial side of knee.

Bulge of fluid appears on medial side of knee with a small amount of joint effusion.

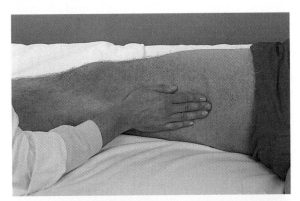

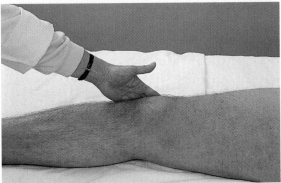

Performing the "bulge" knee test: stroking the knee (*top*), observing the medial side for bulging (*bottom*). (© B. Proud.)

(continued)

ASSESSMENT PROCEDURE	NORMAL FINDINGS	ABNORMAL FINDINGS
The ballottement test helps to detect large amounts of fluid in the knee. With the client in a supine position, firmly press your nondominant thumb and index finger on each side of the patella. This displaces fluid in the suprapatellar bursa located between the femur and patella. Then, with your dominant fingers, push the patella down on the femur. Feel for a fluid wave or a click.	No movement of patella noted. Patella rests firmly over femur.	Fluid wave or click palpated with large amounts of joint effusion.

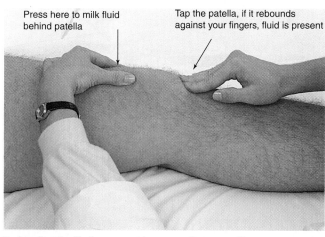

Press here to milk fluid behind patella

Tap the patella, if it rebounds against your fingers, fluid is present

Performing the "ballottement" knee test. (© B. Proud.)

Test ROM

Ask the client to:
• Bend each knee up (flexion) toward buttocks or back.
• Straighten knee (extension/hyperextension).
• Walk normally.
Repeat these maneuvers against resistance.
	Normal ranges: 120 degrees to 130 degrees of flexion; 0 degrees of extension to 15 degrees of hyperextension.
	    Client should have full ROM against resistance.
		Osteoarthritis is characterized by a decreased ROM with synovial thickening and crepitation. Flexion contractures of the knee are characterized by an inability to extend knee fully.
		    Decreased muscle strength against resistance is seen in muscle and joint disease.

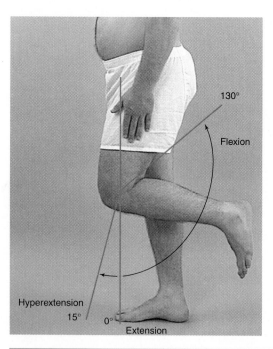

130°

Flexion

Hyperextension 15°

0°

Extension

Normal range of motion of the knee. (© B. Proud.)

(continued)

ASSESSMENT PROCEDURE	NORMAL FINDINGS	ABNORMAL FINDINGS

Test for Pain and Injury

If the client complains of a "giving in" or "locking" of the knee, perform McMurray's test. With the client in the supine position, ask the client to flex one knee and hip. Then, place your thumb and index finger of one hand on either side of the knee. Use your other hand to hold the heel of the foot up. Rotate the lower leg and foot laterally. Slowly extend the knee, noting pain or clicking. Repeat, rotating lower leg and foot medially. Again, note pain or clicking.

No pain or clicking noted.

Pain or clicking is indicative of a torn meniscus of the knee.

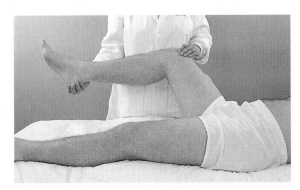

Performing McMurray's test. (© B. Proud.)

ANKLES AND FEET

Inspect and Palpate

With the client sitting, standing, and walking, inspect position, alignment, shape, and skin.

Toes usually point forward and lie flat; however, they may point in (pes varus) or point out (pes valgus). Toes and feet are in alignment with the lower leg. Smooth, rounded medial malleolar prominences with prominent heels and metatarsophalangeal joints. Skin is smooth and free of corns and calluses. Longitudinal arch; most of weight bearing is on foot midline.

A laterally deviated great toe with possible overlapping of the second toe and possible formation of an enlarged, painful, inflamed bursa (bunion) on the medial side is seen with hallux valgus. Common abnormalities include feet with no arches (pes planus or "flat feet"), feet with high arches (pes cavus); painful thickening of the skin over bony prominences and at pressure points (corns); nonpainful thickened skin that occurs at pressure points (calluses); and painful warts (verruca vulgaris) that often occur under a callus (plantar warts; Display 22-5).

Palpate ankles and feet for tenderness, heat, swelling, or nodules.

No pain, heat, swelling, or nodules

Tender, painful, reddened, hot, and swollen metatarsophalangeal joint of the great toe is seen in gouty arthritis. Nodules of the posterior ankle may be palpated with rheumatoid arthritis. Pain and tenderness of the metatarsophalangeal joints are seen in inflammation of the joints, rheumatoid arthritis, and degenerative joint disease.

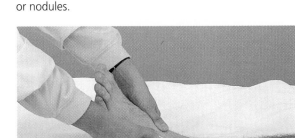

Palpating the ankles and feet. (© B. Proud.)

(continued)

ASSESSMENT PROCEDURE	NORMAL FINDINGS	ABNORMAL FINDINGS

Test ROM

Ask the client to:

Point toes upward (dorsiflexion) and then downward (plantar flexion).

Turn soles outward (eversion) and then inward (inversion).

Rotate foot outward (abduction) and then inward (adduction).

Turn toes under foot (flexion) and then upward (extension).

Repeat these maneuvers against resistance.

Normal ranges: 20 degrees dorsiflexion of ankle and foot; 45 degrees plantar flexion of ankle and foot.

20 degrees of eversion; 30 degrees of inversion.

10 degrees of abduction; 20 degrees of adduction.

40 degrees of flexion; 40 degrees of extension.

Client has full ROM against resistance.

Decreased strength against resistance is seen in muscle and joint disease.

Hyperextension of the metatarsophalangeal joint and flexion of the proximal interphalangeal joint is apparent in hammer toe (see Display 22-5).

Decreased strength against resistance is common in muscle and joint disease.

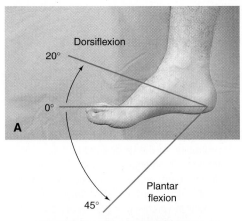

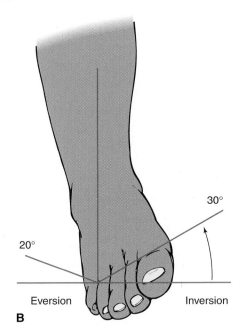

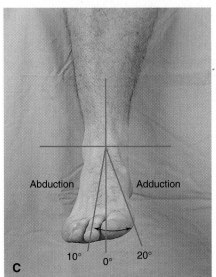

Normal range of motion of the feet and ankles: (*A*) dorsiflexion/plantar flexion; (*B*) eversion/inversion; (*C*) abduction/adduction. (Photos © B. Proud.)

DISPLAY 22-3. Abnormal Spinal Curvatures

ABNORMAL
FINDINGS

FLATTENING OF THE LUMBAR CURVE

Flattening of the lumbar curvature may be seen with a herniated lumbar disc or ankylosing spondylitis.

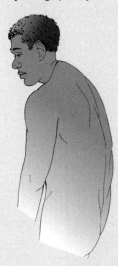

KYPHOSIS

A rounded thoracic convexity (kyphosis) is commonly seen in older adults.

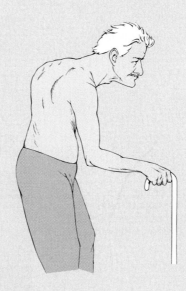

LUMBAR LORDOSIS

An exaggerated lumbar curve (lumbar lordosis) is often seen in pregnancy or obesity.

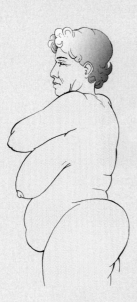

SCOLIOSIS

Lateral curvature of the spine with an increase in convexity on the side that is curved is seen in scoliosis.

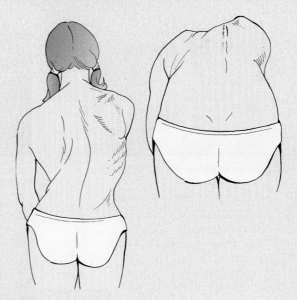

ABNORMAL FINDINGS

DISPLAY 22-4. Abnormalities Affecting the Wrists, Hands, and Fingers

The following abnormalities are commonly associated with the upper extremities. Early detection is important because early intervention may help to preserve dexterity and daily function.

ACUTE RHEUMATOID ARTHRITIS

Tender, painful, swollen, stiff joints are seen in acute rheumatoid arthritis.

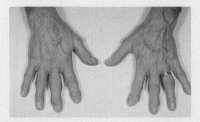

(© 1991 National Medical Slide Bank/CMSP.)

CHRONIC RHEUMATOID ARTHRITIS

Chronic swelling and thickening of the metacarpophalangeal and proximal interphalangeal joints, limited range of motion, and finger deviation toward the ulnar side are seen in chronic rheumatoid arthritis.

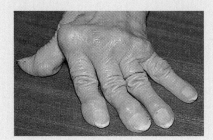

(© 1995 Science Photo Library.)

BOUTONNIÈRE AND SWAN-NECK DEFORMITIES

Flexion of the proximal interphalangeal joint and hyperextension of the distal interphalangeal joint (boutonnière deformity) and hyperextension of the proximal interphalangeal joint with flexion of the distal interphalangeal joint (swan-neck deformity) are also common in chronic rheumatoid arthritis.

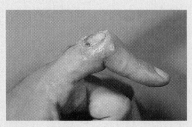

Boutonnière deformity. (© 1990 CMSP.)

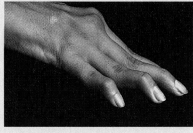

Swan neck deformity. (© 1991 National Medical Slide Bank/CMSP.)

GANGLION

Nontender, round, enlarged, swollen, fluid-filled cyst (ganglion) is commonly seen at the dorsum of the wrist.

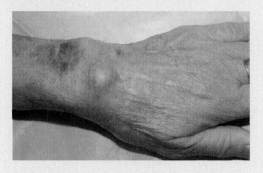

OSTEOARTHRITIS

Hard, painless nodules over the distal interphalangeal joints (Heberden's nodes) and over the proximal interphalangeal joints (Bouchard's nodes) are seen in osteoarthritis.

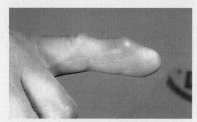

Heberden's nodes. (© 1991 National Medical Slide Bank / CMSP.)

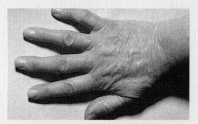

Bouchard's nodes. (© 1991 National Medical Slide Bank / CMSP.)

TENOSYNOVITIS

Painful extension of a finger may be seen in acute tenosynovitis (infection of the flexor tendon sheathes).

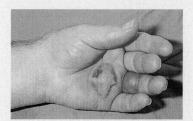

(© 1995 Michael English. MD/CMSP.)

THENAR ATROPHY

Atrophy of the thenar prominence due to pressure on the median nerve is seen in carpal tunnel syndrome.

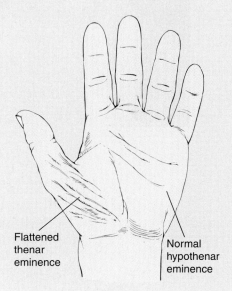

Flattened thenar eminence

Normal hypothenar eminence

ABNORMAL
FINDINGS

DISPLAY 22-5. Abnormalities of the Feet and Toes

The following abnormalities affect the feet and toes, typically causing discomfort and impeding mobility. Early detection and treatment can help to restore or maximize function.

ACUTE GOUTY ARTHRITIS

In gouty arthritis, the metatarsophalangeal joint of the great toe is tender, painful, reddened, hot, and swollen.

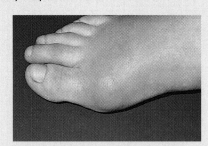

(© 1995 Science Photo Library/CMSP.)

CALLUS

Calluses are nonpainful, thickened skin that occur at pressure points.

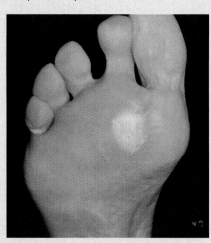

CORN

Corns are painful thickenings of the skin that occur over bony prominences and at pressure points.

FLAT FEET

A flat foot (pes planus) has no arch and may cause pain and swelling of the foot surface.

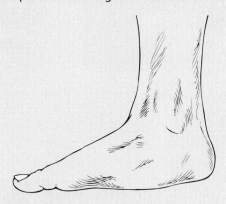

HALLUX VALGUS

Hallux valgus is an abnormality in which the great toe is deviated laterally and may overlap the second toe. An enlarged, painful, inflamed bursa (bunion) may form on the medial side.

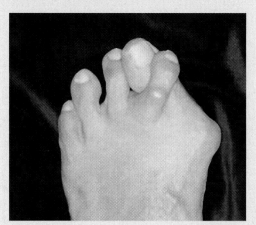

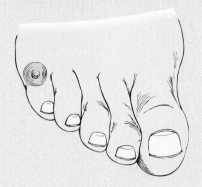

(continued)

DISPLAY 22-5. Abnormalities of the Feet and Toes (Continued)

HAMMER TOE

Hyperextension at the metatarsophalangeal joint with flexion at the proximal interphalangeal joint (hammer toe) commonly occurs with the second toe.

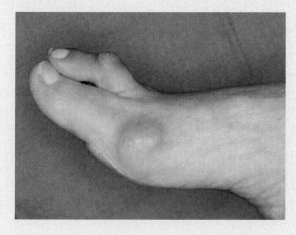

PLANTAR WART

Plantar warts are painful warts (verruca vulgaris) that often occur under a callus, appearing as tiny dark spots.

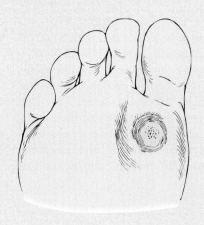

Validation and Documentation of Findings

Validate the musculoskeletal assessment data that you have collected. This is necessary to verify that the data are reliable and accurate.

EXAMPLE OF SUBJECTIVE DATA

No history of past problems with joints or muscles. "Broke right arm as child, had cast for 6 weeks." No problems with that arm since that time. Walks 1 mile four times a week; plays golf twice a week; likes being outside when not at work. Polio immunization as child; last tetanus immunization 3 years ago after cutting foot with garden tiller. Recalls grandmother as having rheumatoid arthritis. Does not smoke or drink alcohol. Drinks two caffeinated colas per day. Consumes food from all food groups; drinks milk daily. Client is 5 feet, 6 inches, weighs 140 lb, with no recent weight gain or loss. Occupation requires long hours sitting working at a computer. Has good supportive chair. Has not had any back problems.

EXAMPLE OF OBJECTIVE DATA

Gait smooth, with equal stride and good base of support. Full ROM of TMJ with no pain, tenderness, clicking, or crepitus. Sternoclavicular joint midline without swelling or redness. Normal curves of cervical, thoracic, and lumbar spine. Paravertebral area nontender. Full, smooth ROM of cervical and lumbar spine. Upper and lower extremities symmetric without lesions, nodules, deformities, tenderness, or swelling. Full, smooth ROM against gravity and resistance.

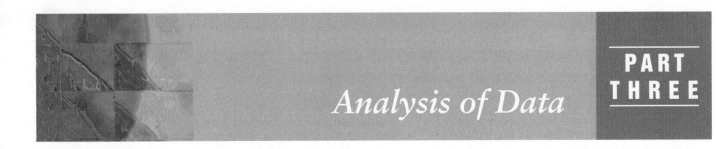

After you have collected your assessment data, you will need to analyze the data, using diagnostic reasoning skills. The section titled Diagnostic Reasoning: Possible Conclusions presents an overview of common conclusions that you may reach after musculoskeletal assessment. The case study that follows shows you how to analyze the assessment data for a specific client. You also have an opportunity to analyze data in the critical thinking exercise that is included in the study guide/lab manual available for this textbook.

Diagnostic Reasoning: Possible Conclusions

Below are some possible conclusions that you may reach after assessing the client's musculoskeletal system.

SELECTED NURSING DIAGNOSES

After collecting subjective and objective data pertaining to the musculoskeletal system, you will need to identify abnormalities and cluster the data to reveal any significant patterns or abnormalities. These data will then be used to make clinical judgments (nursing diagnoses: wellness, risk, or actual) about the status of the client's musculoskeletal system. Following is a listing of selected nursing diagnoses that you may identify when analyzing data for this part of the assessment.

Nursing Diagnoses (Wellness)

- Opportunity to Enhance Activity and Exercise Patterns

Nursing Diagnoses (Risk)

- Risk for Trauma related to repetitive movements of wrists or elbow with recreation or occupation
- Risk for Injury: Pathologic fractures related to osteoporosis
- Risk for Injury to joints, muscles, or bones related to environmental hazards
- Risk for Disuse Syndrome
- Risk for Urinary Tract Infection related to urine stasis secondary to immobility

Nursing Diagnoses (Actual)

- Impaired Physical Mobility related to impaired joint movement, decreased muscle strength, or fractured bone
- Activity Intolerance related to muscle weakness or joint pain
- Constipation related to decreased gastric motility and muscle tone secondary to immobility
- Ineffective Sexuality Patterns related to lower back pain
- Acute (or Chronic) Pain related to joint, muscle, or bone problems
- Impaired Skin Integrity related to prolonged pressure on the skin secondary to immobility
- Impaired Social Interaction related to depression or immobility
- Disturbed Body Image related to skeletal deformities

After grouping the data, it may become apparent that certain collaborative problems emerge. Remember that collaborative problems differ from nursing diagnoses in that they cannot be prevented with nursing interventions alone. However, these physiologic complications of medical conditions can be detected and monitored by the nurse. In addition, the nurse can use physician- and nurse-prescribed interventions to minimize the complications of these problems. The nurse may also have to refer the client in such situations for further treatment of the problem.

Following is a list of collaborative problems that may be identified when assessing the musculoskeletal system. These problems are worded as Potential Complications (or PC), followed by the problem.

SELECTED COLLABORATIVE PROBLEMS

- PC: Osteoporosis
- PC: Joint dislocation
- PC: Compartmental syndrome
- PC: Pathologic fractures

MEDICAL PROBLEMS

After grouping the data, it may become apparent that the client has signs and symptoms that may require medical diagnosis and treatment. Referral to a primary care provider is necessary.

Diagnostic Reasoning: Case Study

The case study presents assessment data for a specific client. It is followed by an analysis of the data, working out the seven key steps to arrive at specific conclusions.

Frances Funstead has come to the occupational health nurse's office asking for help with her back problem. During the interview, she states that she has recently experienced burning in her lower back in an area just below the waist and has pain in her shoulder muscles. She denies pain in her hips and legs.

Ms. Funstead's job in the manufacturing plant requires her to stand on the assembly line where she puts together small parts from 7:00 AM to 3:00 PM. She has 30 minutes for lunch (11:00 to 11:30 AM), which she eats in the company lunchroom, and two 10-minute coffee breaks. She also states that many life changes are going on right now and she is seeking spiritual counseling in handling these. She is 55 years old and can't retire for another 7 years. Physical examination reveals rigid neck and shoulder muscles with palpable "knots," with strong shoulder shrug and neck rotation against resistance; however, neck rotation ROM is limited, with pain beyond 60-degree rotation bilaterally. A slight right lateral spinal curvature and mild lordosis are noted from T10 to L2. Muscles in this area do not appear swollen, but the area is slightly warmer to touch than the surrounding area.

1 Identify abnormal data and strengths (in both subjective and objective data).

SUBJECTIVE DATA

- Seeks help from occupational health nurse for back problem
- Burning in her lower back, just below the waist area (flank)
- Pain in her shoulder muscles
- Pain with neck rotation beyond 60 degrees bilaterally
- Denies pain in hips or legs
- Stands on the assembly line all day with only three short breaks
- Puts together small parts with her hands
- Many life changes right now
- 55 years old, can't retire for 7 years
- Seeking spiritual counseling for life changes

OBJECTIVE DATA

- Neck and shoulder muscles are rigid with palpable "knots"
- Strong shoulder shrug and neck rotation against resistance
- Neck rotation ROM is limited
- Slight right lateral spinal curvature T10 to L2
- Mild lordosis is noted at T10 to L2
- Muscles in affected area do not appear swollen
- Area is slightly warmer to touch than the surrounding area

2 Cue Clusters	**3** Inferences	**4** Possible Nursing Diagnoses	**5** Defining Characteristics	**6** Confirm or Rule Out
A • Burning in the lower back, just below the waist • Pain in her shoulder muscles • Pain with neck rotation beyond 60 degrees bilaterally • Stands on the assembly line all day with only three short breaks • Puts together small parts with her hands • Many life changes right now • Neck and shoulder muscles are rigid with palpable "knots"	Inflamed muscles and pain in shoulders and mid-lower back could be the result of strain from her spinal curvatures coupled with occupational stress, or the result of poor posture, but a physician referral is needed to rule out arthritic or spinal disc pathology. Her life changes could be causing additional stress, which can result in muscle tension.	Acute Pain: lower back, related to possible improper posture and knowledge deficit of ways to prevent physical strain at work Ineffective Coping related to perceived powerlessness in life situation	*Major:* Communicates pain descriptors *Minor:* Alterations in muscle tone (rigid) *Major:* None *Minor:* Reported (implied) difficulty with life stressors	Confirm Rule out because it does not meet major defining characteristics, but the collection of data may confirm this highly probable diagnosis at a later time.

2 Cue Clusters	**3** Inferences	**4** Possible Nursing Diagnoses	**5** Defining Characteristics	**6** Confirm or Rule Out
• Neck rotation ROM is limited • Slight right lateral spinal curvature—T10 to L2 • Mild lordosis is noted at T10 to L2 • Muscles in affected area do not appear swollen • Area is slightly warmer to touch than the surrounding area				
B • Strong shoulder shrug and neck rotation against resistance • Denies pain in hips or legs	These two negative findings can help rule out problems with cranial nerve XI (spinal accessory) or involvement of the sciatic nerve in lumbar disc problems. Inquire about pain in the arms, which could indicate pinched nerves at the cranial and upper thoracic spinal disc levels.			
C • Seeks help from occupational health nurse for back problem • Many life changes right now • Seeking spiritual counseling for life changes	Client is aware of need for help and appears to have some insight into possible contributing factors to her physical problem because she shares that she is undergoing life changes and is seeking spiritual assistance.	Health-Seeking Behavior	*Major:* Expressed desire to seek information for health promotion *Minor:* Not verbalized, but implied concern about current environmental and personal conditions on health status	Confirm because it meets the major and minor defining characteristics.
		Risk for spiritual distress related to multiple life changes	*Major:* None stated *Minor:* None stated	This is a risk diagnosis and it does not need to meet defining characteristics to be confirmed. Because the client has indicated she is seeking spiritual counseling, it is possible her life changes are putting her at risk for this diagnosis. Accept the risk diagnosis and collect more data to see if complementary nursing interventions are needed.

7 Document conclusions.

Three nursing diagnoses are appropriate for Ms. Funstead at this time:

- Acute Pain: lower back, related to possible improper posture and knowledge deficit of ways to prevent physical strain at work
- Health-Seeking Behaviors
- Risk for spiritual distress related to multiple life changes

Ms. Funstead should be referred to a physician for further evaluation of possible spinal disk dislocations, arthritis, or early tumors. Depending on the findings, she should be referred to a physical therapist for muscle-strengthening exercises and instruction regarding body mechanics to prevent muscle strain. If medical evaluation indicates that this problem is a work-related disability, the nurse should refer Ms. Funstead to the appropriate person to assist with the implementation of rehabilitative measures or disability benefits.

REFERENCES AND SELECTED READINGS

Adkins III, S. B., & Figler, R. A. (2000). Hip pain in athletes. *American Family Physician, 61*(7), 2109–2118.

Arcuni, S. E. (2000). Rotator cuff pathology and subacromial impingement. *The Nurse Practitioner, 25*(5), 58–78.

Baxter, R. E. (1998). *Pocket guide to musculoskeletal assessment.* Philadelphia, PA: W. B. Saunders.

Blackburn, W. D. (1999). *Approach to the patient with a musculoskeletal disorder* (1st ed.). Caddo, OK: Professional Communications, Inc.

Carpenter, D. R., & Hudacek, S. (1994). Polymyalgia rheumatica: A comprehensive review of this debilitating disease. *Nurse Practitioner, 19*(6), 50–51, 55–58.

Cwikel, J., Fried, A. V., Galinsky, D., & Ring, H. (1995). Gait and activity in the elderly: Implications for community falls—prevention and treatment programmes. *Disability and Rehabilitation, 17,* 277–280.

Deathe, A. B., Pardo, R. D., Winter, D. A., Hayes, K. C., & Russell-Smyth, J. (1996). Stability of walking frames. *Journal of Rehabilitation Research and Development, 33*(1), 30–35.

Johnson, M. W. (2000). Acute knee effusions: A systematic approach to diagnosis. *American Family Physician, 61*(8), 2391–2400.

Kerrigan, D. C., Thirunarayan, M. A., Sheffler, L. R., Ribaudo, T. A., & Corcoran, P. J. (1996). A tool to assess biomechanical gait efficiency: A preliminary clinical study. *American Journal of Physical Medicine and Rehabilitation, 75,* 3–8.

Klippel, J. H., Weyand, C. M., & Wortmann, R. (Eds.). (1998). *Primer on the rheumatic diseases: An official publication of the Arthritis Foundation* (11th ed.). Atlanta, GA: Arthritis Foundation.

Mangini, M. (1998). Physical assessment of the musculoskeletal system. *Nursing Clinics of North America, 33*(4), 643–652.

Means, K. M., Rodell, D. E., & O'Sullivan, P. S. (1996). Use of an obstacle course to assess balance and mobility in the elderly: A validation study. *American Journal of Physical Medicine and Rehabilitation, 75,* 88–95.

Mecagni, C., Smith, J. P., Roberts, K. E., & O'Sullivan, S. B. (2000). Balance and ankle range of motion in community-dwelling women aged 64 to 87 years: A correlational study. *Physical Therapy, 80*(10), 1004–1011.

Muirhead, G. (2000). Diagnosing bursitis of the hip. *Patient Care, 34*(5), 196–210.

O'Kane, J. W. (1999). Anterior hip pain. *American Family Physician, 60*(6), 1687–1696.

Padua, L., Padua, R., LoMonaco, M., Aprile, I., & Tonali, P. (1999). Multiperspective assessment of carpal tunnel syndrome: A multicenter study. Italian CTS Study Group. *Neurology, 58*(8), 1554–1559.

Post, W. R. (1998). Patellofemor pain. *The Physician and Sportsmedicine, 26*(1), 68–75.

Quaschnick, M. S. (1996). The diagnosis and management of plantar fasciitis. *The Nurse Practitioner, 21*(4), 50–65.

Snider, R. K., (Ed.). (2001). *Essentials of musculoskeletal care* (2nd ed.). Rosemont, IL: American Academy of Orthopaedic Surgeons.

———. (1997). *Essentials of musculoskeletal care* (1st ed.). Rosemont, IL: American Academy of Orthopaedic Surgeons.

Strand, L. I., & Solveig, L. W. (1999). The sock test for evaluating activity limitation in patients with musculoskeletal pain. *Physical Therapy, 79*(2), 136–145.

Treml, L. A. (1996). Assessing patient mobility: Mobility screening as part of a community-based geriatric assessment. *Home Care Provider, 1*(1), 26–29, 48.

Wexler, R. K. (1998). The injured ankle. *American Family Physician, 57*(3), 474–480.

Woodard, T. W., & Best, T. M. (2000). The painful shoulder: Part I. Clinical evaluation. *American Family Physician, 61*(10), 3079–3088.

Risk Factors—Osteoporosis

International Osteoporosis Foundation (IOF). (2001). Osteoporosis [On-line]. Available: http://www.osteofound.org.

National Institutes of Health (NIH). (2001). NIH Osteoporosis and related bone diseases (ORBD) national resource center [On-line]. Available: http://www.osteo.org.

National Osteoporosis Foundation (NOF). (2001). Prevention: Who's at risk [On-line]. Available: http://nof.org.

Overfield, T. (1995). Biological variation in health and illness: Race, age, and sex differences (2nd ed.). Boca Raton, FL: CRC Press.

For additional information on this book, be sure to visit http://connection.lww.com.

Neurologic Assessment

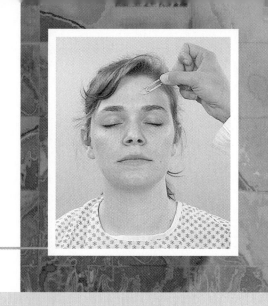

23

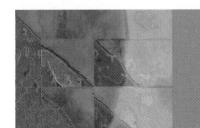
The very complex neurologic system is responsible for coordinating and regulating all body functions. It consists of two structural components: the central nervous system (CNS) and the peripheral nervous system.

Central Nervous System

The CNS encompasses the brain and spinal cord, which are covered by meninges, three layers of connective tissue that protect and nourish the CNS. Surrounding the brain and spinal cord is the subarachnoid space. The subarachnoid space is filled with cerebrospinal fluid, which is formed in the ventricles of the brain and which flows through the ventricles into the space. This fluid-filled space cushions the brain and spinal cords, nourishes the CNS, and removes waste materials. Electrical activity of the CNS is governed by neurons located throughout the sensory and motor neural pathways. The CNS contains upper motor neurons that influence lower motor neurons, located mostly in the peripheral nervous system.

BRAIN

Located in the cranial cavity, the brain has four major divisions: The cerebrum, the diencephalon, the brain stem, and the cerebellum (Fig. 23-1).

Cerebrum

The cerebrum is divided into the right and left cerebral hemispheres, which are joined by the corpus callosum—a bundle of nerve fibers responsible for communication between the hemispheres. Each hemisphere sends and receives impulses from the opposite sides of the body and consists of four lobes (frontal, parietal, temporal, and occipital). The lobes are composed of a substance known as gray matter, which mediates higher-level functions such as memory, perception, communication, and initiation of voluntary movements. Consisting of aggregations of neuronal cell bodies, gray matter rims the surfaces of the cerebral hemispheres, forming the cerebral cortex. See Table 23-1 for the specific functions of each lobe. Damage to a lobe results in impairment of the specific function directed by that lobe.

Diencephalon

The diencephalon lies beneath the cerebral hemispheres and consists of the thalamus and hypothalamus. Most sensory impulses travel through the gray matter of the thalamus, which is responsible for screening and directing the impulses to specific areas in the cerebral cortex. The hypothalamus (which is part of the autonomic nervous system, which is a part of the peripheral nervous system) is responsible for regulating many body functions, including water balance, appetite, vital signs (temperature, blood pressure, pulse, and respiratory rate), sleep cycles, pain perception, and emotional status.

Brain Stem

Located between the cerebral cortex and the spinal cord, the brain stem consists of the midbrain, pons, and medulla oblongata. The midbrain serves as a relay center for ear and eye reflexes and relays impulses between the higher cerebral centers and the lower pons, medulla, cerebellum, and spinal cord. The pons links the cerebellum to the cerebrum and the midbrain to the medulla. It is responsible for various reflex actions. The medulla oblongata has centers that control and regulate respiratory function, heart rate and force, and blood pressure.

Cerebellum

The cerebellum, located behind the brain stem and under the cerebrum, also has two hemispheres. Its primary functions include coordination and smoothing of voluntary movements, maintenance of equilibrium, and maintenance of muscle tone.

SPINAL CORD

The spinal cord (Fig. 23-2) is located in the vertebral canal and extends from the medulla oblongata to the first lumbar vertebra. (Note that the spinal cord is not as long as the vertebral canal.) The inner part of the cord has an H-shaped appearance and is made up of two pairs of columns (dorsal and ventral) consisting of gray matter. The outer part is made up of white matter and surrounds the gray matter (Fig. 23-3). The spinal cord conducts sensory impulses up ascending tracts to the brain, conducts motor impulses down descend-

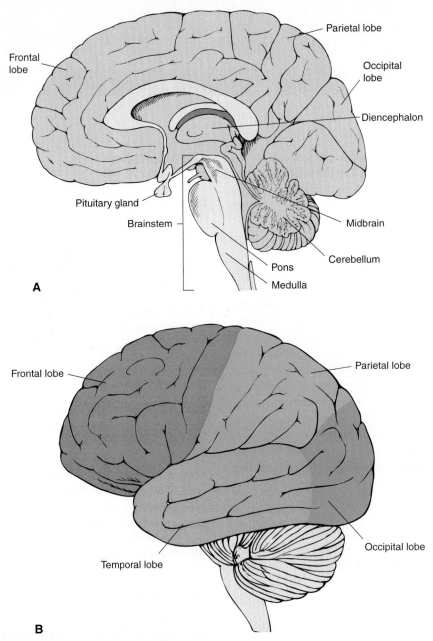

FIGURE 23-1. (*A*) Structures of the brain. (*B*) Lobes of the brain.

ing tracts to neurons that stimulate glands and muscles throughout the body, and is responsible for simple reflex activity. Reflex activity involves various neural structures. For example, the stretch reflex—the simplest type of reflex arc—involves one sensory neuron (afferent), one motor neuron (efferent), and one synapse. An example of this is the knee jerk, which is elicited by tapping the patellar tendon. More complex reflexes involve three or more neurons.

NEURAL PATHWAYS

Sensory impulses travel to the brain by way of two ascending neural pathways (the spinothalamic tract and posterior columns) (Fig. 23-4). These impulses originate in

the afferent fibers of the peripheral nerves and are carried through the posterior (dorsal) root into the spinal cord. Sensations of pain, temperature, and crude and light touch travel by way of the spinothalamic tract, whereas sensations of position, vibration, and fine touch travel by way of the posterior columns. Motor impulses are conducted to the muscles by two descending neural pathways, the pyramidal (corticospinal) tract and extrapyramidal tract (Fig. 23-5). The motor neurons of the pyramidal tract originate in the motor cortex and travel down to the medulla, where they cross over to the opposite side and then travel down the spinal cord, where they synapse with a lower motor neuron in the anterior horn of the spinal cord. These impulses are carried to muscles and produce

TABLE 23-1. Lobes of the Cerebral Hemispheres and Their Function

Lobe	Function
Frontal	Directs voluntary, skeletal actions (left side of lobe controls right side of body and right side of lobe controls left side of body). Also influences communication (talking and writing), emotions, intellect, reasoning ability, judgment, and behavior. Contains Broca's area, which is responsible for speech.
Parietal	Interprets tactile sensations, including touch, pain, temperature, shapes, and two-point discrimination.
Occipital	Influences the ability to read with understanding and is the primary visual receptor center.
Temporal	Receives and interprets impulses from the ear. Contains Wernicke's area, which is responsible for interpreting auditory stimuli.

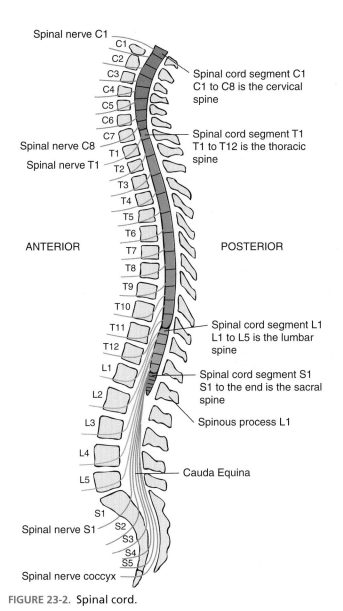

Spinal nerve C1

C1
C2
C3 — Spinal cord segment C1 C1 to C8 is the cervical spine
C4
C5
C6
C7
Spinal nerve C8 — T1 — Spinal cord segment T1 T1 to T12 is the thoracic spine
Spinal nerve T1 — T2
T3
T4
T5
T6
ANTERIOR — T7 — POSTERIOR
T8
T9
T10
T11 — Spinal cord segment L1 L1 to L5 is the lumbar spine
T12
L1 — Spinal cord segment S1 S1 to the end is the sacral spine
L2
L3 — Spinous process L1
L4
L5 — Cauda Equina
S1
Spinal nerve S1 — S2
S3
S4
S5
Spinal nerve coccyx

FIGURE 23-2. Spinal cord.

voluntary movements that involve skill and purpose. The extrapyramidal tract motor neurons consist of those motor neurons that originate in the motor cortex, basal ganglia, brain stem, and spinal cord that are outside the pyramidal tract. They travel from the frontal lobe to the pons, where they cross over to the opposite side and down the spinal cord, where they connect with lower motor neurons that conduct impulses to the muscles. These neurons conduct impulses related to maintenance of muscle tone and body control.

Peripheral Nervous System

Carrying information to and from the CNS, the peripheral nervous system consists of 12 pairs of cranial nerves and 31 pairs of spinal nerves. These nerves are categorized as two types of fibers: somatic and autonomic. Somatic fibers carry CNS impulses to voluntary skeletal muscles, whereas autonomic fibers carry CNS impulses to smooth, involuntary muscles (in the heart and glands). The somatic nervous system mediates conscious, or voluntary, activities, whereas the autonomic nervous system mediates unconscious, or involuntary, activities.

CRANIAL NERVES

Twelve pairs of cranial nerves evolve from the brain or brain stem (Fig. 23-6) and transmit motor or sensory messages. See Table 23-2 for the number, names, type of impulse, and primary functions of the cranial nerves.

SPINAL NERVES

Comprising 8 cervical, 12 thoracic, 5 lumbar, 5 sacral, and 1 coccygeal nerve, the 31 pairs of spinal nerves are named after the vertebrae below each one's exit point along the spinal cord (see Fig. 23-2). Each nerve is attached to the spinal cord by two nerve roots. The sensory (afferent) fiber enters through the dorsal (posterior) roots of the cord, whereas the motor (efferent) fiber exits through the ventral (anterior) roots of the cord. The sensory root of each spinal nerve innervates an area of the skin called a dermatome (Fig. 23-7).

Autonomic Nervous System

Some peripheral nerves have a special function associated with automatic activities; they are referred to as the autonomic nervous system. Autonomic nervous system impulses are carried by both cranial and spinal nerves. These impulses are carried from the CNS to the involuntary, smooth muscles that make up the walls of the heart and glands. The autonomic nervous system, which maintains the inter-

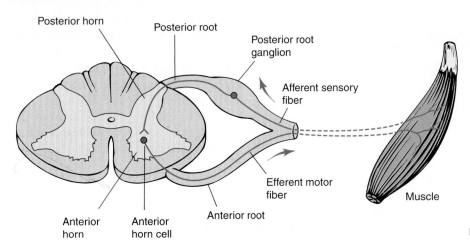

FIGURE 23-3. Cross-section of spinal cord.

nal homeostasis of the body, incorporates the sympathetic and parasympathetic nervous systems. The sympathetic nervous system ("fight-or-flight" system) is activated during stress and elicits responses such as decreased gastric secretions, bronchiole dilatation, increased pulse rate, and pupil dilatation. These sympathetic fibers arise from the thoracolumbar level (T1 to L2) of the spinal cord. The parasympathetic nervous system functions to restore and maintain normal body functions, for example, by decreasing heart rate. The parasympathetic fibers arise from the craniosacral regions (S1 to S4 and cranial nerves III, VI, IX, and X).

(*text continues on page 547*)

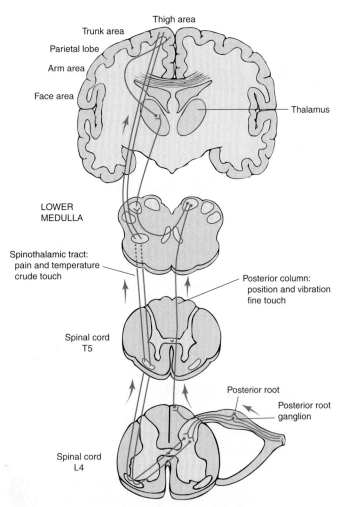

FIGURE 23-4. Sensory (ascending) neural pathways.

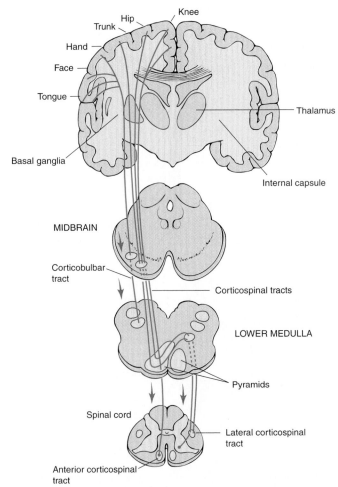

FIGURE 23-5. Motor (descending) neural pathways.

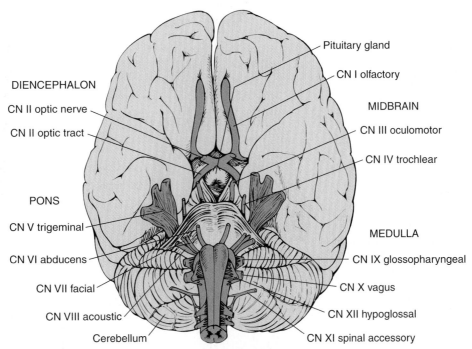

FIGURE 23-6. Twelve cranial nerves and brain landmarks.

TABLE 23-2. Cranial Nerves: Type and Function

Cranial Nerve (Name)	Type of Impulse	Function
I (olfactory)	Sensory	Carries smell impulses from nasal mucous membrane to brain
II (optic)	Sensory	Carries visual impulses from eye to brain
III (oculomotor)	Motor	Contracts eye muscles to control eye movements (inferior lateral, medial, and superior), constricts pupils, and elevates eyelids
IV (trochlear)	Motor	Contracts one eye muscle to control inferomedial eye movement
V (trigeminal)	Sensory Motor	Carries sensory impulses of pain, touch, and temperature from the face to the brain Influences clenching and lateral jaw movements (biting, chewing)
VI (abducens)	Motor	Controls lateral eye movements
VII (facial)	Sensory Motor	Contains sensory fibers for taste on anterior two thirds of tongue and stimulates secretions from salivary glands (submaxillary and sublingual) and tears from lacrimal glands Supplies the facial muscles and affects facial expressions (smiling, frowning, closing eyes)
VIII (acoustic, vestibulocochlear)	Sensory	Contains sensory fibers for hearing and balance
IX (glossopharyngeal)	Sensory Motor	Contains sensory fibers for taste on posterior third of tongue and sensory fibers of the pharynx that result in the "gag reflex" when stimulated Provides secretory fibers to the parotid salivary glands; promotes swallowing movements
X (vagus)	Sensory Motor	Carries sensations from the throat, larynx, heart, lungs, bronchi, gastrointestinal tract, and abdominal viscera Promotes swallowing, talking, and production of digestive juices
XI (spinal accessory)	Motor	Innervates neck muscles (sternocleidomastoid and trapezius) that promote movement of the shoulders and head rotation. Also promotes some movement of the larynx
XII (hypoglossal)	Motor	Innervates tongue muscles that promote the movement of food and talking

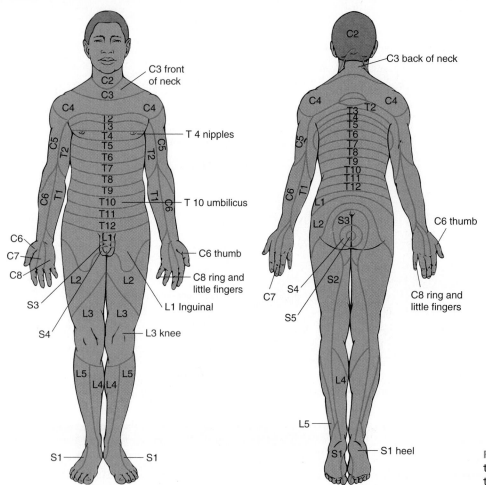

FIGURE 23-7. Anterior (*left*) and posterior (*right*) dermatomes (areas of the skin innervated by spinal nerves).

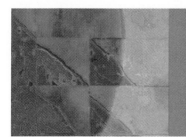

Collecting Subjective Data

Problems with other body systems may affect the neurologic system, and neurologic system disorders can affect all other body systems. Regardless of the source of the neurologic problem, the client's total lifestyle and level of functioning are often affected. Because of their subjective nature, neurologic problems related to activities of daily living are typically detected through an in-depth nursing history. For example, problems with loss of concentration, loss of sensation, or dizziness are usually identified only through precise questioning during the interview with the client. In fact, it is at this point in the interview that the nurse usually finds the COLDSPA mnemonic handy and most useful.

COLDSPA

CHARACTER: Describe the sign or symptom. How does it feel, look, sound, smell, and so forth?

ONSET: When did it begin?

LOCATION: Where is it? Does it radiate?

DURATION: How long does it last? Does it recur?

SEVERITY: How bad is it?

PATTERN: What makes it better: What makes it worse?

ASSOCIATED FACTORS: What other symptoms occur with it?

Clients who are experiencing symptoms associated with the neurologic system (such as headaches or memory loss) may be very fearful that they have a serious condition, such as a metastatic brain tumor or a difficult-to-treat disease such as Alzheimer's. Fear of losing control and independence, along with threatened self-esteem or role performance, are common. The examiner needs to be sensitive to these fears and concerns because the client may decline to share important information with the examiner if these fears and concerns are not addressed.

Nursing History

CURRENT SYMPTOMS

Question Do you experience any numbness or tingling?

Rationale Loss of sensation or tingling may occur with damage to the brain, spinal cord, or peripheral nerves.

Q Do you experience seizures?

R Seizures occur with epilepsy, metabolic disorders, head injuries, and high fevers.

Q Describe what happens before you have the seizure and where on your body the seizure starts. How do you feel afterward? Do you take medications for the seizures? Do you wear medical identification to alert others that you have seizures? Do you take safety precautions regarding driving or operating dangerous machinery?

R In some cases, an aura (an auditory, visual, or motor sensation) forewarns the client that a seizure is about to occur. Where the seizure starts and what occurs before and after can aid in determining the type of seizure (eg, generalized, formerly known as grand mal and affecting both hemispheres of the brain, or absence seizure, also known as petit mal) and its treatment. Antiepileptic medications (anticonvulsants) must be distributed at a therapeutic level in the blood to be effective. Wearing a medical identification tag, such as a MedicAlert bracelet, and the client's knowledge of the medication regimen and the importance of safety measures provide information on the client's willingness to be involved in and adhere to the treatment plan.

Q Do you experience headaches? When do they occur and what do they feel like? (See related questions in Chapter 10.)

R See Chapter 10 for a description of various types of headaches. Morning headaches that subside after arising may be an early sign of a brain tumor.

Q Do you experience dizziness or lightheadedness or problems with balance or coordination? Or have you experienced any falling? Do you have any clumsy movement?

R Dizziness or lightheadedness may be related to carotid artery disease, cerebellar abscess, Meniere's disease, or inner ear infection. Imbalance and difficulty coordinating or controlling movements are seen in neurologic diseases involving the cerebellum, basal ganglia, extrapyramidal tracts, or the vestibular part of cranial nerve VIII (acoustic). Diminished cerebral blood flow and vestibular response may increase the risk of falls.

Q Have you noticed a decrease in your ability to smell or to taste?

R A decrease in the ability to smell may be related to a dysfunction of cranial nerve I (olfactory) or a brain tumor. A decrease in the ability to taste may be related to dysfunction of cranial nerves VII (facial) or IX (glossopharyngeal).

Decreased taste and scent sensation occurs normally in older adults.

Q Have you experienced any ringing in your ears or hearing loss?

R Ringing in the ears and decreased ability to hear may occur with dysfunction of cranial nerve VIII (acoustic).

There is a normal decrease in the older person's ability to hear.

Q Have you noticed any change in your vision?

R Changes in vision may occur with dysfunction of cranial nerve II (optic), increased intracranial pressure, or brain tumors. Damage to cranial nerves III (oculomotor), IV (trochlear), or VI (abducens) may cause double or blurred vision. Transient blind spots may be an early sign of a cerebrovascular accident (CVA).

There is a normal decrease in the older person's ability to see.

Q Do you have difficulty understanding when people are talking to you? Do you have difficulty making others understand you?

R Injury to the cerebral cortex can impair the ability to use or understand verbal language.

Q Do you experience difficulty swallowing?

R Difficulty swallowing may relate to CVA, Parkinson's disease, myasthenia gravis, Guillain-Barré syndrome, or dysfunction of cranial nerves IX (glossopharyngeal), X (vagus), or XII (hypoglossal).

Q Have you lost bowel control or do you retain urine?

R Loss of bowel control or urinary retention and bladder distention are seen with spinal cord injury or tumors.

Q Do you have muscle weakness?

R Unilateral weakness or paralysis may result from CVA, compression of the spinal cord, or nerve injury. Progressive weakness is a symptom of several nervous system diseases.

Q Do you experience any memory loss?

R Recent memory (24-hour memory) is often impaired in amnestic disorders, Korsakoff's syndrome, delirium, and dementia. Remote memory (past dates and historical accounts) may be impaired in cerebral cortex disorders.

Q Do you experience any tremors?

R Tremors are typical in degenerative neurologic disorders, such as Parkinson's disease (three to six per second while muscles are at rest), or in cerebellar disease and multiple sclerosis (variable rate, and especially with intentional movement).

Older adults may experience tremors with movement. Tremors may involve the hands, head (yes or no nodding), and the tongue, which may protrude back and forth. Such tremors are not associated with disease, but they may cause embarrassment or emotional distress.

PAST HISTORY

Q Have you ever had any type of head injury with or without loss of consciousness (eg, sports injury, auto accident, fall)? If so, describe any physical or mental changes that have occurred as a result. What type of treatment did you receive?

R Head injuries, even if minor, can produce long-term neurologic deficits and affect level of functioning.

Q Have you ever had meningitis, encephalitis, injury to the spinal cord, or a stroke? If so, describe any physical or mental changes that have occurred as a result. What type of treatment did you receive?

R These disorders can affect the long-term physical and mental status of the client.

FAMILY HISTORY

Q Do you have a family history of high blood pressure, stroke, Alzheimer's disease, epilepsy, brain cancer, or Huntington's chorea?

R These disorders may be genetic. Some tend to run in families.

LIFESTYLE AND HEALTH PRACTICES

Q Do you take any prescription or nonprescription medications? How much alcohol do you drink? Do you use recreational drugs, such as marijuana, tranquilizers, barbiturates, or cocaine?

R Prescription and nonprescription drugs can cause various neurologic symptoms, such as tremors or dizziness, altered level of consciousness, decreased response times, and changes in mood and temperament.

Q Do you smoke?

R Nicotine, which is found in cigarettes constricts the blood vessels, which decreases blood flow to the brain. Cigarette smoking is a risk factor for CVA. See Risk Factors—Cerebrovascular Accident (Stroke).

Cerebrovascular Accident (Stroke)

OVERVIEW

Cerebrovascular accident (CVA), commonly called stroke, results when the blood supply to an area of the brain is disrupted. This blood supply disruption can be caused by thrombosis, embolism, infarction, or hemorrhage. All four of these may result from underlying cerebrovascular disease (Zuber & Mas, 1992).

Stroke is the leading neurologic problem in the United States and is ranked third overall in cause of death. African Americans have a higher incidence of stroke. They experience stroke at an earlier age, and they are twice as likely to die of stroke as whites or Hispanics (National Stroke Association, 2000; Overfield, 1995). Strokes can also cause serious disability. Approximately 4 million people live with some type of disability caused by a stroke; many of them require help with their activities of daily living (National Stroke Association, 2000).

RISK FACTORS

- Older adulthood—risk doubles each decade after age 55
- Male sex (slightly higher risk)
- History of stroke or transient ischemic attack (TIA)
- Hypertension
- Smoking
- Chronic alcohol intake (more than three drinks per day)
- History of cardiovascular disease, such as coronary artery disease, heart failure, rhythm abnormalities (especially atrial fibrillation), mitral valve prolapse
- Sleep apnea
- High serum levels of fibrinogen, beta-lipoproteins, cholesterol, hematocrit
- Diabetes mellitus
- Drug abuse (especially cocaine)
- Oral contraceptives (especially with coexisting hypertension, smoking, and high estrogen levels)
- High estrogen levels
- Postmenopausal woman not taking estrogen replacement
- Overweight
- African American
- Newly industrializing environment (National Stroke Association, 2000; Overfield, 1995)

RISK REDUCTION TEACHING TIPS

- Monitor blood pressure regularly; exercise regularly
- Stop smoking, especially if taking oral contraceptives
- Limit intake of alcohol to less than three drinks per day
- Schedule regular health care checkups
- Adhere to a diet low in fat and cholesterol; follow cardiovascular disease risk factor modifications
- Have regular blood tests to measure cholesterol, hematocrit levels
- Schedule regular health care checkups
- If diabetic, follow diabetes treatment plan
- Monitor blood sugar regularly, if diabetic
- Avoid use of drugs such as cocaine
- Have regular blood tests to measure estrogen levels
- Take estrogen replacement (postmenopausal women)

 CULTURAL CONSIDERATIONS

Twelve U.S. states and the District of Columbia have a 10% higher stroke rate than the other states. This "stroke belt" (Virginia, North Carolina, South Carolina, Georgia, Florida, Alabama, Mississippi, Louisiana, Arkansas, Tennessee, Kentucky, Indiana, and Washington, DC) may be due to a higher percentage of older adults, a higher percentage of African Americans, and dietary factors (National Stroke Association, 2000).

CVA is declining in many industrialized countries in recent decades. A 30% decrease was noted in France in all age groups of both sexes, except for women younger than 40 years of age (Zuber & Mas, 1992). In Japan, a 5% annual rate of decline has been noted, similar to U.S. white men. However, African Americans have a high rate of CVA, with the mortality rate among black men almost twice that of white men (Spector, 1996).

Q Do you wear your seat belt when riding in vehicles? Do you wear protective head gear when riding a bicycle or playing sports?

R Seat belts and protective head gear can prevent head injury.

Q Describe your usual daily diet.

R Peripheral neuropathy can result from a deficiency in niacin, folic acid, or vitamin B_{12}.

Q Have you ever had prolonged exposure to lead, insecticides, pollutants, or other chemicals?

R Prolonged exposure to these substances can alter neurologic status.

Q Do you frequently lift heavy objects or perform repetitive motions?

R Intervertebral disc injuries may result when heavy objects are lifted improperly. Peripheral nerve injuries can occur from repetitive movements.

Q Can you perform your normal activities of daily living?

R Neurologic symptoms and disorders often negatively affect the ability to perform activities of daily living.

Q Has your neurologic problem changed the way you view yourself? Describe.

R Low self-esteem and body image problems may lead to depression and changes in role functions.

Q Has your neurologic problem added much stress to your life? Describe.

R Neurologic problems can impair ability to fulfill role responsibilities, greatly increasing stress. Stress can increase existing neurologic symptoms.

Collecting Objective Data

A complete neurologic examination consists of evaluating the following five areas:

- Mental status
- Cranial nerves
- Motor and cerebellar systems
- Sensory system
- Reflexes

The examinations may be performed in an order that moves from a level of higher cerebral integration to a lower level of reflex activity.

Mental status examinations provide information about cerebral cortex function. Cerebral abnormalities disturb the client's intellectual ability, communication ability, or emotional behaviors. A mental status examination is often performed at the beginning of the head-to-toe examination because it provides clues regarding the validity of the subjective information provided by the client. For example, if the nurse finds that the client's thought processes are distorted and memory is impaired, another means of obtaining necessary subjective data must be identified.

The *cranial nerve evaluation* provides information regarding the transmission of motor and sensory messages, primarily to the head and neck. Many of the cranial nerves are evaluated during the head, neck, eye, and ear examinations.

The *motor and cerebellar systems* are assessed to determine functioning of the pyramidal and extrapyramidal tracts. The cerebellar system is assessed to determine the client's level of balance and coordination. The motor system examination is usually performed during the musculoskeletal examination.

Examining the *sensory system* provides information regarding the integrity of the spinothalamic tract, posterior columns of the spinal cord, and parietal lobes of the brain, whereas testing *reflexes* provides clues to the integrity of deep and superficial reflexes. Deep reflexes depend on an intact sensory nerve, a functional synapse in the spinal cord, an intact motor nerve, a neuromuscular junction, and competent muscles. Superficial reflexes depend on skin receptors rather than muscles.

If meningitis is suspected, the examiner may try to elicit Brudzinski's and Kernig's signs, which are characteristic of meningeal irritation. Sometimes, a complete neurologic examination is unnecessary. In such cases, the nurse performs a "neuro check"—a brief screening of the client's neurologic status. A neuro check includes the following assessment points:

- Level of consciousness
- Pupillary checks
- Movement and strength of extremities
- Sensation in extremities
- Vital signs

This type of assessment is useful in an emergency situation and when frequent assessments are needed during an acute phase of illness to detect rapid changes in neurologic status. A neuro check is also useful for a client who has already had a complete neurologic examination but needs to be rechecked for changes related to therapy or other conditions.

CLIENT PREPARATION

Prepare for the neurologic examination by asking the client to remove all clothing and jewelry and to put on an examination gown. Initially, have the client sit comfortably on the examination table or bed, but explain to him or her that several different position changes are necessary throughout the different parts of the examination. Assure the client that each position will be explained before the start of the particular examination.

Explain also that the examination will take a considerable amount of time to perform and that you will provide rest periods as needed. If the client is elderly or physically weak, the examination can be divided into parts and performed over two different time periods. Explain that actions the client will be asked to perform, such as counting backward or hopping on one foot, may seem unusual but that these activities are parts of a comprehensive neurologic evaluation.

 Tip From the Experts Demonstrate what you want the client to do—especially during the cerebellar examination, when the client will need to perform several different coordinated movements.

EQUIPMENT AND SUPPLIES

- *General:* Examination gloves
- *Mental status examination:* Annotated Mini-Mental State Examination (optional), pencil, and paper
- *Cranial nerve examination:* Cotton-tipped applicators; newsprint to read; ophthalmoscope; paper clip; penlight; Snellen chart; sterile cotton ball; substances to smell or taste; such as soap, coffee, vanilla, salt, sugar, lemon juice; tongue depressor; tuning fork
- *Motor and cerebellar examination:* Tape measure
- *Sensory examination:* Cotton ball; objects to feel, such as a quarter or key; paper clip; test tubes containing hot and cold water; tuning fork (low-pitched)
- *Reflex examination:* End of cotton-tipped applicator; reflex (percussion) hammer (Display 23-1)

DISPLAY 23-1. How to Use the Reflex Hammer

The reflex (or percussion) hammer is used to elicit deep tendon reflexes. Proceed as follows to elicit a deep tendon reflex:

GUIDELINES

1. Encourage the client to relax because tenseness can inhibit a normal response.
2. Position the client properly.
3. Hold the handle of the reflex hammer between your thumb and index finger so it swings freely.
4. Palpate the tendon that you will need to strike to elicit the reflex.
5. Using a rapid wrist movement, briskly strike the tendon. Observe the response. Avoid a slow or weak movement for striking.
6. Compare the response of one side with the other.
7. To prevent pain, use the pointed end to strike a small area, and the wider, blunt (flat) end to strike a wider area or a more tender area.
8. Use a reinforcement technique, which causes other muscles to contract and thus increases reflex activity, to assist in eliciting a response if no response can be elicited.
9. For arm reflexes, ask the client to clench his or her jaw or to squeeze one thigh with the opposite hand, then immediately strike the tendon. For leg reflexes, ask the client to lock the fingers of both hands and pull them against each other, then immediately strike the tendon.
10. Rate and document reflexes using the following scale and figure:
    - Grade 4+ Hyperactive, very brisk, rhythmic oscillations (clonus); abnormal and indicative of disorder
    - Grade 3+ More brisk or active than normal, but not indicative of a disorder
    - Grade 2+ Normal, usual response
    - Grade 1+ Decreased, less active than normal
    - Grade 0 No response

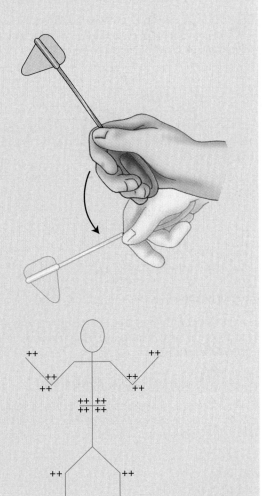

KEY ASSESSMENT POINTS

- Identify the structures and functions of the central and peripheral nervous systems.
- Understand what is meant by mental status and level of consciousness.
- Correctly apply and interpret mental status examinations and the Glasgow Coma Scale (GCS).
- Identify the 12 cranial nerves and their sensory and motor functions.
- Thoroughly assess movement, balance, coordination, sensation, and reflexes during physical examination.
- Coordinate patient education—particularly in regard to risks related to stroke—with the health interview and physical examination.

(*text continues on page 573*)

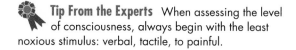

PHYSICAL ASSESSMENT

ASSESSMENT PROCEDURE	NORMAL FINDINGS	ABNORMAL FINDINGS

MENTAL STATUS AND LEVEL OF CONSCIOUSNESS

Observe Level of Consciousness

Call the client's name and noting the response. If the client does not respond, call the name louder. If necessary, shake the client gently. If the client still does not respond, apply a painful stimulus.

> **Tip From the Experts** When assessing the level of consciousness, always begin with the least noxious stimulus: verbal, tactile, to painful.

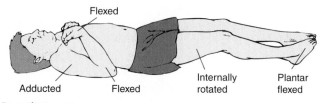

Decorticate posture.

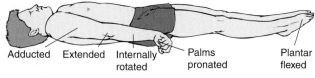

Decerebrate posture.

Use the Glasgow Coma Scale (GCS) for clients who are at high risk for rapid deterioration of the nervous system (Display 23-2).

Observe Posture and Body Movements

Be alert for tense, nervous, fidgety, and restless behavior, which may be seen in anxiety or may simply reflect the client's apprehension during a physical examination.

Client is alert and awake with eyes open and looking at examiner. Client responds appropriately.

GCS score of 14 indicates an optimal level of consciousness.

The client appears to be relaxed, with shoulders and back erect when standing or sitting.

The following levels of consciousness are abnormal:

Lethargy: Client opens eyes, answers questions, and falls back asleep.

Obtunded: Client opens eyes to loud voice, responds slowly with confusion, seems unaware of environment.

Stupor: Client awakens to vigorous shake or painful stimuli, but returns to unresponsive sleep.

Coma: Client remains unresponsive to all stimuli; eyes stay closed. Client with lesions of the corticospinal tract draws hands up to chest (*decorticate* or abnormal flexor posture) when stimulated.

Client with lesions of the diencephalon, midbrain, or pons extends arms and legs, arches neck and rotates hands and arms internally (*decerebrate* or abnormal extensor posture) when stimulated.

GCS score of less than 14 indicates some impairment in the level of consciousness. A score of 3, the lowest possible score, indicates deep coma.

Slumped posture may reflect feelings of powerlessness or hopelessness characteristic of depression or organic brain disease. Prolonged, euphoric laughing is typical of mania. Bizarre body movements and behavior may be noted in schizophrenia or may be a side effect of drug therapy or other activity.

(continued)

ASSESSMENT PROCEDURE	NORMAL FINDINGS	ABNORMAL FINDINGS
Observe Dress, Grooming, and Hygiene		
Keep the examination setting and the reason for the assessment in mind as you note the client's degree of cleanliness and attire. For example, if the client arrives directly from home, he or she may be neater than if he or she comes to the assessment from the workplace.	Skin clean, nails neat and trim, facial hairs shaven or trimmed. Clothes fit and are appropriate for the occasion and weather.	Unusually meticulous grooming and finicky mannerisms may be seen in obsessive-compulsive disorder. Poor hygiene and inappropriate dress may be seen in depression, schizophrenia, dementia, and Alzheimer's disease. One-sided neglect may result from lesion in the opposite parietal cortex, usually the nondominant side.
Observe Facial Expressions		
Note particularly eye contact and affect.	Good eye contact, smiles and frowns appropriately.	Poor eye contact is seen in depression or apathy. Extreme facial expressions of happiness, anger, or fright may be seen in anxious clients. Clients with Parkinson's disease may have a masklike, expressionless face.
Observe Speech		
Observe and listen to tone, clarity, and pace of speech.	Moderate tone; clear with moderate pace.	Slow, repetitive speech is characteristic of depression or Parkinson's disease. Loud, rapid speech may occur in manic phases of bipolar disorder (Table 23-3).
If the client has difficulty with speech, perform additional tests: • Ask the client to name objects in the room. • Ask the client to read from printed material appropriate for his or her educational level. • Ask the client to write a sentence.	Names familiar objects without difficulty. Reads age-appropriate written print. Writes a coherent sentence with correct spelling and grammar.	Client cannot name objects correctly, read print correctly, or write a basic correct sentence. Deficits in this area require further neurologic assessment to identify any dysfunction of higher cortical levels.

Tip From the Experts Speech is largely influenced by experience, level of education, and culture.

Observe Mood, Feelings, and Expressions		
Ask client "How are you feeling today?" and "What are your plans for the future?"	Cooperative or friendly, expresses feelings appropriate to situation, verbalizes positive feelings regarding others and the future, expresses positive coping mechanisms (support groups, exercise, sports, hobbies, counseling).	Expression of prolonged negative, gloomy, despairing feelings is noted in depression. Expression of elation and grandiosity, high energy level, and engagement in high-risk but pleasurable activities is seen in manic phases. Excessive worry may be seen in anxiety or obsessive-compulsive disorders. Eccentric moods not appropriate to the situation are seen in schizophrenia.

Tip From the Experts Moods and feelings often vary from sadness to joy to anger, depending on the situation and circumstance.

(continued)

ASSESSMENT PROCEDURE	NORMAL FINDINGS	ABNORMAL FINDINGS

Observe Thought Processes and Perceptions

Observe thought processes for clarity, content, and perception by inquiring about client's thoughts and perceptions expressed. Use statements such as, "Tell me more about what you just said," or "Tell me what your understanding is of the current situation or your health."

Expresses full, free-flowing thoughts; follows directions accurately; expresses realistic perceptions; is easy to understand and makes sense; does not voice suicidal thoughts.

Abnormal processes include persistent repetition of ideas, illogical thoughts, interruption of ideas, invention of words, or repetition of phrases as in schizophrenia; rapid flight of ideas, repetition of ideas, and use of rhymes and punning as in manic phases of bipolar disorder; continuous, irrational fears, and avoidance of an object or situation as in phobias; delusion, extreme apprehension; compulsions; obsessions; and illusions are also abnormal (see the glossary for definitions).

Tip From the Experts When assessing the mental status of an older client, be sure first to check vision and hearing before assuming the client has a mental problem.

Identify possibly destructive or suicidal tendencies in client's thought processes and perceptions by asking, "How do you feel about the future?" or "Have you ever had thoughts of hurting yourself or doing away with yourself?" or "How do others feel about you?"

Verbalizes positive, healthy thoughts about the future and self.

Clients who are suicidal may share past attempts of suicide, give plan for suicide, verbalize worthlessness about self, joke about death frequently. Clients who are depressed or feel hopeless are at higher risk for suicide.

Use the Yesevage Geriatric Depression Scale if depression is suspected in the older client (Display 23-3). Read the questions to the client if the client cannot read.

Scores 10 or less.

Scores between 10 and 30 may indicate depression.

Observe Cognitive Abilities

Orientation

Ask the client name and names of family members (person), the time, such as hour, day, date, or season (time), and where the client lives or is now (place).

Client is aware of self, others, time, home address, and current location.

Reduced degree of orientation may be seen with organic brain disorders or psychiatric illness such as withdrawal from chronic alcohol use or schizophrenia. (*Note:* Schizophrenia may be marked by hallucinations—sensory perceptions that occur without external stimuli—as well as disorientation.)

Tip From the Experts When assessing orientation to time, place, and person, remember that orientation to time is usually lost first and orientation to person is usually lost last.

Some older clients may seem confused, especially in a new or acute care setting, but most know who and where they are and the current month and year.

Concentration

Note the client's ability to focus and stay attentive to you during the interview and examination. Give the client directions such as, "Please pick up the pencil with your left hand, place it in your right hand, then hand it to me."

Listens and can follow directions without difficulty.

Distraction and inability to focus on task at hand are noted in anxiety, fatigue, attention deficit disorders, and impaired states due to alcohol or drug intoxication.

Some older clients may like to reminisce and tend to wander somewhat from the topic at hand.

Recent Memory

Ask the client "What did you have to eat today?" or "What is the weather like today?"

Recalls recent events without difficulty.

Inability to recall recent events is seen in delirium, dementia, depression, and anxiety.

Some older clients may exhibit hesitation with short-term memory.

(continued)

ASSESSMENT PROCEDURE	NORMAL FINDINGS	ABNORMAL FINDINGS

Remote Memory

Ask the client: "When did you get your first job?" or "When is your birthday?" Information on past health history also gives clues as to the client's ability to recall remote events.

Normal: Correctly recalls past events.

Abnormal: Inability to recall past events is seen in cerebral cortex disorders.

Use of Memory to Learn New Information

Ask the client to repeat four unrelated words. The words should not rhyme and they cannot have the same meaning (eg, rose, hammer, automobile, brown). Have the client repeat these words in 5 minutes, again in 10 minutes, and again in 30 minutes.

Normal: Able to recall words correctly after a 5-, 10-, and 30-minute period.

Clients older than 80 should recall two to four words after 5 minutes and possibly after 10 and 30 minutes with hints that prompt recall.

Abnormal: Inability to recall words after a delayed period is seen in anxiety, depression, or Alzheimer's disease.

Abstract Reasoning

Ask the client to compare objects. For example, "How are an apple and orange the same? How are they different?" Also ask the client to explain a proverb. For example, "A rolling stone gathers no moss" or "A stitch in time saves nine."

Normal: Explains similarities and differences between objects and proverbs correctly. The client with limited education can joke and use puns correctly.

Abnormal: Inability to compare and contrast objects correctly or interpret proverbs correctly is seen in schizophrenia, mental retardation, delirium, and dementia.

> **Tip From the Experts** If clients have limited education, note their ability to joke or use puns, which also requires abstract reasoning.

Judgment

Ask the client, "What do you do if you have pain?" or "What would you do if you were driving and a police car was behind you with its lights and siren turned on?"

Normal: Answers to questions are based on sound rationale.

Abnormal: Impaired judgment may be seen in organic brain syndrome, emotional disturbances, mental retardation, or schizophrenia.

Visual Perceptual and Constructional Ability

Ask the client to draw the face of a clock or copy simple figures.

Normal: Draws the face of a clock fairly well. Can copy simple figures.

Abnormal: Inability to draw the face of a clock or copy simple figures correctly is seen with mental retardation, dementia, or parietal lobe dysfunction of the cerebral cortex.

Figures to be drawn by client.

Mini-Mental State Examination

Perform the Mini-Mental State Examination if time is limited and a quick standard measure is needed to evaluate or reevaluate cognitive function (Display 23-4).

Normal: Scores between 24 and 30.

Abnormal: Scores lower than 21 may be seen in organic brain disease (delirium or dementia) or affective disorders. Scores of 21 to 24 are questionable with regard to disease and require further evaluation.

Caution: Note that potential harm from labeling or identifying clients with possible dementia must be weighed against benefits of assessment (Patterson, 2000).

> **Tip From the Experts** This examination tests level of orientation, memory, speech, and cognitive functions, but not mood, feelings, expressions, thought processes, or perceptions.

(continued)

ASSESSMENT PROCEDURE	NORMAL FINDINGS	ABNORMAL FINDINGS

CRANIAL NERVES

Cranial Nerve I—Olfactory

For all assessments of the cranial nerves, have client sit in a comfortable position at your eye level. Ask the client to clear the nose to remove any mucus then to close eyes, occlude one nostril, and identify a scented object that you are holding, such as soap, coffee, or vanilla. Repeat procedure for the other nostril.

Correctly identifies scent presented to each nostril.

Some older clients' sense of smell may be decreased.

Inability to identify the correct scent may indicate olfactory tract lesion or tumor or lesion of the frontal lobe. Loss of smell may also be congenital or due to other causes such as nasal disease, smoking, and use of cocaine.

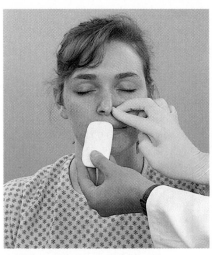

Testing cranial nerve I. (© B.Proud.)

Cranial Nerve II—Optic

Use a Snellen chart to assess vision in each eye (see Chapter 11, for additional information)
.

20/20 vision OD (right eye) and OS (left eye).

Difficulty reading Snellen chart; misses letters, squints.

Ask the client to read a newspaper or magazine paragraph to assess near vision.

Reads print at 14 inches without difficulty.

Reads print by holding closer than 14 inches or holds print farther away as in presbyopia, which occurs with aging.

Assess visual fields of each eye by confrontation.

Full visual fields (see Chapter 11).

Loss of visual fields may be seen in retinal damage or detachment, with lesions of the optic nerve, or with lesions of the parietal cortex (see Chapter 11).

Use an ophthalmoscope to view the retina and optic disc of each eye.

Round red reflex present, optic disc 1.5 mm, round or slightly oval, well-defined margins, creamy pink with paler physiologic cup. Retina pink (see Chapter 11).

Papilledema (swelling of the optic nerve) results in blurred optic disc margins and dilated, pulsating veins. Papilledema occurs with increased intracranial pressure from intracranial hemorrhage or a brain tumor. Optic atrophy occurs with brain tumors (see Chapter 11).

(continued)

ASSESSMENT PROCEDURE	NORMAL FINDINGS	ABNORMAL FINDINGS

Cranial Nerves III—Oculomotor, IV—Trochlear, and VI—Abducens

Inspect margins of the eyelids of each eye.	Eyelid covers about 2 mm of the iris.	Ptosis (drooping of the eyelid) is seen with weak eye muscles, such as in myasthenia gravis.
Assess extraocular movements. If nystagmus is noted, determine the direction of the fast and slow phases of movement (see Chapter 11).	Eyes move in a smooth, coordinated motion in all directions (the six cardinal fields).	Some abnormal eye movements and possible causes follow: Nystagmus: rhythmic oscillation of the eyes), *cerebellar disorders*. Limited eye movement through the six cardinal fields of gaze, *increased intracranial pressure*. Paralytic strabismus, *paralysis of the oculomotor, trochlear, or abducens nerves* (see Chapter 11).
Assess pupillary response to light (direct and indirect) and accommodation in both eyes (see Chapter 11).	Bilateral illuminated pupils constrict simultaneously. Pupil opposite the one illuminated constricts simultaneously.	Unequal pupils may be a normal variation or they may occur with disorders of the CNS. Some abnormalities and their implications follow: Dilated pupil (6–7 mm), *oculomotor nerve paralysis*. Argyll Robertson pupils, *CNS syphilis, meningitis, brain tumor, alcoholism*. Constricted, fixed pupils, *narcotics abuse or damage to the pons*. Unilaterally dilated pupil unresponsive to light or accommodation, *damage to cranial nerve III (oculomotor)*. Constricted pupil unresponsive to light or accommodation, *lesions of the sympathetic nervous system* (see Chapter 11).

Cranial Nerve V—Trigeminal

Motor Function

Ask the client to clench the teeth while you palpate the temporal and masseter muscles for contraction.	Temporal and masseter muscles contract bilaterally.	Bilateral muscle weakness is seen with peripheral or central nervous system dysfunction. Unilateral weakness may indicate a lesion of cranial nerve V (trigeminal).

Tip From the Experts This test may be difficult to perform and evaluate in the client without teeth.

(continued)

ASSESSMENT PROCEDURE	NORMAL FINDINGS	ABNORMAL FINDINGS

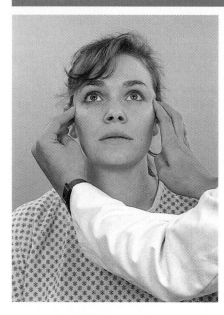

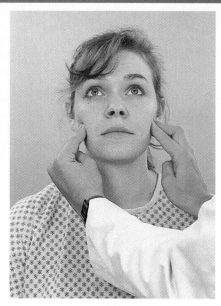

Testing motor function of cranial nerve V: (*left*) palpating temporal muscles; (*right*) palpating masseter muscles. (© B.Proud.)

Sensory Function

Tell the client: "I am going to touch your forehead, cheeks, and chin with the sharp or dull side of this safety pin or paper clip (a paper clip is less hazardous). Please close your eyes and tell me if you feel a sharp or dull sensation. Also tell me where you feel it." Vary the sharp and dull stimulus in the facial areas and compare sides. Repeat test for light touch with a wisp of cotton.

The client correctly identifies sharp and dull stimuli and light touch to the forehead, cheeks, and chin.

Inability to feel and correctly identify facial stimuli occurs with lesions of the trigeminal nerve or lesions in the spinothalamic tract or posterior columns.

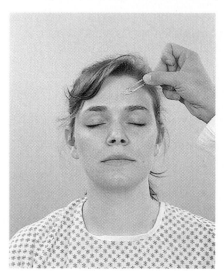

Testing sensory function of cranial nerve V: dull stimulus using a paper clip. (© B.Proud.)

🎗 **Tip From the Experts** To avoid transmitting infection, use a new object with each client. Avoid "stabbing" the client with the object's sharp side.

(continued)

ASSESSMENT PROCEDURE	NORMAL FINDINGS	ABNORMAL FINDINGS

Corneal Reflex

Ask the client to look away and up while you lightly touch the cornea with a fine wisp of cotton. Repeat on the other side.

Eyelids blink bilaterally.

An absent corneal reflex may be noted with lesions of the trigeminal nerve or lesions of the motor part of cranial nerve VII (facial).

Tip From the Experts
This reflex may be absent or reduced in clients who wear contact lenses.

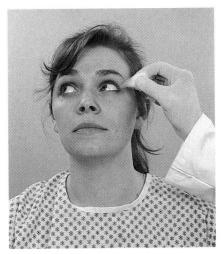

Testing corneal reflex. (© B.Proud.)

Cranial Nerve VII—Facial

Motor Function

Ask the client to:
- Smile
- Frown and wrinkle forehead
- Show teeth
- Puff out cheeks
- Purse lips
- Raise eyebrows
- Close eyes tightly against resistance

Smiles, frowns, wrinkles forehead, shows teeth, puffs out cheeks, purses lips, raises eyebrows, and closes eyes against resistance.

Inability to close eyes, wrinkle forehead, or raise forehead along with paralysis of the lower part of the face on the affected side is seen with Bell's palsy (a peripheral injury to cranial nerve VII [facial]). Paralysis of the lower part of the face on the opposite side affected may be seen with a central lesion that affects the upper motor neurons, such as from CVA.

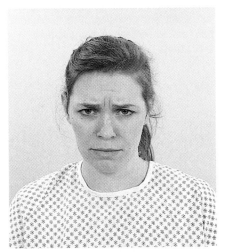 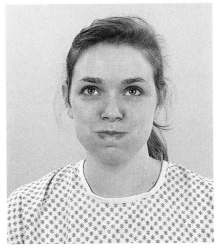

Testing cranial nerve VII: (*left*) frowning and wrinkling forehead; (*right*) puffing out cheeks. © B.Proud.)

(continued)

ASSESSMENT PROCEDURE	NORMAL FINDINGS	ABNORMAL FINDINGS

Sensory Function

Sensory function is not routinely tested. If it is, however, touch the anterior two thirds of the tongue with a moistened applicator dipped in salt, sugar, or lemon juice and ask the client to identify the flavor. If the client is unsuccessful, repeat the test using one of the other solutions. If needed, repeat the test using the remaining solution.

Identifies correct flavor.

In some older clients. the sense of taste may be decreased.

Inability to identify correct flavor on anterior two thirds of the tongue suggests impairment of cranial nerve VII (facial).

> **Tip From the Experts** Make sure the client leaves the tongue protruded to identify the flavor. Otherwise, the substance may move to the posterior third of the tongue (vagus nerve innervation). The posterior portion is tested similarly to evaluate functioning of cranial nerves IX and X. The client should rinse the mouth with water between each taste test.

Cranial Nerve VIII—Acoustic (Vestibulocochlear)

Test the client's hearing ability in each ear and perform the Weber and Rinne tests to assess the cochlear (auditory) component of cranial nerve VIII (see Chapter 12, Ear Assessment, for detailed procedures).

Note: The vestibular component, responsible for equilibrium, is not routinely tested. In comatose clients, the test is used to determine integrity of the vestibular system. (See a neurology textbook for detailed testing procedures.)

Hears whispered words from 1 to 2 feet. *Weber test*: Vibration heard equally well in both ears. *Rinne test*: AC > BC (air conduction is twice as long as bone conduction).

Vibratory sound lateralizes to good ear in sensorineural loss. Air conduction is longer than bone conduction, but not twice as long, in a sensorineural loss (see Chapter 12).

Cranial Nerves IX—Glossopharyngeal and X—Vagus (Test These Nerves Together)

Motor Function

Ask the client to open mouth wide and say "ah" while you use a tongue depressor on the client's tongue.

Uvula and soft palate rise bilaterally and symmetrically on phonation.

Soft palate does not rise with bilateral lesions of cranial nerve X (vagus). Unilateral rising of the soft palate and deviation of the uvula to the normal side are seen with a unilateral lesion of cranial nerve X (vagus).

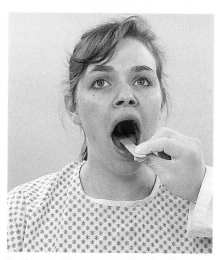

Testing cranial nerves IX and X: checking uvula rise and gag reflex. (© B.Proud.)

(continued)

ASSESSMENT PROCEDURE	NORMAL FINDINGS	ABNORMAL FINDINGS
Test the gag reflex by touching the posterior pharynx with the tongue depressor. Warn the client that you are going to do this and that the test may feel a little uncomfortable.	Gag reflex intact. Some normal clients may have a reduced or absent gag reflex.	An absent gag reflex may be seen with lesions of cranial nerve IX (glossopharyngeal) or X (vagus).
Check the client's ability to swallow by giving the client a drink of water. Also, note the client's voice quality.	Swallows without difficulty. No hoarseness noted.	Dysphagia or hoarseness may indicate a lesion of cranial nerve IX (glossopharyngeal) or X (vagus) or other neurologic disorder.

Cranial Nerve XI—Spinal Accessory

Ask the client to shrug the shoulders against resistance to assess the trapezius muscle.	Symmetric, strong contraction of the trapezius muscles.	Asymmetric muscle contraction or drooping of the shoulder may be seen with paralysis or muscle weakness due to neck injury or torticollis.

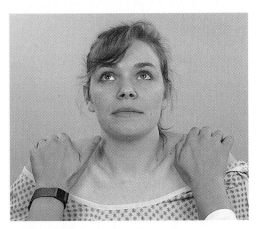

Testing cranial nerve XI: assessing strength of trapezius muscle. (© B.Proud.)

Ask the client to turn the head against resistance, first to the right and then to the left, to assess the sternocleidomastoid muscle.	Strong contraction of sternocleidomastoid muscle on side opposite the turned face.	Atrophy with fasciculations may be seen with peripheral nerve disease.

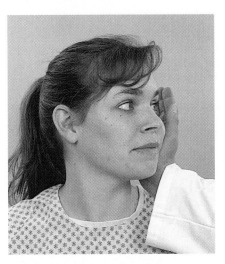

Testing cranial nerve XI: assessing strength of sternocleidomastoid muscle. (© B.Proud.)

Cranial Nerve XII—Hypoglossal

To assess strength and mobility of the tongue, ask the client to protrude tongue, move it to each side against the resistance of a tongue depressor, then put it back in the mouth.	Tongue movement is symmetric and smooth and bilateral strength is apparent.	Fasciculations and atrophy of the tongue may be seen with peripheral nerve disease. Deviation to the affected side is seen with a unilateral lesion.

(continued)

ASSESSMENT PROCEDURE	NORMAL FINDINGS	ABNORMAL FINDINGS

MOTOR AND CEREBELLAR SYSTEMS

Condition and Movement of Muscles

Assess the size and symmetry of all muscle groups (see Chapter 22, Musculoskeletal Assessment, for detailed procedures). Some older clients may have reduced muscle mass from degeneration of muscle fibers.	Muscles fully developed and symmetric in size (bilateral sides may vary 1 cm from each other).	Muscle atrophy may be seen in diseases of the lower motor neurons or muscle disorders (see Chapter 22).
Assess the strength and tone of all muscle groups (see Chapter 22).	Relaxed muscles contract voluntarily and show mild, smooth resistance to passive movement. All muscle groups equally strong against resistance, without flaccidity, spasticity, or rigidity.	Soft, limp, flaccid muscles are seen with lower motor neuron involvement. Spastic muscle tone is noted with involvement of the corticospinal motor tract. Rigid muscles that resist passive movement are seen with abnormalities of the extrapyramidal tract.
Note any unusual involuntary movements such as fasciculations, tics, or tremors.	No fasciculations, tics, or tremors noted. Some older clients may normally have hand or head tremors or dyskinesia (repetitive movements of the lips, jaw, or tongue).	Abnormal findings include • Tic (twitch of the face, head, or shoulder) from stress or neurologic disorder • Unusual, bizarre face, tongue, jaw, or lip movements from chronic psychosis or long-term use of psychotropic drugs • Tremors (rhythmic, oscillating movements) from Parkinson's disease, cerebellar disease, multiple sclerosis (with movement), hyperthyroidism, or anxiety • Slow, twisting movements in the extremities and face from cerebral palsy • Brief, rapid, irregular, jerky movements (at rest) from Huntington's chorea

Balance

To assess gait, ask the client to walk naturally across the room. Note posture, freedom of movement, symmetry, rhythm, and balance. **Tip From the Experts** It is best to assess gait when the client is not aware that you are directly observing his or her gait.	Gait is steady; opposite arm swings. Some older clients may have a slow and uncertain gait. The base may become wider and shorter and the hips and knees may be flexed for a bent-forward appearance.	Gait and balance can be affected by disorders of the motor, sensory, vestibular, and cerebellar systems. Therefore, a thorough examination of all systems is necessary when an uneven or unsteady gait is noted (see Display 23-5 for more information about abnormal gaits).
Ask the client to walk first in heel-to-toe fashion (tandem walking), next on the heels, and then on the toes. Demonstrate the walk first; then stand close by in case the client loses balance.	Maintains balance with tandem walking. Walks on heels and toes with little difficulty. For some older clients, this examination may be very difficult.	An uncoordinated or unsteady gait that did not appear with the client's normal walking may become apparent with tandem walking or when walking on heels and toes.

(continued)

ASSESSMENT PROCEDURE	NORMAL FINDINGS	ABNORMAL FINDINGS

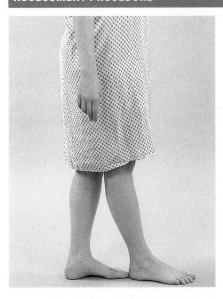

Testing balance: tandem walking. (© B.Proud.)

Perform the Romberg test. Ask the client to stand erect with arms at side and feet together. Note any unsteadiness or swaying. Then, with the client in the same body position, ask the client to close the eyes for 20 seconds. Again, note any imbalance or swaying.

Stands erect with minimal swaying, with eyes both open and closed.

Swaying and moving feet apart to prevent fall is seen with disease of the posterior columns, vestibular dysfunction, or cerebellar disorders.

 Tip From the Experts Stand near the client to prevent a fall should one happen.

Now, ask the client to stand on one foot and to bend the knee of the leg he or she is standing on. Then, ask the client to hop on that foot. Repeat on the other foot.

Bends knee while standing on one foot; hops on each foot without losing balance.

Inability to stand or hop on one foot is seen with muscle weakness or disease of the cerebellum.

This test is often impossible for the older adult to perform because of decreased flexibility and strength. Moreover, it is not usual to perform this test with the older adult because it puts the client at risk.

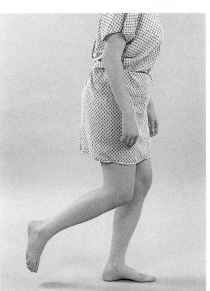

Tandem balance: standing and hopping on one foot. (© B.Proud.)

(continued)

ASSESSMENT PROCEDURE	NORMAL FINDINGS	ABNORMAL FINDINGS

Coordination

Demonstrate the finger-to-nose test to assess accuracy of movements and then ask the client to extend and hold arms out to the side with eyes open. Next, say "Touch the tip of your nose first with your right index finger, then with your left index finger. Repeat this three times." Next, ask the client to repeat these movements with eyes closed.

Touches finger to nose with smooth, accurate movements, with little hesitation.

Loss of positional sense and inability to touch tip of nose are seen with cerebellar disease.

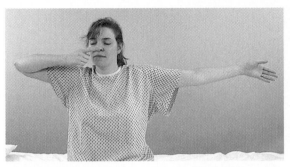

Testing coordination: finger-to-nose test. (© B.Proud.)

> **Tip From the Experts** When assessing coordination of movements, bear in mind that normally the client's dominant side may be more coordinated than the nondominant side.

Next, assess rapid alternating movements. First, ask the client to touch each finger to the thumb and to increase the speed as the client progresses. Repeat with the other side.

Touches each finger to thumb rapidly.

For some older clients, rapid alternating movements are difficult because of decreased reaction time and flexibility.

Inability to perform rapid alternating movements may be seen with cerebellar disease, upper motor neuron weakness, or extrapyramidal disease.

Next, ask the client to put the palms of both hands down on both legs, then turn the palms up, then turn the palms down again. Ask the client to increase the speed.

Rapidly turns palms up and down.

Uncoordinated movements or tremors are abnormal findings. They are seen with cerebellar disease.

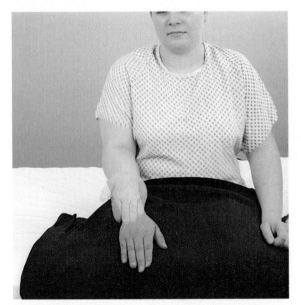

Testing rapid alternating movements: palms. (© B.Proud.)

(continued)

ASSESSMENT PROCEDURE	NORMAL FINDINGS	ABNORMAL FINDINGS
Perform the heel-to-shin test. Ask the client to lie down and to slide the heel of the right foot down the left shin. Repeat with the other heel and shin.	Able to run each heel smoothly down each shin.	Deviation of heel to one side or the other may be seen in cerebellar disease.

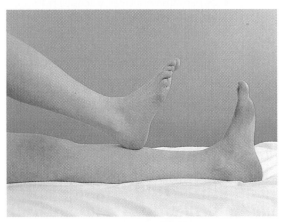

Performing heel-to-shin test. (© B.Proud.)

SENSORY SYSTEM

Light Touch, Pain, and Temperature Sensations

Scatter stimuli over the distal and proximal parts of all extremities and the trunk to cover most of the dermatomes. It is not necessary to cover the entire body surface, unless you identify abnormal symptoms such as pain, numbness, or tingling.

To test light touch sensation, use a wisp of cotton to touch the client.

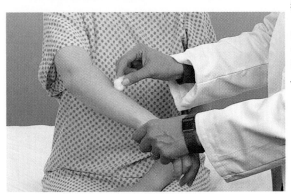

Testing light touch sensation. (© B.Proud.)

Correctly identifies light touch.

In some older clients, light touch and pain sensations may be decreased.

Tip From the Experts
For each test, ask clients to close both eyes and tell you what they feel and where they feel it.

Many disorders can alter a person's ability correctly to perceive sensations. These include peripheral neuropathies (due to diabetes mellitus, folic acid deficiencies, and alcoholism) and lesions of the ascending spinal cord, the brain stem, cranial nerves, and cerebral cortex.

(continued)

ASSESSMENT PROCEDURE	NORMAL FINDINGS	ABNORMAL FINDINGS
To test pain sensation, use the blunt and sharp ends of a safety pin or paper clip. To test temperature sensation, use test tubes filled with hot and cold water	Correctly differentiates between dull and sharp sensations and hot and cold temperatures over various body parts.	Client reports • Anesthesia (absence of touch sensation) • Hypesthesia (decreased sensitivity to touch) • Hyperesthesia (increased sensitivity to touch) • Analgesia (absence of pain sensation) • Hypalgesia (decreased sensitivity to pain) • Hyperalgesia (increased sensitivity to pain)

Tip From the Experts Test temperature sensation only if abnormalities are found in the client's ability to perceive light touch and pain sensations. Temperature and pain sensations travel in the lateral spinothalamic tract, so temperature need not be tested if pain sensation is intact.

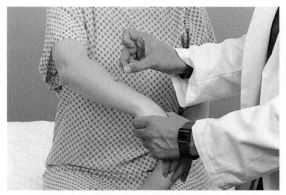
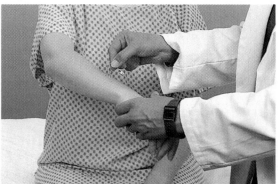

Testing pain sensation: (*left*) dull stimulus and (*right*) sharp stimulus. (© B.Proud.)

Vibratory Sensation

Strike a low-pitched tuning fork on the heel of your hand and hold the base on a bony surface of the fingers or big toe. Ask the client to indicate what he or she feels. Repeat on the other side.

Correctly identifies sensation.

Vibratory sensation at the ankles usually decreases after age 70.

Inability to sense vibrations may be seen in posterior column disease or peripheral neuropathy (eg, as seen with diabetes or chronic alcohol abuse).

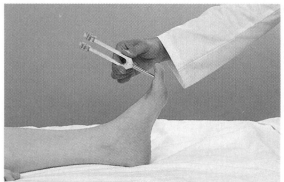

Testing vibratory sensation. (© B.Proud.)

Tip From the Experts If vibratory sensation is intact distally, then it is intact proximally

(continued)

ASSESSMENT PROCEDURE	NORMAL FINDINGS	ABNORMAL FINDINGS

Sensitivity to Position

Ask the client to close both eyes. Then, move the client's toes or a finger up or down. Ask the client to tell you the direction it is moved. Repeat on the other side.

 Tip From the Experts If position sense is intact distally, then it is intact proximally.

Correctly identifies directions of movements.

In some older clients, the sense of position of great toe may be reduced.

Inability to identify the directions of the movements may be seen in posterior column disease or peripheral neuropathy (eg, as seen with diabetes or chronic alcohol abuse).

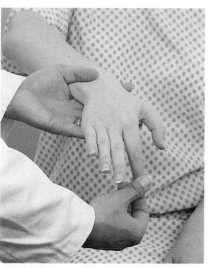

Testing position sense. (© B.Proud.)

Tactile Discrimination (Fine Touch) (or all of these tests, ask the client to close both eyes.)

To test stereognosis, place a familiar object such as a quarter, paperclip, or key in the client's hand and ask the client to identify it. Repeat with another object in the other hand.

Correctly identifies object.

Inability to correctly identify objects, area touched, number written in hand, discriminate between two points, or identify areas simultaneously touched may be seen in lesions of the sensory cortex.

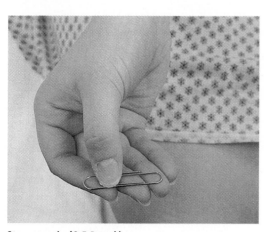

Stereognosis. (© B.Proud.)

(continued)

ASSESSMENT PROCEDURE	NORMAL FINDINGS	ABNORMAL FINDINGS
To test point localization, briefly touch the client and ask the client to identify the points touched.	Correctly identifies area touched.	Same as above.
To test graphesthesia, use a blunt instrument to write a number, such as 2, 3 or 5, on the palm of the client's hand. Ask the client to identify the number. Repeat with another number on the other hand.	Correctly identifies number written.	Same as above.

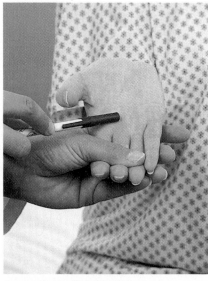

Graphesthesia. (© B.Proud.)

To test two-point discrimination, ask the client to identify the number of points felt when touched with the ends of two applicators at the same time. Touch the client on the fingertips, forearm, dorsal hands, back, and thighs. Note the distance between the applicators.	Identifies two points on: • Fingertips at 2 to 5 mm apart • Forearm at 40 mm apart • Dorsal hands at 20 to 30 mm apart • Back at 40 mm apart • Thighs at 70 mm apart	Same as above.

Two-point discrimination. (© B.Proud.)

To test extinction, simultaneously touch the client in the same area on both sides of the body at the same point. Ask the client to identify the area touched.	Correctly identifies points touched.	Same as above.

(continued)

ASSESSMENT PROCEDURE	NORMAL FINDINGS	ABNORMAL FINDINGS

REFLEXES

Deep Tendon Reflexes

Position client in a comfortable sitting position. Use the reflex hammer to elicit reflexes (see Display 23-1).

✿ Tip From the Experts If deep tendon reflexes are diminished or absent, two reinforcement techniques may be used to enhance their response. When testing the arm reflexes, have the client clench his or her teeth. When testing the leg reflexes, have the client interlock his or her hands. Reinforcement techniques may also help the older client who has difficulty relaxing.

Normal reflex scores range from 1+ (present but decreased) to 2+ (normal) to 3+ (increased or brisk, but not pathologic).

Absent or markedly decreased (hyporeflexia) deep tendon reflexes (rated 0) occur when a component of the lower motor neurons or reflex arc is impaired, and may be seen with spinal cord injuries. Markedly hyperactive (hyperreflexia) deep tendon reflexes (rated 4+) may be seen with lesions of the upper motor neurons and when the higher cortical levels are impaired.

👓 Some older clients may have decreased deep tendon reflexes because of a numeric decrease in nerve axons and increased demyelination of nerve axons. Impulse transmission also may decrease along with a delay in reaction time.

Biceps Reflex

Ask the client partially to bend arm at elbow with palm up. Place your thumb over the biceps tendon and strike your thumb with the reflex hammer. Repeat on the other side. (Evaluates the function of spinal levels C5 and C6.)

Elbow flexes, contraction of the biceps muscle is seen or felt. Ranges from 1+ to 3+.

No response or an exaggerated response is abnormal.

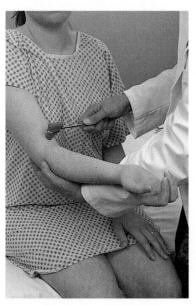

Eliciting biceps reflex. (© B.Proud.)

(continued)

ASSESSMENT PROCEDURE	NORMAL FINDINGS	ABNORMAL FINDINGS

Brachioradialis Reflex

Ask the client to flex elbow with palm down and hand resting on the abdomen or lap. Tap the tendon at the radius about 2 inches above the wrist. Repeat on other side. (Evaluates the function of spinal levels C5 and C6.)

Forearm flexes and supinates. Ranges from 1+ to 3+.

No response or an exaggerated response is abnormal.

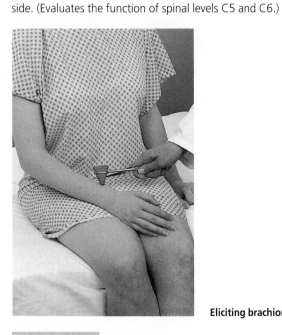

Eliciting brachioradialis reflex. (© B.Proud.)

Triceps Reflex

Ask the client to hang his or her arm freely ("limp like it is hanging from a clothesline to dry") while you support it with your nondominant hand. With the elbow flexed, tap the tendon above the olecranon process. Repeat on the other side. (Evaluates the function of spinal levels C6, C7, and C8.)

Elbow extends, triceps contracts. Ranges from 1+ to 3+.

No response or exaggerated response.

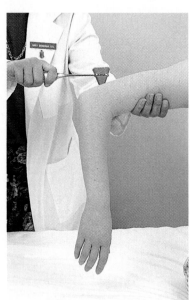

Eliciting triceps reflex. (© B.Proud.)

(continued)

ASSESSMENT PROCEDURE	NORMAL FINDINGS	ABNORMAL FINDINGS

Patellar Reflex

Ask the client to let both legs hang freely off the side of the examination table. Tap the patellar tendon, which is located just below the patella. Repeat on the other side. See the accompanying figure for the client who cannot sit up. (Evaluates the function of spinal levels L2, L3, and L4.)

Knee extends, quadriceps muscle contracts. Ranges from 1+ to 3+.

No response or an exaggerated response is abnormal.

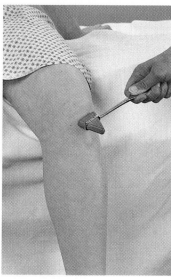

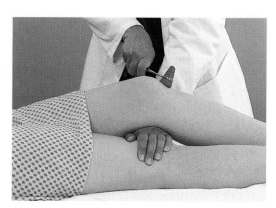

Eliciting patellar reflex. (© B.Proud.)   **Eliciting patellar reflex (supine position). (© B.Proud.)**

Achilles Reflex

With the client's leg still hanging freely, dorsiflex the foot. Tap the Achilles tendon with the reflex hammer. Repeat on the other side. See the accompanying figure for assessing the reflex in the client who cannot sit up. (Evaluates the function of spinal levels S1 and S2).

Plantar flexion of the foot. Ranges from 1+ to 3+.

In some older clients, the Achilles reflex may be absent or difficult to elicit.

No response or an exaggerated response is abnormal.

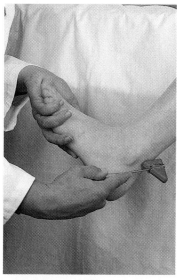

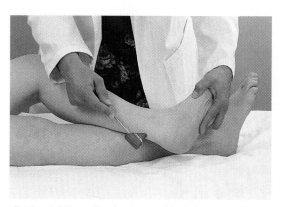

Eliciting Achilles reflex. (© B.Proud.)   **Eliciting Achilles reflex (supine position). (© B.Proud.)**

(continued)

ASSESSMENT PROCEDURE	NORMAL FINDINGS	ABNORMAL FINDINGS

Ankle Clonus

Test when the other reflexes tested have been hyperactive. Place one hand under the knee to support the leg, then briskly dorsiflex the foot toward the client's head. Repeat on the other side.

No rapid contractions or oscillations (clonus) of the ankle.

Repeated rapid contractions or oscillations of the ankle are seen with lesions of the upper motor neurons.

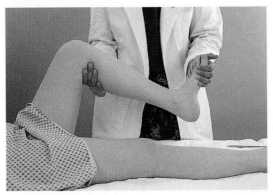

Testing for ankle clonus. (© B.Proud.)

Superficial Reflexes

Plantar Reflex

Tip From the Experts Use the handle end of the reflex hammer to elicit superficial reflexes, whose receptors are in the skin rather than the muscles.

With the end of the reflex hammer, stroke the lateral aspect of the sole from the heel to the ball of the foot, curving medially across the ball. Repeat on the other side. (Evaluates the function of spinal levels L4, L5, S1, and S2).

Flexion of the toes (plantar response).

In some older clients, flexion of the toes may be difficult to elicit and may be absent.

Except in infancy, extension (dorsiflexion) of the big toe and fanning of all toes (positive Babinski response) are seen with lesions of upper motor neurons. Unconscious states resulting from drug and alcohol intoxication or subsequent to an epileptic seizure may also cause it.

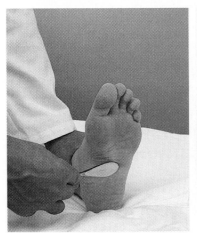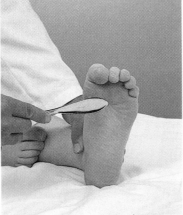

Eliciting plantar reflex (*left*). Normal plantar response (*right*). (© B.Proud.)

(continued)

ASSESSMENT PROCEDURE	NORMAL FINDINGS	ABNORMAL FINDINGS
Abdominal Reflex Lightly stroke the abdomen on each side, above and below the umbilicus. (Evaluates the function of spinal levels T8, T9, and T10 with the upper abdominal reflex and spinal levels T10, T11, and T12 with the lower abdominal reflex.)	Abdominal muscles contract, umbilicus deviates toward the side being stimulated.	Superficial reflexes may be absent with lower or upper motor neuron lesions. *Caution:* The abdominal reflex may be concealed because of obesity or muscular stretching from pregnancies. This is not an abnormality.
Cremasteric Reflex in Male Clients Lightly stroke the inner aspect of the upper thigh. (Evaluates the function of spinal levels T12, L1, and L2).	Scrotum elevates on stimulated side.	Absence of reflex may indicate motor neuron disorder.

TESTS FOR MENINGEAL IRRITATION OR INFLAMMATION

If you suspect the client has meningeal irritation or inflammation from infection or subarachnoid hemorrhage, assess the client's neck mobility. First, make sure there is no injury to the cervical vertebrae or cervical cord. Then, with the client supine, place your hands behind the patient's head and flex the neck forward until the chin touches the chest if possible.	Neck is supple, can easily bend head and neck forward.	Pain in the neck and resistance to flexion can arise from meningeal inflammation, arthritis, or neck injury.
Brudzinski's Sign As you flex the neck, watch the hips and knees in reaction to your maneuver.	Hips and knees remain relaxed and motionless.	Flexion of the hips and knees is a positive Brudzinski's sign and suggests meningeal inflammation.
Kernig's Sign Flex the client's leg at both the hip and the knee, then straighten the knee.	No pain felt. Discomfort behind the knee during full extension occurs in many normal people.	Pain and increased resistance to extending the knee are a positive Kernig's sign. When Kernig's sign is bilateral, the examiner suspects meningeal irritation.

Validation and Documentation of Findings

Validate the neurologic assessment data that you have collected. This is necessary to verify that the data are reliable and accurate. Document the data following the health care facility or agency policy.

Tip From the Experts When documenting your assessment findings, it is better to describe the client's response than to label the behavior.

EXAMPLE OF SUBJECTIVE DATA

No history of head injury, spinal cord injury, seizures, meningitis. No dizziness, tinnitus, severe or chronic headache. No difficulty swallowing or communicating. No memory loss.

EXAMPLE OF OBJECTIVE DATA
Mental Status

Alert, oriented to person, place, day, and time. Good eye contact. Positive about daily activities and the future. Short-term and long-term memory intact. Able to follow directions, compare unlike objects, and explain simple proverbs.

Cranial Nerves

I: Identifies correct scents.

II: Vision 20/20 OS, 20/20 OD, full visual fields intact, red reflex present, optic disc round with well-defined borders. Retinal background pink. No hemorrhages or arteriovenous nicking noted.

III, IV, and VI: No ptosis, full extraocular movements (EOMs), pupils equally round, react to light and accommodation (PERRLA).

V: Temporal and masseter muscles contract bilaterally. Able to identify light, sharp, and dull touch to forehead, cheek, and chin. Corneal reflex present.

DISPLAY 23-2. Using the Glasgow Coma Scale

The Glasgow Coma Scale is useful for rating one's response to stimuli. The client who scores 10 or lower needs emergency attention. The client with a score of 7 or lower is generally considered to be in a coma.

		Score
Eye opening response	Spontaneous opening	4
	To verbal stimuli	3
	To pain	2
	None	1
Most appropriate verbal response	Oriented	5
	Confused	4
	Inappropriate words	3
	Incoherent	2
	None	1
Most integral motor response (arm)	Obeys commands	5
	Localizes pain	4
	Flexion to pain	3
	Extension to pain	2
	None	1
TOTAL SCORE		3 to 15

Teasdale, G., & Jennelt, B. (1974). Assessment of coma and impaired consciousness: A practical scale. *Lancet, 2,* 81.

VII: Able to smile, frown, wrinkle forehead, show teeth, puff out cheeks, purse lips, raise eyebrows, and close eyes against resistance.

VIII: Whispered words heard bilaterally. Vibration heard equally well in both ears; air conduction (AC) greater than bone conduction (BC).

IX and X: Uvula and soft palate rise symmetrically on phonation. Gag reflex present. Swallows without difficulty.

XI: Equal shoulder shrug against resistance; turns head in both directions against resistance.

XII: Protrudes tongue in midline with no tremors, able to push tongue blade to right and left without difficulty.

Motor and Cerebellar Systems

No atrophy, tremors, weakness; full range of motion of all extremities. No fasciculations, tics, or tremors. Gait and tandem walk normal and steady. Negative Romberg test.

Performs repetitive alternating movements, finger-to-nose at smooth, good pace. Runs each heel down each shin with no deviation.

Sensory System

Identifies light touch, dull and sharp sensations to trunk and extremities. Vibratory sensation, stereognosis, graphesthesia, two-point discrimination intact.

Reflexes

Reflexes 2+ bilaterally, except Achilles 1+. No ankle clonus noted. Abdominal reflex present. No Babinski's present.

After you have collected your assessment data, you will need to analyze the data. Refer to the discussion of diagnostic reasoning skills in Chapter 7.

(*text continues on page 579*)

TABLE 23-3. Sources of Voice and Speech Problems

Problem	Description	Source
Dysphonia	Voice volume disorder	Laryngeal disorders or impairment of cranial nerve X (vagus nerve)
Cerebellar dysarthria	Irregular, uncoordinated speech	Multiple sclerosis
Dysarthria	Defect in muscular control of speech (eg, slurring)	Lesions of the nervous system, Parkinson's disease, or cerebellar disease
Aphasia	Difficulty producing or understanding language	Motor lesions in the dominant cerebral hemisphere
Wernicke's aphasia	Rapid speech that lacks meaning	Lesion in the posterior superior temporal lobe
Broca's aphasia	Slowed speech with difficult articulation, but fairly clear meaning	Lesion in the posterior inferior frontal lobe

DISPLAY 23-3. Assessing Geriatric Depression

Choose the best answer for how you felt over the past week

1. Are you basically satisfied with your life?   yes/no
2. Have you dropped many of your activities and interests?   yes/no
3. Do you feel that your life is empty?   yes/no
4. Do you often get bored?   yes/no
5. Are you hopeful about the future?   yes/no
6. Are you bothered by thoughts you can't get out of your head?   yes/no
7. Are you in good spirits most of the time?   yes/no
8. Are you afraid that something bad is going to happen to you?   yes/no
9. Do you feel happy most of the time?   yes/no
10. Do you often feel helpless?   yes/no
11. Do you often get restless and fidgety?   yes/no
12. Do you prefer to stay at home, rather than going out and doing new things?   yes/no
13. Do you frequently worry about the future?   yes/no
14. Do you feel you have more problems with memory than most?   yes/no
15. Do you think it is wonderful to be alive now?   yes/no
16. Do you often feel downhearted and blue?   yes/no
17. Do you feel pretty worthless the way you are now?   yes/no
18. Do you worry a lot about the past?   yes/no
19. Do you find life very exciting?   yes/no
20. Is it hard for you to get started on new projects?   yes/no
21. Do you feel full of energy?   yes/no
22. Do you feel that your situation is hopeless?   yes/no
23. Do you think that most people are better off than you are?   yes/no
24. Do you frequently get upset over little things?   yes/no
25. Do you frequently feel like crying?   yes/no
26. Do you have trouble concentrating?   yes/no
27. Do you enjoy getting up in the morning?   yes/no
28. Do you prefer to avoid social gatherings?   yes/no
29. Is it easy for you to make decisions?   yes/no
30. Is your mind as clear as it used to be?   yes/no

For scoring, reverse the answers for Nos. 1, 5, 7, 9, 15, 19, 21, 27, 29, and 30, then count the total number of "yes" answers.

Scoring: 0–10 = within normal range; 11 or higher = possible indication of depression.

Brink, T. A., et al. (1982). Screening tests for geriatric depression. *Clinical Gerontologist, 1,* 37–44.

DISPLAY 23-4. Annotated Mini Mental State Examination

NAME OF SUBJECT _____ Age _____

NAME OF EXAMINER _____ Years of School Completed __

Approach the patient with respect and encouragement   Date of Examination _____

Ask: Do you have any trouble with your memory?   ☐ Yes ☐ No

May I ask you some questions about your memory?   ☐ Yes ☐ No

SCORE	ITEM
5 ( )	**Time orientation** Ask: What is the year_____(1), season_____(1). month of the year_____(1), date_____(1). day of the week_____(1) ?
5 ( )	**Place orientation** Ask: Where are we now? What is the state_____(1), city_____(1), part of the city_____(1), building_____(1) floor of the building_____(1)?
3 ( )	**Registration of three words** Say: Listen carefully. I am going to say three words. You say them back after 1 stop. Ready? Here they are. . . PONY (wait 1 second), QUARTER (wait 1 second), ORANGE (wait one second). What were those words? _____(1) _____(1) _____(1) Give 1 point for each correct answer, then repeat them until the patient learns all three.
5 ( )	**Serial 7s as a test of attention and calculation** Ask: Subtract 7 from 100 and continue to subtract 7 from each subsequent remainder until I tell you to stop. What is 100 take away 7?_____(1) Say: Keep Going._____(1),_____(1). _____(1),_____(1).
3 ( )	**Recall of three words** Ask: What were those three words I asked you to remember? Give one point for each correct answer_____(1). _____(1),_____(1).
2 ( )	**Naming** Ask: What is this? (show pencil)_____(1). What is this? (show watch)_____(1).
1 ( )	**Repetition** Say: Now I am going to ask you to repeat what I say. Ready? No ifs ands or buts. Now you say that_____(1)
3 ( )	**Comprehension** Say: Listen carefully because I am going to ask you to do something: Take this paper in your left hand (1), fold it in half (1), and put it on the floor. (1)
1 ( )	**Reading** Say: Please read the following and do what it says, but do not say it aloud. (1) **Close your eyes**
1 ( )	**Writing** Say: Please write a sentence. If patient does not respond say: Write about the weather. (1)

(continued)

1 ( )   **Drawing**
Say: Please copy this design.

TOTAL SCORE_____ Assess level of consciousness along a continuum

Alert   Drowsy   Stupor   Coma

	YES	NO		YES	NO	
Cooperative	☐	☐	Deterioration from			FUNCTION BY PROXY
Depressed	☐	☐	previous level of			Please record date when patient
Anxious	☐	☐	functioning	☐	☐	was last able to perform the
Poor vision	☐	☐	Family history of			following tasks.
Poor hearing	☐	☐	dementia	☐	☐	Ask caregiver if patient indepen-
Native language			Head trauma	☐	☐	dently handles.
			Stroke	☐	☐	
			Alcohol abuse	☐	☐	
			Thyroid disease	☐	☐	

	YES	NO	DAT
Money bills	☐	☐	____
Medication	☐	☐	____
Transportation	☐	☐	____
Telephone	☐	☐	____

Used with permission from Folstein, M. F., Folstein, S. E., & McHugh, P. R. (1975). Mini-Mental State: A practical method for grading the cognitive state of patients for the clinician. *Journal of Psychiatric Research, 12*(3), 189–198.

DISPLAY 23-5. Abnormal Gaits

Everyone normally walks a little bit differently from everyone else but sometimes a person's gait is distinctively abnormal suggesting that the person has a neurologic problem. Some common abnormal gaits and their causes follow:

CEREBELLAR ATAXIA

- Wide-based, staggering, unsteady gait
- Romberg test results are positive (client cannot stand with feet together)
- Seen with cerebellar diseases or alcohol or drug intoxication

PARKINSONIAN GAIT

- Shuffling gait, turns accomplished in very stiff manner
- Stooped-over posture with flexed hips and knees
- Typically seen in Parkinson's disease *and drug-induced parkinsonism* because of effects on the basal ganglia

SCISSORS GAIT

- Stiff, short gait; thighs overlap each other with each step
- Seen with partial paralysis of the legs

SPASTIC HEMIPARESIS

- Flexed arm held close to body while client drags toe of leg or circles it stiffly outward and forward
- Seen with lesions of the upper motor neurons in the cortical spinal tract, such as occurs in stroke

FOOTDROP

- Client lifts foot and knee high with each step, then slaps the foot down hard on the ground
- Client cannot walk on heels
- Characteristic of diseases of the lower motor neurons

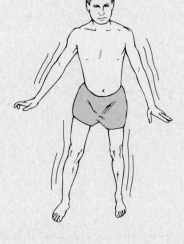

Cerebellar ataxia.

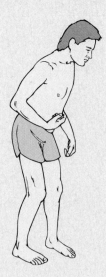

Parkinsonian gait.

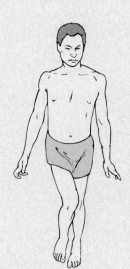

Scissors gait.

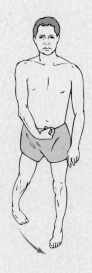

Spastic hemiparesis.

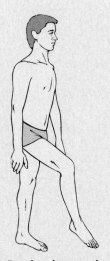

Footdrop (steppage) gait.

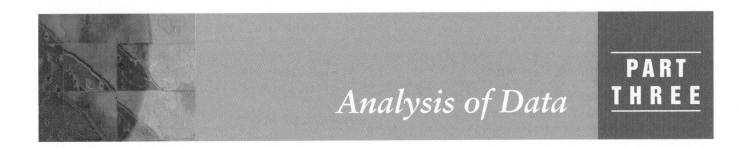
Diagnostic Reasoning: Possible Conclusions

Listed below are some possible conclusions and nursing diagnoses resulting from assessment of the client's neurologic system.

SELECTED NURSING DIAGNOSES

After collecting subjective and objective data pertaining to the neurologic system, you will need to identify abnormalities and cluster the data to reveal any significant patterns or abnormalities. These data will then be used to make clinical judgments (nursing diagnoses: wellness, risk, or actual, or collaborative problems) about the status of the client's neurologic system. Following is a listing of selected nursing diagnoses that you may identify when analyzing data for this part of the assessment.

Nursing Diagnoses (Wellness)

- Opportunity to Enhance Comfort Level
- Opportunity to Enhance Sensory-Perceptual Patterns
- Opportunity to Enhance Spiritual Well-being

Nursing Diagnoses (Risk)

- Risk for Injury related to disturbed sensory-perceptual patterns
- Risk for Aspiration related to impaired gag reflex
- Risk for Self-Directed Violence, related to depression, suicidal tendencies, developmental crisis, lack of support systems, loss of significant others, poor coping mechanisms and behaviors

Nursing Diagnoses (Actual)

- Disturbed Thought Processes related to abuse of alcohol or drugs, psychotic disorder, or organic brain dysfunction
- Impaired Verbal Communication related to aphasia, psychological impairment or organic brain disorder
- Acute or Chronic Confusion related to dementia, head injury, stroke, alcohol or drug abuse
- Impaired Memory related to dementia, stroke, head injury, alcohol or drug abuse

- Sexual Dysfunction
- Impaired Environmental Interpretation Syndrome related to dementia, depression, or alcoholism
- Self-Care Deficit (bathing, hygiene, toileting, or feeding) related to paralysis, weakness, or confusion
- Reflex Urinary Incontinence related to spinal cord or brain damage
- Unilateral Neglect related to poor vision on one side, trauma or neurologic disorder

SELECTED COLLABORATIVE PROBLEMS

After grouping the data, it may become apparent that certain collaborative problems emerge. Remember that collaborative problems differ from nursing diagnoses in that they cannot be prevented with nursing interventions alone. However, these physiologic complications of medical conditions can be detected and monitored by the nurse. In addition, the nurse can use physician- and nurse-prescribed interventions to minimize the complications of these problems. The nurse may also have to refer the client in such situations for further treatment of the problem. Following is a list of collaborative problems that may be identified when assessing the neurologic system. These problems are worded as Potential Complications (or PC), followed by the problem.

- PC: Increased intracranial pressure
- PC: Stroke
- PC: Seizures
- PC: Spinal cord compression
- PC: Meningitis
- PC: Cranial nerve impairment
- PC: Paralysis
- PC: Peripheral nerve impairment
- PC: Increased intraocular pressure
- PC: Corneal ulceration
- PC: Neuropathies

MEDICAL PROBLEMS

After grouping the data, it may become apparent that the client has signs and symptoms that require medical diagnosis and treatment. Referral to a primary care provider is necessary.

Diagnostic Reasoning: Case Study

The case study presents assessment data for a specific client. It is followed by an analysis of the data, working out the seven key steps to arrive at specific conclusions.

Mildred Hutchinson, a 49-year-old divorced woman, had been working as an office manager at a local high school, but recently she began teaching (her first love) language classes (French and German); she also is responsible for teaching two physical education (PE) classes a week.

During the interview, she tells you that she has had multiple sclerosis (MS) for over 20 years but has managed to function at a near-normal level for most of that time. "I had one severe exacerbation during my divorce, but I went into remission after about 6 months." She states that she has come to the clinic for advice about how to prevent another exacerbation. She voices her concerns: "I get so tired by the end of the week that I have difficulty maintaining urinary continence even with my medication (oxybutynin, ie, Ditropan). I feel increasingly weak, and I get pins and needles in my legs. Also, I'm not sleeping well because spasms in my legs keep me awake." She tells you that her vision has not been affected and that, if she rests all weekend, she is "OK" by Monday morning. She goes on to say, "I have no social life, except on the telephone."

Your physical assessment reveals an alert, attractive, well-dressed, thin, middle-aged woman with mildly elevated blood pressure and pulse rate (136/92 and 98), which Ms. H. reports is usually 100/70; PERRLA; extraocular movements intact with conjugate gaze, but slight nystagmus noted when eyes are in extreme lateral positions; mental status intact; grips strong and upper extremity strength good against resistance; unable to walk heel-to-toe without some loss of balance; and 4+ patellar, Achilles, and plantar reflexes with mild clonus.

1 Identify abnormal data and strengths (in both subjective and objective data).

SUBJECTIVE DATA

- Multiple sclerosis for more than 20 years
- Functions at a near-normal level most of that time
- One severe exacerbation during divorce
- Remission after about 6 months
- Seeking advice to prevent another exacerbation
- Concerned because starting new teaching position
- Teaching language classes and two PE classes a week
- "I get so tired by the end of the week."
- Problem maintaining urinary continence with medication (Ditropan)
- Increased weakness and "pins and needles" in legs
- Not sleeping well because of leg spasms
- OK by Monday morning if she rests all weekend
- "But I have no social life, except on the telephone!"
- Vision not affected

OBJECTIVE DATA

- Thin, 49-year-old woman
- BP 136/92 (reported usual 100/70) and pulse rate 98
- PERRLA
- Extraocular movements intact with conjugate gaze, but slight nystagmus noted when eyes in extreme lateral positions
- Mental status intact
- Grips strong and upper extremity strength good against resistance
- Lower extremities show slight weakness against resistance
- Unable to walk heel-to-toe without moderate loss of balance
- 4+ patellar, Achilles, and plantar reflexes with mild clonus

2 Cue Clusters	**3** Inferences	**4** Possible Nursing Diagnoses	**5** Defining Characteristics	**6** Confirm or Rule Out
A • Multiple sclerosis for over 20 years • "I get so tired by the end of the week" • Problem maintaining urinary continence with medication • Increased weakness, "pins and needles," and spasms in legs • OK by Monday morning if rests all weekend	Data point to a confirmation of the diagnosis of multiple sclerosis. Refer to physician (neurologist) for evaluation and management for increase in her symptoms even though she remains somewhat functional. Determine what other medications she is taking to treat her disease. Monitor for collaborative problems.			

2 Cue Clusters	3 Inferences	4 Possible Nursing Diagnoses	5 Defining Characteristics	6 Confirm or Rule Out
A • Slight nystagmus noted when eyes in extreme lateral positions • Mental status intact • Grips strong; upper extremity strength good against resistance; lower extremity slightly weak against resistance • Unable to walk heel-to-toe without moderate loss of balance • 4+ patellar, Achilles, and plantar reflexes with mild clonus				
B • Multiple sclerosis for over 20 years • Functions at a near-normal level most of that time; • One severe exacerbation during divorce • Concerned because starting new teaching position • Teaching language classes and two PE classes a week • "I get so tired by the end of the week" • Problem maintaining urinary continence with medication • Increased weakness, "pins and needles," and spasms in legs • BP 136/92 (reported usual: 100/70) and pulse rate 98	Increase in symptoms possibly due to stress of new position and increased physical requirements of teaching physical education. Increased BP/P could be related to stress or could signify an inability to adapt to increased physical demands—a change that could result in another exacerbation of MS	Activity Intolerance related to fatigue secondary to increased physical demands of new position and long-term MS in remission	*Major:* Increase in diastolic BP by > 15 mm Hg *Minor:* Fatigue and weakness	Confirm because it meets major defining characteristics
		Ineffective Health Maintenance related to increased physical demands and stress of new position	*Major:* None *Minor:* None	Rule out because it does not meet definition of this diagnosis
		Ineffective Coping related to perceived stress of change in work responsibilities	*Major:* None *Minor:* None	Rule out because it does not meet defining characteristics. This might qualify as a risk diagnosis, but the client has not discussed how she copes with stress. Collect more data.
C • Multiple sclerosis for over 20 years • Functions at a near-normal level most of that time • One severe exacerbation during divorce • Remission after about 6 months	Because of past experience, has legitimate concerns about another exacerbation, especially in light of increased symptoms. Positively seeking help to prevent any further deterioration.	Effective Management of Therapeutic Regimen	*Major/Minor:* Verbalized desire to manage illness and prevent complications	Confirm because it meets defining characteristics.
		Powerlessness related to perceived unpredictable nature of illness	*Major:* None expressed *Minor:* Uneasiness/anxiety (expressed concern)	Rule out because it does not meet major defining characteristic, but collect more data because client may be at risk for this diagnosis.

② Cue Clusters	③ Inferences	④ Possible Nursing Diagnoses	⑤ Defining Characteristics	⑥ Confirm or Rule Out
• Seeking advice to prevent another exacerbation • Concerned because starting new teaching position • "I get so tired by the end of the week" • Problem maintaining urinary continence with medication • Increased weakness, "pins and needles," and spasms in legs				
D • Concerned because starting new teaching position • "I get so tired by the end of the week" • Problem maintaining urinary continence with medication • Increased weakness, "pins and needles," and spasms in legs • BP 136/92 and P 98 (reported usual 100/70)	May have anxiety or fear of losing her opportunity to fulfill long-term goal of teaching because she finds herself with an increase in symptoms that have been under control. Increased BP/P support anxiety, although they could reflect physiologic changes.	Anxiety related to possible loss of teaching position secondary to acceleration of illness symptoms Fear related to possible loss of teaching position secondary to acceleration of illness symptoms	*Major/Minor:* Increased BP/P; admits to apprehension (concern) *Major:* None expressed (related to danger) *Minor:* Increased BP/P	Confirm because it meets defining characteristics Rule out because it does not meet major defining characteristic. Although data for both diagnoses are weak, anxiety is the better diagnosis. Collect more data.
E • Not sleeping well because of increased leg spasms • 4+ patellar, Achilles, and plantar reflexes with mild clonus	Discomfort from muscle spasms interferes with sleeping patterns. It is not known if she has any medication or treatment protocols for the muscle spasms. She does not seem to know how to manage the problem.	Disturbed Sleep Pattern related to knowledge deficit of management strategies for muscle spasm	*Major:* Difficulty remaining asleep *Minor:* None	Confirm because it meets major defining characteristic
F • "I get so tired by the end of the week." • Feels OK by Monday morning if rests all weekend • But "I have no social life, except on the telephone."	The need to get extra rest to maintain her new job may interfere with her usual weekend social activities.	Impaired Social Interaction related to fatigue from new job and need for additional rest secondary to multiple sclerosis Risk for Loneliness related to difficulty maintaining social contacts and attending social events due to fatigue	*Major:* Reports inability to maintain stable supportive relationships (implied by statement) *Minor:* None	Confirm because it meets major defining characteristic, but data are weak. Collect more data before accepting this diagnosis. Confirm because this is a risk diagnosis Carpenito (1999) identifies this as a better diagnosis than Impaired Social Interaction.

7 Document conclusions.

The following nursing diagnoses are appropriate for Ms. Hutchinson at this time:

- Activity Intolerance related to fatigue secondary to increased physical demands of new position in conjunction with multiple sclerosis in remission
- Effective Individual Management of Therapeutic Regimen
- Anxiety related to possible loss of teaching position secondary to acceleration of illness symptoms
- Disturbed Sleep Pattern related to knowledge deficit of management strategies for muscle spasms

- Impaired Social Interaction related to fatigue from new job and need for additional rest secondary to multiple sclerosis
- Risk for Loneliness related to difficulty maintaining social contacts and attending social events due to fatigue

Collaborative problems related to her medical diagnosis could include:

- PC: Hypertension
- PC: Urinary incontinence
- PC: Active multiple sclerosis

Ms. Hutchinson should be referred to a neurologist for evaluation of her treatment regimen.

REFERENCES AND SELECTED READINGS

Davis, A. (1996). Critical care extra: Assessing patients with altered consciousness. *American Journal of Nursing, 96,* 16J, 16L.

Dellasega, C., & Cutezo, E. (1994). Initial assessment of patient cognition in a rehabilitation hospital. *Rehabilitation Nurse, 19,* 293–297.

Dellasega, C., & Cutezo, E. (1994). Strategies used by home health nurses to assess the mental status of homebound elders. *Journal of Community Health Nursing, 11*(3), 129–138.

Folstein, M., Anthony, J., Parhad, I., Duffy, B., & Gruenberg, E. (1985). The meaning of cognitive impairment in the elderly. *Journal of the American Geriatrics Society, 33,* 228–235.

Folstein, M. F., Folstein, S. E., & McHugh, P. R. (1975). Mini-Mental State: A practical method for grading the cognitive state of patients for the clinician. *Journal of Psychiatric Research, 12*(3), 89–198.

Geary, S. M. (1995). Nursing management of cranial nerve dysfunction. *Journal of Neuroscience Nursing, 27*(2), 102–108.

Greenberg, M. S. (1997). *Handbook of neurosurgery, Vols. I & II* (4th ed.). Lakeland, FL: Greenberg Graphics.

Jacubowitz, T. R. (1999). Culturally sensitive care for the elderly. *Nurse Practitioner Forum, 10*(1), 8–11.

Kahn, R., Goldfarb, A., Pollack, M., & Peck, A. (1960). Brief objective measures for the determination of mental status in the aged. *American Journal of Psychiatry, 117,* 326–328.

Krach, P. (1995). Assessment of depressed older persons living in a home setting. *Home Health Nurse, 13*(3), 61–64.

Lansinger, T. (1995). Proverb interpretation to assess mental status. *Journal of Nursing Education, 34,* 290–291.

Lewis, A. M. (1999). Neurologic emergency! *Nursing99, 29*(10), 54–56.

Minton, M., & Hickey, J. (1999). A primer of neuroanatomy and neurophysiology. *Nursing Clinics of North America, 34*(3), 555–572.

Neatherlin, J. (1999). Foundation for practice: Neuroassessment for neuroscience nurses. *Nursing Clinics of North America, 34*(3), 573–592.

Nichols, T. O. (1999). Neurologic assessment. *American Journal of Nursing, 99*(6), 44–50.

Patterson, C. (2000). *Screen for cognitive impairment in the elderly.* Canadian Task Force on Preventive Health Care. [On-line]. Available: http://www.ctfphc.org.

Schumacher, L. (2000). Identifying patients "at risk" for alcohol withdrawal syndrome and a treatment protocol. *Journal of Neuroscience Nursing, 32*(3), 158–163.

Solomon, P. R., & Pendleburry, W. W. (1998). Recognition of Alzheimer's disease: The 7-minute screen. *Family Medicine, 30*(4), 265–271.

Solomon, P. R., Hirschoff, A., Bridget, K., et al. (1998). A 7-minute neurocognitive screening battery highly sensitive to Alzheimer's disease. *Archives of Neurology, 55,* 349–355.

Staff. (1995). Cognitive testing helps elderly patients get better care. *Case Management Advisor, 6*(9), 126.

Yesevage, J. (1983). Development and validation of a geriatric depression screening scale: A preliminary report. *Journal of Psychiatric Research, 17,* 38–49.

Risk Factors—Cerebrovascular Accident (Stroke)

de Paula, T., Lagana, K., & Gonzalez-Ramirez, L. (1996). Mexican Americans. In J. Lipson, S. Dibble & P. Minarik (Eds.), *Culture and nursing care: A pocket guide* (pp. 203–221). San Francisco: UCSF Nursing Press.

Kramer, B. J. (1996). American Indians. In J. Lipson, S. Dibble & P. Minarik (Eds.), *Culture and nursing care: A pocket guide* (pp. 11–22). San Francisco: UCSF Nursing Press.

Locks, S., & Boateng, L. (1996). Black/African Americans. In J. Lipson, S. Dibble & P. Minarik (Eds.), *Culture and nursing care: A pocket guide* (pp. 37–43). San Francisco: UCSF Nursing Press.

National Stroke Association. (2000a). *Brain attack statistics* [On-line]. Available: http://www.stroke.org.

———. (2000b). *Stroke risk factors and their impact* [On-line]. Available: http://www.stroke.org.

Overfield, T. (1995). *Biologic variation in health and illness: Race, age, and sex differences* (2nd ed.). Boca Raton, FL: CRC Press.

Spector, R. (1996). *Cultural diversity in health and illness* (4th ed.). Stamford, CT: Appleton & Lange.

Yano, K., Popper, J., Kagan A., Chyou, P., & Grove, J. (1994). Epidemiology of stroke among Japanese men in Hawaii during 24 years of follow-up: The Honolulu Heart Program. *Health Reports, 6*(1), 9–12.

Zuber, M., & Mas, J. (1992). Epidemiology of cerebrovascular accidents. *Revue Neurologique, 148*(4), 243–255.

For additional information on this book, be sure to visit http://connection.lww.com.

Nursing Assessment of Special Groups

Assessment of Infants, Children, and Adolescents

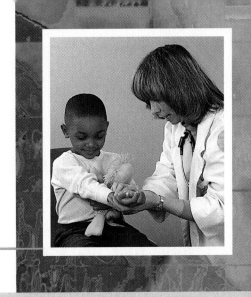

24

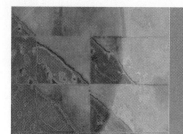

PART ONE

Structure and Function

Skin, Hair, and Nails

At birth, the newborn's skin is smooth and thin. It may appear ruddy because of visible blood circulation through the newborn's thin layer of subcutaneous fat. This thin layer of fat, combined with the skin's inability to contract and shiver, results in ineffective temperature regulation. The skin may appear mottled on the trunk, arms, or legs. The dermis and epidermis are thin and loosely bound together. This increases the skin's susceptibility to infection and irritation and creates a poor barrier, resulting in fluid loss. When the newborn's body temperature drops, the hands or feet or both may appear blue (acrocyanosis).

After birth, the newborn's sebaceous glands are active because of high levels of maternal androgen. Milia develops when these glands become plugged. Eccrine glands function at birth, creating palmar sweating, which is helpful when assessing pain. Apocrine glands stay small and nonfunctional until puberty.

The fine, downy hairs called lanugo, which appear on the newborn's body, shoulders, and/or back at birth, disappear within the first 2 weeks of life. Scalp hair-follicle growth phases occur concurrently at birth but are disrupted during early infancy. This may result in overgrowth or alopecia (hair loss). Regardless, any newborn's scalp hair sheds in 2 to 3 months and is replaced by more permanent hair. During the toddler years, hair grows coarser, thicker, and darker and usually loses curliness. Fine hair becomes visible on the distal portions of the upper and lower extremities.

During early childhood, the skin develops a tighter bond with the dermis, making it more resistant to infection, irritation, and fluid loss. The texture is smooth because the skin has not had years of exposure to the environment and because the hair is less coarse than in adulthood. The sebaceous glands and eccrine glands are minimally active, and, although the eccrine glands function during this time, they produce little sweat.

Skin structure and function remain stable until puberty, when adrenarche (adrenocortical maturation) signals the onset of increased sebum production from the sebaceous glands, a process that continues until late adolescence. Sebum is involved in the development of acne. The apocrine glands also respond more to emotional stimulation and heat, with the end result being body odor.

The development of pubic hair signals the initiation of adrenarche (Tables 24-1 and 24-2; see also Display 19-1).

Pubic hair signifies the onset of puberty in boys; in girls, pubic hair usually develops 2 to 6 months after thelarche (breast development). Axillary hair development occurs late in puberty. It follows definitive penile and testicular enlargement in boys and precedes menarche (first menstrual period) in girls. Facial hair in boys also develops at this time.

Nails are usually present at birth. Missing or short nails usually signify prematurity, and long nails usually signify postmaturity. Nails are usually pink, convex, and smooth throughout childhood and adolescence.

Head and Neck

Head growth predominates during the fetal period. At birth, the head circumference is greater (by 2 cm) than that of the chest. The cranial bones are soft and separated by the coronal, lambdoid, and sagittal sutures, which intersect at the anterior and posterior fontanelle (Fig. 24-1). Ossification begins in infancy and continues into adulthood. The posterior fontanelle usually measures 1 to 2 cm at birth and usually closes at 2 months. The anterior fontanelle usually measures 4 to 6 cm at birth and closes between 12 and 18 months. A full anterior fontanelle may be palpable when the baby cries. Visible pulsations may also appear, representing the peripheral pulse. The sutures and fontanelles allow the skull to expand to accommodate brain growth.

Brain growth is reflected by head circumference (occipital–frontal circumference), which increases six times as much during the first year as it does the second. Half of postnatal brain growth is achieved within the first year of life. The newborn's skull is typically asymmetric (plagiocephaly) because of molding that occurs as the newborn passes through the birth canal. The skull molds easily during birth, allowing for overlapping of the cranial bones.

During infancy, body growth predominates and the head grows proportionately to body size, reaching 90% of its full adult size by age 6 years. Facial bone growth is variable, especially for the nasal and jaw bones. During the toddler years, the nasal bridge is low and the mandible and maxilla are small, making the face seem small compared with the whole skull. During the school-age years, the face grows proportionately faster than the rest of the cranium, and secondary teeth appear too large for the face. In adolescence, the nose and thyroid cartilage enlarge in boys.

TABLE 24-1. Tanner's Sexual Maturity Rating: Male Genitalia Development and Pubic Hair Growth

Developmental Stage	Genitalia	Pubic Hair
Stage 1 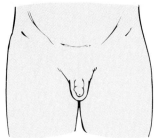	Prepubertal	Prepubertal: No pubic hair; fine vellus hair
Stage 2 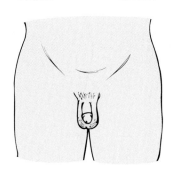	Initial enlargement of scrotum and testes with ruggation and reddening of the scrotum	Sparse, long, straight, downy hair
Stage 3 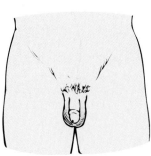	Elongation of the penis; testes and scrotum further enlarge	Darker, coarser, curly; sparse over entire pubis
Stage 4 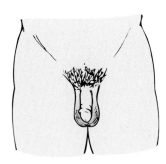	Increase in size and width of penis and the development of the glans; scrotum darkens	Dark, curly, and abundant in pubic area; no growth on thighs or up toward umbilicus
Stage 5 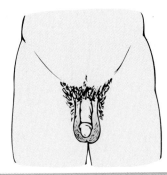	Adult configuration	Adult pattern (growth up toward umbilicus may not be seen); growth continues until mid-20s

TABLE 24-2. Tanner's Sexual Maturity Rating: Female Pubic Hair Growth and Breast Development

Developmental Stage	Pubic Hair	Breast
Stage 1	Prepubertal: No pubic hair; fine vellus hair	Prepubertal: Elevation of nipple only
Stage 2	Sparse, long, straight, downy hair	Breast bud stage; elevation of breast and nipple as small mound, enlargement of areolar diameter
Stage 3	Darker, coarser, curly; sparse over mons pubis	Enlargement of the breasts and areola with no separation of contours
Stage 4	Dark, curly, and abundant on mons pubis; no growth on medial thighs	Projection of areola and nipple to form secondary mound above level of breast
Stage 5	Adult pattern of inverse triangle; growth on medial thighs	Adult configuration; projection of nipple only, areola receded into contour of breast

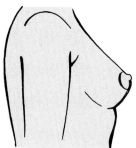
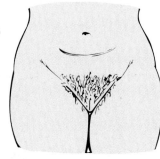

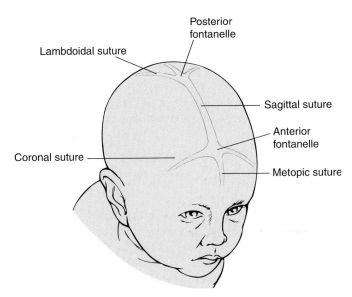

FIGURE 24-1. The infant head.

The neck is usually short during infancy, lengthening at about age 3 or 4 years. Lymphoid tissue is well developed at birth and reaches adult size by age 6 years. Lymphoid tissue continues to grow rapidly until age 10 or 11 years, exceeding adult size before puberty, after which the tissue atrophies and stabilizes to adult dimensions by the end of adolescence.

Eyes and Ears

Eye structure and function are not fully developed at birth. Peripheral vision is developed, but central vision is not. The newborn is farsighted and has a visual acuity of 20/200. The iris shows little pigment, and the pupils are small. The macula, which is absent at birth, develops at 4 months and is mature by 8 months. Tearing and voluntary control over eye muscles begin at 2 to 3 months; by 4 months, infants establish binocular vision and focus on a single image with both eyes simultaneously. These functions are better developed by 9 months. Newborns cannot distinguish between colors; this ability develops by 8 months. During childhood, the eyes are less spherical than adult eyes. In addition, children remain farsighted until age 6 or 7 years, when they achieve an acuity of 20/20.

The inner ear develops during the first trimester of gestation. Therefore, maternal problems during this time, such as rubella, may impair hearing. Newborns can hear loud sounds at 90 decibels and react with the startle reflex. They respond to low-frequency sounds, such as a heartbeat or a lullaby, by decreasing crying and motor movement. They react to high-frequency sounds with an alerting reaction. In infants, the external auditory canal curves upward and is short and straight. Therefore, the pinna must be pulled down and back to perform the otoscopic examination. The eustachian tube is wider, shorter, and more horizontal, increasing the possibility of infection rising from the pharynx. In older children,

the eustachian tube lengthens, but it may become occluded from growth of lymphatic tissue, specifically the adenoids. The canal shortens and straightens as the child ages, and the pinna can be pulled up and back as in the adult.

Mouth, Throat, Nose, and Sinuses

Saliva is minimal at birth, but drooling is evident by 3 months because of the increased secretion of saliva. Drooling persists for a few months until the infant learns to swallow the saliva. Drooling does not signify tooth eruption. The development of both temporary (deciduous) and permanent teeth begins in utero. Deciduous tooth eruption takes place between the ages of 6 and 24 months. Deciduous teeth are lost between the ages of 6 and 12 years. Permanent teeth begin forming in the jaw by age 6 months and begin to replace temporary teeth at age 6 years, usually starting with the central incisors. Permanent teeth appear earlier in African Americans than in Caucasians and in girls before boys.

The tonsils and adenoids are small in relation to body size and hard to see at birth. The pharynx is best seen when the newborn is crying. The tonsils and adenoids rapidly grow, reaching maximum development by age 10 to 12 years. At this point, they may be about twice their adult size. However, as with other lymphoid tissue, they atrophy to stable adult dimensions by the end of adolescence.

Newborns are obligatory nose breathers and, therefore, have significant distress when their nasal passages are obstructed. Nasal cartilage grows during adolescence with the secondary sex characteristics. Growth starts at age 12 or 13 years and reaches full size by 16 years in girls and 18 years in boys. The maxillary and ethmoid sinuses are present at birth, but they are small and cannot be examined until they develop, when the child is much older. The frontal sinuses develop around age 7 to 8 years, and the sphenoid sinuses develop after puberty.

Thorax and Lungs

At term gestation, the fetal lungs should be developed and the alveoli should be collapsed. Gas exchange is performed by the placenta. Immediately after birth, the lungs aerate; blood flows through them more vigorously, causing greater expansion and relaxation of the pulmonary arteries. The decrease in pulmonary pressure closes the foramen ovale, increasing oxygen tension and closing the ductus arteriosus. The lungs continue to develop after birth, and new alveoli form until about 8 years of age. Thus, in a child with pulmonary damage or disease at birth, pulmonary tissue may regenerate and the lungs can eventually attain normal respiratory function.

The chest wall is thin with very little musculature. The ribs are soft and pliable with the xiphoid process movable. The airways of children are also smaller and narrower than in adults; therefore, children are at risk for airway obstruction from edema and infections in the lungs. A child's respiratory rate is much faster than an adult's, and children younger than 7 years old tend to be abdominal breathers. Once children are between 8 and 10 years old, respiratory rates lower and breathing becomes thoracic like the adult's.

Heart

In fetal circulation, the lungs are bypassed and arterial blood is returned to the right side of the heart. Blood is shunted through the foramen ovale and ductus arteriosus into the left side of the heart and out the aorta. At birth, lung aeration causes circulatory changes. The foramen ovale closes within the first hour because of the newly created low pressure in the right side of the heart, and the ductus arteriosus closes about 10 to 15 h after birth.

In children, the heart is positioned more horizontally in the chest. The apical impulse is felt at the fourth intercostal space left of the midclavicular line in young children. By the time the child is 7 years old, the apical pulse reaches the fifth intercostal space and the midclavicular line. Heart sounds are louder, higher pitched, and of shorter duration in children. Physiologic splitting of the second sound, which widens with inspiration, may be heard in the second left intercostal space. A third heart sound (S_3) may be heard at the apex and is present in one third of all children. Sinus arrhythmia is normal and reaches its greatest degree during adolescence. Some children may have physiologic murmurs that do not indicate disease.

The pulse rate is usually between 120 and 160 beats/min in the newborn. The rate decreases as the child ages, usually dropping to about 85 beats/min by 8 years of age. Athletic adolescents may have even lower heart rates. Peripheral pulses should be palpated; weakness or absence of peripheral pulses in the lower extremities may indicate coarctation of the aorta in the newborn.

Breasts

Ventral epidermal ridges (milk lines), which run from the axilla to the medial thigh, are present during gestation. True breasts develop along the thoracic ridge; the other breasts along the milk line atrophy. Occasionally, a supernumerary nipple persists along the ridge track. At birth, lactiferous ducts are present in the nipple, but there are no alveoli. Although the newborn's breasts may be temporarily enlarged from the effects of maternal estrogen, they are usually flat and remain so until puberty.

In girls, breast growth is stimulated by estrogen at the onset of puberty. Between 8 and 13 years of age, the larche may occur and breasts continue to develop in stages (see Table 24-2). Breasts enlarge primarily as a result of fat deposits. However, the duct system also grows and branches, and masses of small cells develop at the duct endings. These masses are potential alveoli. Tenderness and asymmetric development are common, and anticipatory guidance and reassurance are needed.

Gynecomastia, enlargement of breast tissue in boys, may be noted in some male adolescents. This is related to pubertal changes and is usually temporary. However, use of marijuana and anabolic steroids are two of several external causes of gynecomastia.

Abdomen

The umbilical cord is prominent in the newborn and contains two arteries and one vein. The umbilicus consists of two parts—the amniotic portion and the cutaneous portion. The amniotic portion is covered with a gel-like substance and dries up and falls off within 2 weeks of life. The cutaneous portion is covered with skin and draws back to become flush with the abdominal wall.

The abdomen of infants and small children is cylindrical, prominent in the standing position, and flat when supine. The abdomen of toddlers appears prominent and gives the child what is popularly called a pot-belly appearance. The contours of the abdomen change to adult shapes during adolescence. Peristaltic waves may be visible in infants and thin children, and they may also be indicative of a disease or disorder.

Kidney development is not complete until 1 year of age. The tip of the right kidney may be felt in young children, especially during inspiration. Bladder capacity increases with age, and the bladder is considered an abdominal organ in infants because it is located between the symphysis pubis and the umbilicus (higher than in adults). The newborn's liver is palpable at 0.5 to 2.5 cm below the right costal margin, thereby occupying proportionately more space than at any other time after birth. In infants and small children, the liver is palpable at 1 to 2 cm below the right costal margin. The spleen may be palpable below the left costal margin at 1 to 2 cm. Often in older children, these structures are not palpable.

Genitalia

The testes develop prenatally and drop into the scrotum during month 8 of gestation. Each testis measures about 1 cm wide and 1.5 to 2 cm long. Enlargement of the testes is an early sign of puberty in boys, occurring between the ages of 9.5 and 13.5 years. Pubic hair development and penile enlargement are concurrent with testicular growth (see Table 24-1). Development from preadolescence to adulthood averages 2 to 5 years. The onset of spontaneous nocturnal emission of seminal fluid is a sign of puberty similar to menarche in females.

At birth, female genitalia may be engorged. Mucoid or bloody discharge may be noted because of the influence of maternal hormones. The genitalia return to normal size in a few weeks and remain small until puberty, when estrogen stimulates the development of the reproductive tract and secondary sex characteristics. The external genitalia increase in size and sensitivity, whereas the internal reproductive organs increase in weight and mass. Pubic hair begins growing early in puberty and follows a distinct pattern (see Table 24-2). Menarche takes place in the latter half of puberty, after breast and pubic hair begin to develop. Menarche typically begins 2.5 years after the onset of puberty. The menstrual cycle is usually irregular during the first 2 years because of physiologic anovulation.

Anus, Rectum, and Prostate

Meconium is passed during the first 24 hours of life, signifying anal patency. Stools are passed by reflex, and anal sphincter control is not reached until 1.5 to 2 years of age, after the nerves supplying the area have become fully myelinated. In boys, the prostate gland is underdeveloped and not palpable. However, during puberty, it grows rapidly to twice its prepubertal size under the influence of androgens.

Muscles and Bones

The skeleton of infants and small children is made chiefly of cartilage, accounting for the relative softness and malleability of the bones and the relative ease with which certain deformities can be corrected. Bone formation occurs by ossification, beginning during the gestational period and continuing throughout childhood. Bones grow rapidly during infancy. As children grow into adolescence, they will experience a skeletal growth spurt, usually seen in correlation with Tanner's stage 2 for girls and Tanner's stage 3 for boys. Skeletal growth continues throughout Tanner's stage 5 for both sexes.

Bone growth occurs in two dimensions: diameter and length. Growth in diameter takes place predominantly in children and adolescents and slows as the person ages because of the predominance of bone breakdown over bone formation. Growth in length takes place at the epiphyseal plates, vascular areas of active cell division. Bones increase in circumference and length under the influence of hormones, primarily pituitary growth hormone and thyroid hormone.

Muscle growth is related to growth of the underlying bone. Individual fibers, ligaments, and tendons grow throughout childhood. Bone and muscle development is influenced by use of the extremities. If extremities are not used, minimal growth of the muscle will occur. Walking and weight-bearing activities stimulate bone and muscle growth.

The newborn vertebral column differs in contour from the normal adult vertebral column. The spine has a single C-shaped curve at birth. By 3 to 4 months, the anterior curve in the cervical region develops from the infant raising its head when prone. The anterior curve in the lumbar region develops between ages 12 and 18 months, when the infant starts to stand erect and walk.

Muscle growth contributes significantly to weight gain in the child. Individual fibers grow throughout childhood, and growth is considerable during the adolescent growth spurt, which usually peaks at 12 years in girls and 14 years in boys.

Neurologic Structures

The neurologic system is not fully developed at birth. Motor control is maintained by the spinal cord and medulla, and most actions in the newborn are primitive reflexes. As myelinization develops and the number of brain neurons grows rapidly, from the 30th week of gestation through the first year of life, voluntary control and advanced cerebral function appear and the more primitive reflexes diminish or disappear. The nervous system grows rapidly during fetal and early postnatal life, reaching 25% of adult capacity at birth, 50% by age 1 year, 80% by age 3, and 90% by age 7.

Newborns have rudimentary sensation—any stimulus must be strong to cause a reaction, and the response is not localized. A strong stimulus causes a vigorous response of crying with whole-body movements. As myelinization develops, stimulus localization becomes possible and the child responds in a more localized manner. Motor control develops in a head-to-neck to trunk-to-extremities sequence. Development takes place in an orderly progression, but each child develops at his or her own pace. The norms demonstrate wide variation among individuals as well as within a single individual under different circumstances.

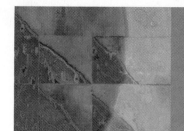

Nursing Assessment

PART TWO

Collecting Subjective Data

Because infants and children are uniquely different from adults, a separate subjective assessment that focuses on questions suited for this population is vital. Subjective assessment of infants and children encompasses interviewing and compiling a complete nursing history.

General interviewing techniques used for the adult are used in the pediatric setting (see Chapter 4). However, in pediatrics, the history may be given by someone other than the client, usually the parent. Thus, the interview becomes the onset of a relational triad between the nurse, the child or adolescent, and the parents. Nurses establish a comfortable, yet professional rapport that forms the foundation for the ongoing therapeutic relationship. Nurses accomplish this by developing communication and interviewing skills that incorporate the needs of both the parent and child or adolescent, treating both as equal partners.

INTERVIEWING PARENTS

The parental interview entails more than just fact gathering. The tone of future contacts is established as parents begin to develop a trusting relationship with the nurse. Parents expect health professionals to be sources of information and education, and they assess professional competence during the initial contact. Therefore, it is important that the nurse use a friendly, nonjudgmental approach while demonstrating proficiency as a practitioner. Rarely is the interview just data gathering; it is also a forum for rapport building, explaining, and health teaching (Fig. 24-2).

Introductory Stage

As with all clients, the nurse–parent relationship begins with the introduction, when nurses explain their roles and the purpose of the interview. Clarification and consistency are crucial from the start because parents may be anxious about the child's condition or uncomfortable about their role, especially if the setting is a hospital. Anxiety may be overt or masked, even demonstrated by negative behaviors such as hostility.

Cultural variations may also affect parental reactions and response. Active listening facilitates the use of leads and better enables nurses to keep the interview focused on specific concerns. It also allows nurses to uncover clues that further the interview, to seek validation of perceptions and

responses that may have alternate meanings, and to provide reassurance for both the expressed and hidden concerns that parents may be experiencing.

Encouraging Talk

By encouraging parents to talk, nurses can identify information that affects all aspects of a child's life. Some parents take the lead without prompting (eg, "He's been pulling up his legs like he's in pain"). Others offer vague concerns (eg, ". . . she's just not acting right") and need more direction. However, all have significant information about their child. Nurses can further encourage verbalization through communication techniques such as open-ended questioning ("How does Jamie behave when she isn't acting just right?") and focus directing ("When does Darryl have the pain?"). Communication skills allow nurses to elicit information in all patient groups, even in the most difficult situations.

The atmosphere should create an exchange of information rather than one directed solely by the nurse. Nurses use problem solving, collaboration, and anticipatory guidance. For example, the parent could be asked, "What do you see as the problem?" Once the problem is identified, the parent can be led through the problem-solving process to arrive at a solution. Parents should also be asked what they found to be effective or ineffective in managing their child's problems. Anticipatory guidance promotes an exchange because parents can better participate in discussions of their child's future developmental trends.

Nurses should also be aware of the barriers to effective nurse–parent communication. These include time constraints, frequent interruptions, lack of privacy, and language differences, as well as provider callousness and cultural insensitivity. Nurses must make every effort possible to avoid these barriers. Adequate time and privacy should be allotted for every interview, with interruptions kept at a minimum. Interpreters can assist when language differences are present. Nurses should always display a warm, professional manner when interacting with clients and families, and they should be sensitive to cultural differences displayed in values, beliefs, and customs.

INTERVIEWING CHILDREN AND ADOLESCENTS

As noted earlier, the child or adolescent and parent are treated as equal partners in the health care triad. The child is included in the introductory stage of the interview and is

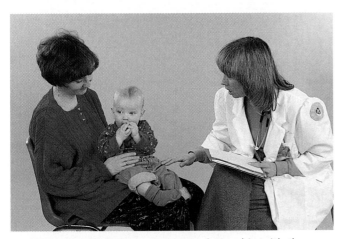

FIGURE 24-2. Developing a trusting relationship with the parent(s) is an essential aspect of the interview process. (© B. Proud.)

observed for signs of readiness to evaluate the level of participation. Readiness evaluation includes questioning the parents about how the child copes with stressful situations and what the child has been told about this particular health encounter.

Play As Communication

Nurses should talk to the child at eye level (be aware of cultural variations in eye contact) and actively engage children through play and verbalization. Play is one of the most valuable communication techniques when working with children, and it allows for the discovery of important cues to children's development and illness behaviors (Display 24-1). Rushing creates anxiety; therefore, time should be taken to listen and to allow children to feel comfortable. Privacy and confidentiality are important in pediatric nursing, especially when assessing the adolescent. Children or adolescents may be anxious, fearful, or embarrassed. Their emotions should be respected.

The interview process and assessment procedures should be explained in terms that are clear and honest. Directions should be stated in a positive manner, and choices should be offered only when available and appropriate. Honest praise is used to reinforce positive behaviors; gratuitous praise is quickly recognized by children and may decrease the child's trust in the nurse.

Touch

Touch is a powerful communication tool, especially for the infant who calms when cuddled or patted. However, the older infant and child may find touch intrusive if the nurse has not yet begun to formulate a relationship with the child. Cultural taboos may also prohibit touch. Therefore, it is

prudent to communicate with the child at a "safe distance" until the relationship begins to form.

Direct communication, such as open-ended and closed-ended questions, age-appropriate humor, and dialogue strategies, is usually more beneficial when used with indirect communication techniques, including sentence completion, mutual story telling, and using drawings, play (the universal language of children), and magic.

Developmental Considerations

Nurses should also be familiar with developmentally oriented approaches to interviewing children. Display 24-2 presents specific developmentally oriented approaches that may be used in interviewing children and adolescents.

These approaches are important to know because barriers can exist when communicating with children. For example, some nurses overestimate the understanding abilities of young children and underestimate those of older children and adolescents. This creates frustration for all involved. Nurses need to be habitually aware of children's cognitive status when interacting with them. Another barrier develops when the child is excluded altogether. Children and adolescents can be eager participants and should be treated as such.

Finally, although many children are eager participants, others need encouragement, especially toddlers and preschoolers who may react with crying and lack of cooperation. Nurses should avoid power struggles and, instead, rely on empathy, developmental strategies, parental assistance, and a good sense of humor.

Adolescent Concerns

Adolescents are neither children nor adults and, therefore, should be treated accordingly. Privacy is essential, as are respect and confidentiality. General health issues may or may not be discussed with the parent present. However, sensitive issues, such as sex, sexuality, drugs, and alcohol, are best handled without parental presence. Trust and genuineness are important; nurses should not "talk down" to adolescents or mimic their language style. The approach should be as a professional, not as a peer, parent, or big sister or brother (Fig. 24-3). Open-ended and specific questions are used to avoid "yes/no" answers, and silence is used sparingly because it may be viewed as threatening to this age group.

Nurses should also be aware of their own nonverbal and facial expressions. Delicate issues should be approached with sensitivity and a nonjudgmental, matter-of-fact manner to keep them from appearing to be focal points. History taking provides an excellent opportunity for health teaching with adolescents, who are eager to learn about their ever-changing bodies. Questions should be encouraged and answered throughout the history.

DISPLAY 24-1. Characteristics of Play Among Children

Play is often called the "work" of children. Play demonstrates how children develop, interact, think and perform. Some typical play characteristics of specific childhood groups follow:

INFANTS

Play reflects infants' development and awareness of the environment. Infants engage in basically solitary (noninteractive) play. They develop sensory and motor skills by manipulating toys and other objects.

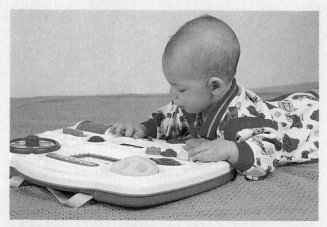

TODDLERS

Toddlers engage in parallel play—they play alongside, not with, others. Imitation is one of the most common forms of play and locomotion skills can be enhanced with push-pull toys. Toddlers change toys frequently because of short attention spans.

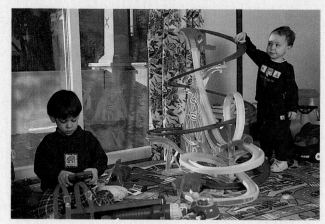

PRESCHOOLERS

Typical preschool play is associative—interactive and co-operative with sharing. Preschoolers need contact with age mates. Activities, such as jumping, running and climbing, promote growth and motor skills. Pre-schoolers are at a typical age for imaginary playmates. Imitative, imaginative, and dramatic play are important. TV and video games should only be a part of the child's play and parents should monitor content and amount of time spent in use. Associative play materials include dress-up clothes and dolls, housekeeping toys, play tents, puppets, and doctor and nurse kits. Curious and active preschoolers need adult supervision, especially near bodies of water and gym sets.

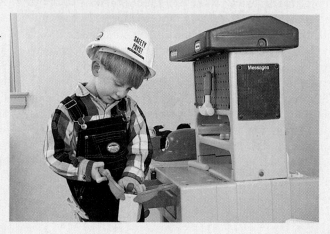

(continued)

DISPLAY 24-1. *Characteristics of Play Among Children* (Continued)

SCHOOL-AGE CHILDREN

Play becomes more competitive and complex during the school-age period. Characteristic activities include joining team sports, secret clubs, and "gangs"; scouting or like activities; working complex puzzles, collecting, playing quiet board games, reading, and hero worshiping. Rules and rituals are important aspects of play and games.

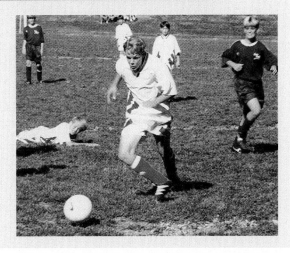

Nursing History

The complete pediatric nursing history is one of the most crucial components of child health care. Many of the materials and questions are unique to this population. The nursing history interview usually provides an opportunity to observe the caregiver– or parent–child interaction and to participate in early detection of health problems and prevention of future difficulties.

Nurses must have the communication skills needed to elicit data about the child and family within a framework that incorporates biographic data, current health status, past history, family history, a review of each body system, knowledge of growth and development, and lifestyle and health practices–related information. It is important to keep in mind that data collected in one category may have relevance to another category. For example, data collected about the condition of the child's skin, hair, and nails may indicate a problem in the area of nutrition.

DEMOGRAPHIC–BIOGRAPHICAL INFORMATION

Gathering this type of information is a good way to begin the health history. It consists of general, easy-to-answer information that puts the parent and child at ease. It also can provide the nurse with important clues that can benefit the rest of the subjective examination. For example, discovering that a 5-year-old child lives in the city with his 40-year-old professional parents and no brothers or sisters may give the nurse clues about his developmental level, activity, relationships, and socioeconomic status. However, the nurse must be careful not to make quick assumptions based on demographic or biographical data.

These types of questions are often asked on a form that the parent fills out before the assessment. However, the nurse should go over the form with the parent and child (if feasible) at the beginning of the assessment. Typical data include the following:

What is the child's name? Nickname?

What are the parents' or caregivers' names?

Who is the child's primary health care provider, and when was the child's last well-child care appointment? (Table 24-3 provides guidelines for primary health care provider visits developed by the Committee on Practice and Ambulatory Medicine and the American Academy of Pediatrics [AAP]).

Where does the child live? (Address)

Do the parents and child live in the same residence?

Who else lives in this residence?

Are the child's parents married, single, divorced, homosexual?

What is the child's age?

What are the parents' ages?

What is the child's date of birth?

Is the child adopted, foster, natural?

What is the child's ethnic origin? Religion?

What do the child's parents do for a living?

CURRENT HEALTH STATUS

As with adults, it is important to obtain information regarding the child's current status of health. Nurses should ask the parent, and child if possible, to describe the child's general state of health and compare it with how it was 1 and 5 years ago (if age appropriate). If the answer is "good," ask what "good" means to them. "Good" could mean "only one cold this year" for a generally healthy child or "only two hospitalizations this year" for a child with a chronic illness such as cystic fibrosis.

Current health status also includes information regarding chronic illnesses and allergies. Chronic illness, such as

DISPLAY 24-2. Age-Specific Interview Techniques

Each child responds differently during the assessment interview according to his or her developmental status, severity and perception of illness, experience with health care, intrusiveness of procedures, and the child's own uniqueness. The following are some guidelines for adapting the interview techniques to the child's status.

INFANTS: SENSORIMOTOR STAGE

Intellect develops and the infant learns about the environment through the senses: Primary infant communication is by nonverbal (crying, smiling) methods and response to the behaviors of others.

- Infant's focus is on the caregiver.
- Use gentle tone of voice and touch with infant. Speak softly. When using touch, remember that older infants are usually wary of strangers.
- Talk to and touch infant before procedures.
- Provide infant with favorite toy.
- Spend time with infant before assessment procedure.
- Infants attend to the human voice and face.
- Be alert to infant's cues (crying, kicking, arm waving).
- Allow child to identify you with parent.

TODDLERS: SENSORIMOTOR TO PREOPERATIONAL STAGES

Trial and error experimentation and relentless exploration are typical in the early toddler stage; later, the toddler uses representational thought in intellectual development. Children under 5 years of age are egocentric. Toddler's attention span ranges between 5 and 10 minutes.

- Encourage parental presence.
- Provide careful and simple explanations just before procedure.
- Use play as a communication technique.
- Tell child it is okay to cry.
- Encourage expression through toys.
- Use simple terminology; child's receptive language is more advanced than his or her expressive language.
- Allow child to be close to parent—be alert for separation anxiety.
- Acknowledge child's favorite toy or a unique characteristic about the child.

PRESCHOOLERS: PREOPERATIONAL STAGE

Preschoolers progress from making simple classifications and associating one event with a simultaneous one to classifying and quantifying and exhibiting intuitive thought processes. A preschooler's attention span ranges between 10 and 15 minutes. Preschoolers use magical thinking.

- Explain why things are as they are, simply.
- Validate child's perceptions.
- Avoid threatening words.
- Use simple visual aids.
- Involve child in teaching by doing something (handling equipment).
- Allow child to ask questions.
- Use child's toys for expression; use miniature equipment on toys.
- Avoid using words that have double meaning.
- Explain sensations that the child will experience.
- Answer "why" questions with simple explanations.
- Be direct and concrete; do not use analogies, abstractions, or words with more than one meaning; avoid slang (such as "laugh your head off"—preschoolers interpret literally).
- Ask simple questions.
- Allow child to manipulate equipment.
- Use the child's active imagination—use toys, puppets, and play.

(continued)

DISPLAY 24-2. Age-Specific Interview Techniques (Continued)

SCHOOL AGE CHILDREN: OPERATIONAL STAGE

Egocentric thinking progresses to objective thinking in school-age children who begin using inductive reasoning, logical operations, and reversible concrete thought. A school-age child's attention span ranges between 30 and 45 minutes. Use books and other visual aids to advance the assessment interview.

- Remember to remain concrete (ie, avoid abstractions).
- Use group discussion to educate children among their peers; also use games.
- Provide health teaching; perform demonstrations.
- Give more responsibility to child.
- School-age children like explanations and need assistance in vocalizing their needs.
- Allow children to engage in discussions.

ADOLESCENTS: FORMAL OPERATIONS STAGE

Abstract thought develops, as does thinking beyond the present and forming theories about everything.

- Give adolescents control whenever possible.
- Use scientific explanations and make expectations clear.
- Explore expected parental level of involvement before initiating it.
- Involve adolescents in planning.
- Clearly explain how body will be affected.
- Anticipate feelings of anger and grief.
- Use peers with common situation to help with teaching.
- Encourage expression of ideas and feelings.
- Maintain confidentiality; facilitate trust.
- Give adolescents your undivided attention.
- Make expectations clear.
- Ask to speak to adolescent alone.
- Encourage open and honest communication.
- Be nonjudgmental; respect views, differences, and feelings.
- Ask open-ended questions.

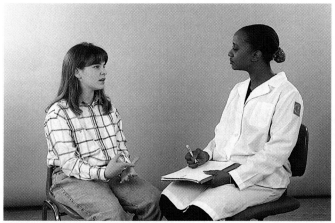

FIGURE 24-3. Handle sensitive issues with adolescents by establishing trust and genuineness. (© B. Proud.)

asthma, or disability, such as cerebral palsy, must be established early in the history to allow for better assessment and teaching strategies. Allergies are very common during childhood. Nurses need to ask what the specific allergen is and how the child reacts to it. Some parents consider medication side effects to be allergic responses (eg, diarrhea that is common after antibiotic use) and need information to differentiate side effects from actual allergies.

Finally, nurses must ask for complete medication and treatment information. This includes prescription and over-the-counter medications, devices and treatments (eg, hot/cold compresses, respiratory therapy, assistive devices, such as orthopedic braces), and home or folk remedies. The child may be taking a combination of medications that are incompatible or a folk remedy that is harmful (eg, azaron, *(text continues on page 602)*

TABLE 24-3. American Academy of Pediatrics—Recommendations for Preventive Pediatric Health Care (RE9939)

Each child and family is unique; therefore, these **Recommendations for Preventive Pediatric Health Care** are designed for the care of children who are receiving competent parenting, have no manifestations of any important health problems, and are growing and developing in satisfactory fashion. Additional visits may become necessary if circumstances suggest variations from normal.

Age[5]	Prenatal[1]	Newborn[2]	2–4 mo[3]	By 1 mo	2 mo	4 mo	6 mo	9 mo	12 mo
History									
Initial/Interval	•	•	•	•	•	•	•	•	•
Measurements									
Height and Weight		•	•	•	•	•	•	•	•
Head Circumference		•	•	•	•	•	•	•	•
Blood Pressure									
Sensory Screening									
Vision		S	S	S	S	S	S	S	S
Hearing		O[7]	S	S	S	S	S	S	S
Developmental Behavioral Assessment[8]		•	•	•	•	•	•	•	•
Physical Examination[9]		•	•	•	•	•	•	•	•
Procedures—General[10]									
Hereditary/Metabolic Screening[11]			←——•——→						
Immunization[12]		•	•	•	•	•	•	•	•
Hematocrit or Hemoglobin[13]								•——→	
Urinalysis									
Procedures—Patient at Risk									
Lead Screening[16]								•——→	
Tuberculin Test[17]									★
Cholesterol Screening[18]									
STD Screening[19]									
Pelvic Exam[20]									
Anticipatory Guidance[21]	•	•	•	•	•	•	•	•	•
Injury Prevention[22]	•	•	•	•	•	•	•	•	•
Violence Prevention[23]	•	•	•	•	•	•	•	•	•
Sleep Positioning Counseling[24]	•	•	•	•	•	•	•		
Nutrition Counseling[25]	•	•	•	•	•	•	•	•	•
Dental Referral[26]									←——

[1] A prenatal visit is recommended for parents who are at high risk, for first-time parents, and for those who request a conference. The prenatal visit should include anticipatory guidance, pertinent medical history, and a discussion of benefits of breastfeeding and planned method of feeding per AAP statement "The Prenatal Visit" (1996).

[2] Every infant should have a newborn evaluation after birth. Breastfeeding should be encouraged and instruction and support offered. Every breastfeeding infant should have an evaluation 48–72 hours after discharge from the hospital to include weight, formal breastfeeding evaluation, encouragement, and instruction as recommended in the AAP statement "Breastfeeding and the Use of Human Milk" (1997).

[3] For newborns discharged in less than 48 hours after delivery per AAP statement "Hospital Stay for Healthy Term Newborns" (1995).

[4] Developmental, psychosocial, and chronic disease issues for children and adolescents may require frequent counseling and treatment visits separate from preventive care visits.

[5] If a child comes under care for the first time at any point on the schedule, or if any items are not accomplished at the suggested age, the schedule should be brought up to date at the earliest possible time.

[6] If the patient is uncooperative, rescreen within 6 months.

[7] All newborns should be screened per the AAP Task Force on Newborn and Infant Hearing statement, "Newborn and Infant Hearing Loss: Detection and Intervention" (1999).

[8] By history and appropriate physical examination: if suspicious, by specific objective developmental testing. Parenting skills should be fostered at every visit.

[9] At each visit, a complete physical examination is essential, with infant totally unclothed, older child undressed and suitably draped.

[10] These may be modified, depending on entry point into schedule and individual need.

[11] Metabolic screening (eg, thyroid, hemoglobinopathies, PKU, galactosemia) should be done according to state law.

[12] Schedule(s) per the Committee on Infectious Diseases, published annually in the January edition of *Pediatrics.* Every visit should be an opportunity to update and complete a child's immunizations.

[13] See AAP *Pediatric Nutrition Handbook* (1998) for a discussion of universal and selective screening options. Consider earlier screening for high-risk infants (eg, premature infants and low-birth-weight infants). See also "Recommendations to Prevent and Control Iron Deficiency in the United States." *MMWR.* 1998;47 (RR-3):1–29.

[14] All menstruating adolescents should be screened annually.

[15] Conduct dipstick urinalysis for leukocytes annually for sexually active male and female adolescents.

[16] For children at risk of lead exposure, consult the AAP statement "Screening for Elevated Blood Levels" (1998). Additionally, screening should be done in accordance with state law where applicable.

[17] TB testing per recommendations of the Committee on Infectious Diseases, published in the current edition of *Red Book: Report of the Committee on Infectious Diseases.* Testing should be done upon recognition of high-risk factors.

These guidelines represent a consensus by the Committee on Practice and Ambulatory Medicine in consultation with national committees and sections of the American Academy of Pediatrics. The Committee emphasizes the great importance of continuity of care in comprehensive health supervision and the need to avoid fragmentation of care.

	Early Childhood[4]					Middle Childhood[4]				Adolescence[4]										
	15 mo	18 mo	24 mo	3 y	4 y	5 y	6 y	8 y	10 y	11 y	12 y	13 y	14 y	15 y	16 y	17 y	18 y	19 y	20 y	21 y
	•	•	•	•	•	•	•	•	•	•	•	•	•	•	•	•	•	•	•	•
	•	•	•	•	•	•	•	•	•	•	•	•	•	•	•	•	•	•	•	•
	•	•	•																	
				•	•	•	•	•	•	•	•	•	•	•	•	•	•	•	•	•
	S	S	S	O[6]	O	O	O	O	O	S	O	S	S	O	S	S	O	S	S	S
	S	S	S	S	O	O	O	O	O	S	O	S	S	O	S	S	O	S	S	S
	•	•	•	•	•	•	•	•	•	•	•	•	•	•	•	•	•	•	•	•
	•	•	•	•	•	•	•	•	•	•	•	•	•	•	•	•	•	•	•	•
	•	•	•	•	•	•	•	•	•	•	•	•	•	•	•	•	•	•	•	•
	★	★	★	★	★	★				◄————————— •[14] ————————————————————————————►										
						•				◄————————————————————— [15] ————————————————————————►										
			★																	
	★	★	★	★	★	★	★	★	★	★	★	★	★	★	★	★	★	★	★	★
			★	★	★	★	★	★	★	★	★	★	★	★	★	★	★	★	★	★
										★	★	★	★	★	★	★	★	★	★	★
										★	★	★	★	★	★	★	◄——★[20]——►			★
	•	•	•	•	•	•	•	•	•	•	•	•	•	•	•	•	•	•	•	•
	•	•	•	•	•	•	•	•	•	•	•	•	•	•	•	•	•	•	•	•
	•	•	•	•	•	•	•	•	•	•	•	•	•	•	•	•	•	•	•	•
	•	•	•	•	•	•	•	•	•	•	•	•	•	•	•	•	•	•	•	•
◄————————————————————— •																			

[18] Cholesterol screening for high-risk patients per AAP statement "Cholesterol in Childhood" (1998). If family history cannot be ascertained and other risk factors are present, screening should be at the discretion of the physician.

[19] All sexually active patients should be screened for sexually transmitted diseases (STDs).

[20] All sexually active females should have a pelvic examination. A pelvic examination and routine Pap smear should be offered as part of preventive health maintenance between the ages of 18 and 21 years.

[21] Age-appropriate discussion and counseling should be an integral part of each visit for care per the AAP Guidelines for Health Supervision III (1998).

[22] From birth to age 12, refer to the AAP injury prevention program (TIPP(r)) as described in A Guide to Safety Counseling in Office Practice (1994).

[23] Violence prevention and management for all patients per AAP Statement "The Role of the Pediatrician in Youth Violence Prevention in Clinical Practice and at the Community Level" (1999).

[24] Parents and caregivers should be advised to place healthy infants on their backs when putting them to sleep. Side positioning is a reasonable alternative but carries a slightly higher risk of SIDS. Consult the AAP statement "Changing Concepts of Sudden Infant Death Syndrome: Implications for Infant Sleeping Environment and Sleep Position" (2000).

[25] Age-appropriate nutrition counseling should be an integral part of each visit per the AAP Handbook of Nutrition (1998).

[26] Earlier initial dental examinations may be appropriate for some children. Subsequent examinations as prescribed by dentist.

Key:
• = to be performed
S = subjective, by history
¬•¬ = the range during which a service may be provided, with the dot indicating the preferred age
★ = to be performed for patients at risk
O = objective, by a standard testing method
NB: Special chemical, immunologic, and endocrine testing is usually carried out upon specific indications. Testing other than newborn (eg, inborn errors of metabolism, sickle disease, etc) is discretionary with the physician.
The recommendations in this statement do not indicate an exclusive course of treatment or serve as a standard of medical care. Variations, taking into account individual circumstances, may be appropriate.
Copyright © 2000 by the American Academy of Pediatrics.

used in Mexico for digestive problems, contains lead). As with adults, children's medication information should include the name of the drug, dosage, frequency, and the reason why the medication is administered.

CURRENT SYMPTOMS

The purpose of asking about the child's current health status is to determine why the child was brought in for an examination. For some examinations, the child and parents may have no symptoms to report. In this case, the parent and child should be asked to describe the general state of the child's health.

If there is a perceived problem with the child's health or if the child or parent notices symptoms, the same focus questions that are asked for each body system for the adult client are used for the child (eg, location, intensity, duration). However, for the child, it is important to ask both the parent and the child (if possible) to get the most accurate information. Conflicting information may clue the nurse in to other areas that may need to be assessed. When asking the child about symptoms, the following techniques are usually helpful:

Ask the child to point with one finger to where the pain or symptom is located.

Use a pain scale developed for children, such as the FACES Pain Rating Scale (six characters ranging from a happy face signifying no pain to a tearful face signifying the worst pain); the Oucher scale (six photographs of children's faces ranging from "no hurt" to "biggest hurt you could ever have"; also comes with scale from 0 to 100); or a numeric scale (straight line with numbers from 0 to 10 representing no pain to worst pain). Figure 24-4 illustrates the FACES and numeric pain-rating scales.

PAST HISTORY

Past history is important information to collect when assessing children. Certain problems and conditions can be associated with a difficult birth experience, whether the child was immunized, genetic conditions acquired from parents, and the like. Obviously, most of this information must come from the birth parent. If the child is a foster child or adopted, some of the information may be obtained from hospital records.

Sample nursing history questions include:

Was your pregnancy planned?
When did you first receive prenatal care?
How was your general health during pregnancy?
Did you have any problems with your pregnancy?
Did you take any medications during pregnancy?
Did you have any accidents during this pregnancy?
Did you use any tobacco, alcohol, or drugs during this pregnancy?
Where was the child born?
What type of delivery did you have?
Were there any problems during the delivery?
What was the child's Apgar score?
What were the child's weight, height, and head circumference?
Did the child have any problems after birth (eg, feeding, jaundice)?
Has the child ever been hospitalized?
Has the child ever had any major illnesses?
Has the child ever experienced any major injuries?
Does the child have a history of allergies?
What immunizations has the child received thus far? (Table 24-4)
Has your child had any reactions to immunizations?

Wong-Baker FACES Pain Rating Scale

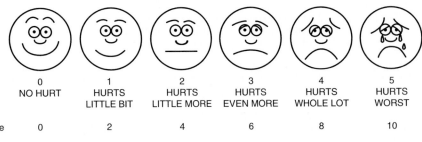

| 0 NO HURT | 1 HURTS LITTLE BIT | 2 HURTS LITTLE MORE | 3 HURTS EVEN MORE | 4 HURTS WHOLE LOT | 5 HURTS WORST |

| Alternative coding | 0 | 2 | 4 | 6 | 8 | 10 |

Explain to the person that each face is for a person who feels happy because he has no pain (hurt) or sad because he has some or a lot of pain. Face 0 is very happy because he doesn't hurt at all. Face 1 hurts just a little bit. Face 2 hurts a little more. Face 3 hurts even more. Face 4 hurts a whole lot. Face 5 hurts as much as you can imagine, although you don't have to be crying to feel this bad. Ask the person to choose the face that best describes how he is feeling.

Rating scale is recommended for persons age 3 years and older.

Brief word instructions: Point to each face using the words to describe the pain intensity. Ask the child to choose face that best describes own pain and record the appropriate number.

FIGURE 24-4. Pain rating scales: numerical scale and FACES pain rating scale (Wong, D. L., Hockenberry-Eaton, M., Wilson D., Winkelstein, M. L., & Schwartz, P. [2001]. *Wong's essentials of pediatric nursing* [6th ed.]. St. Louis: Mosby. Copyrighted by Mosby, Inc. Reprinted by permission.)

TABLE 24-4. Recommended Childhood Immunization Schedule United States, January–December 2001

Vaccines[1] are listed under routinely recommended ages. Bars indicate range of recommended ages for immunization. Any dose not given at the recommended age should be given as a "catch-up" immunization at any subsequent visit when indicated and feasible. Ovals indicate vaccines to be given if previously recommended doses were missed or given earlier than the recommended minimum age.

Age ▶ Vaccine ▼	Birth	1 mo	2 mos	4 mos	6 mos	12 mos	15 mos	18 mos	24 mos	4–6 yrs	11–12 yrs	14–18 yrs
Hepatitis B[2]		Hep B #1										
			Hep B #2			Hep B #3					(Hep B[2])	
Diphtheria, Tetanus, Pertussis[3]			DTaP	DTaP	DTaP		DTaP[3]			DTaP	Td	
H. influenzae type b[4]			Hib	Hib	Hib	Hib						
Inactivated Polio[5]			IPV	IPV		IPV[5]				IPV[5]		
Pneumococcal Conjugate[6]			PCV	PCV	PCV	PCV						
Measles, Mumps, Rubella[7]						MMR				MMR[7]	(MMR[7])	
Varicella[8]						Var					(Var[8])	
Hepatitis A[9]										Hep A-in selected areas[9]		

[1] This schedule indicates the recommended ages for routine administration of currently licensed childhood vaccines, as of 11/1/00, for children through 18 years of age. Additional vaccines may be licensed and recommended during the year. Licensed combination vaccines may be used whenever any components of the combination are indicated and its other components are not contraindicated. Providers should consult the manufacturers' package inserts for detailed recommendations.

[2] *Infants born to HBsAg-negative mothers* should receive the 1st dose of hepatitis B (Hep B) vaccine by age 2 months. The 2nd dose should be at least one month after the 1st dose. The 3rd dose should be administered at least 4 months after the 1st dose and at least 2 months after the 2nd dose, but not before 6 months of age for infants.

Infants born to HBsAg-positive mothers should receive hepatitis B vaccine and 0.5 mL hepatitis B immune globulin (HBIG) within 12 hours of birth at separate sites. The 2nd dose is recommended at 1–2 months of age and the 3rd dose at 6 months of age.

Infants born to mothers whose HBsAg status is unknown should receive hepatitis B vaccine within 12 hours of birth. Maternal blood should be drawn at the time of delivery to determine the mother's HBsAg status; if the HBsAg test is positive, the infant should receive HBIG as soon as possible (no later than 1 week of age).

All children and adolescents who have not been immunized against hepatitis B should begin the series during any visit. Special efforts should be made to immunize children who were born in or whose parents were born in areas of the world with moderate or high endemicity of hepatitis B virus infection.

[3] The 4th dose of DTaP (diphtheria and tetanus toxoids and acellular pertussis vaccine) may be administered as early as 12 months of age, provided 6 months have elapsed since the 3rd dose and the child is unlikely to return at age 15–18 months. Td (tetanus and diphtheria toxoids) is recommended at 11–12 years of age if at least 5 years have elapsed since the last dose of DTP, DTaP or DT. Subsequent routine Td boosters are recommended every 10 years.

[4] Three *Haemophilus influenzae* type b (Hib) conjugate vaccines are licensed for infant use. If PRP-OMP (PedvaxHIB® or ComVax® [Merck]) is administered at 2 and 4 months of age, a dose at 6 months is not required. Because clinical studies in infants have demonstrated that using some combination products may induce a lower immune response to the Hib vaccine component, DTaP/Hib combination products should not be used for primary immunization in infants at 2, 4 or 6 months of age, unless FDA-approved for these ages.

[5] An all-IPV schedule is recommended for routine childhood polio vaccination in the United States. All children should receive four doses of IPV at 2 months, 4 months, 6–18 months, and 4–6 years of age. Oral polio vaccine (OPV) should be used only in selected circumstances. (See *MMWR Morb Mortal Wkly Rep* May 19, 2000/49 (RR-5);1–22).

[6] The heptavalent conjugate pneumococcal vaccine (PCV) is recommended for all children 2–23 months of age. It also is recommended for certain children 24–59 months of age. (See *MMWR Morb Mortal Wkly Rep* Oct. 6, 2000/49(RR-9);1–35).

[7] The 2nd dose of measles, mumps, and rubella (MMR) vaccine is recommended routinely at 4–6 years of age but may be administered during any visit, provided at least 4 weeks have elapsed since receipt of the 1st dose and that both doses are administered beginning at or after 12 months of age. Those who have not previously received the second dose should complete the schedule by the 11–12 year old visit.

[8] Varicella (Var) vaccine is recommended at any visit on or after the first birthday for susceptible children, i.e. those who lack a reliable history of chickenpox (as judged by a health care provider) and who have not been immunized. Susceptible persons 13 years of age or older should receive 2 doses, given at least 4 weeks apart.

[9] Hepatitis A (Hep A) is shaded to indicate its recommended use in selected states and/or regions, and for certain high risk groups; consult your local public health authority. (See *MMWR Morb Mortal Wkly Rep* Oct. 1, 1999/48(RR-12); 1–37).

Approved by the Advisory Committee on Immunization Practices (ACIP), the American Academy of Pediatrics (AAP), and the American Academy of Family Physicians (AAFP).

For additional information about the vaccines listed above, please visit the National Immunization Program Home Page at www.cdc.gov/nip or call the National Immunization Hotline at 800-232-2522 (English) or 800-232-0233 (Spanish).

FAMILY HISTORY AND REVIEW OF SYSTEMS

The questions asked about family history for the child are basically the same types of questions that are asked of the adult client (eg, whether certain diseases/conditions run in the family, the age and cause of death for blood relatives, and family members with communicable diseases). This is an area of the subjective assessment in which the nurse focuses primarily on the parent for the necessary information. An exception might be if the child is older and knows a great deal about his or her family history. As with the past history information, if the child is adopted or a foster child, family history information may not be known. An important reason for collecting these data is to implement preventive teaching at a young age.

It is essential that pertinent subjective data be collected for each body system. Many of the questions for each body system asked of the adult are asked of the parent or child. The additional nursing history questions listed in the following sections for each system are of special concern in children.

Skin, Hair, Nails

Has your child had any changes in hair texture?
Does your child complain of scalp itching? (May indicate lice, seborrhea, allergies, ringworm)
Have you noticed any changes in your child's nails? Color? Cracking? Shape? Lines?
Does your child bite his or her nails?
Has your child been exposed to any contagious diseases such as measles, chickenpox, lice, ringworm, scabies, and the like?
Has your child ever had any rashes? Acne?
Has your child had any excessive bruising?
Does your child use any cosmetics? Have tattoos? Have any pierced body parts?

Head and Neck

Has your child ever had a head injury?
Does your child experience headaches? How frequently?
Has your child ever had swollen neck glands for any significant length of time?
Has your child ever experienced any neck stiffness?

Eyes and Vision

Does your infant have any unusual eye movements?
Does your infant/child excessively cross eyes?
Does your infant blink when necessary?
Is your infant able to focus on moving objects?
Has your infant ever had cloudiness in the eyeball?
Does your child frequent rub his or her eyes or blink repeatedly?
Does your child strain/squint to see distant objects?
Has your child's vision been tested?
Does your child wear glasses or contact lenses?

Ears and Hearing

Does your child appear to be paying attention when you speak? (Infants and children should respond to the human voice.)
Does your child or adolescent listen to loud music? (This is common behavior among adolescents and usually does not indicate hearing deficit. However, it can lead to a hearing deficit.)
Does your child use a hearing aid?
Has your child had frequent ear infections? Tubes in ears?
How frequently does your child have his or her hearing tested?

Mouth, Throat, Nose, Sinuses

Has your child ever had any difficulty swallowing or chewing?
Has your child ever had strep throat or any problems affecting the mouth?
Has your infant had thrush?
Does your child get frequent oral lesions?
Does your child have any dental problems?
Does your child wear any dental devices (braces)?
Does your child experience nosebleeds?
Does your child have any sinus problems?

Thorax and Lungs

Has your child ever had cough, wheezing, shortness of breath, nocturnal dyspnea; if so, when does it occur?
Does your child smoke?
Is your child exposed to second-hand smoke?
(Adolescents and older school-age children should be asked about smoking, including smokeless tobacco, in private.)

Heart and Neck Vessels

Has your child ever experienced chest pain, heart murmurs, congenital heart disease, hypertension?
Does your infant become fatigued or short of breath during feedings?
Has your child ever complained of fatigue?
Does your child have difficulty keeping up with peers when running or exercising?
Has your child ever fainted?
Has your child ever turned "blue" during activity?
Do you believe that your child is meeting the normal growth requirements for his or her age?

Breasts and Lymphatics

Has your daughter started developing breasts (thelarche)? If so, when did development start?
Have you noticed any abnormal breast development in your son or young daughter?

Have you noticed any swollen glands under your child's arms (axillary glands)?

Have you noticed any discharge from your infant's nipples?

Abdomen

Has your child ever had any excessive vomiting? Abdominal pain? Please describe.

Does your child have any digestive problems (ie, irritable bowel)?

Has your child ever experienced any trauma to the abdomen?

Does your child have any hernias?

Genitalia and Sexuality

How often does your child urinate? How many wet diapers do you change per day?

At what age was your child toilet (bladder) trained? Night?

Does your child ever wet his or her pants? (History of enuresis; if positive history, obtain routine that family follows to deal with problem.)

Is there any history of frequency, burning, pain during urination?

Do you have any concerns about your child related to masturbation, asking/answering questions about sex, not respecting other's privacy, wanting too much privacy?

Has anyone ever touched your child in a way that made him or her feel uncomfortable? (Make sure to ask the parent and child this question.)

Does your child engage in any sexually precocious activity/play?

Does your child recognize whether he or she is male or female?

What words does your child use to describe body parts?

Have parents discussed sex/sexuality topics with the child?

Has child started puberty, thelarche, menarche?

Has the child started having wet dreams (nocturnal emissions)?

Who is/are the source(s) of sex/AIDS education? Questions to the adolescent about sexuality and reproductive issues should be asked privately.

Do you know how to perform breast self-examination or testicular self-examination? (see Performing BSE/TSE in Appendix C)

How old were you when you started menstruating?

When was your last menstrual period?

What is your menstrual cycle schedule? Has it always been this way?

What is your bleeding like? Light, moderate, heavy?

Do you experience any cramps? Tell me about them.

Do you experience any other physical or emotional discomfort associated with menstruation?

Do you use tampons? How frequently do you change them?

What is your sexual preference?

What was your age at first intercourse?

Do you experience any discomfort/pain with intercourse?

How many sexual partners do you have/have you had?

What type of contraception do you use and how do you use it?

Do you use condoms? How do you use them? (To ascertain correct condom usage)

Have you ever had a sexually transmitted disease?

Were you ever pregnant? What was the result of that pregnancy?

Have you had or considered having a gynecologic examination? (Should be performed for all sexually active adolescent girls and is suggested as a routine examination for those older than 18 years of age.)

Anus and Rectum

How often does your child have a bowel movement? What does it look like?

At what age was your child toilet trained (bowel)?

Does your child ever soil his or her pants? (History of encopresis; if positive history, obtain routine that family follows to deal with problem.)

Is there any history of bleeding, constipation, diarrhea, rectal itching, or hemorrhoids?

(Hemorrhoids are very unusual in children, unless chronically constipated. They may indicate an intra-abdominal mass or child abuse [sodomy].)

Peripheral Vascular

Does your child ever experience bluing of the extremities?

Does your child's hands and or feet get unusually cold?

Has your child ever had problems with blood clots?

Musculoskeletal

Has your child ever had limited range of motion, joint pain, stiffness, paralysis?

Has your child ever had any fractures?

Has your child ever used any corrective devices (orthopedic shoes, scoliosis brace)?

Describe your child's posture.

Neurologic

Does you child have any learning disabilities?

Does your child have any attention problems at home or at school?

Has your child ever experienced any problems with memory?

Has your child ever had a seizure?

Has your child ever had a head injury?

Has your child ever experienced any problems with motor coordination?

GROWTH AND DEVELOPMENT

Nurses must possess a baseline knowledge of the fundamental principles of growth and development, as well as strategies for assessment and client teaching. Several theories exist regarding the various stages and phases of development. It is suggested that nurses review the basic principles of the major theorists, such as Erikson and Piaget, to refresh their frame of reference. Information about these theorists is readily accessible in any basic or developmental psychology text.

Growth Patterns

Infants. The best indicator of good overall health in an infant is steady growth in height, weight, and head and chest circumference. Birth length usually increases 50% by 12 months (Display 24-3).

Birth weight doubles by 6 months and triples by 12 months. Head circumference (HC) or occipital frontal circumference (OFC) rapidly increases the first 6 months, then growth slows during the second 6-month period. By 12 months of age, the OFC has increased 33% and brain weight has increased two and one half times from birth.

As the OFC diameter increases, the fontanelles begin narrowing. At birth, the posterior fontanelle is triangular and measures 0.5 to 1.0 cm. The anterior fontanelle is diamond shaped and measures 4 to 5 cm at birth. By 18 months, each fontanelle is usually closed.

Toddlers. Height and weight increase in a steplike rather than a linear fashion, reflecting the growth spurts and lags characteristic of toddlerhood (Table 24-5). The toddler's characteristic protruding abdomen results from underdeveloped abdominal muscles. Bow-leggedness typically persists through toddlerhood because the leg muscles must bear the weight of the relatively large trunk. The height at age 2 years approximately equals one half of the child's adult height. The child's birth weight quadruples by age 2.5 years. HC equals chest circumference by 1 to 2 years. Total increase in HC in the second year of life is 2.5 cm, and the rate then increases slowly at 0.5 inch per year until age 5 years. Primary dentition (20 deciduous teeth) is completed by 2.5 years.

Preschoolers. Preschoolers are generally slender, graceful, and agile. The average 4-year-old child is 101.25 cm tall and weighs 16.8 kg (37 lb).

School-Age Children. During the school-age period, girls often grow faster than boys and commonly surpass them in height and weight. During preadolescence, extending from about age 10 to 13, children commonly experience rapid and uneven growth compared with age mates (see Display 24-3). The average 6-year-old child is 112.5 cm tall and weighs 21 kg (46 lb), whereas the average 12-year-old child is 147.5 cm tall and weighs 40 kg (88 lb). Beginning around age 6, permanent teeth erupt, and deciduous teeth are gradually lost. Caries, malocclusion, and periodontal disease become evident.

Adolescents. From 20% to 25% of adult height is achieved in adolescence. Girls grow 5 to 20 cm until about age 16 or 17. Boys grow 10 to 30 cm until about 18 or 20 years of age. From 30% to 50% of adult weight is achieved during adolescence (see Display 24-3). Adolescence encompasses puberty, the period during which primary and secondary sex characteristics begin to develop and reach maturity. In girls, puberty begins between the ages of 8 and 14 years and is completed within 3 years. In boys, puberty begins between the ages of 9 and 16 years and is completed by age 18 or 19. During adolescence, hormonal influence causes important developmental changes.

Body mass reaches adult size, sebaceous glands become active, and eccrine sweat glands become fully functional. Apocrine sweat glands develop, and hair grows in the axillae, areola of the breast, and genital and anal regions. Body hair assumes characteristic distribution patterns, and texture changes (see Tables 24-1 and 24-2).

During puberty, girls experience growth in height, weight, breast development, and pelvic girth with expansion of uterine tissue. Menarche typically occurs about 2.5 years after onset of puberty. Boys experience increases in height, weight, muscle mass, and penis and testicle size. Facial and body hair growth and voice deepening also occur. The onset of spontaneous nocturnal emissions of seminal fluid is an overt sign of puberty, analogous to menarche in girls. Sexual development is evaluated by noting the specific stages that take place in boys and girls. These changes are noted in Tables 24-1 and 24-2.

MOTOR DEVELOPMENT

Infants

Gross Motor. Newborns can turn their heads from side to side when prone unless they are lying on a soft surface. This inability to turn their head while lying on a soft surface makes suffocation a real concern. By 3 months, there is almost no head lag. Infants roll from front to back at 5 months, sit leaning forward by 7 months, and sit unsupported by 8 months (Fig. 24-5). They pull to stand by 9 months, cruise by 10 months, and walk when hand-held by 12 months.

Fine Motor. The grasp reflex is present at birth and strengthens at 1 month. This reflex fades at 3 months, at which time an infant can actively hold a rattle. Five-month-old infants can grasp voluntarily, and 7-month-old infants can hand-to-hand transfer. The pincer grasp develops by 9 months, and 12-month-old infants will attempt to build a two-block tower.

Toddlers

Gross Motor. The major gross motor skill is locomotion. At 15 months, toddlers walk without help (Fig. 24-6). At 18 months, they walk upstairs with one hand held. At

(*text continues on page 617*)

DISPLAY 24-3. Growth Charts: United States

The growth charts on the following pages were developed by the National Center for Health Statistics in collaboration with the National Center for Chronic Disease Prevention and Health Promotion under the auspices of the United States Centers for Disease Control and Prevention (CDC), 2000.

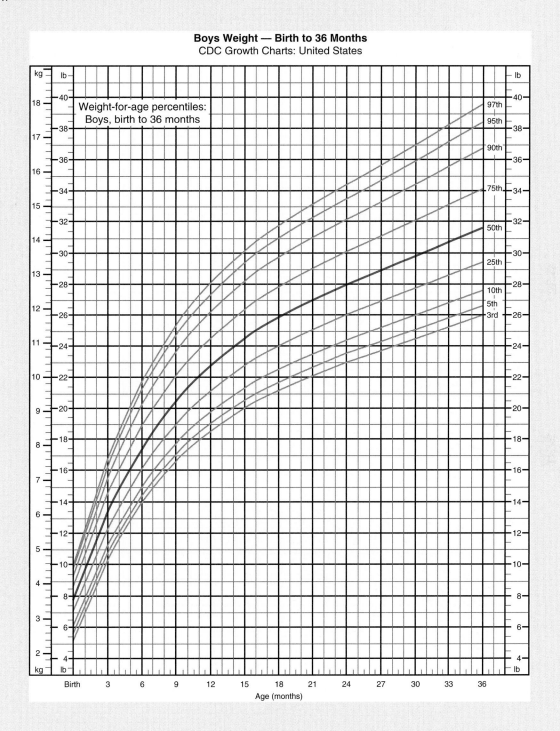

Boys Weight — Birth to 36 Months
CDC Growth Charts: United States

Weight-for-age percentiles:
Boys, birth to 36 months

(continued)

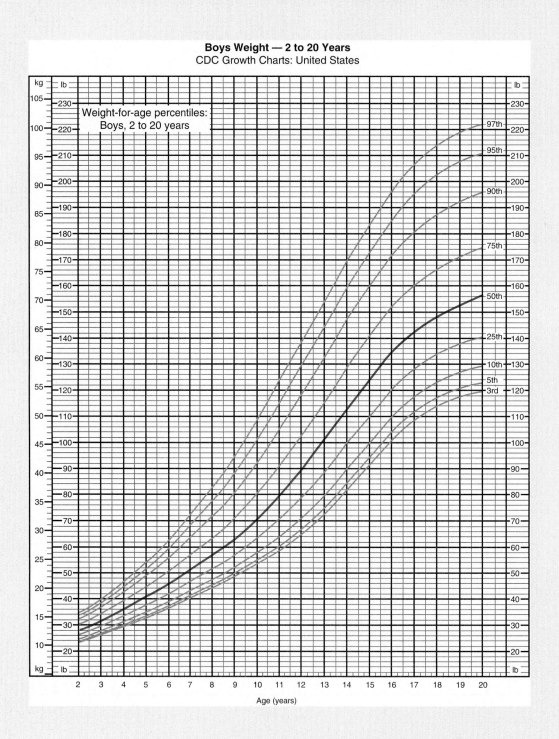

Boys Weight — 2 to 20 Years
CDC Growth Charts: United States

Weight-for-age percentiles:
Boys, 2 to 20 years

Age (years)

(continued)

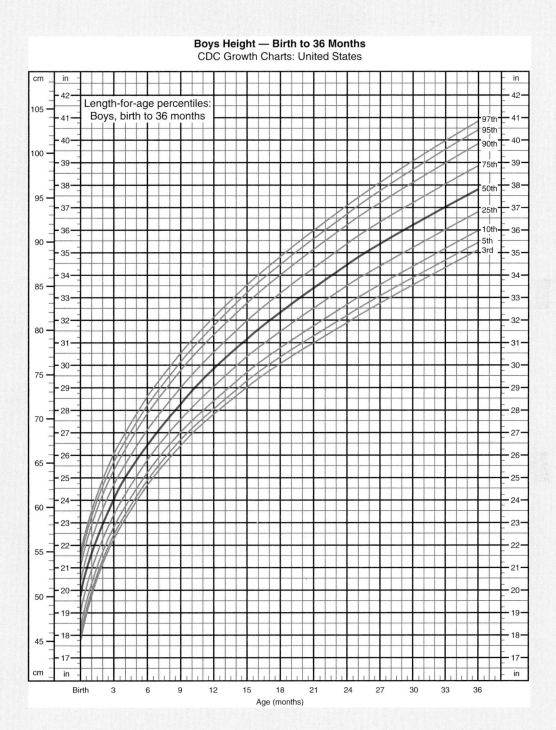

Boys Height — Birth to 36 Months
CDC Growth Charts: United States

Length-for-age percentiles:
Boys, birth to 36 months

Age (months)

(continued)

DISPLAY 24-3. Growth Charts: United States (Continued)

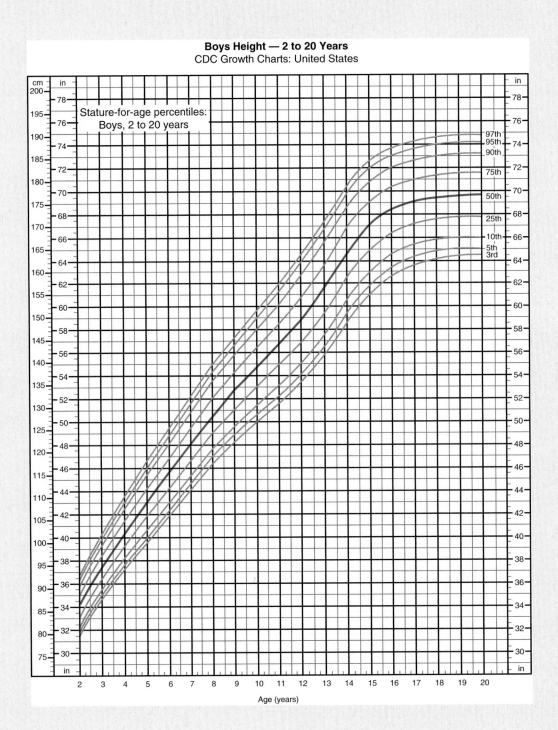

Boys Height — 2 to 20 Years
CDC Growth Charts: United States

Stature-for-age percentiles:
Boys, 2 to 20 years

Age (years)

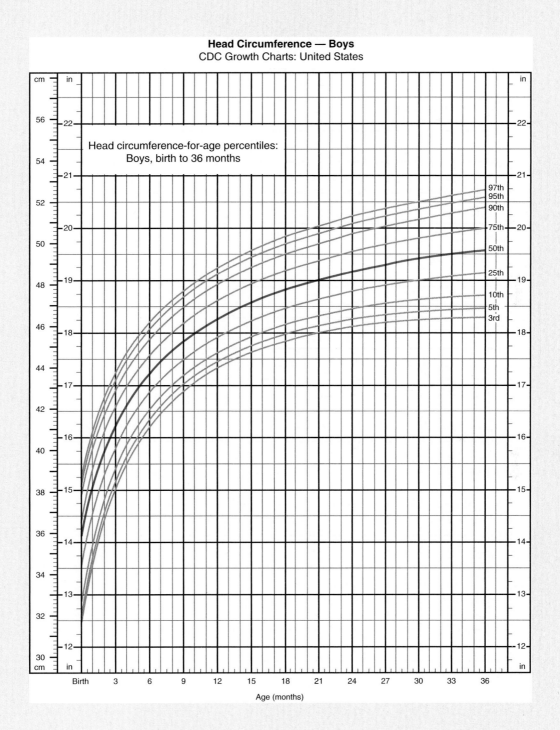

Head Circumference — Boys
CDC Growth Charts: United States

Head circumference-for-age percentiles:
Boys, birth to 36 months

Age (months)

(continued)

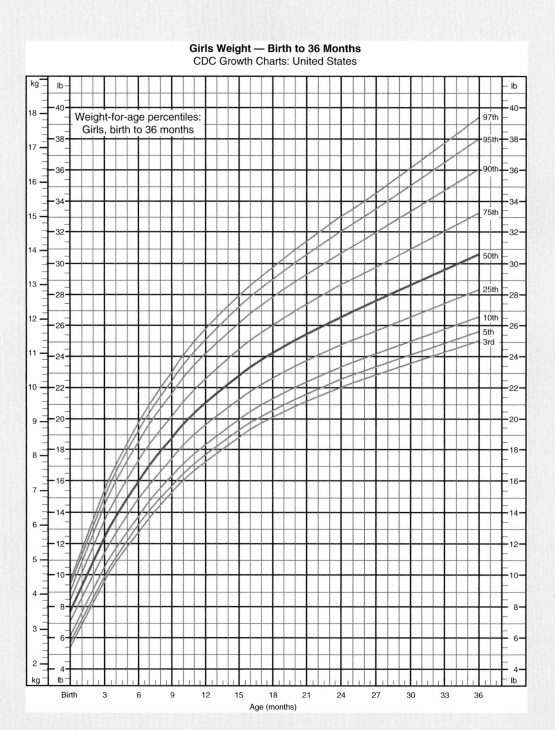

Girls Weight — Birth to 36 Months
CDC Growth Charts: United States

Weight-for-age percentiles:
Girls, birth to 36 months

(continued)

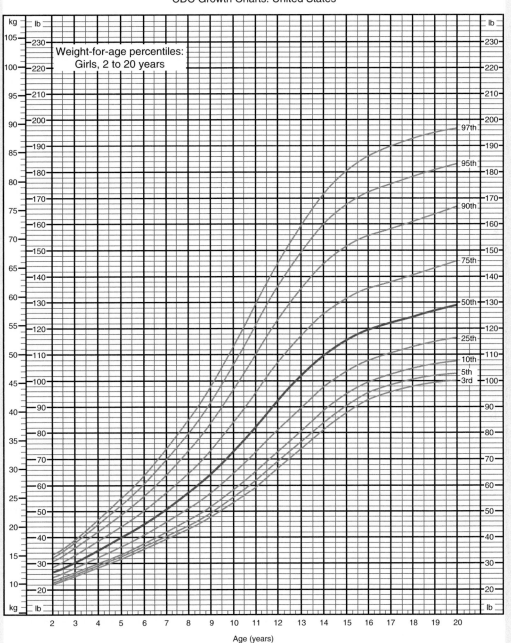

Girls Weight — 2 to 20 Years
CDC Growth Charts: United States

Weight-for-age percentiles:
Girls, 2 to 20 years

Age (years)

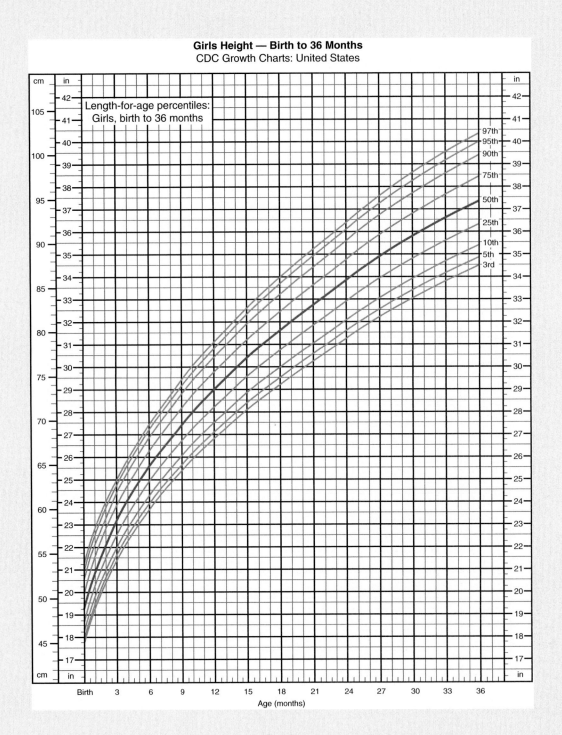

Girls Height — Birth to 36 Months
CDC Growth Charts: United States

(continued)

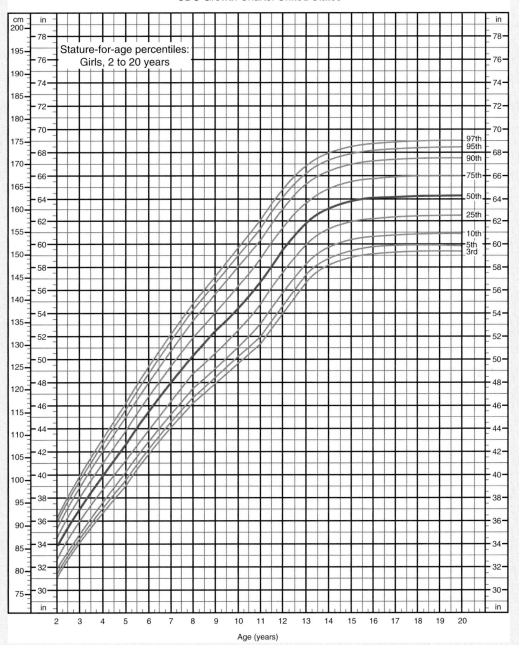

Girls Height — 2 to 20 Years
CDC Growth Charts: United States

Stature-for-age percentiles:
Girls, 2 to 20 years

Age (years)

(continued)

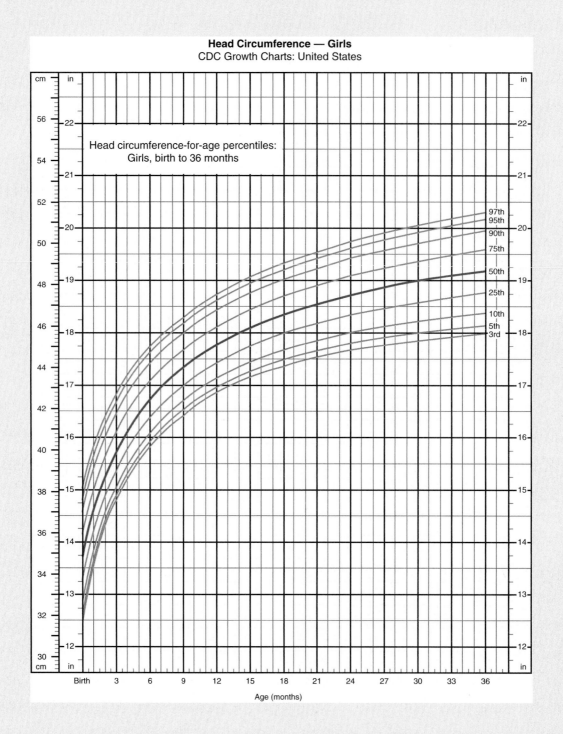

Head Circumference — Girls
CDC Growth Charts: United States

Head circumference-for-age percentiles:
Girls, birth to 36 months

Age (months)

TABLE 24-5. Growth Patterns Through Childhood and Adolescence

Measurement	0 to 6 mo	Toddler	Preschool	School Age	Throughout Adolescence	
					Girls	Boys
Height	2.5 cm/mo	7.5 cm/y	6.2–7.5 cm/y	5 cm/y	5–20 cm	10–30 cm
Weight	1.5 lb/mo	4–6 lb/y	5 lb/y	4–6.5 lb/y	15–55 lb	15–65 lb
Head circumference	1.32 cm/mo	0.5 inch/y				

24 months, toddlers walk up and down stairs one step at a time. At 30 months, they jump with both feet.

Fine Motor. Fifteen-month-old toddlers can build a two-block tower and scribble spontaneously. At 18 months, they can build a three- to four-block tower. Toddlers at 24 months imitate a vertical stroke, and, at 30 months, they build an eight-block tower and copy a cross.

Preschoolers

Gross Motor. At 3 years old, children can ride a tricycle, go upstairs using alternate feet, stand on one foot for a few seconds, and broad jump. Four-year-old children can skip,

hop on one foot (Fig. 24-7), catch a ball, and go downstairs using alternate feet. At 5 years, children can skip on alternate feet, throw and catch a ball, jump rope, and balance on alternate feet with eyes closed.

Fine Motor. Three-year-old children can build a tower of up to 10 blocks, build three-block bridges, copy a circle, and imitate a cross. At 4 years old, children can lace shoes, copy a square shape, trace a diamond shape, and add three parts to a stick figure. Five-year-old children can tie shoelaces, use scissors well, copy diamond and triangle shapes, add seven to nine parts to a stick figure, and print a few letters and numbers and their first name.

School-Age Children

Gross Motor. Skills acquired during the school years include bicycling, roller skating, rollerblading, and skateboarding. Running and jumping improve progressively, and swimming is added to the child's repertoire.

Fine Motor. Printing skills develop in the early school years; script skills in later years (by age 8; Fig. 24-8). School-age

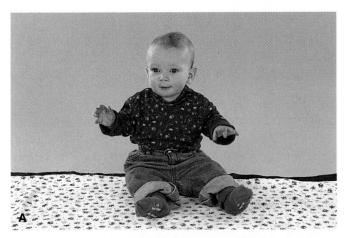

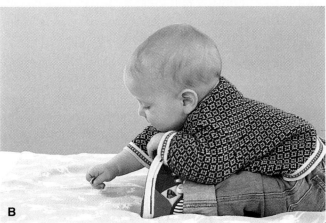

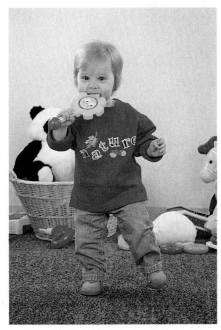

FIGURE 24-5. (**A**) An infant can sit unsupported by 8 months; the pincer grasp (**B**) develops by 9 months. (© B. Proud.)

FIGURE 24-6. At 15 months a toddler can walk without help. (© B. Proud.)

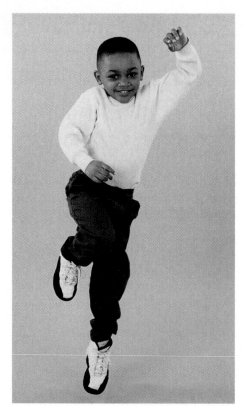

FIGURE 24-7. A 4-year-old preschooler can hop on one foot. (© B. Proud.)

children also develop greater dexterity and competence for crafts, video games, and computers.

Adolescents

Gross motor skills have reached adult levels, and fine motor skills continue to be refined.

Sample nursing history questions for infancy to adolescence include:

Can your infant lift his or her head?
Does your infant roll over? Front to back? Back to front?
Can your infant sit without support?
Can your infant stand without support?
When did your child first walk?
Can your infant successfully reach and grab objects?
Can your toddler walk up and down steps?
Can your toddler jump with both feet?
Does your toddler spontaneously scribble?
Can your preschooler run, hop, and skip?
Can your preschooler lace shoes?
Can your preschooler write his or her first name?
Can your school-age child ride a bicycle?
Can your school-age child write script?
Does your adolescent have a job, hobby, or interest that involves hand skills? If so, how is his or her performance?

SENSORY PERCEPTION (VISION, HEARING, AND OTHER SENSES)

Infants

Visual. The newborn's visual impressions are unfocused, and the ability to distinguish between colors is not developed until approximately 8 months of age. Therefore, stimuli should be bright, simple, moving, and, preferably, black and white (eg, a mobile that consists of black and white circles and cubes; Fig. 24-9).

Auditory. Newborns can distinguish sounds and turn toward voices and other noises. They may be very familiar with their mother's voice, and other sounds gradually gain significance when associated with pleasure.

Olfactory. Smell is fully developed at birth, and a 2-week-old infant can differentiate the smell of his or her mother's milk and parents' body odors.

Tactile. Touch is well developed at birth, especially the lips and tongue. Touch should be used frequently because infants enjoy rocking, warmth, and cuddling.

Toddlers

Visual. Toddlers' visual acuity and depth perception improve, and they are able to recall visual images.

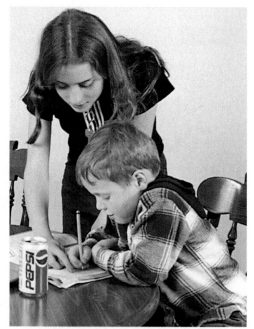

FIGURE 24-8. Printing skills develop in the early school-age years.

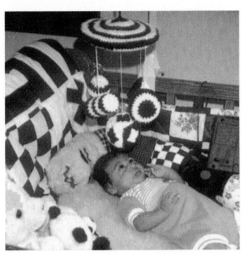

FIGURE 24-9. A black-and-white mobile is a good visual stimulus for an infant. (Courtesy of S. Ludington.)

Auditory. Toddlers begin learning the ability to listen and comprehend. As every parent knows, listening is different from hearing. This ability includes attending to what is heard, discriminating sound qualities, creating cognitive associations with previous learning, and remembering.

Olfactory and Gustatory. Both senses are influenced by voluntary control and are associated with other sensory and motor areas. Therefore, toddlers refuse to eat anything that looks unpleasant to them. Children also begin to learn conditioned reactions to odors at this age.

Preschoolers

Visual. Color and depth perception become fully developed. Preschoolers may be aware of visual difficulties.

Auditory. Hearing reaches its maximum level, and listening further develops. Preschoolers usually enjoy vision and hearing testing.

School-Age Children

Visual. Visual capacity reaches adult level (20/20) by age 6 or 7 years.

Auditory. Hearing acuity is almost complete.

Adolescents

All senses have reached their mature capacity by adolescence.
Sample nursing history questions related to sensory function from infancy to adolescence include:

Does your infant have any unusual eye movements?
Does your infant excessively cross eyes?
Does your infant blink when necessary?

Is your infant able to focus on moving objects?
Has your infant ever had cloudiness in eyeball?
Does your child frequently rub his or her eyes?
Does your child become irritable with close work?
Does your child blink repeatedly?
Does your child ever appear cross-eyed?
Does your child strain to see distant objects or sit close to the TV?
Does your child reverse letters or numbers?
Does your child ever complain of headache?
How frequently does your child have vision tested?
Does your child wear glasses or contact lenses?

Infants normally attend to the human voice; therefore, question parents as to whether their child appears to be paying attention when they speak.

Does your child respond to verbal commands? (Remember, we can only test hearing, not listening.)
Does your child sit too close to the TV?
Does your adolescent blast the stereo? (This may not indicate a hearing deficit, as it is typical behavior; however, it can lead to hearing deficit.)
Does your child have any speech difficulties? (This may suggest hearing impairment.)
Does your child use a hearing aid?
Has your child had frequent ear infections; tubes in ears?
How frequently does your child have his or her hearing tested?
Does your child have any difficulty with smell or taste?
How does your child respond to touch?
Does your child have any pain? If so, analyze pain as a symptom. (Use the COLDSPA mnemonic.)

COLDSPA

CHARACTER: Describe the sign or symptom. How does it feel, look, sound, smell, and so forth?
ONSET: When did it begin?
LOCATION: Where is it? Does it radiate?
DURATION: How long does it last? Does it recur?
SEVERITY: How bad is it?
PATTERN: What makes it better? What makes it worse?
ASSOCIATED FACTORS: What other symptoms occur with it?

If you are interviewing a child who can talk or otherwise participate in the interview, use words that are appropriate for the age of the child. For example, if the child is very young, you could refer to pain as a "booboo," or ask the child to point to where the pain is. Also, use a pain scale developed especially for children, such as the Wong/Baker FACES Pain Rating Scale (see Figure 24-4) or the Oucher scale (six photographs of children's faces ranging from "no hurt" to "biggest hurt you could ever have," which comes with a scale numbered from 0 to 100).

Additional sensory-related questions may focus on smell, taste, or tactile sensation.

Does your child ever complain of having difficulty with his or her sense of smell? Taste?

Does your child ever complain of numbness/tingling?

COGNITIVE AND LANGUAGE DEVELOPMENT (PIAGET)

Infants

The sensorimotor stage, from birth to around 18 months, involves the development of intellect and knowledge of the environment gained through the senses. During this stage, development progresses from reflexive activity to purposeful acts. At the completion of this stage, the infant achieves a sense of object permanence (retains a mental image of an absent object; sees self as separate from others). An emerging sense of body image parallels sensorimotor development.

Crying is the first means of communication, and parents can usually differentiate cries. Cooing begins by 1 to 2 months, laughing and babbling by 3 to 4 months, and consonant sounds by 3 to 4 months. The infant begins to imitate sounds by 6 months. Combined syllables ("mama") are vocalized by 8 months, and the infant understands "no-no" by 9 months. "mama" and "dada" are said with meaning by 10 months, and the infant says a total of 4 to 10 words with meaning by 12 months.

Toddlers

The sensorimotor phase (between ages 12 and 24 months) involves two substages in toddlerhood: tertiary circular reactions (age 12 to 18 months), involving trial-and-error experimentation and relentless exploration, and mental combinations (age 18 to 24 months), during which the toddler begins to devise new means for accomplishing tasks through mental calculations. Toddlers go through a preconceptual substage of the preoperational phase typical of preschoolers. During this time, the child uses representational thought to recall the past, represent the present, and anticipate the future. As toddlers get older, they begin to enter the preoperational phase. This phase is described in the following section on preschoolers.

At 15 months, toddlers use expressive jargon. At 2 years, they say 300 words and use 2- to 3-word phrases and pronouns. At 2.5 years, toddlers give their first and last names and use plurals.

Preschoolers

This stage of preoperational thought (age 2 to 7 years) consists of two phases. In the preconceptual phase, extending from age 2 to 4, the child forms concepts that are not as complete or logical as an adult's; makes simple classifications; associates one event with a simultaneous one (transductive reasoning); and exhibits egocentric thinking.

In the intuitive phase, extending from age 4 to 7, the child becomes capable of classifying, quantifying, and relating objects, but remains unaware of the principles behind these operations; exhibits intuitive thought processes (is aware that something is right but cannot say why); is unable to see viewpoint of others; and uses many words appropriately but without a real knowledge of their meaning. Preschoolers exhibit magical thinking and believe that thoughts are all-powerful. They may feel guilty and responsible for bad thoughts, which, at times, may coincide with the occurrence of a wished event (eg, wishing a sibling were dead and the sibling suddenly needs to be hospitalized).

Three-year-old children can say 900 words, 3- to 4-word sentences, and can talk incessantly. Four-year-old children can say 1,500 words, tell exaggerated stories, and sing simple songs. This is also the peak age for "why" questions. Five-year-old children can say 2,100 words, and they know four or more colors, the names of the days of the week, and the months.

School-Age Children

A child aged 7 to 11 years is in the stage of concrete operations, marked by inductive reasoning, logical operations, and reversible concrete thought. Specific characteristics of this stage include movement from egocentric to objective thinking—seeing other's point of view, seeking validation, and asking questions; focusing on immediate physical reality with inability to transcend the here and now; difficulty dealing with remote, future, or hypothetical matters; development of various mental classifying and ordering activities; and development of the principle of conservation—of volume, weight, mass, and numbers. Typical activities of a child at this stage may include collecting and sorting objects (eg, baseball cards, dolls, marbles); ordering items according to size, shape, weight, and other criteria; and considering options and variables when problem solving. Electronic games (Nintendo, PlayStation) are popular with this age group.

Children develop formal adult articulation patterns by age 7 to 9. They learn that words can be arranged in terms of structure. The ability to read is one of the most significant skills learned during these years (Fig. 24-10).

Adolescents

In the development of formal operations, which commonly occurs from ages 11 to 15 years, the adolescent develops abstract reasoning. This period consists of three substages:

Substage 1—The adolescent sees relationships involving the inverse of the reciprocal.

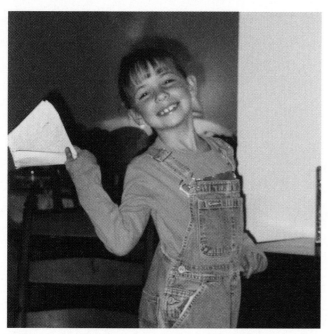

FIGURE 24-10. Reading is a milestone achievement for a school-age child.

Substage 2—The adolescent develops the ability to order triads of propositions or relationships.

Substage 3—The adolescent develops the capacity for true formal thought.

In true formal thought, the adolescent thinks beyond the present and forms theories about everything, delighting especially in considerations of "that which is not." However, adolescents in this age group do not have futuristic thoughts. They do not relate current events "here and now" to long-term results (2 years from now). An example of this includes teenagers who are sexually active and who may not consider the consequences of sexual activity (pregnancy and parenthood).

Sample nursing history questions for infancy to adolescence include:

Does your infant cry when approached by strangers?
When did your infant first say "mama" or "dada?"
What and when was your infant's first word?
Can your toddler name some body parts?
Can your toddler state first and last name?
Does your toddler imitate adults?
Does your toddler put two words together to form sentence? (eg, "me go")
Does your preschooler tell fantasy stories?
Does your preschooler have an invisible friend?
Can your preschooler make simple classifications? (eg, dogs and cats)
Is your preschooler "chatty"? Does your preschooler frequently ask "why?"
Can your preschooler name at least four colors?

Can your school-age child see another's point of view?
Does your school-age child collect things? (eg, baseball cards, dolls)
Does your school-age child try to solve problems?
How well does your school-age child do in school? Also ask school-age child and compare the answers.
How well does your school-age child read?
Do you consider your adolescent to be a problem solver?
How well does your adolescent do in school? Also ask the adolescent and compare the responses.

MORAL DEVELOPMENT (KOLBERG)

Infant

Although Kolberg's theory of moral development begins with toddlerhood, infants cannot be overlooked. Child moral development begins with the value and belief system of the parents, and the infant's own development of trust. Parental discipline patterns may start with the young infant as interventions may take place for crying behaviors. Stern discipline and withholding of love and affection may affect infant moral development. Love and affection are the building blocks of an infant's developing sense of trust.

Toddler

A toddler is typically at the first substage of the preconventional stage, involving punishment and obedience orientation, in which he or she makes judgments on the basis of avoiding punishment or obtaining a reward. Discipline patterns affect a toddler's moral development. For example, physical punishment and withholding privileges tend to give the toddler a negative view of morals; withholding love and affection as punishment leads to feelings of guilt in the toddler. Appropriate disciplinary actions include providing simple explanations why certain behaviors are unacceptable, praising appropriate behavior, and using distraction when the toddler is headed for danger.

Preschooler

A preschooler is in the preconventional stage of moral development, which extends to 10 years. In this phase, conscience emerges, and the emphasis is on external control. The child's moral standards are those of others, and he or she observes them either to avoid punishment or reap rewards.

School-Age Child

A child at the conventional level of the role conformity stage (generally, age 10 to 13 years) has an increased desire to please others. The child observes and, to some extent, externalizes the standards of others. The child wants to be considered "good" by those people whose opinion matters to him or her.

Adolescent

Development of the postconventional level of morality occurs at about age 13, marked by the development of an individual conscience and a defined set of moral values. For the first time, the adolescent can acknowledge a conflict between two socially accepted standards and try to decide between them. Control of conduct is now internal, both in standards observed and in reasoning about right or wrong.

Sample nursing history questions for infancy through adolescence include:

Does your child understand the difference between right and wrong?

Do you discuss family values with your child?

Do you have family rules? How are they implemented?

How are disciplinary measures handled?

Has your child ever had any problems with lying, cheating, or stealing?

Has your child ever required disciplinary action at school?

Has your child ever violated the law?

PSYCHOSOCIAL DEVELOPMENT (ERIKSON)

Infant

The crisis faced by an infant (birth to 1 year) is termed trust versus mistrust. In this stage, the infant's significant other is the "caretaking" person. Developing a sense of trust in caregivers and the environment is a central focus for an infant. This sense of trust forms the foundation for all future psychosocial tasks. The quality of the caregiver–child relationship is a crucial factor in the infant's development of trust. An infant who receives attentive care learns that life is predictable and that his or her needs will be met promptly; this fosters trust. In contrast, an infant experiencing consistently delayed needs gratification develops a sense of uncertainty, leading to mistrust of caregivers and the environment. An infant commonly seeks comfort from a security object (a blanket or a favorite toy) during times of stress.

Toddler

Erikson terms the psychosocial crises facing a child between ages 1 and 3 years *autonomy versus shame and doubt*. The psychosocial theme is "to hold on; to let go." The toddler has developed a sense of trust and is ready to give up dependence to assert his or her budding sense of control, independence, and autonomy (Fig. 24-11). The toddler begins to master the following:

- Individuation—Differentiation of self from others
- Separation from parent(s)
- Control over bodily functions
- Communication with words
- Acquisition of socially acceptable behavior
- Egocentric interactions with others

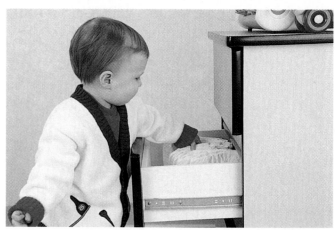

FIGURE 24-11. Toddlers love to assert their sense of control, independence and autonomy.

The toddler has learned that his or her parents are predictable and reliable. The toddler begins to learn that his or her own behavior has a predictable, reliable effect on others. The toddler learns to wait longer for needs gratification. The toddler often uses "no," even when he or she means "yes." This is done to assert independence (negativistic behavior). A sense of shame and doubt can develop if the toddler is kept dependent in areas where he or she is capable of using newly acquired skills or if made to feel inadequate when attempting new skills. A toddler often continues to seek a familiar security object, such as a blanket, during times of stress.

Preschooler

Between ages 3 and 6 years, a child faces a psychosocial crisis that Erikson terms *initiative versus guilt*. The child's significant other is the family. At this age, the child has normally mastered a sense of autonomy and moves on to master a sense of initiative. A preschooler is an energetic, enthusiastic, and intrusive learner with an active imagination. Conscience (an inner voice that warns and threatens) begins to develop.

The child explores the physical world with all his or her senses and powers. Development of a sense of guilt occurs when the child is made to feel that his or her imagination and activities are unacceptable. Guilt, anxiety, and fear result when the child's thoughts and activities clash with parental expectations. A preschooler begins to use simple reasoning and can tolerate longer periods of delayed gratification.

School-Age Child

Erikson terms the psychosocial crisis faced by a child aged 6 to 12 years *industry versus inferiority*. During this period, the child's radius of significant others expands to include school and instructive adults. A school-age child normally has mastered the first three developmental tasks—trust, autonomy, and initiative—and now focuses on mastering industry. A child's sense of industry grows out of a desire for real achievement. The child engages in tasks and activities that he or she can carry through to completion. The child learns rules and how to compete with others and to cooperate to achieve goals. Social relationships with others become increasingly important sources of support. The child can develop a sense of inferiority stemming from unrealistic expectations or a sense of failing to meet standards set for him or her by others. Because the child feels inadequate, his or her self-esteem sags.

Adolescent

Erikson terms the psychosocial crisis faced by adolescents (aged 13 to 18 years) *identity versus role diffusion*. For an adolescent, the radius of significant others is the peer group. To an adolescent, development of who he or she is and where he or she is going becomes a central focus. The adolescent continues to redefine his or her self-concept and the roles that he or she can play with certainty. As rapid physical changes occur, adolescents must reintegrate previous trust in their body, themselves, and how they appear to others. The inability to develop a sense of who he or she is and what he or she can become results in role diffusion and inability to solve core conflicts.

Sample nursing history questions for infancy through adolescence include:

How does your infant respond to comforting?
Does your toddler try to do things for himself or herself? (eg, feed, dress)
Does your toddler have temper tantrums? How are they handled?
Does your toddler frequently use the word "no"?
At what age was your toddler completely toilet trained?
Does your toddler actively explore the environment?
Does your preschooler have an active imagination?
Does your preschooler imitate adult activities?
Does your preschooler engage in fantasy play?
Does your preschooler frequently ask questions?
Does your preschooler enjoy new activities?
What are your school-age child's interests/hobbies?
Does your school-age child interact well with teachers, peers?
Does your school-age child enjoy accomplishments?
Does your school-age child shame self for failures?
What is your school-age child's favorite activity?
Does your adolescent have a peer group?
Does your adolescent have a best friend?
Does your adolescent exhibit rebellious behavior at home?
How does your adolescent see self as fitting in with peers?
What does your adolescent want to do with his or her life?

PSYCHOSEXUAL DEVELOPMENT (FREUD)
Infant

In the *oral stage* of development, from birth to 18 months, the erogenous zone is the mouth and sexual activity takes the form of sucking, swallowing, chewing, and biting. In this stage, the infant meets the world by crying, tasting, eating, and early vocalization; biting, to gain a sense of having a hold on and having greater control of the environment; and grasping and touching to explore texture variations in the environment.

Toddler

In the *anal stage*, typically extending from age 8 months to 4 years, the erogenous zone is the anus and buttocks, and sexual activity centers on the expulsion and retention of body waste. In this stage, the child's focus shifts from the mouth to the anal area, with emphasis on bowel control as he or she gains neuromuscular control over the anal sphincter. The toddler experiences both satisfaction and frustration as he or she gains control over withholding and expelling, containing and releasing. The conflict between "holding on" and "letting go" gradually resolves as bowel training progresses; resolution occurs once control is firmly established. Toilet training is a major task of toddlerhood (Fig. 24-12). Readiness is not usual until 18 to 24 months of age. Bowel training occurs before bladder; night bladder training usually does not occur until 3 to 5 years of age. Masturbation can occur from body exploration. Toddlers learn words associated with anatomy and elimination and can distinguish the sexes.

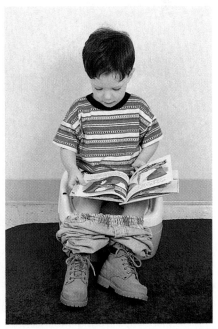

FIGURE 24-12. Toilet training is a major task of toddlerhood.

Preschooler

In the *phallic stage,* extending from about 3 to 7 years of age, the child's pleasure centers on the genitalia and masturbation. Many preschoolers masturbate for physiologic pleasure. The Oedipal stage occurs, marked by jealousy and rivalry toward the same-sex parent and love of the opposite-sex parent. The Oedipal stage typically resolves in the late preschool period with a strong identification with the same-sex parent. Sexual identity is developed during this time. Modesty may become a concern, and the preschooler may have fears of castration. Because preschoolers are keen observers but poor interpreters, the child may recognize but not understand sexual activity. Before answering a child's questions about sex, parents should clarify what the child is really asking, and what the child already thinks about the specific subject. Questions about sex should be answered simply and honestly, providing only the information that the child requests; additional details can come later.

School-Age Child

The *latency period,* extending from about 5 to 12 years, represents a stage of relative sexual indifference before puberty and adolescence. During this period, development of self-esteem is closely linked with a developing sense of industry in gaining a concept of one's value and worth. Preadolescence begins near the end of the school-age years, and discrepancies in growth and maturation between the sexes become apparent. A school-age child has acquired much of his or her knowledge of, and many of his or her

attitudes toward sex at a very early age. During the school-age years, the child refines this knowledge and these attitudes. Questions about sex require honest answers based on the child's level of understanding.

Adolescent

In the *genital stage,* which extends from about age 12 to 20 years, an adolescent focuses on the genitals as an erogenous zone and engages in masturbation and sexual relations with others. During this period of renewed sexual drive, an adolescent experiences conflict between his or her own needs for sexual satisfaction and society's expectations for control of sexual expression. Core concerns of adolescents include body image development and acceptance by the opposite sex. Relationships with the opposite sex are important (Fig. 24-13). Adolescents engage in sexual activity for pleasure, to satisfy drives and curiosity, as a conquest, for affection, and because of peer pressure. Teaching about sexual function, begun during the school years, should expand to cover more in-depth information on the physical, hormonal, and emotional changes of puberty. An adolescent needs accurate, complete information on sexuality and cultural and moral values. Information must include how pregnancy occurs; methods of preventing pregnancy, stressing that male and female partners both are responsible for contraception; and transmission of and protection against sexually transmitted diseases, especially acquired immunodeficiency syndrome (AIDS) and hepatitis.

Sample nursing history questions for infancy to adolescence include:

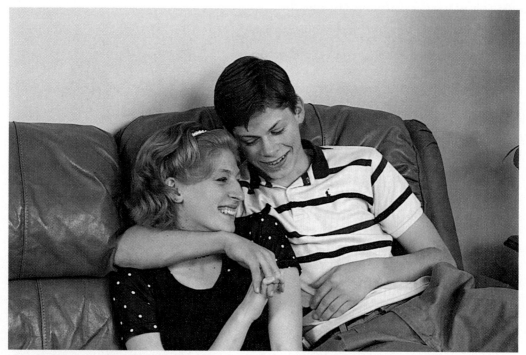

FIGURE 24-13. During adolescence, relationships with the opposite sex are important stepping stones to adulthood.

Does your infant use a pacifier or suck the thumb?

Does your toddler have any problems with toilet training?

Does your toddler masturbate?

Does your preschooler masturbate?

Does your preschooler know what sex he or she is?

Has your preschooler asked questions about sex, childbirth, and the like?

Does your school-age child interact with same-sex peers?

What has your school-age child been told about puberty and sex?

A full, confidential sexual/sexuality history should be obtained from adolescents. This history includes questioning previously noted in the reproductive review of systems as well as:

What is your sexual preference?

How do you feel about becoming a man/woman?

It is also suggested that children of all ages be questioned about sexual abuse. This may be elicited by asking, "Has anyone ever touched you where or when you did not want to be touched?"

LIFESTYLE AND HEALTH PRACTICES

Normal Nutritional Requirements

Proper nutrition is necessary for childhood growth and development. Food and feeding are important parts of growing up, with needs and desires changing as the child grows (Fig. 24-14). Table 24-6 provides several nutritional requirements for each age group. General overviews for each phase of nutritional follow.

Infants. Breast milk is the most desirable complete food for the first 6 months of a child's life. However, commercially prepared, iron-fortified formula is an acceptable alternative. Formula intake varies per infant. Most infants take 100 cal/kg body weight/day. This amount of formula should be offered to the infant every 3 to 4 h, approximately four to six

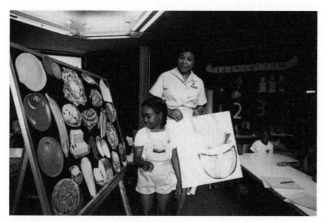

FIGURE 24-14. Children in schools, community centers, and other community groups can learn the importance of eating healthful foods.

times a day. Solids are not recommended before 4 months of age due to the presence of the protrusion or sucking reflexes and the immaturity of the gastrointestinal tract and the immune system. Infant rice cereal is usually the initial solid food given because it is easy to digest, contains iron, and rarely triggers allergy. Additional foods usually include other cereals, followed by fruits and vegetables, and finally meats. Juices may be offered at 6 months of age. Finger foods are introduced at 8 or 9 months. Weaning from breast or bottle to cup should be gradual. The desire to imitate at 8 to 9 months increases the success of weaning. Honey should be discouraged during the first year of life because it may cause infant botulism.

Toddlers. Growth rate slows dramatically during the toddler years, thus decreasing the need for calories, protein, and fluid. Starting at about 12 months, most toddlers are eating the same foods as the rest of the family. At 18 months, many toddlers experience physiologic anorexia and become picky eaters. They experience food jags and eat large amounts one day and very little the next. They like to feed themselves and prefer small portions of appetizing foods. Frequent, nutritious snacks can replace a meal. Food should not be used as a reward or a punishment. Milk should be limited to no more than 1 quart per day to ensure intake and absorption of iron-enriched foods to prevent anemia. Recommendations for screening for anemia should be based on age, sex, and risk of anemia.

Preschoolers. Requirements are similar to those of the toddler. Three- and four-year-old children may still be unable to sit with family during meals. Four-year-old children are picky eaters. Five-year-old children are influenced by food habits of others. A 5-year-old child tends to be focused on the "social" aspects of eating: Table conversation, manners, willingness to try new foods, and help with meal preparation and clean-up.

School-Age Children. A school-age child's daily caloric requirements diminish in relation to body size. Caregivers should continue to stress the need for a balanced diet from the food pyramid because resources are being stored for the increased growth needs of adolescence. The child is exposed to broader eating experiences in the school lunchroom; he or she may still be a "picky" eater but should be more willing to try new foods. Children may trade, sell, or throw away home-packed school lunches. At home, the child should eat what the family eats; the patterns that develop now stay with the child into adulthood.

Adolescents. An adolescent's daily intake should be balanced among the foods in the pyramid; average daily caloric intake requirements vary with sex and age, as noted in Table 24-6. Adolescents typically eat whatever they have at break activities; readily available nutritious snacks provide good insurance for a balanced diet. Milk (calcium) and protein are needed in quantity to aid in bone and muscle growth. Maintaining adequate quality and quantity of daily

TABLE 24-6. Recommended Daily Energy and Nutrient Intake by Age, Average Height, and Weight

	Infants, Toddlers, and Children					Boys and Men			Girls and Women			Pregnant
Age	0–6 mo	6–12 mo	1–3 yr	4–6 yr	7–10 yr	11–14 yr	15–18 yr	19–24 yr	11–14 yr	15–18 yr	19–24 yr	Pregnant
Weight (kg)	6	9	13	20	28	45	66	72	46	55	58	
Height (cm)	60	71	90	112	132	157	176	177	157	163	164	
Nutrient												
Energy (kcal/kg)	108	98	102	90	70	55	45	40	40	38	38	+ 300 kcal/d in second and third trimesters
Protein (g/kg)	2.2	1.6	1.2	1.1	1.0	1.0	0.9	0.8	0.8	0.8	0.8	
Vitamin A, µ RE	375	375	400	500	500	1000	1000	1000	800	800	800	800
Thiamin (B_1), mg	0.3	0.4	0.7	0.9	1	1.3	1.5	1.5	1.1	1.1	1.1	1.5
Riboflavin (B_2), mg	0.4	0.5	0.8	1.1	1.2	1.5	1.8	1.7	1.3	1.3	1.3	1.6
Niacin (mg NE)	5	6	9	12	13	17	20	19	15	15	15	17
Pyridoxine (B_2), mg	0.3	0.6	1	1.1	1.4	1.7	2	2	1.4	1.5	1.6	2.2
Folate, µg	25	35	50	75	100	150	200	200	150	400	400	800
Vitamin B_{12}, µg	0.3	0.5	0.7	1	1.4	2	2	2	2	2	2	2.2
Vitamin C, mg	30	35	40	45	45	50	60	60	50	60	60	70
Vitamin D, µg	7.5	10	10	10	10	10	10	10	10	10	10	10
Vitamin E, mg	3	4	6	7	7	10	10	10	8	8	8	10
Vitamin K, µg	5	10	15	20	30	45	65	70	45	55	60	65
Calcium, mg	400	600	800	800	1200	1300	1300	1200	1300	1300	1200	1200–1500
Fluoride, mg*	0 (If breastfed); 6 (if not breastfed)	0.2–0.5	0.5–1.5	1.0–2.5	1.5–2.5	1.5–2.5	1.5–2.5	1.5–4.0	1.5–2.5	1.5–2.5	1.5–4.0	1.6–2.5
Iron, mg	10	10	10	10	10	12–15	12–15	12–15	15–30	15–30	15–30	30
Zinc, mg	5	5	10	10	10	15	15	15	12	12	12	15

*Fluoride supplement is not necessary if the water supply contains ≥3 ppm (parts per million) fluoridation.

RE, retinol equivalent. 1 retinol equivalent = 1 µg. β-carotene; NE, niacin equivalent. 1 niacin equivalent = 1 mg of niacin or 60 mg of dietary tryptophan.

Adapted with permission from *Recommended Dietary Allowances* 10th ed. Copyright 1989 by the National Academy of Sciences, Washington, DC; *Dietary Reference Intakes for Calcium, Phosphorus, Magnesium, Vitamin D, and Fluoride.* Copyright 1997 by the National Academy Press, Washington DC; and US Public Health Service, 1992.

intake may be difficult because of such factors as busy schedule, influence of peers, and easy availability of fast foods. Family eating patterns established during the school years continue to influence an adolescent's food selection. Female adolescents are very prone to negative dieting behaviors. Common dietary deficiencies include iron, folate, and zinc.

Sample nursing history questions for infancy to adolescence include:

> What does your child eat in a typical day?
> Is your child on any special type of diet? If so, what for?
> What foods does your child like/dislike most?
> Does your child have any feeding problems?
> Is your child allergic to any foods? If so, how does your child react to those foods?
> Does your child take any vitamin or mineral supplements?
> How much fluid does your child drink per day?
> Is your water fluorinated? If not, does your child take supplements?
> Has your child had any recent weight gain or loss?
> Does your child have any concerns with body image?
> Has your child been on any self-imposed diet?
> How often does your child weigh himself or herself?
> Has your child ever used any of the following methods for weight loss: self-induced vomiting? Laxatives? Diuretics? Excessive exercise? Fasting?

The last five questions should be asked directly of adolescents when parents are not present.

Normal Activity and Exercise

Activity and exercise are important components of a child's life and, therefore, should be assessed when a complete subjective examination is being performed. Play, activity, and exercise patterns can give the nurse valuable clues about the overall health of a child. This assessment also allows the examiner to provide health promotion teaching.

Sample nursing history questions for infancy to adolescence include:

> What is your child's activity like during a typical 24-hour day? (including activities of daily living, play, and school)
> What are your child's favorite activities and toys?
> How many hours of television does your child watch per day? What is his or her favorite programs/movies? Do you discuss TV shows/movies with your child? Are there any restrictions on TV watching (content, hours, relationship to chores/homework)?
> What chores does your child do at home (school-age child/adolescent)?
> Does the older child/adolescent work outside the home? What does he or she do?
> How many hours does he or she work during the school year?
> Does the work interfere with school or social life?

> Why does the child work?
> Does your child have any problems that restrict physical activity?
> Does your child require any special devices to manage with activities of daily living/play?
> At what age did your child first walk?
> Can your child keep up with his or her peers?
> Does your child have any hobbies/interests (ages 6 and older)?
> What sports does your child participate in?

Normal Sleep Requirements and Patterns

Sleep is an integral part of health assessment. Lack of sleep can affect all areas of health, including cognitive, physical, and emotional health. Children require varying amounts of sleep based primarily on their age. They also have varying sleep habits that correlate with their developmental status.

Infants. Sleep patterns vary among infants. During the first month, most infants sleep when not eating. By 3 to 4 months, most infants sleep 9 to 11 h at night. By 12 months, most take morning and afternoon naps. Bedtime rituals should begin in infancy to prepare the infant for sleep and prevent future sleep problems. Because of the possibility of SIDS (sudden infant death syndrome), it is suggested that young infants sleep in the supine or side-lying position.

Toddlers. Total sleep requirements decrease during the second year and average about 12 h per day. Most nap once a day until the end of the second or third year. Sleep problems are common and may be due to fears of separation. Bedtime rituals and transitional objects, such as a blanket or stuffed toy, are helpful.

Preschoolers. The average preschooler sleeps 11 to 13 h per day. Preschoolers typically need an afternoon nap until age 5, when most begin kindergarten. Bedtime rituals persist, and sleep problems are common. These include nightmares, night terrors, difficulty settling in after a busy day, and stretching bedtime rituals to delay sleep. Continuing reassuring bedtime rituals with relaxation time before bedtime should help the child settle in. The daytime nap may be eliminated if it seems to interfere with nighttime sleep. For many preschoolers, a security object and night light continue to help relieve anxiety/fears at bedtime (Fig. 24-15).

School-Age Children. School-age children's individual sleep requirements vary, but typically range from 8 to 9.5 h per night. Because the growth rate has slowed, children actually need less sleep now than during adolescence. The child's bedtime can be later than during the preschool period but should be firmly established and adhered to on school nights. Reading before bedtime may facilitate sleep and set up a positive bedtime pattern. Children may be unaware of

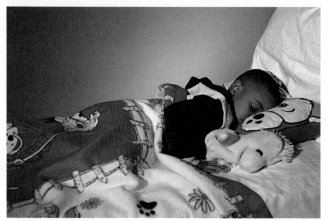

FIGURE 24-15. A security object, such as a favorite toy, can help a preschooler sleep. (© B. Proud.)

fatigue, and, if allowed to remain up, they will be tired the next day.

Adolescents. During adolescence, rapid growth, overexertion in activities, and a tendency to stay up late commonly interfere with sleep and rest requirements. In an attempt to "catch up" on missed sleep, many adolescents sleep late at every opportunity. Each adolescent is unique in the number of sleep hours required to stay healthy and rested.

Sample nursing history questions for infancy to adolescence include:

What position does the infant sleep in?
Where does child sleep; what type of bed?
With whom does the child sleep?
Does child use a sleep aid (blanket, toy, night light, medication, beverage)?
Does the child have a bedtime ritual?
What time does child go to bed at night?
What time does child get up in the morning?
Does child sleep through the night?
Does child require feeding at night, and, if so, what and how is it administered (bottle caries)?
What is child's nap schedule, and how long does child sleep for naps?
Is the child's sleep restful or restless; any snoring or breathing problems?
Does the child sleepwalk or -talk?
Does the child have nightmares or night terrors?
If the child has sleep problems, what do you do for them?

Socioeconomic Situation

A family's socioeconomic situation greatly affects all aspects of a child's life, including development, nutrition, and overall health and functioning. Low socioeconomic status has the greatest adverse effect on health, and many children in this country live below the poverty level. Therefore, it is critical to obtain this assessment to initiate intervention strategies at the earliest opportunity.

Sample nursing history questions for infancy to adolescence include:

Does the child have health care insurance?
Would you seek more medical assistance (eg, in the way of preventive screenings, check-ups, sick visits, medication requests, eyeglass prescriptions) for your child if you had the money to do so?
Do you have any financial difficulties with which you need assistance?
How would you describe the family's living conditions?

Relationship and Role Development

The development of relationships and a role within groups is a crucial aspect of childhood. The ability of children to establish high-quality relationships and form specific roles in the early years significantly determines their ability to form high-quality relationships and roles when adulthood is reached.

Culture is an important factor in a person's relationship and role development. Things to consider include whether the child's culture/ethnicity is a minority within the major cultural group; what the traditional role of children in the particular child's culture is; and whether there is male or female dominance in the particular culture. Another major influence on the child's development of relationships and roles is the structure of the family. Various family structures include two-parent families, single-parent families, blended families, homosexual parent families, families with an adopted child, or families with a foster child.

Early intervention in, and early prevention of poor relationships between the child and his or her caregivers, siblings, peers, and influential adults outside the immediate family, are vital. Therefore, assessment of this aspect of a child's life is extremely important. It is important to ask the parent or caregiver questions as well as the child, because they may have differing views concerning the nature of the child's relationships.

Sample nursing history questions for infancy to adolescence (specifically geared to parent or caregiver) include:

What is your family structure?
With what culture or ethnic group does your family identify?
How would you describe your family support system?
Who is child's primary caretaker (especially for smaller children, not in school)?
What is the child's role in the family?
What are the family occupations and schedules?
How much time do you spend with children, and what activities do you participate in when you are together?
Have there been any changes in family lately—divorce, birth, deaths, moves?
How does child get along with parents, siblings, extended family, teachers, and peers?

Discuss your child's circle of friends.

What disciplinary measures do you use?

Sample nursing history questions for infancy to adolescence (specifically geared to child and/or adolescent) include:

How do you get along with your parents? brothers? sisters?

What activities does the family do together?

What chores do you do around the house?

What would you consider your role in the family?

What are the names of your family members and friends?

Do you have a best friend?

What do you like best about family/friends?

What do you dislike about family/friends?

What do you do/share with your friends?

Do your parents know your friends? Do they like them?

Do you get along with the other kids at school?

Do you get along with your teacher(s)?

Self-Esteem and Self-Concept Development

Childhood is the time when an individual develops the self-esteem and self-concept that shapes him or her in adult life (Table 24-7). Therefore, an assessment of this nature is crucial to provide health promotion teaching, prevent future problems, and intervene with current problems. This is a good time to ask questions regarding the child's values and beliefs because these areas tend greatly to influence a person's self-concept. This assessment requires that the same questions be asked of both the parent and the child, because their opinions may be significantly different. Reassure the parent and child that all answers discussed will be kept confidential.

Sample nursing history questions for infancy to adolescence (questions asked of child appear in italic print) include:

How would you describe your child? *How would you describe yourself?*

What does your child do best? *What do you do best?*

In what areas does your child need improvement? *What do you do that needs improvement?*

Is your child ever overly concerned about his or her weight? *Do you like your present weight? What would you like to weigh?*

Are culture and religion important factors in your home? *Are culture and religion important to you?*

In what religion is the child being reared? *What religion are you?*

How does your child define right and wrong? *How would you decide if something is right or wrong?*

What are your family values? *What values are important to you?*

What are the child's goals in life? *What are your goals in life?*

Coping and Stress Management

Childhood is full of stressors and fears, including the developmental crises of transition to each life stage and common childhood fears such as the dark and being left alone (Tables 24-8 and 24-9). The way that children cope with stress and fear can affect their development and how they will handle subsequent life events. Coping mechanisms vary, depending on developmental level, resources, situation, style, and previous experience with stressful events (Table 24-10). The ability of a child to cope is often influenced by individual temperament. Temperament involves the child's style of emotional and behavioral responses across situations. Temperament is biologic in origin; however, it is influenced by environmental characteristics and patterned by the society. This is significant because short- and long-term psychosocial adjustments are shaped by the goodness of fit between the child's temperament and the social environment.

Sample nursing history questions for infancy to adolescence include (questions asked of a child appear in italic print):

What does your child do when he or she gets angry/frustrated? *What do you do when you get angry or frustrated?*

TABLE 24-7. Self-Concept Development

Infants	Awareness of independent existence as a result of contact with other people
Toddler/Preschoolers	Greater sense of independence
Schoolagers	More aware of differences, norms, and morals; sensitive to social pressures
Adolescents	Self-concept crystallizes in later adolescence when child focuses on physical and emotional changes and peer acceptance

TABLE 24-8. Stressors in Children

Young children	Change in daily structure New sibling Separation
Older children	Starting school Long vacations Moving Change in family structure (remarriage) Christmas
Adolescents	Pregnancy Peer loss Breakup with boy/girl friend
All children	Parental loss (divorce, death, jail)

TABLE 24-9. Common Childhood Fears

Infants	Loud noises; falling and sudden movements in the environment; stranger anxiety begins around age 6 months
Toddlers	Loss of parents—separation anxiety; stranger anxiety; loud noises; going to sleep; large animals; certain people (doctor, Santa Claus); certain places (doctor's office); large objects or machines
Preschoolers	The dark; being left alone, especially at bedtime; animals (particularly large dogs); ghosts and other supernatural beings; body mutilation; pain; objects and people associated with painful experiences
Schoolagers	Failure at school; bullies; intimidating teachers; supernatural beings; storms; staying alone; scary things in TV and movies; consequences related to unattractive appearance; death
Adolescents	Relationships with people of the opposite sex; homosexual tendencies; ability to assume adult roles; drugs; AIDS; divorce; gossip; public speaking; plane and car crashes; death

What does your child do when he or she gets tired? *What do you do when you get tired?*

When your child has a tantrum, how do you handle it?

What things make your child scared? *What things scare you?*

What does he or she do when scared? *What do you do when you're scared?*

What kinds of things does your child worry about? *What kinds of things do you worry about?*

When your child has a problem, what does he or she do? *When you have a problem, what do you do?*

Have there been any big problems or changes in your family lately? *Have there been any big problems or changes in your family lately?*

TABLE 24-10. Coping Mechanisms in Children

Infants	Restlessness, rocking, playing with toys, crying, thumb sucking, sleeping
Toddlers/Preschoolers	Asking questions, wanting order, holding favorite toy, learning by trial and error, tantrums, aggression, thumb sucking, withdrawal, regression
Schoolagers	Trying problem solving; communicating, fantasizing, acting out situations, quiet, denial, regression, reaction formation
Adolescents	Problem solving, philosophical discussions, conforming with peers, asserting control, acting out, using drugs/alcohol, denial, projection, rationalization, intellectualization

Is there a problem with alcohol or drugs? *Do you use tobacco, alcohol, or drugs?*

Has your child ever run away from home? *Have you ever run away from home?*

How does your child react when needs are not met immediately, and what do you do about it? *What do you do when you are sad? What do you do when you are angry?*

Is your child "accident prone," and why do you think he or she is? *Did you ever think about hurting yourself? Did you ever think about killing yourself?* (Display 24-4)

Collecting Objective Data
CLIENT PREPARATION

In most cases, physical assessment involves a head-to-toe examination that encompasses each body system. When examining children, the sequence should be altered to accommodate the child's developmental needs (Display 24-5). Less threatening and least intrusive procedures, such as general inspection and heart and lung auscultation, should be completed first to secure the child's trust. Explain what you will be doing and what the child can expect to feel; allow the child to manipulate the equipment before it is used. Try to perform examination in a comfortable, nonthreatening area. The temperature should be warm, the room well lit, and all threatening instruments out of the child's view. The room should contain age-appropriate diversions, such as toys and cartoons for younger children and posters for adolescents.

If the child is uncooperative, first assess the reason (usually fear), then intervene appropriately. If still unsuccessful, involve parents, use a firm approach, and complete the examination as quickly, but completely, as possible. Involve the child in the physical examination at all times unless it is stressful for him or her.

KEY ASSESSMENT POINTS

- Recognize how techniques and demeanor for interviewing and examining children differ among the age groups and from those used for interviewing and examining adults.
- Be able to state the components of a pediatric health history.
- Evaluate growth and development patterns according to the different pediatric age groups and across body systems.
- Recognize children who are difficult to examine because of anxiety or fear.
- Develop forms of age-appropriate "play" to distract less cooperative children so physical examination can be completed.

DISPLAY 24-4. Suicide Assessment: Risks and Signs

Suicide is a leading killer of young people, particularly teenagers. The nurse can be instrumental in detecting signs of impending suicide and possibly, intervening to prevent it. During the nursing assessment, several interviewing methods and questions may help uncover a young client's suicidal thoughts.

- Ask if the child ever thought of hurting or killing self (hurting is different from killing).
- If the answer is "yes," ask the child when he or she thought of killing self.
- Ask how the child planned to do it.
- Ask if the child ever tried to kill himself or herself before and if any help was received after the incident.
- Ask if the child believes that there are any other options besides suicide to resolve problems.

Children and adolescents who verbalize planned, lethal means to commit suicide, and who feel that they do not have any other options, are at extremely high risk of carrying out their plan—especially if they have attempted suicide in the past. Some risk factors and warning signs of potential suicide include the following:

RISK FACTORS

- Previous attempt
- Suicide of family member or close friend
- History of abuse, neglect, or psychiatric hospitalization
- Persistent depression
- Mental disorder (voices tell child to kill self)
- Substance abuse
- Difficult home situation
- Incarceration
- Few social opportunities; isolated
- Firearms in the home

WARNING SIGNS

- Seems preoccupied with death themes, as in books, music, art, films, or TV shows
- Gives away valued possessions
- Talks about death, especially own
- Acts recklessly or adopts antisocial behavior
- Experiences rapid change in school performance
- Has episode of sudden cheerfulness after being depressed
- Exhibits dramatic change in everyday behaviors, such as sleeping and eating
- Smokes continuously (chain smoking)
- Expresses sense of worthlessness or hopelessness

DISPLAY 24-5. Developmental Approaches to the Physical Assessment

Children in each age group respond differently to the hands-on physical assessment; however, the following guidelines should be kept in mind:

INFANTS

Allow infant to sit in parent's lap; encourage parents to hold infant; use distraction; enlist parent's assistance.

TODDLERS

Allow toddler to sit on parent's lap; enlist parent's aid; use play; praise cooperation.

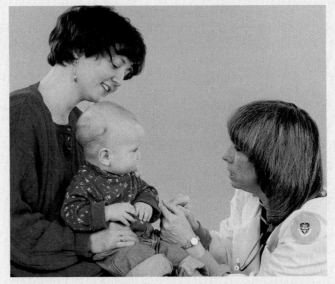

Let an infant sit on parent's lap and provide a toy for distraction. (© B. Proud.)

PRESCHOOLERS

Use story telling; use doll and puppet play; give choices when able.

SCHOOLAGERS

Maintain privacy; use gown; explain procedures and equipment; teach about their bodies.

ADOLESCENTS

Ensure privacy and confidentiality; provide option of having parent present or not; emphasize normality; provide health teaching.

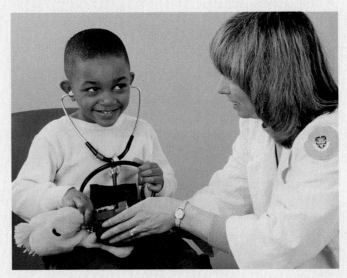

Puppet or doll play is a great way to prepare a preschooler for physical examination. (© B. Proud.)

PHYSICAL ASSESSMENT

ASSESSMENT PROCEDURE	NORMAL FINDINGS	ABNORMAL FINDINGS

GENERAL APPEARANCE AND BEHAVIOR

Observe hygiene, interaction with parents and yourself (and siblings if present). Note also facies (facial expressions), posture, nutritional status, speech, attention span, and level of cooperation

Tip From the Experts Behavioral observation is one of the most important assessments to make with children because alterations usually signify health problems.

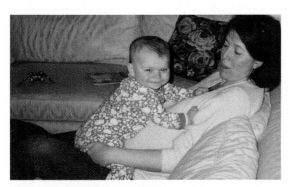
Observe parent–child interaction.

Appears stated age; clean, no unusual body odor, clothing in good condition and appropriate for climate. Child is alert, active, responds appropriately to stress of the situation, and maintains eye contact. Child is appropriately interactive for age, seeks comfort from parent; appears happy or appropriately anxious because of examination. Newborn's arms and legs are in flexed position; toddler is lordotic when standing; preschooler is slightly bowlegged; older child demonstrates straight and well-balanced posture, appears well nourished, is attentive and speech is appropriate for age, follows age-appropriate commands, and is reasonably cooperative.

Lack of eye contact indicates many things, including anxiety or significant psychosocial problems.

Lack of eye contact is normal for certain cultural groups such as Asians and Native Americans.

Deviations from normal that can be discerned from a child's appearance or behavior are listed below.
Facies—Fear, anxiety, anger, allergies, acute illness, pain, mental deficiency, respiratory distress
Posture or movement—Flaccidity or rigidity in newborn may be from neurologic damage or sepsis, pain, low self-esteem, rejection, depression, hostility or aggression
Hygiene—Neglect, poverty, mental illness or retardation, lack of information (teen parent)
Behavior—Neurologic problems (head trauma, cranial lesions), metabolic problems (diabetic ketoacidosis), psychiatric disorders, psychosocial problems
Development—Does not appear stated age (mental retardation, abuse, neglect, psychiatric disorders)

DEVELOPMENTAL ASSESSMENT

Screen for cognitive, language, social, and gross and fine motor developmental delays in the beginning of the physical assessment in infants and preschoolers. Use a standardized assessment tool such as the Draw a Person, Revised Prescreening Developmental Questionnaire, or the Denver Developmental Screening Test II (DDST). Display 24-6 presents the DDST II and directions for its use.

Normal parameters for age. See information contained in subjective data section.

Child lags in earlier stages.

(continued)

| ASSESSMENT PROCEDURE | NORMAL FINDINGS | ABNORMAL FINDINGS |

VITAL SIGNS

Temperature

Use rectal, axillary, skin, or tympanic route when assessing the temperature of an infant. For children older than 4 years of age, the oral route can be used in addition to the other routes.

To take a rectal temperature in a newborn or toddler, lay the child supine and lift lower legs up into the air, bending the legs at the hips. Insert lubricated rectal thermometer no more than 2 cm into rectum. Temperature registers in 3 to 5 min on a rectal thermometer. Lay a school-age child on the stomach on a table. Maintain firm hold on child's hips so child does not raise buttocks up during the procedure. Separate buttocks with thumb and forefinger of nondominant hand and insert thermometer. Axillary and/or tympanic temperature may also be used; however, these methods are less accurate and less reliable than the rectal temperature.

Infants: 99.4°F (because of excess heat production)
Children and adolescents: 98.6°F

🎗 **Tip From the Experts**
Use the rectal route only when absolutely necessary because of the perforation possibility in young infants and increased discomfort in older children. Rectal temperatures are also contraindicated in certain circumstances, such as perforated anus.

Temperature may be altered by exercise, stress, crying, environment, diurnal variation (highest between 4 and 6 PM). Both hyperthermic and hypothermic conditions are noted in children.

Pulse Rate

Count the pulse for a full minute. Children younger than 2 years should have apical pulse measured. Radial pulses may be taken in children over 2 years old.

Awake and resting rates vary with the age of the child:
1 wk–3 mo: 100–160
3 mo–2 y: 80–150
2–10 y: 70–110
10 y–adult: 55–90
Athletic adolescents tend to have lower pulse rates.

Pulse may be altered by apprehension or anxiety, medications, activity, and pain, as well as pathologic conditions. Bradycardia (<100 beats/min) in an infant, is usually an ominous finding.

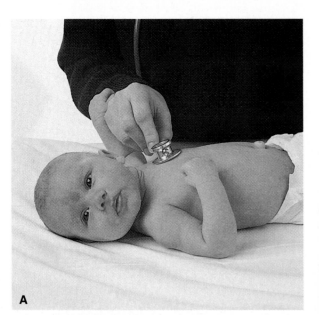

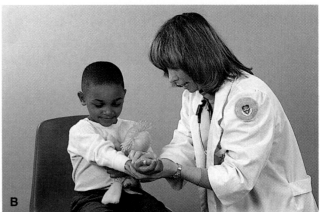

(*A*) Auscultating apical pulse rate in child under 2 years. (*B*) Measuring radial pulse in child over 2 years. (© B. Proud.)

(continued)

ASSESSMENT PROCEDURE	NORMAL FINDINGS	ABNORMAL FINDINGS

Respiratory Rate

Measure respiratory rate and character in infants by observing abdominal movements. Monitor respirations in older children the same as for adults.

Birth–6 mo: 30–50
6 mo–2 y: 20–30
3–10 y: 20–28
10–18 y: 12–20

Respiratory rate and character may be altered by medications, positioning, fever, activity, and anxiety or fear, as well as pathologic conditions.

Blood Pressure

Blood pressure should be measured annually in children 3 years and older, and in all ages when conditions warrant it. The appropriate cuff width is 50% to 75% of the upper arm. The length should encircle the circumference without overlapping. A small diaphragm should be used for the stethoscope. If for some reason the arm cannot be used, a measurement can be taken on the thigh. If children younger than 3 years old require a blood pressure reading, a Doppler stethoscope should be used or an electronic Dynamap machine may be used to record blood pressure readings in the newborn.

Systolic:
1–7 years = age in years + 90
8–18 years = (2 × age in years) + 90
Diastolic:
1–5 years = 56
6–18 years = age in years + 52
(Table 24-11)

Systolic and diastolic BP above 95th percentiles for age and sex after three readings is considered high blood pressure.

🎀 **Tip From the Experts** If the blood pressure reading is too high for age, the cuff may be too small; it should cover two thirds of the child's upper arm. If the blood pressure reading is too low for age, the cuff may be too large. Chapter 8 explains how to take a blood pressure reading.

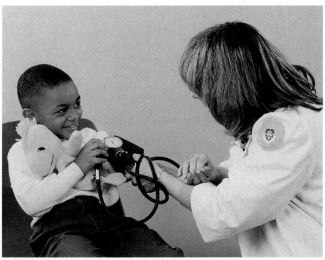

Measuring the child's blood pressure requires a cuff that is appropriately sized. (© B. Proud.)

(continued)

ASSESSMENT PROCEDURE	NORMAL FINDINGS	ABNORMAL FINDINGS

HEIGHT

In a child younger than 2 years, determine height by measuring the recumbent length. Fully extend the body, holding the head in midline and gently grasping the knees and pushing them downward until the legs are fully extended and touching the table. If using a measuring board, place the head at the top of the board and the heels firmly at the bottom. Without a board, use paper under the child and mark the paper at the top of the head and bottom of the heels. Then measure the distance between the two points. Determine an older child's height by having the shoeless child stand as straight as possible with head midline and vision line parallel between the ceiling and floor. Child's back, buttocks, and back of heels should be against the wall; measure height with a stadiometer. Plot height measurement on an age- and gender-appropriate growth chart (birth–36 mo and 2–20 y).

See the growth charts in Display 24-3 for normal findings.

Asian and black newborns are smaller than Caucasian newborns. Asian children are smaller at all ages.

Significant deviation from normal in the growth charts (Display 24-3) would be considered abnormal.

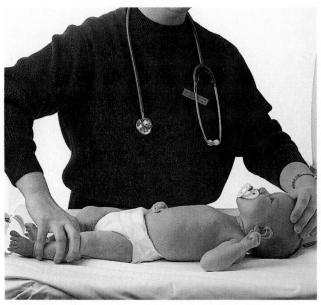
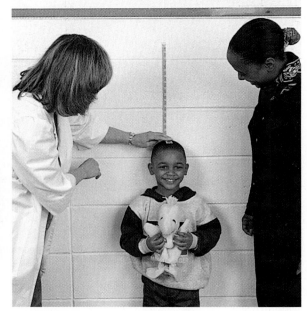

Measuring an infant *(left)* **and a preschooler** *(right).* **(© B. Proud.)**

(continued)

ASSESSMENT PROCEDURE	NORMAL FINDINGS	ABNORMAL FINDINGS

WEIGHT

Measure weight on an appropriately sized beam scale with nondetectable weights. Weigh an infant or small child lying or sitting on a scale that measures to the nearest 0.5 oz or 10 g. Weigh an older child standing on a scale that measures to the nearest 0.25 lb or 100 g. Weigh an infant naked, an older child in underpants or light gown to respect modesty. Plot weight measurement on age- and gender-appropriate growth chart (birth–36 mo and 2–20 y).

See the growth charts in Display 24-3 for normal findings.

Deviation from the wide range of normal weights is abnormal. See growth charts in Display 24-3, and compare differences.

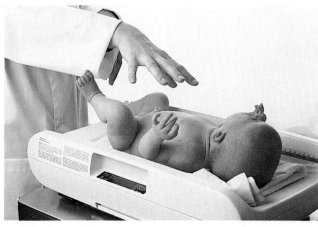

Weighing an infant. (© B. Proud.)

HEAD CIRCUMFERENCE

Measure head circumference (HC) or occipital frontal circumference (OFC) at every physical examination for infants and toddlers younger than 2 years and older children when conditions warrant. Plot the measurement on standardized growth charts specific for gender from birth to 36 months.

HC (OFC) measurement should fall between the 5th and 95th percentiles, and should be comparable to the child's height and weight percentiles.

HC (OFC) not within the normal percentiles may indicate pathology. Those greater than 95% may indicate macrocephaly. Those under the 5th percentile may indicate microcephaly. Increased HC (OFC) in children older than 3 years may indicate separation of cranial sutures due to increased intracranial pressure.

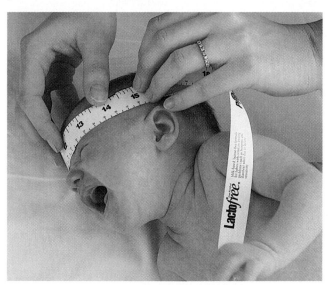

Measuring the circumference of an infant's head. (© B. Proud.)

(continued)

ASSESSMENT PROCEDURE	NORMAL FINDINGS	ABNORMAL FINDINGS

SKIN, HAIR, AND NAIL

Inspect and Palpate Skin

Observe skin color, odor, and lesions.

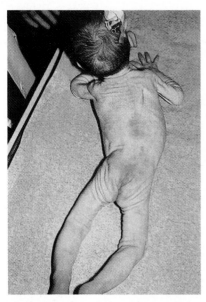

Observe for lesions.

Palpate for texture, temperature, moisture, turgor, and edema.

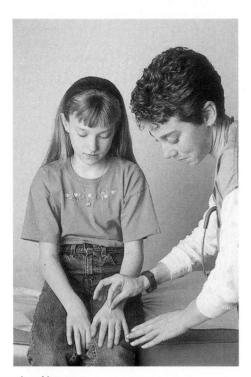

Assessing skin turgor.

Skin color ranges from pale white with pink, yellow, brown, or olive tones to dark brown or black. No strong odor should be evident, and the skin should be lesion free.

Skin should be soft, warm, slightly moist, with good turgor and without edema or lesions.

Common newborn skin variations include:

- Physiologic jaundice
- Birthmarks
- Milia
- Erythema toxicum

Dark-skinned newborns have lighter skin color than their parents. Their color darkens with age. Bluish pigmented areas (Mongolian spots) may be noted on the sacral areas of Asian, black, Native American, and Mexican-American infants (Display 24-7).

Yellow skin may indicate jaundice or intake of too many yellow vegetables in infants (sclera is white in the latter). Blue skin suggests cyanosis, pallor suggests anemia, and redness suggests fever, irritation, or allergies.

Body piercing may be cultural or a fad, but excessive piercing may indicate underlying self-abusive tendencies. If tattoos appear to be "homemade," consider the possibility of contamination with hepatitis B virus or HIV from infected needles.

Urine odor suggests incontinence, dirty diaper, or uremia. Salty sweat may indicate cystic fibrosis (a parent may report that the child's skin tastes salty when the parent kisses the child).

Ecchymoses in various stages or in unusual locations or circular burn areas suggest child abuse although bruising or burning may also be from cultural practices, such as *cupping* or *coining*. Petechiae, lesions, or rashes may indicate serious disorders.

Excessive dryness suggests poor nutrition, excessive bathing, or an endocrine disorder. Flaking or scaling suggests eczema or fungal infections. Poor skin turgor indicates dehydration or malnutrition, edema suggests renal or cardiac disorders; periorbital edema may indicate pathology but may also be due to recent crying, sleeping, or allergies. Russell's sign (abrasion or scarring on joints of index and middle finger) suggests self-induced vomiting. Bite marks may indicate child abuse or self-abusive behavior (psychiatric disorders, mental retardation).

(continued)

ASSESSMENT PROCEDURE	NORMAL FINDINGS	ABNORMAL FINDINGS

Inspect and Palpate Hair

Observe for distribution, characteristics, infestation, and presence of any unusual hair on body.

Hair is normally lustrous, silky, strong, and elastic. Fine, downy hair covers the body.

Adolescents may display a variety of hair styles to assert independence and group conformity.

African-American children usually have hair that is curlier and coarser than white children. Adolescents may color or pierce nails.

Dirty, matted hair may indicate neglect.
Dull, dry, brittle hair may indicate poor nutrition, hypothyroidism, excessive use of chemical hair products (teens).
Grayish, translucent flakes that adhere to hair shaft suggest lice (ova, nits).
Grayish or brown oval bodies suggest ticks.
Balding (alopecia) suggests neglect, trichotillomania (hair pulling), skin diseases, or chemotherapy.
Tufts of hair over spine may indicate spina bifida occulta.
Coarse body hair in prepubertal child or older girl may be from endocrine disorder.
Pubic hair in child younger than 8 years may indicate precocious adrenarche or precocious puberty.

Inspect and Palpate Nails

Note color, texture, shape, and condition of nails.

 Dark-skinned children have deeper nail pigment.

Blue nailbeds—Cyanosis
Yellow nailbeds—Jaundice
Blue-black nailbeds—Nailbed hemorrhage
White color—Fungal infection
Short, ragged nails—Nail biting
Dirty, uncut nails—Poor hygiene
Concave shape, "spoon nails" (koilonychia)—Iron deficiency anemia
Clubbing—Chronic cyanosis
Macerated thumb tip—Thumb sucking
Inflammation at the nail base—Paronychia
Scaly lesions—Fungal infections, especially in adolescents who use artificial nails

HEAD, NECK, AND CERVICAL LYMPH NODES

Inspect and Palpate the Head

Note shape and symmetry. In newborns, inspect and palpate the condition of fontanelles and sutures.

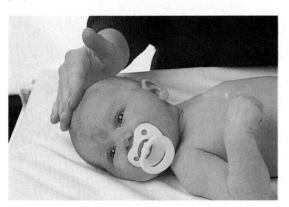

Palpating the anterior fontanelle. (© B. Proud.)

Head is normocephalic and symmetric. In newborns, the head may be oddly shaped from molding (overriding of the sutures) during vaginal birth. The diamond-shaped anterior fontanelle measures about 4 to 5 cm at its widest part. The triangular posterior fontanelle measures about 0.5 to 1 cm at its widest part, and it should close at 2 months of age.

Very large head—hydrocephalus
Oddly shaped head—premature closure of sutures (possibly genetic)
One-sided flattening of the head—prolonged positioning on one side
Third fontanelle between the anterior and posterior fontanelle—Down syndrome
Premature closure of sutures (craniosynostosis), caput succedaneum (edema from trauma) which crosses the suture line, and cephalohematoma (bleeding into the periosteal space) which does not extend across the suture line
Craniotabes—from osteoporosis of the outer skull bone. Palpating too firmly with the thumb or forefinger over the temporoparietal area will leave an indentation of the bone.

(continued)

ASSESSMENT PROCEDURE	NORMAL FINDINGS	ABNORMAL FINDINGS

Premature suture closure may result in (A) caput succedaneum and cephalohematoma. Hydrocephalus (B) in an infant who also has a myelomeningocele is another anomaly.

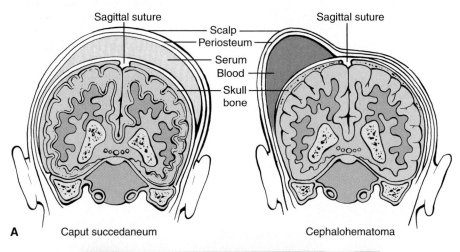

A   Caput succedaneum   Cephalohematoma

Labels: Sagittal suture, Scalp, Periosteum, Serum, Blood, Skull bone, Sagittal suture

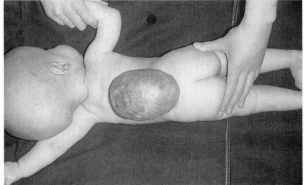

B

© 1991, National Medical Slide Bank/CMSP.

Test head control, head posture, range of motion.	By 4 months, infants should be able to hold head erect and in midline. Full range of motion—up, down, and sideways—is normal.	Head lag after 6 months—Cerebral injury
		   Hyperextension—Opisthotonos or significant meningeal irritation
		   Limited range of motion—Torticollis (wryneck)

(continued)

ASSESSMENT PROCEDURE	NORMAL FINDINGS	ABNORMAL FINDINGS

Inspect and Palpate the Face

Note appearance, symmetry, and movement (have child make faces). Palpate the parotid glands for swelling.

Face is normally proportionate and symmetric. Movements are equal bilaterally. Parotid glands are normal size.

Unusual proportions (short palpebral fissures, thin lips, and wide and flat philtrum, which is the groove above the upper lip) may be hereditary or they may indicate specific syndromes, such as Down syndrome and fetal alcohol syndrome. Other findings may indicate the following:

    Unequal movement—Facial nerve paralysis
    Enlarged parotid gland—Mumps or bulimia
    Abnormal facies—Chromosomal anomaly
    Crease across nose, shiners (dark circles under eyes), and mouth agape—Allergies (allergic facies)

Tip From the Experts Some adolescents may appear to have unusual skin tones or markings from applying makeup as a form of self-expression.

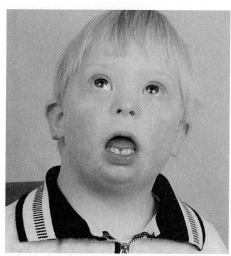

Down's syndrome results from a genetic abnormality. (© B. Proud.)

(continued)

ASSESSMENT PROCEDURE	NORMAL FINDINGS	ABNORMAL FINDINGS

Inspect and Palpate the Neck

Palpate the thyroid gland and the trachea. Also inspect and palpate the cervical lymph nodes for swelling, mobility, temperature, and tenderness.

🎗 **Tip From the Experts** The thyroid is very difficult to palpate in an infant because of the short, thick neck.

The neck is usually short with skin folds between the head and shoulder during infancy. The isthmus is the only portion of the thyroid that should be palpable. The trachea is midline. Lymph nodes are usually non-palpable in infants and adolescents. "Shotty" lymph nodes (small, nontender, mobile) are commonly palpated in children between the ages of 3 and 12 years.

Implications of some abnormal findings include the following:

Short, webbed neck—Anomalies or syndromes

Distended neck veins—Difficulty breathing

Enlarged thyroid or palpable masses—Pathologic processes

Shift in tracheal position from midline—Serious lung problem (eg, foreign body or tumor)

Enlarged firm lymph nodes—Hodgkin's disease or HIV infection

Enlarged, warm, and tender lymph nodes—Lymphadenitis or infection in the head and neck area that is drained by the affected node

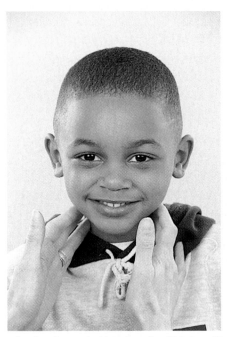

Palpating the cervical lymph nodes. (© B. Proud.)

(continued)

ASSESSMENT PROCEDURE	NORMAL FINDINGS	ABNORMAL FINDINGS

MOUTH, THROAT, NOSE, AND SINUSES

Inspect Mouth and Throat

Note the condition of the lips, palates, tongue, and buccal mucosa.

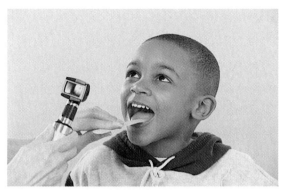

Inspecting the mouth. (© B. Proud.)

Epstein's pearls, small yellow-white retention cysts on the hard palate and gums, are common in newborns and usually disappear in the first weeks of life. In infants, a sucking tubercle (pad) from the friction of sucking may be evident in the middle of the upper lip.

Dry lips may indicate mouth breathing or dehydration. Stomatitis suggests infection or immunodeficiency. Koplik's spots (tiny white spots on red bases) on the buccal mucosa may be a prodromal sign of measles. Cleft lip and/or palate are congenital abnormalities.

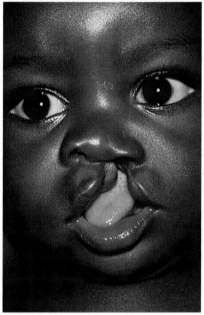

Cleft lip. (© 1991 National Medical Slide Bank/CMSP.)

Observe the condition of the teeth (if present) and gums.

Deciduous teeth begin to develop between 4 and 6 months; all 20 erupt by 36 months; teeth begin to fall out around 6 years, when permanent tooth eruption begins and progresses until all 32 have erupted.

Dental caries may herald "bottle caries syndrome." Enamel erosion may indicate bulimia.

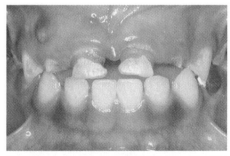

"Bottle caries" syndrome. (© 1992 Edward H. Gill/CMSP.)

(continued)

ASSESSMENT PROCEDURE	NORMAL FINDINGS	ABNORMAL FINDINGS
Note the condition of the throat and tonsils. Also observe the insertion and ending point of the frenulum.	Tonsils are not visible in newborns, but they grow rapidly and are easily seen by age 6 when they increase to adult dimensions. They reach maximum size (about twice adult size) between ages 10 and 12. Atrophy to stable adult dimensions usually occurs by the end of adolescence.	Tonsillar or pharyngeal inflammation suggests infection. Extension of the frenulum to the tip of tongue may interfere with extension of the tongue, which causes speech difficulties.

Inspect Nose and Sinuses

To inspect the nose and sinuses, avoid using the nasal speculum in infants and young children. Instead, push up the tip of the nose and shine the light into each nostril. Observe the structure and patency of the nares, discharge, tenderness, and any color or swelling of the turbinates.	Nose is midline in face, septum is straight, and nares are patent. No discharge or tenderness is present. Turbinates are pink and free of edema.	Choanal atresia is blockage of the posterior nares in the newborn. If the blockage is bilateral, the newborn is at risk for acute respiratory distress. Immediate referral is necessary. Deviated septum may be congenital or caused by injury. Foul discharge from one nostril may indicate a foreign body. Pale, boggy nasal mucosa with or without possible polyps suggests allergic rhinitis. Nasal polyps are also seen in children with cystic fibrosis.

> ✿ **Tip From the Experts** Infants are obligatory nose breathers. Consequently, obstructed nasal passages may precipitate serious health conditions, making it very important to assess the patency of the nares in the newborn. If, after suctioning fluid and mucus from the nares, you suspect obstruction, insert a small-lumen catheter into each nostril to assess patency.

Palpate the sinuses in older children if sinusitis is suspected. The sinuses of infants and young children are not palpable.	No tenderness palpated over sinuses.	Tender sinuses suggest sinusitis.

EYES

Inspect the External Eye

Note the position, slant, and epicanthal folds of the external eye.	Inner canthus distance approximately 2.5 cm, horizontal slant, no epicanthal folds. Outer canthus aligns with tips of the pinnas. 👪 Epicanthal folds (excess of skin extending from roof of nose that partially or completely covers the inner canthus) are normal findings in Asian children, whose eyes also slant upward.	Wide-set position (hypertelorism), upward slant, and thick epicanthal folds suggest Down syndrome. "Sun-setting" appearance (upper lid covers part of the iris) suggests hydrocephalus.

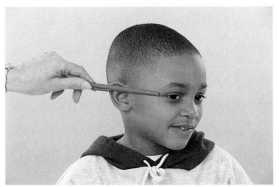

Outer canthus is in alignment with the tip of the pinna. (© B. Proud.)

(continued)

ASSESSMENT PROCEDURE	NORMAL FINDINGS	ABNORMAL FINDINGS
Observe eyelid placement, swelling, discharge, and lesions.	No swelling, discharge, or lesions of eyelids.	Eyelid inflammation may result from blepharitis, hordeolum, or dacryocystis (inflammation or blockage of lacrimal sac or duct). Ptosis (drooping eyelids) suggests oculomotor nerve palsy, congenital syndrome, or a familial trait. A painful, edematous, erythematous area on eyelid may be a hordeolum (style). A nodular, nontender lesion on the eyelid may be a chalazion (cyst). Swelling, erythema, or purulent discharge may indicate infection or blocked tear ducts. Sunken area around eyelids may indicate dehydration. Periorbital edema suggests fluid retention.
Inspect the sclera and conjunctiva for color, discharge, lesions, redness, and lacerations.	Sclera and conjunctiva are clear and free of discharge, lesions, redness, or lacerations. Small subconjunctival hemorrhages may be seen in newborns.	Yellow sclera suggests jaundice, blue sclera may indicate osteogenesis imperfecta ("brittle bone disease"), and redness may indicate conjunctivitis.
Observe the iris and the pupils.	Typically, the iris is blue in light-skinned infants and brown in dark-skinned infants; permanent color develops within 9 months. Brushfield's spots (white flecks on the periphery of the iris) may be normal in some infants. Pupils are equal, round, and reactive to light and accommodation (PERRLA).	Brushfield's spots may indicate Down syndrome. Sluggish pupils indicate a neurologic problem. Miosis (constriction) indicates iritis or narcotic use or abuse. Mydriasis (pupillary dilation) indicates emotional factors (fear), trauma, or certain drug use.
Finally, inspect the eyebrows and eyelashes.	Eyebrows should be symmetric in shape and movement. They should not meet midline. Eyelashes should be evenly distributed and curled outward.	Sparseness of eyebrows or lashes could indicate skin disease or deliberate pulling out of hairs (usually due to anxiety or habit). Corneal abrasions are common during childhood and may not be easily visible to the naked eye.

(continued)

ASSESSMENT PROCEDURE	NORMAL FINDINGS	ABNORMAL FINDINGS

Perform Visual Acuity Tests

Use the following diagnostic tools to perform visual acuity testing:

  Snellen letter chart
  Snellen symbol chart (E chart; used for preschoolers)
  Blackbird Preschool Vision Screening Test (uses modified E that resembles a bird and a story to engage children's attention)
  Faye symbol chart (uses pictures)

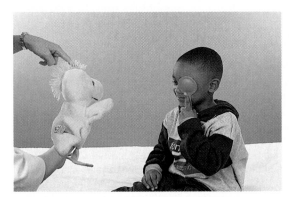

Performing the cover test. (© B. Proud.)

> 🎀 **Tip From the Experts** Fatigue, anxiety, hunger, and distractions interfere with vision testing. Testing should precede procedures that create discomfort.

Visual acuity is difficult to test in infants; it is usually tested by observing the infant's ability to fix on and follow objects. Normal visual acuity is as follows:

  Birth—20/100 to 20/400
  1 year—20/200
  2 years—20/70
  5 years—20/30
  6 years—20/20
Children should be able to differentiate colors by age 5.

Children with a one-line difference between eyes should be referred. Children should also be referred for abnormal visual acuity or inability to distinguish colors. Visual impairment can indicate congenital defects (cataracts), malignant tumors, chronic disease (diabetes), drugs, trauma, enzyme deficiencies, or refractive errors (myopia, hyperopia, astigmatism).

Perform Extraocular Muscle Tests

Cover test: Have the child cover one eye and look at an interesting object. Observe the uncovered eye for any movement. When the child is focused on the object, remove the cover and observe that eye for movement.
Hirschberg test: Shine light directly at the cornea while the child looks straight ahead.

> 🎀 **Tip From the Experts** Use a toy, a puppet, and the parent to focus the child's eyes. Older children, including adolescents, focus better if they are given something to focus on instead of being told to "look straight ahead."

In the cover test, the eyes remain focused.

  In the Hirschberg test, the light reflects symmetrically in the center of both pupils.

Eye movement is present during the cover test; this may indicate strabismus.

  Unequal alignment of light on the pupils in the Hirschberg test signals strabismus.

(continued)

ASSESSMENT PROCEDURE	NORMAL FINDINGS	ABNORMAL FINDINGS

Perform Ophthalmoscopic Examination

The procedure is the same as for adults. Distraction is preferred over the use of restraint, which is likely to result in crying and closed eyes. Careful ophthalmoscopic examination of newborns is difficult without the use of mydriatic medications.

Red reflex present. This reflex rules out most serious defects of the cornea, aqueous chamber, lens, and vitreous humor. When visualized, the optic disc appears similar to an adult's. A newborn's optic discs are pale; peripheral vessels are not well developed.

Absence of the red reflex indicates cataracts. Papilledema is unusual in children under 3 years of age owing to the ability of the fontanelles and sutures to open during increased intracranial pressure. Disc blurring and hemorrhages should be reported immediately.

EARS

Inspect External Ears

Note placement, discharge, or lesions of the ears.

Top of pinna should cross the eye-occiput line and be within a 10-degree angle of a perpendicular line drawn from the eye-occiput line to the lobe. No unusual structure or markings should appear on the pinna.

Low-set ears with an alignment greater than a 10-degree angle suggest mental retardation or congenital syndromes. Abnormal shape may suggest renal disease process, which may be hereditary. Preauricular skin tags or sinuses suggest other anomalies of ears or the renal system.

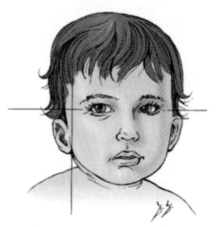

Low-set ears with alignment greater than 10-degree angle.

(continued)

ASSESSMENT PROCEDURE	NORMAL FINDINGS	ABNORMAL FINDINGS

Inspect Internal Ear

The internal ear examination requires using an otoscope and, for infants and toddlers, restraint by (1) having a parent hold the seated child in the lap while holding the child's hands with one hand and the child's head sideways against chest (as shown) or (2) laying the child supine, with the parent holding the child's arms up over head. Then the nurse can gently but firmly hold child's head to the side. Regardless of technique used, the nurse should always hold the otoscope in a manner that allows for rapid removal if the child moves. Because an infant's external canal is short and straight, pull the pinna down and back. Because an older child's canal shortens and becomes less straight, like the adult's, gently pull the pinna up and back.

Normal Findings: No excessive cerumen, discharge, lesions, excoriations, or foreign body in external canal. Tympanic membrane is pearly gray to light pink with normal landmarks. Tympanic membranes redden bilaterally when child is crying or febrile.

Abnormal Findings: Presence of foreign bodies or cerumen impaction. Purulent discharge may indicate otitis externa or presence of foreign body. Purulent, serous discharge suggests otitis media. Bloody discharge suggests trauma, and clear discharge may indicate cerebrospinal fluid leak. Perforated tympanic membrane may also be noted.

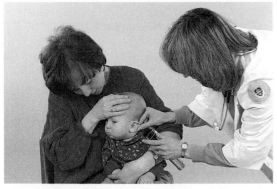

To examine the ears of an infant, restrain the child and pull the pinna down and back. (© B. Proud.)

Assess the mobility of the tympanic membrane by pneumatic otoscopy. This consists of creating pressure against the tympanic membrane using air. To do this, you need to create a seal in the external canal and direct a puff of air against the tympanic membrane. Create the seal by using the largest speculum that will comfortably insert into the ear canal. Cover the tip with rubber for a better and more comfortable seal. Attach a pneumatic bulb to the otoscope and squeeze the bulb lightly to direct air against the tympanic membrane.

Normal Findings: Tympanic membrane is mobile; moves inward with positive pressure (squeeze of bulb) and outward with negative pressure (release of bulb).

Abnormal Findings: Immobility suggests chronic (serous) otitis media; decreased mobility may occur with acute otitis media.

Hearing Acuity

In the infant, test hearing acuity by noting the reaction to noise. Stand approximately 12 inches from the infant and create a loud noise (eg, clap hands, shake/squeeze a noisy toy).

Normal Findings: A newborn will exhibit the startle (Moro) reflex and blink eyes (acoustic blink reflex) in response to noise. Infants 6 months or older try to locate the sound.

Abnormal Findings: No reactions to noise may indicate a hearing deficit.

In an older child, test hearing acuity initially by whispering questions from a distance of approximately 8 feet. If hearing deficit is suspected, complete audiometric testing should be performed. Audiometry measures the threshold of hearing for frequencies and loudness. In addition, all children should have audiometric testing performed before entering school.

Normal Findings: Answers whispered questions. Audiometry results are within normal ranges.

Abnormal Findings: Failure to respond to whispered questions may indicate hearing deficit. Audiometry results outside normal range suggest hearing deficit.

(continued)

ASSESSMENT PROCEDURE	NORMAL FINDINGS	ABNORMAL FINDINGS

THORAX AND LUNGS

Inspect the shape of the thorax.	Infant's thorax is smooth, rounded and symmetric. By age 5 to 6 years, the thoracic diameter reaches the adult 1:2 or 5:7 ratio (anteroposterior to transverse).	Abnormal shapes of the thorax include pectus excavatum and pectus corinatum.
Observe respiratory effort, keeping in mind that newborns and young infants are obligatory nose breathers and older infants and children under 7 years old are abdominal breathers.	Respirations should be unlabored and regular in all ages, except for immediate newborn period when respirations are irregular (see "Vital Signs" section). Some newborns, especially the premature, have periodic irregular breathing, sometimes with apnea (episodes when breathing stops) lasting a few seconds. This is a normal finding if bradycardia does not accompany irregular breathing.	Retractions (suprasternal, sternal, substernal, intercostal) and grunting suggest increased inspiratory effort, which may be due to asthma, atelectasis, pneumonia, or airway obstruction. Periods of apnea that last longer than 20 s and are accompanied by bradycardia may be a sign of a cardiovascular or CNS disease.

Percuss and Auscultate the Lungs

During percussion of the lungs, note tone elicited.	Hyperresonance is the normal tone elicited in infants and young children because of thinness of the chest wall.	A dull tone may indicate a mass, fluid, or consolidation.
Auscultate for breath sounds and adventitious sounds. If a newborn or toddler's lung sounds seem noisy, auscultate the upper nostrils. Infants and toddlers with an upper respiratory infection may transmit noisy breathing from the upper nostrils to the upper lobes of the lungs. Encourage deep breathing in children; try one of the following techniques: blow out light on otoscope, blow cotton ball in air, blow pinwheel, "race" paper off table.	Breath sounds may seem louder and harsher in young children because of their thin chest wall. No adventitious sounds should be heard, although transmitted upper airway sounds may be heard on auscultation of thorax.	Diminished breath sounds suggest respiratory disorders such as pneumonia or atelectasis. Stridor (inspiratory wheeze) is a high-pitched, piercing sound that indicates a narrowing of the upper tracheobronchial tree. Expiratory wheezes indicate narrowing in the lower tracheobronchial tree. Rhonchi and rales (crackles) may indicate a number of respiratory diseases, such as pneumonia, bronchitis, or bronchiolitis.

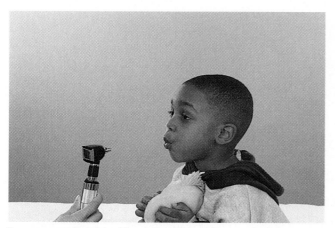

To encourage deep breathing, ask a child to blow out the light on an otoscope or a penlight. (© B. Proud.)

(continued)

ASSESSMENT PROCEDURE	NORMAL FINDINGS	ABNORMAL FINDINGS

BREASTS

Inspect and Palpate Breasts

Note shape, symmetry, color, tenderness, discharge, lesions, and masses.

Breasts are flat and symmetric in prepubertal children. Newborns may have enlarged and engorged breasts with a white liquid discharge resulting from the influence of maternal hormones. This condition resolves spontaneously within days. Obese children may appear to have breast tissue.

Redness, edema, and tenderness indicate mastitis. Enlargement in adolescent boys suggests gynecomastia. Masses in the adolescent female breast usually indicate cysts or trauma.

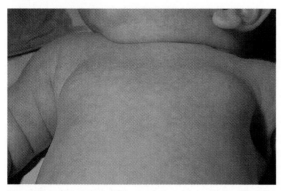

The enlarged breasts of this newborn are normal and result from the influence of maternal hormones. (© 1994 Science Photo Library / CMSP).

Assess stage of breast/sexual development of girl client.

See Tanner's sexual maturity rating in Table 24-2.

Breast development before age 8 may indicate precocious puberty or the larch. Lack of breast development after age 13 may indicate delayed puberty and/or a pathologic process.

HEART

Inspect and Palpate the Precordium

Note lifts, heaves, apical impulse.

The apical pulse is at the 4th intercostal space (ICS) until the age of 7 years, when it drops to the 5th. It is to the left of the midclavicular line (MCL) until age 4, at the MCL between ages 4 and 6, and to the right at age 7.

A systolic heave may indicate right ventricular enlargement. Apical impulse that is not in proper location for age may indicate cardiomyopathy, pneumothorax, or diaphragmatic hernia.

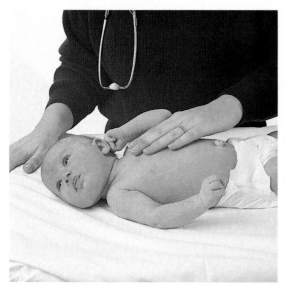

Palpate the infant's chest for lifts and heaves. (© B. Proud.)

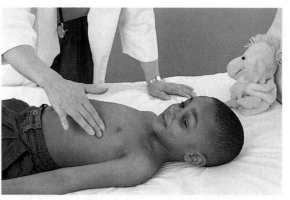

To palpate an infant or preschooler's apical pulse, place your hand at the 4th intercostal space to the left of the midclavicular line. (© B. Proud.)

(continued)

ASSESSMENT PROCEDURE	NORMAL FINDINGS	ABNORMAL FINDINGS

Auscultate Heart Sounds

Listen to the heart. Note rate and rhythm of apical impulse, S_1, S_2, extra heart sounds, and murmurs. Keep in mind that sinus arrhythmia is normal in infants and young children. Heart sounds are louder, higher pitched, and of shorter duration in infants and children. A split S_2 at the apex occurs normally in some infants and children, and S_3 is a normal heart sound in some children. A venous hum also may be normally heard in children.

Normal heart rates are cited in the "Vital Signs" section above. Innocent murmurs, which are common throughout childhood, are classified as systolic; short duration; no transmission to other areas; grade III or less; loudest in pulmonic area (base of heart); low-pitched, musical, or groaning quality that varies in intensity in relation to position, respiration, activity, fever, and anemia. No other associated signs of heart disease.

Murmurs that do not fit the criteria for innocent murmurs may indicate a disease or disorder. Extra heart sounds and variations in pulse rate and rhythm also suggest pathologic processes.

ABDOMEN

Inspect the shape of the abdomen.

In infants and children up to 4 years of age, the abdomen is prominent in standing and supine positions. After age 4, the abdomen appears slightly prominent when standing, but flat when supine, until puberty.

A scaphoid (boat shaped; ie, sunken with prominent rib cage) abdomen may result from malnutrition or dehydration.

Inspect Umbilicus

Note color, discharge, evident herniation of the umbilicus.

Umbilicus is pink, no discharge, odor, redness or herniation. Remnant of cord should appear dried in newborn.

Inflammation, discharge, and redness of umbilicus suggest infection.

Diastasis recti (separation of the abdominal muscles) is seen as midline protrusion from the xiphoid to the umbilicus or pubis symphysis. This condition is secondary to immature musculature of abdominal muscles and usually has little significance. As the muscles strengthen, the separation resolves on its own.

A bulge at the umbilicus suggests an umbilical hernia, which may be seen in newborns; many disappear by the age of 1 year, and most by 4 or 5 years of age.

 Umbilical hernias are seen more frequently in African American children.

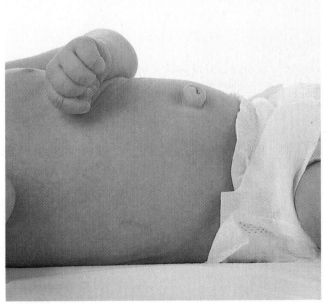
Umbilical hernia.

(continued)

ASSESSMENT PROCEDURE	NORMAL FINDINGS	ABNORMAL FINDINGS
Auscultate Bowel Sounds		
Follow auscultation guidelines for adult clients provided in Chapter 18.	Normal bowel sounds occur every 10 to 30 s. They sound like clicks, gurgles, or growls.	Marked peristaltic waves almost always indicate a pathologic process, such as pyloric stenosis.
Palpate for Masses and Tenderness		
Palpate abdomen for softness or hardness.	Abdomen is soft to palpation and without masses or tenderness.	A rigid abdomen is almost always an emergent problem. Masses or tenderness warrants further investigation.

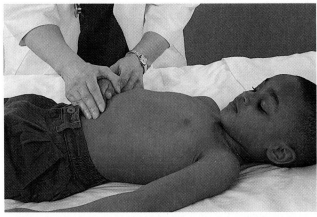

Let a child help palpate his or her abdomen to decrease ticklishness. (© B. Proud.)

Tip From the Experts To decrease ticklishness, have the child help by placing his or her hand under yours, using age-appropriate distraction techniques, and maintaining conversation focused on something other than the examination.

ASSESSMENT PROCEDURE	NORMAL FINDINGS	ABNORMAL FINDINGS
Palpate Liver		
Palpate the liver the same as you would for adults (see Chapter 18).	Liver is usually palpable 1 to 2 cm below the right costal margin in young children.	An enlarged liver with a firm edge that is palpated more than 2 cm below the right costal margin usually indicates a pathologic process.
Palpate Spleen		
Palpate the spleen the same as you would for adults.	Spleen tip may be palpable during inspiration.	Enlarged spleen is usually indicative of a pathologic process.
Palpate Kidneys		
Palpate the kidneys the same as you would for adults.	The tip of the right kidney may be palpable during inspiration.	Enlarged kidneys are usually indicative of a pathologic process.
Palpate Bladder		
Palpate the bladder the same as you would for adults.	Bladder may be slightly palpable in infants and small children.	An enlarged bladder is usually due to urinary retention but may be due to a mass.

(continued)

ASSESSMENT PROCEDURE	NORMAL FINDINGS	ABNORMAL FINDINGS

MALE GENITALIA

Inspect Penis and Urinary Meatus

Inspect the genitalia observing size for age and any lesions.

🏵 **Tip From the Experts** Use distraction or teaching (such as testicular self-examination) when examining the genitalia in older children and adolescents to decrease embarrassment.

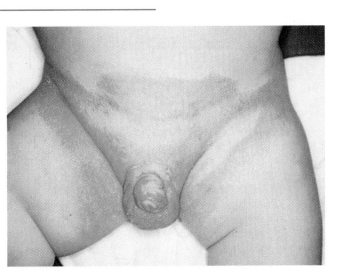

When the examiner inspects the genital area, a common finding is diaper rash in infants. (© Princess Margaret Rose Orthopedic Hospital / Science Photo Library / CMSP.)

Penis is normal size for age, and no lesions are seen. The foreskin is retractable in uncircumcised child. Urinary meatus is at tip of glans penis and has no discharge or redness. Penis may appear small in obese boys because of overlapping skin folds.

An unretractable foreskin in a child older than 3 months suggests phimosis. Paraphimosis is indicated when the foreskin is tightened around the glans penis in a retracted position. Hypospadias, urinary meatus on ventral surface of glans, and epispadias, urinary meatus on dorsal surface of glans, are congenital disorders (see Display 19-2). Discharge, redness, or lacerations may indicate abuse in young children, but may occur from infections or foreign body. Discharge in adolescents may be due to sexually transmitted disease, infection, or irritation.

Inspect and Palpate Scrotum and Testes

To rule out cryptorchidism, it is important to palpate for testes in the scrotum in infants and young boys.

🏵 **Tip From the Experts** When palpating the testicles in the infant and young boy, you must keep the cremasteric reflex in mind. This reflex pulls the testicles up into the inguinal canal and abdomen and is elicited in response to touch, cold, or emotional factors. Block this reflex in infants by placing two fingers at the external inguinal ring. Then palpate down the inguinal ring to the scrotum. Have young boys sit with knees flexed and abducted. This lessens the cremasteric reflex and enables you to examine the testicles.

Scrotum is free of lesions. Testes are palpable in scrotum, with the left testicle usually lower than the right. Testes are equal in size, smooth, mobile, and free of masses. If a testicle is missing from the scrotal sac but the scrotal sac appears well developed, suspect physiologic cryptorchidism. The testis has originally descended into the scrotum but has moved back up into the inguinal canal because of the cremasteric reflex and the small size of the testis. You should be able to milk the testis down into the scrotum from the inguinal canal. This normal condition subsides at puberty.

Absent testicle(s) and atrophic scrotum suggest true cryptorchidism (undescended testicles; see Chapter 6). This suggests that the testicle(s) never descended. This condition occurs more frequently in preterm than term infants because testes descend at 8 months of gestation. It can lead to testicular atrophy and infertility, and increases the risk for testicular cancer. Hydroceles are common in infants. They are fluid-filled masses that can be transilluminated (see Display 19-3). They usually resolve spontaneously. A scrotal hernia is usually caused by an indirect inguinal hernia that has descended into the scrotum. It can usually be pushed back into the inguinal canal. This mass will not transilluminate. A painless nodule on the testis may indicate testicular cancer, which appears most frequently in males aged 15 to 34 years; therefore, testicular self-examination (TSE) should be taught to all boys 14 years old and older.

(continued)

ASSESSMENT PROCEDURE	NORMAL FINDINGS	ABNORMAL FINDINGS
Inspect and Palpate Inguinal Area for Hernias		
Observe for any bulge in the inguinal area. Ask the child to bear down or try to lift something heavy to elicit a possible hernia. Using your pinky finger, palpate up the inguinal canal to the external inguinal ring if a hernia is suspected.	No inguinal hernias are present.	A bulge in the inguinal area or palpation of a mass in the inguinal canal suggests an inguinal hernia. Indirect inguinal hernias occur most frequently in children (see Chapter 19).
Assess Sexual Development		
Note public hair pattern, and size and development of penis and scrotum.	See Tanner's sexual maturity ratings in Table 24-1.	Pubic hair growth, enlargement of the penis to adolescent or adult size, and enlarged testes in a young boy suggest precocious puberty.

FEMALE GENITALIA

Inspect External Genitalia

Note labia majora, labia minora, vaginal orifice, urinary meatus, and clitoris.

> **Tip From the Experts** Have female children assist with genitalia examination by using their hands to spread the labia. This helps to decrease any stress and embarrassment.

Labia majora and minora are pink and moist. Newborn's genitalia may appear prominent because of influence of maternal hormones. Bruises and swelling may be caused by breech vaginal delivery. Young girls have flattened majora, thin minora, small clitoris, and thin hymen. Starting at school age, the labia become fuller and the hymen thickens. This progresses until puberty when the genitalia develop adult characteristics. No discharge from vagina or meatus; no redness or edema present normally.

Enlarged clitoris in newborn combined with fusion of the posterior labia majora suggests ambiguous genitalia. Partial or complete labia minora adhesions are sometimes seen in girls younger than 4 years of age. Referral is necessary to disintegrate the thin, membraneous adhesion. An imperforate hymen (no central orifice) is sometimes seen and is not significant unless it persists until puberty and causes problems with menstruation. Discharge from vagina or urinary meatus, redness, edema, or lacerations may suggest abuse in the young child. However, infections or a foreign body in the vagina may cause these symptoms. Discharge in adolescents suggests sexually transmitted disease, infection, or irritation.

Inspect Internal Genitalia

An internal genitalia examination is not routinely performed in the child although it may be called for if infection, bleeding, a foreign body, disease, or sexual abuse is suspected. The examination should be performed by a pediatric specialist. An internal genital examination consisting of both the speculum and bimanual examinations is recommended for all sexually active adolescents and/or virgins starting at 18 years of age. In addition, an internal examination is indicated in the adolescent who has nonmenstrual bleeding or discharge. The procedure is the same as for the adult. Time and care must be taken for adequate teaching and reassurance.

See Chapter 20 for normal findings.

See Chapter 20 for abnormal findings.

Assess Sexual Development

Note pubic hair pattern.

See Tanner's sexual maturity ratings in Table 24-2 for normal findings.

Growth of pubic hair in young girls (<8 years of age) suggests precocious puberty. Unusual pubic hair distribution in pubertal girls may indicate a disorder. For example, a male pattern of hair growth may suggest polycystic ovary disease.

(continued)

ASSESSMENT PROCEDURE	NORMAL FINDINGS	ABNORMAL FINDINGS

ANUS AND RECTUM

Inspect the Anus

The anus should be inspected in infants, children, and adolescents. Perform quickly at the end of the genitalia examination to limit embarrassment in the older child and adolescent. Spread the buttocks with gloved hands, and note patency of anal opening, presence of any lesions and fissures, and condition and color of perianal skin.

The anal opening should be visible, moist, and hairless. No hemorrhoids or lesions. Perianal skin should be smooth and free of lesions. A mild diaper rash (red papules) may be seen in infants. Perianal skin tags may be noted.

Imperforate anus (no anal opening) should be referred. Hemorrhoids are unusual in children and could be due to chronic constipation, but may be caused by sexual abuse or abdominal pressure from lesion. Bleeding and pain often indicate tears or fissures in the anus, which often cause constipation because of pain of passing stool. Pustules may indicate secondary infection of diaper rash. A dark ring around the anus may indicate heavy metal poisoning. Lacerations, purulent discharge, or extreme apprehension during examination may indicate physical or sexual abuse. Diaper rashes with more than mild red/pink papules suggest problems such as seborrhea, diaper dermatitis, and monilial infection.

Palpate Rectum

This internal examination is not routinely performed in infants, children, or adolescents. However, it should be performed if symptoms suggest a problem. The infant or child should be in a supine position with the legs flexed. Provide reassurance throughout the examination. If the child is old enough, ask him or her to bear down. This helps to relax the sphincter. Slowly insert a gloved, lubricated finger (the pinky finger may be used for comfort, but the index finger is more sensitive) into the anal opening, aiming the finger toward the umbilicus.

Prostate gland is nonpalpable in young boys. Bimanual recto-abdominal exam in girls may reveal small midline mass (cervix).

If other masses are palpated, they are considered abnormal; no other structures are palpable until adolescence.

(continued)

ASSESSMENT PROCEDURE	NORMAL FINDINGS	ABNORMAL FINDINGS

MUSCULOSKELETAL

Assess Feet and Legs

Note symmetry, shape, movement, and positioning of the feet and legs. Perform neurovascular assessment.

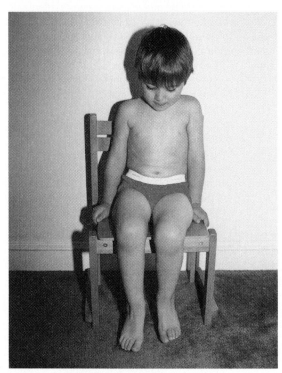

Normally positioned feet and legs.

Feet and legs are symmetric in size, shape, and movement. Extremities should be warm, and mobile with adequate capillary refill. All pulses (radial, brachial, femoral, popliteal, pedal) should be strong and equal bilaterally. A common finding in children (up to 2 or 3 years old) is metatarsus adductus deformity. This is an inward positioning of the forefoot with the heel in normal straight position, and it resolves spontaneously. Tibial torsion, also common in infants and toddlers, consists of twisting of the tibia inward or outward on its long axis, is usually caused by intrauterine positioning, and typically corrects itself by the time the child is 2 years old.

Short, broad extremities, hyperextensible joints, and palmar simian crease may indicate Down syndrome. Polydactyly (extra digits) and syndactyly (webbing) are sometimes found in children with mental retardation. Absent femoral pulses may indicate coarctation of the aorta. Neurovascular deficit in children is usually secondary to trauma (eg, fracture).

Fixed-position (true) deformities do not return to normal position with manipulation. Metatarsus varus is inversion (a turning inward that elevates the medial margin) and adduction of the forefoot.

Talipes varus is adduction of the forefoot and inversion of the entire foot.

Talipes equinovarus (clubfoot) is indicated if foot is fixed in the following position: adduction of forefoot, inversion of entire foot, and equinus (pointing downward) position of entire foot.

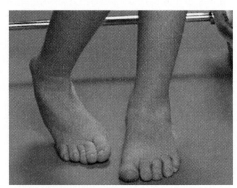

Talipes equinovarus, also called clubfoot. (© 1995. Science Photo Library / CMSP.)

> **Tip From the Experts** If the client is a newborn, keep in mind that the feet may retain their intrauterine position and appear deformed (positioned outward or inward from normal right angle to the leg). This is normal if the foot easily returns to its normal position with manipulation (either scratch along the lateral edge of the affected foot or gently push the forefoot into its normal position).

Assess for Congenital Hip Dysplasia

Assessing for hip dysplasia is an important aspect of the physical examination for infants. The assessment should be performed at each visit until the child is about 1 year old. (Several tests are described below.)

Begin by assessing the symmetry of the gluteal folds. Also assess hip abduction using the maneuvers below.

Equal gluteal folds, and full hip abduction are normal findings

Unequal gluteal folds and limited hip abduction are signs of congenital hip dysplasia.

(continued)

ASSESSMENT PROCEDURE	NORMAL FINDINGS	ABNORMAL FINDINGS
Perform Ortolani's maneuver to test for congenital hip dysplasia. With the infant supine, flex the knees while holding your thumbs on midthigh and your fingers over the greater trochanters; abduct the legs, moving the knees outward and down toward the table.	Negative Ortolani's sign.	Positive Ortolani's sign: A click heard along with feeling the head of the femur slip in or out of the hip.

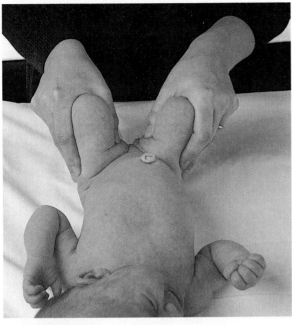

Ortolani's maneuver.

Perform Barlow's maneuvers. With the infant supine, flex the knees while holding your thumbs on midthigh and your fingers over the greater trochanters; adduct legs until thumbs touch.	Negative Barlow's sign.	Positive Barlow's sign: A feeling of the head of the femur slipping out of the hip socket (acetabulum).

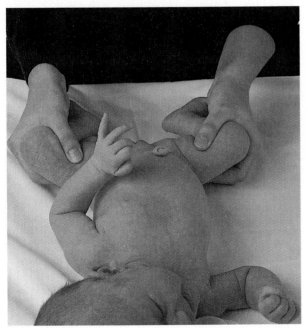

Barlow's maneuver.

(continued)

ASSESSMENT PROCEDURE	NORMAL FINDINGS	ABNORMAL FINDINGS

Assess Spinal Alignment

Observe spine and posture.

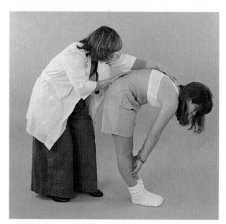

Assessing spinal curvature for scoliosis. (© B. Proud.)

In newborns, the spine is flexible, with convex dorsal and sacral curves. In infants younger than 3 months, the spine is rounded.

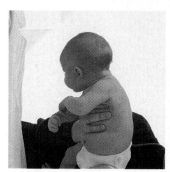

The spine is rounded in infants under 3 months old.

In infants 3 to 4 months, cervical curve develops. By 12 to 18 months, the lumbar curve develops. Newborns are flexed, whereas toddlers display lordotic posture. Findings in older children and adolescents are similar to those in adults.

Kyphosis may result from poor posture or from pathologic conditions. Scoliosis usually is idiopathic and is more common in adolescent girls. In newborns, flaccid or rigid posture is considered abnormal. In older infants and children, abnormal posture suggests neuromuscular disorders such as cerebral palsy. Extremities that are asymmetric in size, shape, and movement indicate scoliosis or hip disease.

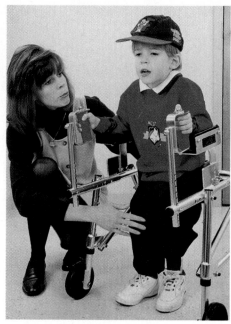

Neuromuscular weakness is a hallmark of cerebral palsy.

(continued)

ASSESSMENT PROCEDURE	NORMAL FINDINGS	ABNORMAL FINDINGS

Assess Gait

Observe gait initially when the child enters the exam room. This enables you to observe the child when he or she is unaware of being observed and gait is most natural. Later, have the child walk to and from the parent (the child should be barefoot), and observe gait.

Toddlers have a wide-based gait and are usually bow-legged (genu varum). Children aged 2 to 7 are usually knock-kneed (genu valgum). Gait in older children is the same as in adults.

"Toeing in" or "toeing out" indicates problems such as tibial torsion or clubfoot. Limping may indicate congenital hip dysplasia (toddlers); synovitis (preschoolers); Legg-Calvé-Perthes disease (school-age children); slipped capital femoral epiphysis, scoliosis (adolescents). When child is wearing shoes, limping usually suggests poorly fitting shoes or presence of a pebble. Many abnormal gaits are noted in cerebral palsy.

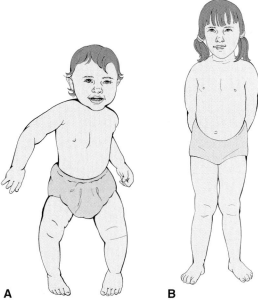

A   **B**

(A) Genu varum (bow legs); *(B)* genu valgum (knock knees).

Assess Joints

Note range of motion, swelling, redness, and tenderness.

Full range of motion and no swelling, redness, or tenderness.

Limited range of motion, swelling, redness, and tenderness indicate problems ranging from mild injuries to serious disorders, such as rheumatoid arthritis.

Assess Muscles

Note size and strength.

Muscle size and strength should be adequate for the particular age and should be equal bilaterally.

Inadequate muscle size and strength for the particular age indicate neuromuscular disorders such as muscular dystrophy.

NEUROLOGIC

Much of the neurologic examination of children older than age 2 years is performed in much the same way as for adults.

Tip From the Experts   As with adults, integrate the neurologic assessment into the overall assessment, observing the child first in the natural state, then purposefully. Playing games such as "Simon Says" can help elicit responses from young children.

(continued)

ASSESSMENT PROCEDURE	NORMAL FINDINGS	ABNORMAL FINDINGS

Perform Newborn Assessment

Assess the newborn's cry, responsiveness, adaptation, and infantile reflexes.

The newborn cries are lusty and strong; responds appropriately to stimuli, and quiets to soothing when held in the *en face* position. Infantile reflexes are present when appropriate and are symmetric.

Inappropriate response to stimuli suggests CNS disorders or problems. An inability to quiet to soothing and gaze aversion is seen in "cocaine babies." Infantile reflexes that are present when inappropriate, are absent when appropriate, or are asymmetric may indicate a CNS problem.

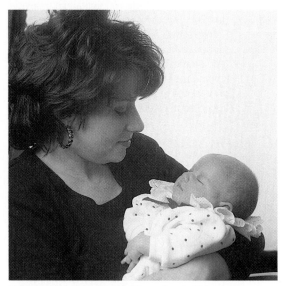
The newborn quiets to soothing when held en face.

Test Cerebral Function

Assess level of consciousness, behavior, adaptation, and speech.

The child should be alert and active, respond appropriately, and relate well to the parent and the nurse. Increased independence will be demonstrated with age. By age 3 years, speech should be easily understood.

Abnormal findings include altered level of consciousness and inappropriate responses. Maladaptation is displayed by an inability to relate well to parent and nurse, lack of independence with age, inappropriate responses to commands, hyperactivity, and poor attention span. Although physiologic dysfluency is normal in preschoolers, unintelligible speech by age 3 years, prolonged stuttering, slurring, and lisping indicate speech disorders or neurologic problems. Slurring may also be indicative of substance abuse, drug toxicity, or conditions such as diabetic ketoacidosis.

Test Cranial Nerve Function

Test cranial nerve function in young people the same way as for adults when possible.

Normal findings are the same as for adults, except extraocular movements in children younger than 6 months old may occur because of immaturity of the eye muscles.

Alterations in cranial nerve function demonstrate problem or pathologic process.

(continued)

ASSESSMENT PROCEDURE	NORMAL FINDINGS	ABNORMAL FINDINGS
Test Deep Tendon and Superficial Reflexes		
Test deep tendon and superficial reflexes in young people the same way as for adults. Display 24–8 discusses reflex testing in newborns.	Normal findings are the same as for adults, except the Babinski response is normal in children younger than 2 years (this response usually disappears between 2 and 24 months), and triceps reflex is absent until age 6. Ankle clonus (rapid, rhythmic plantar flexion) in response to eliciting ankle reflex is common in newborns.	Absence or marked intensity of these reflexes, asymmetry, and presence of Babinski response after age 2 years may demonstrate pathology. Sustained (continuous) ankle clonus is abnormal and suggests CNS disease.
Test Balance and Coordination		
Balance and coordination in a child are tested in much the same way as for an adult. Have the child hop, skip, and jump, when appropriate for developmental age.	School-age children and adolescents should be able to perform most balance and coordination tests.	Abnormal findings include unstable gait, lack of coordination of movements, and positive Romberg. These may indicate a number of problems, including CNS disease and neuromuscular disorders.
Test Sensory Function		
Same as for adults, when possible.	Sensitivity to touch and discrimination should be present. The sensory exam in newborns is limited. The thresholds of touch, pain, and temperature are higher in older children.	Absent or decreased sensitivity to touch and two-point discrimination may indicate paresthesia.
Test Motor Function		
Tests for motor function in children are similar to tests for adults. Also watch for head lag and hand preference.	Gross and fine motor skills should be appropriate for the child's developmental age. Head control should be acquired by 4 months of age. Hand preference is developed during the preschool years.	Gross and fine motor skills that are inappropriate for developmental age and lack of head control by age 6 months may indicate cerebral palsy. Hand preference that is not developed during preschool years may indicate paresis on opposite side.
Observe for "Soft Signs"		
Soft signs of neurologic problems are controversial, because these signs do not always indicate a pathologic process.	Soft signs disappear with age.	Soft signs include, but are not limited to: Short attention span Poor coordination of position Hypoactivity Impulsiveness Labile emotions Distractibility No demonstration of handedness Language and articulation problems Learning problems

DISPLAY 24-6. Using the Denver Developmental Screening Test

The following is an example of the Denver Developmental Screening Test (DDST), which assesses a child's gross motor, language, fine motor, and personal social development according to the child's age. Testing kits, test forms, and reference manuals (which must be used to ensure accuracy in administering the test) may be ordered from Denver Developmental Materials Inc., P.O. Box 6919, Denver, CO 80206-0919. (Reprinted with permission from William K. Frankenburg, M.D.).

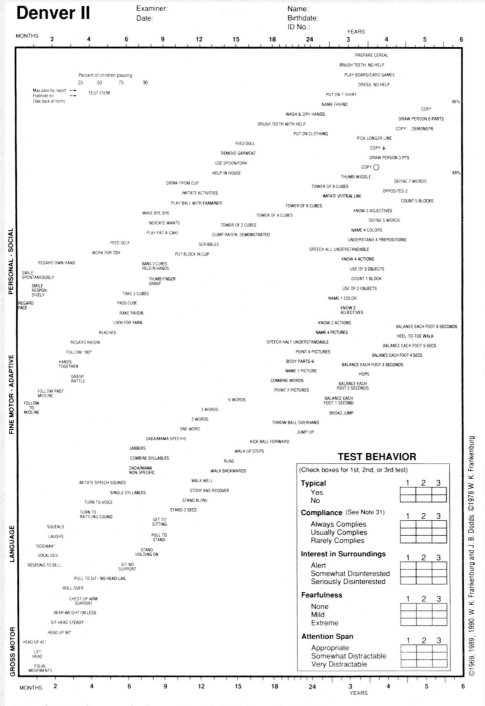

Testing kits, test forms, and reference manuals (which must be used to ensure accuracy in administration of the test) for the DDST may be ordered from Denver Developmental Materials Incorporated, P.O. Box 6919, Denver, CO 80206-0919. (Reprinted with permission from William K. Frankenburg, M.D.)

(continued)

DISPLAY 24-6. Using the Denver Developmental Screening Test (Continued)

DIRECTIONS FOR ADMINISTRATION

1. Try to get child to smile by smiling, talking or waving. Do not touch him/her.
2. Child must stare at hand several seconds.
3. Parent may help guide toothbrush and put toothpaste on brush.
4. Child does not have to be able to tie shoes or button/zip in the back.
5. Move yarn slowly in an arc from one side to the other, about 8" above child's face.
6. Pass if child grasps rattle when it is touched to the backs or tips of fingers.
7. Pass if child tries to see where yarn went. Yarn should be dropped quickly from sight from tester's hand without arm movement.
8. Child must transfer cube from hand to hand without help of body, mouth, or table.
9. Pass if child picks up raisin with any part of thumb and finger.
10. Line can vary only 30 degrees or less from tester's line.
11. Make a fist with thumb pointing upward and wiggle only the thumb. Pass if child imitates and does not move any fingers other than the thumb.

  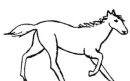   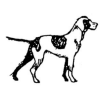

12. Pass any enclosed form. Fail continuous round motions.

13. Which line is longer? (Not bigger.) Turn paper upside down and repeat. (pass 3 of 3 or 5 of 6)

14. Pass any lines crossing near midpoint.

15. Have child copy first. If failed, demonstrate.

When giving items 12, 14, and 15, do not name the forms. Do not demonstrate 12 and 14.

16. When scoring, each pair (2 arms, 2 legs, etc.) counts as one part.
17. Place one cube in cup and shake gently near child's ear, but out of sight. Repeat for other ear.
18. Point to picture and have child name it. (No credit is given for sounds only.)
    If less than 4 pictures are named correctly, have child point to picture as each is named by tester.

    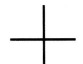 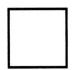 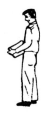

19. Using doll, tell child: Show me the nose, eyes, ears, mouth, hands, feet, tummy, hair. Pass 6 of 8.
20. Using pictures, ask child: Which one flies?… says meow?… talks?… barks?… gallops? Pass 2 of 5, 4 of 5.
21. Ask child: What do you do when you are cold?… tired?… hungry? Pass 2 of 3, 3 of 3.
22. Ask child: What do you do with a cup? What is a chair used for? What is a pencil used for?
    Action words must be included in answers.
23. Pass if child correctly places <u>and</u> says how many blocks are on paper. (1, 5).
24. Tell child: Put block **on** table; **under** table; **in front of** me, **behind** me. Pass 4 of 4.
    (Do not help child by pointing, moving head or eyes.)
25. Ask child: What is a ball?… lake?… desk?… house?… banana?… curtain?… fence?… ceiling? Pass if defined in terms of use, shape, what it is made of, or general category (such as banana is fruit, not just yellow). Pass 5 of 8, 7 of 8.
26. Ask child: If a horse is big, a mouse is __? If fire is hot, ice is __? If the sun shines during the day, the moon shines during the __? Pass 2 of 3.
27. Child may use wall or rail only, not person. May not crawl.
28. Child must throw ball overhand 3 feet to within arm's reach of tester.
29. Child must perform standing broad jump over width of test sheet (8 1/2 inches).
30. Tell child to walk forward, ⊂⊃⊂⊃⊂⊃⊂⊃➤ heel within 1 inch of toe. Tester may demonstrate.
    Child must walk 4 consecutive steps.
31. In the second year, half of normal children are non-compliant.

OBSERVATIONS:

TABLE 24-11. Blood Pressure Levels for the 90th and 95th Percentiles of Blood Pressure for Girls and Boys, Ages 1 to 17

Age	BP Percentile[a]	Systolic BP (mmHg), by Height Percentile from Standard Growth Curves							Diastolic BP (mmHg), by Height Percentile from Standard Growth Curves						
		5%	10%	25%	50%	75%	90%	95%	5%	10%	25%	50%	75%	90%	95%
Girls															
1	90th	97	98	99	100	102	103	104	53	53	53	54	55	56	56
	95th	101	102	103	104	105	107	107	57	57	57	58	59	60	60
2	90th	99	99	100	102	103	104	105	57	57	58	58	59	60	61
	95th	102	103	104	105	107	108	109	61	61	62	62	63	64	65
3	90th	100	100	102	103	104	105	106	61	61	61	62	63	63	64
	95th	104	104	105	107	108	109	110	65	65	65	66	67	67	68
4	90th	101	102	103	104	106	107	108	63	63	64	65	65	66	67
	95th	105	106	107	108	109	111	111	67	67	68	69	69	70	71
5	90th	103	103	104	106	107	108	109	65	66	66	67	68	68	69
	95th	107	107	108	110	111	112	113	69	70	70	71	72	72	73
6	90th	104	105	106	107	109	110	111	67	67	68	69	69	70	71
	95th	108	109	110	111	112	114	114	71	71	72	73	73	74	75
7	90th	106	107	108	109	110	112	112	69	69	69	70	71	72	72
	95th	110	110	112	113	114	115	116	73	73	73	74	75	76	76
8	90th	108	109	110	111	112	113	114	70	70	71	71	72	73	74
	95th	112	112	113	115	116	117	118	74	74	75	75	76	77	78
9	90th	110	110	112	113	114	115	116	71	72	72	73	74	74	75
	95th	114	114	115	117	118	119	120	75	76	76	77	78	78	79
10	90th	112	112	114	115	116	117	118	73	73	73	74	75	76	76
	95th	116	116	117	119	120	121	122	77	77	77	78	79	80	80
11	90th	114	114	116	117	118	119	120	74	74	75	75	76	77	77
	95th	118	118	119	121	122	123	124	78	78	79	79	80	81	81
12	90th	116	116	118	119	120	121	122	75	75	76	76	77	78	78
	95th	120	120	121	123	124	125	126	79	79	80	80	81	82	82
13	90th	118	118	119	121	122	123	124	76	76	77	78	78	79	80
	95th	121	122	123	125	126	127	128	80	80	81	82	82	83	84
14	90th	119	120	121	122	124	125	126	77	77	78	79	79	80	81
	95th	123	124	125	126	128	129	130	81	81	82	83	83	84	85
15	90th	121	121	122	124	125	126	127	78	78	79	79	80	81	82
	95th	124	125	126	128	129	130	131	82	82	83	83	84	85	86
16	90th	122	122	123	125	126	127	128	79	79	79	80	81	82	82
	95th	125	126	127	128	130	131	132	83	83	83	84	85	86	86
17	90th	122	123	124	125	126	128	128	79	79	79	80	81	82	82
	95th	126	126	127	129	130	131	132	83	83	83	84	85	86	86
Boys															
1	90th	94	95	97	98	100	102	102	50	51	52	53	54	54	55
	95th	98	99	101	102	104	106	106	55	55	56	57	58	59	59
2	90th	98	99	100	102	104	105	106	55	55	56	57	58	59	59
	95th	101	102	104	106	108	109	110	59	59	60	61	62	63	63
3	90th	100	101	103	105	107	108	109	59	59	60	61	62	63	63
	95th	104	105	107	109	111	112	113	63	63	64	65	66	67	67
4	90th	102	103	105	107	109	110	111	62	62	63	64	65	66	66
	95th	106	107	109	111	113	114	115	66	67	67	68	69	70	71

(continued)

TABLE 24-11. Blood Pressure Levels for the 90th and 95th Percentiles of Blood Pressure for Girls and Boys, Ages 1 to 17 (Continued)

Age	%ile														
5	90th	104	105	106	108	110	112	112	65	65	66	67	68	69	69
	95th	108	109	110	112	114	115	116	69	70	70	71	72	73	74
6	90th	105	106	108	110	111	113	114	67	68	69	70	70	71	72
	95th	109	110	112	114	115	117	117	72	72	73	74	75	76	76
7	90th	106	107	109	111	113	114	115	69	70	71	72	72	73	74
	95th	110	111	113	115	116	118	119	74	74	75	76	77	78	78
8	90th	107	108	110	112	114	115	116	71	71	72	73	74	75	75
	95th	111	112	114	116	118	119	120	75	76	76	77	78	79	80
9	90th	109	110	112	113	115	117	117	72	73	73	74	75	76	77
	95th	113	114	116	117	119	121	121	76	77	78	79	80	80	81
10	90th	110	112	113	115	117	118	119	73	74	74	75	76	77	78
	95th	114	115	117	119	121	122	123	77	78	79	80	80	81	82
11	90th	112	113	115	117	119	120	121	74	74	75	76	77	78	78
	95th	116	117	119	121	123	124	125	78	79	79	80	81	82	83
12	90th	115	116	117	119	121	123	123	75	75	76	77	78	78	79
	95th	119	120	121	123	125	126	127	79	79	80	81	82	83	83
13	90th	117	118	120	122	124	125	126	75	76	76	77	78	79	80
	95th	121	122	124	126	128	129	130	79	80	81	82	83	83	84
14	90th	120	121	123	125	126	128	128	76	76	77	78	79	80	80
	95th	124	125	127	128	130	132	132	80	81	81	82	83	84	85
15	90th	123	124	125	127	129	131	131	77	77	78	79	80	81	81
	95th	127	128	129	131	133	134	135	81	82	83	83	84	85	86
16	90th	125	126	128	130	132	133	134	79	79	80	81	82	82	83
	95th	129	130	132	134	136	137	138	83	83	84	85	86	87	87
17	90th	128	129	131	133	134	136	136	81	81	82	83	84	85	85
	95th	132	133	135	136	138	140	140	85	85	86	87	88	89	89

Source: Reprinted from National High Blood Pressure Education Program Working Group on Hypertension Control in Children and Adolescents.
ª Blood pressure percentile determined by a single measurement.

Validation and Documentation of Findings

Documentation for children and adolescents is the same as that for adults. Nurses document what they observed, palpated, percussed, and auscultated. Descriptions should be objective, accurate, and concise, yet comprehensive. Terms such as *good, poor,* and *normal* should be avoided. Phrases and standardized abbreviations are preferable to full sentences, and a sequential manner should be followed.

EXAMPLE OF SUBJECTIVE DATA

Biographical data: Caucasian female, age 1 year
Chief complaint: Well-child care
Current health and illness status: Has been well since last health care visit at age 9 months; no current problems, health concerns, or medications
Past history

- Birth FTNSVD (full-term, normal, spontaneous delivery), BW (birth weight) 7 lb; no problems
- Previous illnesses, injuries, or surgeries: Otitis media at age 6 months
- Allergies (and reaction to same): None
- Immunization status: UTD (up to date)
- Growth and developmental milestones: Sat at 6½ months; walked at 11 months; first word ("dada") at 8 months
- Habits: None

REVIEW OF SYSTEMS

- *General:* Well child, three "colds" in first year
- *Integument:* No lesions, bruising
- *Head:* No trauma, headaches
- *Eyes:* Visual acuity, no problems by history; last eye exam (N/A [nonapplicable]); no drainage, infections
- *Ears:* Hearing acuity, no problems by history; last hearing exam (N/A); no drainage; history of (h/o) otitis media at 6 months treated with amoxicillin)

(*text continues on page 672*)

COMMON VARIATIONS

DISPLAY 24-7. Common Skin Variations in Infants and Children

Although most bruises, scars, and rashes are cause for concern, some of the skin markings described below are common and not considered abnormal findings.

STORKBITE

This birthmark is an irregularly shaped, red or pink patch that appears on the face or back of the neck. It usually fades by the time the infant is 12 months old.

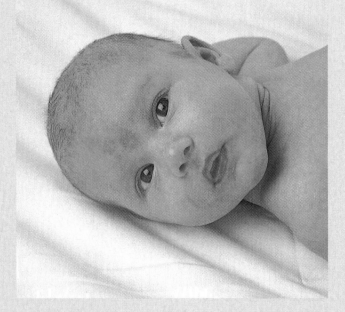

HEMANGIOMA

This skin variation is caused by an increased amount of blood vessels in the dermis.

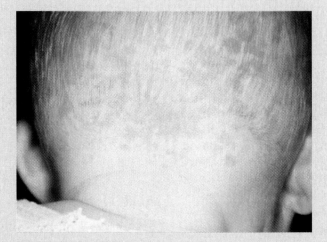

DISPLAY 24-7. Common Skin Variations in Infants and Children (Continued)

PORT-WINE STAIN

This birthmark consisting of capillaries is dark red or bluish and darkens with exertion or temperature exposure. It appears as a large, irregular, macular patch on the scalp or face. Unlike a hemangioma, this birthmark does not fade with time.

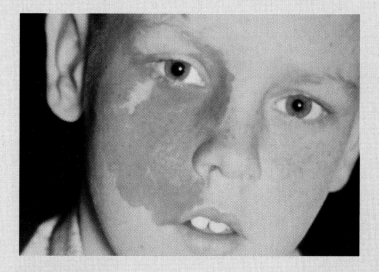

CAFÉ AU LAIT SPOT

This birthmark is a light brown, round or oval patch. If there are more than six separate, large (>1.5 cm) patches, an inherited neurocutaneous disease may be present.

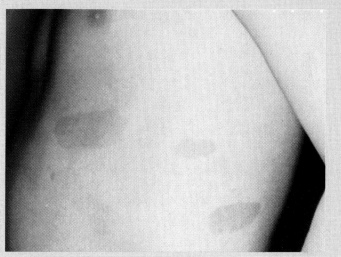

MONGOLIAN SPOTS

These bluish pigmented areas on the buttocks, back, and shoulder are common in dark-skinned infants.

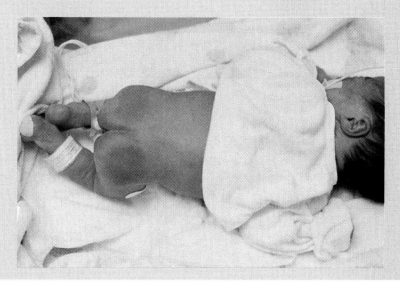

DISPLAY 24-8. Newborn Reflexes: Normal and Abnormal

The reflexes illustrated and described below are the most commonly tested newborn reflexes. These reflexes are present in all normal newborns, and most disappear within a few months after birth. Therefore, absence of a reflex at birth or persistence of a reflex past a certain age may indicate a problem with central nervous system function.

ROOTING REFLEX

To elicit the rooting reflex, touch the newborn's upper or lower lip or cheek with a gloved finger or sterile nipple. The newborn will move the head toward the stimulated area and open the mouth.

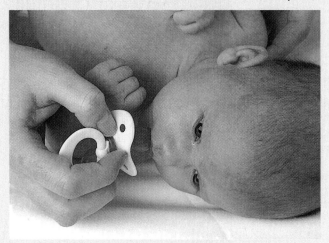

Disappearance of Reflex

The rooting reflex disappears by 3 to 4 months.

Abnormal Findings

Absence of a rooting indicates serious CNS disease.

SUCKING REFLEX

Place a gloved finger or nipple in the newborn's mouth, and note the strength of the sucking response. (A diminished response is normal in a recently fed newborn.)

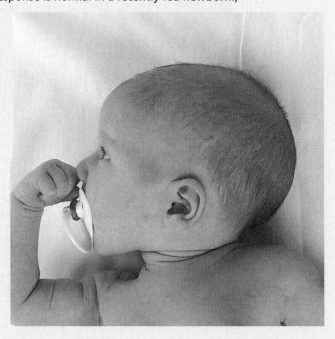

(continued)

Disappearance of Reflex
This reflex disappears at 10 to 12 months.

Abnormal Findings
A weak or absent sucking reflex may indicate a neurologic disorder, prematurity, or CNS depression caused by maternal drug use or medication during pregnancy.

PALMAR GRASP REFLEX
Press your fingers against the palmar surface of the newborn's hand from the ulnar side. The grasp should be strong—you may even be able to pull the newborn to a sitting position.

Disappearance of Reflex
This reflex disappears at 3 to 4 months.

Abnormal Findings
A diminished response usually indicates prematurity; no response suggests neurologic deficit; asymmetric grasp suggests fracture of the humerus or peripheral nerve damage. If this reflex persists past 4 months, cerebral dysfunction may be present.

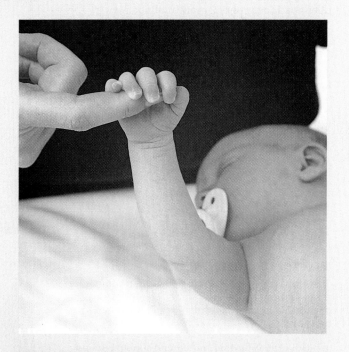

PLANTAR GRASP REFLEX
Touch the ball of the newborn's foot. The toes should curl downward tightly.

Disappearance of Reflex
This reflex disappears at 8 to 10 months.

Abnormal Findings
A diminished response usually indicates prematurity; no response suggests neurologic deficit.

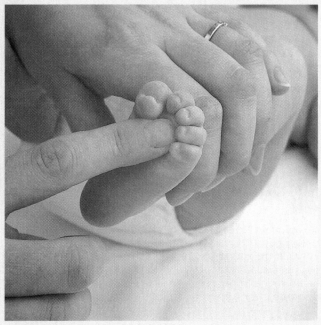

(continued)

DISPLAY 24-8. Newborn Reflexes: Normal and Abnormal (Continued)

TONIC NECK REFLEX

The newborn should be supine. Turn the head to one side with newborn's jaw at the shoulder. The tonic neck reflex is present when the arm and leg on the side to which the head is turned extend and the opposite arm and leg flex. This reflex usually does not appear until 2 months of age.

Disappearance of Reflex

This reflex disappears by 4 to 6 months. The reflex may not occur every time that the examiner tries to elicit it, in which case, repeat stimulus of turning head to one side to re-elicit the response.

Abnormal Findings

If this reflex persists until later in infancy, brain damage is usually present.

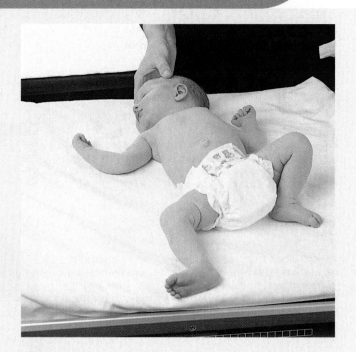

MORO (OR STARTLE) REFLEX

The Moro reflex is a response to sudden stimulation or an abrupt change in position. This reflex can be elicited by using either one of the following two methods:

1. Hold the infant with the head supported and rapidly lower the whole body a few inches.
2. Place the infant in the supine position on a flat, soft surface. Hit the surface with your hand or startle the infant in some way.

The reflex is manifested by the infant slightly flexing and abducting the legs, laterally extending and abducting the arms, forming a "C" with thumb and forefinger, and fanning the other fingers. This is immediately followed by anterior flexion and adduction of the arms. All movements should be symmetric.

Disappearance of Reflex

This reflex disappears by 3 months.

Abnormal Findings

An asymmetric response suggests injury of the slower part. Absence of a response suggests CNS injury. If the reflex was elicited at birth and disappears later, cerebral edema or intracranial hemorrhage is suspected. Persistence of the response after 4 months suggests CNS injury.

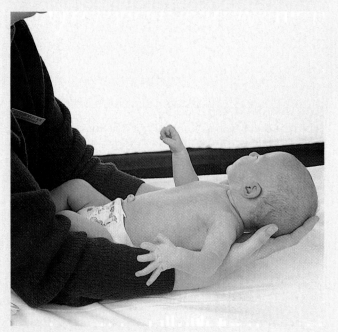

(continued)

DISPLAY 24-8. Newborn Reflexes: Normal and Abnormal (Continued)

BABINSKI REFLEX

Hold the newborn's foot and stroke up the lateral edge and across the ball. A positive Babinski reflex is fanning of the toes. Many normal newborns will not exhibit a positive Babinski reflex; instead, they will exhibit the normal adult response, which is flexion of the toes. Response should always be symmetric bilaterally.

Disappearance of Reflex
This reflex disappears within 2 years.

Abnormal Findings
A positive response after 2 years suggests pyramidal tract disease.

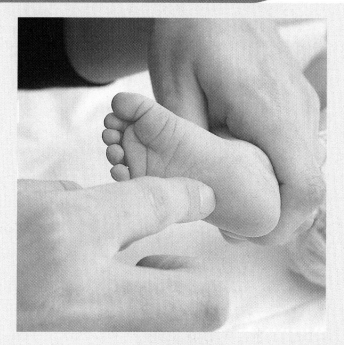

STEPPING REFLEX

Hold the newborn upright from behind, provide support under the arms, and let the newborn's feet touch a surface. The reflex response is manifested by the newborn stepping with one foot and then the other in a walking motion.

Disappearance of Reflex
This reflex usually disappears within 2 months.

Abnormal Findings
An asymmetric response may indicate injury of the leg, CNS damage, or peripheral nerve injury.

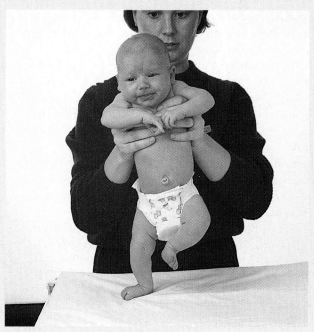

- *Nose:* No bleeding, congestion, discharge
- *Mouth:* No lesions, soreness; no tooth eruption, last dental exam (N/A)
- *Throat:* No sore throats, hoarseness, difficulty swallowing
- *Neck:* No stiffness, tenderness
- *Chest:* No pain, cough, wheezing, shortness of breath, asthma, infections
- *Breasts:* No thelarche, lesions, discharge
- *Cardiovascular:* No history of murmurs, exercise tolerance, dizziness, palpitations, congenital defects
- *Gastrointestinal:* Appetite excellent; bowel habits (one soft, brown BM/day); no food intolerances, nausea, vomiting, pain, history of parasites
- *Genitourinary:* No urgency, frequency, discharge, urinary tract infections
- *Gynecologic:* No discharge
- *Musculoskeletal:* No pain, swelling, fractures, mobility problems
- *Neurologic:* No tremors, unusual movements, seizures
- *Lymphatic:* No pain, swelling or tenderness, enlargement of spleen or liver
- *Endocrine/metabolic:* Growth patterns follow 50%; no polyuria, polydipsia, polyphagia

Psychiatric history: No developmental disorder

Family history: Diabetes (maternal grandmother); hypertension (paternal grandfather)

Nutritional history: Drinks three 8-oz bottles of whole milk/day; eats three meals consisting of mixture of baby and table foods. Likes finger foods; hates strained meats and string beans. No problems with feeding, feeds self with much assistance, uses spoon and cup. Takes multivitamin daily.

Determine the quantity and the types of food or formula ingested daily: use 24-h recall, food diary for 3 days (2 weekdays and 1 weekend day), or food frequency record.

Sleep history: Bedtime is 8 PM, awakens at 6 AM. Takes two brief naps/day. Sleeps with favorite blanket, "Kermie."

Psychosocial history:

- *Home:* Lives with single mother, age 35 years. Mother is vice president at major company; mother completed graduate school. Cultural background is Italian/Irish; religion, Protestant. Mother has no contact with child's father but does have strong network of friends and family members. No financial difficulties.
- *School:* Attends day care while mother works

- *Activities:* Plays with dolls and push toys; mother very safety conscious of toys and uses car seat
- *Discipline:* Mother uses distraction and reinforces word "no"
- *Sex:* N/A
- *Substance use:* N/A
- *Violence:* No history of domestic violence; no guns in household

Developmental Assessment by History

- *Cognitive:* Likes to put things in her mouth to explore them; likes to feel different textures. Knows her name and can point to five body parts. Searches for hidden objects.
- *Language:* Knows 10 words, including "no"
- *Gross motor:* Walks without help, starting to climb
- *Fine motor:* Right-handed, builds two-block tower

EXAMPLE OF OBJECTIVE DATA

General appearance: Alert, active, well-developed, well-nourished 1-year-old girl, in no acute distress

Vital signs: BP 90/50; P 100; T 98.6. Wt: 21 lb. (50%); Ht: 29 in (50%); HC 45 cm (50%).

Skin: Pink, moist, appropriate turgor, no lesions; hair curly with normal distribution; nails pink and hard

Head and neck: Normocephalic, fontanelles not palpable, neck supple, no lymph nodes palpable

Mouth, throat, nose, and sinus: Pharynx clear, no adenopathy, nares patent, turbinates pink with scant clear discharge

Eyes and ears: Sclera clear, pupils equally round, react to light and accommodation (PERRLA), external ear canal free of cerumen impaction, foreign body, discharge, tympanic membrane pink with normal landmarks

Thorax and lungs: Thorax round and symmetric, hyperresonance percussed over lung fields

Heart: 100 beats/min, regular rhythm, no murmurs auscultated

Abdomen: Soft, no masses or organomegaly

Genitalia and rectum: Tanner's 1, no discharge or lesions

Musculoskeletal: Spine straight, no tufts or dimples, FROM, adequate muscle strength and tone

Neurologic: Cranial nerves II to XII intact, deep tendon reflexes 2+, no Babinski, sensitive to touch, coordination, gross and fine motor movement appropriate for age

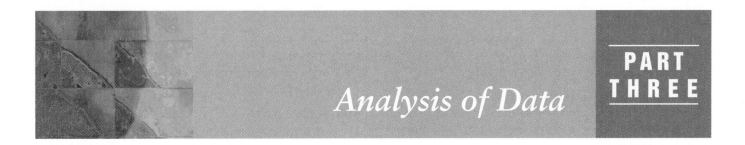

After you have collected your assessment data, you will need to analyze the data, using the diagnostic reasoning skills that you are developing and that you can review in Chapters 6 and 7. After that, in Diagnostic Reasoning: Possible Conclusions, you will see an overview of common conclusions that you may reach after assessment of infants and children. The case study that follows shows you how to analyze the assessment data for a *specific* client. Another opportunity to analyze data is provided in the critical thinking exercise in the study guide and lab manual available with this textbook.

Diagnostic Reasoning: Possible Conclusions

Listed below are some possible conclusions after assessment of infants and children.

SELECTED NURSING DIAGNOSES

After collecting subjective and objective data pertaining to infants and children, you will need to identify abnormalities and cluster the data to reveal any significant patterns or abnormalities. These data will then be used to make clinical judgments (nursing diagnoses: wellness, risk, or actual) about the status of the infant or child. Following is a listing of selected nursing diagnoses that you may identify when analyzing data for this assessment.

Nursing Diagnoses (Wellness)

- Opportunity to enhance knowledge of eye care during the growing years
- Opportunity to enhance nutritional metabolic pattern of child
- Opportunity to enhance sexual function

Nursing Diagnoses (Risk)

- Risk for Impaired Skin Integrity: "diaper rash" to parental knowledge deficit of skin care for diapered infant or child
- Risk for Injury related to open fontanelles
- Risk for Injury to teeth related to developmental age and play activities
- Risk for Injury related to insertion of foreign bodies into nasal cavity
- Risk for Injury related to attempts to insert foreign objects into ear
- Risk for Aspiration related to improper feeding and small size of stomach in newborns
- Risk for Impaired Urinary Elimination related to parental knowledge deficit of toilet-training techniques
- Risk for Injury related to premature physical developmental level
- Risk for Imbalanced Nutrition: Less Than Body Requirements

Nursing Diagnoses (Actual)

- Impaired Skin Integrity: Acne related to developmental changes
- Ineffective Health Maintenance related to lack of proper mouth care
- Ineffective Airway Clearance related to bronchospasm and increased pulmonary secretions
- Deficient Fluid Volume related to vomiting or diarrhea
- Imbalanced Nutrition: More Than Body Requirements

SELECTED COLLABORATIVE PROBLEMS

After grouping the data, it may become apparent that certain collaborative problems emerge. Remember that collaborative problems differ from nursing diagnoses in that they cannot be prevented with nursing interventions alone. However, these physiologic complications of medical conditions can be detected and monitored by the nurse. In addition, the nurse can use physician- and nurse-prescribed interventions to minimize the complications of these problems. The nurse may also have to refer the client in such situations for further treatment of the problem. Following is a list of collaborative problems seen more frequently in the pediatric client. However, other collaborative problems seen in the adult are also seen in pediatric clients. These problems are worded as Potential Complication (or PC), followed by the problem.

- PC: Severe malnutrition/dehydration
- PC: Delayed growth
- PC: Failure to thrive
- PC: Respiratory distress
- PC: Permanently deformed femoral head
- PC: Hydrocephalus/shunt infections

Diagnostic Reasoning: Case Study

Mrs. Carter brings 2½-year-old Michael to the pediatrician's office because he has "been irritable and feverish since last night." Further history reveals that Michael also had a runny nose and cough for 2 days, and that his appetite and fluid intake have decreased since the fever started. Michael is otherwise healthy; this is his first episodic illness. His physical examination reveals slight, irritable, 2½-year-old boy, pulling at ears, temperature of 102°F; nasal congestion with clear discharge, tympanic membranes red and bulging bilaterally, pharynx slightly red without exudate, chest clear, abdomen soft without hepatosplenomegaly (HSM), and no meningeal signs.

The pediatrician diagnoses an upper respiratory infection (URI) and bilateral otitis media (BOM), and orders amoxicillin 250 mg tid for 10 days. You, the office nurse, are to perform the parent teaching for Michael's home care. During your discussion with Mrs. Carter, she tells you that she is concerned that Michael is jealous of his new baby sister because he has occasional tantrums when she holds the baby. She is also concerned about Michael's development because he recently started to refuse using the potty, a skill that is newly acquired. Mrs. Carter is very attentive to both the new baby and Michael throughout the interview, and she asks you for suggestions in how to help Michael cope with the new arrival. While doing so, she points out that her husband has been extra attentive to Michael since his sister was born.

1 Identify abnormal data and strengths (in both subjective and objective data).

SUBJECTIVE DATA

- "Been irritable and feverish since last night"
- Runny nose and cough for 2 days
- His appetite and fluid intake have decreased since the fever started
- Michael is otherwise healthy; this is his first episodic illness
- [Mother] concerned that Michael is jealous of his new baby sister because he has occasional tantrums when she holds the baby
- [Mother] concerned about Michael's development because he recently started to refuse using the potty, a skill that is newly acquired
- [Mother] asks you for suggestions in how to help Michael cope with the new arrival
- Father extra attentive to Michael since new baby was born

OBJECTIVE DATA

- 2½ years old
- Slight irritability
- Pulling at ears
- Temperature of 102°F
- Nasal congestion with clear discharge
- Tympanic membranes red and bulging bilaterally
- Pharynx slightly red without exudate
- Mrs. Carter is very attentive to both the new baby and Michael throughout the interview

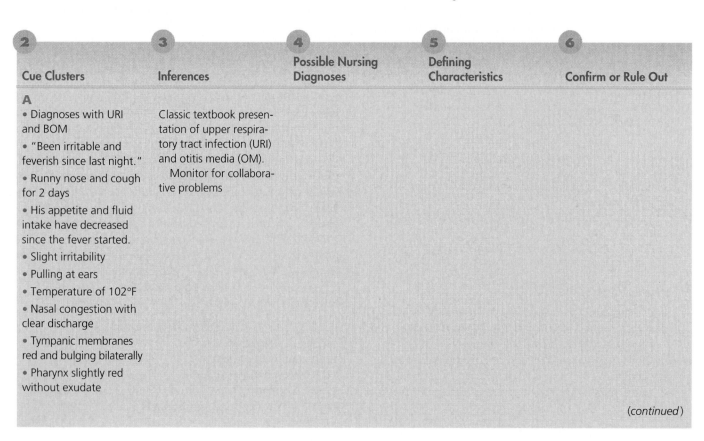

2 Cue Clusters	**3** Inferences	**4** Possible Nursing Diagnoses	**5** Defining Characteristics	**6** Confirm or Rule Out
A • Diagnoses with URI and BOM • "Been irritable and feverish since last night." • Runny nose and cough for 2 days • His appetite and fluid intake have decreased since the fever started. • Slight irritability • Pulling at ears • Temperature of 102°F • Nasal congestion with clear discharge • Tympanic membranes red and bulging bilaterally • Pharynx slightly red without exudate	Classic textbook presentation of upper respiratory tract infection (URI) and otitis media (OM). Monitor for collaborative problems			

(continued)

② Cue Clusters	③ Inferences	④ Possible Nursing Diagnoses	⑤ Defining Characteristics	⑥ Confirm or Rule Out
B • "Been irritable and feverish since last night." • 102° F temperature • Slight irritability • First episodic illness in otherwise healthy child	Child experiencing discomfort from fever and increased tympanic pressure Mother has not had previous experience with child being ill	Acute pain related to (mother's) knowledge deficit of ways to relieve discomfort of ear infection and fever	*Major:* Pulling at ears *Minor:* Irritable	Confirm because it meets major and minor defining characteristics.
C • Decreased fluid intake since illness started • Temp 102° F • Age 2½ years	Child probably does not want to swallow because of pharyngeal irritation and pain	Risk for Fluid Volume Deficit related to poor fluid intake and increased metabolic need secondary to fever	*Major:* Decreased intake; T 102°F	Confirm, although a risk diagnosis does not need to meet defining characteristics. However, a hydration assessment should be completed to monitor for this problem.
		Altered Nutrition: Less than Body Requirements related to possible pain with eating and increased metabolic need	*Major:* None *Minor:* None	Rule out this diagnosis since it does not meet the defining characteristics, but collect more data or make it a risk diagnosis.
D • Refuses to use potty • Had recently learned toilet training • Tantrums when mother holds baby • Mother expresses concern about child being jealous • Mother very attentive to both children • Father giving extra attention to Michael • Mother asks for suggestions on how to help her son cope with the new baby	Child may be exhibiting regressive behaviors in response to feeling displaced from his usual place in the family by a new sibling. He is no longer the only child! Mother and father aware of child's problem with a new sister and are asking for assistance	Ineffective Individual Coping (child) related to change of role/position in family	*Major:* Inappropriate use of defense mechanisms *Minor:* Alterations in social participation	Confirm diagnosis since it meets defining characteristics of behavior as reported by mother. Although the described characteristics are focused on adult behavior, they can be adapted to apply to a small child.
		Altered Family Processes related to stress of older child's behavior changes	*Major:* None *Minor:* None	Rule out since no defining characteristics are present.
		Family Coping: Potential for Growth	*Major:* Family members move in direction of health-promoting lifestyle that supports maturational processes	Confirm since both parents are active in trying to help child grow and adjust to sister, and thus promote growth of whole family.

⑦ **Document conclusions.**

The following diagnoses are appropriate for Michael and the Carter family at this time:

- Acute Pain related to (mother's) knowledge deficit of ways to relieve the discomforts of ear infection and fever
- Risk for Fluid Volume Deficit related to decreased fluid intake secondary to sore throat and increased metabolic need secondary to fever
- Ineffective Individual Coping (child) related to change of role and position in family

- Family Coping: Potential for Growth

Collaborative problems related to his diagnosis include:

- PC: Hyperthermia
- PC: Impairment of hearing
- PC: Pneumonia

Michael should return for follow-up with his pediatrician in 10 to 14 days to check for resolution of his upper respiratory infection and otitis media.

REFERENCES AND SELECTED READINGS

American Academy of Child & Adolescent Psychiatry. (1998). Practice parameters for the assessment and treatment of children and adolescents with substance use disorders. *Journal of the American Academy of Child & Adolescent Psychiatry, 37*(1), 122–126.

———. (1997). Practice parameters for the assessment and treatment of children, adolescents, and adults with ADHD. *Journal of the American Academy of Child & Adolescent Psychiatry, 36*(S10), 85S–121S.

American Academy of Pediatrics, Committee on Nutrition. (1998). *Pediatric nutrition handbook* (4th ed.). Elk Grove Village, IL: Author.

Andrews, M., & Boyle, J. (1999). *Transcultural concepts in nursing care* (3rd ed.). Philadelphia, PA: Lippincott Williams & Wilkins.

Bickley, L. (1999). *Bates' guide to physical examination and history taking* (7th ed.). Philadelphia, PA: Lippincott Williams & Wilkins.

Biederman, J., Wilens, T., Mick, E., Spencer, T., & Faraone, S. V. (1999). Pharmacotherapy of attention-deficit/hyperactivity disorder reduces risk for substance use disorder. *Pediatrics, 104,* e20 [On-line]. Available: *www.pediatrics.org/cgi/contnet/full/104/2/e20.*

Brown, R., & Friedman, S. (2001). Treating the adolescent who might be "out of control." *Pediatric Annals, 30*(2), 81–86.

Burns, C., Brady, M., Dunn, A., & Starr, N. (2000). *Pediatric primary care* (2nd ed.). Philadelphia, PA: WB Saunders.

Carey, W. B. (1998). Let's give temperament its due. *Contemporary Pediatrics, 15,* 91–113.

Cash, J. C., & Glass, C. A. (2000). *Family practice guidelines.* Philadelphia, PA: Lippincott Williams & Wilkins.

Centers for Disease Control and Prevention. (1998, April 3). Recommendations to prevent and control iron deficiency in the US. *MMWR, 47*(No. RR-3).

Dershewitz, R. A. (1999). *Ambulatory pediatric care* (3rd ed.). Philadelphia, PA: Lippincott Williams & Wilkins.

Erickson, S. J., Robinson, T. N., Haydel, F., & Killen, J. D. (2000). Are overweight children unhappy? Body mass index, depressive symptoms, and overweight concerns in elementary school children. *Archives of Pediatric & Adolescent Medicine, 154*(9), 931–935.

Erikson, E. (1986). *Childhood and society* (3rd ed.). New York: W. W. Norton.

Finke, L. M., & Bowman, C. A. (1997). Factors in childhood drug and alcohol use: A review of the literature. *Journal of Child and Adolescent Psychiatric Nursing, 10,* 29–34.

Fox, J. (1997). *Primary health care of children.* St. Louis, MO: C. V. Mosby.

Green, M., & Palfrey, G. (eds.). (2000). *Bright futures guidelines for health supervision of infants, children and adolescents* (2nd ed.). U. S. Department of Health and Human Services, Maternal Child Health Bureau, National Center for Education in Maternal Child Health, Georgetown University, Arlington, VA.

Hoekelman, R. A. (Ed.). (1997). *Pediatric primary care* (3rd ed.). St. Louis, MO: C. V. Mosby.

Huff, R., & Kline, M. (1999). *Promoting health in multicultural populations.* Thousand Oaks, CA: Sage.

Hunt, R., Paguin, A., & Payton, K. (2001). An update on assessment and treatment of complex attention-deficit hyperactivity disorder. *Pediatric Annals, 30*(3), 162–172.

Kenny, K. (2000). Heart murmurs in children. *Advance for Nurse Practitioners, 8*(9) 26–31.

Leonard, H., Freeman, J., Garcia, A., Garvey, M., Snider, L., & Sweden, S. (2001). Obsessive-compulsive disorder and related conditions. *Pediatric Annals, 30*(3), 154–161.

Loewenson, P., & Blum, R. (2001). The resilient adolescent: Implications for the pediatrician. *Pediatric Annals, 30*(2), 76–80.

Luckmann, J. (2000). *Transcultural communication in health care.* Albany, NY: Delmar.

Mayer, B. W., & Burns, P. (2000). Differential diagnosis of abuse injuries in infants and young children. *The Nurse Practitioner, 25*(10), 15–35.

Pillitteri, A. (2002). *Maternal and child health nursing* (4th ed.). Philadelphia, PA: Lippincott Williams & Wilkins.

Purnell, L., & Paulanka, B. (1998). *Transcultural health care.* Philadelphia, PA: FA Davis.

Priess, D. J. (1998). The young child with sickle cell disease. *Advance for Nurse Practitioners, 6*(6), 33–39.

Shoaf, T., Emslie, G., & Mayes, T. (2001). Childhood depression: Diagnosis and treatment strategies in general pediatrics. *Pediatric Annals, 30*(3), 130–137.

Tanner, J. M. (1962). *Growth at adolescence* (2nd ed.). Oxford: Blackwell Scientific Publications.

U. S. Department of Health and Human Services. (2000). *Substance abuse treatment of persons with child abuse and neglect issues:* Treatment Protocol Series, No. 36. Rockville, MD: Author, Public Health Services, Substance Abuse and Mental Health Services Administration Center for Substance Abuse Treatment.

Varley, C., & McCauley, E. (2000). Diagnosis and management of pediatric depression. Presented at the American Academy of Pediatrics Annual Meeting, October 28, 2000.

Weber, J. (2001). *Nurse's handbook of health assessment* (4th ed.). Philadelphia, PA: Lippincott Williams & Wilkins.

For additional information on this book, be sure to visit http://connection.lww.com.

Assessment of the Childbearing Woman

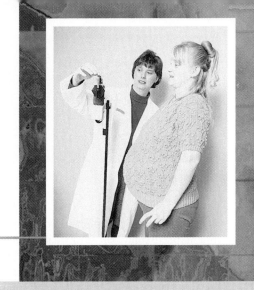

25

The body experiences physiologic and anatomic changes during pregnancy. Most of these changes are influenced by the hormones of pregnancy, primarily estrogen and progesterone. Normal physiologic and anatomic changes during pregnancy are discussed in this chapter.

Skin, Hair, and Nails

During pregnancy, integumentary system changes occur primarily because of hormonal influences. Many of these skin, hair, and nail changes fade or completely resolve after the end of the gestation. As the pregnancy progresses, the breasts and abdomen enlarge and striae gravidarum, or stretch marks, pinkish-red streaks with slight depressions in the skin, begin to appear over the abdomen, breasts, thighs, and buttocks. These marks usually fade to a white or silvery color, but never completely resolve after the pregnancy.

Hyperpigmentation results from hormonal influences (eg, estrogen, progesterone, and melanocyte-stimulating hormone). It is most noted on the abdomen (linea nigra, a dark line extending from the umbilicus to the mons pubis) and face (chloasma, a darkening of the skin on the face, known as the facial "mask of pregnancy"). Some women who take oral contraceptives may also have chloasma because of the hormones in the medication. Other skin changes during pregnancy include darkening of the areolae and nipples, axillae, umbilicus, and perineum. Scars and moles may also darken from the influence of melanocyte-stimulating hormone. Vascular changes, such as spider nevi (tiny red angiomas occurring on the face, neck, chest, arms, and legs), may occur because of elevated estrogen levels. Palmar erythema (a pinkish color on the palms of the hands) may also be noted.

The activity of the eccrine sweat glands and the excretion rate of sebum onto the skin increase in normal pregnancy, whereas the activity of the apocrine sweat glands appears to decrease. The changes that occur in the endocrine system help to maintain optimal maternal and fetal health. Estrogen is primarily responsible for the changes that occur to the pituitary, thyroid, parathyroid, and adrenal glands. The increased production of the hormones, especially triiodothyronine (T_3) and thyroxine (T_4), increases the basal metabolic rate, cardiac output, vasodilation, heart rate, and heat intolerance. The basal metabolic rate increases up to 30% in a term pregnancy.

Growth of hair and nails tends to increase. Some women note excessive oiliness or dryness of the scalp and a softening and thinning of the nails by the 6th week of gestation.

Ears and Hearing

Pregnant women may report a decrease in hearing, a sense of fullness in the ears, or earaches because of the increased vascularity of the tympanic membrane and blockage of the eustachian tubes.

Mouth, Throat, Nose, and Sinus

Some women may note changes in their gums during pregnancy. Gingival bleeding when brushing the teeth and hypertrophy are common. Occasionally, epulis, which are small, irritating nodules of the gums, develop. These nodules usually resolve on their own. Occasionally, the lesion may need to be surgically excised if the nodule bleeds excessively.

Nasal "stuffiness" and epistaxis are common during pregnancy because of the estrogen-induced edema and vascular congestion of the nasal mucosa and sinuses. Vocal changes may be noted because of the edema of the larynx.

Thorax and Lungs

As the pregnancy progresses, progesterone influences the relaxation of the ligaments and joints. This relaxation allows the rib cage to flare, thus increasing the anteroposterior and transverse diameters. This accommodation is necessary as the pregnancy progresses and the enlarging uterus pushes up on the diaphragm. The client's respiratory pattern changes from abdominal to costal. Shortness of breath is a common complaint during the last trimester. The client may be more aware of her breathing pattern and of deep respirations and more frequent sighing. Oxygen requirements increase during pregnancy because of the additional cellular growth of the body and the fetus. Pulmonary requirements increase, with the tidal volume increasing by 30% to 40%. All of these changes are normal and are to be expected during the last trimester.

Breasts

Soon after conception, the surge of estrogen and progesterone begins, causing notable changes in the mammary glands (Fig. 25-1). Breast changes noted by many women include:

- Tingling sensations and tenderness
- Enlargement of breast and nipple
- Hyperpigmentation of areola and nipple
- Enlargement of Montgomery tubercles
- Prominence of superficial veins
- Development of striae
- Expression of colostrum in the second and third trimester

Heart

Significant cardiovascular changes occur during pregnancy. One of the most dynamic changes is the increase in cardiac output and maternal blood volume by approximately 40% to 50%. Because the heart is required to pump much harder, it actually increases in size. Its position is rotated up and to the left approximately 1 to 1.5 cm. The heart rate may increase by 10 to 15 beats/min, and systolic murmurs may be heard.

With the dynamic increase in maternal blood volume, a physiologic anemia (pseudoanemia) commonly develops. This anemia results primarily from the disproportionate in-crease in blood volume compared to the increased red blood cell (RBC) production. Plasma volume increases 40% to 50%, and RBC volume increases 18% to 30% by 30 to 34 weeks' gestation.

As the plasma blood volume increases, the blood vessels must accommodate for this volume, so progesterone acts on the vessels to make them relax and dilate. Clients often complain of feeling dizzy and lightheaded beginning with the second trimester. These effects peak at approximately 32 to 34 weeks. As the pregnancy progresses, the arterial blood pressure stabilizes and symptoms begin to resolve. Prepregnant values return in the third trimester.

Other changes that occur during pregnancy include dependent edema and varicosities. As the expanding uterus applies pressure on the femoral venous area, femoral venous pressure increases. This uterine pressure restricts the venous blood flow return, causing stagnation of the blood in the lower extremities and resulting in dependent edema. Varicose veins in the lower extremities, vulva, and rectum are also common during pregnancy.

Abdomen

In addition to the visible skin changes on the abdomen, the abdominal muscles stretch as the uterus enlarges. These muscles, known as the rectus abdominis muscles, may stretch to the point that permanent separation occurs. This condition is

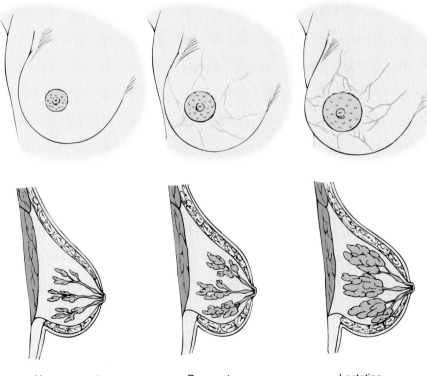

FIGURE 25-1. Breast changes during pregnancy.

Non-pregnant   Pregnant   Lactating

known as *diastasis recti abdominis.* Four paired ligaments (broad ligaments, uterosacral ligaments, cardinal ligaments, round ligaments) support the uterus and keep it in position in the pelvic cavity (Fig. 25-2). As the uterus enlarges, the client may complain of lower pelvic discomfort, which quite commonly results from stretching of the ligaments, especially the round ligaments.

In the abdomen, the expanding uterus exerts pressure on the bladder, kidney, and ureters (especially on the right side), predisposing the client to kidney infection. Urinary frequency is a common complaint in the first and third trimesters. The applied pressure on the kidneys and ureters causes decreased flow and stagnation of the urine. As a result, physiologic hydronephrosis and hydroureter occur. During the second trimester, bladder pressure subsides and urinary frequency is relieved by the uterus enlarging and being lifted out of the pelvic area.

The enlarging uterus also applies pressure and displaces the small intestine. This pressure along with the secretion of progesterone decreases gastric motility. Gastric tone is decreased, and the smooth muscles relax, decreasing emptying time of the stomach. Constipation results from these physiologic events. Heartburn, which may also result, may also be related to the decreased gastrointestinal motility and displacement of the stomach. This causes reflux of stomach acid into the esophagus. Progesterone secretion also relaxes the smooth muscles of the gallbladder, and, as a result, gallstone formation may occur because of the prolonged emptying time of the gallbladder.

Other gastrointestinal symptoms include ptyalism and pica. Ptyalism (excessive salivation) may occur in the first trimester. Pica, a craving for or ingestion of non-nutritional substances such as dirt or clay, is seen in all socioeconomic classes and cultures. Pica can be a major concern if the craving interferes with proper nutrition during pregnancy.

Carbohydrate metabolism is also altered during pregnancy. Glucose use increases, leading to decreased maternal glucose levels. The rise in serum levels of estrogen, progesterone, and other hormones stimulates beta-cell hypertrophy and hyperplasia, and insulin secretion increases. Glycogen is stored, and gluconeogenesis is reduced. In addition, the mother's body tissues develop an increased sensitivity to insulin, thus decreasing the mother's need. As a result, maternal hypoglycemia leads to hypoinsulinemia and increased rates of ketosis. Some well-controlled insulin-dependent diabetic clients have frequent episodes of hypoglycemia in the first trimester. This buildup of insulin ensures an adequate supply of glucose, because the glucose is preferentially shunted to the fetus.

In contrast, during the second half of pregnancy, tissue sensitivity to insulin progressively decreases, producing hyperglycemia and hyperinsulinemia. Insulin resistance becomes maximal in the latter half of the pregnancy.

Genitalia

Before conception, the uterus is a small, pear-shaped organ that weighs approximately 44 g. Its cavity can hold approximately 10 mL of fluid. Pregnancy changes this organ, giving it the capacity of weighing approximately 1,000 g and potentially holding approximately 5 L of amniotic fluid. This dynamic change is mainly due to the hypertrophy of preexisting myometrial cells and the hyperplasia of new cells. Estrogen and the growing fetus are primarily responsible for this growth. Once conception occurs, the

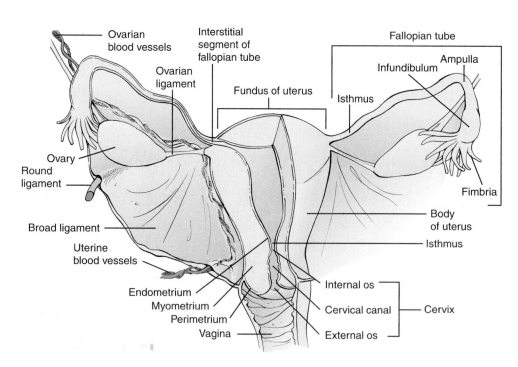

FIGURE 25-2. Anterior cross-section of the female reproductive structures.

uterus prepares itself for the pregnancy: ovulation ceases, the uterine endometrium thickens, and the number and size of uterine blood vessels increase.

With fetal growth, the uterus continues to expand throughout the pregnancy. At approximately 10 to 12 weeks' gestation, the uterus should be palpated at the top of the symphysis pubis. At 16 weeks' gestation, the top of the uterus, known as the fundus, should reach halfway between the symphysis pubis and the umbilicus. At 20 weeks' gestation, the fundus should be at the level of the umbilicus. For the rest of the pregnancy, the uterus grows approximately 1 cm/week, so the fundal height should equal the number of weeks pregnant (eg, at 25 weeks' gestation, the fundal height should measure 25 cm). This formula is known as McDonald's rule. It can be calculated by taking the fundal height in centimeters and multiplying it by 8/7. With a full-term pregnancy, the fundus should reach the xiphoid process. The fundal height measurement may drop the last few weeks of the pregnancy if the fetal head is engaged and descended in the maternal pelvis. This occurrence is known as *lightening*.

Near term gestation, the uterine wall begins thinning out to approximately 5 mm or less. Fetal parts are easily palpated on the external abdomen in the term pregnancy. Braxton Hicks contractions (painless, irregular contractions of the uterus) may occur sporadically in the third trimester. These contractions are normal as long as no cervical change is noted.

Normal changes in the cervix, vagina, and vulva also occur with pregnancy. Cervical softening (Goodell's sign), bluish discoloration (Chadwick's sign), and hypertrophy of the glands in the cervical canal all occur. With these glands secreting more mucus, there is an increase in vaginal discharge, which is acidic. The mucus collects in the cervix to form the mucous plug. This plug seals the endocervical canal and prevents bacteria from ascending into the uterus, thus preventing infection. The vaginal smooth muscle and connective tissue soften and expand to prepare for the passage of the fetus through the birth canal.

Anus and Rectum

Constipation is a common problem during pregnancy. Progesterone decreases intestinal motility, allowing more time for nutrients to be absorbed for the mother and fetus. This also increases the absorption time for water into the circulation, taking fluid from the large intestine and contributing to hardening of the stool and decreasing the frequency of bowel movements. Iron supplementation can also contribute to constipation for those women who take additional iron. As a result, hemorrhoids (varicose veins in the rectum) may develop because of the pressure on the venous structures from straining to have a bowel movement. Vascular congestion of the pelvis also contributes to hemorrhoid development.

Peripheral Vascular System

Two thirds of all pregnant women have swelling of the lower extremities in the third trimester. Swelling is usually noted late in the day after standing for long periods. Fluid retention is caused by the increased hormones of pregnancy, increased hydrophilicity of the intracellular connective tissue, and the increased venous pressure in the lower extremities. Pregnant women are also more prone to development of thrombophlebitis because of the hypercoagulable state of pregnancy. Women who are placed on bedrest during pregnancy are at a very high risk for development of thrombophlebitis.

Musculoskeletal System

Anatomic changes of the musculoskeletal system result from fetal growth, hormonal influences, and maternal weight gain. As the pregnancy progresses, uterine growth pulls the pelvis forward, making the spine curve forward and creating a gradual lordosis (Fig. 25-3). The enlarging breasts influence the shoulders to droop forward. The pregnant client pulls her shoulders back and straightens her head and neck to accommodate for this weight. Progesterone and relaxin (nonsteroidal hormone) influence the pelvic joints and ligaments to relax. The symphysis pubis, sacroiliac and sacrococcygeal joints become more flexible during pregnancy. This flexibility allows the pelvic outlet diameter to increase slightly, which reduces the risk of trauma during childbirth. After the postpartum period, the pelvic diameter will generally remain larger than the size before childbirth.

Hormonal influences also affect the client's gait during pregnancy. The pregnant women's gait is often described as "waddling," and her balance is less stable starting at approximately 24 weeks' gestation. Gait changes are also attributed to weight gain of the uterus, fetus, and breasts. The woman's center of gravity and stance change, causing the woman to lean back slightly to balance herself. Backaches are common. Along with these changes, the woman may also see an increase in shoe size, especially in width.

Neurologic System

Most neurologic changes that occur during pregnancy are discomforting to the client. Common neurologic complaints include:

- Pain or tingling feeling in the thigh—Caused by pressure on the lateral femoral cutaneous nerve.
- Carpal tunnel syndrome—Pressure on the median nerve below the carpal ligament of the wrist causes a tingling sensation in the hand. Because fluid retention occurs during pregnancy, swollen tissues compress the median

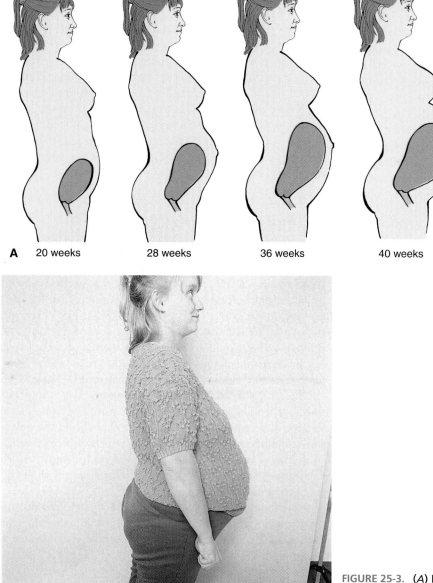

A   20 weeks   28 weeks   36 weeks   40 weeks

B

FIGURE 25-3. (*A*) Postural changes during pregnancy. (*B*) Lordosis in pregnant patient.

nerve in the wrist and produce the tingling sensations. Pain can be reproduced by performing Tinel's sign and Phalen's test. Frequent movement of the wrist up and down aggravates this condition.

- Leg cramps—Caused by inadequate calcium intake.
- Dizziness and lightheadedness—In early pregnancy, dizziness may be experienced because of the blood pres-

sure slightly decreasing as a result of vasodilation and decreased vascular resistance. In later pregnancy, when in the supine position, the client may experience dizziness caused by the heavy uterus compressing the vena cava and aorta. This compression reduces cardiac return, cardiac output, and blood pressure. This is known as *supine hypotensive syndrome.*

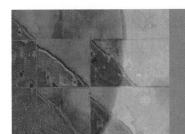

Collecting Subjective Data

A complete health history is necessary to provide high-quality care for the pregnant client. If the examiner does not have access to a recent complete health history for the pregnant client, a complete health history should be performed before focusing on particular questions associated with the pregnancy. The questions discussed in this section are particular questions associated with pregnancy. The first prenatal visit focuses on collection of baseline data about the client and her partner and identification of risk factors.

Nursing History
CURRENT SYMPTOMS

Question What was your normal weight before pregnancy? Has your weight changed since a year ago?

Rationale Optimal weight gain during pregnancy depends on the client's height and weight. Recommended weight gain in pregnancy is as follows: Underweight client, 28 to 40 lb; normal weight client, 25 to 35 lb; overweight client, 15 to 25 lb; twin gestation, 35 to 45 lb (American College of Obstetrician and Gynecologists [ACOG], 1993). Low pregnant weight and inadequate weight gain during pregnancy contribute to intrauterine growth retardation and low birth weight. Figure 25-4 shows typical distribution of weight gain in pregnancy.

Q Do you have any trouble with your throat? Is your nose often stuffed up when you don't have a cold? Have you had a fever or chills, except with a cold, since your last menstrual period?

R Fetal exposure to viral illnesses has been associated with intrauterine growth retardation, developmental delay, hearing impairment, and mental retardation.

Q Do you have a cough that hasn't gone away or do you have frequent chest infections?

R Persistent cough and frequent chest infections may indicate pneumonia or tuberculosis.

Q Do you have nausea or vomiting that doesn't go away? Is your thirst greater than normal?

R Hydration needs to be maintained; the client may be at risk for hyperemesis gravidarum, cholecystitis, or cholelithiasis.

Q Do you ever have bloody stools? Do you have diarrhea or difficulty when trying to have a bowel movement?

R Changes in stool appearance and bowel habits may indicate constipation or hemorrhoids.

Q Do you experience a burning sensation on urination?

R Pregnant women may have asymptomatic bacteruria. Urinary tract infections (UTIs) need to be diagnosed and treated with antibiotics. Untreated UTIs predispose the client to complications such as preterm labor, pyelonephritis, and sepsis.

Q Do you have vaginal bleeding, leakage of fluid, or vaginal discharge?

R Vaginal bleeding, leakage, or discharge may indicate placenta previa, membrane rupture, or vaginal infections (eg, bacterial vaginosis, trichomoniasis, *Chlamydia*). Untreated infections can predispose the client to preterm labor or fetal infections.

Q Have you lost interest in eating? Do you have trouble falling asleep or staying asleep? Do you ever feel depressed or like crying for no reason? Are problems at home or work bothering you? Have you ever thought of suicide? Have you ever had professional counseling (psychiatric/psychological)?

R These symptoms may indicate psychological disorders. If the client has a history of psychological disorders, be aware of these and continually monitor her for signs and symptoms. Collaboration with a psychologist or psychiatrist may be needed. If the client is on medications prescribed for psychological problems, evaluate them in light of their possible teratogenic effects on the fetus.

Q Have you noticed breast pain or lumps, or fluid leakage?

R Breast pain, lumps, or fluid leakage may indicate breast disease. Colostrum secretion, however, is normal during pregnancy. Colostrum varies in color among individuals. Erythematous, painful breasts may indicate a bacterial infection.

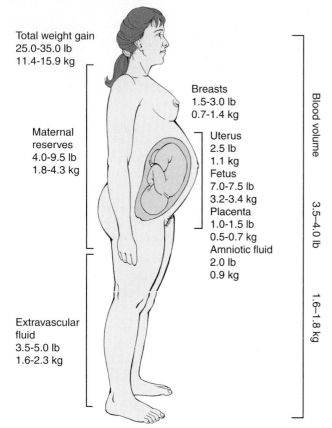

Total weight gain
25.0-35.0 lb
11.4-15.9 kg

Breasts
1.5-3.0 lb
0.7-1.4 kg

Maternal
reserves
4.0-9.5 lb
1.8-4.3 kg

Uterus
2.5 lb
1.1 kg
Fetus
7.0-7.5 lb
3.2-3.4 kg
Placenta
1.0-1.5 lb
0.5-0.7 kg
Amniotic fluid
2.0 lb
0.9 kg

Blood volume

3.5-4.0 lb

1.6-1.8 kg

Extravascular
fluid
3.5-5.0 lb
1.6-2.3 kg

FIGURE 25-4. Distribution of weight gain during pregnancy.

Q Have you thought about breast-feeding or bottle-feeding your infant?

R Discuss advantages of breast-feeding for the client and infant. Supply educational resources for the client.

Q Are there any problems or concerns you may have that we haven't discussed yet?

R Give the client an opportunity to discuss her concerns.

PAST HISTORY

Q Describe your previous pregnancies, including child's name, birth date, birth weight, sex, gestational age, type of delivery (if cesarean section, discuss reason). Did you experience any complications (eg, pregnancy-induced hypertension, diabetes, bleeding, depression, other medical problems) during any of these pregnancies?

R History of previous pregnancies helps identify clients at risk for complications during pregnancy (eg, preterm labor, gestational diabetes).

Q Describe any neonatal complications, such as birth defects, jaundice, infection, or any problems within the first 2 weeks of life. Describe any perinatal or neonatal losses, in-

cluding when the loss occurred and the reason for the loss, if known.

R Previous neonatal complications may be hereditary and may recur in future births. Knowledge of these helps in detecting abnormalities early.

Q Discuss previous abortions (elective or spontaneous), including procedures required and gestational age of fetus.

R Previous history of abortions helps to identify women who have had habitual abortions and who may need medical treatment to maintain the pregnancy.

Q Have you ever had a hydatidiform mole (molar pregnancy)?

R Molar pregnancies occur in 1 of every 2,000 pregnancies. Incidence increases with the woman's age and particularly after age 45. Women who have had a molar pregnancy are at increased risk for a second molar pregnancy. About 10% to 20% of women who have a complete molar pregnancy progress to metastatic choriocarcinoma (Gorrie, McKinney & Murray, 1998).

Q Have you ever had a tubal (ectopic) pregnancy (pregnancy outside of the uterus)?

R A history of previous ectopic pregnancy increases the risk of having a second ectopic pregnancy.

Q When was the first day of your last menstrual period (LMP)? Was this period longer, shorter, or normal? Have you had any bleeding or spotting since your last period? Are your periods usually regular or irregular?

R Menstrual history helps to determine expected date of confinement (EDC).

Q Describe the most recent form of birth control used. If you've used birth control pills in the past, when did you take the last pill?

R Intrauterine devices in place at the time of conception place the client at risk for an ectopic pregnancy. Birth control pills should be discontinued when pregnancy is confirmed.

Q Have you had any difficulty in getting pregnant for longer than 1 year?

R Inability to conceive after trying for more than 1 year may signal reproductive complications, such as infertility.

Q Have you ever had any type of reproductive surgery? Have you ever had an abnormal Pap smear? Have you ever had any treatment performed on your cervix for abnormal Pap smear results? When was your last Pap test, and what were the results?

R Reproductive surgery and instrumentation to the cervix place the client at risk for complications during pregnancy.

Conization of the cervix places the client at risk for an incompetent cervix during pregnancy.

Q Do you have a history of having any type of sexually transmitted infections (STIs), such as a chlamydial infection, gonorrhea, herpes, genital warts, or syphilis? If so, describe when it occurred and the treatment. Does your partner have a history of STI? If so, when was he treated?

R Early identification and treatment of STIs prevent intrauterine complications from long-term exposure to infections.

Q Do you have a history of any vaginal infections such as bacterial vaginosis, yeast infection, or others? If so, when did the infection occur and what was the treatment?

R Vaginal infections need treatment. During pregnancy, nonteratogenic medications, such as clindamycin (Cleocin 2%) intravaginal cream or oral tablets, may be recommended. Metronidazole may be used in the second or third trimester (ACOG, 1996).

Q Do you know your blood type and Rh factor? If you are Rh negative, do you know the Rh factor of your partner?

R Rh-negative mothers should receive Rh_o immune globulin at 28 weeks' gestation and with antepartum testing (chorionic villi sampling, amniocentesis) to prevent isoimmunization.

Q Have you ever received a blood transfusion for any reason? If so, explain reason and provide date.

R Infections (hepatitis, human immunodeficiency virus [HIV], and so forth) and antibodies can be received from contaminated blood during blood transfusions, which can be detrimental to the mother and fetus. Foreign antibodies can be life threatening for the fetus. Positive antibody screens need to be followed up to identify the antibody detected in the blood. Besides Rh antibody, other antibodies include Kell, Duffy, and Lewis. Titers should be followed to prevent fetal complications.

Q Do you have a history of any major medical problem (eg, heart trouble, rheumatic fever, hypertension, diabetes, lung problems, tuberculosis, asthma, trouble with nerves and/or depression, kidney disease, cancer, convulsions or epilepsy, abnormality of female organs [uterus, cervix], thyroid problems, or hearing loss in infancy)?

R Identification of any medical problem is important during pregnancy because the body undergoes so many physiologic changes.

Q Do you have diabetes or has anyone ever told you that you had diabetes?

R The fetus of diabetic clients who have uncontrolled disease and high $HgbA_{1c}$ values at the time of conception have a 6% to 8% incidence of anomalies.

Q Have you had twins or multiple gestation?

R Early identification of multiple gestation is important. Refer clients with multiple gestation to an obstetrician for continued care. Multiple gestation places the client in the "high risk" category during pregnancy.

Q Do you have any medication, food, or other allergies? If so, list the allergies and describe the reactions.

R Identification of medication allergies is necessary to prevent complications.

Q Have you ever been hospitalized or had surgery (not including hospitalizations or surgery related to pregnancy)? If so, discuss the reason for the hospitalization or surgery, the date, and if the problem is resolved today.

R Previous hospitalizations or surgeries must be noted to assess for potential medical complications during the pregnancy.

Q Are you currently taking any medications (either prescription or nonprescription), or have you taken any since you have become pregnant? If so, list the medication, the amount taken, the date you started taking it, and the reason for taking it.

R Some medications are teratogenic to the fetus during pregnancy. All medications taken since the LMP need to be discussed with the practitioner.

GENETIC INFORMATION

Q Will you be 35 years or older at the time the baby is born? Are you and the baby's father related to each other (eg, cousins or other relations)?

R Women who are age 35 or older at the time of delivery should be offered genetic counseling and testing. Obtain genetic information so you can assess fetal risk of abnormal karyotype or genetic disorders.

Q Have you had two or more pregnancies that ended in miscarriage?

R A woman who has had habitual abortions needs medical evaluation for incompetent cervix, systemic lupus erythematosus, and other potential complications.

Q Have you ever had a child that died around the time of delivery or in the first year of life?

R Death of a child in the first year of life may indicate a risk for fetal cardiac disease or other diseases. This information is necessary for assessing fetal risk for birth defects.

Q Do you have a child with a birth defect? Do you have any type of birth defect or inherited disease such as cleft lip or cleft palate, clubfoot, hemophilia, mental retardation, or any others? Are there any members in your family with a birth defect? What is your ethnic or racial group—Jewish, Black/African, Asian, Mediterranean (eg, Greek, Italian), French Canadian?

R Certain inherited disorders occur more often in particular ethnic groups, such as Tay-Sachs disease in the Ashkenazi Jewish population.

FAMILY HISTORY

Q Has anyone in your family (grandparents, parents, siblings, children) had heart trouble before age 50 years or rheumatic fever?

R Cardiovascular disease or heart defects may be inherited.

Q Has anyone in your family had lung problems, diabetes, tuberculosis, or asthma?

R Pulmonary or endocrine disorders may be familial.

Q Has anyone in your family been diagnosed with any type of cancer? If so, what kind?

R There is a genetic component associated with certain types of cancer.

Q Has anyone in your family been born with any birth defects, inherited diseases, blood disorders, mental retardation, or any other problems?

R There is a genetic risk factor for Down syndrome, spina bifida, brain defects, chromosome problems, anencephaly, heart defects, muscular dystrophy, cystic fibrosis, hemophilia, thalassemia, and other inherited diseases.

Q For the African-American client: Is there a history of sickle cell disease?

R Identification of signs and symptoms of sickle cell disease is important to assist in early treatment.

LIFESTYLE AND HEALTH PRACTICES

Q Since the start of this pregnancy, have you had alcohol-containing drinks almost each day or frequently?

R Daily alcohol intake puts the fetus at risk for fetal alcohol syndrome.

Q How much do you smoke per day?

R Maternal cigarette smoking correlates with an increased incidence of perinatal mortality, preterm delivery, premature rupture of membranes, abruptio placentae, stillbirth, and bleeding during pregnancy (Gabbe, Niebyl & Simpson, 1991). *Smoking is also associated with decreased fetal size and weight.* Women who quit smoking during the 9-month gestation quit smoking for the health of themselves and for the

fetus. These women may also have a lower relapse rate of smoking again when compared to women who are not pregnant (ACOG, 1997).

Q Have you used cocaine, marijuana, speed, or any street drug during this pregnancy?

R Women who use cocaine during pregnancy have a higher rate of spontaneous abortions and abruptio placentae. Infants exposed in utero are shown to have poor organizational response to stimuli compared with a control group (Gabbe et al., 1991).

Q Does anyone in your family consider your social habits to be a problem? Do your social habits interfere with your daily living? If so, please explain.

R Women who abuse substances (alcohol, cocaine, marijuana, and so forth) do not always consider their habits to be a problem. They also tend to underestimate the amount of substances used. Family members or friends may give a truer estimate of the substances abused. These habits need to be known to assist the client during pregnancy and to alert neonatal personnel after delivery to prepare for potential neonatal complications.

Q What is your normal baseline weight? Have you lost or gained more than 10 lb in the last year?

R There is a positive linear relationship between maternal weight gain and newborn weight. Low prepregnant weight and inadequate weight gain during pregnancy are dominant contributors to intrauterine growth retardation and low birth weight (ACOG, 1993).

Q What is a normal daily intake of food for you? Are you on any special diet? Do you have any diet intolerances or restrictions? If so, what are they?

R Maternal nutrition has a direct relationship to maternal–fetal well-being. Daily maternal caloric intake, as reflected by weight gain, has a direct relationship to birth weight. The caloric content required to supply daily energy needs and to achieve appropriate weight gain can be estimated by multiplying the client's optimal body weight (in kilograms) by 35 kcal and adding 300 kcal to the total.

Q Do you currently take any vitamin supplements? If so, what are they?

R The client's balanced diet should provide an appropriate supply of vitamins required for pregnancy. Routine multivitamin supplementation for clients is based solely on a needs assessment. The diet selection should be from protein-rich foods, whole-grain breads and cereals, dairy products, and fruits and vegetables. Of the minerals, only iron supplementation is recommended to maintain body stores and minimize the occurrence of iron deficiency anemia (ACOG, 1993). The US Public Health Service recommends all women of childbearing age consume 400 μg of folic acid daily to help prevent neural tube defects in the fetus. This can be achieved by eating fruits, vegetables, and fortified cereals and/or a folic acid supplement. The American College of Obstetricians and Gynecologists (ACOG) also recommends a folic acid supplement daily. Women who have previously had newborns born with spinal cord defects can decrease the risk of neural tube defects in future pregnancies by supplementing the diet with folic acid 2 to 3 months before conceiving.

Activity and Exercise

Q Do you exercise daily? If so, what do you do and for how long?

R Daily exercise is highly recommended as long as it is tolerated well by the pregnant client. Women who are in good physical condition tend to have shorter, less difficult labors compared with women who are not physically fit.

Q Do you perform any type of heavy labor working? If so, please describe.

R Pregnancy places a tremendous amount of stress on the body due to the physiologic changes that occur. Encourage rest periods.

Q Are you easily fatigued? If so, please describe. What are your normal sleeping patterns?

R Regular and routine exercise may be continued as long as tolerated. Caution women not to start *new* forms of exercise during pregnancy.

Q Do you frequently have rest periods? If so, for how long? Has your normal routine or exercise ever had a negative impact on your previous pregnancies? If so, please discuss.

R Regular and routine exercise may be continued as long as tolerated. Caution women not to start new forms of exercise during pregnancy.

Toxic Exposure

Q Have you or your partner ever worked around chemicals or radiation? If so, please explain. Are you exposed to an excessive amount of smoke daily?

R Assessment of toxic exposure can identify potential teratogens to the fetus.

Q Do you have a cat? If so, are you exposed to the cat litter or the cat's feces?

R Education regarding proper handling of cat litter is needed because of risk of infection (toxoplasmosis). Advise clients to have other family members change cat litter. Encourage the patient to wash hands well after petting cats.

Role and Relationships

Q What is the highest level of education you have completed? What is your occupation or major activity? Discuss your feelings about this pregnancy. Is the father of the baby involved with the pregnancy? How does your partner feel about the pregnancy? What type of support systems do you have at home? Who is your primary support person? To what degree do you feel that the father of the baby will be involved with the pregnancy (eg, not involved, interested and supportive, full caretaker of the pregnancy)? List the people living with you, including their names, ages, relationship to you, and any health problems that they may have. Are they aware of your pregnancy? Has anyone close to you ever threatened to hurt you? Has anyone ever hit, kicked, choked, or physically hurt you? Has anyone ever forced you to have sex? Are you afraid of your partner for any reason?

R Assessment of social structures and supportive influences is required to determine potential client needs. If additional needs are noted, contact social services for assistance. Lack of recognition of domestic violence is one of the primary barriers to recognizing domestic violence for women. Universal screening is recommended (ACOG, 1999a).

Q How have you introduced this pregnancy to the siblings? What are their reactions regarding this pregnancy? Do you plan to involve the siblings in any type of education program to enhance the attachment process for the newborn?

R Sibling rivalry can interfere with the bonding process between siblings. Education and preparation for the new family member (the newborn) can alleviate potential problems with sibling rivalry. Encourage siblings to attend sibling class offered at your institution.

Q What is your partner's highest level of education? What is your partner's occupation or major activity? How much alcohol does your partner use daily? List type and amount. How often does your partner smoke? List amount and frequency. How often does your partner use illicit drugs? List drug type, amount, and frequency.

R Exploration of the partner's social or cultural habits may identify needs of the family unit.

Collecting Objective Data
CLIENT PREPARATION

The nurse needs to provide a warm and comfortable environment for the physical assessment. After meeting the client, the nurse should quickly explain the sequence of events for the visit. Note that a full head-to-toe examination will be performed, including a pelvic examination. Pelvic cultures obtained with this examination include a

Pap smear and gonorrhea and chlamydial cultures. Explain that after the examination is complete, the client will go to the laboratory for initial prenatal blood tests, including complete blood count, blood type and screen, Rh status, rubella titer, serologic test for syphilis, hepatitis B surface antigen, and sickle cell anemia screen (for clients of African ancestry). Clients who are at high risk for infection with HIV should be screened for this disease.

The first procedure involves obtaining a clean-catch, midstream urine specimen. After the client has voided, instruct her to undress. Provide adequate gowns and cover-up drapes to ensure privacy.

EQUIPMENT AND SUPPLIES

- Adequate room lighting
- Ophthalmoscope
- Otoscope
- Stethoscope
- Sphygmomanometer
- Speculum
- Light for pelvic examination
- Tape measure
- Fetal Doppler ultrasound device
- Disposable gloves
- Lubricant
- Slides
- KOH (potassium hydroxide)
- Normal saline solution
- Cytology fixative

KEY ASSESSMENT POINTS

- Obtain an accurate and complete prenatal history.
- Understand and recognize cardiovascular changes of pregnancy.
- Recognize skin changes.
- Identify common complaints of pregnancy and explain what causes them.
- Correctly measure growth of uterus during pregnancy.
- Demonstrate the four Leopold's maneuvers and explain their significance.

(*text continues on page 701*)

PHYSICAL ASSESSMENT

ASSESSMENT PROCEDURE	NORMAL FINDINGS	ABNORMAL FINDINGS
GENERAL SURVEY: VITAL SIGNS, HEIGHT, AND WEIGHT		
Have the client sit on the examination table while you measure blood pressure (BP).	Range of 90 to 139/60 to 89. BP decreases during the second trimester because of the relaxation effect on the blood vessels. By 32 to 34 weeks, the client's BP should be back to normal.	Elevated BP at 9 to 11 weeks may be indicative of hydatidiform mole pregnancy or thyroid storm. After 20 weeks, increased BP (>140/90) may be associated with pregnancy-induced hypertension. Decreased blood pressure may indicate supine hypotensive syndrome.
Measure pulse rate.	60 to 90 beats/min; may increase 10 to 15 beats/min higher than prepregnant levels	Irregularities in heart rhythm, chest pain, dyspnea, and edema may indicate cardiac disease.
Take the client's temperature.	97° to 98.6°F	An elevated temperature (above 99°) may indicate infection.

ASSESSMENT PROCEDURE	NORMAL FINDINGS	ABNORMAL FINDINGS
Measure height and weight.	Establish a baseline height and weight. The client should gain 2 to 4 lb in the first trimester and approximately 11 to 12 lb in both the second and third trimesters, for a total weight gain between 25 and 35 lb.	A sudden gain exceeding 5 lb a week may be associated with pregnancy-induced hypertension and fluid retention. Weight gain <2 lb a month may indicate insufficient nourishment.

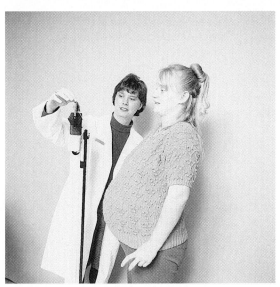

Weighing the pregnant client.

Observe behavior.	*First trimester:* Tired, ambivalent. *Second trimester:* Introspective, energetic. *Third trimester:* Restless, preparing for baby, labile moods (father may also experience these same behaviors).	Denial of pregnancy, withdrawal, depression, or psychosis may be seen in the client with psychological problems.

SKIN, HAIR, AND NAILS

Inspect the skin. Note hyperpigmented areas associated with pregnancy.	Linea nigra, striae, gravidarum, chloasma, and spider nevi may be present.	Pale skin suggests anemia. Yellow discoloration suggests jaundice.
Observe skin for vascular markings associated with pregnancy.	Angiomas and palmar erythema are common.	
Inspect the hair and nails.	Hair and nails tend to increase in growth; softening and thinning are common.	

HEAD AND NECK

Inspect and palpate the neck. Assess the anterior and posterior cervical chain lymph nodes. Also palpate the thyroid gland.	Smooth, nontender, small cervical nodes may be palpable. Slight enlargement of the thyroid may be noted during pregnancy.	Hard, tender, fixed, or prominent nodes may indicate infection or cancer. Marked enlargement of the thyroid gland indicates thyroid disease. Benign and malignant nodules as well as tenderness are noted in thyroiditis.
Inspect the ears.	Tympanic membranes clear: landmarks visible.	Tympanic membrane red and bulging with pus indicates infection.

(continued)

ASSESSMENT PROCEDURE	NORMAL FINDINGS	ABNORMAL FINDINGS

MOUTH, THROAT, AND NOSE

Inspect the mouth. Pay particular attention to the teeth and the gingival tissues, which may normally appear swollen and slightly reddened.	Hypertrophy of gingival tissue is common.	Bleeding may occur due to brushing teeth or dental examinations. Epulis nodules may be present.

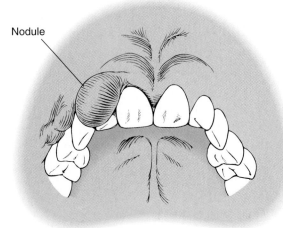

Nodule

Epulis.

Inspect the throat.	Throat pink, no redness or exudate.	Throat red, exudate present, tonsillary hypertrophy indicate infection.
Inspect the nose.	Nasal mucosal swelling and redness may result from increased estrogen production.	Epistaxis is a common variation because of the increased vascular supply to the nares during pregnancy.

THORAX AND LUNGS

Inspect, palpate, percuss, and auscultate the chest.	Normal findings include increased anteroposterior diameter, thoracic breathing, slight hyperventilation; shortness of breath in late pregnancy. Lung sounds are clear to auscultation bilaterally.	Dyspnea, rales, rhonchi, wheezes, rubs, absence of breath sounds, and unequal breath sounds are signs of respiratory distress.

(continued)

ASSESSMENT PROCEDURE	NORMAL FINDINGS	ABNORMAL FINDINGS

BREASTS

Inspect and palpate the breasts and nipples for symmetry and color.

Venous congestion is noted, with prominence of veins. Montgomery's tubercles prominent. Breast size is increased and nodular. Breasts are more sensitive to touch. Colostrum is excreted, especially in the third trimester. Hyperpigmentation of nipples and areolae is evident.

Nipple inversion could be problematic for breast-feeding. Inverted nipples should be identified in the beginning of the third trimester. Breast shields can be inserted in the bra to train the nipple to turn outward.

Localized redness, pain, and warmth could indicate mastitis.

Bloody discharge of the nipple and retraction of the skin could indicate breast cancer.

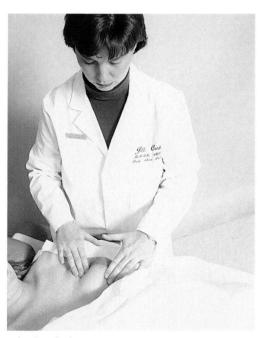

Palpating the breasts.

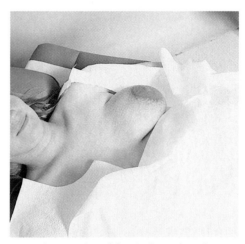

Hyperpigmentation of the nipples and areolae.

HEART

Auscultate the heart.

Normal sinus rhythm.
   Soft systolic murmurs are audible during pregnancy secondary to the increased blood volume.

Irregular rhythm.
   Progressive dyspnea, palpitations, and markedly decreased activity tolerance indicate cardiovascular disease.

ABDOMEN

For this part of the examination, ask the client to recline with a pillow under her head and her knees flexed. Then inspect the abdomen Note striae, scars, and the shape and size of the abdomen.

Striae and linea nigra are normal. The size of the abdomen may indicate gestational age. The shape of the uterus may suggest fetal presentation and position in later pregnancy.

Scars indicate previous surgery; be careful to note cesarean section scars and location. A transverse lie may be suspected by abdominal palpation, noting enlargement of the width of the uterus.

Palpate the abdomen. Note organs and any masses.

The uterus is palpable beginning at 10 to 12 weeks' gestation.

Abnormal masses palpable in the abdomen may indicate uterine fibroids or hepatosplenomegaly.

Palpate for fetal movement after 24 weeks.

Fetal movement should be felt by the mother by approximately 18 to 20 weeks, sooner for multiparous women.

If fetal movement is not felt, the EDC may be wrong or the fetus may not have survived.

(continued)

ASSESSMENT PROCEDURE	NORMAL FINDINGS	ABNORMAL FINDINGS
Palpate for uterine contractions. Note intensity, duration, and frequency of contractions.	The uterus contracts and feels firm to the examiner.	Regular contractions before 37 completed weeks' gestation may suggest preterm labor.

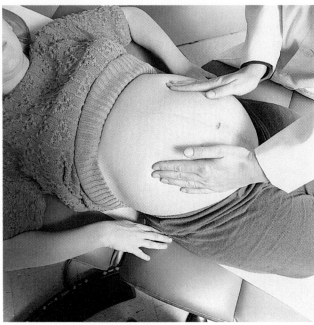

Palpating for uterine contractions.

Palpate the abdomen and notice the difference between the uterus at rest and during a contraction.	Intensity of contractions may be mild, moderate, or firm to palpation.	
Time the length of the contraction from the beginning to the end. Also note the frequency of the contractions, timing from the beginning of one contraction until the beginning of the next.	Contraction may last 40 to 60 seconds and occur every 5 to 6 min.	

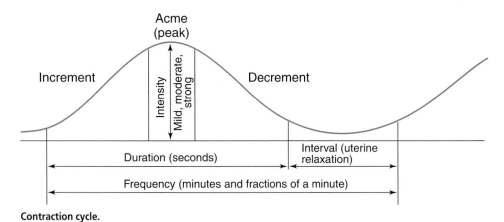

Contraction cycle.

(continued)

ASSESSMENT PROCEDURE	NORMAL FINDINGS	ABNORMAL FINDINGS

Fundal Height

Measure fundal height by placing one hand on each side of the abdomen. Walk hands up the sides of the uterus until you feel the uterus curve, and hands should meet. Take a tape measure and place the zero point on the symphysis pubis and measure to the top of the fundus.

Uterine size should approximately equal the number of weeks of gestation (eg, the uterus at 28 weeks' gestation should measure approximately 28 cm). Measurements may vary by about 2 cm, and examiners' techniques may vary, but measurements should be about the same.

Measurements beyond 4 cm of gestational age need to be further evaluated. Measurements greater than expected may indicate a multiple gestation, polyhydramnios (excess of amniotic fluid), fetal anomalies, or macrosomia (great increase in size similar to obesity). Measurements smaller than expected may indicate intrauterine growth retardation.

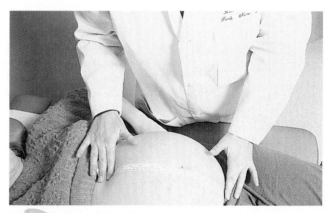

Measuring the fundal height.

Fetal Position

Using Leopold's maneuvers, palpate the fundus, lateral aspects of the abdomen, and the lower pelvic area. Leopold's maneuvers assist in determining the fetal lie (where the fetus is lying in relation to the mother's back), presentation (the presenting part of the fetus into the maternal pelvis), size, and position (the fetal presentation in relation to the maternal pelvis).

A longitudinal lie, in which the fetal spine axis is parallel to the maternal spine axis, is the expected finding. The presentation may be cephalic, breech, or shoulder. The size of the fetus may be estimated by measuring fundal height and by palpation.

Oblique or transverse lie needs to be noted. If vaginal delivery is expected, external version can be performed to rotate the fetus to the longitudinal lie. Breech or shoulder presentations can complicate delivery if it is expected to be vaginal. Fetal positions include right occiput anterior (ROA), left occiput posterior (LOP), left sacrum anterior (LSA), and so on. (Refer to a textbook on obstetrics for further detail.)

36
40
32
26
20
16
12
10

Approximate height of fundus at various weeks of gestation.

(continued)

ASSESSMENT PROCEDURE	NORMAL FINDINGS	ABNORMAL FINDINGS
Perform Leopold's maneuvers. For the first maneuver, face the client's head. Place your hands on the fundal area, expecting to palpate a soft, irregular mass in the upper quadrant of the maternal abdomen.	The soft mass is the fetal buttocks. The fetal head feels round and hard.	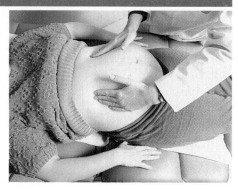

Leopold's maneuvers: First maneuver.

For the second maneuver, move your hands to the lateral sides of the abdomen.	On one side of the abdomen, you will palpate round nodules; these are the fists and feet of the fetus. Kicking and movement are expected to be felt. The other side of the abdomen feels smooth; this is the fetus's back.

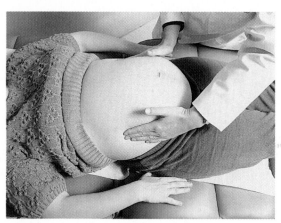

Leopold's maneuvers: Second maneuver.

Third maneuver: Move your hands down to the lower pelvic area and palpate the area just above the symphysis pubis to determine the presenting part. Grasp the presenting part with the thumb and third finger.	The unengaged head is round, firm, and ballottable, whereas the buttocks are soft and irregular.	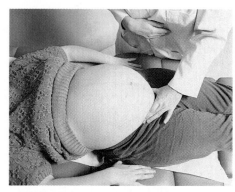

Leopold's maneuvers: Third maneuver.

(continued)

ASSESSMENT PROCEDURE	NORMAL FINDINGS	ABNORMAL FINDINGS
Fourth maneuver: Face the client's feet, place your hands on the abdomen and point your fingers toward the mother's feet. Then try to move your hands toward each other while applying downward pressure.	If the hands move together easily, the fetal head has not descended into the maternal pelvic inlet. If the hands do not move together and stop to resistance met, the fetal head is engaged into the pelvic inlet.	

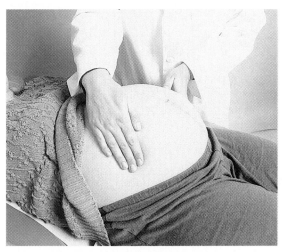

Leopold's maneuvers: Fourth maneuver.

Auscultate the Fetal Heart

Note the location, rate, and rhythm of the fetal heart. Auscultate the fetal heart rate in the left lower quadrant when the fetal back is noted on maternal left, vertex position. When the fetal back is located elsewhere, note other locations illustrated in Display 25-1, for auscultation.	Fetal heart rate ranges from 120 to 160 beats/min. During the third trimester, the fetal heart rate should accelerate with fetal movement.	Inability to auscultate fetal heart tones with a fetal Doppler at 12 weeks may indicate a retroverted uterus, uncertain dates, fetal demise, or false pregnancy. Fetal heart rate decelerations could indicate poor placental perfusion. In breech presentations, fetal heart rate is heard in the upper quadrant of maternal abdomen.

(continued)

| ASSESSMENT PROCEDURE | NORMAL FINDINGS | ABNORMAL FINDINGS |

Tip From the Experts After assessing the fetal position, you can auscultate fetal heart tones best through the back of the fetus. A fetal Doppler ultrasound device can be used after 10 to 12 weeks' gestation to hear the fetal heartbeat. A fetoscope may also be used to hear the heartbeat after 18 weeks' gestation.

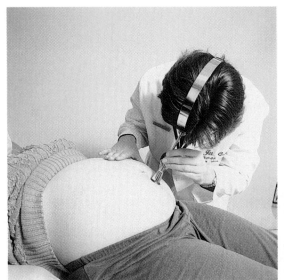 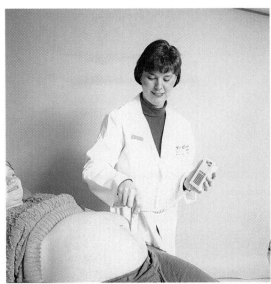

Auscultating the fetal heart rate with *(left)* a fetoscope and *(right)* a Doppler ultrasound device.

GENITALIA

ASSESSMENT PROCEDURE	NORMAL FINDINGS	ABNORMAL FINDINGS
Inspect the external genitalia. Note hair distribution, color of skin, varicosities, and scars.	Normal findings include enlarged labia and clitoris, parous relaxation of the introitus, and scars from an episiotomy or perineal lacerations (in multiparous women).	Labial varicosities, which can be painful
Palpate Bartholin's and Skene's glands.	There should be no discomfort or discharge with examination.	Discomfort and discharge noted with palpation may indicate infection.
Inspect vaginal opening for cystocele or rectocele.	No cystocele or rectocele.	Cystocele or rectocele may be more pronounced because of the muscle relaxation of pregnancy.

Speculum Examination

(Refer to gynecologic examination in textbook.) Insert speculum into the vagina. Visualize the cervix, noting position and color. Obtain Pap smear and cultures if indicated. Withdraw speculum.	Cervix should look pink, smooth, and healthy. With pregnancy, the cervix may appear bluish (Chadwick's sign). In multiparous women, the cervical opening has a slitlike appearance known as "fish mouth." A small amount of whitish vaginal discharge (leukorrhea) is normal.	Gonorrhea infection may present with thick, purulent vaginal discharge. A thick, white, cheesy discharge presents with a yeast infection. Grayish-white vaginal discharge, positive "whiff test" (fishy odor), and clue cells (epithelial cells that have been invaded by disease-causing bacteria) are evidence of bacterial vaginosis.

(continued)

ASSESSMENT PROCEDURE	NORMAL FINDINGS	ABNORMAL FINDINGS

Pelvic Examination

Put on gloves lubricated with water or KY jelly, gently insert fingers into the vagina, and palpate the cervix. Estimate the length of the cervix by palpating the lateral surface of the cervix from the cervical tip to the lateral fornix.

The cervix may be palpated in the posterior vaginal vault. It should be long, thick, and closed. Cervical length should be approximately 2.3 to 3 cm. Positive Hegar's sign (softening of the lower uterine segment) should be present.

An effaced opened cervix may indicate preterm labor or an incompetent cervix if gestation is not at term.

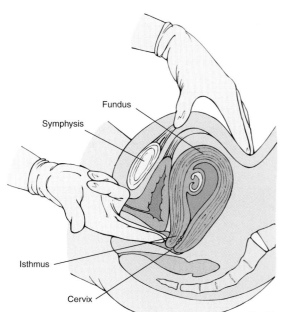

Positive Hegar's sign.

While leaving the fingers in the vagina, place the other hand on the abdomen and gently press down toward the internal hand until you feel the uterus between the two hands.

The uterus should feel about the size of an orange at 10 weeks and about the size of a grapefruit at 12 weeks.

If uterine size is not consistent with dates, consider wrong dates, uterine fibroids, or multiple gestation.

Palpate the left and right adnexa.

No masses should be palpable. Discomfort with examination is due to stretching of the round ligaments throughout the pregnancy.

Adnexal masses may indicate ectopic pregnancy.

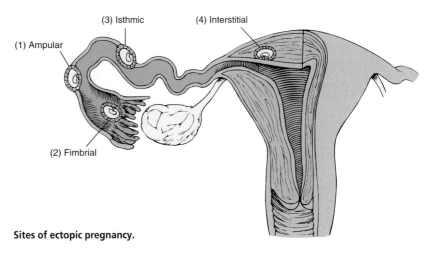

Sites of ectopic pregnancy.

(continued)

ASSESSMENT PROCEDURE	NORMAL FINDINGS	ABNORMAL FINDINGS

ANUS AND RECTUM

Inspect the anus and rectum. Note color, varicosities, lesions, tears, or discharge.	Mucosa should be pink and intact. No varicosities, lesions, tears, or discharge present.	Hemorrhoids or varicose veins may be present. Hemorrhoids usually get bigger and more uncomfortable during pregnancy. Bleeding and infection may occur. Masses may indicate cancer.

PERIPHERAL VASCULAR

Inspect face and extremities. Note color and edema.	During the third trimester, dependent edema is normal. Varicose veins may also appear.	Abnormal findings include calf pain, positive Homan's sign, generalized edema, and diminished pedal pulses. These findings may indicate thrombophlebitis.
Percuss deep tendon reflexes.	Normal reflexes 1 to 2+. Clonus is absent.	Reflexes 3 to 4+ and positive clonus require evaluation for pregnancy-induced hypertension.

MUSCULOSKELETAL

Determine pelvic adequacy for a vaginal delivery by estimating the angle of the subpubic arch.	The subpubic arch should be greater than 90 degrees.	A narrow pubic arch displaces the presenting part posteriorly and impedes the fetus from passing under the pubic arch.

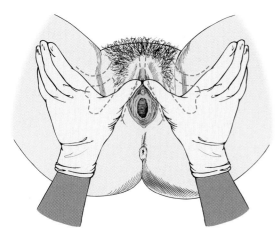

Estimating the angle of the subpubic arch.

ASSESSMENT PROCEDURE	NORMAL FINDINGS	ABNORMAL FINDINGS
Determine the height and inclination of the symphysis pubis.	The height and inclination of the symphysis pubis should be short and gradual, respectively.	A long or steeply inclined symphysis pubis may interfere with a successful vaginal delivery.

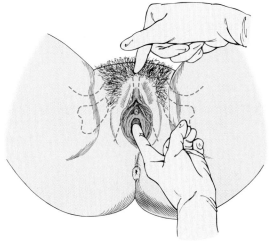

Determining the height and incline of the symphysis pubis.

Palpate the lateral walls of the pelvis.	Lateral walls should be straight or divergent.	Lateral walls that narrow as they approach the vagina may be problematic with vaginal delivery.
To palpate the ischial spines, sweep the finger posteriorly from one spine over to the other spine.	Ischial spines are small, not prominent. Interspinous diameter is at least 10.5 cm.	Prominent spines. Interspinous diameter less than 10.5 cm.

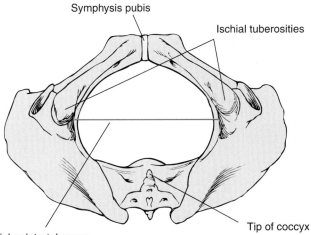

Symphysis pubis

Ischial tuberosities

Tip of coccyx

Bi-ischial or intertuberous diameter (11 cm)

Ischial spines.

Examine the sacrum and coccyx. Sweep fingers down the sacrum. Gently press back on the coccyx to determine mobility.	Gynecoid pelvis is most common. Mobile coccyx increases ease of delivery by expansion, enlarging the area in the pelvis.	Anthropoid or platypoid pelvis with an immobile coccyx may interfere with vaginal birth.

(continued)

ASSESSMENT PROCEDURE	**NORMAL FINDINGS**	**ABNORMAL FINDINGS**
Measure the diagonal conjugate. The diagonal conjugate measures the anteroposterior diameter of the pelvic inlet, through which the fetal head passes first. Measure the diagonal conjugate by pressing internal hand into the sacral promontory and up; mark the spot on your hand directly below the symphysis pubis.	Pelvic adequacy is expected if diagonal conjugate measures 12.5 cm or greater. If the middle finger cannot reach the sacral promontory, space is considered adequate.	A diagonal conjugate measuring less than 12.5 cm may impede vaginal delivery process.

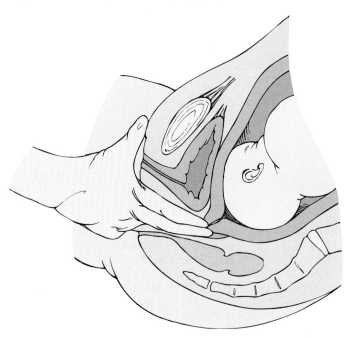

Measuring the diagonal conjugate.

Calculate the obstetric conjugate. The obstetric conjugate is the smallest opening through which the fetal head must pass. To calculate it, subtract 1.5 cm from the diagonal conjugate measurement.	Measurement of the obstetric conjugate should be 10.5 to 11 cm.	An obstetric conjugate measuring less than 10.5 cm may pose difficulty with vaginal delivery.

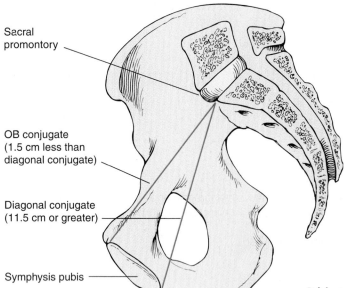

Sacral promontory

OB conjugate (1.5 cm less than diagonal conjugate)

Diagonal conjugate (11.5 cm or greater)

Symphysis pubis

Pelvic structure: Obstetric (OB) conjugate, diagonal conjugate.

(continued)

ASSESSMENT PROCEDURE	NORMAL FINDINGS	ABNORMAL FINDINGS
To measure the transverse diameter of the pelvic outlet, make a fist and place it between the ischial tuberosities.	The measurement between ischial tuberosities is usually 10 to 11 cm.	Diameters of less than 10 cm may inhibit fetal descent toward the vagina.

Tip From the Experts Know the measurement of your own hand to estimate the measurement.

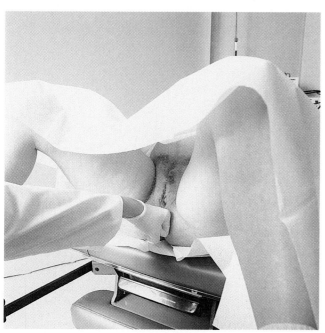

Using the fist to measure the pelvic outlet.

Validation and Documentation of Findings

Validate the assessment data on the childbearing woman that you have collected. This is necessary to verify that the data are reliable and accurate. Document the assessment data following the health care facility or agency policy.

EXAMPLE OF SUBJECTIVE DATA

- Client is a 25-year-old white, married, obstetric patient at 10 weeks' gestation by LMP.
- Prepregnancy weight 125 lb. No recent change in weight.
- No s/s cold or illness since LMP.
- Has occasional nausea and vomiting. Drinks fluids well.
- No change in stools or urinary pattern.
- Denies vaginal bleeding or discharge.
- Eats well.
- No history of psychological problems.
- Reports normal breast exam.

Past History

- Gravida 1—First pregnancy; denies previous deliveries, miscarriages, or molar pregnancy.
- LMP 8/20/02. Normal period—28-day cycle. No spotting.
- Last form of contraception—Oral contraceptive pill; stopped pill 4 months ago.
- Denies history of reproductive or fertility problems.
- Denies history of vaginal infections or STIs; partner also negative for STIs.
- Patient blood type A positive; no history of blood transfusion.
- Medical history—Unremarkable.
- Allergies—No known drug allergies.
- Surgeries—None. Hospitalizations—None.
- Current medications: Prenatal vitamin—One daily.
- Father not related to client.
- Primigravida—No history of past pregnancies.
- Race—White.

DISPLAY 25-1. Where to Auscultate Fetal Heart Rate

The illustrations below represent the best locations for auscultating the fetal heart rate: Left occiput anterior (LOA), right occiput anterior (ROA), left occiput posterior (LOP), right occiput posterior (ROP), left sacrum anterior (LSA), and right sacrum posterior (RSP).

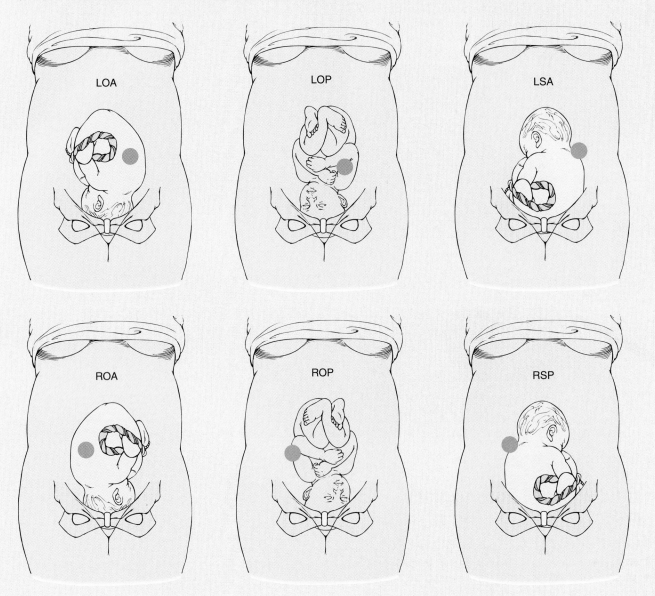

Family History

- No history of early deaths, diabetes, tuberculosis, asthma, cancer, birth defects, blood disorders, or mental retardation.

Lifestyle and Health Practices

- No alcohol, cigarettes, or drug use since LMP.
- No family members consider habits a problem.

- Diet consists of three meals a day and snacks (primarily meats, vegetables, fruits, bread, water).
- Prepregnant weight is 125 lb with no significant weight changes.
- Current vitamins—Prenate ultra-vitamin daily.

Activity and Exercise

- Exercises three to five times/week. Walks 30 min, occasional weight lifting with aerobics.

- Denies heavy lifting or heavy labor.
- Denies exposure to toxic substances.
- Has cats but does not change litter. Washes hands well after petting cat.

Role and Relationships

- Highest level education—MS.
- Occupation—RN.
- Lives with husband who is delighted about pregnancy.
- Additional support—Parents, in-laws, sister, and friends.
- Partner—Highest level education BS in business administration; current occupation—CPA; nonsmoker, drinks alcohol occasionally on weekends with friends; no history of illicit drug use.

EXAMPLE OF OBJECTIVE DATA

- B/P 100/60; pulse 90; temp 98.6°; height 5 feet 4 inches; weight 128 lb.
- Behavior—Ambivalent, excited.
- Skin—No hyperpigmentation yet.
- Hair/nails—Soft, smooth, clean.
- Neck—Supple; thyroid—No masses or enlargement noted.
- Ears—TM clear; landmarks visible.
- Mouth/throat/nose—Pink, no exudate, no hypertrophy.
- Thorax/lungs—CTA bilaterally.
- Breasts—No masses palpable, no discharge, symmetric, no nipple inversion.
- Heart—NSR without murmur.
- Abdomen—Soft, nontender, no hepatosplenomegaly; fundal height palpable above symphysis pubis, approx. 10 weeks' size, no contractions. Leopold's maneuvers—Inappropriate for 10 weeks' gestation.
- Fetal heart tones—Audible with fetal Doppler, rate 158 b/min.
- Genitalia—External: No scars or varicosities; Bartholin's and Skene's glands negative; no cystocele or rectocele noted.
- Speculum: Chadwick's sign present; no vaginal discharge or bleeding; Pap smear performed.
- GC and *Chlamydia* cultures taken and sent to lab.
- Pelvic—Cervix: posterior, closed, long and thick. Uterus: Approx. 10 weeks' size. No masses palpable.
- Adnexa—Negative R and L.
- Anus/rectum—Negative for lesions or varicosities.
- Peripheral vascular—Face/extremities—No edema; pink, well perfused; pulses equal bilaterally, Homans' sign, DTRs 1–2 +, -clonus.
- Pelvis—Subpubic arch >90°; symphysis pubis—short, gradual inclination. Lateral walls straight.
- Ischial spines—Blunt. Interspinous diameter >10.5 cm.
- Pelvis—Gynecoid, coccyx mobile.
- Diagonal conjugate—>12.5 cm.
- Obstetric conjugate—>10.5 cm.
- Transverse diameter—>11 cm.
- *Assessment:* Healthy obstetric physical examination.
- *Plan:* Routine obstetric care.

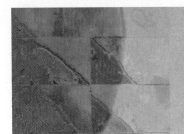 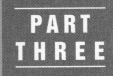
After you have collected your assessment data, you will need to analyze the data, using diagnostic reasoning skills presented in Chapter 7. In Diagnostic Reasoning: Possible Conclusions, you will see an overview of common conclusions that you may reach after assessment of the childbearing woman. Next, Diagnostic Reasoning: Case Study shows you how to analyze assessment data for a *specific* childbearing client. Finally, you have an extra opportunity to analyze data in the critical thinking exercise presented in the lab manual study guide available with the textbook.

Diagnostic Reasoning: Possible Conclusions

Listed are some possible conclusions after assessing a childbearing woman.

SELECTED NURSING DIAGNOSES

After collecting subjective and objective data pertaining to the assessment of the childbearing woman, you will need to identify abnormalities and cluster the data to reveal any significant patterns or abnormalities. These data will then be used to make clinical judgments (nursing diagnoses: wellness, risk, or actual) about the status of the client's pregnancy. Following is a listing of selected nursing diagnoses that you may identify when analyzing data for this part of the assessment.

Nursing Diagnoses (Wellness)

- Deficient Knowledge: self-care during pregnancy
- Imbalanced Nutrition: Less Than Body Requirements
- Disturbed Body Image, related to pregnancy

Nursing Diagnoses (Risk)

- Risk for Deficient Fluid Volume (related to excessive nausea/vomiting)

- Risk for Injury (maternal) (related to elevated arterial pressure)
- Risk for Injury (fetal) (related to decreased placental perfusion due to blood loss)

Nursing Diagnoses (Actual)

- Anxiety (related to fear of loss of pregnancy)

SELECTED COLLABORATIVE PROBLEMS

After grouping the data, certain collaborative problems may emerge. Remember that collaborative problems differ from nursing diagnoses in that they cannot be prevented with nursing interventions alone. However, these physiologic complications of medical conditions can be detected and monitored by the nurse. In addition, the nurse can use physician- and nurse-prescribed interventions to minimize the complications of these problems. The nurse may also have to refer the client in such situations for further treatment of the problem. Following is a list of collaborative problems that may be identified when assessing the childbearing woman. These problems are worded as Potential Complication (or PC) followed by the problem.

- PC: Anemia
- PC: Advanced maternal age
- PC: Gestational diabetes

MEDICAL PROBLEMS

After grouping the data, it may become apparent that the client has signs and symptoms that may require medical diagnosis and treatment. Referral to a primary care provider is necessary.

Diagnostic Reasoning: Case Study

The case study presents assessment data for a specific client. It is followed by an analysis of the data, working out the seven key steps to arrive at specific conclusions.

Mrs. Mary Farrow is a 29-year-old Caucasian woman, gravida 3, para 2, who presents to the clinic today for her initial prenatal examination. She states that her last menstrual period (LMP) was on September 15, approximately 16 weeks ago. Because she was unable to get transportation to the clinic, she did not come in for prenatal care earlier in this pregnancy. "I do know how important early prenatal care is, but I just couldn't get here. And I feel good—no problems so far." Mrs. Farrow lives with her husband and two sons in a two-bedroom trailer on land owned by her in-laws. She states that her in-laws are very supportive and help out during tough times by not charging rent. Her husband works full time at a fast-food chain restaurant, but is looking for a job that pays more money. It is often hard for them to meet their financial responsibilities; however, they believe it is important for her to stay home with the children so she does not contribute financially. She reports that, in general, she encourages healthful practices for herself and family, but because her husband gets a discount on food and soda from his work, they don't eat as well as she knows they should. "But I am eating less so I don't gain so much weight this time."

Mrs. Farrow's past medical history is unremarkable; her two pregnancies were term gestations and deliveries were vaginal. However, during the last pregnancy, she was diagnosed with pregnancy-induced hypertension and gestational diabetes and labor was induced at 38 weeks' gestation. She states that she gained 60 lb with that pregnancy and that her son weighed 9 lb, 2 oz.

Your physical assessment of Mrs. Farrow reveals BP 100/60 right arm, sitting; pulse rate 86, regular and strong; respirations 18, regular and moderately shallow; temperature 36.7 degrees centigrade. Her apical beat is also 86 and strong; heart sounds: S_1 and S_2 with no murmurs or clicks. Skin is warm and dry, slightly pale with light pink nail beds, pale palpebral conjunctiva and oral mucous membranes. Abdomen moderately rounded with striae; fundal height 20 cm; fetal heart rate 158 per Doppler, right lower quadrant. Current weight 138 lb at 5 feet 9 inches tall, 2 lb less than her stated usual weight. Lab values show hemoglobin (Hgb) 10.2 g/dL; hematocrit (Hct) 29.9%; red blood cell (RBC) count $3.20 \times 10^{-6}/mm^3$. The remainder of the blood values are within normal limits. Urinalysis results are negative for protein and glucose.

1 Identify abnormal data and strengths (in both subjective and objective data).

SUBJECTIVE DATA

- LMP 9/15—16 weeks ago
- Gravid 3, para 2
- Unable to come in earlier for prenatal care
- No transportation to clinic
- "I know the importance of early prenatal care."
- "I feel good—no problems so far."
- Lives with husband and children in trailer on land owned by in-laws
- In-laws supportive (not specific how, except financially)
- Husband works in fast-food restaurant; looking for higher paying job
- Difficult to meet financial responsibilities
- In-laws help out by not charging rent when times are tough
- Client stays home with children
- Believes in healthful practices but eats fast food and sodas for financial reasons
- "I am eating less so I don't gain so much weight this time."
- First pregnancy and delivery unremarkable
- Pregnancy-induced hypertension and gestational diabetes with last pregnancy; gained 60 lb, infant weight 9 lb, 2 oz

OBJECTIVE DATA

- BP: 100/60, pulse 86 regular, respirations 18, temperature 36.7°C
- Cardiac assessment WNL (within normal limits)
- Skin warm, dry, pale with light pink nail beds
- Pale palpebral conjunctiva and oral mucous membranes
- Abdomen moderately rounded with striae
- Fundal height: 20 cm
- FHR: 158 per Doppler, RLQ
- Hgb 10.2 g/dL; Hct 29.9%; RBC 3.2
- Weight 138 lb, 2 lb below usual weight
- Urine: Negative

2 Cue Clusters	**3** Inferences	**4** Possible Nursing Diagnoses	**5** Defining Characteristics	**6** Confirm or Rule Out
A • Sixteen weeks pregnant by report • Unable to come for care due to no transportation	Came in for prenatal care as soon as transportation available	Health-Seeking Behaviors	None specific but implied because client monitored her status and sought care as soon as possible	Confirm and support efforts
• Knows importance of early prenatal care • Difficulty meeting financial responsibilities	Unstable/inadequate financial resources to meet own/family health needs	Risk for Ineffective Health Maintenance related to inadequate financial resource	Reported lack of financial resources	Confirm

② Cue Clusters	③ Inferences	④ Possible Nursing Diagnoses	⑤ Defining Characteristics	⑥ Confirm or Rule Out
		Risk for Compromised Family Coping related to inadequate resources to support another child	None noted at this time, but not needed for a risk diagnosis	Confirm and collect more data regarding family's plans to manage an additional family member
B • Diet consists mostly of fast foods and sodas because husband gets a discount • Hgb 10.2; Hct 29.9; RBC 3.2 • Eating less to decrease weight gain • Weight 138 lb—down 2 lb • Pale skin, conjunctiva, mucous membranes	Mild anemia from inadequate diet and not eating enough to support expected weight gain for 16+ weeks of pregnancy	Imbalanced Nutrition: Less Than Body Requirements related to inadequate finances to provide proper nutrition for client/fetus and knowledge deficit of appropriate weight gain for current stage of pregnancy	Abnormal hematology values Pale conjunctiva and mucous membranes Reported lack of proper food	Confirm
C • History of pregnancy-induced hypertension and diabetes • Late entry into care • Weight loss from beginning of pregnancy • Hgb 10.2; Hct 29.9	Risk for complications this pregnancy	Risk for Injury, Mother/Baby related to past history of pregnancy complications and unhealthful eating behaviors (high salt/sugar)	None	Rule out: Does not meet definition for Risk for Injury. This information points to collaborative diagnoses where the nurse will monitor for signs and symptoms of complications.
		Fear related to lack of understanding of why previous complications occurred	None stated or observed	Rule out, but collect more data
D • Fundal height greater than dates would suggest	Possible incorrect dates, multiple gestations, or fetal anomalies	Collaborative diagnoses		

  Document conclusions.

The following diagnoses are appropriate for Mrs. Farrow at this time:

- Health-Seeking Behavior
- Risk for Ineffective Health Maintenance related to inadequate financial resources
- Risk for Interrupted Family Coping related to inadequate resources to support another child
- Imbalanced Nutrition: Less Than Body Requirements related to inadequate finances to provide proper nutrition and knowledge deficit of appropriate weight gain for current stage of pregnancy

Collaborative problems related to pregnancy could include the following:

- PC: Pregnancy-induced hypertension
- PC: Fetal compromise
- PC: Multiple gestation
- PC: Hyperglycemia
- PC: Fetal abnormality

REFERENCES AND SELECTED READINGS

American College of Obstetricians and Gynecologists (ACOG). (2000a). *Breastfeeding: Maternal and Infant Aspects.* Educational Bulletin: No. 258. Washington, DC: Author.

———. (2000b). *Genetic Screening for Hemoglobinopathies.* Committee Opinion: No. 238. Washington, DC: Author.

———. (1999a). *Domestic Violence.* Educational Bulletin: No. 257. Washington, DC: Author.

———. (1999b). *Nutrition and Women.* Educational Bulletin: No. 229. Washington, DC: Author.

———. (1997). *Smoking and Women's Health.* Educational Bulletin: No. 240. Washington, DC: Author.

———. (1996). *Vaginitis.* Technical Bulletin: No. 226. Washington, DC: Author.

Gabbe, S., Niebyl, J., & Simpson, J. (1999). *Pocket companion to obstetrics.* New York: Churchill Livingstone.

Gorrie, T., McKinney, E., & Murray, S. (1998). *Foundations of maternal–newborn nursing.* Philadelphia: WB Saunders.

Hacker, N., & Moore, J. (1998). *Essentials of obstetrics and gynecology* (3rd ed.). Philadelphia: WB Saunders.

Olds, S., London, M., & Ladewig, P. (1999). *Maternal–newborn nursing.* Upper Saddle River, NJ: Prentice-Hall.

Seltzer, V., & Pearse, W. (2000). *Women's primary health care: Office practice and procedures* (2nd ed.). New York: McGraw-Hill.

For additional information on this book, be sure to visit http://connection.lww.com.

Assessment of the Frail Elderly Client

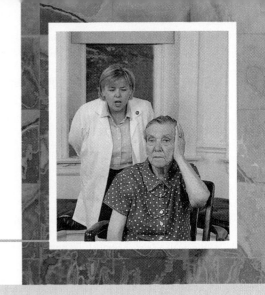

26

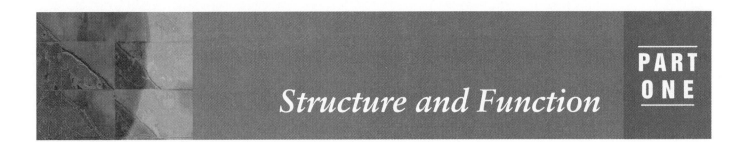

Structure and Function

PART ONE

A major challenge in physical assessment of the older person is differentiating findings related to the usual "wear and tear" of aging from those that indicate a pathologic process. Many of the signs and symptoms of disease and common physical findings in elderly clients have been identified throughout this book. Correctly identifying the manifestations of disability and treatable conditions in the elderly is the key to maintaining their health and vitality. Although the vast majority of older adults lead active, independent lives, they often do so despite multiple chronic conditions. It is not the physiologic changes of aging, per se, that warrant a special approach to assessment of the elderly client. It is, rather, the tendency that advancing age has to place a person at greater risk for chronic illness and disability that has led to using the term *frail elderly*. The term describes the vulnerability of those age 85 and older to be in poorer health, to have more chronic disabilities, and to function less independently. Because the 85 and older age group is the most rapidly growing age group in the United States, the caregiving needs of this age group also have a significant impact on society.

Frail elderly clients may be living at home alone or with the assistance of a caregiver, in a residential care setting with minimal assistance, or in a long-term care facility. They are often living with multiple chronic illnesses and some level of functional disability. As a result, health complaints or abnormalities disclosed during physical examination are not readily attributable to a specific disease. In fact, the symptoms of disease often present differently in this age group.

Because poor management of chronic illness and the inability to correctly identify and treat acute illness increase the risk of frailty among the oldest people, prompt assessment and management are often the key to quality of life. The combination of physiologic changes and the tendency for multiple chronic illnesses in the elderly client makes it difficult to attribute health complaints or abnormalities to a specific disease. The unique way in which disease presents in the frail elderly has been identified as the "geriatric syndromes." Assessment of the frail elderly client, therefore, involves a more integrated approach as well as an awareness of the unique ways in which illness may present and a heightened sensitivity to the meaning that functional disability will have on an older person's quality of life.

Assessment of the frail elderly person also requires a systematic, interdisciplinary approach and an awareness of the effect that chronic pain, increasing dependency, death of loved ones, and end-of-life decisions may have on overall life satisfaction. To some clients, the ability to function independently enough to stay in their own homes may be of paramount importance. To others, being able to afford long-term care and avoid "being a burden" to a son or daughter may be the ultimate goal. The combination of physical frailty and adjustments mandated by living into the advanced years necessitates an integrated assessment of psychosocial, functional, and physical health.

Functional assessment is an evaluation of the person's ability to carry out the basic self-care activities of daily living (ADLs) such as bathing, eating, grooming, and toileting. In addition, it includes those activities necessary for well-being and survival as an individual in a society. These activities known as instrumental ADLs focus primarily on household chores (eg, cooking, cleaning, laundry), mobility-related activities (eg, shopping and transportation), and cognitive abilities (money management, using the telephone, and ability to make decisions affecting basic safety and social needs). Functional ability is determined by the dynamic interplay of the frail elder's physiologic status, emotional and cognitive status, and the physical, interpersonal, and social environment. Thus, an evaluation of the frail elder's physical and social environment and the degree to which these resources are able to compensate for physiologic frailty is essential for assisting the frail elderly person to achieve maximal quality of life.

Physical and Functional Changes Related to Aging

Even in the absence of disease, aging involves an overall general decline in tissues throughout the body. This decline reaches about 50% by the time a person is age 80 or older. However, decline in tissue mass does not necessarily correlate with functional decline. The body is designed with a great deal of physiologic reserve. For example, renal failure is not generally apparent until approximately 75% to 80% of renal function has been lost. In the absence of strenuous activity, the body's need for blood and oxygen can be met with nearly half the normal cardiac output. The significance of physical decline with aging often becomes evident only when acute or chronic illness places a demand on the body and no physiologic reserve is available.

Additionally, the structural changes and general decline in various body systems brought about by aging do not

709

necessarily cause a decrease in function. However, they do generally diminish the body's ability to protect itself and to compensate for internal and external stress. In assessing the frail elderly client, the nurse needs to understand how the structural changes of aging may be expected to change physical examination findings. However, whether a structural change is normal or abnormal to the degree that it warrants intervention is best determined by whether it changes the older person's ability to function and derive satisfaction in the activities of daily living (ADLs). Some major concerns regarding age and related dysfunction are identified by the acronym SPICES, which stands for:

- **S**kin impairment
- **P**oor nutrition
- **I**ncontinence
- **C**ognitive impairment
- **E**vidence of falls or functional decline
- **S**leep disturbances (Francis, Fletcher & Simon, 1998)

Body system changes contributing to SPICES are discussed from head to toe in the pages that follow.

SKIN, HAIR, AND NAILS

The major anatomic change in elderly skin is the gradual replacement of elastic collagen with more fibrous tissue and the loss of subcutaneous tissue. Although this does not pose a life-threatening problem, the skin can be easily torn by shearing forces. Vascular fragility can also add to the fragility of the skin, and purpura (purple patches) may be present. Epidermal cells regenerate at only about 25% the rate of those cells in young adults. Compromised by the weakening of the dermal blood vessels and less efficient capillary microcirculation, the skin's repair system is significantly impaired, which has serious consequences for wound healing. As fat is redistributed to the abdomen and thighs in advanced age, bony surfaces, such as the hands, face, and sacrum, are especially prone to injury. A decrease in the number of surveillance cells of the immune system, such as the Langerhans' cells in the epidermis, and a decrease in eccrine, sebaceous, and apocrine glands leaves the skin of the aged poorly protected from exposure to the sun, heat, cold, and infectious organisms. Decreased sebaceous gland function causes the common complaint of dryness.

Despite a decrease in the total number of melanocytes, hyperpigmentation occurs in skin exposed to sunlight (eg, neck, face, and arms), which manifests as brown pigmented areas called *lentigenes,* which are commonly referred to as *liver or age spots.* Functional changes that place the older person at risk of hypothermia and hyperthermia are largely due to the decreased vascularity and diminished neurologic response to temperature changes as well as general loss of subcutaneous tissue. Atrophy of eccrine sweat glands increases the risk of hyperthermia. Although some increased cold intolerance is expected, sudden and sharp intolerance should be investigated to detect possible hypothyroidism.

Increased dermatologic lesions are common, affecting up to 95% of the hospitalized elderly. Fortunately, many lesions are benign. They include venous lakes, which occur on ears or other facial areas; skin tags, which are flesh colored; and seborrheic keratoses, which occur most commonly in fair-skinned persons in sun-exposed areas and which are tan, brown, or reddish.

Conversely, some lesions are not benign, and they signify more serious conditions. The combination of environmental exposure and diminished immunodeficiency with aging greatly increases the risk of skin cancer. Premalignant lesions include actinic keratoses, which appear as round or irregularly shaped tan scaly lesions that may be inflamed or bleed around the edges, and leukoplakia, which has a 20% to 30% progression rate to squamous cell carcinoma. Because the prevalence of malignancy is so high in elderly clients, the client should be referred for biopsy and any suspicious looking lesion should be analyzed. Factors that increase the need for concern are any new pigmented or asymmetric lesions, border irregularities, color variations, increase in size, or elevation of a previously flat lesion.

In addition, the potential for the growth of *Candida* lesions in the mouth, vagina, and nail beds increases as a result of decreasing numbers of Langerhans' cells and predisposing conditions, such as diabetes mellitus, malnutrition, and steroid and antibiotic use. Also more common with age are the clear vesicles that erupt from herpes zoster (shingles), a reactivation of the latent virus in the dorsal root ganglion. The outbreak may be complicated if postherpetic neuralgia persists longer than 4 weeks after the resolution of the skin lesions. This occurs in more than half of affected individuals over age 65.

Scalp, axillary, and pubic hair gradually becomes thinner and coarser. Loss of hair pigment is the cause of graying. Appearance of facial hair on an older woman may occur after menopause because of a decrease in the ratio of estrogen to testosterone. Toenails usually thicken, but fingernails may become thin and split. They may also appear yellowish and dull.

EYES AND VISION

Decreased tear production by the lacrimal glands often results in dry eyes that are described as irritated or having a scratchy sensation to them. Because eyelid skin is the thinnest skin of the body, it tends to stretch over time. In the upper eyelid, this stretched skin may limit the peripheral field of vision and may produce a feeling of heaviness and a tired appearance. In the lower eyelid, "bags" form.

Some older adults also experience excessive tearing. The tearing may be from impaired tear drainage as a result of ectropion, a turning out of the lower eyelid. In such cases, stretching of the lower eyelid causes it to droop downward and keeps it from shutting completely. Ectropion can also cause dryness, redness, or sensitivity to light and wind. The opposite condition, entropion (a turning in of the lower eyelid) occurs most commonly in the aged. This causes the lower eyelashes to touch the conjunctiva and cornea, which may result in an ulcerous corneal infection. Surgical correction may be necessary to restore the normal position of the eyelid.

A loss of transparency in the crystalline lens of the eye occurs as the natural process of aging. This cloudiness is known as a *cataract*, which is a milky to a yellowish or brownish discoloration. Cataracts most commonly affect people after age 55, although they can also be caused by injury, inherited tendencies, certain diseases, or birth defects. After age 75, about 92% of the populace has some degree of cataract formation with nearly 50% experiencing a significant vision loss (Kennedy-Malone, Fletcher & Plank, 2000). There is growing evidence that exposure to ultraviolet light (sunlight) and cigarette smoking may speed their development. The degree to which a person's vision is affected by cataract formation depends on the location and degree of clouding. If the area of the clouding initially starts on the side of the lens, a person's vision may not be drastically affected for years because peripheral vision is not as useful as central vision. Although cataracts typically develop in both eyes, the rate of progression varies with each eye.

With age, there is an overall decrease in the size of the pupil and its ability to dilate in the dark. The slower ability of the pupils to constrict in response to bright light also makes the older adult more sensitive to glare. Older adults generally require two to three times more diffuse light as well as light that is directed on the task at hand. Many eye disorders of the aged can potentially result in significant visual loss or even blindness. These more potentially damaging conditions include glaucoma, macular degeneration, detached or torn retina, and diabetic retinopathy (Display 26-1).

EARS AND HEARING

Structural changes in the outer ear begin in middle adulthood. The earlobes elongate, and the pinna increases in length and width. The hairs become coarser. Cerumen pro-

---

ABNORMAL
FINDINGS

DISPLAY 26-1. Age-Related Abnormalities of the Eye

Common age-related abnormalities of the eye include glaucoma, macular degeneration, retinal detachment, and diabetic retinopathy.

GLAUCOMA

The client with glaucoma is usually symptom free. In elderly people, diabetes and atherosclerosis are conditions that increase the risk of glaucoma. The disorder is caused by increased pressure that can destroy the optic nerve and cause blindness if not treated properly. An acute form of glaucoma can occur at any age and is a true medical emergency because blindness can result in a day or two without treatment. Rainbow-like halos or circles around lights, severe pain in the eyes or forehead, nausea, and blurred vision may occur with the acute form of glaucoma.

MACULAR DEGENERATION

Macular degeneration, a gradual loss of central vision, is caused by aging and thinning of the microthin membrane in the center of the retina called the macula. Most cases begin to develop after age 50, but damage may be occurring for months to years before symptoms occur. Peripheral vision is not affected, and the condition may occur initially in only one eye. Only about 10% of all age-related macular degeneration leaks occur in the small blood vessels in the retinal pigment epithelium. This type accounts for the most serious loss of vision.

RETINA DETACHMENT

Retinal detachment occurs at a greater frequency with aging as the vitreous pulls away from its attachment to the retina at the back of the eye, causing the retina to tear in one or more places. A retinal detachment is always a serious problem. Blindness will result if the detachment is not treated.

DIABETIC RETINOPATHY

Many older adults have diabetes, which can lead to cataracts, glaucoma, and diabetic retinopathy. Of those with diabetes mellitus, about 90% will develop diabetic retinopathy to some degree. The more serious of the two forms of the disease, proliferative diabetic retinopathy, occurs most often among those who have had diabetes for more than 25 years. People with the advanced form of the disease usually experience a noticeable loss of vision, including cloudiness, distortion of familiar objects, and, occasionally, blind spots or floaters. If not treated, diabetic retinopathy will lead to connective scar tissue, which over time can shrink, pulling on the retina and resulting in a retinal detachment. In the early stages of the milder form of the disease, background diabetic retinopathy, the person may be unaware of problems because the loss of sight is usually gradual and mainly affects peripheral vision.

duction decreases, leading to dryness and the increased tendency toward impaction.

The most common type of hearing loss associated with aging is called *presbycusis*. It involves the diminished ability to hear high-frequency sounds and is due to degeneration in the hair cells of the inner ear. Soft consonant sounds, such as S, Z, T, F, and G, or background noises, such as television or music, that compete with voices may make speech discrimination especially challenging. Because the frequency of the voice increases with volume, raising one's voice to someone with presbycusis will only make it more difficult for them to hear. Conductive losses in hearing also occur because the tympanic membrane thickens or, more commonly, ear wax accumulates.

MOUTH AND THROAT

Periodontal disease, swallowing abnormalities, and dry mouth contribute to nutritional problems, which are a major concern for many frail elderly people. There is some decrease in saliva production with aging. However, the major cause of xerostomia (dry mouth) in the elderly is from using medications that have anticholinergic effects (eg, dry mouth, blurred vision, increased heart rate, constipation). Because saliva has antibacterial, antifungal, and tooth-cleansing properties, decreased production may promote dental caries. Dental caries in the frail elderly person can increase the risk for pneumonia, a common problem that may have serious consequences.

Nutrition

Problems contributing to poor nutrition include alterations in taste due largely to disease and the effects of medications used to treat disease rather than a significant decline in taste bud function or the ability to discriminate sweet, sour, salty, and bitter at usual concentrations. However, taste preferences typically change with age and, with an overall age-related decrease in appetite, the person tends to prefer sweeter or spicier foods and may tend to add salt and sugar to foods. The occurrence of lactose intolerance increases with age and may result in bloating, abdominal discomfort, and increased flatus.

Swallowing and Dysphagia

In older adults, esophageal motility is slower and more disorganized, giving rise to dysphagia, a swallowing dysfunction involving the transfer of a bolus of food from the mouth to the stomach. Dysphagia can have a mechanical or neurologic basis. Stroke, multiple medical diagnoses, advanced age, and residing in a nursing home are all risk factors for dysphagia. Symptoms of dysphagia (Display 26-2) may range from choking to subtle signs, such as pocketing of food or a weak or hoarse voice (especially after drinking or eating). Periodic nutritional assessments are recommended for all people who are diagnosed with dysphagia and who have an altered diet (tube-feeding or pureed).

NOSE AND SINUSES

Olfactory function gradually decreases with aging and may lead to a decreased ability to detect odors. This does not generally lead to problems other than a heightened concern about the need for smoke detectors or routine home checks for gas leaks. Diminished smell, however, may also lead to a decline in appetite.

Allergic rhinitis, vasomotor rhinitis, and infectious sinusitis are common problems in the elderly. Newly constructed buildings in which new carpeting or cabinetry made of fiberboard is present can elicit an allergic response in an atopic (allergic) person. Fumes from paint may elicit a nonallergic vasomotor response as well as an allergic response. Relocation into a newly constructed residential or long-term care facility should be investigated as a possible

---

DISPLAY 26-2. Signs and Symptoms of Dysphagia

COMMONLY REPORTED COMPLAINTS
- "Food catches in my throat."
- "I choke on water."
- "I feel like I'm choking."

PHYSICAL SIGNS
- Coughing after food or fluid intake
- Drooling
- Pocketing of food
- Spitting out food
- Drooping mouth
- Chronic congestion
- Weak or hoarse voice (especially change in voice quality after drinking or eating)

exacerbating factor when symptoms of allergic or nonallergic rhinitis appear in a frail elderly person. Additionally, a nasogastric feeding tube or nasal polyps also place the elder at risk for sinusitis. Sinusitis, like any other infection, can be the cause of delirium in a frail older adult.

THORAX AND LUNGS

The decrease of collagen and elastin associated with aging causes the lungs to recoil less during expiration. This increases the energy needed for breathing and requires the active use of accessory muscles. The alveoli are also less elastic and contain fewer functional capillaries. The loss of skeletal muscle strength in the thorax and diaphragm, combined with the loss of resilience that holds the thorax in a slightly contracted position, contributes to the slight barrel chest seen in many older adults.

The physiologic effect of these structural changes is decreased vital capacity and increased residual volume. The decrease in vital capacity (the amount of air exhaled after a deep breath) can be measured as the forced expiratory volume in 1 second (FEV_1). For a nonsmoker, the decrease is approximately 30 mL/year after age 30 (Fitzpatrick, Fulmer, Wallace & Flaherty, 2000, p. 81).

Because anatomic changes result in an increased use of abdominal and diaphragmatic breathing, elders are more sensitive to intra-abdominal pressure changes. Total lung capacity, however, remains unchanged, although there is a normal decrease in arterial oxygen levels. Age adjustments in normal values for the partial pressure of oxygen in arterial blood can be expressed as $PaO_2 = 109 - 0.043$ (age) $+ 4.0$ (Lonergan, 1996). The decrease in arterial oxygen saturation levels should not be misconstrued as an indication of pulmonary disease in healthy elders (Fitzpatrick et al., 2000).

To what degree the structural changes of aging in the pulmonary system will result in functional declines in aerobic capacity and dyspnea with exertion largely depends on the exposure that a person has had over a lifetime to pollutants, smoke, and infectious agents and the resistance they have developed through physical conditioning and exercise. For example, it is now known that kyphosis is less prevalent in women who maintain an adequate level of physical fitness throughout their life (Cutler, Friedman & Genovese-Stone, 1993); the disorder is not entirely due to postmenopausal osteoporosis.

Respiratory Infections

A major threat to the health of a frail elderly person is respiratory infection. Pneumonia is the most common cause of infection-related deaths in elderly clients and is characterized as a "silent killer." Age-related diminished ciliary function and cough reflex increase the risk of pulmonary infection. Pulmonary infection in the elderly client seldom presents as the classic triad of cough, fever, and pleuritic pain. Instead, subtle changes, such as increased respiration

and sputum production, confusion, loss of appetite, and hypotension, may be the presenting signs and symptoms (Fitzpatrick et. al., 2000). In fact, the client may already have sepsis and accompanying hypothermia at initial presentation and diagnosis.

Frail elderly clients who are malnourished, immunocompromised, and institutionalized are at greater risk for tuberculosis (TB), and a high percentage of active TB found in elderly people is reactivated from a prior infection. Symptoms are commonly insidious and of long duration. Elderly people with neurologic impairments from Parkinson's or Alzheimer's disease or cardiovascular accident (CVA, or stroke) are at particular risk for aspiration pneumonia. Another common problem is the increased risk of a pulmonary embolism in elderly people who undergo major abdominal or thoracic surgery.

HEART AND BLOOD VESSELS

Heart failure is the leading cause of hospitalization, and coronary artery disease is the leading cause of death in the elderly. The effect of cardiovascular disease on mortality and functional status is due to a complex interplay of genetics, behavioral risk factors, age-related changes, and comorbid conditions such as diabetes. Only a few of the common findings are due to aging alone. As in almost all body tissues, the heart undergoes an increase in fibrotic tissue and a decrease in elastic tissue.

Valvular Changes

The primary significance of these tissue changes is a calcification, stiffening, and dilation of the aortic and mitral valves. Such changes to the aortic valves are evidenced as a soft systolic murmur, which is heard best at the base of the heart and is found in at least 20% of older people. A fourth heart sound (S_4) often accompanies an aortic murmur. It is most likely due to decreased ventricular compliance and is not considered to be an abnormality unless symptoms of heart failure are present. There is a slight increase in the atria as a compensatory response to the diminished ventricular compliance. When the age-related degenerative changes in valve structure are compounded by some valvular damage caused by rheumatic fever or atherosclerosis, the soft systolic murmur of aortic sclerosis may become aortic stenosis. Aortic stenosis can precipitate heart failure and is best differentiated from sclerosis by echocardiography.

Dysrhythmias

The accumulation of lipofuscin, amyloid, collagen, and fats in the pacemaker cells of the heart predispose the older adult to dysrhythmias, even in the absence of heart disease. People with transient tachycardia are more prone to heart failure, and sustained tachycardia will generally lead to a decompensatory response much sooner in the frail elderly than in younger people. Loss of pacemaker cells in the sinus node and fibers in the bundle of His may also lead to sick sinus syndrome, atrioventricular (AV) block, and bundle branch block. Atrial fibrillation is very common in elderly people and can be a contributing factor to syncope, heart failure, and blood clots or emboli. The greater the exercise intolerance of the older adult, the less the heart rate will increase with exercise and the longer it will take to return to the pre-exercise rate.

Blood Pressure

Both systolic and diastolic pressure rise with age due to a loss of elasticity of the aorta and arteries. There is generally a greater increase in the systolic pressure, resulting in a widening of the pulse pressure. Because of the higher pressure required to overcome the more noncompliant vessels, there is controversy about the definition and treatment of hypertension in the frail elderly client. The combination of some decreased baroreceptor sensitivity and the widespread use of antihypertensives, diuretics, and drugs with anticholinergic side effects makes orthostatic hypotension a common problem. One of the most serious concerns related to orthostatic hypotension is the potential for light-headedness and dizziness, both of which may precipitate falls, which carry with them the risk for hip fracture and head trauma among other injuries.

Heart Diseases

Assessment of cardiovascular disease processes is similar for all ages of adults with two major exceptions: Myocardial infarction (MI) and heart failure. MIs generally produce much less demonstrable symptoms in the very old. It is not uncommon for mild confusion or nausea to be the only symptom. Secondly, functional status is an important prognostic factor in the elderly person after MI with early or mild impairments to be significant for subsequent functional dependence (Gill, Williams, Mendes de Leon & Tinetti, 1997). Heart failure remains a leading cause of disability and diminished quality of life. The importance of correlating physical assessments with functional status is essential to managing cardiovascular conditions in the very old person.

BREASTS

The aged breasts, particularly in women, are often described as pendulous. This is because fat and elastic tissue decreases and the existing tissue becomes more fibrotic. Overall, breast tissue mass declines with aging, but the incidence of breast cancer increases with age, which is why aged clients are more likely to have had mastectomies.

Because the general rate for detection and treatment of tumors in the early stages is 95%, yearly clinical examination and mammography as well as breast self-examination are recommended. Elderly women who are breast cancer survivors and who have been on estrogen replacement therapy (ERT) for many years are at greater risk. Any history of estrogen-dependent breast neoplasia, however, is a contraindication to ERT.

ABDOMEN

With advancing age, abdominal structures undergo changes in size and function. For example, the liver decreases in size; the formation of gallstones increases; and the kidneys lose nephrons and cortical mass while interstitial tissue increases.

Renal Changes

The kidneys are also affected by glomerular degeneration, thickening of glomerular and tubular basement membranes, and decrease in length and volume of the proximal and distal tubules. Cardiac output typically decreases, and renal artery atherosclerosis is more prevalent with aging, resulting in an approximate 50% decrease in renal blood flow between the ages of 20 and 90. By age 80, the glomerular filtration rate is approximately 60% to 70% of the normal adult value. A concurrent rise in serum creatinine level is seldom seen in the elderly because the loss of muscle mass from which creatinine is derived is diminished. Thus, a 24-hour urinalysis for creatinine clearance more accurately reflects renal function. Diminished renal function must always be a consideration in the dosing and administration of drugs in the frail elderly person. Chronic conditions such as congestive heart failure, hypertension, and diabetes mellitus precipitate acute and chronic renal failure in the elderly.

Gastrointestinal Changes

Motility throughout the intestinal structures is generally reduced. This results not only from a general loss of muscle tone and atrophy but also from multiple pathologic conditions such as CVA, diabetes mellitus, and Parkinson's disease, which occur with increased frequency among frail elderly people. The decrease in motility increases the propensity for constipation and a slight delay in esophageal motility. The incidence of hiatal hernia is also much greater in older people.

Insufficient dietary fiber may also increase the risk of diverticula, chronic constipation, and impaction. Most diverticula are in the sigmoid colon and present no problems except for the occasional complaint of colic-type pain and constipation. However, the diverticula can become inflamed. Referred to as *diverticulitis*, this inflammation may require emergency treatment to prevent perforation and sepsis.

Atrophy of antral cells in the stomach is common among the elderly and results in decreased secretion of hydrochloric acid and intrinsic factor with the possibility of impaired protein digestion and vitamin B_{12} absorption. The atrophy of intestinal villi is the basis for lactose intolerance, which may occur for the first time in old age. A decrease in gastric emptying time occurs with aging and is exacerbated also by Parkinson's disease and diabetes. It may be characterized by early satiety (fullness), vomiting of undigested food, or high residual stomach content in the tube-fed patient. It should be suspected whenever good blood glucose control deteriorates in an elderly diabetic client.

GENITALIA
Women

Because reproductive and breast tissues depend on estrogen for growth, many atrophic changes begin in women at menopause. The size of the ovaries, uterus, and cervix decreases. The pubic hair thins and becomes more brittle. A loss of elastic tissue and vascularity in the vagina results in a thin, pale epithelium. Loss of elasticity and reduced vaginal lubrication from diminishing levels of estrogen can cause dyspareunia (painful intercourse). The vagina also narrows and shortens, and the labia flatten due to loss of subcutaneous fat. Sexual desire and pleasure are not necessarily diminished by these structural changes, nor do women lose the capacity for orgasm with age. Some research has shown that when sexuality is investigated from a more holistic perspective, the pleasure derived from intimate physical relationships may increase in the later years.

Men

The decline in testosterone production brings about similar atrophic changes in men. However, this decline occurs at a later age than that of menopause in women. By the age of 80 or 90, a man's sperm count may decrease by as much as 50% and sperm motility slows. Some degree of prostatic enlargement (known as benign prostatic hypertrophy [BPH]) almost always occurs by age 85 and accounts for a decrease in the amount and viscosity of seminal fluid. Orgasm may be briefer, and the time to obtain an erection may increase. These changes, however, do not usually result in any loss of satisfaction or libido.

ANUS, RECTUM, AND PROSTATE
Prostate Disorders

BPH is the benign growth of the prostate from exposure to androgen hormones. It occurs in 80% of men over age 70. It may result in urinary frequency, nocturia, urinary retention with overflow incontinence, increased prevalence of urinary tract infections, or difficulty starting a stream of urine. Over-the-counter drugs with anticholinergic side effects (eg, cold and sinus preparations and sleeping medications) may contribute to urinary retention or add to obstructive symptoms.

Difficult or painful urination may also occur from prostatitis, an inflammation or infection of the prostate gland. Fever and pain are common with acute prostatitis. Chronic bacterial prostatitis is seen most frequently in older men and may require prolonged antibiotic therapy. Irritative voiding is common in chronic prostatitis. Acute bacterial prostatitis is seen less frequently in older men, and nonbacterial prostatitis, although not common, is often caused by *Chlamydia*.

Obstructive urinary symptoms may also be a sign of prostate cancer, which is often asymptomatic in early stages. About 83% of prostate cancer cases are found in men over age 64 (Kennedy-Malone et al., 2000) and are generally detected as hard irregular nodules upon digital rectal examination (DRE).

Elimination

Although constipation is not a normal process of aging, factors relating to the aging process may contribute to it. For instance, as peristalsis decreases, stools have a longer transit time. This allows more water to be reabsorbed and, thereby, produces a harder stool that is more difficult to evacuate. The risk of constipation is compounded by diminished physical activity, lower fluid intake, reduced bulk and fiber in the diet, and medications with a constipating effect.

Lower gastrointestinal (GI) bleeding must be investigated and must always be suspected when an older person is anemic or complains of weakness and fatigue. Causes may include hemorrhoids, neoplasia, ischemia, diverticula, infections, or inflammatory bowel disease. Lower GI bleeding also may be a harbinger of a life-threatening emergency or may indicate the need for managing chronic constipation. For example, minor rectal hemorrhage may be a complication of manual removal of impacted feces.

MUSCLES AND BONES

The structural changes of the musculoskeletal system illustrate very clearly how difficult it is to differentiate physiologic changes of aging from those of disease or disuse. For example, it is now apparent that a general decline in exercise tolerance is not as much a function of aging, per se, as it is of disuse. Exercise may slow the rate of decline in cardiac reserve to 5% per decade as opposed to the 10% seen in sedentary people. Thus, a key aspect of health promotion for elderly people includes an assessment of exercise and fitness to identify those people who could benefit most greatly from a moderate exercise program. It is now known that loss of muscle mass and functional decline in mobility can be greatly ameliorated by regular aerobic exercise three times weekly. In general, muscle strength declines by 30% to 40% between the ages of 30 and 80.

Bone Loss

In addition, a general thinning and drying of the intervertebral disks occurs with age and results in a loss of height of up to several inches. In the very advanced years, it is not uncommon for bone loss to progress to the point where minimal trauma such as a vigorous sneeze or step down from a curb results in a hip or vertebral fracture (Display 26-3). Osteoporosis results in reduced volume of cancellous bone and a loss of reserve capacity of the bone marrow.

Bone loss is also associated with curvatures of the spine, such as kyphosis, lordosis, or scoliosis. As stated previously, bone and muscle mass loss depends on various factors. Bone loss in postmenopausal women can be ameliorated by exercise and supplemental estrogen therapy. The degree of muscle loss can be ameliorated by exercise. Because men start out adulthood with greater bone and muscle mass, their loss with aging is not as great.

Muscle Weakness

A decrease in type II muscle fibers accompanied by an increase in small type I fibers also contributes to muscle atrophy with aging. Loss of muscle strength attributable to aging should be the same on both left and right sides. Malnutrition, CVAs, and neurologic disorders frequently exacerbate the loss of muscle strength in the very old. As muscle tissue degenerates, the proportion of adipose tissue to lean mass typically increases, decreasing total body water and increasing the risk of dehydration. Tendons shrink and sclerose with aging. The result may be more muscle cramping.

Joint Disease

Limitations in joint range of motion, stiffness, and deformities are due to a combination of aging, disuse, obesity, and diseases such as degenerative joint disease (DJD), rheumatoid arthritis, carpal tunnel syndrome, and Parkinson's disease. DJD is a common age-related condition involving joints throughout the body. Most commonly affected joints include the hips, knees, spine, and fingers. The stress of joint use gradually breaks down the cartilage, resulting in protrusions of bone into the joint capsule. These bony overgrowths can cause pain that worsens with activity, limited joint mobility, and structural deformities. In the spine, these overgrowths are called *osteophytes*. In the distal and proximal joints of the fingers, they are called *Heberden's nodes* and *Bouchard's nodes*, respectively.

Pain

Assessing the pain connected with joint and muscle deterioration and subsequent disuse is exceedingly important in preventing depression and functional decline. In the frail elderly client, for example, functional decline can begin within 24 to 48 h of confined bedrest. Moreover, issues related to pain management become especially important in frail elderly clients because they are at greater risk for drug-induced complications, such as GI bleeding, hepatic and renal toxicity, and mental status changes, resulting from taking nonsteroidal anti-inflammatory drugs (NSAIDs) to relieve joint and muscle pain. They are also at greater risk for septic joints resulting from various intra-articular corticosteroid injections used to treat arthritis. Ongoing assessment and documentation of joint swelling, heat, and redness are important for differentiating bleeding or infection from the inflammatory process.

NEUROLOGIC FUNCTION

Starting in early adulthood, a predicted loss of several thousand neurons a day occurs. The brain shrinks, the sulci widen, and neurotransmitter levels change. For example,

DISPLAY 26-3. Causes and Consequences of Hip Fractures

Hip fracture and the risk for hip fracture in frail elderly clients are serious concerns. The effect of hip fracture on level of function is devastating for most elderly adults because they may never return to baseline levels of function. The consequences of a hip fracture in a frail elderly person frequently include prolonged immobility and associated complications, such as pressure ulcers (also called decubiti), thrombophlebitis, pulmonary emboli, urinary tract infection, wound infection, loss of independence, and even death.

Most hip fractures result from falls, so it is vital that a thorough assessment of the cause or potential source of a fall be undertaken. The elderly client's environment should be assessed for hazardous obstacles, such as clutter or slippery throw rugs. Often, the earliest signs of certain illnesses are falling episodes, which are referred to as *prodromal falls*. Illnesses that usually interfere with postural stability include cardiac dysrhythmias, electrolyte disorders, stroke, seizures, infections (eg, urinary tract infections, pneumonia), syncope, hypotension, and acute exacerbations of underlying chronic diseases, such as kidney failure, heart failure, and chronic obstructive pulmonary disease (Tideiksaar, 1998).

Additional important assessment parameters include monitoring for other conditions that may complicate hip fracture. These include malnutrition, delirium, incontinence, urinary tract infection, dehydration, skin breakdown, and anemia. Many of the complications of hip fractures are due to the pathologic process causing the fall (eg, dysrhythmia, drug toxicity, infection) rather than the fracture itself.

norepinephrine levels fall and serotonin levels rise. However, mental function is not mainly determined by numbers of neurons or quantity of neurotransmitters, but rather by the function of complex neural pathways. The common changes in cognition and motor function attributed to aging are slower impulse transmission, which manifests as a decrease in reaction time cognitively and reflexively. A loss of short-term memory is sometimes attributed to aging; however, it is suggested that this results from a combination of slowed neural impulses and more stored information rather than a decline in function.

Mobility and Motor Function

Related motor signs of advanced age include a reduced rate and amount of motor activity, slowed reaction time, decreased agility and fine motor coordination, and changes in posture and gait. To compensate for a stooped posture and less flexible knee, hip, and shoulder joints, the elderly person often walks with the feet farther apart from each other and the knees slightly bent. Swaying, shuffling, dragging, or a "waddling" type of gait is a sign of neurologic or musculoskeletal conditions and not aging. The decrease in postural stability seen in advanced age is usually attributed to diminished vibratory sensations and slowed motor responses, which are necessary for making the fine adjustments in posture needed to maintain postural stability. This places the frail elderly person at a disadvantage in avoiding obstacles quickly, negotiating uneven surfaces, or in situations necessitating fast movements.

Dystonias and dyskinesias are more frequent because of neural deterioration. Degenerative motor diseases such as Parkinson's disease and amyotrophic lateral sclerosis (ALS) are associated with advancing age. The primary symptoms of Parkinson's disease are related to movement problems: stiffness and rigidity, bradykinesia, slowness and unpredictability of movement, postural instability, and tremor. The "pill rolling" tremor that occurs both at rest and with movement affects approximately 75% of those with Parkinson's disease. Handwriting is usually affected and may become difficult to read. Concurrent depression is more common when symptoms of Parkinson's begin in old age. Late onset Parkinson's also tends to have a shorter, more severe course than Parkinson's disease that begins from age 40 to 60.

The diminished efficiency of the autonomic nervous system in regulating temperature and blood pressure manifests as impaired thermoregulation and postural hypotension in elderly adults. The complaint of dizziness (the sensation of lightheadedness, weakness, or spinning) is a common one and has multiple causes, which can range from head trauma or inner ear disease to cardiovascular disease (discussed previously) to transient ischemic attacks (TIAs), or minor strokes, to sinusitis or medication toxicity. Decreased alertness, somnolence, disorientation, or amnesia is commonly associated with TIAs. Typically, the client should be referred to a neurologist for diagnosis and treatment.

Mental and Emotional Status

The very old are at great risk for various other neurologic abnormalities including delirium (because almost any acute health problem, such as hypoglycemia, fever, dehydration, or infection can cause sudden and dramatic deficits in oxygenation and nutritional needs of brain tissue) and dementia, which is a progressive decline in memory, abstract thinking, judgment, and perception to the extent that the client cannot carry out daily activities or function within the family or community (Display 26-4). Another change in mental state is depression (sometimes called "pseudodementia" because it so frequently mimics the signs and symptoms of dementia. A screening tool, such as the Geriatric Depression Scale (Display 26-5), can be used to detect signs of an elderly client's decreasing satisfaction with quality of life.

DISPLAY 26-4. Causes of Delirium and Dementia

Various disease states, some diagnosed and some undetected, may contribute to delirium or dementia or both in frail elderly clients.

DISORDERS CONTRIBUTING TO DELIRIUM
- Brain tumors
- Dehydration
- Toxic drug levels or interactions
- Infections
- Electrolyte imbalances
- Liver or kidney disease
- Hypoxia secondary to respiratory or circulatory disorders
- Hyperthermia or hypothermia
- Metabolic disorders (especially thyroid and blood glucose abnormalities)
- Nutritional deficiencies (especially folate, vitamin B_{12}, and iron deficiencies)

(continued)

DISPLAY 26-4. Causes of Delirium and Dementia (Continued)

DISORDERS CONTRIBUTING TO DEMENTIA

Infections
- Creutzfeldt-Jakob disease
- Human immunodeficiency virus (HIV)
- Syphilis

Degenerative Neurologic Disorders
- Alzheimer's disease
- Pick's disease
- Huntington's disease
- Parkinson's disease

Vascular Disorders
- Ministrokes
- Cardiovascular accidents (CVA)

Structural and Traumatic Disorders
- Normal pressure hydrocephalus
- Subdural hemotoma
- Head injury
- Tumors

Adapted from Johnson, B. P. 1998. The elderly. In N. C. Frisch & L. E. Frisch (Eds). *Psychiatric mental health nursing* (pp. 524–557). Albany, NY: Delmar Publishers.

DISPLAY 26-5. Geriatric Depression Scale

1. Are you basically satisfied with your life? (no)
2. Have you dropped many of your activities and interests? (yes)
3. Do you feel that your life is empty? (yes)
4. Do you often get bored? (yes)
5. Are you in good spirits most of the time? (no)
6. Are you afraid that something bad is going to happen to you? (yes)
7. Do you feel happy most of the time? (no)
8. Do you often feel helpless? (yes)
9. Do you prefer to stay home at night, rather than go out and do new things? (yes)
10. Do you feel that you have more problems with memory than most? (yes)
11. Do you think it is wonderful to be alive now? (no)
12. Do you feel pretty worthless the way you are now? (yes)
13. Do you feel full of energy? (no)
14. Do you feel that your situation is hopeless? (yes)
15. Do you think that most persons are better off than you are? (yes)

Score 1 point for each response that matches the yes or no answer after each question.

Reprinted with permission from Yesavage, J. A., & Brink, T. I. (1983). Development and validation of a geriatric depression screening scale: A preliminary report. *Journal of Psychiatric Research, 17*, 37–49. Oxford, England: Elsevier Science Ltd. Pergamon Imprint.

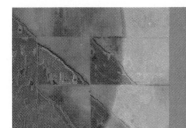
Collecting Subjective Data

Adapting basic assessment principles and techniques for any particular age group assumes that there are certain physical and psychosocial similarities that must be taken into consideration when making clinical judgments. This is one of the great challenges of geriatric health care because elderly adults are a very heterogenous group. Individual, family, and cultural variations in diet, recreational and work activities, the physical and social environment, educational and spiritual beliefs all have a tremendous impact on a person's genetic predisposition to health or illness. Thus, older people tend to have less in common than do younger people.

ADAPTING INTERVIEW TECHNIQUES

In today's youth-oriented culture, it is not uncommon to think of physical frailty as a serious problem. If older people experience some degree of declining health, fear of increasing dependency may be paramount in their minds. Most elderly clients approach clinicians with well-deserved hesitation because they have known friends and family members who have become sicker or died as a result of intervention. They may also be reluctant to admit problems because they fear being admitted to a hospital or nursing home. Thus, it is essential that the nurse adapt routine interviewing techniques and approach the assessment from the perspective that, regardless of the extent of disability and illness being experienced by the older adult, there is always something positive that the older person is doing. Otherwise, the client couldn't have lived to advanced age. This survivorship mentality is often expressed by the very old as both a blessing and a "badge of honor." (It can also be seen as a curse for the very old who have outlived spouses, friends, and even adult children.)

For example, it is important to look for good nutritional habits as well as to identify which foods are to be avoided or normal, everyday activities that keep an older person moving to whatever degree may be possible as well as identifying those people at risk for falls. Health among the elderly means supporting activities, relationships, and honoring the accomplishments that have made life meaningful over time.

DETERMINING FUNCTIONAL STATUS

A major purpose of assessing the frail elderly person is to maximize function and limit disability by correctly identifying and describing that person's ability to perform daily activities. Approximately 45% of people over age 75 have limitations in daily activities as compared with 23% of people aged 45 to 64 (National Academy on an Aging Society, 1999). The ultimate goal of assessment and intervention should be to empower a person to maintain the relationships, activities, and events that they find meaningful. Thus, the goal of assessment for the older person may not be as focused on disease prevention as it is on minimizing the disability associated with chronic illness and preventing complications and exacerbations of chronic maladies.

Because the symptoms of disease may be more subtle in advanced age, recognizing changes in functional ability as harbingers of a potential health problem is often crucial for prompt and accurate management of both acute and chronic illness in this age group. A functional assessment is the benchmark against which acute changes must be profiled to accurately identify the causes as well as to understand the significance of the symptoms. Early and appropriate treatment and referral of illness are essential for diminishing morbidity, mortality, and disability. Treating disease at its onset is most essential in the frail elderly people who lack the physiologic reserve to overcome the physical stress that illness places on their fragile bodies. Equally important in preventing a rapid decline, which may quickly lead to severe disability and total dependence, is the identification and procurement of the psychosocial and environmental resources that may be used to maintain health and independence and to achieve the greatest possible quality of life while living with physical frailty and chronic illness.

RECOGNIZING GERIATRIC SYNDROMES

The classic diagnostic features of illness are based on the more flamboyant responses of the young and middle-aged. A toddler may have a temperature of 103°F in response to the common cold or rhinovirus in contrast to an 85-year-old person who may be unable to develop a respectable fever in response to a fatal pneumonia. In general, pain, fever, and physiologic parameters as measured by laboratory test values become less reliable indicators of disease in frail elderly adults. Symptoms of disease and disability more frequently present as "geriatric syndromes." These include incontinence, falls, weakness and lethargy, confusion, sleep disturbances, and loss of appetite or weight loss.

Not only do these syndromes describe the common and most recognizable ways in which disease often presents itself in the frail elderly, but they also describe the consequences of physiologic stress in the frail elderly person. For example, in the frail elderly person, incontinence and confusion are more often signs of infection than is a fever. The incontinence and confusion can easily lead to a fall when the older person attempts to walk to the bathroom, but on the way experiences some lightheadedness caused by dehydration and postural hypotension. The fall results in a hip fracture and immobility. The immobility leads to a pressure ulcer, urinary tract infection, and delirium. In such cases, the "slippery slope" of unfortunate events leads a frail, but independent elder living at home to near total dependence and disability.

Risk screening tools, such as SPICES (Francis et al., 1998), may be used to monitor the population of high-risk frail aged for some of the more common nonspecific indicators of disease that are known to be indicators of potential disability. Because the oldest people have the highest prevalence of chronic illness and comorbidity, one disease may mask the symptoms of another. For example, the fatigue and dyspnea of severe congestive heart failure may mask the anemia caused by a duodenal ulcer. A severe illness is more likely to affect multiple organ systems as the body's reserves and ability to respond to physiologic stress are impaired. For instance, pneumonia will typically precipitate congestive heart failure.

To complicate the assessment and management of illness even more, the treatment of disease primarily with drugs has a greater chance of resulting in a significant adverse effect than of improving the symptoms in the frail elderly. Often, a drug is used to treat the adverse drug effect and the problems spiral into a nearly indecipherable multiplicity of symptoms. Thus, an approach to assessment of the frail elderly client may begin with a discussion of the common geriatric syndromes. Regardless of whether a nurse practices in home health, intensive care, or long-term care, identifying an acute illness or an exacerbation of chronic illness is the key to making an appropriate referral and preventing the complications of both the disease and the adverse effects of drugs used to treat the disease.

Subjective data about the frail elderly person must take into consideration the more common ways in which diseases and disorders present in elderly people. The subjective data collected with regard to falls, weakness, incontinence, confusion, sleep disturbances, and loss of appetite combined with the more traditional review of symptoms from a functional perspective provide the type of thorough baseline data and history needed for early detection of conditions warranting referral or intervention. It is essential that the rather unique presentation of illness in the frail elderly person be compared with that person's ability to function in everyday activities (eg, eating, walking, driving, socializing, and communicating). Finally, the family and/or residential context within which symptoms arise must be explored to identify not only environmental precipitants (isolation, physical barriers, neglect) but also family, social, and economic resources that can serve as a buffer to physiologic and functional decline and enhance the client's quality of life.

Nursing History

The subjective data collection process that is similar for every client regardless of age involves further exploring any sign or symptom of illness or functional decline detected by the nurse or reported by the client. In such cases, the mnemonic COLDSPA can be a helpful guide to compiling significant information. In many instances, the nurse will continue to collect health history data during the head-to-toe assessment.

COLDSPA

CHARACTER: Describe the sign or symptom. How does it feel, look, sound, smell, and so forth?

ONSET: When did it begin?

LOCATION: Where is it? Does it radiate?

DURATION: How long does it last? Does it recur?

SEVERITY: How bad is it?

PATTERN: What makes it better? What makes it worse?

ASSOCIATED FACTORS: What other symptoms occur with it?

CURRENT SYMPTOMS

Skin, Hair, and Nails

Question Over the past year, what changes have you noticed in your skin, hair, and nails? Have any rashes developed after you took a new medication? If so, what was the medication?

Rationale Certain changes, including rashes, result from allergic reactions; others, such as inflammation, may result from infection or cancer.

Q Do you have a problem with dry or itchy skin? What is your routine in bathing? What type of moisturizers do you use?

R Dry, itchy skin may result from the drying properties of soaps or alcohol-based after-bath preparations.

Q Do you have a history of ulcers (open wounds) on your feet or lower legs?

℞ Elderly clients with skin ulcerations, such as those related to diabetes or peripheral vascular disease, should be monitored for infection. They should be referred to a podiatrist every 3 to 6 months to have nails clipped and any corns or calluses removed professionally to prevent infection and other complications. Smoking cessation should be encouraged for anyone with ulcers resulting from arterial insufficiency (see Chapter 17 for more information).

Eyes and Vision

℀ Do you see better with one eye than another? Have you noticed any change in your vision? If so, describe.

℞ Better vision in one eye is a warning sign of macular degeneration, a leading cause of blindness in elderly people. In chronic forms of macular degeneration, the client may need a referral to a low-vision specialist or may benefit from visual aids, such as magnifying devices, large-print reading materials, or talking books. Early laser treatment may retard the loss of vision.

℀ Do you ever see small specks or "clouds" moving across your field of vision?

℞ With aging, tiny clumps of gel may develop within the eye. These are referred to as "floaters." New floaters, an increase in frequency, or floaters associated with flashes of light, may be a sign of retinal detachment, which is an indication for immediate referral to an ophthalmologist. Early detection and treatment may be crucial in preventing blindness.

℀ Do your eyes feel dry or irritated? Do they tear excessively?

℞ Physical examination may validate ectropion or entropion. Referral to an ophthalmologist may be warranted depending on the severity of symptoms.

Ears and Hearing

℀ How well do you hear? Have you noticed any hearing loss recently? Do you have difficulty hearing someone if there is a lot of noise in the background? Have you ever had to have ear wax removed?

℞ Thickening of the tympanic membrane and accumulation of ear wax may result in conductive hearing loss. If accumulated cerumen accounts for hearing loss, the loss is usually gradual.

Tip From the Experts Irrigation and ceruminolytic agents are contraindicated for clients with a perforated tympanic membrane or an ear infection.

℀ Do you ever feel especially uncomfortable or confused because you cannot hear as well as you would like?

℞ Many elderly people—especially those with dementia—are at risk for becoming withdrawn, anxious, or increasingly confused as hearing impairment progresses.

Head and Neck

℀ Do you have intermittent or continuous pain in the head or neck region?

℞ Various disorders associated with frail elderly adults, such as arthritis, are accompanied by pain in the head and neck area.

℀ When was your last dental examination? Do you have a problem with dry mouth?

℞ Dental caries are more likely to occur in clients with dry mouth from decreased saliva production, which is more prevalent among frail elderly adults.

Mouth and Throat

℀ Do you ever feel like you're choking when you drink water or feel like food is catching in your throat?

℞ Dysphagia (inability to swallow easily) is an age-related problem.

Tip From the Experts Caregivers of dysphagic people may assist with swallowing by preparing semisolid foods and fluids of pudding consistency, alternating solid food with thickened foods, and encouraging the client to lean slightly forward and tuck the chin under to prevent gagging.

Nutrition

℀ Have you experienced any change in your appetite in the past 6 months? (If the response indicates a decline in appetite, continue with the following questions.) When did you first notice a decline in appetite? Did you have any other health problem at about this same time? Did you start taking any new medication at this time?

℞ A loss of appetite is a nearly universal cofactor of both physical and mental disease in the elderly. Because the aged body is housing a "smaller engine," the minimum caloric intake does decrease in old age. Even healthy older adults consume only an estimated 1,200 to 1,600 calories per day. This has led to the general consensus that older adults need nutrient-dense foods to ingest enough essential nutrients. There is less consensus with regard to how dietary recommendations should vary for the 75+ age group than as to what the indicators and factors place an older adult at risk of malnutrition and dehydration.

℀ Besides appetite loss, additional questions to consider when assessing nutritional status include: Is the client in pain, which diminishes appetite? Is the client's mobility limited? Do limitations affect shopping for and preparing food? Is the client impoverished? Has there been a recent loss of a spouse or other close relative or friend? Is the client housebound? Institutionalized? Cognitively impaired? Is feeding assistance required? Do other factors, such as depression, chronic illness, dementia, fever, diarrhea, vomiting, dysphagia, or infection, affect nutritional status?

R Certain problems—dysphagia, immobility, and cognitive impairment—are more common among the very old than among middle-aged adults. Certain chronic diseases, such as cancer and rheumatoid arthritis, enjoy an increased incidence in the elderly. These chronic diseases cause an increase in inflammatory cellular components that are associated with anorexia and fatigue. Any illness or medication that causes nausea and fatigue, then, can contribute to loss of appetite. This is why the very old are especially vulnerable to the bias of an acute care medical system that inadequately manages pain caused by chronic disease (eg, osteoarthritis and osteoporosis). A certain degree of anorexia always accompanies pain—especially chronic pain. Toxic levels of drugs must always be suspected when appetite loss is sudden and severe.

Q Can you describe what you eat in an average day? On a day when your appetite is less, how would your eating habits change?

R Assessment of nutritional status has a twofold purpose in the very old person. You should ask about eating habits and any recent changes in them when older adults are seeking care for an acute, episodic illness or as part of a comprehensive baseline assessment. When there is a sudden loss of appetite, it is most often a symptom of disease or an adverse medication effect. As part of a comprehensive assessment, a nutritional screening tool (see Appendix E) can be used to identify the need for treatment recommendations with regard to specific dietary adjustments, assistance with eating, shopping, or meal preparation, or further assessment of specific conditions such as dysphagia or cognitive impairment.

Hydration

Q How much fluid do you think you drink each day?

R Loss of appetite almost always coexists with inadequate hydration. Decreased thirst sensation is common with aging. And decreased mobility makes it less possible for the frail elderly person to respond to an already diminished sense of thirst. Drug use may contribute to dehydration as well. For example, diuretics are widely used in treating cardiovascular and renal disease as are fluid restrictions. Unfortunately, when the body's need for fluid increases, as it does with infection and the concomitant increase in metabolic rate, adjustments are not always appropriately made for functionally dependent frail elderly people. Thus,

loss of appetite is both a symptom of an acute or chronic medical condition as well as a risk factor for malnutrition and dehydration, which pose a threat to overall health and well-being. Functional risk factors that signal the need for a hydration assessment are the same as for malnutrition with the addition of urinary incontinence.

Thorax and Lungs

Q Do you ever experience shortness of breath? If so, is it related to activity? (Specific questions about endurance, stair climbing, or activities of daily living are necessary for quantifying the extent of the problem.) Does it occur at rest or when lying down? How many pillows are used?

R Dyspnea is the most common reason for emergency room visits (Parshall, 1999) and is a frequently reported symptom associated with common illnesses among elderly clients. These illnesses include COPD, asthma, lung cancer, and heart failure. Older adults with chronic respiratory or cardiac problems who experience some constant degree of dyspnea are unlikely to seek care or note dyspnea unless there is a change in functional capabilities related to breathing. Therefore, it is important to ascertain to what degree dyspnea affects daily function.

Q Do you seem to be breathing faster? Sweating? Do you experience anorexia (loss of appetite) or fatigue?

R In the frail elder, an increase in respirations, sweating, or overall malaise may be the only indication of a respiratory problem (Kennedy-Malone et al., 2000).

Q Do you have a recurrent cough? Does it ever have blood in it? Do you use tobacco or have you in the past?

R A recurrent cough, fatigue, weight loss, shortness of breath, and productive cough (sometimes blood-tinged) are hallmarks of lung cancer. It is the most common cause of cancer-associated deaths in the United States, and the incidence increases with aging (second most common type of cancer in men over age 75, with incidence rising in women).

Q Have you experienced weight loss or changes in your health along with your cough?

R Weight loss, night sweats, or changes in respiratory status, such as coughing, may be signs of tuberculosis (TB). Debilitated elderly people are at increased risk of TB. In addition, glucocorticosteroid therapy and the nutritional deficiencies depress the immune system, thereby exacerbating the chances of reactivating a dormant TB infection.

Q Have you received the pneumococcal vaccine within the past 6 years? Do you get annual flu vaccines?

R Pneumonia is the most common cause of infection-related deaths in the elderly. The pneumovax is recommended once a lifetime for those over age 65 and every

6 years for high-risk patients. Debilitated and institutionalized elders are particularly at risk for serious influenza-related illness.

Heart and Blood Vessels

Impaired circulation and other conditions related to aging increase the elderly client's risk for falls. Relevant questions to ask when compiling health history data follow:

Q Do you ever feel lightheaded or dizzy when you get up from a chair or the bed?

R If the client reports dizziness, you may need to perform a safety assessment to evaluate a fall history or potential for falls. Also indicated is a "Get Up and Go" test (see Physical Assessment section), which helps assess gait and balance, or a Performance Oriented Environmental Mobility Screen (POEMS; Display 26-6).

Q Do you have any discomfort in your legs with activity? Would you describe the discomfort as pain, cramping, aching, fatigue or weakness in the calf? Do your hips, thighs, and/or buttocks hurt with ambulation? If so, how far can you walk before the pain occurs? Does the pain go away with rest?

R These symptoms are associated with intermittent claudication, a circulatory disorder affecting the peripheral blood vessels of the leg. As the distance the client needs to walk before incurring pain decreases, the amount of arterial insufficiency is generally worsening. Symptoms affecting the calf muscles suggest femoral or popliteal stenosis; buttock, hip, and thigh symptoms suggest arterioiliac stenosis. Symptoms are usually bilateral and progressive (Brown, Bedford & White, 1999).

Q Do you think it takes an excessively long time for you to stop bleeding after you get a cut or scratch?

R Some medications used for cardiovascular disease and some coagulation disorders are associated with extended bleeding times and decreased clotting ability.

Abdomen

Q Do you ever have heartburn? Indigestion? Chest pain? Hiccups? Belching? Gas?

R Heartburn, also called gastroesophageal reflux disease (GERD) in its most severe form, can mimic angina pectoris and can irritate vocal cords and cause hoarseness, coughing, and wheezing. Heartburn, hiccups, belching, gas, vomiting, and sour or bitter taste generally occur after a meal and may be worse if the client lies down. Decreased esophageal motility is commonly related to central nervous system (CNS) disease, diabetes mellitus, or thyroid disor-

DISPLAY 26-6. Performance Oriented Environmental Mobility Screen (POEMS)

LOCATION	MANEUVER	NORMAL	IMPAIRED
Bedroom	Ambulation		
	Straight line	❑	❑
	Turning	❑	❑
	Chair transfer		
	Onto	❑	❑
	Off	❑	❑
	Standing balance		
	Eyes open	❑	❑
	Eyes closed	❑	❑
	Sternal nudge	❑	❑
	Bending down	❑	❑
	Bed transfer		
	Onto	❑	❑
	Off	❑	❑
Bathroom	Ambulation		
	Straight line	❑	❑
	Turning	❑	❑
	Toilet transfer		
	Onto	❑	❑
	Off	❑	❑
	Toilet hygiene	❑	❑
Hallway	Ambulation		
	Straight line	❑	❑
	Turning	❑	❑
	Distance	❑	❑

Adapted from Tideiksaar, R. (1998). *Falls in older persons: Prevention and management* (2nd ed.). Baltimore: Health Professions Press, Inc.

ders. Reflux may result from decreased lower esophageal sphincter (LES) pressure as a result of age or alcohol, nicotine, or other drug use including nitrates, calcium channel blockers, theophylline, anticholinergics, antidepressants, and benzodiazepines.

Q Do you have any trouble with digestion? Vomiting?

R Early satiety or vomiting of undigested food may indicate an excessive delay in gastric emptying. This may be seen in Parkinson's disease and diabetes mellitus. (Note: A warning sign may be deteriorating blood glucose control in an elderly diabetic patient.)

Tip From the Experts Bulk-forming agents taken before meals may contribute to early satiety. Acute gastrointestinal abnormalities such as cholecystitis and peritonitis often produce much less severe symptoms (eg, pain and mild changes in lab values) in the very old—often delaying a timely diagnosis. Once again, the more subtle symptoms as discussed in the section on "Geriatric Syndromes" may be the presenting symptoms of life-threatening problems such as peritonitis or sepsis.

Q Do you suffer with any pain in the upper right portion of the abdomen?

R Pain may be related to cholecystitis and the formation of gallstones, which occurs more frequently in the aged. However, only mild right upper quadrant pain, vomiting, and elevation in bilirubin and hepatic enzyme levels may be seen. Fever is seldom a symptom of cholecystitis.

Urinary Continence

Incontinence can be a manifestation of a chronic problem or an acute, reversible one. It can, also, be multifactorial and the result of a combination of factors such as immobility, dehydration, medication, infection, altered cognition, or weakness and lethargy.

Q Many illnesses and medications can cause problems with urine control. This is not something that is normal just because one is getting older, but it is a common problem. Have you ever experienced anything like this?

R Loss of bladder function or control can be an embarrassing and demeaning problem, so it is sometimes best to introduce the topic with a question such as this. Many older adults subscribe to the predominant myth that problems with bladder control are a normal and expected part of aging. Yet this is not an expected part of aging. Incontinence is often associated with chronic conditions, such as stroke, multiple sclerosis, prostatitis, and urinary tract infection. It may also be the result of a fecal impaction, constipation, an adverse drug effect, or urinary tract infection (UTI). Without a systematic method of identifying and evaluating incontinence, many people live with the underlying condition undiagnosed

and untreated. The first step, therefore, involves recognizing that incontinence is an abnormality and requires assessment.

Q Do you ever have any urine leakage or problems controlling your urine flow?

R Urinary incontinence is an involuntary loss of urine with or without warning, which is sufficient enough to be a problem. Between 15% and 30% of older adults living at home and up to 50% of nursing home residents are incontinent. The success of treatment measures depends on a comprehensive assessment for the purpose of determining all of the etiologic factors responsible. Although incontinence is most successfully approached from a multidisciplinary perspective, the nurse plays a major role in assessment, collaboration, and management.

Q How long has the leakage (or use client's descriptive words) been going on? Has it ever suddenly gotten worse?

R Any new onset of incontinence or exacerbation of it should most definitely raise a question about infection. In the hospitalized elder, UTI ranks high as a suspected cause for any new onset of incontinence (UTI is the most common hospital-acquired bacterial infection). UTI must also be a concern for elders at home or in long-term care because it is the most frequent source of bacteremia for these people. A UTI is particularly perplexing in elderly clients because it presents in such an atypical way (ie, without fever, or elevation in white blood cell counts, or dysuria, or urinary frequency). Even more common symptoms of a UTI in the frail elderly person may be confusion, lethargy, anorexia, and nocturia.

Q What activities are associated with your loss of urine control?

R The client's activities during an episode of incontinence may help to determine the type of incontinence and, therefore, its treatment. See Display 26-7 for a description of the kinds of urinary incontinence.

Bowel Elimination

Q Do you have any problems with bowel elimination, such as diarrhea or constipation?

R As people age, GI motility decreases because of a loss of muscle tone and atrophy. Many older adults complain of constipation.

Q Describe a typical day. What kinds of foods, beverages, and exercise do you enjoy each day?

R Adequate fluid intake, dietary fiber, and moderate exercise are key factors in maintaining efficient elimination.

Q Have you had a change in bowel habits recently? Have you ever had blood in your stools? Have you had your stools tested for blood? What medications do you take?

DISPLAY 26-7. Understanding Urinary Incontinence: Assessment and Intervention

TYPES OF INCONTINENCE

The signs and symptoms associated with the involuntary loss of urine have been clustered into three categories: urge, stress, and overflow incontinence. Any one or a combination of all three types may be present in an individual. Voiding diaries are useful for determining the type of incontinence that is occurring based on the amount, timing, and associated symptoms of incontinent episodes.

Voiding Diary

Time	Drinks		Voiding	
	Kind	How much	How many times	How much
6–7 AM	coffee	2 cups	I	medium
7–8 AM	orange juice	1 glass	II	lots
8–9 AM	———	———	I ———	little
9–10 AM	———	———	———	———
10–11 AM	water	1 glass	I	medium

Time	Leaks/Accidents	Strength of urge	Activity at the time of leak
6–7 AM		strong	no leak
7–8 AM		strong	
8–9 AM	I		frying eggs
9–10 AM			
10–11 AM			

Urge Incontinence

Urge incontinence is the involuntary loss of urine associated with an abrupt and strong desire to void. It is frequently caused by a neurologic disorder such as a cerebrovascular accident (CVA) or multiple sclerosis (MS), which impairs the ability of the bladder or urinary sphincter to contract and relax.

Stress Incontinence

Stress incontinence is the involuntary loss of urine during coughing, sneezing, laughing, or other physical activities that increase abdominal pressure. In women, stress incontinence may result from weakened and relaxed muscles from the combined effects of aging superimposed on the effects of childbirth.

Note: Atrophic vaginitis from estrogen deficiency usually results in symptoms of urge incontinence as well as stress incontinence (mixed incontinence).

Overflow Incontinence

Overflow incontinence is the involuntary loss of urine associated with overdistention of the bladder. Prostatic hypertrophy is a common cause in men, and diabetic neuropathy is a common cause in both sexes.

Functional Incontinence

Functional incontinence is the inability to get to the bathroom in time or to understand the cues to void due to problems with mobility or cognition.

STEPS OF ASSESSMENT

The nursing assessment varies somewhat depending on the client's general health status and whether the problem is an acute or chronic one. In general, however, a comprehensive nursing assessment can be described as a five-step process that includes screening for an infection with a

(continued)

DISPLAY 26-7. Understanding Urinary Incontinence (continued)

urinalysis, obtaining a voiding diary, evaluating functional status, compiling a health history, and performing a physical examination. Key features within the five steps follow:

● Record all incontinent and continent episodes for 3 days in a voiding diary.
● Review medication for any newly prescribed drugs that may be triggering incontinence. Follow up with physician regarding need to discontinue therapy or change medication.
● Rule out constipation or fecal impaction as a source of urinary incontinence. If client has had no bowel movement within last 3 days or is oozing stool continuously, check for impaction by digital examination or abdominal palpation. Problem should be treated if identified.
● Assess functional status along with signs and symptoms as they relate to incontinence. Contributors to incontinence may include immobility, insufficient fluid intake, and confusion. Accompanying signs and symptoms include polyuria, nocturia, dysuria, hesitancy, poor or interrupted urine stream, straining, suprapubic or perineal pain, urgency and characteristics of incontinent episodes (precipitated by walking, coughing, getting in and out of bed and so forth).
● Consult physician regarding physical examination and need to measure postvoid residual volume by straight catheterization (particularly if client dribbles, reports urgency, has difficulty starting stream). Components of the physical examination include direct observation of urine loss using a cough stress test; abdominal, rectal, genital and pelvic examination; and identification of neurologic abnormalities. Abdominal and vaginal examinations are performed to detect prolapse or a palpable bladder after micturition.

INTERVENTIONS

The physician is responsible for identifying and treating the conditions causing reversible or chronic incontinence. A physical therapist may play a role in identifying specific activities that are associated with incontinent episodes. Either a nurse or physical therapist may be involved in teaching Kegel exercises to help relieve stress incontinence. When functional incontinence and urgency have been identified, the expertise of an occupational therapist in appropriate dressing and undressing and for choosing incontinence aids may be beneficial.

R The guaiac stool test to detect occult blood is a common test administered to detect abnormalities of the GI tract. Clients with a past history of polyps, adenomas, and inflammatory bowel disease are at increased risk for colorectal cancer in old age. Warning signs include rectal bleeding, unexplained weight loss, and a change in bowel habits. NSAIDs, such as aspirin and naproxen (Aleve), corticosteroids, and anticoagulants, such as warfarin (Coumadin) may promote GI bleeding.

Genitalia

In some situations, the physical assessment of genital structures may be the time for the client to voice concerns with aspects of sexual function. When gathering historical data, keep in mind that older clients, like younger clients, may feel uncomfortable and hesitant to discuss sexual function, whereas others just need to be assured that the information they contribute will remain private and confidential. Examples of possible questions follow.

Q How satisfied are you with your sexual function? Do you have any physical problems that you perceive to be impediments to satisfying function?

R If the client is comfortable with this topic, questions like these offer an opportunity to discuss an existing prob-

lem, investigate what may be causing it, and refer the client for counseling. For example, clients with musculoskeletal or cardiovascular disorders may benefit from alternative positions for intercourse. Premedication with nitrates or inhalers may be advisable for those with coronary artery disease or COPD. If the client is taking Viagra, education and monitoring for adverse effects are warranted.

Tip From the Experts Privacy issues in extended care and the complex emotional needs of clients and their partners in various stages of dementia should not be overlooked. Referrals for counseling should be made only if the expertise of counselors regarding sexuality and geriatrics is known.

Q Do you have any complaints about erectile function?

R With aging, an erection may be less firm, require a longer period of time to achieve, and have a longer refractory period. Ejaculation may be less forceful, and the volume may be reduced. Approximately 25% of men over the age of 65 are impotent (Brown et al., 1999). Impotence may have physiologic or psychogenic causes (*Note:* Physiologic causes should be ruled out before treating as psychogenic unless an evident stressor is identified from the client's history (Brown et al., 1999).

Q What medications are you taking at this time?

R Antihypertensives, antipsychotics, muscle relaxants, antidepressants, digoxin, cimetidine, anticonvulsants, narcotics, alcohol, and nicotine should be investigated as possible contributors to arousal dysfunction.

Q Do you have any vaginal itching, discomfort, or blood-tinged discharge (especially after intercourse), or dyspareunia?

R Many years of estrogen deprivation lead to atrophy of the vaginal and vulvar epithelium. Sexual abstinence or infrequent intercourse intensifies atrophic changes. Short intermittent courses of hormone replacement are usually adequate for treatment (Kennedy-Malone et al., 2000).

Muscles and Bones

Q Do you have problems with grasping, reaching, or activities that use your hands, arms, back, or legs? Do you have pain? If so, is the pain worse with activity? Relieved by rest? Have you ever had joint replacement surgery?

R Functional limitations and pain are common consequences of inflammatory joint disease in the frail elderly person. Inflamed joints may require rest, movement, or a delicate balance to prevent loss of function. Occupational therapy referrals may be indicated for instruction on task or environmental modification or assistive devices to reduce joint stress when performing ADLs. Physical therapy referrals may be indicated for an exercise treatment plan, assistive ambulatory devices, splints, and braces. A multidisciplinary approach to pain management with pharmacologic and non-pharmacologic therapies such as heat or ice or both, ultrasound, and transcutaneous electrical nerve stimulation (TENS) is advisable for maximizing the efficacy of analgesics and reducing the potential for drug-induced side effects. The combination of pain and functional impairment may predispose the client to social isolation and depression. Thus, a dual approach is needed to prevent a downward spiral of pain and increasing immobility leading to more isolation and depression (Display 26-8).

When assessing a frail elderly client, nurses always need to keep in mind that the subjective and objective findings are meaningful only when compared with the way in which such findings affect functional abilities and overall life satisfaction.

Q Do you have any difficulty when getting up out of bed or from sitting in a chair? Does stiffness and soreness inhibit your ability to move about? Do you ever feel like your legs are going to "give way" or that they are weak? If so, describe. What is your usual daily pattern of activity? Exercise routine?

R Clients may benefit from exercises to improve flexibility, fitness, and endurance and to delay functional decline. Exercises can benefit even people in their 70s and 80s and those who have led sedentary lifestyles or who already have some functional deficits.

Q Have your living quarters been checked for safety recently?

R Controlling the environment is one way to help prevent falls. Furniture arranged in an orderly fashion, nonskid rugs, unobstructed pathways and the use of assistive devices, such as hand rails, grab bars, and raised toilet seats can make activities of daily living safer and more enjoyable for frail elderly people. Supportive devices, such as canes and walkers, may also improve the gait and reduce the risk of falls.

Fall Assessment

Q Do you ever need to grab onto something because you feel like you're going to stumble or fall?

R A fall is an unintentional slip, trip, or drop to the floor from an upright position, and a new fall occurs when an object or person prevents the person from landing on the floor. Risk factor assessment for falls is important because the fall can be a symptom of another problem needing attention. A fall can be the symptom of a treatable medical condition, the result of an adverse response to a medication, or a problem associated with chronic illness and frailty. The highest incidence of falling occurs in the 80- to 89-year-old age group and is a reflection of illness and frailty (Tideiksaar, 1998). It is estimated that for people over age 85, one in every five falls results in death (Rubenstein, Josephson & Osterwell, 1996).

Gait instability and fear of falling can lead to self-imposed restrictions in activity and a downward spiral of immobility, which greatly increases the risk of falling. The most successful interventions in reducing the rate of falls in nursing homes and the community are multifactorial and include exercise, identifying and treating pathologic conditions, and environmental modifications. The most frequent interventions initiated by fall risk and prevention assessments, however, focus on removing hazards from the environment, instructing the person to ask for help when ambulating or transferring, and using motion monitors that signal staff when the person moves. However, these programs do not address the factors that place a person at risk for falls and are not an adequate substitute for a multidimensional assessment and management program.

In undertaking a fall assessment, the nurse must be very sensitive to an older person's fears and anxieties elicited by falls or the threat of falls and the ways in which these feelings pose a threat to the client's self-esteem and sense of well-being. Loved ones are also concerned with the safety threat imposed by falls and the possible guilt associated with not being available at the time that a fall occurs. Although the fear of falling is a realistic and common fear, the need to stay active both before and after a fall is even

DISPLAY 26-8. Assessment of Pain in Frail Elderly Clients

Herr and Mobily (1993) tested five pain assessment tools with an elderly population. They found them all to be appropriate, depending on the specific abilities and preferences of the client. In general, the elderly people in this study preferred the Verbal Descriptor Scale (VDS) for ease of use. The Visual Analog Scale (VAS), however, was also found to be reliable and valid.

The elderly people in this study tended to prefer the vertical over the horizontal form of the VAS. This study suggests that clinicians should collaborate with each elderly patient to choose a pain intensity scale that is best suited to individual needs and preferences.

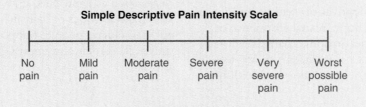

Simple Descriptive Pain Intensity Scale

No pain | Mild pain | Moderate pain | Severe pain | Very severe pain | Worst possible pain

Visual Analog Scale (VAS)

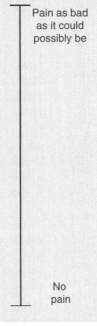

Pain as bad as it could possibly be

No pain

greater. Falling is not a normal part of aging. Limitations in activity are not the appropriate response to a positive fall assessment. The risk of falling can be minimized by a comprehensive assessment followed by appropriate medical, exercise, and adaptive environmental interventions.

Q What time of day have your falls occurred? What were you doing when the fall occurred? What other kinds of feelings or symptoms do you have when you fall?

R Taking a fall history consists of asking about the location, time of day, and activity at the time of the fall. Any associated symptoms such as trips, legs "giving way," dizziness or "blacking out," loss of consciousness or balance must be explored. Signs of trauma such as bruising, headache, or diminished alertness should be investigated. The history should

determine the circumstances surrounding any previous falls of the past 3 months to determine whether a pattern exists. The pattern and circumstances surrounding the fall can provide valuable clues with regard to the physical, medication, or environmental basis for the fall. For example, falls occurring with standing up and associated with dizziness may point to orthostatic hypotension and an adverse reaction to medication. If the client reports tripping or slipping in the absence of stiffness or weakness and any symptoms, an environmental basis such as shoes or floors with a slick surface or loose carpeting or rugs may be suspected.

If a history of falls or a fear of falling is indicated by the subjective assessment, objective measures of gait and exercise tolerance such as the "Get Up and Go" test (Podsindlo & Richardson, 1991) or a screening test to identify risk factors such as the Performance-Oriented Environmental Mobility Screen (POEMS; see Display 26-6) can be done. The POEMS is designed to take approximately 10 min to complete and can be used to help design environmental and rehabilitative interventions and to monitor clinical changes or outcomes over time. It can also be incorporated into the full or quarterly assessments of the minimum data set (MDS) used by long-term care facilities. In long-term care, any decline in mobility could be a sign of disease or an increased risk for fall.

Neurologic Function and Mental Status

Q Have you noticed any changes in your ability to concentrate or think clearly enough to keep up with your daily activities? If so, about when did this begin and describe what you have noticed?

Tip From the Experts If the older person is too lethargic, agitated, or medically unstable to respond, family or professional caregivers should be queried with regard to how current cognition and behavior compares with the client's prior level of function. If the client appears to be excessively distracted during the interview or has revealed multiple inconsistencies or the inability to describe daily activities or to answer specific questions, it is generally advisable to speak with a family member/caregiver when the client is not present about noted changes in cognition or behavior.

R Although intellectual capacity does not diminish with advancing age, the brain as it ages does become more susceptible to injury. Reversible abnormalities such as infection, dehydration, or drug toxicities are common causes of acute changes in the older adult's level of consciousness and cognition.

Although delirium occurs most commonly in hospitals, mental status changes in older adults living in a nursing home or in their own home may be the first sign of an acute illness. Thus, family members or professional caregivers may report sudden and dramatic changes in the person's mental status. When such a change in cognition develops over a short period of time and is characterized by a change in level of alertness, ranging from extreme lethargy to agitation, it is called delirium (see Display 26-4). Delirious people may continuously shift attention from one stimulus to another. Their speech is often difficult to understand because they shift abruptly and inappropriately from one thought to another. It may be difficult to engage such persons in conversation because of their inability to focus or sustain attention on any certain stimulus.

Disorientation is more often to time and place rather than to self. Speech may be rambling or incoherent, and the person often experiences disturbances in perceptions, such as illusions or hallucinations. Psychomotor activity often fluctuates from restlessness to lethargy, and emotions fluctuate from fear and irritability to apathy and anger. Changes in

cognition that develop suddenly over a matter of days are always the result of temporary injury to brain tissue. Unfortunately, unless the specific cause is identified and reversed, permanent brain damage can result. For the very old person, this is a situation that happens all too frequently when changes in orientation, alterations in attention, or agitation are seen not as symptomatic of a physical illness, but as the untreatable consequence of old age or "senility."

Rather than triggering the response to sedate or restrain, behavior associated with delirium and acute confusional states should elicit in-depth assessment, medical consultation, environmental manipulation, and collaborative interventions to reverse physical pathophysiology. The risk of permanent brain damage can only be decreased if there is a timely and competent response to confusion as a symptom of pathology.

Q Do you believe that you have more problems with memory than most? Do you believe that life is empty? Have you recently had to drop many of your activities and interests?

R Depression is not more common in old age. However, symptoms of depression in the elderly more commonly manifest as changes in cognition (memory deficits, paranoia, and agitation) and physical symptoms (muscle aches, joint pains, gastrointestinal disturbances, headache, and weight loss) than they do in younger adults. Depression in the elderly has even been called "pseudodementia." It can also be a symptom of certain physical disorders, especially endocrine disorders such as hypothyroidism, pancreatic and adrenal disorders, and cancers of all types.

Certain antihypertensives, antianxiety drugs, and hormones may also precipitate depressive symptoms. Once again, the first step in treating the problem is to differentiate the memory loss and changes in cognition as a symptom of depression rather than an irreversible dementia or a normal consequence of growing older. Without treatment, there may be significant consequences such as social isolation, substance abuse, physical disability, and even suicide.

Generally, open-ended questions will yield the most beneficial information when screening for depression in the elderly. However, when time is limited or whenever warning signs are noted, a screening instrument such as the short version of the Geriatric Depression Scale (Yesavage & Brink, 1983) should be used for further validation (see Display 26-5). When more than five questions are answered as indicated on the tool, a high probability of depressive symptoms exist. The purpose of a screening tool is not to confirm a diagnosis, but rather to point out the need for a more in-depth assessment or referral.

Because the elderly have the highest rate of suicide of any age group, assessing the risk of suicide should be a high priority. Because cognitive impairments are a common symptom of depression in the elderly, the risk of suicide may be greater when judgment and inhibitions are impaired. The importance of independence and interpersonal relationships for bringing meaning to an older person's life is manifested in a variety of ways. The inability to give meaning to life by moving outside and beyond oneself during times of crisis, change, or suffering has been found to be a risk factor for suicide in older adults (Buchanon, Farran & Clark, 1995). Elderly caregivers often become socially isolated and are also at risk for depressive symptomatology.

Q Are you concerned about changes in your memory? Are you bothered by anger or inability to control your frustrations with day-by-day living?

R By the age of 85, nearly half the population will be exhibiting signs of the most common type of dementia, Alzheimer's disease (AD). Dementia is a broad diagnostic category that includes multiple physical disorders characterized by alterations in memory, abstract thinking, judgment, and perception (see Display 26-4). Unlike delirium, dementias are characterized by gradual onset, usually over months or years. Although memory impairment is generally characterized as the key diagnostic criteria for AD, the earliest signs may more often be behavioral and characterized by irritability, aggression or angry outbursts, suspiciousness, or even withdrawal.

The common factor in all of the dementing disorders is a significant degree of memory loss and a progressive decline in intellectual functioning to the extent that daily function is affected. Although forgetfulness is a very common complaint of older adults, memory problems severe enough to cause decreased abilities to function in everyday family and social life are not normal at any age. Although affected persons are often aware of their declining abilities, they are often not able to judge the consequences of the loss of memory and cognition. The poor judgment and poor insight that are a result of the dementia often result in uncharacteristic outbursts and suspicious behaviors. This presents a great challenge to family members or caregivers faced with figuring out how to curtail activities such as driving or the control over banking and finances for an older person who may be completely unaware of the risks involved and who is accustomed to being independent in such matters for more than 50 years.

The Mini-Mental Status Examination (MMSE) is a commonly used questionnaire to screen for dementia. The MMSE, however, is designed to be used solely as a screening device. The diagnosis of dementia must be based on a comprehensive medical, functional, and psychological battery of tests that rules out any reversible pathologic conditions responsible for the cognitive changes.

To care for an older adult experiencing a change in cognitive abilities, the nurse must understand as much as possible about the basis for these impairments. To maximize quality of life, the nurse must differentiate between the reversible cognitive impairments for which medical intervention is warranted and those that cannot be reversed and for which assistance with managing the deficits is indicated. Outcomes will be determined mainly by the extent to which the impairment in cognition may be arrested or reversed. After all attempts have been made to correct physiologic abnormalities and treat cognitive impairments resulting from

depression, nursing care must be directed toward preserving the dignity and integrity of a person's selfhood and the well-being of the family structure to the fullest extent possible.

Collecting Objective Data

There is often a fine line between deterioration of function from aging and deterioration from disease. For this reason, it is crucial to integrate the subjective, functional, and physical assessments. The significance of a physical finding is often determined by the effect that it is having on the person's level of comfort and ability to function. A medical pathology should be suspected whenever any physical or functional change has occurred suddenly (days to weeks).

An efficient and effective way to determine the significance of physical findings in an older person is to collect subjective data while you are conducting a physical examination. Because medication is the primary method of treating disease in this country and polypharmacy is such a common occurrence in the elderly, sudden changes or abnormalities noted in the physical examination must always be analyzed for the possibility of being the result of an adverse drug effect. Because many diseases have a "silent" presentation in the elderly, an in-depth, comprehensive physical examination is especially important to detect and treat disease in a timely way.

CLIENT PREPARATION

Most importantly, the examiner must take care to approach the frail elderly client without assumptions with regard to mental status or physical ability. Attitudes or stereotypical assumptions based on a person's age will limit the willingness of the older adult to share concerns or reveal functional limitations. It is essential that the frail elderly person be approached as an individual, that adjustments be made to accommodate the client's specific functional limitations, and that the nurse be sensitive to the client's need for privacy as well as his or her wishes for a caregiver to remain in the room during all or parts of the assessment.

The examination of a frail elderly adult usually takes longer than that of a younger adult because of the chronic conditions, disabilities, and ensuing discomfort that many frail elderly people experience. It is best to limit the length of the examination. This may mean that a complete assessment may require several sessions over a period of time. The client may feel less hurried if paperwork, such as a health questionnaire, can be completed at home either by the client alone or with the help of a caregiver. Some modifications and techniques appropriate for an examination of the frail elderly person include:

- Keep the temperature of the examination room warmer than may be comfortable for younger adults.
- Eliminate background noise as much as possible.

- When interacting with an elderly client, remember that it may be more acceptable to be more formal than informal. For example, address the client by first name only if the client specifically requests that you do so.
- Keep your voice volume down even if you anticipate the client has difficulty hearing. Speaking clearly and at a moderate pace is more beneficial in cases of hearing loss. Remember to face the client when speaking with him or her.
- Do not assume that the client cannot answer questions if he or she has a cognitive impairment. However, if the impairment has significantly impaired function or verbal expression, give only one-step directions and avoid questions that require two responses. The cognitively impaired elderly person with few remaining verbal abilities may have no or only minimal loss of the ability to comprehend nonverbal cues.
- If you need to question caregivers or collateral sources to validate or clarify information, avoid consulting them in the presence of the client.
- Elderly people with physical disabilities may need assistance with dressing and with parts of the examination. Allow additional time in deference to the client's need for independence as well as your need to know how much the client can do independently.

EQUIPMENT AND SUPPLIES

In addition to the equipment needed for performing a complete adult physical examination, the following items will be needed for assessing the functional capacity of the frail elderly adult:

- Newspaper or book and lamp light for vision testing
- Lemon slice or mint for sense of smell test

- Pudding or food of pudding consistency and spoon for swallowing examination. A teacup may also be used.
- Food and fluid diary sheets or forms
- Two or three pillows for client comfort and positioning
- Straight-backed chair for "Get Up and Go" test

KEY ASSESSMENT POINTS

- Health complaints or abnormalities are as likely to be the result of an adverse reaction to drug therapy as they are to a disease process. Compiling a profile of prescription and over-the-counter medications is an essential component of any assessment of the frail elderly person—whether it is being performed to treat a specific health complaint or for compiling baseline data of the client's health status.
- Abnormalities in physiologic parameters are less reliable guides for diagnostic and treatment decisions than are the ways in which abnormalities affect the elderly person's ability to function in everyday life.
- Keep in mind that it is very difficult to attribute health complaints or abnormalities to a specific disease process. Comorbidity and the more generalized way in which disease presents creates the need for an integrated assessment of psychosocial, functional, and physical health.
- Astute assessments are crucial for diminishing morbidity and disability in the frail elderly person who is living with less physiologic reserve in most body systems. An important determinant of treatment efficacy is how early in the disease interventions have been implemented so that remaining physiologic reserves are preserved as much as possible and the risks of adverse effects resulting from overly aggressive treatments are minimized.

(*text continues on page 748*)

PHYSICAL ASSESSMENT

ASSESSMENT PROCEDURE	NORMAL FINDINGS	ABNORMAL FINDINGS
SKIN, HAIR, AND NAILS		
Inspect and palpate skin lesions. (Note whether they are flat or raised, palpable or nonpalpable. Also note color, size, and exudates, if any.) 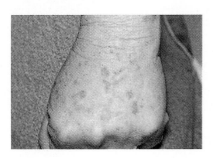 Solar lentigines are very common on aging skin.	Lentigenes—Hyperpigmentation in sun-exposed areas appear as brown, pigmented, round or rectangular patches. Venous lakes—Reddish vascular lesions on ears or other facial areas resulting from dilation of small, red blood vessels. Skin tags—Acrochordons, flesh-colored pedunculated lesions.	Mole that bleeds or has changed in shape or color or with a diameter wider than a pencil eraser (see Chapter 9 for a discussion of skin cancers and other abnormalities of the skin) Irregularly shaped lesion or scaly, elevated lesion (squamous cell carcinoma) Actinic keratoses (proliferative form) Waxy or raised lesion, especially on sun-exposed (basal cell carcinoma) Large vesicles or bulla overlying erythema, pruritic

(continued)

ASSESSMENT PROCEDURE	NORMAL FINDINGS	ABNORMAL FINDINGS
	Seborrheic keratoses—Tan, brown, or reddish, flat lesions commonly found on fair-skinned persons in sun-exposed areas. Cherry angiomas—Small, round, red spots. Senile purpura—Vivid purple patches (lesion should not blanch to touch)	Herpes zoster vesicles (shingles) draining clear fluid or pustules atop an erythematous base following a clear linear pattern and accompanied by pain Ringworm (dermatomycosis)—Reddish rings with vesicles and scaling (generally accompanied by itching and some pain) Pinpoint-sized, red-purple, nonblanchable petecchia (common sign of platelet deficiency) Large bruises may result from anticoagulant therapy, a fall, renal or liver failure, or elder abuse.
Note color, texture, integrity, and moisture of skin and sensitivity to heat or cold. **Tip From the Experts** Room humidifiers, avoidance of harsh deodorants or soaps, and use of lanolin-containing products after bathing (while skin is still moist) may help relieve effects of dry skin.	Somewhat transparent, pale, skin with an overall decrease in body hair on lower extremities. Skin may wrinkle and tent when pinched. *Note:* Pinching skin is not an accurate test of turgor in the elderly.	Torn skin (possibly the result of abrasive tape used to hold bandages or tubes in place) Extremely thin, fragile skin (friable skin) with excessive purpura (possibly from corticosteroid use) Dry, warm skin, furrowed tongue, and sunken eyes from dehydration (especially when the client has decreased urinary output, increased serum sodium, BUN and creatinine levels, increased osmolality, and hematocrit values, tachycardia; and mental confusion)
Inspect and palpate hair and scalp.	Thinning and graying of scalp, axillary, and pubic hair. Mild hair growth on upper lip of women.	Patchy or asymmetric hair loss

HEAD AND NECK

Inspect head and neck for symmetry and movement. Observe facial expression. 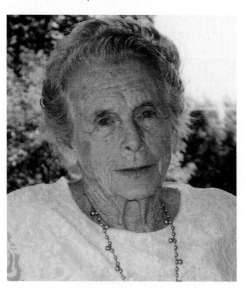 **Observe facial expression.**	Atrophy of face and neck muscles Reduced range of motion of head and neck Shortening of neck due to vertebral degeneration and development of "buffalo hump" at top of cervical vertebrae	Asymmetry of mouth or eyes possibly from Bell's palsy or CVA Marked limitation of movement or crepitation in back of neck from cervical arthritis Involuntary facial or head movements from an extrapyramidal disorder, such as Parkinson's disease or some medications Reported episodic, unilateral, shocklike or burning pain of the face or continuous pain, which may be postherpetic or caused by a dental caries or abscess. *Note:* In cognitively impaired elders, sleep disturbances or agitation may be the only sign of neuropathic pain.

(continued)

ASSESSMENT PROCEDURE	NORMAL FINDINGS	ABNORMAL FINDINGS

MOUTH AND THROAT

ASSESSMENT PROCEDURE	NORMAL FINDINGS	ABNORMAL FINDINGS
Inspect the gums and buccal mucosa for color and consistency.	Decreased salivary gland secretion is commonly seen in the elderly client. Gums and mucosa should be pink and without swelling, bleeding, or lesions.	Saliva-depressing medications include antihistamines, antipsychotics, antihypertensives, and any drug with anticholinergic side effects.
If the client is wearing dentures, inspect them for fit. Then ask the client to remove them for the rest of the oral examination.	Resorption of gum ridge commonly results in poorly fitting dentures	Loose-fitting dentures or inability to close mouth completely may also be the result of a significant weight gain or loss. Foul-smelling breath may indicate periodontal disease. Whitish or yellow-tinged patches in mouth or throat may be candidiasis from use of steroid inhalers or antibiotics.
Examine the tongue. Observe symmetry and size.	The tongue should be pink and moist.	A swollen, red, and painful tongue may indicate vitamin B or riboflavin deficiency.
Observe the client swallowing food or fluids.	Mild decrease in swallowing ability	Coughing, drooling, pocketing, or spitting out of food after intake are all possible signs of dysphagia. A drooping mouth, chronic congestion, or a weak or hoarse voice (especially after eating or drinking) also suggests dysphagia. Observed swallowing difficulties, in which case a nutritional assessment should be completed and the client referred for a barium swallow examination.

Assessing for swallowing problems. (© B. Proud.)

Tip From the Experts   Help the client who reports dysphagia to lean slightly forward with the chin tucked in toward the neck when swallowing and offer food of pudding consistency to minimize the risk of aspiration.

ASSESSMENT PROCEDURE	NORMAL FINDINGS	ABNORMAL FINDINGS
Depress the posterior third of the tongue, and note gag reflex.	Slightly sluggish in some older adults.	Absence of a gag reflex may be the result of a neurologic disorder and indicates the need to be alert for signs of aspiration pneumonia.

(continued)

ASSESSMENT PROCEDURE	NORMAL FINDINGS	ABNORMAL FINDINGS

NOSE AND SINUSES

Inspect the nose for color and consistency. Evaluate the sense of smell. Have the client close the eyes and smell a common substance, such as mint, lemon, or soap.

Nose and nasal passages are not inflamed, and skin and mucous membranes are intact.
   Slightly diminished sense of smell and ability to detect odors

Edema, redness, swelling, or clear drainage, which may indicate allergies or rhinitis. Client cannot identify strong odor.

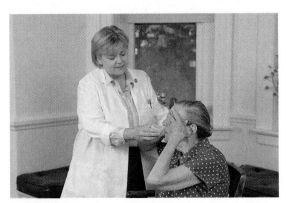

Assessing sense of smell. (© B. Proud.)

🏵️ **Tip From the Experts**   Alert clients with diminished smell to the importance of smoke alarms and routine inspections of stoves and furnaces.

Test nasal patency by asking the client to breathe while blocking one nostril at a time.

Client can breathe with reasonable ease.

Reported feeling of inadequate breath intake, which may result from nasal polyps, a deviated septum, or allergic or infectious rhinitis or sinusitis.

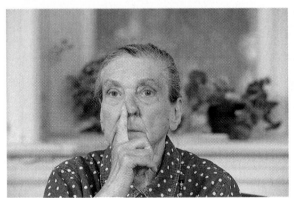

© B. Proud.

(continued)

ASSESSMENT PROCEDURE	NORMAL FINDINGS	ABNORMAL FINDINGS
Palpate the frontal and maxillary sinuses for consistency and to elicit possible pain.	Area is free of lesions and pain.	Client reports pain and dryness; inflammation evident.

Tip From the Experts Elderly clients with nasogastric feeding tubes are at increased risk for sinusitis related to the obstruction.

Tip From the Experts Elderly clients may self-treat sinus pain and/or nasal congestion with decongestants and antihistamines, which may further dry the nasal passages and prevent normal sinus drainage. These drugs may also aggravate hypertension (in clients taking antihypertensive drugs) and exacerbate cardiac dysrhythmias. In clients taking antibiotics for sinusitis, watch for adverse effects on renal function. Because antibiotics also may kill normal bacteria, watch for signs of candidal or *Clostridium difficile* infection in the GI tract, mouth, or vagina.

EYES AND VISION

Inspect eyes, eyelids, eyelashes, and conjunctiva. Also observe eye and conjunctiva for dryness, redness, tearing, or increased sensitivity to light and wind.	The skin around the eyes becomes thin, and wrinkles appear normally with age. Eyelids close easily, and eyelashes turn outward. Client may have some dryness resulting from diminished tear production that occurs with aging.	Eyelids that droop downward and do not shut completely suggest ectropion. Eyelids that turn inward may cause eyelashes to rub against the eyeball and suggest entropion, which may be complicated by infection and drainage. Abnormalities in blinking may result from Parkinson's disease; dull or blank staring may be a sign of hypothyroidism.
Inspect the cornea and lens. Also ask the client when he or she last had an eye and vision examination.	An arcus senilis, a cloudy or grayish ring around the iris, and decreased pigment in iris are age-related changes.	A yellowish or brownish discoloration of the lens is usually a cataract. Common symptoms include painless blurring of vision, glare and haloes around lights, poor night vision, colors that look dull or brownish, and frequent eyeglass prescription changes. The extent of visual impairment (especially central vision) determines the point at which a cataract needs to be removed. A thickening of the bulbar conjunctiva that grows over the cornea (called pterygium) may interfere with vision.

Tip From the Experts Tonometry should be performed every 1 to 2 years on everyone older than 35 to detect glaucoma. Elevated intraocular pressure indicates the need for referral to an ophthalmologist and confirmation with applanation tonometry.

(continued)

ASSESSMENT PROCEDURE	NORMAL FINDINGS	ABNORMAL FINDINGS

Observe the pupils. With a penlight or similar device, test pupillary reaction to light.

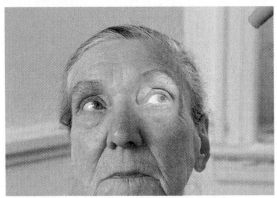

© B. Proud.

Overall decrease in size of pupil and ability to dilate in dark and constrict in light may occur with advanced age; this results in poorer night vision and decreased tolerance to glare.

An irregularly shaped pupil, which may indicate removal of a cataract

Asymmetric response, which may be due to a neurologic condition

Test vision. Ask the client to read from a newspaper or magazine. Use only room lighting for the initial reading. Use task lighting for a second reading.

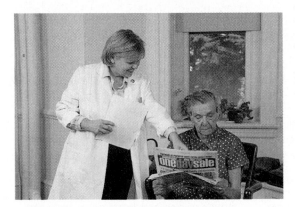

Reading with room lighting. (© B. Proud.)

Impaired near vision is indicative of presbyopia (farsightedness), a common finding in older adults. Also common are slight decreases in peripheral vision and difficulty in differentiating blues from greens.

🎗 **Tip From the Experts** If client has difficulty reading or doing handwork, suggest additional task lighting.

A significant decrease in central vision, to the extent needed for activities of daily living, may signal a cataract in one or both eyes.

Macular degeneration (thin membrane in the center of the retina) is suspected if the client has difficulty in seeing with one eye. The disorder almost always becomes bilateral. Related abnormal findings include blurry words in the center of the page or door frames that don't appear straight.

A noticeable loss of vision, including cloudiness, distortion of familiar objects, and, occasionally, blind spots or floaters are common symptoms of diabetic retinopathy.

EARS AND HEARING

Inspect the external ear. Observe shape, color, and hair growth. Also look for lesions or drainage.

Hairs may become coarser and thicker in the external ear, especially in men.

Inflammation, drainage, or swelling may be from infection.

Perform an otoscopic examination to determine quantity, color, and consistency of cerumen.

Cerumen accumulation increases.

Hard, dark brown cerumen signals impaction of the auditory canal.

A darkened hole in the tympanic membrane or patches indicate perforation or scarring of the tympanic membrane.

(continued)

ASSESSMENT PROCEDURE	NORMAL FINDINGS	ABNORMAL FINDINGS
Perform the *voice–whisper test*, a functional examination to detect obvious (conversational) hearing loss. Instruct the client to put a hand over one ear and to repeat the sentence you say. Stand approximately 2 feet away from the client and whisper a sentence.	The inability to hear high-frequency sounds or to discriminate a variety of simultaneous sounds results from degeneration of the hair cells of the inner ear and is called *presbycusis*.	Inability to hear the whispered sentence indicates a hearing deficiency and the need to refer the client to an audiologist for testing.

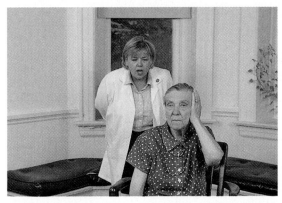

Assessing hearing with the voice-whisper test. (© B. Proud.)

Tip From the Experts

Assess hearing acuity before as well as after the otoscopic examination, if cerumen is removed during the examination. If you are facing the client, hold your hand close to your mouth so the client cannot read your lips.

THORAX AND LUNGS

ASSESSMENT PROCEDURE	NORMAL FINDINGS	ABNORMAL FINDINGS
Inspect shape of thorax and also respiratory rate, rhythm, and quality of breathing.	Increase in normal respiratory rate of 16 to 25 (Pierson & Kacmarek, 1992) Increased reliance on diaphragmatic breathing and increased work of breathing related to the anatomic changes in the costal cartilage, respiratory muscles, and lung tissue	Respiratory rate exceeding 25 breaths/min may signal a pulmonary infection along with increased sputum production, confusion, loss of appetite, and hypotension (McGann, 2000). Respiratory rate of less than 16 breaths/min may be a sign of neurologic impairment, which may lead to aspiration pneumonia.
Percuss lung tones as you would in a younger adult.	In general, the normal sound to percussion is the same in an older adult as it is in a younger adult—resonant. However, in the presence of structural changes such as kyphosis or a slight barrel chest, resonance may increase.	Consolidation of infection will cause dullness to percussion; alveolar retention of air, as occurs in emphysema, results in hyperresonance. *Note:* Supine positioning, shallow breathing, and poor dental hygiene increase the risk of pulmonary infection.
Auscultate lung sounds as you would in a younger adult.	Vesicular sounds should be heard over all areas of air exchange. However, because lung expansion may be diminished, it may be necessary to emphasize taking deep breaths with the mouth open during the exam. This may be very difficult for those with dementia.	Breath sounds may be distant over areas affected by kyphosis or the barrel chest of aging. Rales and rhonchi are heard only with diseases, such as pulmonary edema, pneumonia, or restrictive disorders. Diminished breath sounds, wheezes, crackles, rhonchi that do not clear with cough, and egophony are common signs of consolidation caused by pneumonia.

(continued)

ASSESSMENT PROCEDURE	NORMAL FINDINGS	ABNORMAL FINDINGS

HEART AND BLOOD VESSELS

Take blood pressure to detect actual or potential orthostatic hypotension and, therefore, the risk for falling. Measure pressure with the client in lying, sitting, and standing positions. Also measure pulse rate. Have the client lie down for 5 min; take the pulse and blood pressure; at 1 min, take blood pressure and pulse after client is sitting and again at 1 min after client stands.

An elderly person's baroreceptor response to positional changes is slightly less efficient.

Blood pressure increases as elasticity decreases in arteries with proportionately greater increase in systolic pressure resulting in a widening of pulse pressure.

More than 10 mmHg drop in systolic or diastolic pressure and an increase in heart rate of 20 beats or more per minute indicates orthostatic hypotension, which places the client at risk for falls.

Tip From the Experts If dizziness occurs, instruct client to sit a few minutes before attempting to stand up from a supine or reclining position.

Tip From the Experts Some sources of orthostatic hypotension include medications, such as antihypertensives, diuretics, and drugs with anticholinergic side effects (anxiolytics, antipsychotics, hypnotics, tricyclic antidepressants, and antihistamines.

Any client with blood pressure exceeding 160/90 mmHg should be referred to the health care provider for follow up.

A sudden and increasingly widened pulse pressure, especially in combination with other neurologic abnormalities and a change in mental status is a classic sign of increased intracranial pressure (which in elderly clients may be due to a hemorrhagic stroke or hematoma).

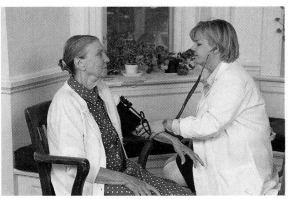

© B. Proud.

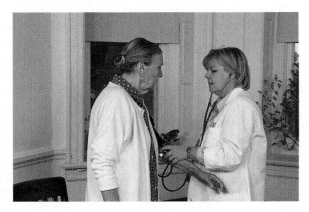

(continued)

ASSESSMENT PROCEDURE	NORMAL FINDINGS	ABNORMAL FINDINGS
Evaluate exercise tolerance, either by reviewing results of stress testing or by observing the client's ability to move from a sitting to a standing position, or to flex and extend fingers rapidly. Both tests may be used to measure activity tolerance.	The maximal heart rate with exercise is less than in a younger person. The heart rate will also take longer to return to its pre-exercise rate. Normally, the rise in pulse rate should be no greater than 10 to 20 beats/min. The pulse rate should return to the baseline rate within 2 min.	A rise in pulse rate greater than 20 beats/min and a rate that does not return to baseline within 2 min is an indicator of exercise intolerance. Cardiac dysrhythmias as determined by stress testing are also indicative of exercise intolerance.

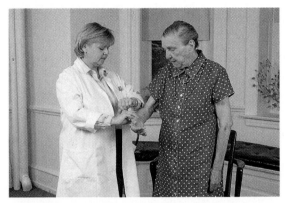

Assessing heart rate after the client rises from a sitting position provides clues to his or her tolerance of physical exertion. (© B. Proud.)

Tip From the Experts Poor lower body strength, especially in the ankles, may impair the ability of the frail elderly person to rise from a chair to a standing position. Poor upper body strength, especially in the shoulders, may impede the ability to push up from a bed or chair or to extend and flex fingers.

Determine adequacy of blood flow by palpating the arterial pulses in all locations (carotid, brachial, radial, femoral, popliteal, posterior tibial, and dorsalis pedis) for strength and quality.	Proximal pulses may be easier to palpate due to loss of supporting surrounding tissue. However, distal lower extremity pulses may be more difficult to feel or even nonpalpable. The dorsalis pedis pulse is absent in approximately 20% of older persons (Mezey, Rauckorst & Stokes, 1993, p. 90).	Insufficient or absent pulses are a likely indication of arterial insufficiency. Partially obstructed blood flow increases the risk of ulcers and infection; completely obstructed blood flow is a medical emergency requiring immediate intervention to prevent gangrene and possible amputation.

Tip From the Experts Palpate carotid arteries gently and one side at a time to avoid stimulating vagal receptors in the neck, dislodging existing plaque, or causing syncope or a stroke.

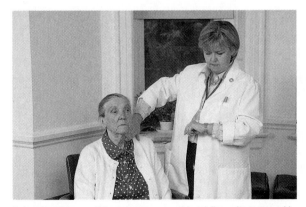

Palpating the carotid artery to assess blood flow. (© B. Proud.)

(continued)

ASSESSMENT PROCEDURE	NORMAL FINDINGS	ABNORMAL FINDINGS
Auscultate the carotid, abdominal, and femoral arteries.	No unusual sounds should be heard.	A bruit is abnormal, and the client needs a prompt referral for further care because of the high risk of CVA from a carotid embolism or an abdominal or femoral aneurysm.

Use the bell of the stethoscope to listen for bruits. (© B. Proud.)

ASSESSMENT PROCEDURE	NORMAL FINDINGS	ABNORMAL FINDINGS
Evaluate arterial and venous sufficiency of extremities by elevating the legs above the level of the heart and observing color, temperature, size of the legs, and skin integrity. 🌸 **Tip From the Experts** Client reports of leg pain associated with walking and descriptions of burning or cramping are symptoms of arterial insufficiency. Signs of arterial insufficiency include duskiness or mottling when the leg is in a dependent position; paleness with elevation; cool, thin, shiny skin; thickened, brittle nails; and diminished pulses (often in association with atherosclerosis and diabetes mellitus).	Hair loss occurs normally with advanced age and cannot be used singly as an indicator of arterial insufficiency.	Client reports of aching or pain not particularly associated with activity are characteristic of venous insufficiency. Elevation of the leg may relieve discomfort. Dependent rubor and elevation pallor with rest pain or claudication indicates arterial disease. Arterial ulcers are usually located at ends of toes and are often round and covered with black eschar, with very little drainage. Peripheral pulses will be diminished. Irregularly shaped wound edges located on the medial aspect of the lower leg (typically just above the medial malleolus) with some drainage and normal pedal pulses are generally venous ulcers. Peripheral edema and hemosiderin deposits are usually also present. These ulcers are often very sensitive or painful. Diffuse erythema may be from cellulites.
Inspect and palpate veins while client is standing.	Prominent, bulging veins are common. Varicosities are considered a problem only if ulcerations, signs of thrombophlebitis, or cords, are present. Cords are nontender, palpable veins having a rubber tubing consistency.	Unilateral warmth, tenderness, and swelling may be indications of thrombophlebitis.
Inspect and palpate the precordium.	The precordium is still and without thrills, heaves, or visible, palpable pulsations (noted exception may be the apex of the heart if close to the surface).	Heaves—Felt with an enlarged right or left ventricular aneurysm Thrills—Indicate aortic, mitral, or pulmonic stenosis and regurgitation, which may originate from rheumatic fever Pulsations—Suggest an aortic or ventricular aneurysm, right ventricular enlargement, or mitral regurgitation

(continued)

ASSESSMENT PROCEDURE	NORMAL FINDINGS	ABNORMAL FINDINGS

BREASTS

Auscultate heart sounds.	Extra heart sounds (low-intensity, systolic murmur and an S_4) resulting from normal age-related calcification of heart valves and vessels and fibrotic changes in the heart muscle.	Abnormal heart sounds are generally considered to be disease related only if there is additional evidence of compromised cardiovascular function. However, any previously undetected extra heart sound warrants further investigation. S_3 and S_4 sounds may reflect the cardiac and fluid overload of heart failure, aortic stenosis, cardiomyopathy, or myocardial infarction.
Inspect and palpate breast and axillae. When viewing axillae and contour of breasts, assist a client with arthritis to raise the arms over the head. Do this gently and without force and only if it is not painful for the client. If the breasts are pendulous, assist the client to lean slightly so the breasts hang away from the chest wall, enabling you to best observe symmetry and form.	The breasts of elderly women are often described as pendulous due to the atrophy of breast tissue and supporting tissues, and the forward thrust of the client brought about by kyphosis. Decreases in fat composition and increase in fibrotic tissue may make the terminal ducts feel more fibrotic and palpable as linear, spoke-like strands. Nipples may retract due to loss in musculature. Unlike nipple retraction due to a mass, nipples that are retracted because of aging can be everted with gentle pressure (Mezey et al., 1993)	Pain upon palpation may indicate an infectious process or cancer. Or breast tenderness, pain, or swelling may be side effects of hormone replacement therapy and an indication that a lower dosage is needed. Male breast enlargement (gynecomastia) may result from a decrease in testosterone.

Tip From the Experts If the client has an obvious abnormality in one breast, begin the examination on the unaffected breast. (Zembruzski, 2001).

Inspect skin under breasts.	Skin is intact without lesions or rashes.	Macerated skin under the breasts may result from perspiration or fungal infection (usually seen in an immunocompromised client).

ABDOMEN

Assess Nutritional Status

Elderly clients typically report gastrointestinal problems related not only to elimination but also to diet and nutrition. Therefore, measure and record the client's height and weight, noting weight changes and problems with swallowing or chewing. Review laboratory test values (complete blood count, and vitamin B_{12}, cholesterol, albumin, and prealbumin levels). In addition, compile a 24-hour food and fluid diary noting food preferences and cravings, vitamin and food supplement intake, and dietary restrictions (eg, salt).	Antral cells and intestinal villi atrophy, and gastric production of hydrochloric acid decreases with age.	Indicators of malnutrition include: Client weighs less than 80% ideal body weight. Client has had 10% loss in body weight over past 6 months or 5% loss in body weight over past month. Hemoglobin level is lower than 12 g/dL. Hematocrit is lower than 35. Vitamin B_{12} level is lower than 100 pg/mL. Indicators of poor nutritional status include: Serum cholesterol level lower than 160 mg/dL. Serum albumin level lower than 3.5 g/dL. Serum prealbumin levels (used to monitor improvement of nutritional status) that do not increase 1 mg/dL/day.

Tip From the Experts Suspect drug toxicity in clients taking medications, such as digoxin, theophylline, quinidine, or antibiotics if client reports nausea or diarrhea.

(continued)

ASSESSMENT PROCEDURE	NORMAL FINDINGS	ABNORMAL FINDINGS

Assess Hydration Status

Because, muscle mass decreases and fatty tissues increase, the elderly client is at increased risk for dehydration. Evaluate hydration status as you would nutritional status. Begin with accurate serial measurements of weight, careful review of laboratory test findings (serial serum sodium level, hematocrit, osmolality, BUN level, and urine-specific gravity), and a 2- to 3-day diary of fluid intake and output.

Normal findings include stable weight and stable mental status.

Tip From the Experts Increases over time in laboratory values are usually indicators of deteriorating hydration (even though values may be within normal limits).

Sudden weight loss; fever; dry, warm skin; furrowed, swollen, and red tongue; decreased urine output; lethargy and weakness are all signs of dehydration.

An acute change in mental status (particularly confusion), tachycardia, and hypotension may indicate severe dehydration, which may be precipitated by certain medications, such as diuretics, laxatives, tricylic antidepressants, or lithium.

Fluid intake of fewer than 1500 mL daily (excluding caffeine-containing beverages) is a possible indicator of dehydration.

ASSESS MOTILITY

Assess GI motility and auscultate bowel sounds.

5–30 sounds/min.

Absence of bowel sounds

Determine absorption or retention problems in elderly clients receiving enteral feedings.
Note: An abdominal x-ray, flatplate, should be taken to check for correct placement of newly inserted nasogastric tubes.

Fewer than 100 mL residual is a normal finding for intermittent feedings.

More than 100 mL residual measured before a scheduled feeding is a sign of insufficient absorption and excessive retention.

Abdominal distention, diarrhea, fluid overload, aspiration pneumonia, or fluid/electrolyte imbalances may also be indicators of excessive retention although mental status changes may be the first or only sign.

Inspect and percuss abdomen in same manner as for younger adults.

Tip From the Experts The loss of abdominal musculature that occurs with aging may make it easier to palpate abdominal organs.

Liver, pancreas, and kidneys normally decrease in size, but the decrease is not generally appreciable upon physical examination.

Anorexia, abdominal pain and distention, impaired protein digestion, and vitamin B_{12} malabsorption suggest inflammatory gastritis or a peptic ulcer.

Abdominal distention, cramping, and diarrhea are signs of lactose intolerance, which may occur for the first time in old age.

Bruits over aorta suggest an aneurysm. If present, do not palpate because this could rupture the aneurysm.

Guarding upon palpation, rebound tenderness, or a friction rub (sounds like pieces of sandpaper rubbing together) often suggests peritonitis, which could be secondary to ruptured diverticuli, tumor, or infarct.

Palpate the bladder, but ask client to empty bladder before the examination. If the bladder is palpable, percuss from symphysis pubis to umbilicus. If the client is incontinent, postvoid residual content may also need to be measured.

Empty bladder is not palpable or percussable.

Full bladder sounds dull. More than 100 mL drained from bladder is considered abnormal for a postvoid residual. A distended bladder with an associated small-volume urine loss may indicate an overflow incontinence (see Display 26-7).

(continued)

ASSESSMENT PROCEDURE	NORMAL FINDINGS	ABNORMAL FINDINGS

GENITALIA

Female

Assist the client into the lithotomy position; inspect the urethral meatus and vaginal opening.	Pubic hair is usually sparse, and labia are flattened.	White, glistening particles attached to pubic hair may be a sign of lice. Redness or swelling from the urethral meatus indicates a possible urinary tract infection.
Tip From the Experts Arthritis may make the lithotomy position particularly uncomfortable for the elderly woman, necessitating changes. If the client has breathing difficulties, elevating the head to a semi-Fowler's position may help.		
Ask the client to cough while in the lithotomy position.	No leakage of urine	Leakage of urine that occurs with coughing is a sign of stress incontinence and may be due to lax pelvic muscles from childbirth, surgery, obesity, cystocele, rectocele, or a prolapsed uterus. *Note:* In noncommunicative patients, an excoriated perineum may be the result of incontinence, which warrants further investigation.
Tip From the Experts Incontinence is not a normal part of aging. If embarrassment or acceptance is preventing the client from acknowledging the problem, the genital examination may be a more acceptable time to introduce the topic.		
To test for prolapse, ask the client to bear down while you observe the vaginal opening.	No prolapse evident	A protrusion into the vaginal opening may be a cystocele, rectocele, or uterine prolapse, which is a common sequelae of relaxed pelvic musculature in older women.
Perform a pelvic examination. Put on disposable gloves and use a small speculum if the vaginal opening has narrowed with age.	Vaginal secretions should be white, clear, and odorless. The vaginal epithelium is thinner, drier, and may be pale and shiny. Atrophic changes are intensified by infrequent intercourse. Because the ovaries, uterus, and cervix shrink with age, the ovaries may not be palpable.	Malignancy, vulvar dystrophies, urinary tract infections, and other infections, such as *Candida albicans,* bacterial vaginosis, gonorrhea, or *Chlamydia,* can mimic atrophic vaginitis (Kennedy-Malone et al, 2000).
Test pelvic muscle tone by asking the woman to squeeze muscles while the examiner's finger is in the vagina. Assess perineal strength by turning fingers posterior to the perineum while the woman squeezes muscles in the vaginal area.	The vaginal wall should constrict around the examiner's finger, and the perineum should feel smooth.	If the client has a cystocele, the examiner's finger in the vagina will feel pressure from the anterior surface of the vagina. In clients with uterine prolapse, protrusion of the cervix is felt down through the vagina. A bulging of the posterior vaginal wall and part of the rectum may be felt with a rectocele.

(continued)

ASSESSMENT PROCEDURE	NORMAL FINDINGS	ABNORMAL FINDINGS
Male		
Inspect the male genital area with the client in standing position if possible.	Pubic hair is thinner. Scrotal skin is slightly darker than surrounding skin and is smooth and flaccid in the older man. Testicular size decreases.	Scrotal edema may be present with portal vein obstruction or heart failure. Lesions on the penis may be a sign of infection. Associated symptoms frequently include discharge, scrotal pain, and difficulty with urination.
Observe and palpate for inguinal swelling or bulges suggestive of hernia in the same manner as for a younger male.	No swelling or bulges	Masses or bulges are abnormal, and pain may be a sign of testicular torsion. A mass may be due to a hydrocele, spermatocele, or cancer.
Auscultate the scrotum if a mass is detected; otherwise palpate the right and left testicle using the thumb and first two fingers.	No detectable sounds or masses	Bowel sounds heard over the scrotum may suggest an indirect inguinal hernia. Masses are abnormal, and the client should be referred to a specialist for follow-up examination.

ANUS, RECTUM, AND PROSTATE

Inspect the anus and rectum.	The anus is darker than the surrounding skin.
	    Bluish, grapelike lumps at the anus are indicators of hemorrhoids.
		Lesions, swelling, inflammation, and bleeding are abnormalities.
		    If hemorrhoids account for discomfort, the degree to which bleeding, swelling, or inflammation interferes with bowel activity generally determines whether treatment is warranted.

Put on gloves to palpate the anus and rectum. Also palpate the prostate in the male client. 🎗 **Tip From the Experts** The left side-lying position with knees tucked up toward the chest is the preferred one for comfort. Pillows may be needed for positioning and client comfort.	The prostate is normally soft or rubbery-firm and smooth, and the median sulcus is palpable.	Palpation of internal masses could indicate polyps, internal hemorrhoids, rectal prolapse, cancer, or fecal impaction. Obliteration of the median sulcus is felt with prostatic hyperplasia. A hard, asymmetrically enlarged, and nodular prostate is suggestive of malignancy (Mezey et al., 1993). A tender and softer prostate is more common with prostatitis.

MUSCULOSKELETAL SYSTEM

Balance, Posture, and Gait		
Observe the client's posture and balance upon standing, especially the first 3 to 5 s. 🎗 **Tip From the Experts** The ability to reach for everyday items without losing balance can be assessed by asking the client to remove an object from a shelf that is high enough to require stretching or standing on the toes and to bend down to pick up a small object, such as a pen, from the floor.	Client stands reasonably straight with feet positioned fairly widely apart to form a firm base of support. This stance compensates for diminished sense of proprioception in lower extremities. Body usually bends forward as well.	A "humpback" curvature of the spine, called kyphosis, usually results from osteoporosis. The combination of osteoporosis, calcification of tendons and joints, and muscle atrophy makes it difficult for the frail elderly person to extend the hips and knees fully when walking. This impairs the ability to maintain balance early enough to prevent a fall. Client cannot maintain balance without holding onto something or someone. Postural instability increases the risk of falling and immobility from the fear of falling.

(continued)

ASSESSMENT PROCEDURE	NORMAL FINDINGS	ABNORMAL FINDINGS
Observe the client's gait by performing the timed "Get Up and Go" test: 1. Have the client rise from a straight-backed arm chair, stand momentarily, and walk about 3 m toward a wall. 2. Ask the client to turn without touching the wall and walk back to the chair; then turn around and sit down. 3. Using a watch or clock with a second hand, time how long it takes the client to complete the test. 4. Score performance on a 1–5 scale: 1 = normal; 2 = very slightly abnormal; 3 = mildly abnormal; 4 = moderately abnormal; 5 = severely abnormal.	Widening of pelvis and narrowing of shoulders Client walks steadily without swaying, stumbling, or hesitating during the walk. The client does not appear to be at risk of falling. Elderly clients without impairments in gait or balance can complete the test within 10 s.	Shuffling gait, characterized by smaller steps and minimal lifting of the feet, increases the risk of tripping when walking on uneven or unsteady surfaces. Abnormal findings from the timed "Get Up and Go" test include hesitancy, staggering, stumbling, and abnormal movements of the trunk and arms. People who take more than 30 s to complete the test tend to be dependent in some activities of daily living, such as bathing, getting in and out of bed, or climbing stairs.

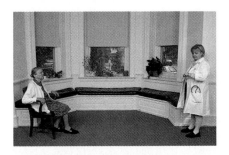
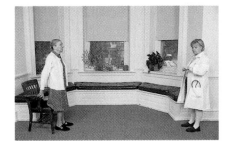
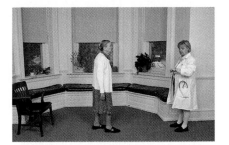

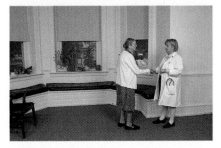
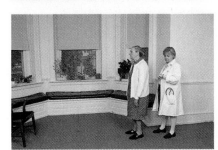
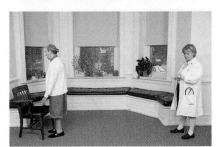

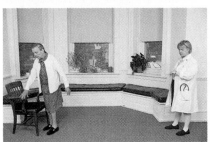
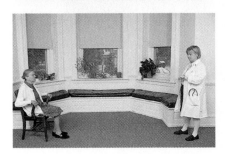

© B. Proud.

(continued)

ASSESSMENT PROCEDURE	NORMAL FINDINGS	ABNORMAL FINDINGS

Inspect the general contour of limbs, trunk, and joints. Palpate wrist and hand joints.

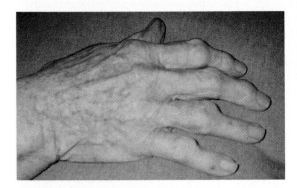

Enlargement of the distal, interphalangeal joints of the fingers, called Heberden's nodes, are indicators of degenerative joint disease (DJD), a common age-related condition involving joints in the hips, knees, and spine as well as the fingers.

With accumulated damage and loss of cartilage, bony overgrowths protrude from the bone into the joint capsule, causing deformities, limited mobility, and pain.

Hand deformities such as ulnar deviation, swan-neck deformity, and boutonniere deformity are of concern because of the limitations they impose on activities of daily living and related pain.

Range of Motion

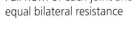

Assess ROM by asking client to touch each finger with the thumb of the same hand, to turn wrists up toward the ceiling and down toward the floor, to push each finger against yours while you apply resistance, and to make a fist and release it.

Full ROM of each joint and equal bilateral resistance

Limitations in ROM or strength may be due to degenerative disk disease (DJD), rheumatoid arthritis, or a neurologic disorder, which, if unilateral, suggests CVA.

Signs of pain such as grimacing, pulling back, or verbal messages are indicators of the need to do a pain assessment (see Display 26–8).

Grating, popping, crepitus, and palpation of fluid are also abnormalities. Crepitus and joint pain that is worse with activity and relieved by rest in the absence of systemic symptoms is often associated with DJD.

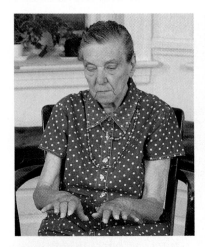
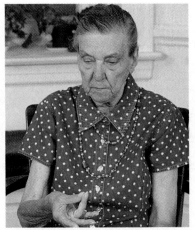
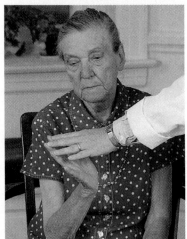
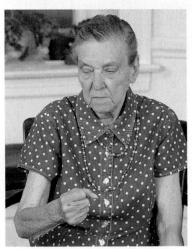

© B. Proud.

(continued)

ASSESSMENT PROCEDURE	NORMAL FINDINGS	ABNORMAL FINDINGS

Similarly, assess ROM and strength of shoulders (left) and elbows (right).

Tenderness, stiffness, and pain in the shoulders and elbows (and hips), which is aggravated by movement, are common signs associated with polymyalgia rheumatica (PMR).

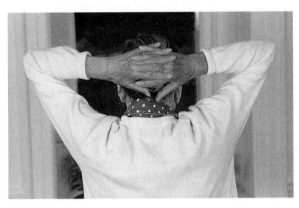

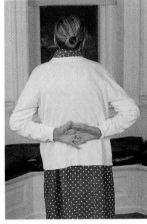

© B. Proud.

Assess hip joint for strength and ROM in the same manner as for a younger adult.

Intact flexion, extension, and internal and external rotation

Hip pain that is worse with weight bearing and relieved with rest may indicate DJD. There is usually also an associated crepitation and decrease in ROM.

Complaints of hip or thigh pain, external rotation and adduction of the affected leg, and an inability to bear weight are the most common signs of a hip fracture. Much less common signs may be mild discomfort and minimal shortening of the leg. (Burke & Walsh, 1997).

Inspect and palpate knees, ankles, and feet. Also assess comfort level particularly with movement (flexion, extension, rotation).

The common problems associated with the aged foot, such as soreness and aching, are most frequently due to improperly fitting footwear.

A great toe overriding or underlying the second toe may be halluces valgus (bunion).

Other abnormal findings may be enlargement of the medial portion of the first metatarsal head and inflammation of the bursae over the medial aspect of the joint.

Bunions are associated with pain and difficulty walking.

NEUROLOGIC SYSTEM

Assess the elderly client's mental status, including level of consciousness, orientation, judgment and insight, short-term and long-term memory. Ability to recall events or data and calculate are core elements of a mental status exam. (An explanation of the Mini-Mental Status Examination is presented in Display 23-4.) The test is used in various settings as a screening tool to measure insight, judgment, calculation ability, short-term and long-term memory as well as recall.

No observable change in cognition or motor function in the absence of disease; the usual loss of neurons and brain mass as well as increased response time seen in advanced age does not manifest as any abnormality.

Date and time may become a less significant indicator of orientation for the older person who lacks a routine, relies on others for the daily routine, or has significant deficits in vision or hearing.

A slight decline in short-term memory is common with aging.

Acute fluctuations in level of alertness (restlessness to lethargy) and difficulty concentrating are hallmarks of delirium. Speech may be rambling or incoherent, and the person often experiences disturbances in perception, such as illusions or hallucinations.

Difficulties with memory or cognition severe enough to cause problems in everyday activities, family and social life are abnormal at any age.

Decreased alertness, somnolence, disorientation, or amnesia possibly from transient ischemic attacks

Aphasia

(continued)

ASSESSMENT PROCEDURE	NORMAL FINDINGS	ABNORMAL FINDINGS
Observe for tremors and involuntary movements.	Resting tremors increase in the aged. In the absence of an identifiable disease process, they are not considered pathologic.	The tremors of Parkinson's may occur when the client is at rest. They usually diminish with voluntary movement. They usually begin in the hand and may affect only one side of the body (especially early in the disease). The tremors are accompanied by muscle rigidity.
Inspect client's muscle bulk, tone, and strength. On a scale of 0 to 5, evaluate tone and strength in biceps and triceps; grip; finger abduction; opposition of the thumb; flexion, extension abduction, and adduction of the hip; flexion and extension of the knee and dorsiflexion and plantar flexion of the foot.	Atrophy of the hand muscles may occur with normal aging.	Muscle atrophy can result from rheumatoid arthritis, muscle disuse, malnutrition, motor neuron disease, or diseases of the peripheral nervous system. Increased resistance to passive range of motion is a classic sign of Parkinson's disease especially in clients with bradykinesia. Decreased resistance may also suggest peripheral nervous system disease, cerebellar disease, or acute spinal cord injury.
Test sensation to pain, temperature, touch position and vibration as you would for a younger adult.	Touch and vibratory sensations may diminish normally with aging.	Unilateral sensory loss suggests a lesion in the spinal cord or higher pathways; a symmetric sensory loss suggests a neuropathy that may be associated with a condition such as diabetes.
Assess positional sense by using the Romberg test as presented in Chapter 22. The exception to the test are clients who must use assistive devices such as a walker.	Minimal swaying without loss of balance	Significant swaying with appearance of a potential fall

Validation and Documentation of Findings

The prevalence of chronic conditions in the frail elderly redefines the meaning of normalcy. The ability of the elderly person to function in everyday activities, albeit with environmental and pharmacologic intervention, is a more meaningful measure of normalcy than are physical findings alone. Thus, the objective and subjective data must reflect a functional and physical assessment.

EXAMPLE OF SUBJECTIVE DATA

Client is an 86-year-old female who moved to a residential care facility 2 years ago because of difficulty climbing stairs and maintaining her home of 43 years. Eats two meals a day in dining room and has had gradually improving appetite since moving into the care facility where meals are provided. Reports occasional episodes (about once every 2 to 3 weeks) of some difficulty swallowing, especially food that is dry or meat that is tough. Takes Metamucil to keep bowel movements regular and soft. Current prescription medications are Sinemet 1 tid and sodium Diuril 500 mg qd.

Has regular dental examinations and sucks on hard candy to alleviate dry mouth. Until last 5 to 10 years was 5 foot 5 inches and weighed approximately 130 lb. Denies any recent falls, syncopal episodes, or dyspnea with daily activities. However, client reports that she tries to sit for 5 to 10 minutes before standing to avoid becoming lightheaded. Client has yearly mammograms and Pap smears done. She is a breast cancer survivor and stopped taking supplemental estrogen when diagnosed and treated 20 years ago. She reports no bleeding or change in moles or skin lesions. Client receives B_{12} injections once a month and reports that she always has more energy for 2 to 3 weeks after that. Client reports that she has had to get new eyeglasses twice in the last 4 years and that she sees occasional halos around lights. She can still read the newspaper if she shines a bright light directly on it, and she enjoys quilting. Client states that she is contented with her life and keeps in touch with family and friends with frequent phone calls and occasional visits. She also has made several new friends since moving into the care facility.

EXAMPLE OF OBJECTIVE DATA

Client is 5 foot 3 inches, 122 lb; no orthostatic BP (lying = 150/85, HR = 88; sitting = 148/84, HR = 90; standing = 148/84, HR = 90); RR = 22. Client is independent in transfers and uses a walker for ambulating. She has a pill-rolling tremor at rest. She completes the "Get Up and Go" test with no noted abnormalities. Physical examination reveals a soft systolic murmur, absent pedal pulses, and soft and nondistended abdomen. She has no pedal edema; toenails are thick and yellowish; no ulcerations or discoloration of skin on lower extremities. No abdominal or carotid bruits noted on auscultation; lungs are clear to auscultation. The client's tongue is pink and moist. Her skin is thin and transparent. Numerous moles and brown, pigmented flat lesions (lentigenes) are noted on her hands, lower arms, and neck. Her fingernails are yellowish and brittle. A yellowish discoloration is noted for the lens of both eyes. Slight accumulation of dry earwax in outer ear; tympanic membrane is pink and intact. Mini Mental Status exam is normal. Client has no noted difficulties in conversation with memory, judgment, comprehension, or word recall.

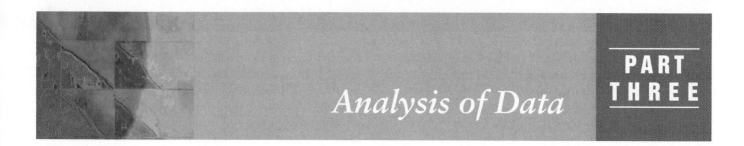

Once you have compiled the assessment data, use the diagnostic reasoning skills you have been practicing to analyze the information (see Chapter 7). Next, refer to Diagnostic Reasoning: Possible Conclusions below, which presents an overview of common conclusions that you may reach after assessing a frail elderly client. Then, review the case study that follows for help with analyzing the assessment data for a *specific* client. Also, consult the critical thinking exercise in the study guide/laboratory manual that can be purchased with this textbook.

Diagnostic Reasoning: Possible Conclusions

Listed below are some possible conclusions that may be drawn after assessment of a frail elderly adult.

SELECTED NURSING DIAGNOSES

From the collected subjective and objective data pertaining to the frail elderly client, identify abnormalities and cluster the data to disclose significant patterns or abnormalities. You will use these data to make clinical judgments (nursing diagnoses: wellness, risk, or actual) about the status of the client. Following is a listing of selected nursing diagnoses that you may identify.

Nursing Diagnoses (Wellness)

- Opportunity to Enhance Effective Caregiving

Nursing Diagnoses (Risk)

- Risk for Caregiver Role Strain, related to complexity of illness and lack of resources
- Risk for Ineffective Family Coping related to emotional conflicts secondary to chronic illness of parent
- Risk for Social Isolation related to inability to communicate effectively, decreased mobility, effects of chronic illness
- Risk for Imbalanced Nutrition, Less Than Body Requirements related to dysphagia, or decreased desire to eat secondary to altered level of consciousness
- Risk for Constipation related to decreased physical mobility, decreased intestinal motility, lower fluid intake, reduced fiber and bulk in diet, and effects of medications

- Risks for Impaired Skin Integrity related to loss of subcutaneous tissue, immobility, malnutrition
- Risk for Ineffective Thermoregulation related to loss of subcutaneous tissue, atrophy of eccrine sweat glands, decreased functioning of sebaceous glands
- Risk for Disturbed Sensory Perception: Visual—related to dry eyes, loss of lens transparency, slow pupil constriction—and Auditory—related to presbycusis
- Risk for Violence related to history of dysfunctional relationships within family structure and current stress of chronic condition
- Risk for Impaired Gas Exchange related to diminished recoil of lungs, less elastic alveoli, and loss of skeletal muscle strength
- Risk for Loneliness related to changing role and decreasing functional status

Nursing Diagnoses (Actual)

- Caregiver Role Strain related to severity of illness, complexity of caregiving tasks
- Diversional Activity Deficit related to impaired mobility or impaired thought processes
- Fatigue related to compromised circulatory or respiratory system and/or effects of medications
- Grieving related to debilitating effects of chronic illness
- Hopelessness related to deteriorating physical condition
- Chronic Sorrow of parent, caregiver, or individual client related to chronic physical or mental disability of client
- Ineffective Therapeutic Regimen Management related to lack of community resources
- Impaired Physical Mobility related to pain, age, pathologic changes in joints, or neuromuscular impairment
- Powerlessness related to unpredictability of complex disease processes and complex treatments
- Ineffective Protection related to decreased immunity
- Activity Intolerance related to weakness, fatigue, or pain related to joint and muscle deterioration and subsequent disuse of joints
- Ineffective Role Performance related to chronic illness
- Functional Urinary Incontinence related to immobility
- Wandering related to cognitive impairment, disorientation, and sedation
- Bathing/Hygiene Self-Care Deficit related to impaired physical or cognitive functioning

- Dressing/Grooming Self-Care Deficit related to impaired physical or cognitive functioning
- Acute Confusion related to adverse effects of medication, infection, or dehydration

SELECTED COLLABORATIVE PROBLEMS

After grouping the data, certain collaborative problems may emerge. Remember that collaborative problems differ from nursing diagnoses in that nursing interventions cannot prevent them. However, these physiologic complications of medical conditions can be detected and monitored by the nurse. In addition, the nurse can use physician- and nurse-prescribed interventions to minimize the complications of the problems. The nurse may also have to refer the client in such situations for further treatment of the problem. Following is a list of collaborative problems that may be identified when assessing the frail elderly client. These problems are worded as Potential Complications, or PC, followed by the problem.

- PC: Ankylosis
- PC: Joint contractures
- PC: Respiratory distress
- PC: Joint degeneration
- PC: Congestive heart failure
- PC: Myocardial infarction
- PC: Cerebrovascular accidents
- PC: Infections
- PC: Renal failure
- PC: Hypertension
- PC: Skin cancer
- PC: Osteoporosis
- PC: Pneumonia
- PC: Complications secondary to side effects, interactions, or adverse reactions to medications

MEDICAL PROBLEMS

After grouping the data, you may identify signs and symptoms that may require medical diagnosis and treatment. Referral to a primary care provider is necessary.

Diagnostic Reasoning: Case Study

You are doing the intake assessment on Mrs. Doris Miller, a 79-year-old Caucasian widow who lives with her daughter, Delores Ralston, in the daughter's large home in the suburb of a large city. Delores has a small greeting card business that she operates from her home. Also at home are her husband and two teenage children. After a recent hospitalization for bronchitis, Mrs. Miller was referred to the home health agency by her physician because the medication that she takes for diagnosed Parkinson's disease may need monitoring and Mrs. Miller's family needs to learn more about the disease.

Your assessment reveals a thin, fragile-appearing, pale woman who does not communicate verbally and sits hunched over in a wheelchair. She leans to the left. Mrs. Miller attempts to follow commands but cannot straighten her arms for you to apply a blood pressure cuff. Nor can she lift her head to look at you. She has a resting tremor of her hands, extreme flexion rigidity of her arms and legs, and a deformity of her feet which you identify as a "striatal foot." You notice that she has redness and cracking in the corners of her mouth, especially on the left; her daughter has placed a towel on the pillow her mother leans on "to catch the drool." While it is difficult to measure Mrs. Miller's blood pressure because of her arm flexion rigidity and because the sound is so soft, you finally hear 85/45 rt and 80/41 lt. Mrs. Miller's heart sounds are distant at 64 regular. Her lung sounds are clear but only heard in the upper lobes. Her height is reported at 5 feet 0 inches and her weight taken 2 weeks ago is 79 lb. Although her skin is pale, thin, and dry in most areas, it appears intact and well cared for. However, some redness is noted on the elbows and the antecubital spaces are moist with some beginning maceration.

Delores reports that Mrs. Miller cannot walk but does transfer from bed to chair with much help, it takes her "hours" to eat, she does not consume very much, and she tends to choke on fluids. She says that her mother has gotten progressively worse over the last year and rarely talks since her recent hospitalization for bronchitis. Delores expresses concern that she is unable to communicate with her mother because she gets so little feedback. "I don't know how much Mom hears or understands. I'm concerned that she is lonely, even with all the activity that goes on in this house."

1 Identify abnormal data and strengths (in both subjective and objective data).

SUBJECTIVE DATA (FROM DAUGHTER)
- Lives with daughter and family in a large home
- Daughter has small business in home
- Client has gotten progressively worse over the last year
- Can't walk but transfers with help
- Rarely talks
- Takes hours to eat—doesn't consume much
- Chokes on fluids
- Daughter questions ability to communicate with mother because of minimal feedback
- "I don't know how much Mom hears or understands."
- "I'm concerned that she is lonely, even with much activity."

OBJECTIVE DATA
- Diagnosed with Parkinson's disease
- Recent hospitalization with bronchitis
- Thin, fragile-appearing

- Hunched over, unable to lift head
- Wheelchair-bound
- Attempts but unable to follow commands
- Extreme flexion rigidity of arms and legs
- Resting tremor of hands
- Striatal foot deformity

- Cannot straighten arms
- Skin thin and dry, mostly intact and well cared for
- Redness of elbows
- Antecubital spaces moist with beginning maceration
- Weight 79 lb; height 5 foot 0 inches
- Lungs CTA, decreased in lower lobes

2 Cue Clusters	3 Inferences	4 Possible Nursing Diagnoses	5 Defining Characteristics	6 Confirm or Rule Out
A Can't walk, transfers with assistance • Wheelchair bound • Tremor, flexion rigidity • Cannot lift head • Attempts to follow commands	Manifestation of disease inhibits ability to walk, move self, and perform self-care	Impaired Physical Mobility related to loss of coordinated movements and rigidity	*Major:* Compromised ability to move purposefully within the environment. ROM limitations	*Confirm:* Meets major criteria
		Self-Care Deficit Syndrome, related to immobility due to Parkinson's disease	*Major:* Unable to bring food to mouth; unable to wash body or body parts; unable to dress/undress self; unable to get to toilet; unable to do any household activities	*Confirm:* Meets major defining characteristics for all self-care areas
B Takes hours to eat • Doesn't consume much • Thin, frail appearance • Weight 79 lb; height 5' • BP, 80–85/41–45 • Chokes on fluids	Difficulty swallowing and possible chewing result in decreased nutritional intake. Also client can't feed self or express preferences. Low BP could be due to medication or a sign of dehydration.	Imbalanced Nutrition: Less Than Body Requirements related to caregiver (CG) knowledge deficit regarding ways to increase caloric/nutritional density and promote increased intake	*Major:* Inadequate food intake *Minor:* Weight about 25% below ideal body weight for age, height, frame	*Confirm:* Meets major and minor defining characteristics, but major are by report of caregiver. Important to collect data regarding actual intake.
		Deficient Fluid Volume related to difficulty swallowing fluids	*Major:* Insufficient oral fluid; weight loss	Confirm, but evaluate hydration status more specifically to ascertain if client is actually dehydrated or if low BP and weight loss are due to other causes.
C • Chokes on fluids • Lungs CTA but decreased in bases • Recent hospitalizations for bronchitis	Difficulty swallowing and moving put client at risk for aspiration as well as decreased respiratory excursion secondary to weakness or the disease process.	Risk for Aspiration related to deficient knowledge of prevention strategies	*Major:* Impaired swallowing secondary to Parkinson's disease	*Confirm:* Meets major criteria
		Ineffective Breathing Pattern related to immobility and loss of energy	*Major:* None *Minor:* None	Rule out but monitor as a collaborative problem

Cue Clusters	Inferences	Possible Nursing Diagnoses	Defining Characteristics	Confirm or Rule Out
D • Skin thin and dry • Mostly intact, cared for • Redness of elbows • Moistness/macerations of antecubital spaces • Drools • Redness and cracking of corners of mouth	Caregiver providing good skin care but may lack the knowledge of how to manage skin care in moist areas of arms and mouths.	Impaired Skin Integrity related to caregiver's deficient knowledge of management for moist skin areas because of arm rigidity and drooling	*Major:* Disruptions of epidermal tissue	*Confirm:* Meets both major and minor defining characteristics
E Lives with daughter and family	Lack of communication may result in client not having socialization needs met. Daughter seems to need feedback. This may create stress especially because daughter has responsibilities related to work and other family members. Difficult to evaluate client's social needs or desires at this time.	Impaired Verbal Communication related to unknown causes	*Major:* Meets part of criteria but not all	Rule out because uncertain of client's ability to understand but collect more data because client does seem to try to follow commands.
		Caregiver Role Strain related to perceived inability to meet client's needs	*Major:* None expressed	Rule out for now, but consider as a risk diagnosis and collect more information regarding the effect of client's care needs on client and family members.
		Risk for Loneliness related to inability to participate in family activities	Not needed for risk diagnosis	Confirm, but collect more information about client's previous social behaviors.

7 Document conclusions.

The following nursing diagnoses are appropriate for Mrs. Miller and her daughter at this time:

- Impaired Physical Mobility related to loss of coordinated movement and to rigidity
- Self-Care Deficit Syndrome related to immobility due to Parkinson's disease
- Imbalanced Nutrition: Less Than Body Requirements related to caregiver knowledge deficit regarding ways to increase caloric and nutritional density and promote increased intake
- Deficient fluid volume related to difficulty swallowing fluids

- Risk for Aspiration related to caregiver knowledge deficit of prevention strategies
- Impaired Skin Integrity related to caregiver's deficient knowledge of management of moist skin areas related to arm rigidity and drooling
- Risk for Loneliness related to inability to participate in family activities

Collaborative problems related to Mrs. Miller's medical diagnosis and drug treatment could include:

- PC: Pneumonia
- PC: Constipation

REFERENCES AND SELECTED READINGS

Brown, J., Bedford, N., & White, S. (1999). *Gerontological protocols for nurse practitioners.* Philadelphia: Lippincott Williams & Wilkins.

Buchanon, D., Farran, C., & Clark, D. (1995). Suicidal thought and self-transcendence in older adults. *Journal of Psychosocial Nursing and Mental Health Services, 33*(10), 31–34.

Burke, M., & Walsh, M. (1997). *Gerontologic nursing: Wholistic care of the older adult* (2nd ed.). St. Louis, MO: Mosby.

Fitzpatrick, J., Fulmer, T., Wallace, M., & Flaherty, E. (Eds.). (2000). *Geriatric nursing research digest.* New York: Springer.

Folstein, M., Folstein, S., & McHugh, P. (1975). Mini-mental state: A practical method for grading the cognitive state of patients for the clinician. *Journal of Psychiatric Research, 12,* 189–198.

Francis, D., Fletcher, K., & Simon, L. (1998). The geriatric resource nurse model of care. *Nursing Clinics of North America, 33*(3), 482–496.

Gill, T. M., Williams, C. S., Mendes de Leon, C. F., & Tinetti, M. E. (1997). The role of change in physical performance in determining risk of dependence in ADLs among nondisabled community–living elderly persons. *Journal of Clinical Epidemiology, 60,* 765–772.

Herr, K. A., & Mobily, P. R. (1993). Comparison of selected pain assessment tools for use with the elderly. *Applied Nursing Research, 6*(1), 39–46.

Johnson, B. P. (1998). The elderly. In N. C. Frisch & L. E. Frisch (Eds.), *Psychiatric mental health nursing* (pp. 524–557). Albany, NY: Delmar.

Kennedy-Malone, L., Fletcher, K., & Plank, L. (2000*). Management guidelines for gerontological nurse practitioners.* Philadelphia: F. A. Davis.

Lonergan, E. (Ed.). (1996). *Geriatrics.* Stanford, CT: Appleton and Lange.

McGann, E. (2000). Pulmonary changes in elders. In J. Fitzpatrick, T. Fulmer, M. Wallace & E. Flaherty (Eds.), *Geriatric nursing research digest* (pp. 80–84). New York: Springer.

Mezey, M., Rauckhorst, L., & Stokes, S. (1993). *Health assessment of the older individual* (2nd ed.). New York: Springer.

National Academy on an Aging Society. (1999). *Chronic conditions: A challenge for the 21st century.* Washington, DC: Author.

Parshall, M. (1999). Adult emergency visits for chronic cardiorespiratory disease: Does dyspnea matter? *Nursing Research, 48*(2), 62–70.

Podsindlo, D., & Richardson, S. (1991). The timed "Get Up and Go": A test of basic functional mobility for frail elderly persons. *Journal of the American Geriatric Society, 39,* 142–148.

Rubenstein, L. Z., Josephson, K. P., & Osterwell, D. (1996). Falls and fall prevention in the nursing home. *Clinics in Geriatric Medicine, 12*(4), 881–902.

Tideiksaar, R. (1998). *Falls in older persons: Prevention and management.* Baltimore, MD: Health Professions Press.

Yesavage, J. A., & Brink, T. L. (1983). Development and validation of a geriatric depression screening scale: A preliminary report. *Journal of Psychiatric Research, 17,* 37–49.

Zembrzuski, C. (2001). *Clinical companion for assessment of the older adult.* Albany, NY: Delmar.

For additional information on this book, be sure to visit http://connection.lww.com.

Assessment of
the Family

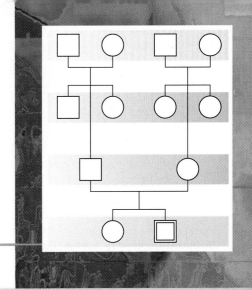

27

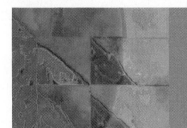

Structure and Function

PART ONE

Family assessment varies with the nurse's level of education in family nursing. It also varies with the type of family nursing care to be provided.

What Is Family Assessment?

The usual approach to family assessment taken by nurses who are not specialists in family nursing is to focus on the individual as client and the family as context for the client's illness and care. This type of family assessment focuses on determining strengths and problem areas within the family's structure and function that influence the family's ability to support the client.

A more advanced knowledge of family nursing is required to care for the family as client. Using this approach, the nurse views the family unit as a system and does not focus on any one family member. Instead, the nurse works at all times simultaneously with a mental picture of the family system and the individuals in the system. The nurse caring for the family system can still provide care to the individual when necessary, but the primary assessment and interventions are directed toward the family as a dynamic system.

To meet the needs of all nurses who assess the family, the information provided in this chapter is relevant to either approach. In addition, the step-by-step assessment of the family can be used with either the usual approach or the family systems approach (Display 27-1). To assess a family, the nurse must first determine who constitutes a family. The traditional definition of family was based on relationships of blood, marriage, or adoption. This definition has evolved over the years, and a number of different groups of people living together are now considered to be families (eg, single-parent families, extended families, communes, gay and lesbian couples, multigenerational families). Therefore, at the turn into the 21st century, those involved in family nursing incorporated a broader definition of family, thought to be more relevant to the times. This definition is: "The family is a social system composed of two or more persons who co-exist within the context of some expectations of reciprocal affection, mutual responsibility, and temporal duration. The family is characterized by commitment, mutual decision making and shared goals." (Department of Family Nursing, Oregon Health Sciences University, 1985, quoted in Hanson & Boyd, 1996, p. 6)

Based on this definition, it is relatively simple for the nurse to determine who constitutes a family—*the family is whoever they say they are.* If there is disagreement within a family about who is a part of the family and who is not, the nurse should note this difference of opinion and determine that the family for the assessment consists of those people who interact the most frequently.

Why Assess Families?

Among the many reasons for nurses to understand the concepts of family assessment, three stand out as important to a nursing assessment text:

- An ill person's family is an essential part of the context in which the illness occurs.
- The family members, the ill person, and even the illness itself interact in such a way that no one can be really separated from the rest.
- The statistics on family caregiving show that families are very much involved in providing care for an ill family member. (For an overview of the many people involved in caring for ill, chronically ill, or disabled family members in the United States, see Display 27-2).

The dynamic interactions of the ill family member, the illness, and the other family members will become clear as the elements of family assessment are described throughout this chapter.

Components of Family Assessment

In recent years, a variety of nursing models or frameworks have been developed as tools for assessing the family. Nurses have developed these models on the basis of family theories because none of the non-nursing fields has captured the necessary elements of the nursing of families. The framework used in this chapter for assessing the family is a modified combination of the Calgary Family Assessment Model (Wright & Leahey, 1994) and Friedman's (1992) Family Assessment Model. Regardless of which model or framework you use to assess the family, there are three essential components of family assessment especially prominent in all family assessment models:

- Structure
- Development
- Function

DISPLAY 27-1. Family Beliefs About Illness

In 1996, Wright, Watson, and Bell developed an Illness Beliefs Model focused on family members' beliefs about their illness experience. The beliefs that nurses commonly assess are:

- Beliefs about etiology
- Beliefs about treatment and healing
- Beliefs about prognosis and outcome
- Beliefs about the role of family members
- Beliefs about the role of health professionals
- Beliefs about spirituality and religion (Wright, Watson & Bell, 2000.)

Wright, Watson, and Bell (1996) note that the ultimate goal of this exploration of beliefs, used in their advanced clinical practice approach to family systems nursing, "is to enable healing for family members through the telling of their illness stories and the relief of emotional, physical, and/or spiritual suffering from their illness experience" (p. 1). Although the nurse without preparation above the baccalaureate level will be unable to use the Illness Beliefs Model in depth, a discussion of the family's beliefs and responses to illness may provide an opportunity for both the nurse and family to better understand the family's experience with ill health.

DISPLAY 27-2. Family Caregiving Statistics*

- More than one quarter (26.6%) of the adult population has provided care for a chronically ill, disabled or aged family member or friend during the past year. Based on current census data, that translates into more than 54 million people. (Source: National Family Caregivers Association (NFCA) Random Sample Survey of 1000 Adults, Funded by CareThere.com, Summer, 2000.)
- Caregiving is no longer predominantly a women's issue. Men now make up 44% of the caregiving population. (Source: National Family Caregivers Association (NFCA) Random Sample Survey of 1000 Adults, Funded by CareThere.com, Summer, 2000.)
- The value of the services family caregivers provide for "free" is estimated to be $196 billion a year. (Source: Health Affairs March/April 1999.)
- Virtually one half of the US population has a chronic condition. Of these, 41 million were limited in their daily activities. Twelve million are unable to go to school, to work, or to live independently. (Source: Chronic Care in America [Institute for Health & Aging, Univ. of CA/SF for the Robert Wood Johnson Foundation], 1996.)
- People over 85 years of age are the fastest-growing segment of the population. Half of them need some help with personal care. (Source: US Bureau of the Census Statistical Brief, *Sixty Five Plus in the United States,* May 1995.)
- Elderly caregivers with a history of chronic illness themselves who are experiencing caregiving-related stress have a 63% higher mortality rate than their non-caregiving peers. (Source: *Journal of the American Medical Association,* December 15, 1999, Vol. 282, No. 23.)
- The pool of family caregivers is dwindling. In 1990 there were 11 potential caregivers for each person needing care. In 2050 that ratio will be 4:1. (Source: Chronic Care in America—as above.)
- Sixty-one percent (61%) of "intense" family caregivers (those providing at least 21 hours of care a week) have suffered from depression. Some studies have shown that caregiver stress inhibits healing. (Source: National Family Caregivers Association/Fortis Long Term Care [Caregiving Across the Life Cycle] 1998; *Lancet* 1995;346) (Slowing of Wound Healing by Psychological Stress—Kiecolt-Glaser, JK et al.)
- Heavy-duty caregivers, especially spousal caregivers, do not get consistent help from other family members. One study has shown that as many as three fourths of these caregivers are "going it alone." (Source: Caregiving Across the Life Cycle—as above.)
- Approximately 80% of home care services are provided by family caregivers. (Source: US General Accounting Office [GAO/HEHS 95-26, "Long-Term Care: Diverse, Growing Population Includes Millions of Americans of All Ages"], 1994.)
- A recent study calculated that American business loses between $11 billion and $29 billion each year due to employees' need to care for loved ones 50 years of age and older. (Source: National Alliance for Caregiving/Met Life [Met Life Study of Employer Costs for Working Caregivers].)
- Fifty-nine percent of the adult population either is or expects to be a family caregiver. (Source: National Family Caregivers Association [Random Sample Survey of 1,000 Adults Sponsored by Aleve].)

*Compiled by the National Family Caregivers Association.

Environmental components, cultural-ethnic variations, and areas of family coping, family stress, and family communication are usually incorporated into these three essential components. However, some models of family assessment may address them separately.

FAMILY STRUCTURE

Family structure has three elements: internal structure, external structure, and context. Some theorists focus on a structural-functional framework that, when applied to family assessment, examines the interaction between the family and its internal and external environment (Friedman, 1992). Other theorists separate the assessment of family structure from assessment of family function within the structural component. This chapter focuses on the interaction between the family structure and its internal and external environment.

Internal Structure

The internal structure of a family refers to the ordering of relationships within the confines of that family. It consists of all the details in the family that define the structure of the family. Elements of internal structure include:

- Family composition (chartered in a genogram)
- Gender (and gender roles)
- Rank order
- Subsystems
- Boundaries
- Power structure

FAMILY COMPOSITION

Family composition can be illustrated by recording the family tree graphically as a genogram. A genogram helps the nurse view the whole family as a unit. It shows names, relationships, and other information such as ages, marriages, divorces, adoptions, and health data. Behavior and health–illness patterns can be examined using the genogram because both of these patterns tend to repeat through the generations. Figure 27-1 illustrates the format and symbols used for a simple three-generation family genogram.

GENDER

A family member's gender often determines his or her role and behavior in the family. Beliefs about male and female roles and behaviors vary from one family to another. Also, there may be female or male subsystems that share common interests or activities.

RANK ORDER

Rank order refers to the sibling rank of each family member. For instance, families treat the oldest child differently from the way they treat the youngest child. The rank order and gender of each family member in relation to

other siblings' rank order and gender make a difference in how the person will eventually relate to a spouse and children. For example, an older sister of a younger brother may bring certain expectations of how women relate to men into a marriage. If the older sister marries a man who is an older brother to a younger sister, there may be conflict or competition because each may expect to be the responsible leader.

SUBSYSTEMS

Each member of a family may belong to several subsystems. Subsystems may be related to gender, generational position (parents, grandparents, children), shared interests or activities (eg, music, sports, hobbies), or to function (work at home; work away from home). Examples of subsystems are parent–child, spousal, sibling, grandmother–granddaughter, mother–daughter, and father–son. Subsystems in a family relate to one another according to rules and patterns, which are often not perceived by the family until pointed out by an outsider.

BOUNDARIES

Boundaries keep subsystems separate and distinct from other subsystems. They are maintained by rules that differentiate the particular subsystem's tasks from those of other subsystems. The most functional families have subsystems with clear boundaries; however, some connection between subsystems is maintained along with the boundaries. According to a theory by the family therapist Salvator Minuchin, the family and its subsystems may have problems with connectedness, so that boundaries are either too rigid or too diffuse. Disengaged families have rigid boundaries, which leads to low levels of effective communication and support among family members. Enmeshed families have diffuse boundaries, which make it difficult for individuals to achieve individuation from the family.

POWER STRUCTURE

Power structure has to do with the influences each member has on the family processes and function. Some distribution of power is necessary to maintain order so the family can function. There is usually a power hierarchy, with the parents having more authority than the children. In the most functional families, parents have a sense of shared power and children gain increasing power as they mature and become more responsible.

A tool to help the nurse and family examine family structure, and function within the structure, is the Family Attachment Diagram. This is a diagram of the family members' interactions. It represents the reciprocal nature and quality of interactions. Figure 27-2 represents both a nuclear family with close and balanced relationships and a family with some conflicting, negatively attached relationships.

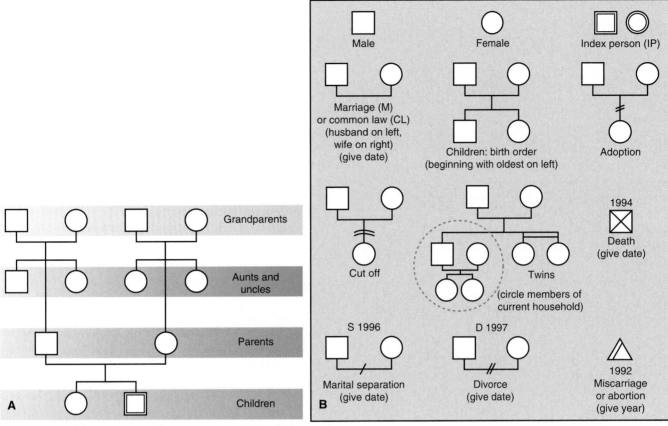

FIGURE 27-1. **(A)** Format used for genogram. **(B)** Symbols used in genogram.

External Structure

External structure refers to those outside groups or things to which the family is connected. External structures may influence aspects of the internal structure of the family. Two elements of external structure include extended family and external systems.

EXTENDED FAMILY

Extended family may consist of family members not residing in the home but with whom the family interacts frequently, such as grandparents or an aunt and uncle who live only 5 minutes away. It also may include family members with whom the family interacts infrequently, such as a first cousin who lives across the country and with whom the family communicates only through Christmas cards and a visit once every few years. However, the family feels confident that this cousin would be supportive in time of need. Another type of extended family is the "cut off" family member. An example would be a brother who left home 10 years ago and with whom there is no contact at all. This brother may still be considered extended family.

EXTERNAL SYSTEMS

External systems are those systems that are larger than the family and with which the family interacts. These systems include institutions, agencies, and significant people outside the family. Some specific examples of external systems include a family's health center, school, jobs, volunteer agency, church, recreational organizations, friends, neighbors, coworkers, and extended family (only those with whom interaction is frequent).

An ecomap can be used to assess the family members' interactions with the systems outside the family. The diagram, illustrated in Figure 27-3, is similar to the attachment diagram and shows the positive or conflicting nature of the family's relationships with outside groups or organizations.

Context

The context of a family refers to the interrelated conditions in which the family exists—it is the family's setting. Four elements make up the context of the family structure:

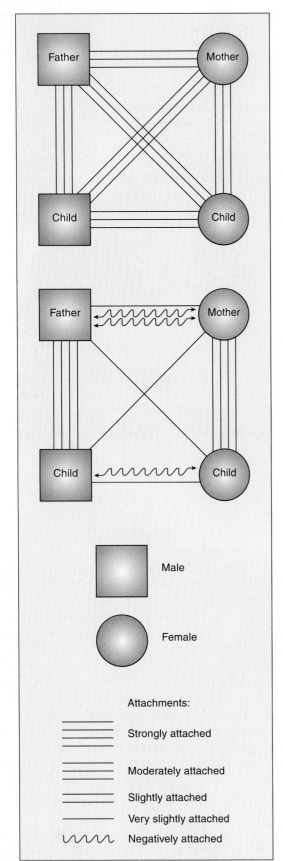

FIGURE 27-2. Family attachment diagram. **(Top)** Nuclear family with close, balanced relationship. **(Bottom)** Nuclear family with some conflicting, negatively attached relationships.

- Race-ethnicity
- Social class
- Religion
- Environment

Race or ethnicity may influence family structure and interactions. Assessment should include how much the family identifies with and adheres to traditional practices of a particular culture, whether the family's practices are similar to those of the neighborhood of residence, and whether the family has more than one ethnic or racial makeup.

The effects of *social class* and *religion* provide context for the family structure and lifestyle.

Environmental characteristics of the residence, neighborhood, and family–neighborhood interactions also clarify the context for the family structure and interactions.

FAMILY DEVELOPMENT

Like individuals, families go through stages of growth and development. These stages of development are as important to the health and well-being of the family as they are to the individual. In fact, a static family structure is dysfunctional. Friedman (1992) developed theories about family life-cycle stages and associated tasks. Three of these stages—the traditional nuclear family, divorced family, and remarried family stages and tasks—are described by Wright and Leahey (1994) and are presented in Displays 27-3, 27-4, and 27-5.

FAMILY FUNCTION

Friedman (1992) defined five basic family functions: Affective, socialization and social placement, reproductive, economic, and health care. For purposes of this chapter's approach to family assessment, however, the components of family function are organized into four areas:

- *Instrumental*—Instrumental function is the ability of the family to carry out activities of daily living in normal circumstances and in the presence of a family member's illness.
- *Affective and socialization*—Affective function refers to the family's response to all members' needs for support, caring, closeness, intimacy, and the balance of needs for separateness and connectedness. Socialization function refers to the family's ability to bring about healthy socialization of children.
- *Expressive*—Expressive function refers to communication patterns used within the family. Members of well-functioning families are able to express a broad range of emotions; clearly express feelings and needs; encourage feedback; listen attentively to one another; treat one another with respect; avoid displacing, distorting, or masking verbal messages; avoid negative circular com-

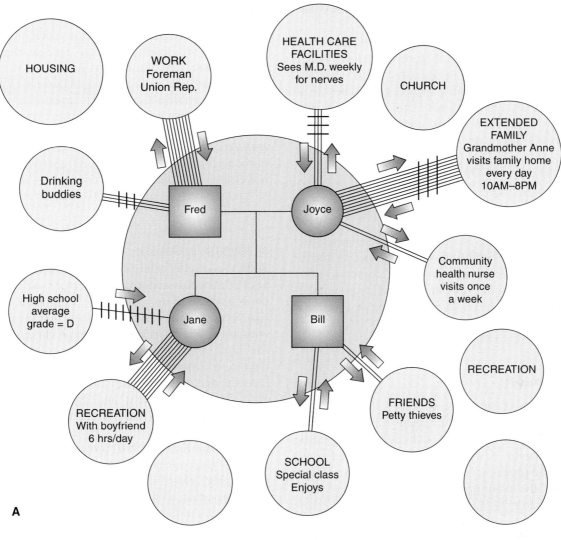

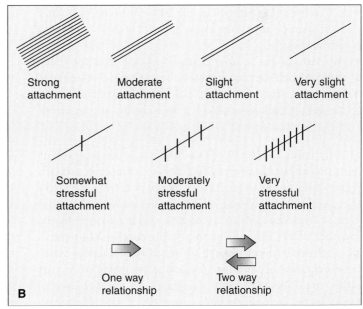

FIGURE 27-3. (A) An ecomap is used to assess family members' interactions with systems outside the family. (B) Symbols used in ecomap.

munication patterns; and use encouraging versus punishment methods to influence behavior.

- *Health care*—Assessment of health care function is useful for the nurse. It refers to family members' beliefs about a health problem; its etiology, treatment, and prognosis; and the role of professionals. Whether all family members agree or some members disagree with the beliefs helps the nurse to understand the family. The family's health promotion practices are also assessed.

THEORETICAL CONCEPTS OF FAMILY FUNCTION

Some of the components of family function discussed previously are based on theoretical concepts found in systems theory, Bowen's family system theory, and communication theory. It is important for the nurse to have a good understanding of these concepts before performing an assessment of family function.

Systems Theory

Systems theory holds that a system is composed of subsystems that are interconnected to the whole system and to each other by means of an integrated and dynamic self-regulating feedback mechanism. Systems theory can be applied to any group with reciprocal dynamic interaction. According to Boyd (1996), the major principles of systems theory as applied to family are:

- Each system has its own characteristics.
- The whole is greater than the sum of the parts (rather than just the sum of the characteristics of individual parts of the system).
- All parts of the system depend on one another (even though each part has its own role within the system).
- There are mechanisms for exchange of information within the system (subsystems) and within the broader environment (suprasystem).

Wright and Leahey (1994) list the major concepts of systems theory that they apply to families: A family is part of a larger suprasystem and is also composed of many subsystems (eg, parent–child, sibling, marital); the family as a whole is greater than the sum of its parts; a change in one family member affects all family members; the family is able to create a balance between change and stability; and family members' behaviors are best understood from a view of circular rather than linear causality. For example, any behavior of family member A affects family member B, and B's behavior then affects A. Therefore, rather than an individual causing a family problem, the behavior pattern or system causes another behavior.

Bowen's Family System Theory

The family therapist Bowen (discussed in Shepard & Moriarty, 1996) developed several concepts that are widely used to assess family function. Bowen views the nuclear family as part of a multigenerational extended family with patterns of relating that tend to repeat over generations. When the pattern of projecting anxiety onto a child continues across generations, it is called the *multigenerational transmission process*. Bowen theorizes that familial emotional and interaction patterns are reflected in eight interwoven concepts. Two of these concepts—differentiation of self and triangles—are especially important to grasp for assessment of family function.

DIFFERENTIATION OF SELF

Differentiation of self is assessed in relation to the boundaries of the subsystems in the structure of the family. This concept is based on a balance of emotional and intellectual levels of function. The emotional level, associated with lower brain centers, relates to feelings. The intellectual level, associated with the cerebral cortex, relates to cognition. How connected these levels, or systems, are affects the person's social functioning. The greater the balance between thinking and feeling, the higher the differentiation of self and the better the person is at managing anxiety.

Frisch and Kelley (1996) provide a summary of key elements of the concept of differentiation of self. The family with highly differentiated adult members is flexible in its interactions, seeks to support all members, understands each member as unique, and encourages members to develop differently from one another. Family roles are assigned on the basis of knowledge, skill, and interest.

The family with low levels of differentiation has adult members who demonstrate impulsive actions, who have difficulty delaying gratification, who cannot analyze a situation before reacting, and who cannot maintain intimate interpersonal relationships (similar to the developmental level of a 2-year-old child). Intense, short-term relationships are the norm, and emotionally based reactions can escalate into violence. Family roles are assigned on the basis of family tradition.

A moderately differentiated person is less dominated by emotions, but personal relationships are often emotion-dominated. Life is rule-bound, and thinking is usually dualistic (things and people are black and white, good or bad, smart or stupid). A situation cannot be perceived from any but a personal perspective. The person tends to "fuse" or become enmeshed with another in emotional relationships, losing himself or herself in the efforts to please the other. Families with moderately differentiated members exhibit rigid patterns of interactions that are rule-bound and have defined roles and acceptable behaviors.

DISPLAY 27-3. The Middle-Class North American Family Life Cycle

STAGE ONE: LAUNCHING THE SINGLE YOUNG ADULT

Tasks

Differentiating self

Developing intimate peer relationships

Establishing self in work and financial independence

STAGE TWO: MARRIAGE: THE JOINING OF FAMILIES

Tasks

Establishing couple identity

Realigning relationships with extended families to include spouse

Making decisions about parenthood

STAGE THREE: FAMILIES WITH YOUNG CHILDREN

Tasks

Making space for child

Joining in child-rearing, financial, and household tasks

Realigning relationships to include parenting and grandparenting roles

STAGE FOUR: FAMILIES WITH ADOLESCENTS

Tasks

Shifting parent–child relationships to permit adolescents to move in or out of system

Refocusing on midlife marital and career issues

Beginning shift toward joint caring for older generation

STAGE FIVE: LAUNCHING CHILDREN AND MOVING ON

Tasks

Renegotiating marital system as a dyad

Developing adult-to-adult relationships between grown children and their parents

Realigning relationships to include in-laws and grown children

Dealing with disabilities and death of grandparents

STAGE SIX: FAMILIES IN LATER LIFE

Tasks

Maintaining own or couple functioning and interest in the face of physiologic decline

Making room in the system for the wisdom and experience of the seniors

Dealing with loss of spouse, siblings, and other peers

Preparing for death

Adapted from Friedman, M. (1992). *Family nursing: Theory and practice* (3rd ed., pp. 82–105). Norwalk, CT: Appleton & Lange.

TRIANGLES

Triangles are discussed in relation to subsystems of family structure. Shepard and Moriarty (1996) describe Bowen's triangle as a relational pattern or emotional configuration that exists among one or two family members and another person, object, or issue. Triangles exist in all families; who makes up a triangle can change depending on the situation.

However, when two people avoid dealing with emotional closeness or an issue that produces anxiety, the two people may use a third person to evade the stress. For instance, a wife may pull in a child as a third person in the couple's relationship; the husband may distance himself from the conflict by deeper involvement in work. As the intensity of the relationship changes, the amount of interaction is usually

DISPLAY 27-4. The Divorce and Postdivorce Family Life Cycle

DIVORCE STAGE ONE: DECIDING TO DIVORCE

Issues

Accepting one's own part in the failure of the marriage

DIVORCE STAGE TWO: PLANNING THE BREAK-UP OF THE SYSTEM

Issues

Working cooperatively on problems of custody, visitation, and finances

Dealing with extended family about the divorce

DIVORCE STAGE THREE: SEPARATION

Issues

Mourning loss of nuclear family

Restructuring marital and parent–child relationships and finances; adaptation to living apart

Realigning relationships with extended family; staying connected with spouse's extended family

DIVORCE STAGE FOUR: DIVORCE

Issues

Retrieving hopes, dreams, and expectations from the marriage

POSTDIVORCE STAGE: SINGLE-PARENT (CUSTODIAL)

Issues

Making flexible visitation arrangements with ex-spouse and his or her family

Rebuilding own financial resources

Rebuilding own social network

POST-DIVORCE STAGE: SINGLE-PARENT (NONCUSTODIAL)

Issues

Finding ways to continue effective parenting relationship with children

Maintaining financial responsibilities to ex-spouse and children

Rebuilding own social network

Adapted from Friedman, M. (1992). *Family nursing: Theory and practice* (3rd ed., pp. 82–105). Norwalk, CT: Appleton & Lange.

---

balanced, so that as two members move closer, the third withdraws.

Communication Theory

Communication theory concerns the sending and receiving of both verbal and nonverbal messages. The focus is on how individuals interact with one another. According to Wright and Leahey (1994), the major concepts of communication theory applied to families are (1) all nonverbal communication is meaningful; (2) all communication has two major channels for transmission (verbal and non-

verbal, including body language, facial expression, voice tone, music, poetry, painting, and so forth); (3) a dyadic (two-person) relationship has varying degrees of symmetry and complementarity (both of which may be healthy depending on context); and (4) all communication consists of two levels—content (what is said) and relationship (of those interacting).

CYBERNETICS

Cybernetics combines communication and general systems theory. Wright and Leahey (1994) state that the major concepts of cybernetics as applied to families are

DISPLAY 27-5. The Remarried Family Life Cycle

STAGE ONE: ENTERING THE NEW RELATIONSHIP; CONCEPTUALIZING AND PLANNING THE NEW MARRIAGE AND FAMILY

Issues

Recommitting to marriage and to forming a family

Developing openness in the new relationship

Planning financial and coparental relationships with ex-spouse

Planning to help children deal with fears, loyalty conflicts, and membership in two systems

Realigning relationships with extended family to include new spouse and children

Planning maintenance of connections for children with extended family of ex-spouse(s)

STAGE TWO: REMARRIAGE AND FAMILY RECONSTITUTION

Issues

Restructuring family boundaries to allow for inclusion of new spouse/step-parent

Realigning relationships and financial arrangements throughout subsystems

Making room for relationships of all children with custodial and noncustodial parents and grand-parents

Sharing memories and histories to enhance step-family integration

Adapted from Friedman, M. (1992). *Family nursing: Theory and practice* (3rd ed., pp. 82–105). Norwalk, CT: Appleton & Lange.

that families possess self-regulating abilities through the process of feedback (Fig. 27-4), and feedback processes can occur simultaneously at different systems' levels within families.

CIRCULAR COMMUNICATION

One example of a feedback system in communications is circular communication. Circular communication is a reciprocal communication between two people. Wright and Leahey (1994) note that most relationship issues have a pattern of circular communication. One person speaks and the other person interprets what is heard, then reacts and speaks on the basis of the interpretation, creating a circular feedback loop based on the individuals' perceptions and reactions.

Circular communication can be positive or negative. An example of negative circular communication is as follows: An angry wife criticizes her husband; the husband feels angry and withdraws; the wife becomes even angrier and criticizes more; the husband becomes angrier and withdraws further. Each person sees the problem as the other's, and each person's communication influences the other person's behavior. Positive and negative circular communication patterns are illustrated in Figure 27-4.

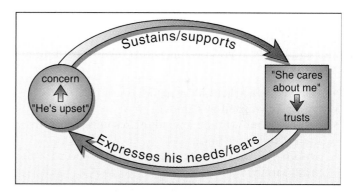

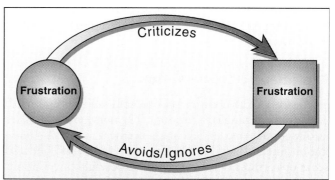

FIGURE 27-4. **(Top)** Positive circular communication. **(Bottom)** Negative circular communication.

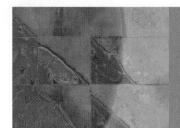

Family History and Dynamics

Wright and Leahey (2000) believe that family nursing knowledge can be obtained and applied even in very brief meetings with a family. They provide a guide to a 15-minute (or shorter) family interview (pp. 275–288). Key elements of the interview, which occurs only in the context of a therapeutic relationship, are manners, therapeutic conversation, family genogram (and ecomap as appropriate), therapeutic questions, and commendations. See Display 27-6 for a summary of the interview technique.

FAMILY INTERVIEW TECHNIQUES

The brief interview consists of several elements, which are described thoroughly by Wright and Leahey in the context of the Calgary Family Assessment Model and the Calgary Family Intervention Model. Essential points follow:

Manners

The simple acts of good manners that invite a trusting relationship are:

- Always call the client(s) by name.
- Introduce yourself by name.
- Examine your attitude and adjust responses to convey interest and acceptance.
- Explain your role for the time you will spend with the client/family.
- Explain any procedure before entering the room with equipment to perform the procedure.
- Keep appointments and promises to return.
- Be honest.

Therapeutic Conversation

Therapeutic conversation is purposeful and time-limited. The art of listening is paramount. The nurse *not only* makes information giving and client involvement in decision making an integral part of the care delivery process but also seeks opportunities to engage in purposeful conversations with families. Nurse–family therapeutic conversations can include such basic ideas as:

- Invitations to accompany the client to the unit, clinic, or hospital

- Inclusion of family members in health care facility admission procedures
- Encouragement to ask questions during client orientation to a health care facility
- Acknowledgment of client and family's expertise in managing health problems by asking about routines at home
- Presentation of opportunities to practice how client will handle different interactions in the future, such as telling family members and others that they cannot eat certain foods
- Consultation with families and clients about their ideas for treatment and discharge (Wright & Leahey, 2000, p. 280)

Family Genograms and Ecomaps

The genogram posted clearly in the client documentation acts as a continuous visual reminder to caregivers to "think family."

Therapeutic Questions

In a very brief family interview, key questions can be asked to involve family members in family health care. Wright and Leahey suggest that the nurse think of at least three key questions to routinely ask all family members (modified to fit the particular setting or context). Examples offered are:

- With which of your family (or friends) would you like us to share information? With which ones do you prefer not to share information (indicates alliances, resources, and possible conflictual relationships)?
- How can we be helpful to you and your family during your stay in this health care facility (clarifies expectations, increases collaboration)?
- What has been most helpful (least helpful) in your past experience with health care facilities (identifies past strengths to repeat and problems to avoid) (Wright & Leahey, 2000, pp. 281–282)?
- What is the greatest challenge facing your family during this illness (indicates actual or potential suffering, roles, and beliefs)?
- Who do you believe is suffering most by this illness (identifies the family member most in need of support and intervention)?

DISPLAY 27-6. **Tips for Conducting the 15-Minute Family Interview**

- Introduce yourself and use good manners in interactions.
- Seek opportunities to involve family in care delivery and decision making.
- Use active listening, create family genograms (ecomaps), and ask key therapeutic questions to help family members (and the nurse) better understand the family's needs and beliefs about themselves and the illness.
- Seek opportunities to commend individuals and the family.

Commendations

Offer at least one or two commendations during each meeting with the family. The individual or family can be commended on strengths, resources, or competencies observed or reported to the nurse. Commendations are observations of behavior. Look for patterns, not one-time occurrences to commend. Examples include: "Your family shows much courage in living with your wife's cancer for 5 years"; "Your son is so gentle despite feeling so ill" (Wright & Leahey,

2000, p. 282). The commendations offer family members a new view of themselves. Wright and Leahey propose that many families experiencing illness, disability, or trauma have a "commendation-deficit disorder" (p. 282). Changing the view of themselves helps the family members to look differently at the health problem and more toward solutions.

As appropriate, incorporate some of these interview techniques in your practice. Also refer to Display 27-7, which offers options for assessing families and helping them make caregiving decisions.

DISPLAY 27-7. **Guide for Family Caregivers**

A helpful tool for exploring family beliefs and functioning during illness is the Options, Outcomes, Values, Likelihoods (OOVL) Decision-Making Guide for Patients and Their Families (Lewis, Hepburn, Corcoran-Perry, Narayan & Lally, 1999). The OOVL Guide recognizes that family caregivers faced with daily decision making for an ill family member may feel burdened, frustrated, and in conflict with other family members, and offers a strategy to guide caregivers thinking about factors involved in decision making.

In addition, the OOVL Guide supports nurses as advocates in affirming clients' values and preferences and offers decision makers structures and procedures. To help caregivers understand family beliefs about decision making, the OOVL Guide suggests asking six questions focused on options, outcomes, values, and likelihoods:

1. What do you need to make a decision about?
2. What actions are you considering (options)?
3. What would you like to have happen as a result of your choice (outcomes)?
4. How important is each outcome to you (values)?
5. How likely is it that each option will lead to each outcome (likelihoods)?
6. What option is most likely to achieve the best outcome?

(A) Decision-making grid.

Besides questions, the OOVL Guide provides a decision-making grid. Options are listed on the left side and outcomes on the top. The grid allows you to work out the level of likelihood (low, moderate, or high) for each option. If, for instance, the caregiver desires a specific outcome as opposed to other possible outcomes, then possible options are determined and the relative likelihood of the possible outcomes are determined. Once the outcome likelihoods are determined for each option (choice of behavior), a decision to act can be made.

(continued)

DISPLAY 27-7. Guide for Family Caregivers (continued)

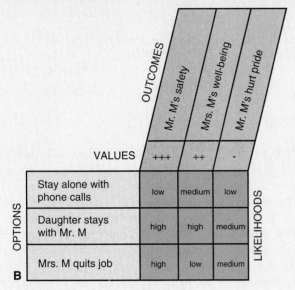

(B) Example of completed decision grid.

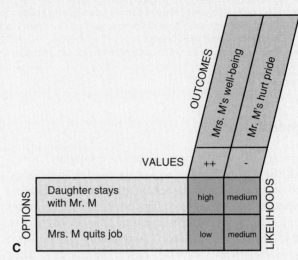

(C) Example of simplified decision grid.

ASSESSMENT OF THE FAMILY

ASSESSMENT PROCEDURE	NORMAL FINDINGS	ABNORMAL FINDINGS

INTERNAL FAMILY STRUCTURE

Composition

Assess family composition. Use a genogram and fill in as much information as possible. Ask the following questions:

- What is the family type (nuclear, three generation, single-parent)?
- Who does the family consider to be family?
- Has anyone recently moved in or out? Has anyone recently died?

New baby born into family or young adult moving out reflects normal life cycle tasks. Death is also a normal part of life, but it is not often viewed as a family strength.

A new baby or a young adult moving out may cause excessive stress for family. Death of a family member often causes a variety of different reactions including denial, extreme grief, depression, and even relief. Serious family problems may result when family members react to, and deal with, the death differently.

Gender Role

Gender often determines an expected family role. Ask each family member the following question:

What are the expected behaviors for men in your family? For women?

Family members understand and agree on expected gender-related behaviors; expected behaviors are flexible.

Rigid, traditional gender-related behaviors reduce the family's flexibility for meeting family needs. One or more family members have different beliefs about expected behaviors for men and women, which can lead to family conflict.

> **Tip From the Experts** It is important to ask both the men and women what they perceive to be the role of men and women in the family because they may perceive the roles differently.

(continued)

ASSESSMENT PROCEDURE	NORMAL FINDINGS	ABNORMAL FINDINGS
Rank Order		
Spousal rank order often plays a significant role in family harmony. Ask spouses: What rank order did you have in your childhood family (eg, older sister, youngest brother)? Using the family's answers and information you know concerning birth order, ask yourself: Are spouses' birth rank orders likely to be complementary or competitive?	Complementary birth order of spouses can support each spouse's interaction with the other based on past experiences with siblings (eg, older brother marries younger sister).	Competitive birth order of spouses may result in problems. For example, if an older brother marries an older sister, both may be used to being the responsible leader.
Subsystems		
Ask the family questions about attachments within the family. For example, is there a mother–daughter relationship? How strong is it? Use a family attachment diagram to determine family subgroups. Assessment of the function of family subgroups is covered under assessment of family function.	Family subgroups are present and appear healthy.	Family subgroups are absent or appear excessively strong, excluding other family members. For instance, a strong female subgroup of mother and daughters may work to exclude the father/husband from important family activities or decision making. Or an overly strong spousal subsystem may impose an emotional distance between parents and children.
Family Boundaries		

Boundaries separate family subsystems. Ask the family questions about how the subsystems are fixed within the family. For example, is the mother–daughter subsystem totally separated from the father–son subsystem? Based on the family's answers, ask yourself the following questions:
 	
   Are there boundaries between subsystems?
   What types of boundaries are present?
     Note: Assessment of the function of family boundaries is covered under "Family Function."
	Permeable boundaries are present.	Rigid or diffuse boundaries are present.

Family Power Structure		
Ask the family to rate the structure of the family on a scale with chaos (no leader) at one end, equality in the middle, and domination by one individual at the other end. If the family is dominated by one individual, ask the client who that person is.	A power hierarchy with parents equally in control, but tending toward egalitarian and flexible power shifts, is considered normal. This type of structure demonstrates respect for all family members and encourages family development and effective functioning.	Chaotic or authoritarian power structures tend to prevent effective family functioning and individual development.

EXTERNAL STRUCTURE

Assess extended family by asking, "Are extended family members available to help support your immediate family?"	Extended family can provide emotional and other support to the family.	Lack of extended family or no contact with extended family results in no support for immediate family.
To assess external systems, ask the family questions about relationships with external systems (eg, agencies and people outside immediate family). Use an ecomap to record and view these relationships. Then ask yourself the following questions based on the ecomap: What relationship is there between the family and external systems?	Positive relationships with external systems are beneficial to the family.	Conflictual relationships with external systems add stress to the family.

(continued)

ASSESSMENT PROCEDURE	NORMAL FINDINGS	ABNORMAL FINDINGS
Are external systems over-involved or underinvolved with the family?	Balanced involvement with external systems adds to the health of the family.	Too little or too much involvement with external systems can prevent the family from effectively using resources to meet its needs. In addition, either over-involvement or under-involvement with external systems can add great stress to the immediate family.

Context

To assess context, ask questions that relate to ethnicity, social class, religion, and environment.
    How does the family's race or ethnicity affect the family structure and function?
    How does the family's race or ethnicity affect interactions with neighbors?
    How does the family's race or ethnicity affect interactions with external systems?
	A family that has a strong ethnic identity and lives in a similar ethnic society will usually have plentiful support.	Racial or ethnic difference from the neighborhood or larger society can produce misunderstanding and negatively affect communications and interactions.

What social class is most representative of the family? Do social class factors affect the family's ability to meet its needs?	Cultural, social, and economic factors of the family's social class support the family's ability to meet its needs.	Cultural, social, and economic resources associated with social class may be inadequate to meet family needs.
Is religion important to the family?	Religion provides the family with supportive spiritual beliefs.	Religious controversies among family members may produce family conflict.
Are environmental characteristics of the residence and neighborhood adequate to meet family needs?	The residence and neighborhood are safe, and necessary resources are available.	The residence or neighborhood is not safe. Resources are not readily available.

FAMILY DEVELOPMENT: LIFE-CYCLE STAGES AND TASKS

Ask the family questions about the family's life-cycle stage(s). Can the family meet the tasks of the current life-cycle stage(s) with which it is dealing?	The family has successfully met the tasks of previous life-cycle stages and can meet the tasks of its current life-cycle stage.	The family has not adequately met tasks of previous life-cycle stages and may be unable to meet tasks of the current stage.

FAMILY FUNCTION

Instrumental Function

Evaluate whether the family can carry out routine activities of daily living.	The family has successfully met routine daily living needs of all family members.	The family cannot carry out one or more activities of daily living.
Does a family member's illness affect the family's ability to carry out activities of daily living?	The family can continue to carry out activities of daily living even with the added stress of an ill family member.	The added stress of caring for an ill family member prevents the family from adequately carrying out one or more activities of daily living.

Affective and Socialization Function

Observe family interactions and ask questions to determine if family members provide mutual support and nurturance to one another.	Families that can meet psychological needs for support and nurturance of family members provide an opportunity for each individual adequately to self-differentiate and reach emotional maturity.	Families that cannot provide for psychological needs for support and nurturance make self-differentiation and emotional health of the members unlikely.

(continued)

ASSESSMENT PROCEDURE	NORMAL FINDINGS	ABNORMAL FINDINGS
Are parenting practices appropriate for healthy socialization of the children?	Parenting practices based on respect, guidance, and encouragement (rather than punishment) encourage socialization.	Parenting practices based on control, coercion, and punishment discourage socialization.
What function do subgroups serve within the family?	Subgroups are flexible and assist family to meet changing needs.	Rigid subgroups do not easily change to meet individual needs.
Are there alliances that produce triangles?	Flexible alliances and triangles form to maintain family functioning.	Rigid alliances and triangles are formed to balance negative forces and stress. They are a coping mechanism.
What function do boundaries serve within the family?	Permeable boundaries encourage emotional development and self-differentiation of family members.	Rigid or diffuse boundaries discourage emotional development and self-differentiation.
Are family members enmeshed? Disengaged?	Adequate involvement of family members without enmeshment or disengagement serves as support for family function and individual development.	Enmeshed or disengaged family members cannot adequately self-differentiate.

EXPRESSIVE FUNCTION

Ask the family and observe interactions to *assess emotional communication:* Do all family members express a broad range of both negative and positive emotion?	Open expression and acceptance of feelings and emotions within a family encourages positive family functioning.	Lack of acceptance of emotional expression, or acceptance of emotional expression by only some family members, tends to prevent effective family development and functioning.
Assess verbal communication: Are verbal messages clearly stated? Displaced? Masked? Distorted?	Clear verbal messages increase open communication.	Displaced, masked, or distorted messages obstruct open communication and may reflect underlying problems in family functioning.
Assess nonverbal communication: Do nonverbal communications match verbal content?	Clear and open communications have verbal and nonverbal elements that match.	Nonverbal communications that do not match verbal content suggest a lack of honesty or openness in the communication.
Assess circular communication: Is there an evident pattern of circular communication? If so, is it negative or positive?	Positive circular communication helps to build up the participants.	Negative circular communication reinforces interpersonal conflict and prevents an understanding of the intended message.

Health Care Function

To assess the family's health care function, ask the following questions:
    What do family members believe about the etiology, treatment, prognosis of the health problem?
    What do family members believe about the role of professionals, role of the family, and level of control the family has relative to the health problem? Are family members' beliefs in agreement or discord?
	Agreement among family members reduces conflict.	Disagreement among family members produces conflict and draws on energy and emotional resources needed to handle the health problem.

(continued)

ASSESSMENT PROCEDURE	NORMAL FINDINGS	ABNORMAL FINDINGS
What strengths does the family believe it has for coping with the health problem?	If the family perceives strengths, it will be more likely to cope effectively.	If the family does not perceive strengths, it will have difficulty coping with the health problem.
Are the family's health promotion practices supportive of family health?	A pattern of health promotion practices provides a basis for building in health care for a particular health problem.	A family that has little practice of health promotion behaviors will have difficulty incorporating health care practices for a particular problem into its routines.

Multigenerational Patterns

Look back over the assessment and determine if there are any multigenerational patterns evident in any categories.	Multigenerational patterns of positive behaviors are often seen in effectively functioning families.	Multigenerational patterns of ineffective or destructive behaviors make change more difficult.

Validation and Documentation of Findings

Validate the family assessment data that you have collected. This is necessary to verify that the data are reliable and accurate. Document the assessment data following the health care facility or agency policy.

EXAMPLE OF SUBJECTIVE AND OBJECTIVE DATA

Family is composed of two parents, one grown child, and one grandmother—a three-generation family. The family also considers two other grown children and their spouses as immediate family. The second-oldest child was married recently and moved away, and the family views the event positively. Family members agree on expected gender-related behaviors, which are flexible. The wife is the youngest daughter of her family, and the husband is the oldest son of his family. Subgroups and triangles between family members are flexible. The boundaries between subgroups are permeable.

The two parents are equally in control, but the grown child and grandmother share equally in decisions that affect the family. The grandmother's other daughter and family live close by and provide emotional and financial support in caring for her. The family is positively involved in the local church, the grown child has a group of supportive friends, the grandmother goes to the local senior center 3 days a week, and the parents enjoy being involved with the local garden club. Time spent with groups outside the family is balanced evenly with time spent with the immediate family.

The family lives in a safe home and in a neighborhood with people of similar ethnicity. The family's cultural, social, and economic factors support their ability to live well. The family is currently able to meet the tasks of its life cycle stage. The family has met routine activities of daily living needs of its members, despite the fact that the grandmother needs care because of arthritis and macular degeneration. Family meets the psychological needs for support and nurturance of all family members. Family members feel free to express and accept feelings and emotions openly. The family, including the extended family, is in agreement about caring for the grandmother's health conditions and feels confident that they can meet her needs. Multigenerational patterns of positive behaviors are seen in this family.

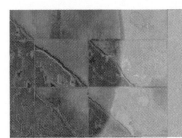

PART THREE

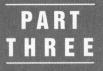

Analysis of Data

After you have collected your assessment data, you will need to analyze the data, using diagnostic reasoning skills, which you can practice as you read through the case study (below) about a specific client. Another opportunity to analyze data is presented in the critical thinking exercise included in the accompanying laboratory manual/study guide available with this textbook.

Diagnostic Reasoning: Possible Conclusions

Listed below are some possible conclusions following assessment of the family.

SELECTED NURSING DIAGNOSES

After collecting subjective and objective data pertaining to the family, you will need to identify abnormal data and cluster the data to reveal any significant patterns or abnormalities. These data will then be used to make clinical judgments (nursing diagnoses: wellness, risk, or actual) about the status of the family. Following is a list of selected nursing diagnoses that you may identify when analyzing data for this part of the assessment.

Nursing Diagnoses (Wellness)

- Opportunity to Enhance Family Coping
- Health-Seeking Behaviors
- Opportunity to Enhance Spiritual Well-Being
- Opportunity to Enhance Parenting
- Opportunity to Enhance Home Maintenance
- Opportunity to Enhance Family Processes

Nursing Diagnoses (Risk)

- Risk for Caregiver Role Strain
- Risk for Impaired Parent/Infant/Child Attachment
- Risk for Impaired Parenting
- Risk for Compromised Family Coping
- Risk for Dysfunctional Family Processes
- Risk for Impaired Home Maintenance

Nursing Diagnoses (Actual)

- Caregiver Role Strain
- Compromised Family Coping
- Ineffective Family Coping: Disabling
- Dysfunctional Family Processes: Alcoholism
- Interrupted Family Processes
- Impaired Home Maintenance
- Ineffective Family Therapeutic Regimen Management
- Parental Role Conflict
- Impaired Parenting
- Impaired Social Interaction
- Social Isolation
- Spiritual Distress
- Ineffective Role Performance

SELECTED COLLABORATIVE PROBLEMS

After grouping the data, it may become apparent that certain collaborative problems emerge. Remember, collaborative problems differ from nursing diagnoses in that they cannot be prevented by nursing interventions. However, these physiologic complications of medical conditions can be detected and monitored by the nurse. In addition, the nurse can use physician- and nurse-prescribed interventions to minimize the complications of these problems. The nurse may also have to refer the client in such situations for further treatment of the problem. Following is a list of collaborative problems that may be identified when assessing the family. These problems are worded as Potential Complications, or (PC), followed by the problem.

- PC: Marital conflict
- PC: Child abuse
- PC: Spouse abuse

MEDICAL PROBLEMS

After grouping the data, it may become apparent that the family has signs and symptoms that may require medical or mental health professional diagnosis and treatment. Referral to a primary care provider is necessary.

773

Diagnostic Reasoning: Case Study

The case study presents assessment data for a specific family. It is followed by an analysis of the data to arrive at specific conclusions.

The Ross family has returned to the clinic for help with dealing with Dan's recent diagnosis and treatment for type 1 diabetes mellitus. Dan is a 17-year-old high school senior who is not following the diet–exercise–insulin protocol prescribed 4 months ago. The physician refers the Ross family to the nurse to help the family address the identified problem of Dan's refusal to follow the protocol. Because the diet and food preparation affect the whole family, sister Jenna attends the family session as well.

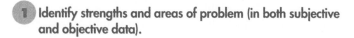 **Identify strengths and areas of problem (in both subjective and objective data).**

SUBJECTIVE DATA

- Identified problem is Dan's refusal to follow prescribed diabetes protocol.
- Parents express concern and caring for Dan's well-being and request assistance with dealing with Dan's diagnosis and treatment.
- Parents express frustration with inability to get Dan to follow the doctor's orders.
- Dan expresses frustration at having a disease and at being asked to follow a protocol that makes him different from his friends and unable to do the things that they do (eg, diet, exercise, partying).
- Dan expresses frustration at having his parents tell him what to do.
- Jenna expresses frustration at Dan for upsetting the family, especially at mealtime, particularly in regard to what family members eat and how they interact.

OBJECTIVE DATA

- Family members appear tense when describing the effect of trying to deal with Dan's disease and his refusal to follow the protocol.
- Dan is a 17-year-old high school senior who is scheduled to leave for college in 6 months. He was diagnosed with type 1 diabetes mellitus 4 months ago.
- Dan has been seen by the physician and in the emergency room five times in the past 4 months for complications resulting from not following the protocol.
- Dan and his parents describe a good understanding of the disease and reasons for the protocol.
- Review of the genogram reveals a multigenerational pattern of very responsible, accomplished males who are leaders in their families and in their communities (Figure 27-5).
- The family is in the life-cycle stage of family with adolescents, with a task of shifting parent–child relationships to permit an adolescent to move out of the system.
- A circular pattern of communication has developed: Between the parents and between the father and Dan. Dan is not following the protocol, which increases the parents' anxiety and frustration. In addition, the parents' expressions of displeasure cause Dan's sense of loss of control, anxiety, and frustration to increase.

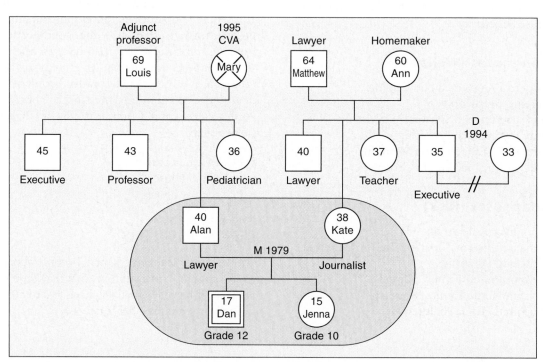

FIGURE 27-5. Genogram of the Ross family.

2 Cue Clusters	3 Inferences	4 Possible Nursing Diagnoses	5 Defining Characteristics	6 Confirm or Rule Out
A • Family asks for assistance with dealing with Dan's diagnosis and treatment	Family recognizes the role of family interactions and seeks to improve these to meet better family and son's needs.	(Family) Health-Seeking Behaviors: request for assistance to improve the ability to deal with son's diagnosis and treatment	*Major:* Expressed desire to seek information for (family) health promotion *Minor:* Expression of desire for increased control of health practice (family)	Rule out diagnosis. The request for assistance originated with the family, but the pattern of interaction for which assistance is sought is already a problem.
B • Dan has returned to doctor and ER five times in 4 months • Parents express frustration at inability to get Dan to follow treatment protocol • Life-cycle stage of family with adolescents • Family members appear tense • Circular communication pattern increasing anxiety	Parents' and Dan's separateness and togetherness needs and needs for control are in conflict. This is increasing family anxiety, which affects Dan's self-care practices and parents' care for Dan.	Risk for Impaired Home Maintenance related to interaction of disease protocol, family life-cycle stage, and family communication patterns	*Major:* Outward expression of difficulty by family in caring for a family member at home *Minor:* Impaired caregivers: anxious. Negative response to ill family member (regarding level of self-care responsibility)	Confirm the diagnosis because building anxiety and stress place the family at risk for inability to care for ill member.
C • Multigenerational male gender role expectations for high level of personal responsibility identified by family • Circular communication pattern increasing parents' and Dan's anxiety • Dan is not following diabetes treatment protocol	Dan may be perceived as not living up to family role for males. Circular communication pattern preventing parents and Dan from listening to and understanding each other. Puts Dan at physical risk for complications.	Interrupted Family Processes related to interaction of disease, treatment protocol, family life-cycle stage, multigenerational gender roles, and family communication process	*Major:* Family system cannot or does not adapt constructively to crisis Family system does not support open and effective communication among family members. *Minor:* Family system cannot or does not meet physical/emotional needs of all its members	Confirm diagnosis
D • Dan is a senior in high school and ready to move out of family to college soon • Family members state anxiety increasing • Parents state anxiety and concern about inability to get Dan to follow protocol • Circular communication pattern increasing anxiety	Family life-cycle tasks for Dan's separation needs are not being met because of threat of dependency and treatment protocol's intrusion into peer relationships. Family is succumbing to pattern of increasing anxiety, which is blocking Dan's desire to care for himself. Separation and togetherness needs of life-cycle stage are increasing family stress.	Ineffective Family Coping related to intrusion of son's diagnosis and treatment, family life-cycle stage, and increasingly ineffective communication patterns	*Major:* None *Minor:* None	Rule out this diagnosis because it does not meet the defining characteristics for this diagnosis

2 Cue Clusters	**3** Inferences	**4** Possible Nursing Diagnoses	**5** Defining Characteristics	**6** Confirm or Rule Out
• Dan has visited doctor and ER five times in four months for complications • Family life-cycle stage of family with adolescents **E** • Significant disease diagnosed 4 months ago • Five subsequent visits to doctor and ER for complications • Dan not following diet–exercise–insulin protocol • Dan reports frustration at having protocol that makes him different and unable to do things his friends do • Family describes frustration and anxiety over Dan's refusal to follow protocol, putting self at risk, and not taking responsibility for self-care	Dan is grieving over loss of health and sense of identity with peers. Family is grieving over loss of youthful member's health. Family's and Dan's adaptation to the loss is not progressing because of increasing frustration and anxiety.	Risk for Dysfunctional Grieving (family) related to loss of health status of youthful family member	*Major:* Unsuccessful adaptation to loss Prolonged denial, depression *Minor:* Failure to restructure life after loss	Loss of health status present; adaptation to the loss incomplete and compromised Diagnosis of Risk for Dysfunctional Grieving confirmed

7 **Document conclusions.**

Three family nursing diagnoses are appropriate at this time. Two are risk diagnoses, and one is an actual problem diagnosis.

- Risk for Impaired Home Maintenance
- Risk for Dysfunctional Grieving (family)
- Interrupted Family Processes

The collaborative problems for which the nurse will monitor and refer, if necessary, to the appropriate mental health or family therapist are:

- PC: Depression
- PC: Marital conflict

REFERENCES AND SELECTED READINGS

Bomar, P., & McNeely, G. (1996). Family health nursing role: Past, present, and future. In P. Bomar (Ed.). *Nursing and family health promotion* (2nd ed., pp. 3–21). Philadelphia: W. B. Saunders.

Boyd, S. (1996). Theoretical and research foundations of family nursing. In S. Hanson & S. Boyd (Eds.). *Family health care nursing* (pp. 41–53). Philadelphia: F. A. Davis.

Duvall, E. (1979). *Marriage and family development* (5th ed.). Philadelphia: J. B. Lippincott.

Friedman, M. (1992). *Family nursing: Theory and practice* (3rd ed.). Norwalk, CT: Appleton & Lange.

Frisch, N., & Kelley, J. (1996). *Healing life's crises.* Albany, NY: Delmar.

Hanson, S., & Boyd, S. (1996). *Family health care nursing.* Philadelphia: F. A. Davis.

Lewis, M., Hepburn, K., Corcoran-Perry, S., Narayan, S., & Lally, R. M. (1999). Options, outcomes, values, likelihoods decision making guide for patients and their families. *Journal of Gerontological Nursing, 25* (12), 19–25.

Shepard, M., & Moriarty, H. (1996). Family mental health nursing. In S. Hanson & S. Boyd (Eds.). *Family health care nursing* (pp. 303–326). Philadelphia: F. A. Davis.

Wright, L., & Leahey, M. (2000). *Nurses and families: A guide to family assessment and intervention* (3rd ed.). Philadelphia: F. A. Davis.

———. (1994). *Nurses and families: A guide to family assessment and intervention* (2nd ed.). Philadelphia: F. A. Davis.

Wright, L., Watson, W., & Bell, J. (2000). Family nursing unit: Therapeutic approach [On-line]. Available: http://www.ucalgary.ca/nu/.

For additional information on this book, be sure to visit http://connection.lww.com.

Community
Assessment

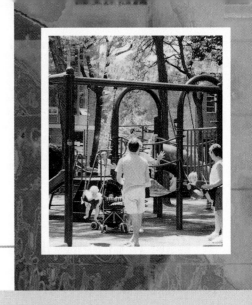

28

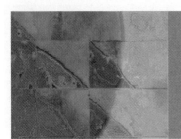

PART ONE

Structure and Function

What Is Community Assessment?

A thorough assessment of a community first requires an understanding of the concept of community. *Community* may be defined several ways, depending on the conceptual view of the term. It may be defined from a sociologic perspective as "a collection of people in a place who interact with one another and whose common interests and goals give them a sense of belonging" (Stackhouse, 1998, p 79). Another definition of *community* is an "open social system characterized by people in a place over time who have common goals" (Smith & Maurer, 2000).

Classification of community depends on the definition. For purposes of assessment, communities are classified according either to location or social relationship. The first classification is a geopolitical community in which people have a time-and-space relationship. Geopolitical communities may be determined by natural boundaries, such as rivers or lakes or mountain ranges. For example, the Mississippi River separates the states of Missouri and Illinois, and the Great Lakes serve as a boundary between Canada and the United States. Geopolitical boundaries also may be manmade—counties, cities, and voting districts. Another example of this type of community is a census tract, which is determined by the government to organize demographic data collection.

Communities also may be classified by relationships among a group of people. These communities are usually centered on a specific goal or function. For example, a group such as Mothers Against Drunk Drivers (MADD) may center on eliciting support for a new ordinance regulating hours of bars and taverns. These types of communities can be organized to address a common interest or problem, such as a state student nurses' association or a support group for family and friends of Alzheimer's patients. Another example of this type of community would be those with similar religious or political beliefs. Any number of social communities may exist within the boundaries of a geopolitical community.

The purpose of community assessment is to determine the health-related concerns of its members, regardless of the type of the community. The nurse gets to know the community, its people, its history, and its culture through the assessment process. A thorough and accurate assessment provides the foundation for diagnosis and for planning appropriate nursing interventions.

MODELS OF COMMUNITY ASSESSMENT

A number of different models or frameworks have been used to provide the structure for assessing both geopolitical and social communities. Wilson (2000) used the Neuman Systems model as the conceptual framework for a comprehensive community assessment from which cardiovascular disease was determined to be of primary concern. The Roy Adaptation model was expanded by Dixon (1999) to provide the framework for community health practice in which comprehensive assessments were performed using the four adaptive modes of physiologic needs, role function, group identity, and interdependence. The Lundeen Community Nursing Center model was the basis for a continuous community assessment emphasizing health promotion (Lundeen, 1999). Eshlemann and Davidhizar (2000) used the Community As Partner model as a guide for baccalaureate nursing students assigned to assess the health needs of a local community.

The Community As Partner model provides a comprehensive guide for data collection based on Betty Neuman's model (Neuman, 1972). Central to the model are the people, or core, of the community. This component includes demographic information as well as information about the history, the culture, and the values and beliefs of the people. Also identified are eight subsystems that are affected by the people of the community and that directly contribute to the health status of the community. These include housing, fire and safety, health, education, economics, politics and government, communication, and recreation.

The Community As Partner model has been adapted for use in this chapter. The nursing assessment section (below) is a step-by-step assessment of the community; it has three categories: People, environment, and health. What to assess in each category and how to assess it are discussed. The nursing component is inherent throughout each category.

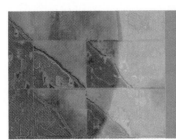

Community assessment involves both subjective and objective data collection using a variety of methods. Subjective data collection includes perceptions of the community by the nurse as well as by members of the community. The nurse should spend time in the community to "get to know" the people and get a sense of their values and beliefs. Through the process of participant observation, the nurse hopes to become accepted as a member of the community. This method of data collection allows the nurse to partici-

pate in the daily life of the community, to make observations, and to obtain information about the structures and influences that affect the community. The nurse should ask key members or leaders of the community as well as "typical" residents to provide further information and insight about the community. Objective methods of data collection include using surveys and analyzing existing data, such as census information, health records, and other public documents.

ASSESSMENT OF THE COMMUNITY

ASSESSMENT PROCEDURE	NORMAL FINDINGS	ABNORMAL FINDINGS
COMMUNITY HISTORY		
Study the history of the community to gain insights into the health practices and belief systems of its members. Look for this information at the local library or ask local residents.	The community history should include initial development, any specific ethnic groups that may have settled there, past economic trends, and past population trends.	The history of some communities may include episodes that have had a disruptive influence on the people of the community, such as relocation because of repeated flooding or a history of racial or ethnic problems.
DEMOGRAPHIC INFORMATION		
Age and Gender		
Obtain age and gender information from census data. Age is the most important risk factor for health-related problems. Gender may be another important risk factor.	A healthy community has a distribution of individuals in various age ranges: >5, 5–19, 30–34, 35–54, 55–64, and 65+ years as well as no significant difference between percentages of males and females.	Communities with a large percentage of elderly people or very young children generally have more health-related problems. Communities with a preponderance of women of child-bearing age may need to improve access to or expand family planning and prenatal services as well as well-baby programs.
Racial and Ethnic Groups		
Study census figures and state and local population reports to learn about racial and ethnic groups that reside in the community.	The lack of significant numbers of racial or ethnic groups suggests that special screenings or programs to meet their needs may not be required.	A large percentage of ethnic or racial minorities may indicate that certain health concerns exist within these groups of individuals. For example, Native Americans often have a higher incidence of diabetes or alcohol-related health problems, and sickle cell anemia is prevalent among African Americans. Therefore, special screenings and programs to meet the needs of particular racial or ethnic groups become more important to these communities.

(continued)

ASSESSMENT PROCEDURE	NORMAL FINDINGS	ABNORMAL FINDINGS

Vital Statistics

Obtain vital statistics data from the National Center for Health Statistics, state and local agencies, and from hospital records. These include birth and death records as well as crude death rates (age and cause), specific death rates, and infant–maternal mortality. Morbidity (disease) data also are important indicators of the health status of the community.

Expected birth, death, and morbidity data should generally reflect overall rates for the United States. See Displays 28-1, 28-2 and 28-3 for age-related causes of mortality.

Higher-than-expected birth, death, and morbidity rates, especially age- and cause-specific rates, may indicate a lack of services or programs in critical areas. For example, higher-than-expected teen birth rates may be related to a lack of family planning services or education; high mortality rates associated with motor vehicles, especially when alcohol is involved, indicate that alcohol awareness programs should be instituted; and greater-than-expected rates of tuberculosis or sexually transmitted infections indicate that primary and secondary prevention efforts should be increased.

Household Size, Marital Status, Mobility

Refer to the US Census Bureau for the following information: Number of people per household, their marital status, and the stability of the population.

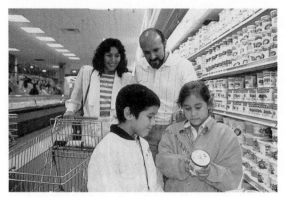

One of the three types of households cited by the Bureau of the Census is a married couple with children.

The Census Bureau identifies three major types of households: Married couple, female householder (no husband present), and male householder (no female present). The nature and size of households in the United States have changed significantly in the last 50 years. Household size has decreased from 3.3 to 2.6 persons per household. The number of divorced people has quadrupled since 1970. Married couples currently make up only 54% of all households, and the number of children living with one parent has more than doubled. It is expected that the number of households with children will continue to decrease (Clemen-Stone, Eigsti & McGuire, 1998). Americans also are a mobile population, moving for education, jobs, or retirement. A healthy community adjusts to these changes and organizes to meet the needs of the population.

Single parents (teenage mothers and fathers, in particular) are at greater risk for health problems, especially those related to role overload. This occurs because single parents often have to assume the role of the missing parent in addition to their own role. Single mothers report a higher incidence of children's academic and behavioral problems than mothers in two-parent families. Unmarried people have a higher mortality rate than do married people. Elderly people living alone also are at higher risk for health problems. In addition, some immigrant groups, such as migrant farm families, are at higher risk. Communities that do not adapt to meet the needs of the mobile population compromise the continuity and quality of care for these people.

(continued)

ASSESSMENT PROCEDURE	**NORMAL FINDINGS**	**ABNORMAL FINDINGS**

Values and Religious Beliefs

Obtain data to determine values and religious beliefs of the community from the local Chamber of Commerce, community directories, surveys, and personal observation and interview. Each community's values are unique, rooted in tradition, and exist to meet the needs of the population (Anderson & McFarlane, 2000). Religious beliefs and culture are closely related to the community's values.

Certain religious beliefs directly affect health practices, such as use of family planning services. Healthy communities demonstrate an awareness and respect for different values and religions. There is a deliberate effort among various subgroups to communicate and to work together. Many communities form ministerial alliances, in which various denominations collaborate to meet the needs of the community. They may provide emergency shelters, operate soup kitchens or food pantries, and provide help for special populations.

Some communities exhibit conflict among subgroups. Different values, beliefs, and practices are seen as a threat to one group's own values and beliefs. An unhealthy community may fail to recognize the existence of cultural or religious differences and believe that all members of the community should conform to one set of values. In such communities, anyone who does not fit the accepted norm is "suspect." Such an atmosphere does not enhance the overall health status of the community, which makes it difficult or even impossible for members to collaborate on problem solving.

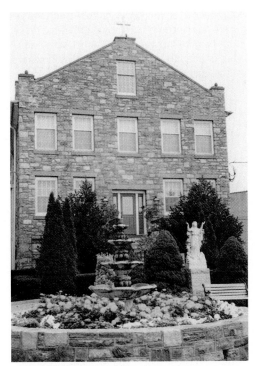

Community values and religious beliefs are unique and rooted in tradition.

PHYSICAL ENVIRONMENT

Geographic Boundaries

Identify geographic boundaries of the community by obtaining information from the library or local assessor's office. Geographic boundaries are determined in a number of different ways. They can be man-made—bridges, highways, railroads—or natural landmarks—rivers, lakes, and so forth. Boundaries also can be determined by census tracts, congressional districts, or school districts.

Boundaries of a community should be clear, uncontested, and accepted by all members.

Boundaries may not always be clearly identified, and communities may not be able to resolve disputes without legal action. One community may seek to annex part of another because of access to certain resources, or a group or neighborhood may attempt to separate legally from the larger community because of ideologic differences, zoning regulations, or other issues. Disagreement about such issues may disrupt delivery of services.

(continued)

ASSESSMENT PROCEDURE	NORMAL FINDINGS	ABNORMAL FINDINGS
Neighborhoods Neighborhoods have specific populations and boundaries and may vary a great deal in culture, leadership, and ties to the larger community. They may be composed of certain ethnic groups, economic classes, or age groups.	Neighborhoods should be cohesive with a sense of identity, yet have strong ties to the larger community.	Some neighborhoods may seek to isolate themselves from the larger community or may be resistant to others who wish to move into the neighborhood. In such situations, conflicts often arise and mistrust may be widespread.
Housing Obtain housing information from census documents, local housing authority, and local realtors. A community should provide a variety of housing options.	A healthy community can provide enough safe, affordable housing to meet the needs of its members.	A lack of adequate housing may be a serious problem in some communities. A shortage of safe, low-income housing contributes directly to the growing number of homeless individuals and families. Other communities may have a serious shortage of adequate rental property or special housing for the elderly or disabled. Inadequate housing contributes to various health problems related to safety, lead poisoning, and communicable diseases.
Climate and Terrain Determine climate and geographic terrain of the area. This information may be obtained from the local library, government agencies, and direct observation. Climate varies from region to region, as does geographic terrain. Both have a direct effect on the health of the community.	Healthy communities have the resources to deal with whatever problems climate and terrain present. Such problems include extreme cold or heat, floods, fires, blizzards, tornadoes, and earthquakes. Certain health problems may be more prevalent in particular geographic areas (eg, Lyme disease, Hanta virus). Safety programs, civil defense and disaster plans, and health education programs should be in place.	Communities inadequately prepared to deal with disasters or health problems related to climate or terrain do not adequately meet the needs of their members. This may result in a higher incidence of the following problems: heat exhaustion, deaths due to overexposure to cold, myocardial infarctions related to shoveling snow, skin cancers, infectious diseases, and deaths and injuries related to other natural disasters.

(continued)

ASSESSMENT PROCEDURE	NORMAL FINDINGS	ABNORMAL FINDINGS

HEALTH AND SOCIAL SERVICES

Hospitals, Clinics, Emergency Care, Private Practitioners

Determine the number of health care facilities and providers available to the community. Information about health services can be obtained from the Chamber of Commerce, local professional organizations, telephone directories, and from personal interview and observation.

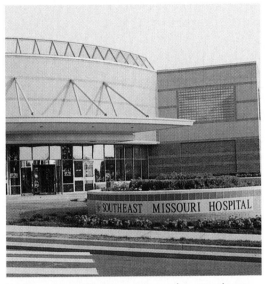

Healthy communities have access to adequate primary health care services.

A healthy community provides adequate primary care services. These include private and non-profit facilities staffed with physicians, nurse practitioners, and nurses who provide medical/surgical, obstetric/gynecologic, pediatric, emergency, and various diagnostic and preventive services. Specialty services, such as neonatal intensive care, should be easily accessible to the community. In addition to physicians and nurses, the health care delivery system should include dentists, physical therapists, and dietitians, among others. Facilities and providers should accept third-party reimbursement including insurance, workers' compensation, Medicare, and Medicaid.

Many communities (particularly rural ones) cannot provide needed services, especially in obstetric care. It is not unusual for a person to be 100 miles or more away from the nearest services. In addition, funding problems have caused many small rural hospitals to close, leaving residents miles away from any health care at all. Ambulance service also may be of concern for some communities. Accessibility may be limited because fewer health care providers are willing to accept some types of third-party reimbursement, especially Medicaid.

(continued)

ASSESSMENT PROCEDURE	NORMAL FINDINGS	ABNORMAL FINDINGS

Public Health and Home Health Services

Obtain data concerning public health and home health services from local directories, the Chamber of Commerce, and personal interviews. Local public health agencies have the responsibility for protecting the health of the general population. Program objectives are related to primary prevention and early diagnosis and are directed toward meeting health objectives of the federal program Healthy People 2010. Home health care is the fastest-growing component of the health care system as hospital stays become briefer while the need for skilled care remains.

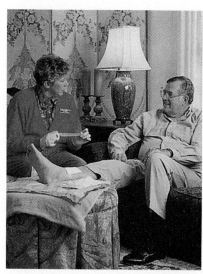

Healthy communities have adequate and available home health and skilled nursing care, among other services.

Local public health services are usually delivered through county or city health departments. Wellness programs also may be offered through nonofficial agencies such as hospitals. Home health services may be provided through a number of different agencies, such as a Visiting Nurses Association (VNA), official agencies, and free-standing proprietary agencies. Services provided include skilled nursing care, homemaker and home health aides, medical social services, nutritional consultation, and rehabilitation services.

Many public health services are supported through local tax revenues. Therefore, small rural communities may not be able to provide the types of services needed, and limited access to these services may be another problem. Certain services may not be offered by home health agencies, and funding to cover visits for people who are not eligible for third-party reimbursement may be limited.

(continued)

ASSESSMENT PROCEDURE	NORMAL FINDINGS	ABNORMAL FINDINGS

Social Service Agencies

Determine what level of social services is available in the community. Information may be obtained through local directories, the Chamber of Commerce, or personal interviews.

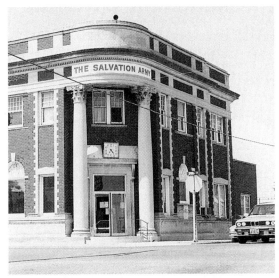

The Salvation Army is a voluntary agency that provides full-scale community services.

A community should provide agency social services—both public and voluntary—for people of all ages. Official agencies include mental health facilities and children and family services, such as Medicaid, Medicare, and Aid to Families with Dependent Children. Other agencies may be substance abuse treatment facilities, centers for abused women, hospices, and shelters for the homeless. Volunteer agencies (Meals on Wheels, Salvation Army) also offer community services. Additional social programs may come from groups such as the YMCA and Parents Without Partners. Safe and certified day care facilities for children and the elderly should also be available.

Access to social service agencies may be an obstacle in urban areas. In addition, funding may limit the number of programs and people these agencies serve. Availability of programs may be limited in rural areas. For example, homeless shelters and shelters for abused women are nonexistent in many rural areas. Lack of transportation in rural areas may also make programs inaccessible. The cost of certain treatment programs can limit accessibility for those who are uninsured.

Long-Term Care Services

Determine if long-term care services are available in the community to meet the needs of elderly members, those with a chronic disabling illness, and those who have suffered disabilities due to accidents. Information can be obtained from local directories and the Chamber of Commerce.

A community should provide services for long-term care assistance in the home as well as extended care for those who can no longer function in their homes. For example, personal care assistance or a visiting nurse and skilled nursing and intermediate care facilities for those needing certain levels of nursing care should be available. Rehabilitation centers, boarding homes, continuing care, and retirement centers are other types of long-term care facilities.

The capacity of available agencies may not meet the needs of the community. Facilities that provide care for special concerns (eg, Alzheimer's disease) may not be available. Facilities in urban areas may be inaccessible because of cost. Rural areas, in general, are likely to have inadequate long-term care resources. This is especially true in areas such as respite care and personal care assistance in the home.

(continued)

ASSESSMENT PROCEDURE	NORMAL FINDINGS	ABNORMAL FINDINGS

Economics

Gather the following types of data from census records, Department of Labor, the Chamber of Commerce, and local and state unemployment offices: median household income, per capita income, percentage of households or individuals below the poverty level, percentage of people on public assistance, and unemployment statistics. In addition, collect data about local business and industry, types of occupations/jobs in which people are employed, and occupational health risks associated with certain occupations.

Income has a direct relationship to the health of the residents of the community. The income of the members of the community determines its tax base and, therefore, the ability of the community to provide needed services (Clark, 1999). Businesses and other local employment opportunities are key factors in economic well-being. Businesses provide not only jobs but also goods and services such as groceries, pharmaceuticals, and clothing.

Economic instability in a community can lead to a number of health-related concerns. Poverty is associated with higher morbidity and mortality rates. High unemployment creates a stressful environment and a threat to the psychological well-being of the community.

Occupationally related death and injuries cost the nation billions of dollars a year, with lung diseases and musculoskeletal injuries being the most frequent causes.

Safety: Fire, Police, Environmental Protection

Gather information regarding fire, police, and environmental services from local and regional police departments, fire departments, environmental agencies, and state health departments. Fire, police, and environmental services also are given the responsibility to protect the community from direct and indirect threats to its health and safety. These services have both a direct and an indirect relationship to a community's well-being in knowing that it is safe from a variety of threats.

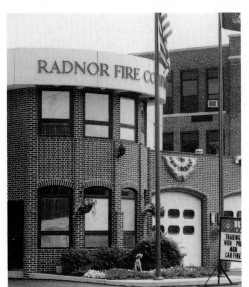

Adequate fire and police department protection are hallmarks of healthy communities.

Police should be equipped with personnel, equipment, and facilities to protect the community. Education programs, such as Drug Abuse Resistance Education; property and personal identification programs; support programs, such as Neighborhood Watch; and animal control programs may also be run by the police department. Numbers of firemen, equipment, response time, and education programs contribute to adequate fire protection services. Environmental protection includes a wide range of programs, such as water and air quality, solid and hazardous waste disposal, sewage treatment, food/restaurant inspection, and monitoring of public swimming pools, motels, and other public facilities.

Violent crimes, such as homicide, rape, robbery, and assault, or increases in loss of life and property due to fires may indicate that police and fire protection services are inadequate. This also contributes to a general sense of fear or uneasiness throughout the community and can lead to increased levels of stress and a loss of a sense of well-being. Poor environmental protection can result in repeated cases of illnesses, injuries, and even death. A number of health problems can be linked to the environment (eg, waterborne illnesses and lead poisonings).

(continued)

ASSESSMENT PROCEDURE	NORMAL FINDINGS	ABNORMAL FINDINGS

Transportation

Determine transportation options available in the community. Obtain information from local business, through interviews, from county and state highway departments, and direct observation.

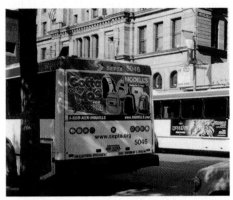

Access to transportation has a direct relationship to access to health care and other essential services.

The most common means of transportation in most communities is the private automobile. Other sources of transportation locally, in addition to walking, are taxis, buses, subways, and trains. Long-distance transportation, in addition to the car, includes air, rail, and bus service. Roads, highways, and sidewalks should be kept in good repair, and communities should have adequate programs for snow and ice removal. Special transportation needs include school transportation and transportation for the elderly or disabled people.

Lack of a private automobile is a particular problem in rural areas where public means of transportation are often nonexistent. Personal safety or cost may make public transportation inaccessible for many in urban areas. Inability to access health care services because of transportation difficulties is a particular problem for the elderly and for mothers with young children

Education

Review levels of education, current school enrollment, and education resources in the community. Information may be obtained from census reports, local school districts, and state education agencies.

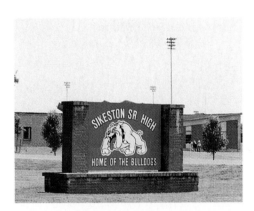

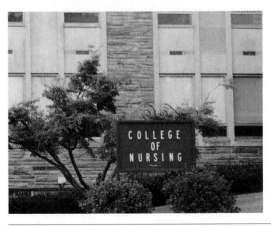

(Top) Secondary schools (high schools) need to be up-to-date and safe with qualified staff and programs that meet the needs of students and the community. **(Bottom)** Schools at higher level (community colleges and universities) offer the community significant opportunities for learning and vocational fulfillment.

In general, the higher the community's education level, the healthier the community. Resources needed to meet community educational needs include preschool and early intervention programs, public or private elementary and secondary schools, and access to advanced education. Adequate supply of qualified educators, up-to-date facilities and equipment, and programs that meet the needs of those with special problems are keys to a successful education system. Low absenteeism and higher-than-average scores on standardized achievement tests are indicators of effectiveness. Adult education, including GED classes, should be available. Additionally, comprehensive school health programs directed by nurses, school meal programs, and after-school programs contribute to the health of a community. Public libraries are an important community supplement to the school system.

Funding for school systems is a growing problem for many communities, especially those in areas where the economy is weak. Many school districts are supported in part by property taxes, so in an area where the tax base is low and unemployment is a problem, schools may struggle to maintain even minimum standards. As a result, many districts must cut equipment purchases, special programs, and extracurricular activities such as music and athletics. School violence is a growing problem for many communities. Another indication that there are problems in the school system is a high dropout rate and a low graduation rate. Availability of post-high school colleges or technical programs may be limited in rural areas. Access may be limited because of lack of financial resources. Libraries often depend on local taxes, and so, in times of economic difficulty, these facilities often face cutbacks.

(continued)

ASSESSMENT PROCEDURE	NORMAL FINDINGS	ABNORMAL FINDINGS

Government and Politics

Review the government and political structure of the community. Information may be obtained from local government agencies, local political organizations, and from local directories. Government agencies are often directly involved in planning and implementing programs that affect the health of the community. In addition, the political system is responsible for health-related legislation. It is important to assess both the formal and informal power structure in the community.

The government of a community and its leaders should be responsible and accessible to the community. Members should participate in the governance of the community, as evidenced by voter registration and percentage of registered voters who actually vote in elections. Open community meetings should be held to allow citizens a forum in which they may express their views. Political organizations should represent the differing views of the citizens, and there should be an atmosphere of tolerance among the different groups.

If the government is not responsive to the views of the citizens, members of the community will become increasingly apathetic, and, as a result, the formal power structure becomes ineffective in meeting the needs of the community. Low voter turnout and little representation of groups with different views and interests may be indicative of an unresponsive or unrepresentative government.

Communication

Determine both the formal and informal means of communication in the community. Sources of information include the Chamber of Commerce, telephone book, and personal interviews and observations.

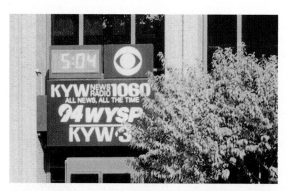

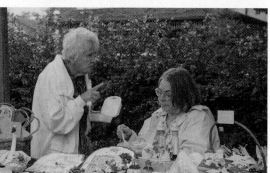

Communication: News travels (*top*) over the airways and (*bottom*) by word of mouth.

Open channels of communication are an important factor in maintaining the health of the community. Larger communities usually have many types of formal communication sources, including local television and radio stations, local cable access, and one or more daily newspapers. Smaller communities usually have access to fewer television and radio stations, and newspapers are typically published weekly. Mail delivery may also be limited. However, on-line services are usually available in all communities. Informal communications include word of mouth, newsletters, and bulletin board notices at community centers, stores, businesses and churches and fliers distributed by mail or door-to-door.

Traditional means of communication may not be sufficient for some people in the community. Those who do not speak or understand English may not be able to obtain necessary information through either formal or informal means. Some people may not have access to telephone or other means of communication. Elderly people and others who are isolated also may be at a disadvantage.

(continued)

| ASSESSMENT PROCEDURE | NORMAL FINDINGS | ABNORMAL FINDINGS |

Recreation

Determine availability of community recreation and leisure programs for individuals and groups in all age ranges. Information may be obtained from the Chamber of Commerce, park and recreation departments, churches, schools, businesses, and personal interview.

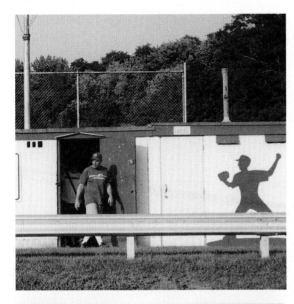

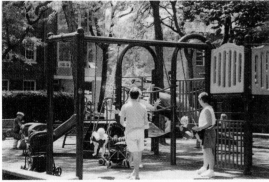

Recreational and leisure activities are directly related to a community's health status in that they connect people in the community and provide opportunities to socialize.

Schools in the area should have a regular program of physical education in which all students must participate. In addition, schools should provide equipment and programs for extracurricular activities, including both team and individual sports (eg, tennis, softball), art, music, and foreign language programs, and other types of recreational programs. Churches may provide recreational programs, senior citizen dinners and outings, youth programs, church festivals, and special holiday activities. A comprehensive, community-based program is essential. Indoor or outdoor facilities (eg, swimming pools, ball fields) should be available to all citizens, easily accessible, and kept in good repair. Organized activities for individuals and groups of all ages, genders, social status, and physical abilities should be available at minimal or no cost.

Communities with a poor economic base or those with a large percentage of rural residents may not be able to provide adequate programs for recreation. Finding funds for building and maintaining recreational facilities is difficult. Lack of transportation may seriously limit access. Social isolation may become a problem for these people. In a community where there are no programs available for young people, gang activity and alcohol/drug abuse may develop. In communities where activities such as water sports or snow sports are common, lack of programs related to safety issues could result in serious injury or even death.

DISPLAY 28-1. Causes of Infant Mortality—United States

1. Congenital anomalies
2. Disorders related to short gestation/low birth weight
3. Sudden infant death syndrome
4. Newborn affected by maternal complications of pregnancy
5. Respiratory distress syndrome

(US DHHS/CDC (2000b.) *National Vital Statistics Reports*, *48*(12), 20. (Accessed through www.cdc.gov/nchs/data/nvs4812pdf.)

DISPLAY 28-2. Causes of Childhood Mortality—United States

AGES 1–4

1. Accidents and adverse effects (motor vehicle, other)
2. Congenital anomalies
3. Homicide and legal intervention
4. Malignant neoplasms

AGES 5–14

1. Accidents and adverse effects (motor vehicle, other)
2. Malignant neoplasms
3. Homicide and legal interventions
4. Congenital anomalies

(US DHHS/CDC (2000a.) *National Vital Statistics Reports*, *48*(11), 26. (Accessed through www.cdc.gov/nchs/data/nvs4811pdf.)

DISPLAY 28-3. Causes of Teen and Adult Mortality—United States

AGES 15–24

1. Accidents and adverse effects (motor vehicle, other)
2. Homicide and legal interventions
3. Suicide
4. Malignant neoplasms

AGES 25–44

1. Accidents and adverse effects (motor vehicle, other)
2. Malignant neoplasms
3. Heart diseases
4. Suicide

AGES 45–64

1. Malignant neoplasms
2. Heart diseases
3. Accidents and adverse effects (motor vehicle, other)
4. Cerebrovascular diseases

AGES 65 AND OLDER

1. Heart diseases
2. Malignant neoplasms
3. Cerebrovascular diseases
4. Chronic obstructive pulmonary diseases and allied conditions

(US DHHS/CDC (2000a.) *National Vital Statistics Reports*, *48*(11), 26–27. (Accessed through www.cdc.gov/nchs/data/nvs4811pdf.)

Validation and Documentation of Findings

Validate the community assessment data that you have collected. This is necessary to verify that the data are reliable and accurate. Document the assessment data following the health care facility or agency policy.

EXAMPLE OF SUBJECTIVE AND OBJECTIVE DATA

The community developed 100 years ago and has grown steadily in economic status and population over the years. There is an even age and gender population distribution. There is a large Hispanic population group in the community (80% white non-Hispanic, 20% Hispanic). Birth, death, and morbidity data reflect the overall rates for the United States. Most households consist of married couples with and without children. Religious organizations are predominantly Methodist, Catholic, and Jewish, and they work closely together to provide services to all community members. Boundaries are clear and uncontested, neighborhoods are cohesive but linked to larger community, and housing needs are met for all community members.

The geographic terrain is mountains and desert, and the climate is hot and dry. The community provides teaching about sun- and heat-related health problems. There is a community hospital that provides medical–surgical, obstetric–gynecologic, and emergency care. A large urban hospital with a trauma unit and specialized programs is 20 miles away, accessible by the community ambulance service. Other health services, such as physical therapy, nutrition consultation, dentistry, and ophthalmology, are available in the community. Most health care facilities accept third-party reimbursement. The public health service is well funded, and home health agencies provide extensive services. Most social service needs of the community are through official, nonofficial, and voluntary health services. Some are located 20 miles away in the urban area, but a shuttle is provided for those requiring the services. Long-term care is available in the home and in four skilled nursing and rehabilitation facilities.

The median income of the community is slightly higher than the national average. A variety of local businesses adequately meet the needs of the community. The police, fire, and environmental agencies are adequately staffed and supplied with equipment to provide protection to the community. There is a bus system, a rail station, and a small airport; most people own at least one car. The public school system for the community is well funded; therefore, many programs are available for the children and adolescents. In addition, there is a 2-year college in the community, and several 4-year colleges are within 40 miles.

The community government is representative of the views of the people, community meetings occur once a month, and most community members vote regularly. There are several local network affiliate television stations, a variety of radio stations, and a daily newspaper that focuses primarily on community news. The local public school system offers a variety of recreational programs, and the community churches offer activities for people of all ages. Many of the local companies (including the hospital) offer recreation and exercise facilities and sponsor community programs. The community itself offers an extensive recreation program. There are teams for all sports and all ages. Activities are also available at minimal cost to all members of the community. Several clubs and associations in the area offer unique recreational activities, such as mountain climbing, a nature club, and a runners' club.

Analysis of Data

After you have collected your assessment data, you will need to analyze the data, using diagnostic reasoning skills. Review the general steps of the process (Chapter 7). After that, in Diagnostic Reasoning: Possible Conclusions you will see an overview of common conclusions that you may reach after community assessment. Next, Diagnostic Reasoning: Case Study shows you how to analyze community assessment data for a *specific* community. Finally, you are given an opportunity to analyze data in the critical thinking exercise in the study guide/laboratory manual companion to this textbook.

Diagnostic Reasoning: Possible Conclusions

Below are some possible conclusions after a community assessment.

SELECTED NURSING DIAGNOSES

After collecting subjective and objective data pertaining to the community, you will need to organize and group the data to reveal any significant patterns of abnormalities. These data will then be used to make clinical judgments (nursing diagnosis: wellness, risk, or collaborative problems) about the status of the client. Following is a list of selected nursing diagnoses that you may identify when analyzing data for this part of the assessment.

Nursing Diagnoses (Wellness)

- Opportunity to Enhance Community Coping
- Health-Seeking Behaviors: initiation of comprehensive wellness program for elderly

Nursing Diagnoses (Risk)

- Risk for Violence related to insufficient police protection

- Risk for Impaired Community Processes related to subgroup of non-English–speaking people
- Risk for Social Isolation related to a lack of recreational activities and facilities
- Risk for Trauma related to climate

Nursing Diagnoses (Actual)

- Ineffective Community Therapeutic Regimen Management related to the presence of occupational health hazards
- Ineffective Community Therapeutic Regimen Management related to lack of substance abuse treatment programs
- Ineffective Community Coping related to increased unemployment
- Ineffective Community Coping related to inadequate resources for day care
- Fear related to rising incidence of crime

SELECTED COLLABORATIVE PROBLEMS

After grouping the data, certain collaborative problems may emerge. Remember, collaborative problems differ from nursing diagnoses in that they cannot be prevented by nursing interventions. However, these physiologic or other complications of medical or other conditions can be detected and monitored by the nurse. In addition, the nurse can use physician- and nurse-prescribed interventions to minimize the complications of these problems. The nurse may also have to refer the client in such situations for further treatment of the problem. Following is a list of collaborative problems that may be identified when assessing the community. These problems are worded as Potential Complications (or PC), followed by the problem.

- PC: Post-traumatic stress syndrome, community

Diagnostic Reasoning: Case Study

The case study presents assessment data for a specific community. It is followed by an analysis of the data, working through the seven key steps to arrive at specific conclusions.

The following is an abbreviated case study of an assessment of a small town. In actual practice, a thorough assessment of a community would require more in-depth data collection than is described in this vignette. Such assessments may be quite lengthy, which is beyond the scope of this book.

History

The area in and around Maple Grove was first inhabited by Native American hunters and trappers. Later, German immigrants settled in the region and the lumber/logging industry became the economic base of the community. The town derived its name from the large stands of hardwood trees, especially maples, that grew in the area.

Demographics

The total population for the town of Maple Grove, as of the year 2000, was 2352, a decrease of 13.6% from the 1990 census. Of the total number of residents, 56% are female and 26.3% are 65 years of age or older. Racial distribution includes 94.5% white, 3% African American, 1.3% Hispanic, and 1.2% other. Most residents aged 15 years and older are married (65.4%), 10.1% are either separated or divorced, 12.3% are single, and 12.2% are widowed. The leading cause of death in Maple Grove is cardiovascular disease. The German immigrants who originally settled the area brought with them their Lutheran faith, and over 80% still practice that religion. There is also a small Baptist congregation in Maple Grove, as well as small Methodist and Catholic churches.

Physical Environment

Maple Grove is situated in a very rural area and is bordered on the north by national forest land. The Cache River runs along its western border and an interstate highway lies 2 miles from the city limits on the east. The southern edge of the town is surrounded by farmland. Average temperature in January is 31.2° F, and in June 87.3° F.

Health and Social Services

Maple Grove has no hospital, and the nearest facility is 25 miles away and is an 85-bed, full-service facility. It is the only hospital in the county. A family practice physician and a nurse practitioner have an office in Maple Grove. The office is open 4 days a week. The county health department has a branch office in Maple Grove and offers immunizations, Special Supplemental Nutrition Program for Women, Infants and Children (WIC), sexually transmitted disease (STD) screening, family planning, and environmental services. A local Visiting Nurse Association (VNA) office offers home health services as well as hospice care. The nearest mental health center is approximately 25 miles away, as are many other services, including county government offices. There is a 50-bed skilled nursing facility in Maple Grove that is operating at full capacity. Several residents have expressed their concern about

this to the nurse. A committee has been formed to examine ways in which the capacity of the facility could be increased.

Economics

The median household income for Maple Grove is $23,480, which is lower than the national average, and the median per capita income is $11,310, also below the national average. Of the nearly 2,400 people living in Maple Grove, 15.1% live below the poverty level. The single largest employer in the community is a minimum-security state correctional facility. Other areas of employment include forestry-related occupations, farming, and local businesses such as automobile sales, farm implement sales, grocery, and the like. The unemployment rate is 7.8%, which is higher than the state average.

Safety and Transportation

Maple Grove maintains a small local police force of five full-time officers, two part-time policemen, and one dispatcher/office worker. The community also receives services from the county sheriff's office and the state police. Maple Grove has a fire department with seven part-time firemen and a small group of volunteer firemen. There are no trained emergency medical personnel working with the fire department. The equipment is slightly outdated but still functional. Environmental services are provided through the county health department. The crime rate is relatively low, with the incidence of violent crime below the state average.

There is no public transportation except for a small taxi service (one taxicab) and a van supported by the area Agency on Aging, which provides transportation for senior citizens. There is an interstate bus service available on a limited basis. The nearest airport is 70 miles away.

Education

Maple Grove supports an elementary school and a high school with a total of approximately 450 students in grades K through 12. There is no school nurse available. School administrators expressed some concern about this. Although health-related problems are referred to the local health department, they have difficulty in getting the required screenings completed, and school immunization records are not up to date. The school principals also are concerned that there is no one available to care for injuries or illness when they occur. The high school provides a limited number of extracurricular activities, including boys' and girls' basketball, baseball, softball, and track. The closest junior college is 30 miles away, and the university is 55 miles from Maple Grove. There is a small library that is open in the afternoons and on Saturday. The community residents are proud of their library because it is entirely funded through contributions. They often hold chili suppers, raffles, and other fund-raising events to support it.

Politics and Government

Maple Grove has a mayor/city council form of government. The mayor was more than willing to meet with the nurse and invited her to attend the city council meeting on the first Monday of the month. Those members of the community with whom the nurse talked indicated that they felt comfortable with their elected officials and that they were free to voice concerns and opinions at any time. Both the Democratic and Republican parties are active in the town. The number of registered voters who voted in the last election was higher than the state average.

Communication

A radio station is located approximately 25 miles away, and the nearest television station is 50 miles from Maple Grove. The town has cable television service and a post office. A small local newspaper is published weekly.

Recreation

Maple Grove has a small city park equipped with playground equipment, three ball fields, and a picnic shelter. There are softball and baseball leagues for ages 7 to 18 and Boy Scout and Girl Scout troops. Other organized recreation activities, such as senior citizen programs, are offered through the churches.

1 Identify abnormal data and strengths (in both subjective and objective data).

SUBJECTIVE DATA

- Expressed concern about insufficient number of long-term care beds
- Expressed concern regarding lack of school nurse
- Members feel comfortable with city government
- Difficulty in meeting requirements for school screenings
- Expressed concern that no one is available to care for injuries or illnesses that occur during school hours

OBJECTIVE DATA

- Maintain a community library through volunteer efforts
- Long-term care facility at full capacity
- Committee formed to increase capacity of long-term care facility
- No school nurse employed by district
- School immunization records not complete
- Median household and per capita income below national average
- Unemployment above state average
- Family practice physician and nurse practitioner available 4 days a week
- No emergency medical technicians available through the fire department

2 Cue Clusters	3 Inferences	4 Possible Nursing Diagnoses	5 Defining Characteristics	6 Confirm or Rule Out
A • Citizens comfortable with government • Organized effort to maintain community library • Committee formed to increase long-term care bed capacity	Community has open system of communication and has the necessary resources to work together and solve problems.	Opportunity to Enhance Community Coping	*Major:* Successful coping with previous crisis or problem. *Minor:* Positive communication Active problem solving by community.	Confirm. Meets defining characteristics.
B • No school nurse • Immunization records not up-to-date • Expressed difficulty in meeting requirements for school screenings • Physician and nurse practitioner available only 4 days/week • No EMT with fire department	School health program inadequate. Physician and emergency care limited	Ineffective Management of Therapeutic Regimen, Community, related to lack of school nurse and availability of emergency care	*Major:* Verbalized difficulty in meeting health needs *Minor:* None	Confirm, based on defining characteristics.

2 Cue Clusters	3 Inferences	4 Possible Nursing Diagnoses	5 Defining Characteristics	6 Confirm or Rule Out
C				
• Per capita and household income below average • Unemployment rate above average	Community may be facing economic crisis.	Risk for Ineffective Community Coping related to low income and high unemployment	*Major:* None *Minor:* None	Does not need to meet defining characteristics for risk diagnosis. Community has a lot of internal support but should be monitored for changes in ability to meet own needs.

7 Document conclusions.

The following diagnoses are appropriate for the Maple Grove community at this time:

- Opportunity to Enhance Community Coping
- Ineffective Management of Therapeutic Regimen, Community, related to lack of school nurse
- Risk for Ineffective Community Coping related to low income, high unemployment, and availability of emergency care

REFERENCES AND SELECTED READINGS

Anderson, E., & McFarlane, J. (2000). *Community as partner*. Philadelphia: Lippincott-Raven Publishers.

Clark, M. J. (1999). *Nursing in the community*. Stamford, CT: Appleton & Lange.

Clemen-Stone, S., Eigsti, D., & McGuire, S. (1998). *Comprehensive community nursing*. St. Louis, MO: C. V. Mosby.

Dixon, E. L. (1999). Community health nursing practice and the Roy Adaptation Model. *Public Health Nursing, 16*(4), 290–300.

Eshlemann, J., & Davidhizar, R. (2000). Community assessment: An RN–BSN partnership with community. *ABNF Journal, 11*(2), 28–31.

Lundeen, S. P. (1999). An alternative paradigm from promoting health in communities: The Lundeen Community Nursing Center model. *Family and Community Health, 21*(4), 15–28.

Neuman, B. N. (1972). A model for teaching total person approach to patient problems. *Nursing Research, 21,* 264–269.

Smith, C., & Maurer, F. (2000). *Community health nursing: Theory and practice*. Philadelphia: W. B. Saunders.

Stackhouse, J. (1998). *Into the community: Nursing in ambulatory and home care*. Philadelphia: Lippincott Williams & Wilkins.

United States Department of Health and Human Services, Centers for Disease Control and Prevention. (2000a). *National Vital Statistics Reports, 48*(11), 26–27.

———. (2000b). *National Vital Statistics Reports, 48*(12), 20.

Wilson, L. C. (2000). Implementation and evaluation of church-based health fairs. *Journal of Community Health Nursing, 17*(1), 39–48.

For additional information on this book, be sure to visit http://connection.lww.com.

Sample Adult Nursing Health History and Physical Assessment

A

Complete Nursing Health History

BIOGRAPHIC DATA

Client's Name (use initials): S. L.
Data provided by: Client
Date and Place of Birth: 4/10/28; St. Louis, Missouri
Gender: Female
Marital Status: Married
Nationality, Culture, Ethnicity: African American
Religion/Spiritual Practices: Baptist
Who Lives With Client: Husband
Significant Others: Husband, two daughters, one son
Education Level: College degree
Occupation (active/laid off/retired): Retired elementary school teacher
Primary language (written/spoken): English
Secondary language: None

REASONS FOR SEEKING HEALTH CARE PROVIDER

Client states: "The main reason I am here today is to get a check-up, I haven't had one in 8 years. I probably should have had one sooner because I have non-insulin-dependent diabetes mellitus (NIDDM), or type 2 diabetes. I think I have it under control, but I want to make sure. Another reason I am here is because I have started to have some pain in my right hip and fingers. It is starting to really bother me, and I thought I should have it examined."

HISTORY OF PRESENT HEALTH CONCERN

Client states that pain started 1 year ago and has been getting progressively worse. Says that pain is worse in AM right after getting out of bed but that it subsides in the afternoon, "after I have been moving around for several hours." Pain started gradually—client cannot think of any event that may have caused it. Client expressed that she thought it was arthritis and that it just happens when "you get old."

States pain is not aggravated by anything that she can think of but that it is relieved with exercise, warm baths, and aspirin. "I try not to let the pain affect my life—but I have trouble making the bed in the morning and I can't write letters until later in the day." Client says she is concerned about the pain getting progressively worse—"My husband and I are very self-sufficient and active; I don't want to have to cut back too much."

PAST HEALTH HISTORY

Client says she had a normal childhood—"all the childhood illnesses." Had an appendectomy at age 18 and a left arm fracture at age 20. Was hospitalized for 1 week with the birth of each child—"Can you believe I could stay in for a whole week for a normal delivery? My daughters had to leave with their babies after 24 hours!" Had a cholecystectomy at age 56 that was performed for complaint of gas pains after eating fatty foods. Satisfied with care received at local hospital. Denies food, drug, and environmental allergies.

Had polyuria and polydipsia before diagnosis of diabetes. Developed urinary tract infection (UTI) at age 60, at which time she sought medical advice and was diagnosed with NIDDM.

FAMILY HISTORY/GENOGRAM

Client states that there is a history of heart attack and high blood pressure in her family and that her father had insulin-dependent diabetes mellitus (IDDM), also called type 1 diabetes.

REVIEW OF BODY SYSTEMS FOR CURRENT HEALTH PROBLEMS

Skin, Hair, Nails: Describes skin and scalp as dry. Uses lotions frequently. Denies easy bruising, pruritus, or nonhealing sores. Nails are hard and brittle. Hair is fine and soft. Denies intolerance to heat or cold.
Head and Neck: Denies neck stiffness, swelling, difficulty swallowing, sore throat, or enlarged lymph nodes. "I get a headache occasionally, but I just put a cool washcloth on my head and lie down for a bit—it usually goes away without having to take medicine."

Eyes: Has worn glasses "all my life." Cannot recall age at which they were prescribed. Prescription change from bifocals to trifocals August 1984. Complains of blurred vision without glasses. Denies diplopia, itching, excessive tearing, discharge, redness, or trauma to eyes.

Ears: Believes she is "a little slow to grasp, and I think it may be because of my hearing." Does not wear hearing aid. Cannot recall last hearing test. Denies tinnitus, pain, discharge, or trauma to ears. Does not ask for questions to be repeated.

Mouth, Throat, Nose, and Sinuses: Wears dentures. Last dental examination October 1984. Denies problems with proper fit, eating, chewing, swallowing, sore throat, sore tongue. Complains of "canker sore" if she eats strawberries. Denies difficulty with smell, pain, postnasal drip, sneezing, or frequent nosebleeds. No difficulty tasting foods.

Breasts: Denies pain, lumps, dimpling, retraction, discharge.

Thorax and Lungs: Denies chest pain, trouble breathing, coughing, or fatigue with activity.

Heart and Neck Vessels: Denies palpitations, chest pain and pressure, fatigue, or edema.

Peripheral Vascular: Denies claudication, cramping, sores on legs, or swelling/edema of legs and feet. Denies intolerance to heat or cold. States "occasionally my feet feel numb," subsides on own.

Abdomen: Denies nausea, vomiting, abdominal pain, or excessive gas. Complains of dyspepsia approximately two times per month. Voices no dislikes or food intolerances.

Genitalia: Voids four to five times per day, clear yellow urine. Denies current problem with dysuria, hematuria, polyuria, hesitancy, incontinence, or nocturia. Complains of urgency during the colder months with no increase in frequency. Age of menarche: Approximately 12 yr; age of menopause: 50 yr. States "going through my change of life wasn't difficult for me physically or emotionally." Described menstrual period as regular, lasting 4 days with moderate flow. Denies postmenopausal spotting at this time. Client is gravida 3, Para 3. No complications with pregnancy or childbirth. Has never used any form of contraception. Client states she is sexually active—"My husband and I have good relations." Denies pain, discomfort, or postcoital bleeding. Denies history of any sexually transmitted diseases. Denies problem with vaginal itching. Last Pap smear: negative in 1976.

Anus/Rectum: Soft, formed, medium brown BM every third day after Dulcolax supplement. States she becomes constipated without use of laxative. Denies mucous, bloody, or tarry stools. States discomfort with BMs starting in September 1984. When having to strain with BMs, felt "some kind of mass" prolapsing from rectum. Consulted her doctor, who explained to her "it was a piece of my colon slipping out." No surgical treatment or exercises prescribed. Gently reinserts tissue when this happens. Denies rectal bleeding, change in color, consistency, or habits.

Musculoskeletal: Pain in right hip and finger joints. Denies stiffness, joint pain, or swelling with activity—"Activity helps my hip and finger pain." Occasionally has lower back pains when carrying large amounts of food or when carrying large trays (see *Activity Level* under *Lifestyle and Health Practices*).

Neurologic: Speech clear without slur or stutter. Follows verbal cues. Expresses ideas and feelings clearly and concisely. States she has a gradual loss of memory over past 5 to 6 years. Believes long-term memory is better than short-term memory. She can recall past weekly events but has trouble recalling dates, times, and places of events. Learns best by writing information down and then reviewing it. Makes major decisions jointly with husband after prayer.

LIFESTYLE AND HEALTH PRACTICES

Typical Day

A typical day for client is to arise at 6:00 AM, eat breakfast, and perform light housekeeping. Client goes to community center in early afternoon to eat lunch, quilt, and visit. Goes home around 2:00 PM. Walks about four blocks with a friend every day. Cleans own house daily for one 2-h period (includes dusting, vacuuming, washing). After walking, returns home and relaxes with crafts and visiting with husband. Attends church-related activities in the evening. Bedtime is around 10:00 PM.

Nutrition Habits and Weight Management

Client states she is on an 1,800-calorie American Diabetic Association–approved diet. Eats breakfast of whole wheat toast, one boiled egg, orange juice, and decaffeinated coffee. Her lunch meal varies, but today she had tuna; salad with lettuce, tomatoes, and broccoli; an apple; and milk. Typical dinner includes small serving of broiled meat, green vegetables, piece of fruit, and glass of milk. Tries not to snack but will have fruit if she feels the urge. Drinks two 8-oz glasses of water a day. Drinks decaffeinated coffee—no tea or colas. Voices no food dislikes or intolerances.

Client expresses desire to maintain current weight. Weight tends to fluctuate ±5 lb/month—"I've always had to watch what I eat because I gain so easily."

Medication/Substance Use

No prescribed medications, takes the following OTC medications: ASA gr prn for "hip and finger joint pain." Takes about two times per month. Denies nausea, abdominal pains, or evidence of bleeding while taking ASA. Mylanta prn for "gas pains." Dulcolax suppository 3 times per week for past 4 years. Multivitamin l qd for past 4 years. Denies use of alcohol, tobacco, and illicit drugs.

Activity Level/Exercise-Fitness Plan

Client performs housekeeping for a couple of hours and walks four blocks a day. Is retired from being an elementary school teacher and part-time caterer. Volunteers to cook for church social functions. Client expresses satisfaction with activity and believes she functions above the level of the average person her age.

Sleep/Rest

Goes to bed at 10:00 PM. Denies difficulty falling asleep or sleeping. Feels well rested when she arises at 6:00 AM. Never used sleep medications. Denies orthopnea and nocturnal dyspnea. Enjoys reading one to two pages of Bible history each evening.

Self-Concept, Self-Esteem, Body Image

Describes self as normal person. Talkative, outgoing, and likes to be around people but hates noisy environments. Happy with the person she has become and states, "I can definitely live with myself." States a weakness is that she worries about "little things" more now than she used to and tends to be irritated more easily. Cannot place specific onset of these feelings. Feels good about self-management of diabetes. Client rates own health as an 8 on a scale of 1 (worst) to 10 (best). Five years ago, she rated health as a 10 and predicts that 5 years in the future health will be a 6. Sees health deterioration as normal aging process and states, "I feel really good when I look at a lot of people my age with all their problems and the medicine they take."

Self-Care Responsibilities

Client seeks health care only in emergencies. Last medical examination was September 1984. Does not check own blood sugar or perform breast self-exam. Always wears seat belt, asks husband to test smoke alarm monthly, uses a sturdy step stool to reach objects out of reach.

Social Relationships

Describes relationship with other members of the church and community groups as friendly and "family-like." Has casual relationship with neighbors. Visits community center every day to socialize, attends church functions several evenings a week. Walks with a friend every day.

Family Relationships

Client has been married 55 years. Describes relationship as the best part of her life right now. Two daughters live in Texas with their husbands and children. Her son and his wife and baby boy live in Minnesota. All the children and their families come home once a year, and the client and her husband visit each family once a year. She expresses desire to visit her children and grandchildren more often and states, "I wish my babies lived nearby. I love being a grandma and miss them so much." Communicates with each of them several times a month by phone. Client was the fourth of five children in her family. Had a happy childhood, describes family as close and loving—"my daddy was very strict though."

Education and Work

Client went to college to be a teacher. Taught elementary school for 30 years. After her children were grown, she would work during the summer as a caterer—"I love to cook." Is retired now but still volunteers to cook for church social functions.

Stress Level and Coping Styles

States that husband's high blood pressure has never been a source of stress to her. Shares confidences with husband and with a few close friends. Most stressful time in life was losing two brothers and a sister, all in 1982. States that with support of husband, children, and church, she handled it "better than most people would have." States she prays and eats when under stress. Cannot identify any major stresses that have occurred in the last year.

Environmental Hazards

Is not aware of any environmental hazards in area where she lives.

DEVELOPMENTAL LEVEL
Integrity Versus Despair

Describes childhood as a very happy time for her. Becomes excited and smiles as she relates stories of her childhood on the farm. States she was an average child and ran and played like all the others. Companions were brothers and sisters. Has been married for 55 years. Describes relationship with husband as close and sharing. Taught elementary school for 30 years and catered in the summers for several years. Lived in a large house until 1976. Currently lives in small two-bedroom bungalow. Active in church and society. Volunteers at church functions. States she enjoys being retired and lives a "comfortable" life. Does not voice financial concerns. Has begun to write will and distribute personal heirlooms to children and grandchildren. States she is not afraid of death and wished to have the "business part taken care of" in order to enjoy the rest of her life together with her husband.

Physical Assessment

GENERAL SURVEY

Ht: 5 foot 4 inches; Wt: 145 lb; Radial pulse: 71; Resp: 16; B/P: R arm—120/72, L arm—120/72; Temp: 98.6. Client alert and cooperative. Sitting comfortably on table with arms crossed and shoulder slightly slouched forward. Smiling with mild anxiety. Dress is neat and clean. Walks steadily with posture slightly stooped.

Skin, Hair, Nails

Skin: Light brown, warm, and dry to touch. Skinfold returns to place after 1 s when lifted over clavicle. Darker "age spots" on posterior hands bilaterally in clusters of four to five and evenly distributed over lower extremities. 3-cm nodule with 2-mm macule in center noted in right axilla; indurated, nontender, and nonmobile. No evidence of vascular or purpuric lesions. No edema.

Hair: Slightly curly, pulled back in a bun at nape of neck, clean, black with white and gray streaks, thin and dry in texture. No scalp lesions or flaking. Fine black hair evenly distributed over arms bilaterally and sparsely on legs bilaterally. No hair noted on axilla or on chest, back, or face.

Nails: Fingernails medium length and thickness, clear. Splinter hemorrhages noted on right thumb near fingertip in midline. No clubbing or Beau's lines.

Head and Neck

Head symmetrically rounded, neck nontender with full ROM. Neck symmetric without masses, scars, pulsations. Lymph nodes nonpalpable. Trachea in midline. Thyroid nonpalpable.

Eyes

Eyes 2 cm apart without protrusion. Eyebrows sparse with equal distribution. No scalines noted. Lids light brown without ptosis, edema, or lesions, and freely closeable bilaterally. Lacrimal apparatus nonedematous. Sclera white without increased vascularity or lesions noted. Palpebral and bulbar conjunctiva slightly reddened without lesions noted. Iris uniformly blue. PERRLA, EOMs intact bilaterally. Peripheral vision is equal to examiner's. Visual acuity: Snellen chart—with glasses off vision is 20/70 OD, OS; with glasses on vision is 20/20 OD, OS. Rosenbaum vision screener—with glasses off vision is blurred at 14 inches away but can identify number of fingers held up. With glasses on vision is clear at 14 inches. Funduscopic examination: Red reflex present bilaterally. Optic disk round with well-defined margins. Physiologic cup occupies disc. Arterioles

smaller than venules. No AV nicking, no hemorrhages, or exudates noted. Macula not seen.

Ears

Left auricle without deformity, lumps, or lesions. Right auricle with tag at top of pinna. Auricles and mastoid processes nontender. Bilateral auditory canals contain moderate amount of dark brown cerumen. Tympanic membrane difficult to view due to wax. Whisper test: Client identifies one out of two words in four attempts. Weber test: No lateralization of sound to either ear. Rinne test: AC is greater than BC in both ears.

Mouth, Throat, Nose, and Sinuses

Lips moist, no lesions or ulcerations. Buccal mucosa pink and moist with patchy areas of dark pigment on ventral surface of tongue, gums, and floor of mouth. No ulcers or nodules. Gums pink and moist without inflammation, bleeding, or discoloration. Hard and soft palates smooth without lesions or masses. Tongue midline when protruded, no lesions, or masses. No lesions, discolorations, or ulcerations on floor of mouth, oral mucosa, or gums. Uvula in midline and elevates on phonation. Tonsils present without exudate, edema, ulcers, or enlargement. External structure without deformity, asymmetry, or inflammation. Nares patent. Turbinates and middle meatus pale pink, without swelling, exudate, lesions, or bleeding. Nasal septum midline without bleeding, perforation, or deviation. Frontal and maxillary sinuses nontender.

Thorax and Lung

Skin light brown without scars, pulsations, or lesions. No hair noted. Thorax expands evenly bilaterally without retractions or bulging. Slope of ribs = 40 degrees. No use of auxiliary respiratory muscles and no nasal flaring. Mild kyphosis. Respirations even, unlabored, and regular (16/min). No cough noted. No tenderness, crepitus, or masses. Tactile fremitus decreases below T5 bilaterally posteriorly, and 4th ICS anteriorly bilaterally. Thorax resonance throughout. Diaphragmatic excursion: Left—on inspiration diaphragm descends to T11, and on expiration diaphragm ascends to T9. Right—on inspiration diaphragm descends to T12, and on expiration diaphragm ascends to T9. Vesicular breath sounds heard in all lung fields. No rales, rhonchi, friction rubs, whispered pectoriloquy, bronchophony, or egophony noted.

Breasts

Breasts moderate size, round, and symmetrical bilaterally. Skin light brown with dark brown areola. No dimpling or retraction. Free movement in all positions. Engorged vein noted running across UOQ to areola in right breast. Nipples inverted bilaterally. No discharge expressed. No thickening or tenderness noted. Hard, immobile 2 cm round mass noted in left breast in LOQ. Client denies ever noticing this. Nontender to palpation. Lymph nodes nonpalpable. Client does not know how to do SBE.

Heart and Neck Vessels

No pulsations visible. No heaves, lifts, or vibrations. Apical Impulse: 5th ICS to LMCL. Clear, brief heart sounds throughout. Physiologic S_2. No gallops, murmurs, or rubs. AP = 72/min and regular.

Abdomen

Abdomen rounded, symmetric without masses, lesions, pulsations, or peristalsis noted. Abdomen free of hair, bruising, and increased vasculature. Healed with appendectomy scar. Umbilicus in midline, without herniation, swelling or discoloration. Bowel sounds low pitched and gurgling at 22/min × 4 quads. Aortic, renal, and iliac arteries auscultated without bruit. No venous hums or friction rubs auscultated over liver or spleen. Tympany percussed over all 4 quads. 8 cm. Liver span percussed in R MCL. Area of dullness percussed at 9th ICS in left postaxillary line. No tenderness or masses noted with light and deep palpation in all 4 quadrants. Liver and spleen nonpalpable.

Genital

Labia pink with decreased elasticity and vaginal secretions. No bulging of vaginal wall, purulent foul drainage, or lesions. Skene's gland not visible. 1-cm nodule palpated in R groin.

Anus/Rectum

Anal area pink with small amount of hair. Rectal mucosa bulges with straining.

Peripheral Vascular

Arms: Equal in size and symmetry bilaterally; pale pink; warm and dry to touch without edema, bruising, or lesions noted. Radial pulses = in rate and amplitude and strong. Allen's test: right = 2-s refill, left = 2-s refill. Brachial pulses strong, equal, and even. Epitrochlear nodes nonpalpable.

Legs: Legs large in size and bilaterally symmetric. Skin intact, light brown; warm and dry to touch without edema, bruising, lesions, or increased vascularity. Superficial inguinal, horizontal, and vertical lymph nodes nonpalpable. Femoral pulses strong and equal without bruits. Popliteal pulse nonpalpable with client supine or prone. Dorsalis pedal and posterior tibial pulses strong and equal. No edema palpable. Homans' sign negative bilaterally. No retrograde filling noted when client stands. Toenails thick and yellowed. Special maneuver for arterial insufficiency: Feet regain color after 4 s and veins refilled in 5 s.

Musculoskeletal

Posture slightly stooped with mild kyphosis. Gait steady, smooth, and coordinated with even base. Limited ROM of lateral flexion and extension of spine. Paravertebrals equal in size and strength; upper extremities and lower extremities with full ROM. Muscles moderately firm bilaterally. No deviations, inflammations, or bony deformities. Small callus on left heel. Moves upper and lower extremities freely against gravity and against resistance. Rheumatoid nodule noted on dorsal surface of left hand.

Neurologic

Mental Status Examination: Pleasant and friendly. Appropriately dressed for weather with matching colors and patterns. Clothes neat and clean. Facial expressions symmetric and correlate with mood and topic discussed. Speech clear and appropriate. Follows through with train of thought. Carefully chooses words to convey feelings and ideas. Oriented to person, place, time, and events. Remains attentive and able to focus on examination during entire interaction. Short-term memory intact, long-term memory before 1980 unclear—especially cannot recall dates and sequencing of events. General information questions answered correctly 100% of the time. Vocabulary suitable to educational level. Explains proverb accurately. Gives semiabstract answers and enjoys joking. Is able to identify similarities 5 seconds after being asked. Answers to judgment questions in realistic manner.

Cranial Nerve Examination: CN I: Correctly identifies scent. CN II: 20/70 vision OD and OS; blurred vision at 14 inches w/o glasses; full visual fields. CN III, IV, and VI: Lid covers 2 mm of iris; bilateral eye movement, bilateral pupil response. CN V: Identifies light touch and sharp touch to forehead, cheek, and chin. Bilateral corneal reflex intact. Masseter muscles contract equally and bilaterally. Jaw jerk +1. CN VII: Identifies sugar and salt on anterior 2/3 of tongue. Smiles, frowns, shows teeth, blows out cheeks, and raises eyebrows as instructed. CN VIII: Hears whispered words from 1 to 2 feet; Weber test: Vibration heard equally well in both ears; Rhine test: AC > BC. CN IX and X: Gag reflex intact, and client identifies sugar and salt on posterior of tongue. Uvula in midline and elevates on phonation. CN XI: Shrugs shoulders and moves head to right and left against resistance. CN XII: Tongue midline when protruded without fasciculations.

Motor and Cerebellar Examination: Muscle tone firm at rest, abdominal muscles slightly relaxed. Muscle size adequate for age. No fasciculations or involuntary movements noted. Muscle strength moderately strong and equal bilaterally. Alternates finger to nose with eyes closed; occasionally tends to hit opposite side of nose. Rapidly opposes fingers to thumb bilaterally without difficulty. Alternates pronation and supination of hands rapidly without difficulty. Heel to shin intact bilaterally. Romberg: Minimal swaying. Tandem walk: Steady. No involuntary movements noted.

Sensory Status Examination: Superficial light and deep touch sensation intact on arms, legs, neck, chest, and back. Position sense of toes and fingers intact bilaterally. Identifies point localization correctly. Identifies coin placed in hand and number written on back correctly.

Two-Point Discrimination	Right	Left
(in mm):		
Fingertips	6	6
Dorsal hand	15	15
Chest	45	49
Forearm	39	35
Back	45	45
Upper arm	40	45
Reflexes		
Biceps	2+	2+
Triceps	2+	2+
Patellar	3+	3+
Achilles	2+	2+
Abdominal	1+	1+
Babinski	negative	negative

CLIENT'S STRENGTHS

- Positive attitude and outlook on life
- Motivation to comply with prescribed diet
- Strong support systems; husband and spiritual beliefs
- No physical limitations

NURSING DIAGNOSES

- Risk for Altered Maintenance related to lack of knowledge concerning importance of regular medical checkups, ie: lesion in UOQ of left breast not seen by physician, no Pap smear, and no follow-up with diabetes

- Acute right hip pain
- Constipation related to lack of bowel routine and laxative overuse
- Knowledge Deficit: Signs and symptoms and treatment of hyperglycemia/hypoglycemia
- Knowledge Deficit: Management and causes of constipation
- Knowledge Deficit: Self breast exam technique
- Knowledge Deficit: Importance of self-blood glucose monitoring

COLLABORATIVE PROBLEMS

- Potential complications: Hyperglycemia, hypoglycemia
- Potential complication: Hypertension

B Collaborative Problems*

Potential Complication: Cardiac/Vascular

PC: Decreased cardiac output
PC: Dysrhythmias
PC: Pulmonary edema
PC: Cardiogenic shock
PC: Thromboemboli/deep vein thrombosis
PC: Hypovolemia
PC: Peripheral vascular insufficiency
PC: Hypertension
PC: Congenital heart disease
PC: Endocarditis
PC: Pulmonary embolism
PC: Spinal shock
PC: Ischemic ulcers
PC: Angina

Potential Complication: Gastrointestinal/Hepatic/Biliary

PC: Paralytic ileus/small bowel obstruction
PC: Hepatic failure
PC: Hyperbilirubinemia
PC: Evisceration
PC: Hepatosplenomegaly
PC: Curling's ulcer
PC: Ascites
PC: GI bleeding

Potential Complication: Metabolic/Immune/Hematopoietic

PC: Hypoglycemia/hyperglycemia
PC: Negative nitrogen balance

(Carpenito, L. J. [2002]. *Nursing diagnosis: Application to clinical practice* [9th ed.]. Philadelphia: Lippincott Williams & Wilkins.)

* Frequently used collaborative problems are represented on this list. Other situations not listed here could qualify as collaborative problems.

PC: Electrolyte imbalances
PC: Thyroid dysfunction
PC: Hypothermia (severe)
PC: Hyperthermia (severe)
PC: Sepsis
PC: Acidosis (metabolic, respiratory)
PC: Alkalosis (metabolic, respiratory)
PC: Hypo/hyperthyroidism
PC: Allergic reaction
PC: Donor tissue rejection
PC: Adrenal insufficiency
PC: Anemia
PC: Thrombocytopenia
PC: Opportunistic infection
PC: Polycythemia
PC: Sickling crisis
PC: Disseminated intravascular coagulation

Potential Complication: Neurologic/Sensory

PC: Increased intracranial pressure
PC: Stroke
PC: Seizures
PC: Spinal cord compression
PC: Meningitis
PC: Cranial nerve impairment (specify)
PC: Paralysis
PC: Peripheral nerve impairment
PC: Increased intraocular pressure
PC: Corneal ulceration
PC: Neuropathies

Potential Complication: Muscular/Skeletal

PC: Osteoporosis
PC: Joint dislocation
PC: Compartmental syndrome
PC: Pathologic fractures

Potential Complication: Renal/Urinary

PC: Acute urinary retention
PC: Renal failure
PC: Bladder perforation
PC: Renal calculi

Potential Complication: Reproductive

PC: Fetal distress
PC: Postpartum hemorrhage
PC: Pregnancy-associated hypertension
PC: Hypermenorrhea
PC: Polymenorrhea
PC: Syphilis
PC: Prenatal bleeding
PC: Preterm labor

Potential Complication: Respiratory

PC: Hypoxemia
PC: Atelectasis/pneumonia
PC: Tracheobronchial constriction

PC: Pleural effusion
PC: Tracheal necrosis
PC: Ventilator dependency
PC: Pneumothorax
PC: Laryngeal edema

Potential Complication: Multisystem

PC: Medication therapy adverse effects
PC: Adrenocorticosteroid therapy adverse effects
PC: Antianxiety therapy adverse effects
PC: Antiarrhythmia therapy adverse effects
PC: Anticoagulant therapy adverse effects
PC: Anticonvulsant therapy adverse effects
PC: Antidepressant therapy adverse effects
PC: Antihypertensive therapy adverse effects
PC: Beta-adrenergic blocker therapy adverse effects
PC: Calcium channel blocker therapy adverse effects
PC: Angiotensin-converting enzyme therapy adverse effects
PC: Antineoplastic therapy adverse effects
PC: Antipsychotic therapy adverse effects

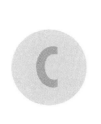

Self-Assessment: Breast and Testicular Self-Examinations

Breast Self-Examination (BSE)

STEP 1

1. Stand before a mirror.
2. Check both breasts for anything unusual.
3. Look for discharge from the nipple, puckering, dimpling, or scaling of the skin.

The next two steps are done to check for any changes in the contour of your breasts. As you do them, you should be able to feel your muscles tighten.

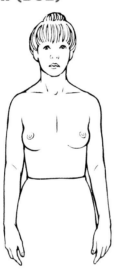

STEP 2

1. Watch closely in the mirror as you clasp your hands behind your head and press your hands forward.
2. Note any change in the contour of your breasts.

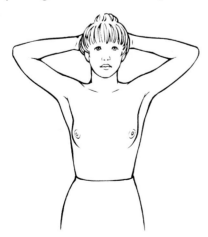

STEP 3

1. Next, press your hands firmly on your hips and bow slightly toward the mirror as you pull your shoulders and elbows forward.
2. Note any change in the contour of your breasts.

Some women do the next part of the examination in the shower. Your fingers will glide easily over soapy skin, so you can concentrate on feeling for changes inside the breast.

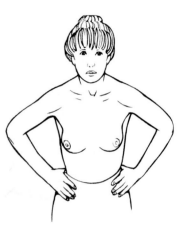

STEP 4

1. Raise your left arm.
2. Use three or four fingers of your right hand to feel your left breast firmly, carefully, and thoroughly.
3. Beginning at the outer edge, press the flat part of your fingers in small circles, moving the circles slowly around the breast.
4. Gradually work toward the nipple.
5. Be sure to exam the whole breast.
6. Pay special attention to the area between the breast and the underarm, including the underarm itself.
7. Feel for any unusual lumps or masses under the skin.

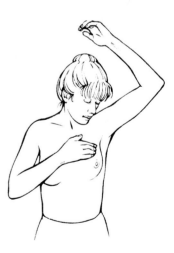

STEP 5

1. Gently squeeze the nipple and look for a discharge.
2. If you have any discharge during the month—whether or not it is during your BSE—see your doctor.
3. Repeat the examination on your right breast.

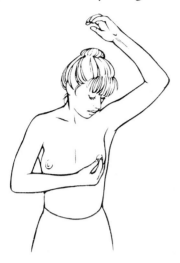

STEP 6

1. Steps 4 and 5 should be repeated lying down.
2. Lie flat on your back with your left arm over your head and a pillow or folded towel under your left shoulder. (This position flattens your breast and makes it easier to check.)
3. Use the same circular motion described above.
4. Repeat on your right breast.

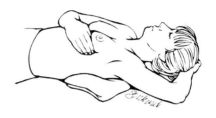

Testicular Self-Examination (TSE)

Testicular self-examination (TSE) is to be performed once a month; it is neither difficult nor time consuming. A convenient time is often after a warm bath or shower when the scrotum is more relaxed.

1. Use both hands to palpate the testis; the normal testicle is smooth and uniform in consistency.
2. With the index and middle fingers under the testis and the thumb on top, roll the testis gently in a horizontal plane between the thumb and fingers (*A*).

3. Feel for any evidence of a small lump or abnormality.
4. Follow the same procedure and palpate upward along the testis (*B*).
5. Locate the epididymis (*C*), a cordlike structure on the top and back of the testicle that stores and transports sperm.
6. Repeat the examination for the other testis. It is normal to find that one testis is larger than the other.
7. If you find any evidence of a small, pealike lump, consult your physician. It may be due to an infection or a tumor growth.

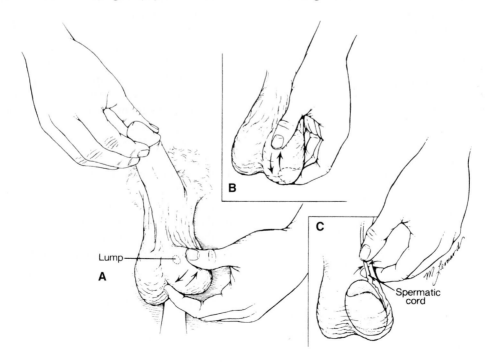

Lump

A

B

C

Spermatic cord

Mini-nutritional Assessment (MNA)

Last name:		First name:		Sex:		Date:
Age:	Weight, kg:		Height, cm:		I.D. Number:	

Complete the screen by filling in the boxes with the appropriate numbers.
Add the numbers for the screen. If score is 11 or less, continue with the assessment to gain a Malnutrition Indicator Score.

Screening

A Has food intake declined over the past 3 months due to loss of appetite, digestive problems, chewing or swallowing difficulties?
0 = severe loss of appetite
1 = moderate loss of appetite
2 = no loss of appetite ☐

B Weight loss during last months
0 = weight loss greater than 3 kg (6.6 lbs)
1 = does not know
2 = weight loss between 1 and 3 kg (2.2 and 6.6 lbs)
3 = no weight loss ☐

C Mobility
0 = bed or chair bound
1 = able to get out of bed/chair but does not go out
2 = goes out ☐

D Has suffered psychological stress or acute disease in the past 3 months
0 = yes   1 = no ☐

E Neuropsychological problems
0 = severe dementia or depression
1 = mild dementia
2 = no psychological problems ☐

F Body Mass Index (BMI) (weight in kg)/(height in m²)
0 = BMI less than 19
1 = BMI 19 to less than 21
2 = BMI 21 to less than 23
3 = BMI 23 or greater ☐

Screening score (subtotal max. 14 points) ☐ ☐

12 points or greater   Normal—not at risk—no need to complete assessment

11 points or below   Possible malnutrition—continue assessment

Assessment

G Lives independently (not in a nursing home or hospital)
0 = no   1 = yes ☐

H Takes more than 3 prescription drugs per day
0 = yes   1 = no ☐

I Pressure sores or skin ulcers
0 = yes   1 = no ☐

J How many full meals does the patient eat daily?
0 = 1 meal
1 = 2 meals
2 = 3 meals ☐

K Selected consumption markers for protein intake
• At least one serving of dairy products
  (milk, cheese, yogurt) per day?   yes ☐   no ☐
• Two or more servings of legumes
  or eggs per week?   yes ☐   no ☐
• Meat, fish or poultry every day   yes ☐   no ☐
0.0 = less than 3 cups
0.5 = if 2 yes
1.0 = if 3 yes ☐

L Consumes two or more servings of fruit or vegetables per day?
0 = no   1 = yes ☐

M How much fluid (water, juice, coffee, tea, milk…) is consumed per day?
0.0 = less than 3 cups
0.5 = 3 to 5 cups
1.0 = more than 5 cups ☐

N Mode of feeding
0 = unable to eat without assistance
1 = self-fed with some difficulty
2 = self-fed without any problem ☐

O Self view of nutritional status
0 = view self as being malnourished
1 = is uncertain of nutritional state
2 = views self as having no nutritional problem ☐

P In comparison with other people of the same age, how does the patient consider his/her health status?
0.0 = not as good
0.5 = does not know
1.0 = as good
2.0 = better ☐

Q Mid-arm circumference (MAC) in cm
0.0 = MAC less than 21
0.5 = MAC 21 to 22
1.0 = MAC 22 or greater ☐

R Calf circumference (CC) in cm
0.0 = CC less than 31   1.0 = CC 31 or greater ☐

Assessment (max. 16 points) ☐ ☐

Screening score ☐ ☐

Total Assessment (max. 30 points) ☐ ☐

Malnutrition Indicator Score

17 to 23.5 points   at risk of malnutrition

Less than 17 points   malnourished

Ref.: Guigoz Y, Vellas B and Garry PJ. 1994. Mini Nutritional Assessment. A practical assessment tool for grading the nutritional state of elderly patients. *Facts and Research in Gerontology.* Supplement #2:15–59.
Rubenstein LZ, Harker J, Guigoz Y and Vellas B. Comprehensive Geriatric Assessment (CGA) and the MNA: An Overview of CGA, Nutritional Assessment, and Development of a Shortened Version of the MNA. In: "Mini Nutritional Assessment (MNA) Research and Practice in the Elderly". Vellas B, Garry PJ and Guigoz Y, editors. Nestlé Nutrition Workshop Series. Clinical & Performance Programme, vol. 1. Karger, Bale, in press.

Glossary

A

ADLs—activities of daily living

adrenarche—adrenocortical maturation, which occurs during puberty

adventitious breath sounds—abnormal breath sounds heard during auscultation of the lung fields; may include rales (crackles), rhonchi (wheezes), or pleural friction rubs

alopecia—hair loss

AMB—as manifested by

anorexia—loss of appetite for food

anthropometer—a type of caliper used for measuring elbow breadth and other body parts

anthropometric measurements—measurements of the human body (eg, height and weight, head circumference, waistline, percentage of body fat, and so forth)

anticholinergic effects—responses to anticholinergic medications, which inhibit the parasympathetic nervous system; in older adults, symptoms are associated with increased or decreased heart rate (depending on dosage), constipation, urinary retention, dilated pupils and vision problems, dry mouth, and drowsiness

anxiety—apprehensiveness related to an unknown source; occurs in different degrees

apical impulse—a normal visible pulsation in the area of the midclavicular line in the left fifth intercostal space; impulse can be seen in about half of the adult population

apnea—cessation of breathing

Argyll Robertson pupils—small, irregular pupils unresponsive to light

arthritis—inflammation of a joint

articulation—place of union or junction between two or more bones of the skeleton

atelectasis—collapse of a lung

atopic—allergic

atrial gallop—low-frequency heart sound known as S_4; occurs at the end of diastole when the atria contract and produced by vibrations from blood flowing rapidly into the ventricles after atrial contraction; S_4 has the rhythm of the word "Ten-nes-see" and may increase during inspiration

auscultation—assessment technique that uses a stethoscope to hear body sounds inaudible to the naked ear (eg, heart sounds, movement of blood through the vessels, bowel sounds, and air moving through the respiratory tract)

AV—atrioventricular

B

BCP—birth control pills

benign breast disease—nonmalignant disease of the breast, such as fibrocystic breast disease

biologic variation—changes in physical status as a result of genetics and/or environment and/or the interaction of genetics and environment; human variation of a biologic and physiologic nature

Biot's respiration—breathing pattern marked by several short breaths followed by long irregular periods of apnea; may be seen with IICP or head trauma

bipolar disorder—mood disorder categorized as a psychosis and characterized by emotional ups and downs ranging from extreme depression to extreme elation

BP—blood pressure

bradycardia—heart rate less than 60 beats per minute

bradypnea—slow breathing pattern less than 10 breaths per minute

Braxton Hicks contractions—painless, irregular contractions of the uterus

Brudzinski's sign—flexion of the hips and knees in response to neck flexion; a sign of meningeal inflammation

bruit—abnormal sound; blowing, swishing, or murmuring sound caused by turbulent blood flow; heard during auscultation

bruxism—grinding the teeth

Buerger's disease—obliterative vascular disease marked by inflammation in small and medium-sized blood vessels.

bursa—small sac filled with synovial fluid that lubricates and cushions a joint

C

calcium—chemical element (Ca^{++}) that is a major component of bone structure and a necessary element for muscle contractions

capillary refill time—time it takes for reperfusion to occur after circulation has been stopped; test for capillary refill involves pressing on a fingernail firmly enough to stop circulation to the digit (signaled by blanching of the underlying tissue), releasing the pressure, and measuring the time it takes for color to return to the tissue; test is used to assess cardiac output

cardiac conduction—process of excitation initiated in the SA node, resulting in contraction of the heart muscle

cardiac cycle—cyclic filling and emptying of the heart

carotid artery—major coronary vessel that transports blood from the heart to the rest of the body

cataract—loss of transparency or cloudiness in the crystalline lens of the eye

Cheyne-Stokes respiration—breathing pattern characterized by a period of apnea of 10 to 60 seconds, followed by increasing, then decreasing rate, followed by another period of apnea

chloasma—darkening of the skin on the face, known as the "mask of pregnancy"

chorionic villi sampling—test to detect birth defects

closed-ended question—question that can be answered with a yes, no, maybe, or other one- or two-word answers; typically used to clarify or specify information contributed in answers to open-ended questions; often begins with the words Are? Do? Did? Is? or Can?

clubbing—enlargement of fingertips and flattening of the angle between the fingernail and nailbed, as a result of heart and/or lung disease

CO—cardiac output

collaborative problems—physiologic complications that nurses monitor to detect their onset or changes in status (Carpenito, 2000)

colonoscopy—internal examination and visualization of the colon performed by a physician with a colonoscope, a fiberoptic endoscope with a miniature camera attachment

compulsion—repetitive act that the client must perform and over which he or she has no control

crepitus—a crackling sound/tactile sensation due to air under the skin; may also be heard in joints

critical thinking—complex thought process that has many definitions; in this textbook, critical thinking is best described as a thinking process used to arrive at a conclusion about information that is available; necessary when trying to reason or analyze what a client's diagnosis is or is not; investigational process or inquiry used to examine data in order to arrive at a conclusion

culture—as defined by Purnell and Paulanka, "the totality of socially transmitted behavioral patterns, arts, beliefs, values, customs, lifeways, and all other products of human work and thought characteristic of a population or people that guide their worldview and decision making"; all verbal and behavioral systems that transmit meaning

culture-bound syndrome—condition or state defined as an illness by a specific cultural group but not interpreted or perceived as an illness by other groups; may have a mental illness component or a spiritual cause

CVA—cerebrovascular accident, stroke

CVS—*see* chorionic villi sampling

cyanosis—bluish or gray coloring of the skin due to decreased amounts of hemoglobin in the blood suggesting reduced oxygenation

cystocele—herniation of the urinary bladder through the vaginal wall

D

delirium—potentially reversible alteration in mental status that has developed over a short time and is characterized by a change in level of alertness

delusion—false feelings of self that are unreal; may be symptoms of psychotic disorders, delirium, or dementia

dementia—diagnostic category that includes multiple physical disorders characterized by slowly deteriorating memory and alterations in abstract thinking, judgment and perception to the degree that the person's ability to perform everyday activities is affected

diastole—period when the heart relaxes and the ventricles fill with blood; in blood pressure measurements, the "bottom" value represents diastole

diastolic blood pressure—pressure between heartbeats (the pressure when the last sound is heard)

dimpling—indentation or retraction of subcutaneous tissue

direct percussion—direct tapping of a body part with one or two fingertips to elicit tenderness

documentation—committing findings in writing to the client's record

DRE—digital rectal examination

drug resistance—phenomenon that occurs when microorganisms develop a resistance to the effects of drug therapy, particularly antibiotic therapy

dyskinesia—incoordination marked by darting movements of the tongue and jerking movement of the arms and legs

dysphagia—difficulty swallowing solids or liquids

dystonia—abnormal muscle tone

E

ectopic pregnancy—pregnancy outside of the uterus; also called tubal pregnancy

ectropion—eversion of the lower eyelid

edema—accumulation of fluid in body tissues, which may cause swelling

ejection click—high-frequency heart sound auscultated just after S_1; produced by a diseased valve in mid-to-late systole

embryonic milk line—line formed during embryonic development; line starts in the axillary area, runs through the nipple, and extends down the abdomen on the outer side of the umbilicus down onto the upper, inner thigh; supernumerary breasts may occur along this line

entropion—inversion of the lower eyelid

epistaxis—nasal bleeding

ethnicity—identification with a socially, culturally, and politically constructed group of people with common characteristics not shared by others with whom the group members come in contact

ethnocentrism—perception that our worldview is the only acceptable truth and that our beliefs, values, and sanctioned behaviors are superior to all others

exophthalmos—protruding eyes

extrapyramidal tract—descending pathway of the nervous system outside of the pyramidal tract and responsible for conducting impulses to the muscles for maintaining muscle tone and body control

F

fasciculations—fine tremors

fibroadenoma—abnormal formation of tissue or tumor of the glandular epithelium-forming fibrous tissue

FOBT—fecal occult blood test; examination of a stool specimen to detect bleeding of unknown origin

fremitus—tactile vibration felt in neck and over the upper thorax from the transmission of vocal sounds from the airways to the surface of the chest wall

friction rub—auscultatory sound resulting from inflammation of the pericardial sac as with pericarditis

fundus—top of the uterus

G

GCS—Glasgow Coma Scale, an instrument for evaluating level of consciousness

geriatric syndrome—symptoms that are common harbingers of disease and disability in a frail elderly person

graphesthesia—ability to identify letters and numbers and drawing by touch and without sight

H

heart murmur—sounds made by turbulent blood flow through the valves of the heart

hemorrhoids—varicose veins in the rectum

hepatomegaly—enlargement of the liver

Homans' sign—aching or cramping pain in the calf felt with passive dorsiflexion of the foot; sign of thrombosis of deep veins in the calf

HR—heart rate

hyperemesis gravidarum—severe and lengthy nausea with pregnancy

I

ICS—intercostal space

illusion—false interpretation of actual stimuli

indirect percussion—also known as mediate percussion; most common percussion method in which tapping elicits a tone that varies with the density of underlying structures (eg, as density increases, the tone decreases)

induration—hardening

inframammary transverse ridge—firm compressed tissue that may be palpated below the mammary gland in the lower edges of the breasts especially in large breasts; normal variation and not a tumor

inspection—physical examination technique using the senses (vision, smell, and hearing) to observe the condition of various body parts, including normal and abnormal findings

intercostal spaces—spaces between the ribs; the first intercostal space is directly below the first rib, the second intercostal space is below the second rib, and so forth

J

jaundice—yellowness of the skin, eye whites, or mucous membranes due to a deposit of bile pigments related to excess bilirubin in the blood; often seen in clients with liver or gallbladder disease, hemolysis, and some anemias

joint—place where two or more bones meet, providing a variety of ranges of motion; a joint may be classified as fibrous, cartilaginous, or synovial

jugular veins—major neck vessels that transport blood from the head and neck to the heart

K

keratin—protein that is the chief component of skin, hair, and nails

Kernig's sign—pain and resistance to extension of the knee in response to flexion of the leg at the hip and the knee; bilateral pain and resistance are signs of meningeal irritation

Korsakoff's syndrome—psychosis induced by excessive alcohol use and characterized by disorientation, amnesia, hallucinations and confabulation

kyphosis—abnormally increased forward curvature of the upper spine

L

lanugo—fine, downy hairs that cover newborn's body

leading statement—statement made to elicit more information from the client; statements may begins with Explain, Describe, Tell, or Elaborate

lentigines—benign, spotty, brown skin discolorations, known as age spots or liver spots

lesion—abnormal change of tissue usually from injury or disease

leukoplakia—thick white patches of cells that adhere to oral tissues; condition is precancerous

ligament—strong dense band of fibrous connective tissue that joins the bones in synovial joints

linea nigra—dark line associated with pregnancy that extends from the umbilicus to the mons pubis

lordosis—exaggerated lumbar concavity often seen in pregnancy or obesity

M

macular degeneration—thinning or torn membrane in the center of the retina

mania—hyperexcitation; "manic" stage of manic–depressive disorder currently known as bipolar disorder

MCL—midclavicular line

melanin—pigment responsible for hair and skin color

menarche—first menstrual period

mucous plug—clump of mucus that seals the endocervical canal and prevents bacteria from ascending into the uterus

N

NANDA—North American Nursing Diagnosis Association

nonverbal communication—communication through body language including stance or posture, demeanor, facial expressions, and so forth

norms—learned behaviors that are perceived to be appropriate or inappropriate

NSR—normal sinus rhythm

nursing diagnosis—clinical judgment about individuals, family, or community responses to actual and potential health problems and life processes (North American Nursing Diagnosis Association, 2001–2002); provides the basis for selecting nursing interventions to achieve outcomes for which the nurse is accountable

nystagmus—rhythmic oscillation of the eyes

O

objective data—findings that are directly or indirectly observed through measurements; data can be physical characteristics (eg, skin color, rashes, posture), body functions (eg, heart rate, respiratory rate), appearance (eg, dress, hygiene), behavior (eg, mood, affect), measurements (eg, blood pressure, temperature, height, weight), or the results of laboratory testing (eg, platelet count, x-ray findings)

obsession—uncontrollable thought or thoughts that are unacceptable to client; characteristic of some neurotic disorders

OD—right eye (from the Latin *oculus dexter*)

open-ended question—question that cannot be answered with a yes, no, or maybe; usually requires a descriptive or explanatory answer; often begins with the words What? How? When? Where? or Who?

opening snap—extra heart sound occurring in early diastole and resulting from the opening of a stenotic or stiff mitral valve; often mistaken for a split S_2 or an S_3

orthopnea—difficulty breathing unless in a sitting or standing position; not uncommon in severe cardiac and pulmonary disease

orthostatic hypotension—drop in blood pressure when client arises from a sitting or lying position

OS—left eye (from the Latin *oculus sinister*)

osteoporosis—low bone density that occurs when bone-forming cells cannot keep pace with bone-destroying cells

OU—each eye (from the Latin *oculus uterque*)

P

PAD—peripheral artery disease

pallor—paleness, lack of color

palpation—examination technique in which the examiner uses the hands to touch and feel certain body characteristics, such as texture, temperature, mobility, shape, moisture, and motion

PAOD—peripheral arterial occlusive disease

paralytic strabismus—eyes deviate from normal position depending on the direction of gaze

parkinsonism—symptoms of Parkinson's disease that are secondary to another condition such as cerebral trauma, brain tumor, infection, or an adverse drug reaction

Parkinson's disease—chronic progressive degeneration of the brain's dopamine neuronal systems that is characterized by muscle rigidity, tremor, and slowed movements

PC—potential complication

percussion—tapping a body chamber with fingers to elicit the sounds from underlying organs and structures

perforator vein—vein that connects a superficial vein with a deep vein; also called communicator vein

PERRL—pupils equally reactive and responsive to light

pica—a craving for non-nutritional substances such as dirt or clay

pneumothorax—accumulation of air in the pleural space

point localization—ability to identify points touched on body without seeing the points touched

polyhydramnios—excessive amniotic fluid associated with multiple gestation or fetal abnormalities

postural hypotension—orthostatic hypotension characterized by dizziness or lightheadedness upon rising from a lying or sitting position

precordium—anterior surface of the body overlying the heart and great vessels

presbycusis—inability to hear high-frequency sounds or to discriminate a variety of simultaneous sounds caused by degeneration of the hair cells in the inner ear

presbyopia—farsightedness; person can see print and objects from farther away than considered normal

primary pain—original source of pain

proctosigmoidoscopy—internal examination and visualization of the sigmoid colon performed by a physician with a sigmoidoscope, a fiberoptic endoscope with miniature camera attachment

prodromal—precursor or early warning symptom of disease (eg, aura before a migraine headache or seizure)

proprioception—sensory faculties mediated by sensory nerves located in tissues such as the muscles and tendons

prostatic hyperplasia—enlargement of the prostate gland

PSA—prostate-specific antigen

pseudodementia—depressive symptoms that are commonly mistaken in the elderly for a dementia

pterygium—thickening of the bulbar conjunctiva that grows over the cornea and may interfere with vision

ptosis—drooping eyelids

ptyalism—excessive salivation

pulse amplitude—strength of the pulse

pyramidal tract—descending pathway of the nervous system; carries impulses that produce voluntary movements requiring skill and purpose

R

range of motion—natural distance and direction of movement of a joint

referral problem—problem that requires the attention or assistance of other health care professionals besides nurses

referred pain—pain perceived in an area that is not related to its original source (eg, gallbladder pain may radiate to the right shoulder and pancreatic pain may radiate to the back)

reinforcement technique—presentation of a stimulus so as to modify a response; increasing of a reflex response by causing the person to perform a physical or mental task while the reflex is being tested

retraction—indentation

r/t—related to

ruga—wrinkle, or fold, of skin or mucous membrane

S

SA—sinoatrial

satiety—fullness, satisfaction commonly associated with meals

scleroderma—degenerative disease characterized by fibrosis and vascular abnormalities in the skin and internal organs

scoliosis—lateral curvature of the spine with an increase in convexity on the side that is curved

splenomegaly—enlargement of the spleen

stereognosis—ability to identify an object by touch rather than sight

sternal retraction—pulling in of sternum during respiration in a physiologic attempt to take in more oxygen; seen in hypoxia or air hunger

STI—sexually transmitted infection; also called sexually transmitted disease

subjective data—descriptive rather than measurable information; symptoms, sensations, feelings, perceptions, desires, preferences, beliefs, ideas, values, and personal information contributed by a client or other person and verifiable only by the client or other person

supernumerary nipple—more than two nipples

SV—stroke volume; the volume of blood pumped with each contraction of the heart

synovitis—inflammation of the synovial membrane; synovial membrane surrounds the joint space and contains synovial fluid that lubricates the joint and enhances movement; characterized by painful movement of the joint

system—interacting whole formed of many parts

systole—cardiac phase during which the ventricles contract and eject blood into the pulmonary and circulatory systems

systolic blood pressure—pressure of the blood flow when the heart beats (the pressure when the first sound is heard).

T

tachycardia—heart rate exceeding 100 beats per minute

tachypnea—rapid, shallow breathing pattern exceeding 20 breaths per minute

temporal event—relating to a particular time of day or activity

tendon—strong fibrous cord of connective tissue continuous with the fibers of a muscle; tendon attaches muscle to bone or cartilage

TENS—transcutaneous electrical nerve stimulation; treatment modality associated with muscle pain, particularly low back pain

thelarche—time during puberty when breasts develop in females

thrill—palpable vibration over the precordium or an artery; usually the result of stenosis or partial occlusion

TIA—transient ischemic attack; minor stroke, sometimes called mini-stroke

TMJ syndrome—temporomandibular joint problems; limited range of motion, swelling, tenderness, pain, or crepitation in the jaw area

torus palatinus—bony protuberance on the hard palate where the intermaxillary transverse palatine sutures join

trigger factors—factors (eg, touch, pressure and/or chemical substances) that initiate or stimulate a response such as pain

turgor—normal skin tone, tension, and elasticity

U

uterine prolapse—protrusion of the cervix down through the vagina

UTI—urinary tract infection

V

validation—verification

values—learned beliefs about what is held to be good or bad

varicocele—varicose veins of the scrotum, which feels like a bag of worms upon palpation

venous hum—benign chest sound like roaring water caused by turbulence of blood in the jugular veins; common in children

ventricular gallop—another term for S_3, the third heart sound, which has low frequency and is often accentuated during inspiration; sound has rhythm of the word "Kentucky" and results from vibrations produced as blood hits the ventricular wall during filling

verbal communication—conversation with words, either spoken or written

viscera (solid, hollow)—internal organs; may consist of solid tissue (eg, liver) or be hollow to fill with fluids or other substances (eg, stomach or bladder)

visual field—what a person sees with one eye; field has four parts or quadrants—upper temporal, lower temporal, upper nasal, and lower nasal

vital signs—measurable signs of cardiopulmonary and thermoregulatory health status; signs include pulse rate, respiratory rate and character, blood pressure, and temperature. (*Note:* Some experts do not consider temperature a vital sign.)

voluntary guarding—person's willful attempt to protect body against pain by holding breath or tightening muscles

Index

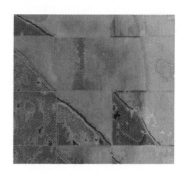

Note: Page numbers followed by f indicate figures; those followed by t indicate tables.

CD-ROM to Accompany Weber and Kelley's Health Assessment in Nursing, *Second Edition*

PROGRAM LICENSE AGREEMENT

Read carefully the following terms and conditions before using the Software. Use of the Software indicates you and, if applicable, your Institution's acceptance of the terms and conditions of this License Agreement. If you do not agree with the terms and conditions, you should promptly return this package to the place you purchased it and your payment will be refunded.

DEFINITIONS

As used herein, the following terms shall have the following meanings:

"Software" means the software program contained on the diskette(s) or CD-ROM or preloaded on a workstation and the user documentation, which includes all accompanying printed material.

"Institution" means a nursing or professional school, a single academic organization that does not provide patient care and is located in a single city and has one geographic location/address.

"Geographic location" means a facility at a specific location; geographic locations do not provide for satellite or remote locations that are considered a separate facility.

"Facility" means a health care facility at a specific location that provides patient care and is located in a single city and has one geographic location/address.

"Publisher" means Lippincott Williams & Wilkins, Inc., with its principal office in Philadelphia, Pennsylvania.

"Developer" means the company responsible for developing the software as noted on the product.

LICENSE

You are hereby granted a nonexclusive license to use the Software in the United States. This license is not transferable and does not authorize resale or sublicensing without the written approval or an authorized officer of Publisher.

The Publisher retains all rights and title to all copyrights, patents, trademarks, trade secrets, and other proprietary rights in the Software. You may not remove or obscure the copyright notices in or on the Software. You agree to use reasonable efforts to protect the Software from unauthorized use, reproduction, distribution or publication.

SINGLE-USER LICENSE

If you purchased this Software program at the Single-User License price or a discount of that price, you may use this program on one single-user computer. You may not use the Software in a time-sharing environment or otherwise to provide multiple, simultaneous access. You may not provide or permit access to this program to anyone other than yourself.

INSTITUTIONAL/FACILITY LICENSE

If you purchased the Software at the Institutional or Facility License Price or at a discount of that price, you have purchased the Software for use within your Institution/Facility on a single workstation/computer. You may not provide copies of or remote access to the Software. You may not modify or translate the program or related documentation. You agree to instruct the individuals in your Institution/Facility who will have access to the Software to abide by the terms of this License Agreement. If you or any member of your Institution fail to comply with any of the terms of this License Agreement, this license shall terminate automatically.

NETWORK LICENSE

If you purchased the Software at the Network License Price, you may copy the Software for use within your Institution/Facility on an unlimited number of computers within one geographic location/address. You may not provide remote access to the Software over a value-added network or otherwise. You may not provide copies of or remote access to the Software to individuals or entities who are not members of your Institution/Facility. You may not modify or translate the program or related documentation. You agree to instruct the individuals in your Institution/Facility who will have access to the Software to abide by the terms of this License Agreement. If you or any member of your Institution/Facility fail to comply with any of the terms of this License Agreement, this license shall terminate automatically.

LIMITED WARRANTY

The Publisher warrants that the media on which the Software is furnished shall be free from defects in materials and workmanship under normal use for a period of 90 days from the date of delivery to you, as evidenced by your receipt of purchase. The Software is sold on a 30-day trial basis. If, for whatever reason, you decide not to keep the software, you may return it for a full refund within 30 days of the invoice date or purchase, as evidenced by your receipt of purchase by returning all parts of the Software and packaging in saleable condition with the original invoice, to the place you purchased it. If the Software is not returned in such condition, you will not be entitled to a refund. When returning the Software, we suggest that you insure all packages for their retail value and mail them by a traceable method.

The Software is a computer assisted instruction (CAI) program that is not intended to provide medical consultation regarding the diagnosis or treatment of any specific patient.

The Software is provided without warranty of any kind, either expressed or implied, including but not limited to any implied warranty of fitness for a particular purpose of merchantability. Neither Publisher nor Developer warrants that the Software will satisfy your requirements or that the Software is free of program or content errors. Neither Publisher nor Developer warrants, guarantees, or makes any representation regarding the use of the Software in terms of accuracy, reliability or completeness, and you rely on the content of the programs solely at your own risk.

The Publisher is not responsible (as a matter of products liability, negligence or otherwise) for any injury resulting from any material contained herein. This Software contains information relating to general principles of patient care that should not be construed as specific instructions for individual patients.

Manufacturers' product information and package inserts should be reviewed for current information, including contraindications, dosages and precautions.

Some states do not allow the exclusion of implied warranties, so the above exclusion may not apply to you. This warranty gives you specific legal rights and you may also have other rights that vary from state to state.

LIMITATION OF REMEDIES

The entire liability of Publisher and Developer and your exclusive remedy shall be: (1) the replacement of any CD which does not meet the limited warranty stated above which is returned to the place you purchased it with your purchase receipt; or (2) if the Publisher or the wholesaler or retailer from whom you purchased the Software is unable to deliver a replacement CD free from defects in material and workmanship, you may terminate this License Agreement by returning the CD, and your money will be refunded.

In no event will Publisher or Developer be liable for any damages, including any damages for personal injury, lost profits, lost savings or other incidental or consequential damages arising out of the use or inability to use the Software or any error or defect in the Software, whether in the database or in the programming, even if the Publisher, Developer, or an authorized wholesaler or retailer has been advised of the possibility of such damage.

Some states do not allow the limitation or exclusion of liability for incidental or consequential damages. The above limitations and exclusions may not apply to you.

GENERAL

This License Agreement shall be governed by the laws of the State of Pennsylvania without reference to the conflict of laws provisions thereof, and may only be modified in a written statement signed by an authorized officer of the Publisher. By opening and using the Software, you acknowledge that you have read this License Agreement, understand it, and agree to be bound by its terms and conditions. You further agree that it is a complete and exclusive statement of the agreement between the Institution/Facility and the Publisher, which supersedes any proposal or prior agreement, oral or written, and any other communication between you and Publisher or Developer relative to the subject matter of the License Agreement.

NOTE

Attach a paid invoice to the License Agreement as proof of purchase.

Performing a Head-to-Toe Assessment CD-ROM to Accompany Health Assessment in Nursing
2nd Edition

MINIMUM SYSTEM REQUIREMENTS

- Pentium 100 CPU (Pentium 3 or higher recommended for highest quality video playback)
- 32 MB RAM (64 or higher recommended)
- Windows 98 or higher
- SVGA display supporting 16 million colors
- Sound card
- 12X CD-ROM drive
- 800x600 monitor resolution
- 5 MB of hard-disk space

Note: In order to view these video clips, you must have Internet Explorer 4.0 or higher with Windows Media Player 7.1 or higher. If you do not currently have this version of Windows Media Player installed, it is a free download available at: http:windowsmedia.com/download/download.asp. (If you have a 56k modem, downloading Windows Media Player will take about twenty-five minutes.)

RUNNING THE PROGRAM

The program should automatically start a few seconds after you have inserted the CD-ROM into your CD-ROM drive. If the program does *not* automatically start, follow these steps:

1. Open the Start menu and select Run.
2. In Open box, type **d:\Head-to-Toe.html**, where d is the letter representing your CD-ROM drive, and press Enter. (If your CD-ROM drive is a letter other than d, substitute that letter.)

Note: Program will automatically play in quarter-screen size. If you choose to view the video in full screen size, you may do so by clicking **"View"** on the Media Player menu bar and selecting **"Full Screen."** The video will be of lower quality in full screen size. To revert back to quarter-screen size, hit the escape key on keyboard.